AF412456

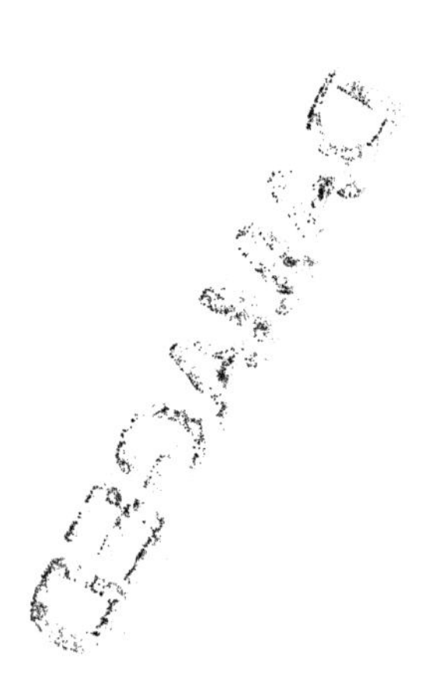

Rapid Eye Movement Sleep

Regulation and Function

Spanning over half a century of investigation into rapid eye movement (REM) sleep, this volume provides comprehensive coverage of a broad range of topics in REM sleep biology. World-renowned researchers and experts are brought together to discuss past and current research and to set the foundation for future developments. Key topics are covered in six sections from fundamental topics (historical context and general biology) to cutting-edge research on neuronal regulation, neuroanatomy and neurochemistry, functional significance, and disturbance in the REM sleep-generating mechanism. A reference source for all aspects of REM sleep research, it also incorporates chapters on neural modeling, findings from non-human species, and interactions between brain regions. This is an invaluable resource, essential reading for all involved in sleep research and clinical practice.

Birendra N. Mallick is Professor of Neurobiology and J. C. Bose National Fellow at Jawaharlal Nehru University, New Delhi, India.

S. R. Pandi-Perumal is President and Chief Executive Officer of Somnogen Inc, Toronto, Canada.

Robert W. McCarley is Professor and Chair of the Harvard Department of Psychiatry and Associate Director of Mental Health at the VA Boston Healthcare System, Boston, USA.

Adrian R. Morrison is Professor Emeritus of Behavioral Neuroscience at the School of Veterinary Medicine, University of Pennsylvania, PA, USA.

Rapid Eye Movement Sleep

Regulation and Function

Birendra N. Mallick
Jawaharlal Nehru University, New Delhi, India

S. R. Pandi-Perumal
Somnogen Inc, Toronto, Canada

Robert W. McCarley
Harvard University, Boston, USA

Adrian R. Morrison
University of Pennsylvania, PA, USA

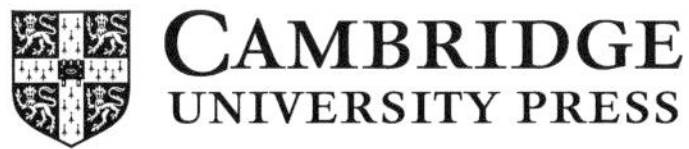

CAMBRIDGE
UNIVERSITY PRESS

CAMBRIDGE UNIVERSITY PRESS
Cambridge, New York, Melbourne, Madrid, Cape Town,
Singapore, São Paulo, Delhi, Tokyo, Mexico City

Cambridge University Press
The Edinburgh Building, Cambridge CB2 8RU, UK

Published in the United States of America by Cambridge
University Press, New York

www.cambridge.org
Information on this title: www.cambridge.org/
9780521116800

First published 2011

Printed in the United Kingdom at the University Press,
Cambridge

*A catalog record for this publication is available from the
British Library*

Library of Congress Cataloging in Publication data
Rapid eye movement sleep : regulation and function /
[edited by] Birendra N. Mallick ... [et al.].
p. ; cm.
Includes bibliographical references and index.
ISBN 978-0-521-11680-0 (hardback)
1. Sleep–Physiological aspects.   2. Rapid eye movement
sleep.   3. Dreams.   I. Mallick, B. N. (Birendra Nath)
[DNLM: 1. Sleep, REM–physiology.   2. REM Sleep
Parasomnias–physiopathology. WL 108]
QP425.R316 2011
612.8′21dc22   2011011502

ISBN 978-0-521-11680-0 Hardback

At last when I woke from my slumber
and opened my eyes, I saw thee standing by me,
flooding my sleep with thy smile.
How I had feared that the path was long and wearisome,
and the struggle to reach thee was hard!

from "*Gitanjali*"
Rabindranath Tagore
The first Asian Nobel Prize winner (1913)

Contents

Section I – Historical context

Section II – General biology

Section III – Neuronal regulation

Section VI – Disturbance in the REM sleep-generating mechanism

Color plates are found between pages 222 and 223.

Contributors

Daniel Aeschbach, PhD,
Division of Sleep Medicine, Department of Medicine, Brigham and Women's Hospital, Boston, MA, USA, and Division of Sleep Medicine, Harvard Medical School, Boston, MA, USA.

Md. Noor Alam, PhD,
Research Service (151A3), Veterans Affairs Greater Los Angeles Healthcare System, Sepulveda, CA, USA; and Department of Psychology, University of California, Los Angeles, CA, USA.

Isabel de Andrés, PhD,
Departamento de Anatomía, Histología y Neurociencia, Universidad Autónoma de Madrid, Spain.

Helen A. Baghdoyan, PhD,
Department of Anesthesiology, University of Michigan, Ann Arbor, MI, USA.

Nishidh Barot, MD,
Stanford Sleep Disorders Clinic, Stanford Center for Human Sleep Research, Stanford University Medical Center, Redwood City, CA, USA.

Radhika Basheer, PhD,
VA Boston Healthcare System and Harvard Medical School, Department of Psychiatry, West Roxbury, MA, USA.

Sudipta Biswas, PhD,
Behavioral Neuroscience Division, Department of Psychology, Arizona State University, Tempe, AZ, USA.

Carlos Blanco-Centurion, PhD,
VA Boston Healthcare System and Harvard Medical School, MA, USA.

Mark S. Blumberg, PhD,
Department of Psychology and Delta Center, The University of Iowa, Iowa City, IA, USA.

Victoria Booth, PhD,
Department of Mathematics and Department of Anesthesiology, University of Michigan, Ann Arbor, MI, USA.

Lichao Chen, PhD,
VA Boston Healthcare System and Harvard Medical School, Department of Psychiatry, Brockton, MA, USA.

Olivier Clement, PhD,
UMR5167 CNRS, Faculté de Médecine RTH Laennec, Institut Fédératif des Neurosciences de Lyon (IFR 19), Université de Lyon, France.

Thien Thanh Dang-Vu, MD, PhD,
Cyclotron Research Centre, University of Liège, Belgium; and Department of Neurology, Massachusetts General Hospital, Harvard Medical School, Boston, MA, USA.

Subimal Datta, PhD,
Laboratory of Sleep and Cognitive Neuroscience, Departments of Psychiatry, Neuroscience, and Neurology, Boston University School of Medicine, Boston, MA, USA.

Martin Desseilles, MD, PhD,
Department of Neuroscience, Geneva Center for Neuroscience, University of Geneva, Switzerland; and Cyclotron Research Centre, University of Liège, Belgium.

Samuel C. Engemann, BS,
Department of Neurology, University of Missouri, Harry Truman Memorial VA Hospital, University of Missouri, Columbia, MO, USA.

Luigi Ferini-Strambi, MD,
Sleep Disorders Center, Department of Neuroscience, Università Vita-Salute San Raffaele, Milan, Italy.

Ariane Foret, MSc,
Cyclotron Research Centre B30, University of Liège – Sart Tilman, Belgium.

Patrice Fort, PhD,
UMR5167 CNRS, Faculté de Médecine RTH Laennec,
Institut Fédératif des Neurosciences de Lyon (IFR 19),
Université de Lyon, France.

Jimmy J. Fraigne, PhD,
Department of Cell and System Biology, University of
Toronto, ON, Canada.

Marcos G. Frank, PhD,
University of Pennsylvania School of Medicine,
Department of Neuroscience, Philadelphia, PA,
USA.

Damien Gervasoni, PhD,
UMR5167 CNRS, Faculté de Médecine
RTH Laennec, Institut Fédératif des
Neurosciences de Lyon (IFR 19), Université
de Lyon, France.

Anupama Gopalakrishnan, PhD,
Technical Services, Promega Corporation, Madison,
WI, USA.

Claude Gottesmann, PhD,
Département de Biologie, Faculté des Sciences,
Université de Nice-Sophia Antipolis, Nice, France.

Sushil K. Jha, PhD,
School of Life Sciences, Jawaharlal Nehru University,
New Delhi, India.

Akihiro Karashima, PhD,
Graduate School of Information Sciences, Tohoku
University, Japan.

Norihiro Katayama, PhD,
Graduate School of Information Sciences, Tohoku
University, Japan.

Tohru Kodama, MD, PhD,
Department of Psychology, Tokyo Metropolitan
Institute for Neuroscience, Fuchu, Tokyo, Japan.

Yoshimasa Koyama, PhD,
Faculty of Symbiotic Systems Science, Fukushima
University, Japan.

Milton Kramer, MD,
Clinical Professor of Psychiatry, University of Illinois
at Chicago, Chicago, IL, USA; and Emeritus Professor
of Psychiatry, University of Cincinnati, Cincinnati,
OH, USA.

Clete Kushida, MD, PhD, RPSGT,
Stanford Sleep Disorders Clinic, Director, Stanford
Center for Human Sleep Research, Stanford
University Medical Center, Redwood City, CA, USA.

Yuan-Yang Lai, PhD,
Neurobiology Research 151A3, VAGLAHS Sepulveda,
North Hills, CA, USA.

John A. Lesku, MSc,
Max Planck Institute for Ornithology – Seewiesen
Sleep & Flight Group, Eberhard-Gwinner-Strasse,
Seewiesen, Germany.

Pierre-Hervé Luppi, PhD,
UMR5167 CNRS, Faculté de Médecine RTH Laennec,
Institut Fédératif des Neurosciences de Lyon (IFR 19),
Université de Lyon, France.

Ralph Lydic, PhD,
Department of Anesthesiology, University of
Michigan, Ann Arbor, MI, USA.

Vibha Madan, PhD,
Department of Animal Biology, School of Veterinary
Medicine, University of Pennsylvania, PA, USA.

Birendra N. Mallick, PhD,
School of Life Sciences, Jawaharlal Nehru University,
New Delhi, India.

Pierre Maquet, MD, PhD,
Cyclotron Research Centre B30, University of Liège –
Sart Tilman, Belgium.

Dolores Martinez-Gonzalez, MD, PhD,
Max Planck Institute for Ornithology – Seewiesen
Sleep & Flight Group, Eberhard-Gwinner-Strasse,
Seewiesen, Germany.

Laura Mascetti, MSc,
Cyclotron Research Centre B30, University of Liège –
Sart Tilman, Liège, Belgium.

Luca Matarazzo, MSc, PhD,
Cyclotron Research Centre B30, University of Liège –
Sart Tilman, Belgium.

Robert W. McCarley, MD,
VA Boston Healthcare System and Harvard Medical
School, Harvard Department of Psychiatry, Brockton,
MA, USA.

Dennis McGinty, PhD,
Research Service (151A3), Veterans Affairs Greater Los Angeles Healthcare System, Sepulveda, CA, USA; and Department of Psychology, University of California, Los Angeles, CA, USA.

James T. McKenna, PhD,
VA Boston Healthcare System and Harvard Medical School, Department of Psychiatry, Brockton, MA, USA.

Mónica Méndez-Díaz, PhD,
Grupo de Neurociencias: Laboratorio de Canabinoides, Depto de Fisiología, Fac. de Medicina, Universidad Nacional Autónoma de México.

Jaime M. Monti, MD,
Department of Pharmacology and Therapeutics, School of Medicine Clinics Hospital. Montevideo, Uruguay.

Adrian R. Morrison, DVM, PhD,
Department of Animal Biology, School of Veterinary Medicine, University of Pennsylvania, Philadelphia, PA, USA.

Asok K. Mukhopadhyay, MD,
Department of Laboratory Medicine, All India Institute of Medical Sciences, New Delhi, India.

Harald Murck, MD,
Discovery Medicine & Clinical Pharmacology (DMCP), Bristol-Myers Squibb Co., Pennington, NJ, USA; and Clinic of Psychiatry and Psychotherapy, Philipps-University of Marburg, Germany.

Vincenzo Muto, MPsy,
Cyclotron Research Centre B30, University of Liège – Sart Tilman, Belgium.

Mitsuyuki Nakao, Dr Eng,
Graduate School of Information Sciences, Tohoku University, Japan.

Seiji Nishino, MD, PhD,
Sleep and Circadian Neurobiology Laboratory, Center for Narcolepsy, Department of Psychiatry & Behavioral Sciences, Stanford University School of Medicine, Palo Alto, CA, USA.

John M. Orem, PhD,
Texas Tech University School of Medicine, Department of Cell Physiology and Molecular Biophysics, Lubbock, TX, USA.

Edward F. Pace-Schott, PhD,
Department of Psychology, University of Massachusetts, Amherst, MA, USA; and Department of Psychiatry, Massachusetts General Hospital, Harvard Medical School.

James F. Pagel, MS, MD,
Associate Clinical Professor, University of Colorado School of Medicine, Southern Colorado Family Medicine Residency Program; Director Rocky Mt. Sleep & Sleep Disorders Center of Southern Colorado, USA.

Dinesh Pal, PhD,
Department of Anesthesiology, University of Michigan, Ann Arbor, MI, USA.

S. R. Pandi-Perumal, MSc,
President and Chief Executive Officer, Somnogen Inc, Toronto, Canada.

Pier Luigi Parmeggiani, MD,
Dipartimento di Fisiologia Umana e Generale, Università di Bologna, Italy.

Marcel Pérez-Morales, PhD,
Grupo de Neurociencias: Laboratorio de Canabinoides, Depto de Fisiología, Fac. de Medicina, Universidad Nacional Autónoma de México.

Gina R. Poe, PhD,
Department of Anesthesiology and Department of Molecular and Integrative Physiology, University of Michigan, Ann Arbor, MI, USA.

Oscar Prospéro-García, MD, PhD,
Grupo de Neurociencias: Laboratorio de Canabinoides, Depto de Fisiología, Fac. de Medicina, Universidad Nacional Autónoma de México.

Niels C. Rattenborg, PhD,
Max Planck Institute for Ornithology – Seewiesen Sleep & Flight Group, Eberhard-Gwinner-Strasse, Seewiesen, Germany.

Richard J. Ross, MD, PhD,
Behavioral Health Service (116 MHC), Philadelphia VA Medical Center, Philadelphia, PA, USA; Department of Psychiatry, University of Pennsylvania School of Medicine, Philadelphia, PA, USA.

Alejandra E. Ruiz-Contreras, PhD,
Laboratorio de Neurogenómica Cognitiva, Depto. de Psicofisiología, Fac. de Psicología. Universidad Nacional Autónoma de México, Mexico.

Pradeep Sahota, MD,
Department of Neurology, University of Missouri, Harry Truman Memorial VA Hospital, University of Missouri, Columbia, MO, USA.

Denise Salvert,
UMR5167 CNRS, Faculté de Médecine RTH Laennec, Institut Fédératif des Neurosciences de Lyon (IFR 19), Université de Lyon, France.

Larry D. Sanford, PhD,
Division of Anatomy, Department of Pathology and Anatomy, Eastern Virginia Medical School, Norfolk, VA, USA.

Emilie Sapin, PhD,
UMR5167 CNRS, Faculté de Médecine RTH Laennec, Institut Fédératif des Neurosciences de Lyon (IFR 19), Université de Lyon, France.

Sophie Schwartz, PhD,
Department of Neuroscience and Geneva Center for Neuroscience, University of Geneva, Switzerland.

Kazue Semba, PhD,
Department of Anatomy & Neurobiology, Faculty of Medicine, Dalhousie University, Halifax, NS, Canada.

Anahita Shaffii, DVM,
Cyclotron Research Centre B30, University of Liège – Sart Tilman, Belgium.

Rishi Sharma, PhD,
Department of Neurology, University of Missouri, Harry Truman Memorial VA Hospital, University of Missouri, Columbia, MO, USA.

Priyattam J. Shiromani, PhD,
VA Boston Healthcare System and Harvard Medical School, West Roxbury, MA, USA.

Jerome M. Siegel, PhD,
Neurobiology Research 151A3, VAGLAHS Sepulveda, North Hills, CA, USA.

Axel Steiger, MD,
Max Planck Institute of Psychiatry, Department of Psychiatry, Munich, Germany.

Virginie Sterpenich, PhD,
Department of Neuroscience and Geneva Center for Neuroscience, University of Geneva, Switzerland.

Robert Stickgold, PhD,
Center for Sleep and Cognition, Beth Israel Deaconess Medical Center and Department of Psychiatry Harvard Medical School, Boston, MA, USA.

Deborah Suchecki, PhD,
Department of Psychobiology, Universidade Federal de São Paulo, Brazil.

Ronald Szymusiak, PhD,
Research Service, Veterans Affairs Greater Los Angeles Healthcare System, Sepulveda, CA, USA; Departments of Medicine and Neurobiology, School of Medicine, University of California, Los Angeles, CA, USA.

Yuichi Tamakawa, MSc,
Graduate School of Information Sciences, Tohoku University, Japan.

Mahesh M. Thakkar, PhD,
Department of Neurology, University of Missouri, Harry Truman Memorial VA Hospital, University of Missouri, Columbia, MO, USA.

Sergio Tufik, MD, PhD,
Department of Psychobiology, Universidade Federal de São Paulo, Brazil.

Giancarlo Vanini, MD,
Department of Anesthesiology, University of Michigan, Ann Arbor, MI, USA.

Robert P. Vertes, PhD,
Center for Complex Systems and Brain Sciences, Florida Atlantic University, Boca Raton, FL, USA.

Jaime R. Villablanca, MD,
Department of Psychiatry and Biobehavioral Sciences, Department of Neurobiology, Intellectual and Developmental Disabilities Research Center, and Brain Research Institute. University of California, Los Angeles, CA, USA.

Matthew P. Walker, PhD,
Sleep and Neuroimaging Laboratory, Department of Psychology and Helen Wills Neuroscience Institute, University of California, Berkeley, CA, USA.

Christopher J. Watson, PhD,
Department of Anesthesiology, University of Michigan, Ann Arbor, MI, USA.

Preface

Since the publication of the first edition of *Rapid Eye Movement Sleep* (Mallick and Inoue, 1999), the advances in the field of sleep research have been phenomenal; in particular, those concerning rapid eye movement (REM) sleep. The emphasis on REM sleep may be gauged by the fact that recently a conference exclusively devoted to this subject was organized in France to celebrate 50 years since the discovery of REM sleep as well as to honor Professor Michel Jouvet, a pioneer and one of the doyens in this field.

Interest in an update to the earlier book led to the preparation of this volume. We used this opportunity to revise considerably the earlier content. Although the overall scientific organization of this volume reflects the philosophy of the editors, the content and comment in each of the chapters depends on the expertise and views of respective author(s). The broad scientific concepts reflected in this book suggest that mastery of basic sleep processes, especially that of REM sleep, are essential in order to become skilled sleep clinicians as well as researchers.

Though recent years have witnessed unprecedented advances in sleep medicine, many sleep physicians and basic sleep researchers may not be aware of all these advances. One may wonder that since many books dealing with the science of sleep are available why this book? It is our opinion that while many books deal with sleep in general (e.g., Steriade and McCarley, 2005), no recent book to our knowledge has focused in such detail on the biology of REM sleep.

The increased importance of REM sleep may be appreciated more broadly by considering the increasing coverage being given in current neuroscience and biology texts. Also, research on REM sleep has significantly increased in recent years as may be seen by the increased number of publications shown in Figure 1. The data were obtained by a Pub-Med search over the past half century, using the keywords "REM sleep and/or paradoxical sleep". Obviously knowledge of REM sleep has increased to such an extent that it cannot be covered in a single review or chapter. Hence, there was an urgent need to have a comprehensive summary of this subject, with as much relevant detail as possible.

Rapid Eye Movement Sleep: Regulation and Function covers various aspects of REM sleep, a phase found definitively in most of the homeotherms: mammals and birds (Pandi-Perumal *et al.*, 2010). Initially waking was considered to be an active state and sleep, a passive one. The latter view was abandoned about forty years ago. Likewise, the idea that sleep was a homogeneous phenomenon had to be abandoned with the recognition of REM sleep by Aserinsky and Kleitman in 1953.

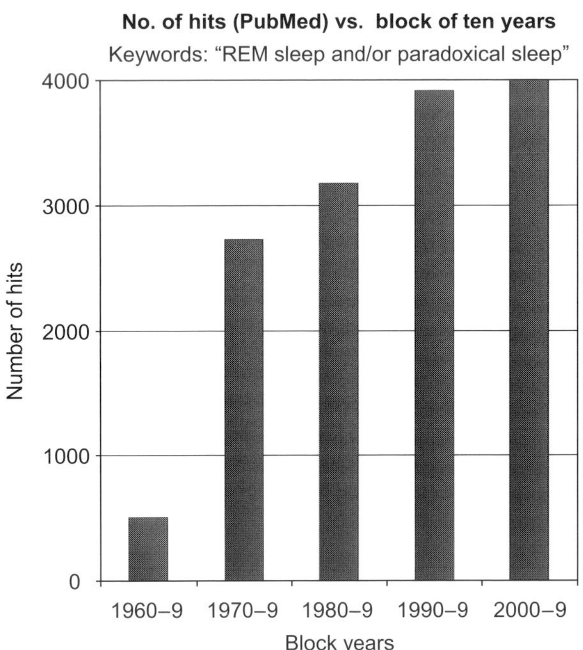

Figure 1

Thus, the foundation for modern sleep research and ultimately sleep medicine was laid when Eugene Aserinsky and Nathaniel Kleitman pioneered the use of electrophysiological recordings of REM sleep signals for monitoring sleep states, opening up a new era of scientific interest in the biology of sleep. It was then observed that REM sleep is usually associated with dreams; the latter phenomenon as such was not new to human knowledge, though. A dream state of sleep has been mentioned in most ancient medical, scientific, and philosophical literature as well as in novels and plays, but definitive scientific recognition awaited the discovery by Aserinsky and Kleitman.

The editors have chosen to be somewhat selective in that the research included deals primarily with studies of the physiological, neurological, and some applied medical aspects of REM sleep, excluding studies that are exclusively clinical and psychological in nature; the latter merits separate review.

References

Aserinsky, E. & Kleitman, N. (1953) Regularly occurring periods of eye motility and concomitant phenomenon during sleep. *Science*, **118**, 273–4.

Mallick, B. N. & Inoue, S. (eds) (1999) *Rapid Eye Movement Sleep*. New York: Marcel Dekker.

Pandi-Perumal, S., Spence, D., Brown, G. M. & Thorpy, M. J. (2010) Great challenges to sleep medicine: problems and paradigms. *Front Neurol*, 1:7. doi:10.3389/fneur.2010.00007.

Steriade, M. & McCarley, R. W. (2005) *Brain Control of Wakefulness and Sleep*. New York: Kluwer Academic/Plenum.

Acknowledgments

This volume owes its final shape and form to the assistance and hard work of many talented people. Creating a volume such as this one, involves the collaborative scholarship of all such individuals. We express our profound gratitude to each of those many people who have given small or big help in this endeavor.

In editing this volume, we have been extremely privileged to have had the opportunity to work with such distinguished colleagues, who have accepted and written on topics that fall within the domain of their expertise. It has been a pleasure, and we have learned a great deal from the contributors. Many of the authors have worked within tight page constraints to conform to the space limitations of the volume (e.g., restriction on reference numbers) and at the same time to infuse their creativity and knowledge into their contributions. We are thankful to all of them, who in spite of their busy schedules, kindly accepted our request and agreed to contribute. Thanks are also due to all others who either could not accept our request because of prior commitments or were forced to give up in between after accepting our request to contribute due to health or other reasons; still, we were very much enthused by their encouragement and support.

We are grateful to our respective organizations, University and Institution, which have given us the freedom to undertake such a project. We would like to thank secretarial and administrative staffs of our respective institutions, for helping us to stay on task, and for their attention to detail. Birendra N. Mallick would like to express his sincere thanks to all his present lab members (2009 and 2010 students and trainees) who came forward and helped him whenever he asked during the course of preparation of this book.

We acknowledge with gratitude the work of the editorial department of Cambridge University Press (CUP), England. We are especially indebted to Dr. Martin Griffiths, Commissioning Editor – Life Sciences, who was an enthusiastic and instrumental supporter from the start. Our gratitude is offered to Ms. Megan Waddington, Assistant Editor – Life Sciences, and Ms. Abigail Jones, Production Editor – Science, Technology and Medicine, who also deserve special recognition and whose equally dedicated efforts promoted a smooth completion of this project. We have thoroughly enjoyed the efficient help and invaluable advice from and constant interactions with the editorial and production department colleagues at CUP for their meticulous work. Their guidance, technical expertise, and commitment to excellence were invaluable.

Finally, on a personal note, the editors as individuals would like to acknowledge the close cooperation they have received from each other. We think that we made a good team, even if we say so ourselves. Thus, this volume is the result of a team working together for more than a year with close cooperation and mutually constructive criticism among the editors so that the best results could be obtained.

Lastly, and certainly not least, it is not possible adequately to thank our wives and families, without whose untiring support none of this work would have proceeded so smoothly. They provided invaluable support and unqualified encouragement and quietly sacrificed much. We appreciate their cheerful forbearance and cherish their support as we have seen this volume through to its realization.

To all these people goes our sincere gratitude.

Birendra N. Mallick, New Delhi, India
S. R. Pandi-Perumal, Toronto, Canada
Robert W. McCarley, Boston, USA
Adrian R. Morrison, Philadelphia, USA

Organization

This volume consists of 44 chapters written by leading scientists from around the globe and covers a broad range of topics related to REM sleep. The chapters have been grouped under six major sections: Section I – Historical context; Section II – General biology; Section III – Neuronal regulation; Section IV – Neuroanatomy and neurochemistry; Section V – Functional significance; Section VI – Disturbance in REM sleep-generating mechanisms.

Section I includes chapters that address REM sleep from historical and philosophical perspectives: the discovery of REM sleep, its relationship with dreams, and if there can be a neurophysiological explanation for the coexistence of dreams and REM sleep.

Section II addresses the general biology of REM sleep. Topics included are the ontogeny and evolutionary perspective of REM sleep. It also includes a systems-level approach to human REM sleep and its relationship with circadian rhythms and homeostatic regulation.

Section III addresses our fundamental understanding of the neuronal regulation of REM sleep from past to present. The topics covered include the initial knowledge gathered from brain lesion studies, modulation and regulation of REM sleep by different anatomical as well as functional brain areas. In this section, readers will find topics, such as preoptic and basal forebrain modulation of REM sleep, amygdalar regulation of REM sleep, pontomedullary-mediated REM sleep atonia, phenomenology and functions of myoclonic twitching, the pontine-wave generator, and hippocampal theta rhythm of REM sleep. Respiration during REM sleep and modulation of REM sleep by non-REM sleep and waking areas of the brain are also covered in this section.

Section IV covers the topical organization of neurons containing neurotransmitters for REM sleep regulation. In this section one will learn the details of the regulation of REM sleep by aminergic neurons (including adrenergic and histaminergic) as well as cholinergic, GABAergic, glutamatergic, hypocretinergic/orexinergic, adenosinergic, and glycinergic neurons. This section also has chapters dealing with changes in levels of neurotransmitters in specific brain regions in relation to REM sleep and, finally, on evolving concepts of neuronal models for the regulation of REM sleep.

Section V deals with the functional significance of REM sleep and the effects of REM sleep loss on physiological parameters. It covers chapters on the significance of REM sleep-deprivation studies and the effects due to stress to the subject induced by such deprivation. Further, the section includes chapters on the role of REM sleep in memory consolidation and processing, in oxidative stress, and in maintenance of brain excitability. The other chapters in this section deal with the relationship of REM sleep to thermoregulation, depression, and changes in several neuropeptides in the body.

Section VI includes chapters dealing with some selected disorders in which REM sleep is significantly altered (e.g., narcolepsy, mood, and other psychosomatic, emotional, and behaviorally altered states). Lastly, it ends with computational modeling of neural circuits for REM sleep regulation and on a theory of dreaming.

In summary, it is our hope that this volume will enable interested basic scientists and medical researchers to develop a better understanding of the regulation of basic mechanisms and functions of REM sleep and their relationship to the practice of sleep medicine. We also hope that this volume will generate new ideas that lead to improvements in the care of patients who suffer from sleep disorders.

Birendra N. Mallick
S. R. Pandi-Perumal
Robert W. McCarley
Adrian R. Morrison

Chapter

1

The sleep–dream state: historic and philosophic perspectives

James F. Pagel

> Who so regardath dreams is like him that catcheth
> at a shadow, and followeth after the wind.
>
> *Ecclesiasticus 34.2*

Summary

Dream study is an ancient science dating to at least 6,000 years ago when dreams perceived as messages from gods were written on the clay codas of Mesopotamia. For the Ancient Greeks and Egyptians it was necessary to distinguish between the "true dreams" of kings and priests (potential messages from god) and other "false dreams" reported even by women and children. Several thousand years later, Rene Descartes, focusing on methods of elucidating such "truths," developed his scientific method while attempting to differentiate dreaming from external reality. At the turn of the twentieth century, Freud developed his psychoanalytic theories of mental functioning from his approach to dream interpretation. In the 1960s, the apparent realization that REM sleep (REMS) was dreaming destroyed 500 years of belief in Cartesian Dualism and led us into this modern age of unitary activation–synthesis theory. If REMS is dreaming, in neuro-scientific actuality, mind equals brain. The literature is replete with such grand theories purporting to explain the dream state, and it is only recently that experimentally testable scientific approaches have been applied to the study of dreaming. Now, most scientists and philosophers accept that research overwhelmingly demonstrates that REMS occurs without dreaming and dreaming without REMS. It is currently unclear as to how much of the highly developed REMS neurocognitive model presented in this book is applicable to the cognitive state of dreaming.

Introduction

No cognitive state has been more extensively studied yet remains more poorly understood than dreaming. During the 4th millennium B.C. in Ladak, a city of ancient Samaria, the king had one of his dreams inscribed upon a clay coda telling the story of how god came to him in a dream and gave him instructions of how to position his temple according to cardinal points. Archaeologists have found multiple imprints of this dream inscribed upon fire-hardened rolls of soft river clay, recording one of our species' first documented attempts at written language. Guttenberg's first printed book was the Bible, but his second was the Oneirocritica, an interpretation of the meaning of dream symbols (Artemidorus, 1500s, trans 1975). Mankind's focus on dreaming, however, pre-dates the development of either printing or writing (Furst, 1994). The argument can cogently be made that the structure and narrative form of language itself is derived from dream (States, 1993).

It is only the rare individual (0.38% of sleep laboratory patients) that never recalls mentation from sleep, what some call a dream (Pagel *et al.*, 2001; Pagel, 2003). Anecdotal reports of individual dreams are often included in chapters documenting the role of dreams in specific stories of creativity or scientific breakthroughs. However, the roles that dreams have played in history and philosophy are more profound, lying at the basis of our species' attempts to understand both ourselves and the outside world. Dreams have been part of the seminal process in the development of the worlds' major religions, philosophies, literature, and science. While currently there are few researchers, limited funding, and a restricted focus of attempts to scientifically and directly approach the process of dreaming, we continue

REM Sleep: Regulation and Function, eds. Birendra N. Mallick, S. R. Pandi-Perumal, Robert W. McCarley, and Adrian R. Morrison. Published by Cambridge University Press. © Cambridge University Press 2011.

to dream, and that same mental activity during sleep recalled on awakening continues to actively influence contemporary religions and philosophy, literature, and even modern science.

Dreams and narrative story

Most dreams are narratives occurring and often presented without applied organization, grammar, or expectation of critique. In the dream we can literally observe the "thinking of the body," and, with it, the birth of the literary process. Our dreams can be considered an exercise in pure storytelling whose end is nothing more (or less) than the organization of experience into set patterns that help to maintain order for the thinking system. Narrative is a perceptual activity that organizes data into a special pattern representing and explaining experience that can be used as a way of organizing experience, drawing together aspects of spatial, temporal, and causal perception into story. Narrative becomes a way of globally interpreting a set of relationships involved in an experience or a sequence of actions (Brannigan, 1992). The relevance of a dream's content to the dreamer's personal life may be less important than this function that dreaming serves as a structuring principle for life (States, 1993).

As dreams progress they begin to obtain a conceptual framework that includes the preconditions for a narrative or story structure. Dreams are inherently self-organized in the structure of thought, with the dreamer requiring no training or critique to learn to present a dream as a narrative. Dreams have a logical sequence of associations, a situational dynamic, in which each dream incidence occurs in response to the incidents that are already there in the dreamer's memory of waking experience. Dreams foreshorten and expand stories as is typical of waking narratives. Yet dreams may not even have plots. It is as if dreams are trying to become genuine stories but typically fall a bit short (Hunt, 1991).

Dreams are often organized in literary forms. These structural forms can be classified as dramatic, epic, or lyric. That these modes of story organization are characteristic of both dreaming and literature implies that these structural forms of organizing dreams may be essential combinational strategies, or ways of bracketing the world. When dreams tell stories, these stories are scripts made out of universal concerns, much as in literature. There is a series of consistent almost universally experienced dreams of flying, chase/ attack, drowning, poor test performance, nakedness, and dreams of being trapped (Garfield, 1991). Plot in literary fiction is a continually evolving pattern of imagery and events (States, 1997). These same structures utilized to organize waking thought, may be the only organizational structures available to organize experience for the order-prone mind (States, 1994). The narrative of dream reflects our attempts at comprehension of our world. It may be that this reflects a basic tenet of what is required of us in being human, "learning to understand and to be able to tell stories" (Foulks, 1985).

Elaine Scarry (1995) has analyzed the techniques that the great sensory writers, including Marcel Proust, Thomas Hardy, John Keats, and Seamus Heaney, use to incite the reader to experience mental images that resemble less the daydream and more the perception of actual experience. These writers do not achieve this goal by an intense description of a scene or experience. It is the scientist, the expert at description, who can obtain reams of data that describe the functioning of both body and brain – EEG, EMG, EKG, EOG, oxygen and CO_2 levels, respiratory function and drive, body position, and if we wish, data on neuron firing, ionic flux, glucose use, and metabolism in the brain. But as the observers in the control room looking at all this data, we have little personal sense of the person or experience that is being described. It is rather the writer who has the capacity to recreate another's experience. The writer accomplishes this not by description, but by creating for the reader a dream-like construct that gives rise to the perceptions that make the described experience look, sound, or feel the way that it would if occurring in the exterior world. Dreams are visually experienced as imagery framed within a narrative storyline formally organized in ways that are more associative and perhaps more bizarre than focused waking. As Harry Hunt (1991) points out, "the creative tension required to produce novel, emergent forms of self-knowledge requires a staged collision between subjectivity and objectivity that may characterize the dream." This process available to every dreamer is what the novelist tries to recreate.

Dreams in religion and philosophy

The dreams of kings, prophets, and priests were sometimes considered to be messages from god. These dreams became the stuff of religion, scripted into walls of Egyptian tombs, the Torah, the Bhagavad-Gita, the

Bible, and the Koran. In many cultures of the ancient world, the study of dreams was a major preoccupation. The remains of temples have been excavated that were devoted to the worship of Serapis, the Egyptian god of dreams (Van de Castle, 1994). The sacred Indian books of wisdom, the Vedas written between 1500 BC and 1000 BC, include descriptions of favorable and unfavorable dreams, as well as speculations concerning the expected realization of prophecies based on the time of night of the dream experience. Chou Kung's *Book of Auspicious and Inauspicious Dreams* is part of the T'sung Shu, an ancient *Chinese Almanac of Life* dating back to 1020 BC (Teillard, T'sung Shu, trans. 1986). In the Torah, God famously proclaims, "If any one among you is a prophet, I will make myself known to him in a vision, I will speak to him in a dream" (Numbers 12:6). Joseph in Egypt explained the Pharaoh's dreams, and Daniel in Babylon gained political power as a dream interpreter for Nebuchadnezzar (Genesis 41; Daniel 2:1–34). In the New Testament, Joseph was told the miraculous basis of Mary's pregnancy and that the child should be named Jesus in a dream (Matthew 1). This same concept of immaculate conception as revealed in a dream is part of Buddhist literature describing the birth of Buddha (Teillard, 1961). Much of the Koran was revealed to Muhammad in dreams, and dream visitations from the angel Moroni led Joseph Smith to find and reveal the Book of Mormon (Van de Castle, 1994).

But not every dream can be a message from god. It is not just the kings and priests who dream. Children, atheists, criminals, the mentally ill, and even women have dreams. In most cases it was not considered politically or religiously correct in the ancient world to attribute such dreams as being messages from god. For the founders of states and religions that were based at least in part on dreams, the first studies of dreams helped determine the true and important dreams so that they could be divined from the false. For the Egyptians and early Greeks, this attempt to divine "true dreams" from false lies at the basis of their logic, philosophy, and science. This focus led the greatest of the ancient philosophers to address basic and continuing aspects of the human experience that remain profound. Plato in *Theaetetus* has Socrates asking, "What proof could you give if anyone should ask us now, at the present moment, whether we are asleep and our thoughts are a dream, or whether we are awake and talking to each other in the waking condition?" (Plato, trans. 1987).

Dreams and science

A series of major conceptual breakthroughs in science are derived from attempts to understand dreaming. Early Greek dream analysis became the science of medicine. In the third century, physician/priests required their patients to sleep at the foot of the god in the temple of Asclepios "incubating" a dream that was to be reported the next morning. The physician's task was to interpret that dream and prescribe a cure based on his interpretation of the dream's significance. Today the Asclepios Temples are littered with stone tablets describing these recorded dreams and the subsequent attempts at cure. These are historical examples of early scientific method as applied to medicine, in which symptoms, dreams, and attempts at treatment, both successes and failures, are recorded for further analysis. Even surgical instruments have been recovered from temple excavations, the products of what were probably very interesting dreams. The rare successes of the physician–priests that were recorded include the surgical removal of the bladder stone and the trepanome – a hole bored through the skull to relieve cranial pressure – for the treatment of debilitating headaches resulting from intracranial bleeding. Later, and even into our days of modern medical technology, these same approaches may be used on patients with similar symptoms (Pagel, 2008).

In the seventeenth century, Rene Descartes developed the process of logic that we now call the scientific method based on a series of dreams: "And finally, taking into account the fact that the same thoughts we have when we are awake can also come to us when asleep, without any of the later thoughts being true, I resolved to pretend that everything that had ever entered my mind was no more true than the illusions of my dream. For how does one know that the thoughts that come to us in our dreams are more false than the others, given that they are no less vivid or expressed?" (Descartes, 1641; p. 17). Working from that original description of "self," Descartes went on to differentiate his dreaming world from his reality without having to rely on the sometimes undependable evidence of his senses. " I should no longer fear lest those things that are daily shown me by my senses are false; rather the hyperbolic doubts of the last few days ought to be rejected as worthy of derision – especially the principal doubt regarding sleep, which I did not distinguish from being awake. For I now notice that a very great difference exists between these two; dreams are never joined with all the other actions of life by the memory, as is the case with those actions that occur when one is awake" (Descartes, 1641; p. 100).

Early in the twentieth century, Sigmund Freud and his adherents developed the psychoanalytic techniques of free association and dream analysis that could be utilized in diagnosing and treating individuals with psychiatric illnesses. Freud utilized dreams as a window into understanding and analyzing the problems and processes of psychiatric illness (Freud, 1907). An individual's psychic structure and dynamic could be inferred by the psychoanalyst from information derived from the associative interpretation of dreams and utilized in developing a therapeutic plan for the treatment of psychiatric symptoms. "...the study of dreams is not only the best preparation for the study of the neuroses, but dreams are themselves a neurotic symptom, which, moreover, offers us the priceless advantage of occurring in all healthy people" (Freud, 1933). Freud viewed psychoanalysis as an attempt to extend the scientific method into the investigation of the mind. For the first half of the twentieth century, psychoanalysis was the primary approach used to describe underlying structural dysfunctions of the mind leading to psychiatric illness. As Freud stated, "Psychoanalysis is related to psychiatry approximately as histology is related to anatomy." (Freud, 1917). For more than a generation, psychiatrists were trained in psychoanalysis, with the data derived from psychoanalytic techniques, such as free association and dream interpretation, used to make diagnoses and form treatment plans. Psychoanalysis was utilized with some success in treating psychiatric illness. However, most of the evidence attesting to the therapeutic efficacy of psychoanalysis has been anecdotal and subjective, and there have been repeated failures to show that clinical outcomes achieved based on psychoanalysis differ from the outcomes achieved through supportive psychotherapy (Grunbaum, 1984; Wallerstein, 1986). The psychoanalytic era of psychiatry turned out to be one of long-term institutionalized therapy. Other psychodynamic and medical approaches to the treatment of these illnesses have proven both cheaper and more efficacious. Today many in the fields of psychology and psychiatry are skeptical that psychoanalysis is a method that is useful in the diagnosis and treatment of psychiatric disease.

With the loss of such basic underpinnings to the field, it would not be surprising if psychoanalytic theories collapsed, and fell into disrepute. The outcome has been quite different. During the same period in which applied psychoanalysis has been in serious decline as a method utilized in treating illness, psychoanalysis has become one of the primary techniques utilized by individuals without diagnosed illness, in their attempts to understand the structure and function of the mind. The psychoanalytic perspective has moved to other fields outside psychiatry that are also focused on attempting to understand aspects of higher cognitive functioning. Psychoanalytic constructs of mind are commonly used to understand the associative thought of creative process, the bidirectionality of cinema, and the impulsive power of art (Pagel, 2008).

Psychoanalysis does differ from most other psychotherapeutic techniques in its attempt to offer insight into the basic psychodynamics of disease. Through analysis of associative thought and dream content, Freud attempted to derive information about the structure of the brain from the study of aspects of the mind. It was Freud's contention that the psychoanalyst could use the associative thought of dreams to describe the brain. In some of the first polysomnographs (PSGs) recorded at the University of Chicago, William Dement noted the strange phenomena of repetitious conjugate eye movements occurring periodically during the night. When he awakened test subjects during this REMS state, most reported dreaming (Dement and Vaughan, 1999). For many, this finding was the psychoanalytic "smoking gun" that demonstrated a biological basis for postulated psychoanalytical brain constructs. It seemed apparent that the brain stem-based REMS state was the dream state – Freud's mythical "id."

Hobson and McCarley incorporated this perspective in their theory of activation–synthesis, proposing that all cognitive behaviors, both conscious and non-conscious, reflect the biological and physiological activity occurring in the central nervous system (CNS) (McCarley and Hobson, 1975). Their proof for this theory was this apparent finding that REMS is the CNS dreaming state. They postulated that the cognitive activity of dreaming is based on the CNS activation associated with REM sleep. According to this theory, dreaming is an upper-cerebral cognitive process utilizing the CNS activation associated with a primitive electrophysiologic state of activation that we call REMS. "REMS = dreaming" was proof of the correlate between psychoanalysis and brain structure. The clear evidence that dreaming occurs outside REMS, and that REMS occurs without dreaming, has been conceptually devastating for psychoanalytic-based theories based on evidence that psychoanalytic constructs reflect actual neuroanatomic brain structures or electrophysiological states.

Contemporary dream use in story, religion, and science

The role of dream in story, religion and philosophy, and science is not restricted to history. Interest and current use of dreaming continues in all these fields. Recent studies of the modern process of filmmaking indicate that dreams are utilized at high frequency in actualizing the process of creative story telling. The filmmaker produces a visual storyline composed of associated images able to interact with the personal memories and emotions of the viewer to create an almost complete cognitive experience, fully outside the viewer's control, and using cognitive processes utilized in dream. Almost all of the successful directors report high levels of dream integration into their waking lives and creative process, and utilization of dreams in the filmmaking process to help in adapting to change and stress (Pagel and Kwiatkowski, 2003). In creating their alternative realities, screenwriters often turn to their dreams to make decisions and to find alternatives to the approaches they develop during waking. Many screenwriters continue to utilize the ancient creative process of dream incubation in developing and writing their scripts. Before sleep they mull over problems confronting them in their writing. Answers to these conundrums can sometimes come in the dreams of sleep, at sleep onset, or during periods of disconnection when awake. Actors incorporate dreams at high levels into all facets of waking life using their dreams in developing character roles, and in achieving a connection with dream visualizations in their acting roles (Pagel and Kwiatkowski, 2003).

Despite a general acceptance in Judeo–Christian tradition that direct dream prophecy may have ended with the writing of the Bible, dreams continue to have roles in religious worship and in achieving religious understanding. That this perspective remains open to interpretation was perhaps best explained by Rabbi Solomon Almoli in his fifteenth century *Pitron Chalomot*, "Since the time of our exile from our homeland Israel, prophecy came to an end and the oracle was hidden from us. Yet even so, we have retained our ability to be inspired by dreams, which tell us of all that will come to pass." Most modern religions have sects that accept that dreams can provide direct access to their deity. In the Eastern Orthodox tradition, such dreams are referred to as "manifestations of the divine." Evangelicals and Pentecostals may refer to such dreams as the "prophetic word of the Lord." Many Catholic and Protestant sects believe that dreams can provide a "divine epiphany," an awareness of the "mysterium tremendum" of the holy presence. Hindus refer to "darshan" a glimpse or vision of the divine that can occur in dream. Mormons speak of the "direct revelation" available in prophetic dreams. Some theologians have adapted psychoanalytic dream theory in the attempt to use dreams in understanding biblical scripture (Sanford, 1970).

It is only recently that experimentally testable scientific approaches have been applied to the study of dreaming, yet the scientific literature is replete with grand theories purporting to explain the dream state. In the last 50 years the scientific focus on dreaming has been on REM sleep as the correlate of dreaming. "REMS = dreaming" is a confounding postulate lying at the basis of modern theories of dream including AIM (activation–input–modulation), the most fully developed and widely accepted theory of CNS functioning (Hobson *et al.*, 2003). It is a primary postulate of AIM that the neurons and neurochemicals that modulate REMS alter dreaming and other conscious states in a similar manner. The AIM model has been adopted and extended into proposals that REMS dreaming is what organizes neural nets in higher cortical regions (Crick and Mitchenson, 1983; Churchland 1986). The search–attention model also relies on the example of REMS as the primary state during which dreaming occurs. Multiple studies have demonstrated the REMS occurs without dreaming and dreaming without REMS (Foulks, 1985; Domhoff, 2003; Solms, 2003). It is unclear as to whether a special association exists between REMS and dreaming. Sleep onset and REMS, both states that are close to waking, have similar recall frequency and content when length of report is taken into account (Domhoff, 2003). REMS can be understood within the context of sleep without invoking the quasi-conscious processes of dreaming (Pagel, 2004, 2005). Proponents of psychoanalytic-based theories such as AIM have been reluctant to accept that dreaming occurs throughout sleep, with REMS but one of the electophysiological brain states associated with dreaming (Nielsen, 2003).

In conclusion, despite such theoretical, structural, and methodological constraints, the study of dreaming continues to attract interested scientists. The progress that researchers have made in understanding dreams has been incremental, and is not nearly as exciting as the breakthrough insights into the process of consciousness that were attributed to dreaming in the last centuries. Despite its incremental nature, this work is revolutionary, reflecting an increase in actual scientific knowledge of the dream state, knowledge based on evidence rather than grand theory. Dreams when not defined as REMS, require a dream report that in most cases is from a human. Studies of such cognitive, behaviorally defined states are affected by a wide variety of medical, psychological, sleep, and social variables. The different aspects of dreaming that can be studied include dream and nightmare recall frequency, methodologically controlled studies of dream content, and dreaming effects on waking behaviors such as emotional expression, and learning and memory. A long history of study has led us to only a limited understanding of dreaming. It is perhaps not surprising that after just fifty years of scientific focus, the association between REMS and dreaming remains as intangible as a shadow, blown by the wind.

References

Almoli, S. (1500s) *Pitron Chalomot Artemidorus*.

Artemidorus (1500s) *Oneirocritica: The Interpretation of Dreams*, trans. R. White (1975) Torance, California: Original Books.

Brannigan, E. (1992) *Narrative Comprehension and Film*. London and New York: Routledge, pp. 3–4.

Churchland, P. (1986) *Neurophilosophy: Toward a Unified Science of the Mind/Brain*. Cambridge: MIT Press, p. 272.

Crick, F. & Mitchenson, G. (1983) The function of dream sleep. *Nature* **304**: 111–14.

Dement, W. & Vaughan, C. (1999) *The Promise of Sleep*. New York: Dell, pp. 35–6.

Descartes, R. (1641) Objections against the Meditations and Replies. In *Great Books of the Western World: Bacon, Descartes and Spinoza* (1993) ed. M. J. Adler. Chicago: Encyclopaedia Britannica, Inc., pp. 17 & 100.

Domhoff, G. W. (2003) *The Scientific Study of Dreams: Neural Networks, Cognitive Development and Content Analysis*. Washington DC: American Psychological Association.

Ecclesiasticus 34.2, from The Inclusive Hebrew Scriptures – Vol III, (2000) Lanham, Maryland: Altimira Press.

Foulks, D. (1985) *Dreaming: A Cognitive-Psychological Analysis*. Hillsdale NJ: Lawrence Erlbaum Associates.

Freud, S. (1907) The interpretation of dreams. In *The Standard Editions of the Complete Psychological Works of Sigmund Freud, Vol. IV and V*. (1953) ed. J Strachey. London, England: Hogarth Press.

Freud, S. (1917) Psychoanalysis and psychiatry general theory of the neuroses. In *Introductory Lectures on Psychoanalysis* (1966) trans. & ed. J. Strachey. New York: W. W. Norton, p. 255.

Freud, S. (1933/1973) *New Introductory Lectures on Psychoanalysis*. Harmondsworth: Penguin, p. 83.

Furst, P. (1994) An overview of shamanism. In *Ancient Traditions: Shamanism in Central Asia and the Americas*, eds. G. Seaman & J. Day. Denver: Colorado, University Press, p. 7.

Garfield, P. (1991) *The Healing Power of Dreams*. New York: Simon and Schuster, p. 26.

Grunbaum, A. (1984) *The Foundations of Psychoanalysis: A Philosophical Critique*. Berkeley: University of California Press.

Hobson, J., Pace-Schott, E. & Stickgold, R. (2003) Dreaming and the brain: toward a cognitive neuroscience of conscious states. In *Sleep and Dreaming: Scientific Advances and Reconsiderations*, eds. E. Pace-Schott, M. Solms, M. Blagrove & S. Harnad. Cambridge: Cambridge University Press, pp. 1–50.

Holy Bible: Dictionary/Concordance – authorized King James Version. USA, Collins World.
a. Daniel 2:1–34. p 543.
b. Genesis 41, p. 29
c. Matthew 1, New Testament, p. 1.
d. Numbers 12:6, p. 101.

Hunt, H. (1991) Dreams as literature/science: an essay. *Dreaming* **1**: 235–42.

McCarley, R. & Hobson, J. (1975) Neuronal excitability modulation over the sleep cycle: a structural and mathematical model. *Science* **189**: 58–60.

Neilsen, T. (2003) A review of mentation in REM and NREM sleep: "covert" REM sleep as a possible reconciliation of two opposing models. In *Sleep and Dreaming: Scientific Advances and Reconsiderations*, eds. E. Pace-Schott, M. Solms, M. Blagrove & S. Harnad. Cambridge: Cambridge University Press, pp. 59–74.

Pagel, J. F. (2003) Non-dreamers. *Sleep Med* **4**: 235–41.

Pagel, J. F. (2004) Drug induced alterations in dreaming: an exploration of the dream data terrain outside activation–synthesis. *Behav Brain Sci* **27**(5): 10–14.

Pagel, J. F. (2005) Neurosignals: incorporating CNS electrophysiology into cognitive process. *Behav Brain Sci* **28**(1): 75–6.

Pagel, J. F. (2008) *The Limits of Dream: A Scientific Exploration of the Mind/Brain Interface*. Oxford UK: Academic Press (Elsevier).

Pagel, J. F. & Kwiatkowski, C. F. (2003) Creativity and dreaming: correlation of reported dream incorporation into awake behavior with level and type of creative interest. *Creativ Res J* **15**(2/3): 199–205.

Pagel, J. F., Blagrove, M., Levin, R. *et al.* (2001) Defining dreaming: a paradigm for comparing disciplinary specific definitions of dream. *Dreaming* **11**(4): 195–202.

Plato. *Theaetetus.* trans. R. Waterfield (1987) Penguin Books.

Sanford, J. (1970) *The Kingdom Within.* San Francisco: Harper, pp. 12–13.

Scarry, E. (1995) On vivacity: the difference between daydreaming and imagining-under-authorial-instruction. *Representations* **52**: 1–26.

Solms, M. (2003) Dreaming and REM sleep are controlled by different brain mechanisms. In *Sleep and Dreaming: Scientific Advances and Reconsiderations* eds. E. Pace-Schott, M. Solms, M. Blagrove & S. Harnad. Cambridge: Cambridge University Press, pp. 51–8.

States, B. O. (1993) *Dreaming and Storytelling.* Ithaca, NY: Cornell University Press, p. 53.

States, B. O. (1994) Authorship in dreams and fictions. *Dreaming* **4**(4): 237–53.

States, B. O. (1997) *Seeing in the Dark: Reflections on Dreams and Dreaming.* New Haven: Yale University Press, p. 206.

Teillard, A. (1961) *Spiritual Dimensions.* London: Routledge and Keegan Paul.

Teillard, A. *T'sung Shu: The Ancient Chinese Almanac of Life,* trans. M. Palmer (1986) Boston: Shambala.

Van de Castle, B. (1994) *Our Dreaming Mind.* New York: Ballantine Books, pp. 41 & 55.

Wallerstein, R. (1986) *Forty-two Lives in Treatment.* New York: Guilford, pp. 304–5.

Chapter

2

REM sleep and dreaming

Edward F. Pace-Schott

Summary

Among sleep stages, awakenings from rapid eye movement (REM) sleep produce the greatest number and reported intensity of dream reports. Dreaming is a conscious state that lacks the insight and cognitive control typical of healthy waking but allows the remarkable emergence of coherent narrative, vivid visual imagery, strong emotion, and sometimes never-before-experienced elements. Similar to waking, ascending activation from the brain stem, basal forebrain, and diencephalon produces the brain-activated state of REM and its associated dream consciousness. However, in REM, the neuromodulatory influences producing this arousal are largely cholinergic and lack the aminergic activation accompanying cholinergic modulation in waking. Positron emission tomography (PET) studies have shown that in REM vs. waking, lateral cortical areas subserving cognitive control and higher order cognition are relatively less activated whereas midline anterior limbic cortical and subcortical structures are equally or more active. Such differences in neuromodulation and regional brain activity help shed light on the neural processes producing phenomenological differences between dream and waking consciousness. Advances in neuroimaging techniques including functional magnetic resonance imaging (fMRI) and electromagnetic source localization are providing new details on the tonic conditions and phasic neural events during REM that may contribute to dream experience.

Dreaming and REM sleep

Following the discovery of REM sleep, there was widespread speculation that this sleep state, in which high- and mixed-frequency low-amplitude electroencephalogram (EEG) activity resembled waking, was the unique substrate of dreaming (Dement and Kleitman, 1957). Although REM sleep yielded dream reports following a high percentage of sleep laboratory awakenings, when awakenings were performed from other sleep stages, dreams were also reported (Foulkes, 1962; also see chapter by Mallick and Mukhopadhyay in this volume). Subsequent studies have showed that, in addition to a higher frequency of dream reports following REM vs. non-REM (NREM) awakenings, REM reports are more visually vivid, motorically animated and emotional, and contain a higher amount of bizarre features (see for review Hobson *et al.*, 2000). A meta-analysis of 29 awakening studies by Nielsen (2000) revealed that about 82% of awakenings from REM result in recall of a dream whereas this frequency following NREM awakenings is lower at 42%. Nielsen speculated that brain activity resembling that of REM but failing to produce the full complement of physiological features required for polysomnographic scoring of REM may underlie NREM dreams and he termed such activity "covert REM." Experimental evidence for "covert REM" processes include enhancement of sleep onset dreams by prior REM deprivation (Nielsen *et al.*, 2005) and a greater frequency of NREM dreaming in round-the-clock, ultra-short (40:20 minutes wake:sleep) sleep cycles during NREM sleep bouts occurring at circadian times with the greatest REM propensity (Suzuki *et al.*, 2004).

Dreaming and the sleep EEG

Recent studies of waking cognition using electroencephalography (EEG) and magnetoencephalography (MEG) have linked the faster, gamma ranges of neuronal oscillations (low gamma, 30 to 80 Hz; high gamma, 80 to 150 Hz) to exteroceptive attention and other effortful cognitive activity such as working memory (Jensen *et al.*,

---

REM Sleep: Regulation and Function, eds. Birendra N. Mallick, S. R. Pandi-Perumal, Robert W. McCarley, and Adrian R. Morrison. Published by Cambridge University Press. © Cambridge University Press 2011.

2007). Synchronization of oscillatory activity between different brain regions has been proposed as one mechanism by which representations processed by disparate regions of the brain can be bound together to form a coherent percept or memory (Singer, 2001). Scalp EEG, intra-cranial EEG (iEEG), and MEG studies have shown that the prevalence and spectral power of gamma oscillations during sleep is greatest in REM (Corsi-Cabrera *et al.*, 2003, 2008). Investigators have speculated that gamma oscillations during REM are associated with cognition and perception (Jouny *et al.*, 2000), memory processing (Cantero *et al.* 2004), and temporal binding of dream imagery (Kahn *et al.*, 1997).

In rats, gamma activity is coupling to and modulated by hippocampal theta-frequency (4–8 Hz) oscillations, which may facilitate cortical information processing during both waking and REM sleep (Montgomery *et al.*, 2008). In human waking, coupling of gamma and theta rhythms may similarly enhance information processing (Canolty *et al.*, 2006) although theta oscillators may originate from anterior midline (anterior cingulate) oscillators instead of or in addition to the hippocampus (Mitchell *et al.*, 2008). In human REM, a slower hippocampal rhythmic activity in the delta frequency (1.5–3 Hz) range may similarly modulate gamma power (Clemens *et al.*, 2009).

In contrast to REM, slow oscillatory rhythms linked to thalamocortical and cortico-cortico circuits predominate in human slow-wave sleep (SWS). These include the characteristic delta and spindle oscillations as well as the cortically generated slow (<1 Hz) oscillation (Achermann and Borbely, 1997; Massimini *et al.*, 2004). These synchronized slow thalamocortical rhythms during NREM correlate with diminished cortical activation (Dang-Vu *et al.*, 2005; Kaufmann *et al.*, 2006) and may attenuate the mental activity that leads to dreaming during the desynchronized, activated REM state (Hobson *et al.*, 2000). The cortical slow oscillation, however, reflects alternation in cortical neurons between brief periods of rapid firing (up-states) and a longer hyperpolarized condition (down-states) (Destexhe *et al.*, 2007) and high levels of neuronal activity have been reported during such up-states in human SWS (Dang-Vu *et al.*, 2008).

Dreaming and cortical connectivity in sleep

During REM sleep relative to waking, attenuated synchrony of high-frequency neuronal oscillations between different brain regions may produce unique dream qualities in the conscious experience resulting from the REM-activated brain (Corsi-Cabrera *et al.*, 2003, 2008). Oscillatory synchrony can be quantified in EEG or MEG as "coherence," a quantity that estimates functional coupling at specific EEG frequencies between brain regions underlying different scalp recording sites. Coherence at gamma frequencies is relatively desynchronized between frontal and posterior regions during REM as compared to both waking and NREM (Corsi-Cabrera *et al.*, 2003, 2008). It has been suggested that the decreased interaction between frontal and posterior areas, suggested by their diminished gamma coherence, may indicate diminished executive control of perceptual processes that, in turn, may contribute to dream bizarreness (Cantero *et al.*, 2004; Corsi-Cabrera *et al.*, 2003, 2008). Interestingly, also during REM, gamma coherence *increases* between posterior regions possibly reflecting enhanced perceptual processing accompanying REM dreaming (Corsi-Cabrera *et al.*, 2003). The use of iEEG has allowed additional sleep-related declines in gamma coherence to be observed between localized cortical regions as well as between cortex and hippocampus (Cantero *et al.*, 2004; Fell *et al.*, 2003).

Interhemispheric coherence at slow EEG frequencies such as delta (1–3 Hz) and theta (4–7 Hz) are typically greater in sleep than in waking due to the synchronizing influence of intrinsic, sleep-related thalamocortical and cortico-cortical oscillations (Steriade, 2006). Nonetheless, progressively lower alpha (8–12 Hz) coherence from waking, through NREM to REM has been reported between fronto-frontal and fronto-occipital sites (Cantero and Atienza, 2005). At still slower, theta-range frequencies, fronto-posterior coherence is significantly lower for REM than for NREM stage 2 sleep (Corsi-Cabrera *et al.*, 2003). However, also in REM vs. NREM stage 2, these frequencies are significantly higher between different posterior sites, a finding that Corsi-Cabrera *et al.* (2003) link with reduced executive control but heightened perceptual intensity during REM vs. NREM dreaming.

Transcranial magnetic stimulation (TMS) allows direct demonstration of the influence of one brain region on another. Such studies have shown reduced functional interaction between brain regions during sleep vs. waking (Bertini *et al.*, 2004; Massimini *et al.*, 2005). For example, Bertini *et al.* (2004) demonstrated that, following REM sleep awakenings as compared with stage 2 NREM awakenings or waking itself, transcallosal inhibition of motor-evoked potential by contralateral TMS is greatly reduced. Similarly, Massimini *et al.* (2005) have shown that premotor TMS stimulation during NREM sleep does not propagate as far or persist as long as it does in waking, suggesting that reduced cortical "effective connectivity" may underlie the attenuation of consciousness in sleep.

The PGO wave, phasic activity in sleep, and its relation to dreaming

During REM sleep in the cat, rapid eye movements are immediately preceded by activation of the thalamic lateral geniculate nucleus (LGN) and occipital cortex via a characteristic ascending potential that originates in the pontine brainstem – the ponto-geniculo-occipital (PGO) wave (reviewed in Hobson *et al.* 2000). The PGO wave was central to the activation–synthesis hypothesis of dreaming (Hobson and McCarley, 1977), which suggests that the forebrain interprets this ascending stimulation from a dedicated visual pathway as visual sensory input leading to the hallucinations of dreaming.

Since discovery of the PGO wave in the cat, there have been continual efforts to demonstrate its existence in humans. In this search, the distinction between tonic and phasic sleep states (Pivik, 1991) has been an organizing concept. During both REM and NREM, phasic (transient, periodic events) are interspersed with tonic (longer duration, less variable) states. The phasic events of REM (and also at certain times in NREM) represent the likely peripheral manifestations of PGO potentials, the most widely studied of which are the rapid eye movements (REM saccades) themselves, but also include peri-orbital integrated potentials, middle ear muscle activity, and skeletal muscle twitches (Pivik, 1991) that often coincide with REM saccades. The REM sleep state, therefore, is frequently subdivided into phasic REM, periods containing single or clustered saccades, and tonic REM during which atonia and desynchronized EEG persists in the absence of saccades.

Early studies attempting to correlate features of dream reports with such phasic events reported mixed findings (reviewed in Pivik, 1991); however, more recent studies have provided clearer linkages. For example, Conduit *et al.* (2004) showed that dream reports from NREM stage 2 awakening that were preceded by eyelid movements (ELMs) more often contained reports of visual imagery than those without

preceding ELMs. These investigators also showed that ELMs correlated with other putative human peripheral PGO signs and, like PGO waves in cats, their rate of occurrence was low in NREM increasing just prior to REM when their frequency was maximal (Conduit *et al.*, 2002). Conduit *et al.* (2002) initially suggested that PGOs and ELMs were indirectly associated via their shared linkage with transient CNS arousals. However, recent work by this group has shown that sub-waking-threshold auditory stimuli that produce EEG arousals during REM suppress both rapid eye movements and post-awakening reports of visual imagery suggesting a direct linkage between central (PGO) and peripheral (saccade) events (Stuart and Conduit, 2009).

Evidence that REMs are associated with perceptual experiences comes from an event-related potential (ERP) study in which brain potentials accompanying voluntary waking saccades were compared with those accompanying REM saccades (Ogawa *et al.*, 2005). In waking, voluntary saccades were preceded by a centro-parietal readiness potential and were then followed by a parieto-occipital "lambda response" believed to reflect visual processing of the saccade target. In contrast, although no readiness potential occurred prior to REM saccades, these saccades were followed by potentials at the same parieto-occipital sites where lambda responses were seen in waking. Ogawa *et al.* (2005) therefore suggest that REM saccades may trigger visual experiences that contribute to dream construction as suggested by the activation–synthesis model.

The distinction between tonic and phasic REM has also been shown to predict changes in the above-described gamma frequency oscillations. Gamma frequency spectral power is greater during phasic vs. tonic REM in scalp EEG (Corsi-Cabrera *et al.*, 2008; Jouny *et al.*, 2000) and MEG (Corsi-Cabrera *et al.*, 2008). Increased gamma power along with decreased power at lower frequencies during phasic vs. tonic REM has been localized to specific areas such as the orbito-frontal cortex using iEEG (Nishida *et al.*, 2005). In the brief (62.5 msec) time window immediately preceding a REM saccade, gamma power is further increased (Corsi-Cabrera *et al.*, 2008) and enhanced prefrontal gamma power in the period following REM saccades further suggests that phasically enhanced forebrain activation accompanies such saccades (Abe *et al.*, 2008a). Corsi-Cabrera *et al.* (2008) report that during phasic REM, there is additional loss of coherence, relative to tonic REM, between frontal and parietal association cortices. These investigators suggest that such phasically decreased frontal control of posterior, perceptual cortical regions may, in turn, phasically increase cognitive or perceptual distortions associated with dream mentation.

The human PGO wave

Early studies identified potential EEG correlates of PGO waves via scalp and intracranial recordings synchronized with REMs (reviewed in Miyauchi *et al.*, 2009). Later EEG dipole tracing in REM recordings showed activity in the pons, midbrain, thalamus, hippocampus, and visual cortex consistent with PGO activity (Inoue *et al.*, 1999). Very recently, human REM sleep recordings from depth electrodes implanted in the pedunculopontine nucleus (a pontine brain stem structure that initiates PGO waves in the cat) of a patient with Parkinson's disease have shown phasic discharges with temporal and morphological characteristics closely resembling the feline PGO wave (Lim *et al.*, 2007).

Neuroimaging techniques also give evidence for human PGO waves. Correlations of REM density with regional brain activity in REM have identified regions that correspond to the PGO network in the cat. For example, using $H_2{}^{15}O$ PET, Peigneux *et al.* (2001) correlated REM density with activation of the rostral brain stem, LGN, and occipital cortex. Similarly, using fMRI, Wehrle *et al.* (2005) correlated REM density with LGN and occipital cortex activity. Electromagnetic tomography achieves the temporal resolution necessary to associate brain activity with phasic events such as REMs albeit with poorer spatial resolution. For example, using MEG tomography, Ioannides and colleagues (Ioannides *et al.*, 2004) identified correlated activity in the pons and frontal eye fields (FEF) that precedes REM saccades. This activity begins 600 msec before saccade onset and intensifies with greater temporal proximity to the saccade suggesting that increasing neuronal excitability leads to the actual REMs (Ioannides *et al.*, 2004). These researchers also suggested that this accumulation of excitability is driven by the pons in which this pre-saccadic activity is greatest.

Most recently, using event-related fMRI, Miyauchi *et al.* (2009) have demonstrated that activity in the pontine tegmentum, ventroposterior thalamus, and primary visual (and, sometimes, extrastriate) cortex takes place in the few seconds prior to REM saccades. These regions and their activation relative to the REM saccade correspond to the neural pathway traversed and the time course, respectively, of the feline PGO wave (Miyauchi *et al.*, 2009). Notably, average pre-saccade onset of activity in these regions was temporally graded in the same sequence as the feline PGO, i.e., pontine tegmentum (−4.7 sec), ventroposterior thalamus (−3.8 sec) and primary visual cortex (−2.8 sec). Voluntary saccades performed in total darkness activated FEF, supplementary eye fields, anterior cingulate, and putamen but not the primary visual cortex (Miyauchi *et al.*, 2009). Miyauchi and colleagues (2009) therefore suggested that their findings show clear evidence for the existence of PGO waves during human REM sleep.

Miyauchi *et al.* (2009) further suggested that because primary visual cortex (V1) activation occurred before REM saccades, this V1 activation cannot be triggered by efferent copies of neural activity in the FEF associated with the saccade (as has been shown in some waking studies) but that REM saccades may be in response to PGO-initiated dreamed visual imagery. They therefore suggested a sequence of events partially consistent with the scanning hypothesis (Roffwarg *et al.*, 1962). Citing earlier findings, Hong *et al.* (2009) suggest that support for the scanning hypothesis is evidenced by correlations between REM density and [18]fludeoxyglucose ([18]FDG) PET activity in the FEF and in midline and parietal attentional systems as well as by correlations between REM density and the visual imagery in dream reports. In additional support of the scanning hypothesis, Hong *et al.* (2009) also cite their most recent fMRI finding that activation of visual primary and association as well as oculomotor control cortices are time-locked to REM saccades. These findings do not exclude the possibility that primary visual cortex activation and REM saccades are both triggered by pontine activity that simultaneously excites oculomotor nuclei and the PGO network (discussed in Hobson *et al.*, 2000).

Limbic activation in association with REM saccades

In addition to pontine, thalamic, and V1 activation preceding REM saccades, Miyauchi *et al.* (2009) showed that activation of parahippocampal and anterior cingulate cortices, amygdala, and putamen coincided with REM (but not voluntary waking) saccade onset. Similar limbic activations in proximity to REM saccades have been reported using MEG and EEG current source localization (Abe *et al.*, 2008b; Ioannides *et al.*, 2004). Using MEG tomography, Ioannides *et al.* (2004) reported current sources in the amygdala as well as orbito-frontal and parahippocampal cortices that become active during the last 150 msec prior to an REM saccade (for potentially related physiology in animals, see Chapter 12 by Sanford and Ross in this volume). Similarly, using standardized low-resolution brain electromagnetic tomography (sLORETA), Abe *et al.* (2008b) estimated that the current sources of a negative potential occurring 150 to 20 msec before REM saccade (pre-REM negativity) were located in anterior limbic regions that included the ventromedial prefrontal (VMPFC), anterior cingulate, insular, temporopolar, and parrahippocampal cortices as well as the basal forebrain and uncus. These investigators suggested that such limbic activity represents phasically enhanced emotional processing occurring prior to REM saccades (Abe *et al.*, 2008b; Corsi-Cabrera *et al.*, 2008; Ioannides *et al.*, 2004). Additionally, using fMRI, Wehrle *et al.* (2007) reported that an expanded network of thalamic, cortical, striatal, and limbic regions are uniquely associated with phasic vs. tonic REM periods. They also suggested that increased activity in this network reflects enhanced emotional and mnemonic processing that is possibly associated with phasically intensified dreaming. Notably, emergence of activity in this network was accompanied by attenuated responses of auditory cortex to sub-waking threshold acoustic stimulation, residual responses to which were, however, seen in tonic REM.

Neuroimaging of REM sleep

Across longer timescales, PET studies comparing REM sleep to waking and NREM have demonstrated distinct regional activation differences between these behavioral states. Decreased activity in frontal brain regions relative to the awake state begins at sleep onset (Kjaer *et al.*, 2002) persists through NREM (Braun *et al.*, 1997; Maquet *et al.*, 1997; Nofzinger *et al.*, 2002) and REM (Braun *et al.*, 1997; Maquet *et al.*, 1996, 2005) as well as during the post-awakening period (Balkin *et al.*, 2002). In addition to lateral frontal deactivation, with deepening NREM sleep following sleep onset, deactivation extends to the brain stem, diencephalon, basal ganglia, and midline cortical and posterior lateral cortices (Braun *et al.*, 1997; Dang-Vu *et al.*, 2005; Maquet *et al.*, 1997; Nofzinger *et al.*, 2002). Findings that both lateral and medial frontal cortices deactivate with sleep onset and deepening NREM have also now been demonstrated using fMRI (Kaufmann *et al.*, 2006).

With the onset of REM, however, midline limbic and paralimbic areas reactivate (Braun *et al.*, 1997; Maquet *et al.*, 1996, 2005; Nofzinger *et al.*, 1997, 2004) whereas lateral frontal and parietal areas remain deactivated (Braun *et al.*, 1997; Maquet *et al.*, 1996, 2005). The midline limbic and paralimbic regions activated during REM have been termed by Nofzinger and colleagues the "anterior paralimbic REM activation area" (APRA) (Nofzinger *et al.*, 1997, 2004). Brain regions thus activating in REM include the pons and midbrain (Braun *et al.*, 1997; Maquet *et al.*, 1996), thalamic areas and hypothalamus (Braun *et al.*, 1997; Nofzinger *et al.*, 2004), basal forebrain, (Nofzinger *et al.*, 1997), basal ganglia including ventral striatum and pallidum (Braun *et al.*, 1997; Nofzinger *et al.*, 1997, 2004), hippocampal formation, uncus, and temporal pole (Braun *et al.*, 1997), as well as rostral, subcallosal, and paracingulate (BA32) anterior cingulate (Braun *et al.*, 1997; Maquet *et al.*, 1996) insular and caudal orbitofrontal (Braun *et al.*, 1997; Nofzinger *et al.*, 2004) medial prefrontal (BA10) (Braun *et al.*, 1997) and visual association (Braun *et al.*, 1998) cortices. In direct comparisons using PET, certain APRA areas have been shown to activate in REM to levels exceeding those of the waking conditions to which they were compared (Braun *et al.*, 1997; Maquet *et al.*, 1996; Nofzinger *et al.*, 1997, 2004).

Investigators reporting these PET findings have suggested functional correlates of REM-related activations and deactivations. Because APRA regions encompass limbic areas subserving emotion and social cognition, Maquet and colleagues have suggested that activity during REM involves processing of memories related to emotion (Maquet and Franck, 1997; Maquet *et al.*, 1996) and social cognition (Maquet *et al.*, 2005). Because these regions encompass cortical and subcortical portions of the mesolimbic reward system, Nofzinger *et al.* (1997) suggest that, during REM, motivational processes become integrated with neocortical functions (Nofzinger *et al.*, 1997) – processes that become dysregulated in depression in which REM-related activity in the APRA is also altered (Nofzinger *et al.*, 2004). Because REM involves activation of visual association and limbic regions concurrent with primary visual and frontal cortical deactivation, Braun and colleagues (1998) have suggested information is being internally processed by the former regions in the absence of sensory input and motor output from the latter. As further discussed below, these functional theories of brain activity during REM have direct relevance to the neurobiology of dreaming.

REM neuromodulation and dreaming

A pioneering biological theory on the association of REM sleep and dreaming, the activation–synthesis model of Hobson and colleagues (Hobson and McCarley, 1977; Hobson *et al.*, 2000) extrapolated from animal data to human dreaming by drawing not only on the PGO-wave findings described above, but also on animal data showing profound differences in the neuromodulation of the two activated brain states, waking and REM. The ascending reticular activating system (ARAS) underlies forebrain activation in both waking and REM (Steriade and McCarley, 2005). However, in waking, a suite of activating neuromodulators including the monoamines norepinephrine (NE), serotonin (5-HT), and histamine (HIST) in addition to acetylcholine (ACh) participate in this activation whereas, during REM, activation of the forebrain is primarily cholinergic. Hobson and colleagues' activation–synthesis model of dreaming and its successor, AIM (activation–input–modulation), suggest that this shift in aminergic/cholinergic balance contributes to the unique features of REM vs. waking mental activity (Hobson *et al.* 2000).

Over the past several decades, numerous micro-injection studies in animal models have demonstrated that augmenting ACh levels in the brain stem increases, whereas aminergic stimulation decreases, REM (reviewed in Hobson *et al.*, 2000, and Chapters by McKenna *et al.*; Gottesmann; and Jha & Mallick in this volume). Cholinergic activation of the forebrain in REM involves stimulation of the thalamus and basal forebrain by the cholinergic pedunculopontine and laterodorsal tegmental (PPT/LDT) nuclei of the mesopontine brain stem (Chapters by McKenna *et al.*; Gottesmann; and Jha & Mallick in this volume). Such stimulation interrupts the intrinsic thalamocortical oscillations of NREM (Steriade, 2000a) and triggers additional cholinergic stimulation of the cortex by cholinergic cells of the basal forebrain (Lu *et al.*, 2006). Cholinergic drugs, such as the cholinesterase inhibitor physostigmine, can trigger REM sleep and dreaming as well as induce nightmares in dementia patients and, in addition, nicotine and its partial agonist varenicline can also intensify dreams (reviewed in Pace-Schott, 2011).

Cholinergic forebrain stimulation in REM may promote hallucinations in dreams by inhibiting the thalamic reticular nucleus' GABAergic inhibition of thalamocortical relay neurons (Steriade, 2000a). In the absence of external sensory input to the thalamus, activity of thalamocortical afferents may then lead to hallucinations (Perry and Perry, 1995). Direct stimulation of nicotinic receptors, which are especially numerous on thalamocortical projection neurons, might further increase excitatory glutamatergic thalamocortical stimulation of the cortex and further promote dreaming (Perry and Perry, 1995). Combined cholinergic stimulation and fMRI has shown that, during a working memory task, ACh increases activity of posterior regions while also decreasing prefrontal activity (Furey *et al.*, 2000). During REM, enhanced cholinergic modulation may similarly favor posterior cortical activity and diminish prefrontal cognitive control thereby further intensifying dream hallucinosis.

Changes in aminergic neuromodulation may also favor REM dreaming. In addition to lowered aminergic tone in REM disinhibiting the PPT/LDT's cholinergic stimulation of the thalamus and basal forebrain, the monoamine dopamine (DA) may intensify REM and its associated dreams. Indeed two neurochemical models of dreaming, unlike AIM's emphasis on cholinergic effects, invoke dopaminergic influence. In one model, Gottesman proposes that, during REM, continued dopaminergic stimulation of the cortex without the inhibitory influences of NE and 5-HT may result in a psychotomimetic state from which dreaming emerges (Gottesmann, 2002). In another model, Solms suggests that dopaminergic stimulation of the mesolimbic reward system during both REM and NREM creates appetitive drives that instigate dreaming (Solms, 1997). Enhancing DA-ergic activity via DA precursors and agonists in Parkinson's disease patients can induce both nightmares and psychotic, hallucinatory states. Additionally, recent cellular neurochemical studies in rats have associated REM with increased dopaminergic activity relative to NREM (Gottesmann, 2002). For example, REM deprivation enhances both REM sleep intensity and c-Fos expression in the dopaminergic ventral tegmental area (VTA), dopamine concentrations increase during REM in the medial prefrontal cortex (MPFC) and nucleus accumbens and, during REM, VTA neurons transition from a tonic to a burst-firing mode that releases more DA from presynaptic terminals at their striatal and cortical targets (see Pace-Schott, 2011, for review and references). The VTA receives major excitatory input from the cholinergic PPT (Oakman *et al.*, 1999). Such cholinergic VTA stimulation is likely to occur during REM thereby linking increased cholinergic and dopaminergic influences on the forebrain in REM.

Unlike DA and ACh, the effects of 5-HT on dreaming may arise from its changing levels with transitions between sleep states (reviewed in Pace-Schott, 2011). Serotonergic drugs such as the selective serotonin reuptake inhibitors (SSRIs) and tramadol enhance dreaming (reviewed in Pace-Schott, 2008). Although within-night REM rebound may explain SSRI dream enhancement, studies on the effects of serotonergic hallucinogens suggest that changing levels of serotonin may also promote dream-like experiences. Serotonergic hallucinogens act at 5-HT$_{2A}$ receptors on presynaptic terminals of glutamatergic excitatory inputs targeting apical dendrites of pyramidal neurons in cortical layer V (Aghajanian and Marek, 1999). In doing so, hallucinogens abnormally prolong the release of glutamate from these presynaptic terminals following its normal pulsatile release triggered by action potentials; this prolonged release of glutamate, in turn, prolongs excitatory postsynaptic potentials (EPSPs) producing altered cognition and perception. Further, the authors showed that in rats, prolonged EPSPs also occur under conditions of low or fluctuating 5-HT levels (Aghajanian and Marek, 1999). Such conditions occur in REM and during transitions into and out of REM respectively (Hobson et al., 2000). Fluctuations and low levels of 5-HT may therefore promote naturally occurring REM-related hallucinations.

Additional evidence that alterations of both serotonergic and cholinergic neuromodulation result in hallucinations comes from studies of peduncular hallucinosis in which damage to ARAS projections from brain-stem nuclei producing these two neuromodulators also leads to hallucinosis (Manford and Andermann, 1998). It is important, however, to stress that just as many neurotransmitters and neuromodulators can influence REM physiology (see Section IV in this volume), neurochemical influences supporting dreaming are also undoubtedly multifactorial.

Neuronal networks generating dream phenomenology

Drawing upon findings reviewed above, a speculative account of how the brain produces dreaming can be constructed. As described above, conditions favoring dreaming in REM relative to NREM result from activation of the forebrain by cholinergic pathways of the

PPT/LDT extending to the thalamus and basal forebrain and that, in turn, activate the cortex via glutamatergic and cholinergic projections respectively (Lu et al., 2006; Steriade, 2000a). Cholinergic activation of the thalamus interrupts the intrinsic thalamocortical oscillations that may attenuate consciousness in NREM, especially SWS (Steriade, 2000a). Among other thalamic nuclei targeted by this ascending cholinergic activation are the intralaminar nuclei (Steriade et al., 1984) that are known to be essential for consciousness (Jones, 1998; Laureys et al., 2000). Differences in formal features between this conscious state, REM, and the other conscious state, waking, may be due to their differing aminergic/cholinergic balance (Hobson et al., 2000).

Phasic elevations in forebrain activation occur through PGO waves (see Chapter by Datta in this volume). These, as well as possibly other phasic ARAS potentials arriving via sensory dedicated pathways through the thalamus, may be interpreted by the cortex as sensory input thereby instigating hallucinated percepts that are incorporated into dreaming (Hobson et al., 2000). In addition to (or in concert with) visual input from PGO waves, emotions may be triggered by phasic activation of paralimbic structures (Abe et al., 2008b; Ioannides et al., 2004; Miyauchi et al., 2009), and complex percepts triggered by projections to visual association cortices (Braun et al., 1998). Enhanced conscious processing during phasic activation may be associated with activation of specific networks (Hong et al., 2009; Miyauchi et al., 2009; Wehrle et al., 2007), phasic elevations of gamma activity (Corsi-Cabrera et al., 2008) and phasic declines in fronto-posterior gamma synchrony (Corsi-Cabrera et al., 2003, 2008).

It is important to note that dream reports have been obtained from NREM as well as REM and, rather than being a quiescent state, SWS contains the slow oscillatory rhythm consisting of intense firing of neuronal populations (cortical "up-state") alternating with their prolonged hyperpolarization ("down-state") (Destexhe et al., 2007; Steriade, 2000a). The cortical up-state has been hypothesized to be a transient wake-like state (Destexhe et al., 2007) and high levels of cortical activation observed during SWS using fMRI have been attributed to these cortical up-states (Dang-Vu et al., 2008), activity that may support NREM dreaming (Steriade, 2000b).

The emotional nature of dreaming can be attributed to activity in the APRA regions described above. As noted, these regions include areas involved in the acquisition, memory, and expression of conditioned fear and its extinction including the amygdala, VMPFC, and hippocampus (Milad *et al.*, 2006). Sleep has been shown to influence processing of conditioned fear and its extinction in both the rat and human (reviewed in Pace-Schott *et al.*, 2009). Levin and Nielsen (2007) have suggested that extinction memories contributing to emotional regulation in waking are formed during REM dreaming when the amygdala, hippocampal, and VMPFC regions subserving extinction in waking are activated. They further suggest that dysregulation of this system may lead to nightmares in post-traumatic stress disorder.

The APRA also encompasses forebrain master nuclei of the autonomic nervous system (ANS) such as the hypothalamus, central nucleus of the amygdala, and bed nucleus of the stria terminalis as well as regions controlling the somatic expression of emotion such as the periaqueductal gray (Ulrich-Lai and Herman, 2009). Activity in forebrain regions of the ANS may account for the occurrence of instinctual programs such as sexual behavior as well as rage and panic states during dreaming (see Jouvet, 1999). Similarly, regions activated during REM encompass the subcortical and many of the cortical elements of the mesolimbic reward system such as the VTA, nucleus accumbens, insula, and VMPFC (Berridge and Kringelbach, 2008). Hence it is not surprising that appetitive behaviors are common in dreams (Solms, 1997).

The hippocampal formation (hippocampus, para-hippocampal gyrus, entorhinal and perirhinal cortices) is also included in the APRA. Unique features of memory in dreaming may result from differences in the way these structures are activated in REM relative to waking. For example, although there is extensive incorporation of semantic features of autobiographical memory in dreams, episodic memory may be largely inaccessible due to REM-specific constraints on hippocampal–neocortical information exchange (Fosse *et al.*, 2003). Nonetheless, recognition memory and its initial emotional verification ('feeling-of-rightness') may operate at a high level due to the activity of perirhinal and VMPFC regions respectively (Brown and Aggleton, 2001; Moscovitch and Winocur, 2002), both of which are encompassed in the APRA. Such activity may account for the frequent strong sense of familiarity during dreaming despite features of persons and places often being incongruous with waking experience (Pace-Schott, 2011). Enhanced familiarity processing may account for the observation that a large percentage of dream characters are identified on the basis of

"just knowing" (Kahn *et al.*, 2000). Dream bizarreness may, in turn, arise when elements in memory as well as *de-novo* dream constructs are uncritically accepted as familiar. Such credulity in dreams may be due to the activated VMPFC confirming feeling-of-rightness in the absence of the anterior and lateral frontal cortical activity that is involved in both the strategic search for memories and their critical cognitive verification (Moscovitch and Winocur, 2002).

Anterior midline areas activated in REM overlap with some regions activated in tasks involving social cognition and theory of mind (ToM, the ability to deduce feelings, thoughts, and intentions of others) (Ioannides *et al.*, 2009; Maquet *et al.*, 2005; Pace-Schott, 2001). Anterior paralimbic REM activation area regions overlapping with those subserving ToM include the paracingulate cortex (BA 32), amygdala, and temporal poles whereas an additional area active in ToM tasks, the superior temporal sulcus, is not part of the APRA (brain correlates of social cognition and ToM are reviewed in Amodio and Frith, 2006). Studies of dream phenomenology have documented the ubiquity of ToM phenomena in dreams (MacNamara *et al.*, 2007) accompanying the ubiquitous social interactions with dream characters. Additionally, portions of the APRA overlap with VMPFC areas involved in self-referential thought (Northoff *et al.*, 2006) and decision-making affectively guided by "somatic markers" (Bechara *et al.*, 2005).

Anterior paralimbic REM activation areas activated in common with ToM and self-referential cognition also overlap with anterior portions of the brain's "default mode," a network of primarily midline cortical areas that consistently deactivate in response to effortful (e.g., working memory) or exteroceptive tasks (Raichle *et al.*, 2001). The default network includes anteriorly the VMPFC and dorsomedial PFC (DMPFC), as well as, posteriorly, the hippocampal formation and, in the parietal lobe, the precuneus, posterior cingulate, and retrosplenial cortex medially and the inferior parietal lobe laterally (Buckner *et al.*, 2008; Raichle *et al.*, 2001). The default network broadly overlaps with areas consistently activated in studies of autobiographical memory as well as prospective imagining (Buckner *et al.*, 2008). This network is believed to carry out self-related adaptive functions such as projective simulation of one's thoughts, emotions, and behavior into future contingencies, behavioral rehearsal, and integrating autobiographical memory with interoceptive, emotional, and self-related cognition (Buckner *et al.*, 2008; Northoff *et al.*, 2006).

Integrated activity in the full complement of default regions (as measured by coherence of very slow oscillations in the blood oxygen level dependent, BOLD, signal of fMRI) persists into stages 1 and 2 of NREM but, in SWS, activity in frontal regions becomes uncoupled from the rest of the network (Horovitz *et al.*, 2009). Based upon PET studies cited above, the portions of this network that then reactivate in REM are those in the VMPFC, DMPFC, and hippocampal formation. However, posterior regions (e.g., the posterior cingulate and inferior parietal cortex) have been found to remain in the deactivated conditions seen in SWS (Maquet *et al.*, 2005). Interestingly, parsing of the default network using fMRI reveals that activity in distinct anterior prefrontal (DMPFC) and hippocampal components are uncorrelated with one another but are both correlated with activity in a core medial parietal component (Buckner *et al.*, 2008). Therefore, in REM dreams, both deficits in episodic memory (Fosse *et al.*, 2003) and frequent illogic vis-à-vis personal reality (Hobson *et al.*, 2000) may arise because self-projection by the medial PFC is dissociated from autobiographical memory retrieved by the hippocampal formation due to inactivity in the core medial parietal portion of the default network.

The inactivity of lateral PFC and parietal regions during REM has been widely speculated to underlie executive deficits in dreaming such as illogic, disorientation, poor working memory, uncritical acceptance of bizarreness, and the above-described inability to perform strategic memory retrieval (Hobson *et al.*, 2000; Maquet *et al.*, 2005; Schwartz and Maquet, 2002). Because the PFC exerts top-down control over activity in the posterior perceptual cortices (Stuss *et al.*, 2002), lateral frontal inactivity in REM may remove constraints acting upon both the generation of fictive dream percepts and their critical appraisal (e.g., see Hobson *et al.*, 2000; Schwartz and Maquet, 2002). One manifestation of working memory deficits may be that successive dream elements evoke subsequent elements with only a limited ability to retrospect resulting in dream narratives that are coherent but illogical and tangential (Pace-Schott, 2005). Notably, however, a recent study of lucid dreaming during REM has shown wake-like gamma activity and coherence in lateral prefrontal areas (Voss *et al.*, 2009).

Hallucinosis in dreaming is predominantly visual but sometimes also includes fictive movement and vestibular sensations, audition, and somatosensory experiences. Visual hallucinosis may be associated both with phasic transmission of pseudosensory input from the LGN to the occipital cortex (see above) and activity in the visual association cortex (Braun *et al.*, 1998). Evidence that this is the case includes the non-visual dreams that have been reported in patients with damage to visual association cortex (Solms, 1997). Fictive movement may arise from REM activation of basal ganglia (Braun *et al.*, 1997) and brain-stem motor pattern generators (Hobson *et al.*, 2000). Cerebellar activity during REM (Braun *et al.*, 1997) may generate vestibular sensations (e.g., falling). Lastly, dreams may require a fictive space in which dream events unfold and, as in waking, such spatial cognition may be subserved by the right inferior parietal lobe. Paradoxically, however, this region is among those reported most consistently deactivated in REM (Maquet *et al.*, 2005), while at the same time being one of the few regions in which destructive lesions can cause global dream cessation (Solms, 1997).

Dynamic interactions of brain networks during REM sleep dreaming

During REM, medial networks integrate activity in anterior paralimbic, medial temporal, and visual association cortices with the hippocampus, amygdala, basal ganglia, brain stem, and cerebellum to generate the experience of dreaming. Other regions including those that, in PET studies, appear deactivated or similarly activated in REM vs. waking are, however, undoubtedly also recruited, perhaps phasically, to support aspects of dreaming. Evidence that this is the case include the fact that, in REM sleep behavior disorder, complex motor activity closely corresponding to dream content is enacted indicating that commands from pre-motor and motor cortices have taken place. Additional evidence is the above-described necessity of the inferior parietal cortex for dreaming, despite its being among the areas consistently deactivated in $H_2^{15}O$ PET studies of REM (Maquet *et al.*, 2005). Similarly, activity in large areas of sensory and multimodal association cortices has been associated with REM saccades using fMRI (Hong *et al.*, 2009) and lateral prefrontal areas are sometimes seen activated during REM using [18]FDG PET (Nofzinger *et al.*, 1997). Most recently, lucidity during REM has been shown to be accompanied by electrophysiological features in frontal regions, including high gamma power and coherence, that are normally seen in waking suggesting that lucidity is a "hybrid" of these two states (Voss *et al.*, 2009).

Despite other techniques showing more widespread neuronal activity in REM than was initially shown in the pioneering PET studies, it remains true that activity in the APRA is consistently observed during REM thus providing a putative physiological basis for the phenomenological feature of dreaming. Such features and their associated neural substrates in the APRA and specific posterior areas include emotional and motivational salience (amygdala, ventral striatum, VMPFC), frequent conflictual (anterior cingulate) and social (VMPFC, DMPFC) themes, fictive movement and vestibular sensations (striatum, brain stem, cerebellum), visual hallucinosis (ventral stream visual association cortex), and instinctual programs (hypothalamus) all of which occur along with deficiencies (relative to waking) in working memory, orientation, and logic (relative deactivation of lateral prefrontal and parietal regions).

Activity in the above regions suggests that the following features of wide-range integrative brain networks occur during REM sleep dreaming. (1) There is activity in circuits linking ventral stream visual association areas with medial temporal areas involved in processing, storage, and retrieval of memories as well as VMPFC areas providing affective verification of such memories or *de-novo* hallucinations. (2) Anterior and medial temporal but not parietal elements of the default network are active possibly producing dream experiences that are analogous to the proposed projective imaginative reality simulation function of the default mode but are missing important elements in episodic memory. (3) Multiple interactions occur in circuits linking the amygdala, medial prefrontal and orbitofrontal cortices, and the hippocampal formation for the memory, regulation, and expression of emotions. (4) There is higher activity in "affective" (orbitofrontal–ventral caudate) and "motivational" (anterior cingulate–nucleus accumbens) fronto-striatal-thalamocortical circuits than in cognitive circuits (that link lateral frontal cortices with dorsal striatum). (5) There is greater activity in cortico-ponto-cerebello-thalamocortical loops that link limbic-related regions of the cerebellum (e.g., vermis) and cortex (e.g., MPFC) relative to similar loops linking the cerebellum with motor and lateral multimodal association cortices.

Future directions

To date, no published functional neuroimaging report has described the brain activity during sleep prior to an awakening with a specific dream report. As such techniques advance, however, this will undoubtedly be achieved and one might look forward to a time when the specific content features of dreams (e.g., visual imagery, movement, emotion) might be correlated with regional brain activity in the same manner as has been done in the past with the EEG's phasic events and power spectrum but with far greater power to explain the neural bases of dreaming. Particularly exciting in this regard are EEG and MEG source localization technologies (e.g., Abe *et al.*, 2008b; Ioannides *et al.*, 2004, 2009) that may provide both spatial and temporal fine-gained resolution as well as localization of the sources of specific oscillatory rhythms that can then be associated with the presence or intensity of reported dream experiences. Until this (hopefully not-far-off) time much can be inferred about the brain's mechanisms for dream construction from rapidly advancing cognitive neuroscience of the more experimentally accessible waking state.

Acknowledgments

National Institute on Drug Abuse (DA11744) and the National Institute of Mental Health (MH48832).

References

Abe, T., Ogawa, K., Nittono, H. & Hori, T. (2008a) Gamma band EEG activity is enhanced after the occurrence of rapid eye movement during human REM sleep. *Sleep Biol Rhythms* **6**: 26–33.

Abe, T., Ogawa, K., Nittono, H. & Hori, T. (2008b) Neural generators of brain potentials before rapid eye movements during human REM sleep: a study using sLORETA. *Clin Neurophysiol* **119**: 2044–53.

Achermann, P. & Borbely, A. A. (1997) Low-frequency (< 1 Hz) oscillations in the human sleep electroencephalogram. *Neuroscience* **8**: 213–22.

Aghajanian, G. K. & Marek, G. J. (1999) Serotonin and hallucinogens. *Neuropsychopharmacol* **21**: 16S-23S.

Amodio, D. M. & Frith, C. D. (2006) Meeting of minds: the medial frontal cortex and social cognition. *Nat Rev Neurosci* **7**: 268–77.

Balkin, T. J., Braun, A. R., Wesensten, N. J. *et al.* (2002) The process of awakening: a PET study of regional brain activity patterns mediating the re-establishment of alertness and consciousness. *Brain* **125**: 2308–19.

Bechara, A., Damasio, H., Tranel, D. & Damasio, A. R. (2005) The Iowa Gambling Task and the somatic marker hypothesis: some questions and answers. *Trends Cogn Sci* **9**: 159–62; discussion 162–4.

Berridge, K. C. & Kringelbach, M. L. (2008) Affective neuroscience of pleasure: reward in humans and animals. *Psychopharmacol* (Berl) **199**: 457–80.

Bertini, M., De Gennaro, L., Ferrara, M. *et al.* (2004) Reduction of transcallosal inhibition upon awakening from REM sleep in humans as assessed by transcranial magnetic stimulation. *Sleep* **27**: 875–82.

Braun, A. R., Balkin, T. J., Wesenten, N. J. *et al.* (1997) Regional cerebral blood flow throughout the sleep–wake cycle: an $H_2^{(15)}O$ PET study. *Brain* **120**(Pt 7): 1173–97.

Braun, A. R., Balkin, T. J., Wesensten, N. J. *et al.* (1998) Dissociated pattern of activity in visual cortices and their projections during human rapid eye movement sleep. *Science* **279**: 91–5.

Brown, M. W. & Aggleton, J. P. (2001) Recognition memory: what are the roles of the perirhinal cortex and hippocampus? *Nat Rev Neurosci* **2**: 51–61.

Buckner, R. L., Andrews-Hanna, J. R. & Schacter, D. L. (2008) The brain's default network: anatomy, function, and relevance to disease. *Ann N Y Acad Sci* **1124**: 1–38.

Canolty, R. T., Edwards, E., Dalal, S. S. *et al.* (2006) High gamma power is phase-locked to theta oscillations in human neocortex. *Science* **313**: 1626–8.

Cantero, J. L. & Atienza, M. (2005) The role of neural synchronization in the emergence of cognition across the wake–sleep cycle. *Rev Neurosci* **16**: 69–83.

Cantero, J. L., Atienza, M., Madsen, J. R. & Stickgold, R. (2004) Gamma EEG dynamics in neocortex and hippocampus during human wakefulness and sleep. *Neuroimage* **22**: 1271–80.

Clemens, Z., Weiss, B., Szucs, A. *et al.* (2009) Phase coupling between rhythmic slow activity and gamma characterizes mesiotemporal rapid-eye-movement sleep in humans. *Neuroscience* **163**: 388–96.

Conduit, R., Crewther, S. G., Bruck, D. & Coleman, G. (2002) Spontaneous eyelid movements during human sleep: a possible ponto-geniculo-occipital analogue? *J Sleep Res* **11**: 95–104.

Conduit, R., Crewther, S. G. & Coleman, G. (2004) Spontaneous eyelid movements (ELMs) during sleep are related to dream recall on awakening. *J Sleep Res* **13**: 137–144.

Corsi-Cabrera, M., Guevara, M. A. & del Rio-Portilla, Y. (2008) Brain activity and temporal coupling related to eye movements during REM sleep: EEG and MEG results. *Brain Res* **1235**: 82–91.

Corsi-Cabrera, M., Miro, E., del-Rio-Portilla, Y. *et al.* (2003) Rapid eye movement sleep dreaming is characterized by uncoupled EEG activity between frontal and perceptual cortical regions. *Brain Cogn* **51**: 337–45.

Dang-Vu, T. T., Desseilles, M., Laureys, S. *et al.* (2005) Cerebral correlates of delta waves during non-REM sleep revisited. *Neuroimage* **28**: 14–21.

Dang-Vu, T. T., Schabus, M., Desseilles, M. *et al.* (2008) Spontaneous neural activity during human slow wave sleep. *Proc Natl Acad Sci U S A* **105**: 15,160–5.

Dement, W. & Kleitman, N. (1957) The relation of eye movements during sleep to dream activity: an objective method for the study of dreaming. *J Exp Psychol* **53**: 339–46.

Destexhe, A., Hughes, S.W., Rudolph, M. & Crunelli, V. (2007) Are corticothalamic 'up' states fragments of wakefulness? *Trends Neurosci* **30**: 334–42.

Fell, J., Staedtgen, M., Burr, W. *et al.* (2003) Rhinal-hippocampal EEG coherence is reduced during human sleep. *Eur J Neurosci* **18**: 1711–16.

Fosse, M. J., Fosse, R., Hobson, J. A. & Stickgold, R. J. (2003) Dreaming and episodic memory: a functional dissociation? *J Cogn Neurosci* **15**: 1–9.

Foulkes, W. D. (1962) Dream reports from different stages of sleep. *J Abnorm Soc Psychol* **65**: 14–25.

Furey, M. L., Pietrini, P. & Haxby, J. V. (2000) Cholinergic enhancement and increased selectivity of perceptual processing during working memory. *Science* **290**: 2315–19.

Gottesmann, C. (2002) The neurochemistry of waking and sleeping mental activity: the disinhibition-dopamine hypothesis. *Psychiatry Clin Neurosci* **56**: 345–54.

Hobson, J. A. & McCarley, R. W. (1977) The brain as a dream state generator: an activation–synthesis hypothesis of the dream process. *Am J Psychiatry* **134**: 1335–48.

Hobson, J. A., Pace-Schott, E. F. & Stickgold, R. (2000) Dreaming and the brain: toward a cognitive neuroscience of conscious states. *Behav Brain Sci* **23**: 793–842; discussion 904–1121.

Hong, C. C., Harris, J. C., Pearlson, G. D. *et al.* (2009) fMRI evidence for multisensory recruitment associated with rapid eye movements during sleep. *Hum Brain Mapp* **30**: 1705–22.

Horovitz, S. G., Braun, A. R., Carr, W. S. *et al.* (2009) Decoupling of the brain's default mode network during deep sleep. *Proc Natl Acad Sci U S A* **106**: 11,376–81.

Inoue, S., Saha, U. K. & Musha, T. (1999) Spatio-temporal distribution of neuronal activities and REM sleep. In *Rapid Eye Movement Sleep.* ed. B. N. Mallick & S. Inoue. New York: Marcel Dekker, pp. 214–20.

Ioannides, A. A., Corsi-Cabrera, M., Fenwick, P. B. *et al.* (2004) MEG tomography of human cortex and brainstem activity in waking and REM sleep saccades. *Cereb Cortex* **14**: 56–72.

Ioannides, A. A., Kostopoulos, G. K., Liu, L. & Fenwick, P. B. (2009) MEG identifies dorsal medial brain activations during sleep. *Neuroimage* **44**: 455–68.

Jensen, O., Kaiser, J. & Lachaux, J. P. (2007) Human gamma-frequency oscillations associated with attention and memory. *Trends Neurosci* **30**: 317–24.

Jones, E. G. (1998) A new view of specific and nonspecific thalamocortical connections. *Adv Neurol* **77**: 49–71; discussion 72–3.

Jouny, C., Chapotot, F. & Merica H. (2000) EEG spectral activity during paradoxical sleep: further evidence for cognitive processing. *Neuroreport* **11**: 3667–71.

Jouvet, M. (1999) *The Paradox of Sleep: the Story of Dreaming*. Cambridge: MIT Press.

Kahn, D., Pace-Schott, E. F. & Hobson, J. A. (1997) Consciousness in waking and dreaming: the roles of neuronal oscillation and neuromodulation in determining similarities and differences. *Neuroscience* **78**: 13–38.

Kahn, D., Stickgold, R., Pace-Schott, E. F. & Hobson, J. A. (2000) Dreaming and waking consciousness: a character recognition study. *J Sleep Res* **9**: 317–25.

Kaufmann, C., Wehrle, R., Wetter, T. C. *et al.* (2006) Brain activation and hypothalamic functional connectivity during human non-rapid eye movement sleep: an EEG/fMRI study. *Brain* **129**: 655–67.

Kjaer, T. W., Law, I., Wiltschiotz, G., Paulson, O.B. & Madsen, P. L. (2002) Regional cerebral blood flow during light sleep: a H$_{(2)}$$^{(15)}$O-PET study. *J Sleep Res* **11**: 201–7.

Laureys, S., Faymonville, M. E., Luxen, A. *et al.* (2000) Restoration of thalamocortical connectivity after recovery from persistent vegetative state. *Lancet* **355**: 1790–1.

Levin, R. & Nielsen, T. A. (2007) Disturbed dreaming, posttraumatic stress disorder, and affect distress: a review and neurocognitive model. *Psychol Bull* **133**: 482–528.

Lim, A. S., Lozano, A. M., Moro, E. *et al.* (2007) Characterization of REM-sleep associated ponto-geniculo-occipital waves in the human pons. *Sleep* **30**: 823–7.

Lu, J., Sherman, D., Devor, M. & Saper, C. B. (2006) A putative flip-flop switch for control of REM sleep. *Nature* **441**: 589–94.

MacNamara, P., McLaren, A., Wowalczyk, S. & Pace-Schott, E. F. (2007) "Theory of Mind" in REM and NREM dreams. In *The New Science of Dreaming, Vol 1 Biological Aspects*. ed. D. Barrett & P. MacNamara. Westport, CT: Praeger, Greenwood Press, pp. 201–20.

Manford, M. & Andermann, F. (1998) Complex visual hallucinations. Clinical and neurobiological insights. *Brain* **121**(10): 1819–40.

Maquet, P., Degueldre, C., Delfiore, G. *et al.* (1997) Functional neuroanatomy of human slow wave sleep. *J Neurosci* **17**: 2807–12.

Maquet, P. & Franck, G. (1997) REM sleep and amygdala. *Mol Psychiatry* **2**: 195–6.

Maquet, P., Peters, J., Aerts, J. *et al.* (1996) Functional neuroanatomy of human rapid-eye-movement sleep and dreaming. *Nature* **383**: 163–6.

Maquet, P., Ruby, P., Maudoux, A. *et al.* (2005) Human cognition during REM sleep and the activity profile within frontal and parietal cortices: a reappraisal of functional neuroimaging data. *Prog Brain Res* **150**: 219–27.

Massimini, M., Ferrarelli, F., Huber, R. *et al.* (2005) Breakdown of cortical effective connectivity during sleep. *Science* **309**: 2228–32.

Massimini, M., Huber, R., Ferrarelli, F., Hill, S. & Tononi, G. (2004) The sleep slow oscillation as a traveling wave. *J Neurosci* **24**: 6862–70.

Milad, M. R., Rauch, S. L., Pitman, R. K. & Quirk, G. J. (2006) Fear extinction in rats: implications for human brain imaging and anxiety disorders. *Biol Psychol* **73**: 61–71.

Mitchell, D. J., McNaughton, N., Flanagan, D. & Kirk, I. J. (2008) Frontal-midline theta from the perspective of hippocampal "theta". *Prog Neurobiol* **86**: 156–85.

Miyauchi, S., Misaki, M., Kan, S., Fukunaga, T. & Koike, T. (2009) Human brain activity time-locked to rapid eye movements during REM sleep. *Exp Brain Res* **192**: 657–67.

Montgomery, S. M., Sirota, A. & Buzsaki, G. (2008) Theta and gamma coordination of hippocampal networks during waking and rapid eye movement sleep. *J Neurosci* **28**: 6731–41.

Moscovitch, M. & Winocur, G. (2002) The frontal cortex and working with memory. In *Principles of Frontal Lobe Function*, ed. D. T. Stuss & R. T. Knight. New York: Oxford University Press, pp. 392–407.

Nielsen, T. A. (2000) A review of mentation in REM and NREM sleep: "covert" REM sleep as a possible reconciliation of two opposing models. *Behav Brain Sci* **23**: 851–66; discussion 904–1121.

Nielsen, T., Stenstrom, P., Takeuchi, T. *et al.* (2005) Partial REM-sleep deprivation increases the dream-like quality of mentation from REM sleep and sleep onset. *Sleep* **28**: 1083–9.

Nishida, M., Uchida, S., Hirai, N. *et al.* (2005) High frequency activities in the human orbitofrontal cortex in sleep–wake cycle. *Neurosci Lett* **379**: 110–5.

Nofzinger, E. A., Buysse, D. J., Germain, A. *et al.* (2004) Increased activation of anterior paralimbic and executive cortex from waking to rapid eye movement sleep in depression. *Arch Gen Psychiatry* **61**: 695–702.

Nofzinger, E. A., Buysse, D. J., Miewald, J. M. *et al.* (2002) Human regional cerebral glucose metabolism during non-rapid eye movement sleep in relation to waking. *Brain* **125**: 1105–15.

Nofzinger, E. A., Mintun, M. A., Wiseman, M., Kupfer, D. J. & Moore, R. Y. (1997) Forebrain activation in REM sleep: an FDG PET study. *Brain Res* **770**: 192–201.

Northoff, G., Heinzel, A., de Greck, M. *et al.* (2006) Self-referential processing in our brain: a meta-analysis of imaging studies on the self. *Neuroimage* **31**: 440–57.

Oakman, S. A., Faris, P. L., Cozzari, C. & Hartman, B. K. (1999) Characterization of the extent of pontomesencephalic cholinergic neurons' projections to the thalamus: comparison with projections to midbrain dopaminergic groups. *Neuroscience* **94**: 529–47.

Ogawa, K., Nittono, H. & Hori, T. (2005) Brain potentials before and after rapid eye movements: an electrophysiological approach to dreaming in REM sleep. *Sleep* **28**: 1077–82.

Pace-Schott, E. F. (2001) "Theory of mind," social cognition and dreaming. *Sleep Research Society Bulletin* **7**: 33–6.

Pace-Schott, E. F. (2005) Complex hallucinations in waking suggest mechanisms of dream construction, Commentary on: Why people see things that are not there: A novel perception and attention deficit model for recurrent complex visual hallucinations by D. Collerton, E. Perry & I. McKeith. *Behav Brain Sci* **28**: 771–2.

Pace-Schott, E. F. (2008) Serotonin and dreaming. In *Serotonin and Sleep: Molecular, Functional and Clinical Aspects*, ed. J. M. Monti, S. R. Pandi-Perumal, B. Jacobs & D. Nutt. Basel: Birkhauser-Verlag, pp. 307–24.

Pace-Schott, E. F. (2011) The neurobiology of dreaming. In *Principles and Practice of Sleep Medicine*, 5th edition, ed. M. H. Kryger, T. Roth & W. C. Dement. Philadelphia: Elsevier, pp. 562–75.

Pace-Schott, E. F., Milad, M. R., Orr, S.P. *et al.* (2009) Sleep promotes generalization of extinction of conditioned fear. *Sleep* **32**:19–26.

Peigneux, P., Laureys, S., Fuchs, S. *et al.* (2001) Generation of rapid eye movements during paradoxical sleep in humans. *Neuroimage* **14**: 701–8.

Perry, E.K. & Perry, R. H. (1995) Acetylcholine and hallucinations: disease-related compared to drug-induced alterations in human consciousness. *Brain Cogn* **28**: 240–58.

Pivik, T. (1991) Tonic and phasic events in relation to sleep mentation. In *The Mind in Sleep*, 2nd edn, ed. S. Ellman & J. Antrobus. John Wiley and Sons, pp. 214–47.

Raichle, M.E., MacLeod, A.M., Snyder, A.Z. *et al.* (2001) A default mode of brain function. *Proc Natl Acad Sci U S A* **98**: 676–82.

Roffwarg, H. P., Dement, W. C., Muzio, J. N. & Fisher, C. (1962) Dream imagery: relationship to rapid eye movements of sleep. *Arch Gen Psychiatry* **7**: 235–58.

Schwartz, S. & Maquet, P. (2002) Sleep imaging and the neuro-psychological assessment of dreams. *Trends Cogn Sci* **6**: 23–30.

Singer, W. (2001) Consciousness and the binding problem. *Ann N Y Acad Sci* **929**: 123–46.

Solms, M. (1997) *The Neuropsychology of Dreams: a Clinico-anatomical Study*. Mahwah, NJ: Lawrence Erlbaum Associates.

Steriade, M. (2000a) Corticothalamic resonance, states of vigilance and mentation. *Neuroscience* **101**: 243–76.

Steriade, M. (2000b) Neuronal basis of dreaming and mentation during slow wave (non-REM) sleep. *Behav Brain Sci* **23**: 1009–11.

Steriade, M. (2006) Grouping of brain rhythms in corticothalamic systems. *Neuroscience* **137**: 1087–106.

Steriade, M. & McCarley, R.W. (2005) *Brain Control of Wakefulness and Sleep*. New York, NY: Kluwer Academic/ Plenum.

Steriade, M., Sakai, K. & Jouvet, M. (1984) Bulbo-thalamic neurons related to thalamocortical activation processes during paradoxical sleep. *Exp Brain Res* **54**: 463–75.

Stuart, K. & Conduit, R. (2009) Auditory inhibition of rapid eye movements and dream recall from REM sleep. *Sleep* **32**: 399–408.

Stuss, D.T., Alexander, M.P. & Floden, D. *et al.* (2002) Fractionalization and localization of distinct frontal lobe processes: evidence from focal lesions in humans. In *Principles of Frontal Lobe Function*, ed. D. T. Stuss & R. T. Knight RT. Oxford: Oxford University Press, pp. 392–407.

Suzuki, H., Uchiyama, M., Tagaya, H. *et al.* (2004) Dreaming during non-rapid eye movement sleep in the absence of prior rapid eye movement sleep. *Sleep* **27**: 1486–90.

Ulrich-Lai, Y. M. & Herman, J. P. (2009) Neural regulation of endocrine and autonomic stress responses. *Nat Rev Neurosci* **10**: 397–409.

Voss, U., Holzmann, R., Tuin, I. & Hobson, J. A. (2009) Lucid dreaming: a state of consciousness with features of both waking and non-lucid dreaming. *Sleep* **32**(9): 1191–2000.

Wehrle, R., Czisch, M., Kaufmann, C. *et al.* (2005) Rapid eye movement-related brain activation in human sleep: a functional magnetic resonance imaging study. *Neuroreport* **16**: 853–7.

Wehrle, R., Kaufmann, C., Wetter, T. C. *et al.* (2007) Functional microstates within human REM sleep: first evidence from fMRI of a thalamocortical network specific for phasic REM periods. *Eur J Neurosci* **25**: 863–71.

Chapter 3

REM sleep and dream sleep: are they identical?

Exploring the conceptual developments in the Upanishads and the present knowledge based on the neurobiology of sleep

Birendra N. Mallick and Asok K. Mukhopadhyay

Summary

Dreams have been known to mankind from time immemorial, while rapid eye movement sleep (REMS) has been objectively defined by characteristic electrophysiological signals since the mid twentieth century only. In the absence of better objective criteria, modern experimental sleep neurobiologists have objectively identified the dream state of a subject with REMS; thus, the dream state and REMS have often been used synonymously. There are reasons to believe that those states are not exclusively correlated to each other, rather they are independent phenomena that are often expressed simultaneously; however, neurobiological explanations are still lacking. In an attempt to better understand the relationship between them, we combined findings from objective science such as non-locality in physics with that of subjective science such as the phenomenon of consciousness. We explored the wisdom in the *Upanishads*, especially those instances where these ancient writings refer to sleep, dream, and states of consciousness, and attempted to offer an explanation based on modern experimental science. Our search led us towards a conceptual novelty in proposing the existence of an all-inclusive basal ground state (*T* or *Turiya*), which possibly equates to very slow waves in the electroencephalogram (EEG), during which *waking, dream, non-REM (NREMS)*, and *REMS* express apparently as independent phenomena, though overlapping to various degrees on many occasions. The proposed hypothesis and model, unlike several other earlier ones, is based on known and rational physiological principles, and hence is amenable to experimental verification.

Background and introduction

It is generally accepted that what can be perceived must exist; however, that does not necessarily imply that the opposite must also be true, i.e., what cannot be perceived does not or cannot exist. We are only aware of a fraction of that which exists, a state of affairs which is due to the limited bandwidth and threshold of our perception; as a consequence, it would be unwise and extremely difficult to comment on what does not exist. Knowledge of the existence of any object and/or information depends not only on the quality of the information, but also on the sensitivity of our perception. To investigate these, it is important to carry out experimental studies that are both objective and repeatable. It is an accepted fact that in higher mammals having an evolved brain, information is processed in the brain; however, it is an open question if similar perceptual processing capabilities can be attributed to species or organisms that do not possess a highly developed central nervous system. We tend to take a position that such a possibility cannot be ignored. For the sake of our understanding especially relevant to and in the context of the present volume, we restrict our discussions on the appreciation, perception, and expression by, and of, the brain. For any signal or information to be appreciated by the brain, the latter has to remain in a state so that the signal can be perceived optimally. Technically it may be said that the signal needs to be effectively and optimally absorbed by the perceiver, the brain or its fundamental unit, the neuron in this instance. This property in terms of physical science terminology most closely matches (analogous) with the impedance matching function/property. Therefore, it is no wonder that the brain must

<hr>

REM Sleep: Regulation and Function, eds. Birendra N. Mallick, S. R. Pandi-Perumal, Robert W. McCarley, and Adrian R. Morrison. Published by Cambridge University Press. © Cambridge University Press 2011.

exhibit different states at least in relation to its perception and expression.

Classically and grossly, the living organism remains in at least two states, sleeping and waking. Every organism undergoes rest and activity, which has been termed as the basic rest and activity cycle (BRAC). Apparently, the sleep and waking states in the higher forms of life are thought to be an evolutionary advancement of the fundamental process, the BRAC. Further, the organisms in higher order of evolution possess brain in addition to the other tissues present in the lower species. Thus, in the higher order species the state changes can be in two spheres, the physical level (BRAC) and the mental or the conscious level; the latter due to the presence of the brain. Since in evolution the neuron (the basic unit of brain) and the brain are of later development, the physical state change should be present in all species, whereas the consciousness state changes, an expression due to the additional presence of the brain, will be seen in higher order species of later origin in evolution. Thus, it is reasonable to predict and propose that the physical and conscious state changes may be expressed simultaneously or independently, being causally or acausally related to each other.

The changes in the states and levels of consciousness are appreciated by its various expressions, which correlate often very subtly with the physico-chemical status of the brain, its experience, age, and several other macro- or micro-level functions, which may be known or yet unknown factors. As a simple example and as an analogy it may be said that although many people may get exposed to and/or may harbor an infective agent, only a few may actually suffer from disease, which, however, is identified by a single symptom or a set of symptoms expressed by the body. Interestingly several of the symptom(s) may be common to several infections. Also, although several individuals may be affected, barring a few common gross symptoms, several symptoms and their intensities may vary among individuals; however, we pick up a few symptoms, often ignoring others. Therefore it is quite likely that brain would express various symptoms and signs associated with various states; in other words various conscious states have been identified based on different associated signs and symptoms.

Most simply in the absence of any better definition, a living organism exists in two states: the rest and activity in lower species, the BRAC; while wake and sleep, in higher species. These states are associated with various behavioral and associated external expressions.

Apparently, during waking different external physical expressions associated with it were considered to define physical states. However, there was very limited expression to define objectively the state of the brain except the expression as *mental states* and *thought processes*, which still continues to be a subjective expression. Notwithstanding, the brain receives inputs from within as well as from external sources, hence, to know the expressions of the brain one needed to study it in its totality and also during both the conditions, i.e., when it receives or is capable to receive inputs from external surroundings (outside the body) and when it is isolated from receiving external inputs. This concept led to the transection, lesion, and stimulation studies carried out from the early twentieth century onwards (Moruzzi, 1972 for review). In contrast to waking, during sleep the appreciable expressions by the brain of a subject are only in the form of dream(s) and hence that was the matter of study. There was a need to find a physical equivalence to objectively analyze the dream state. After the discovery of electrical signaling by the brain, neurons, and other body tissues, the physical, mental, and conscious states could be objectively defined and classified. In classifying such states, in the absence of any better defining characteristic, several physical expressions such as movements and the accompanying or associated electrophysiological changes in the brain were considered expressions of mental and conscious state changes.

Rapid eye movement sleep and dream sleep

Sleep and dreams have always fascinated the human mind and it is very common to find discussions on both of them by scientists, poets, novelists, or philosophers throughout the ages (Vedic, Greek, and Roman) (Lokeswarananda, 1995, 1998; Barbera, 2008). It was necessary to objectively define and classify the state of an individual or the brain during dreaming, which apparently does not have associated appreciable physical expressions, unlike that of the awake and sleep states, to be objectively perceived by a third person. In this enthusiasm, several electrophysiological signals were often found to remain associated with the dream state. In the absence of any better criteria, association of expressions of electrophysiological signals from the brain (the electroencephalogram, EEG), muscle atonia and rapid eye movements, the characteristics of REMS were observed to be associated with the majority of the dream episodes and hence they have been considered to define the dream state of the brain, which is a state of consciousness (Hobson, 2009). However, the researchers found that (1) the behavioral expressions were read mostly as subjective descriptions, and hence may lack objectivity; (2) all the signs and symptoms may not be expressed during every stage of the dream; and (3) sometimes such expressions may not be associated with dream, e.g., during some stages of waking. Therefore, there is a component of *masking* of expressions, which we will discuss later.

Although several functions have been assigned to REMS or dream sleep (Kuiken 2009; readers are also encouraged to consult various chapters in this volume), arguments not supporting some such functions have also been put forward intermittently (Siegel, 2001, 2009). However, since the dream state has a significant component of revelation, realization, and philosophic outcome, to gain an insight into this unique state of consciousness in this chapter we have attempted to explore the knowledge available in the *Vedas* and the *Upanishads*, probably the oldest philosophical literature available to mankind. We have attempted to correlate and possibly connect the ancient (the *Vedic* and the *Upanishadic*) wisdom with the present-day knowledge on dream sleep and REMS states to understand the brain in those states, avoiding the possibility of re-inventing the wheel and to steer future studies in a logical direction. Readers are also encouraged to read other chapters in this volume including that by Pagel.

Although modern-day understanding on the neurobiology of REMS and its possible relation to dream sleep is a little over fifty years old, the human experience of subjective and behavioral wakefulness, sleep, dream, and imagination is as old as cognitive evolution. Since the time human beings started remembering and recording history, one can find accounts on sleep, dreams, and wakefulness in the form of stories in their philosophical, mythological, and historical records. Based on the modern objective electrophysiological criteria the sleep stage has been divided into NREMS and REMS. It is generally accepted that dreams appear during sleep, although it is not uncommon to find in the literature mention of dream during NREMS, dreamless sleep, as well as daydreaming and their patho-physiological effects and correlates. Throughout human history several mentions can be found of "*good*" dreams and "*bad*" dreams and their consequences on health and in shaping the future reality. Co-founder of Microsoft, Bill Gates, and pop-star,

Michael Jackson, had dreams to accomplish; in recent history Alexander the Great and Napoleon Bonaparte both had dreams to fulfill; and there are several stories of scientists solving problems in dreams. Also in the spiritual literature one can find the mention of dreams that preceded the conception in reality of a godly offspring by the mother (the Virgin Mary before conceiving Jesus, and in the recent past the mothers of Sri Ramakrishna and of Swami Vivekananda before conceiving). Many spiritual leaders have been reported to have been initiated by their respective *guru* during a dream.

One of the finest periods of early documented evidence on the progress of cognitive knowledge and associated subjects, including consciousness in humans, is the era of the *Upanishads*, when in spite of not possessing modern techniques, the issues of "*consciousness*" were debated philosophically and extensively to find a reasonable understanding. Although much has been philosophically discussed and debated about REMS and dreams, in order to receive classical experimentalists' scientific acceptance and sanctity we need to find a neural substrate for their expression and regulation. Before we attempt to address this, the fundamental question is, should there be a materialistic substrate for every expression? The answer is that it is generally accepted that most energy, including life processes, needs material substrate to get expressed, especially to be perceived and comprehended by the same or another material human being. In that sense significant advancement has been made in the past three decades toward the understanding of the neural substrate for the regulation of REMS; however, such cannot be said about our understanding of dreams. Therefore the question is whether dream and REMS are identical. The motivation to write this chapter is to reflect briefly on the knowledge of ancient human wisdom, scripted in the *Upanishads*, with a view to possibly finding some leads, if at all, on dream and REMS states especially with a neurobiological perspective.

What are the *Upanishads*?

The author Abbe J. A. Dubois writes, in the introduction of his book titled *Hindu Manners, Customs and Ceremonies*, "It is impossible to doubt for a moment that science and art flourished amongst these nations at an epoch when our most civilized countries of the West were still plunged in the dark abyss of ignorance" (Beauchamp, 2007). During this era, six systems of philosophy existed with the people who lived in the eastern part of the world, primarily the ancient Indian peninsula. They were (1) *Nyaya* of *Gotama*, which deals with reasoning and logic; (2) *Vaisesika* of *Kanada*, which deals with the notions of space, time, matter, and causation; (3) *Samkhya* of *Kapila*, which deals with creation based on 25 different elements; (4) *Yoga* of *Patanjali*, which deals with the eight-fold path of union of body, mind, and soul; (5) *Mimamsa* (also called Purva Mimamsa) of *Jaimini*, which deals with righteousness in action, ethics, and aesthetics in rituals; and (6) *Vedanta* (also called Uttara Mimamsa) of *Vyasa*, which deals with the pathway to supreme knowledge. The *Upanishads* constitute *Uttara Mimamsa*, whereas *Purva Mimamsa* deals with mainly Vedic rituals. The essence of the knowledge of the *Vedas* was named *Vedanta*, which comprises the *Upanishads* (Sri Aurobindo, 1972; Lokeswarananda, 1995, 1998). The *Upanishads*, as literature, are believed to have originated from about 1000 BC; the Vedas originated much earlier. There are 108 *Upanishads* of which 10 are part of *Rig Veda*, 16 are part of *Sama Veda*, 51 are part of *Yajur Veda*, and 31 are part of *Atharva Veda*. The *Upanishads* are a revelation to the conscious being, which keeps on fertilizing the mind and transforms the life in reality.

Upanishads on dreams

There are four important *Upanishads*, namely *Mandukya Upanishad, Brihadaranyaka Upanishad, Prasna Upanishad*, and *Chandogya Upanishad*, in which descriptions of sleep, dream, and wakefulness can be found.

Mandukya Upanishad is the shortest of all *Upanishads*. Stanzas 3 to 7 mention four states of consciousness in the following sequence: wakefulness, dream, sleep (*susupti*), and *Turiya*; unlike our classical knowledge of three states in the following sequence: wakefulness, sleep, and dream. Interestingly, the *Upanishad* says the waking state gives way to dreaming, and the dream state dissolves into deep sleep. In deep sleep, the mind and intellect enter into quiescent phase of consciousness (*pragnya*). The *Turiya* state is beyond the classical three states, however, at the same time encompassing all of the three states: outward-knowing of waking state; inward-knowing of dream state; and knowing of both physical and mental objectless *pragjna*. Thus, there is scope for reinterpretation of the meaning of the words in context. Perhaps we need to dream and sleep since we cannot remain in a fully awakened state of *Turiya* for ever. It has been suggested that the *Turiya* state links the rest of the three states and regulates them, otherwise how would one know how and when to get into and out of any one of these states, a property of being alive (Radhakrishnan, 2006).

Brihadaranyaka Upanishad is the longest of all the *Upanishads*. In the third *Brahamana*, chapter IV of this *Upanishad*, the sage *Yagnavalkya* responds to queries of king *Janaka* regarding the state of self in dream and deep sleep. It is stated that in the dream state, the subtle body of self has experiences through a fine thread of *Nadi* (finer than a thousandth part of a hair) carrying different "hues" of varying intensity. Not only do the old impressions within the memory keep on working during dream but the mind remains "open" to outside influence in the dream state. The consequences of this outside influence may be indifferent; sometimes, however, this may be disturbing and tormenting.

Prasna Upanishad is in response to six profound questions; the fourth being on sleep, dream, and waking. What slumbers? Who dreams? Who remains awake in the sleep state? Who is the master of the awakened, dream, and sleep state? The answers are, respectively, as follows: the senses slumber; the mind dreams; only *prana* (the life principle) remains awake in a dreamless sleep state and all these rest in *Brahaman*, the supreme *Atman*. Thus, the *Prasna Upanishad* makes distinctions between the expressions of senses, mind, self, life principle (*prana*), and consciousness at least in relation to dreams.

According to the *Chandogya Upanishad*, the waking individual and the dreaming individual act differently. It says (translation) "*he who moves about freely like a lord in the state of dream is the self, the Atman; the self in the state of deep sleep is Atman, immortal and fearless. It is the Atman who experiences and it works independent of the body which may be damaged, diseased and dead.*" Therefore, the gateway to the knowledge of larger *self* seems to be beyond the dream state.

Where does the *Vedic* and *Upanishadic* knowledge lead us?

The writings in the *Upanishads* are revelations, which have the power to rejuvenate a person's life with refreshing new energy; the moot point we would like to highlight here is as follows. Could these revelations be made use of in modern scientific approaches to find structural correlates and neural substrates to investigate the relationship between dream and REMS, in particular, and sleep–waking and consciousness, in general? Could the revelations and the modern experimental REMS signs overlap or meet? Perhaps, Yes!

It is a historical fact that experimental science looks for structural and functional bases and correlation between them to explain observations; however, should that be applicable to philosophical concepts and revelations? Since biological processes are derived from and expressed in or through the physical medium, the mortal body, ultimately they cannot disobey physico-chemical principles, which may be very complex, though, and sometimes we may not understand them based on prevailing concepts and knowledge. Hence, how much do we know and understand about the physico-chemico-structural substrates, and how much are we capable of demystifying the unknown realm and then finding structural and functional integration between them to decide the completeness of our knowledge?

Grossly sleep, REMS, and wakefulness are observable objective states of consciousness. The ways in which we appreciate them today based on their physico-chemico-structural substrates and other correlates, especially in terms of modern objective parameter(s), the electrophysiological signals, were unknown to mankind until the early twentieth century. However, the ancient concepts based on wisdom and revelations do not appear illogical. Hence there is a need to look at them again in the light of present-day knowledge, some of which has been explained below as examples.

Ancient wisdom and present objective knowledge: can they meet?

According to the ancient *Vedic* and *Upanishadic* literatures there are four states of consciousness in humans, namely wakefulness, dream, sleep, and *Turiya*; as compared to the present classification of three states based on electrophysiological criteria, all except the *Turiya* state are common. The levels of consciousness of a being, to put it in scientific terminology in concurrence with MacLean's (1990) concept of the triune brain, may be expressed as brain-stem consciousness, limbic consciousness, and cortical consciousness. Finally, when it goes beyond the bounds (!) of the brain we may call it supracortical consciousness (Mukhopadhyay, 1985). The level of consciousness with distinct describable properties when personified, characterizes the being respectively as brain-stem being, limbic being, cortical being, and supracortical being. The *Turiya* state is the unique description of the *Upanishad*. Supracortical

being is the first behavioral expression of the *Turiya* state being biologized (Mukhopadhyay, 2006). To these concepts we need to find the association of neurotransmitter(s) and their related correlates, in line with modern-day science, which might then help us in defining and correlating the levels with the states of consciousness of an individual.

Further, the modern electrophysiological signal-based classification defines the states as exclusive to each other, i.e., an individual is in any of the three states, awake, sleep, or dream. In other words, such classification does not allow the existence of a background basal state on which all other states are expressed one at a time, or more than one state may run simultaneously, or can there be overlap of states or what will be the state(s) under conditions of states overlapping by different degrees. In general, under normal circumstances, although one does not find so, there are instances of such overlap of expressions, which often are termed as disordered states, e.g., split personality and so on. Arguably, it is very unlikely that any expression may come up *de novo* during an altered state, including disease(s), if the expression is inherently absent, which might have remained suppressed though during normal conditions. It is likely that normally such overlap between the *states* of consciousness such as wake, NREMS and REMS, and the non-exclusive relationship between them should exist, which, however, need re-defining, irrespective of *levels* of consciousness of the being.

Can the *Turiya* state provide some explanation?

In the *Vedic* and *Upanishadic* literature one finds mention of an apparently metaphysical state, the *Turiya*. The *Turiya* state has been defined as the fourth state of pure consciousness when the self merges with that of the infinite consciousness (Parthasarathy, 2007). The fundamental question in principle is: does it make sense to look into it and find an analogous correlate in the context of present-day knowledge? The answer certainly is yes, because, other states leading to and following the *Turiya* are explainable. To clarify, based on present-day knowledge, although we find partial explanation for initiation and termination of sleep, waking, and REMS (Moruzzi, 1972; Mallick and Inoue, 1999), we do not have any concept about which state holds them in place so that they keep recurring. Further, the states are non-rhythmic suggesting that they are not autochthonous by nature. It is important conceptually because even if we consider wake, sleep, and REMS/dream sleep as a linear or cyclic sequence, they do not follow the same sequence of events while going into one or the other direction.

Although sleep and waking have been divided into subtypes, we do not know what will be the nature of the state(s) if, on one hand, we extrapolate and extend the deep sleep in one direction (say backward) and the active awake, on the other hand, to the other direction (say forward) or vice versa? Based on the existing classification and sequence of events neither may lead to so-called REMS because backward extension (extrapolation) of NREMS may lead to an analogous condition (as per electrophysiological signals) such as coma, while based on the present-day criteria we do not know what will be the equivalence to more waking than active wake state, if we extend (extrapolate) the latter state. Further, if both these states are open ended, how would they be regulated? On the other hand, if the awake, NREMS and REMS are considered part of a circle, then they should be expressed in a cyclic sequence, it doesn't matter even if they were aperiodic. In that case every NREMS episode must enter into REMS and every REMS must enter into waking, which we know is incorrect based on the appearance of electrophysiological signals and also because dreams have been reported in states other than REMS. Thus, these arguments favor the concept that there should be an interlinking all-inclusive basal or ground state on which the other states, wake, NREMS, and REMS, would play around to express themselves and these states are not all-or-none phenomenon, meaning therefore that there will always be some overlap of states.

Masking and unmasking of expressions defining various states

Based on the discussions above, it may be said that there is likely to be an all-inclusive basal state of the brain, which remains an inherent property of the functional brain caused due to, by and for the matter brain. Obviously there is likely to be some basal level of expression and a corresponding state say "T", which so far has not been defined in the existing sleep science literature, and it needs to be identified, defined, and described. Such basal expression may be isolated, or it may remain floating on, and which the external inputs play or act upon. This basal expression is likely to correlate with the basal uniform activity of the whole brain and is

therefore uniformly distributed all through the brain. We propose that the state "T" is the *Turiya* state; however, it needs to be objectively identified and defined. In the *Upanishads*, this *Turiya* state has been described as the experience of the ground state, devoid of any content or information or even a sense of self, still retaining its overwhelming manipulating power on self, quality of information, and content of consciousness. This is the experience of unconditional consciousness, i.e., consciousness not conditioned by the presence of informational content or even sense of self.

Perturbation of this "T" state induces wake, dream, and NREMS. Perturbation by either localized or generalized input induces waking and when the external (waking) signals are actively ignored or inhibited by the brain areas (the sleep or hypnogenic areas) NREMS ensues. However, perturbation of the "T" state importantly from within the brain substrate and at the same time when the external inputs are functionally disconnected or blocked in a reversible manner, dream appears which is likely to be specific to perturbation of specific functional brain locations, e.g., dreams of sound, vision, smell, pleasure, pain, and so on. Thus, it may be said that the state "T" encompassing all states is ever present; it will be present when one transits from one state to the other and then arguably we can very well consider the overlapping of states.

Further, in this model, since expression of any one of the states including the overlap or junction between two states is expressed on and due to modulation of the state "T", it overcomes the hurdle and difficulty of explaining the exclusive and discrete nature of different states. It also explains the possibility of having dreams during waking, which remain masked due to strong peripheral inputs; however, they get expressed through disorders, e.g., narcolepsy, split personality, hallucination, etc. Similarly, in principle, dreaming during NREMS may be associated to NREMS onset or REMS depending on which part of the brain gets activated and modulates which aspect of the state "T". It is true that present neurobiological knowledge does not know or explain how the activation and/or deactivation of specific parts of the brain takes place for the generation of various types of dreams and during which behavioral state they get expressed. However, in principle it is not difficult to comprehend if the olfactory, or the visual, or the auditory, or any other area or combination thereof, becomes activated to give such dreams provided they act on a uniform system, the "T" state. However, the question to be raised is why does dream normally appear primarily during REMS? We hypothesize that during REMS not only the inputs to the brain are maximally reduced, all other non-essential outputs including to the antigravity muscles (which maintains the posture) are also actively inhibited and therefore dreams are more pronounced, if at all (at least in relation to during wake and NREMS states) and also we remember them. In such a scenario, since the brain substrates are more active the EEG becomes desynchronized.

The *Turiya* state is a non-local expression

In the backdrop of the discussions above it is not difficult to conceptualize the *Turiya* state; however, the challenge is to find the neural correlates of this state. The *Turiya* state is all-inclusive, omnipresent across the brain, perhaps exclusively expressed by the brain, of the brain, and for the brain. This nature of unconditional state of consciousness has been described as *non-local* (Mukhopadhyay, 2008), quite unlike the NREMS and waking centers in the brain, which have been localized, although in more than one region within the brain, and therefore *local* in nature. If we accept such an explanation, one should in principle accept that there should be dreaming center(s) as well, which is yet to be experimentally localized by modern science, although it (they) may be localized in several discrete regions in the brain; use of modern techniques such as PET and fMRI may provide some answers to such questions. Like other states of sleep and waking, since dreams are also expressed in the *Turiya* or "*T*" state, we argue that normally unless all other specific inputs (external or internal from within) to the "*T*" state are reduced to a minimum, dream will not be expressed. Since the inputs are highest during waking, high during NREMS, and least during REMS, normally dream is expressed during REMS. Furthermore, if dream outputs overcome the threshold of, or overlap with, the wake or NREMS state, dreams appear during those respective states.

At present, although several hypotheses and models have been proposed for the regulation of REMS and we know that normally REMS appears only after a state of NREMS and not during waking, we do not know how then one enters into and gets out of this state. In other words, unless there is a basal state, if one of the waking, NREMS, or REMS states fails to get into the following state, what will happen? The *Turiya*, or "*T*" state, as a concept appears a reasonable explanation; however, we need to find a neural substrate to understand and explain the same. In an attempt to find a neural substrate for the *Turiya* or "*T*" state, although it may be extremely difficult, as a first step we need to find an analogous state to that of the basal level. In fact, the existence of slow electrical oscillations and DC potentials from the intact brain and also from isolated cortex has long been recognized (Moruzzi, 1972; Steriade *et al.*, 1993; Lörincz *et al.*, 2009). Can the slow electrical oscillations of the brain, or their variation, offer help or leads to explain the *Turiya* or "*T*" state? Not only the neurons but the glia may also play a significant role in the generation of the slow oscillations, as has been shown very recently (Fellin *et al.*, 2009).

As per the description in the *Upanishads* the brain during dream and sleep acts as an informationally open system. Information can behave both *locally* and *non-locally*. Some important information, which has been termed in the *Upanishads* as "*Prarabdha*", *sanchit karma*, may get purged during the dream state leading to its permanent loss. We may find comparable and/or variations of such concepts put forward in the present era as well by Crick and Mitchison (1983) explaining the removal or shedding of unwanted information during REMS. On the other hand, it has been expressed in the *Upanishads* that entirely new information may get imbibed into the system, the brain, during the dream state of mind, which may lead to the creation of new space and new time for the being, which has not been proposed in the existing REMS literature. It may be argued, at least in terms of the electrical impedance function, that the brain is always in a dynamic state where the impedance gets continuously reset and that state decides the direction of information flow to or from the brain, or if the information flows to and fro simultaneously, the state of impedance would decide the proportion of energy absorbed or reflected. In the state of dream we find a possibility for the merger of the science of *locality* and *non-locality*. In simple terms, the former defines those which can be localized in space in discrete physical terms; while the latter refers to global presence, omnipresence, interwoven all-linking, and all-encompassing. The science of *non-locality* as a concept and terminology, although recognized in physical science (Aspect *et al.*, 1982), is yet to be acknowledged in life sciences in general and in neuroscience in particular (Grinberg-Zylberbaum *et al.*, 1994). Thus, there is an urgent need to develop and define a science of equivalence, the science of information (Mukhopadhyay, 2008).

Another important fact is that, at present, sleep science apparently associates REMS with dreaming. Often these terms have been synonymously used, the former by and large by the neuroscientists (sleep biologists) and the latter by the psychologists and philosophers, because they can be identified by such manifestations. However, that may not be necessarily true, which may find support from several quarters. For instance, the older literatures including the *Vedas* and the *Upanishads*, do not have an analogous term as REMS; however, they do mention sleep with and without dream, dream during waking, and also a state of dreaming when one is neither in sleep nor awake. Additionally, REMS with or without associated dream as well as dreaming during NREMS have been reported (Antrobus and Wamsley, 2009; McNamara *et al.*, 2005; Manni, 2005; Smith *et al.*, 2004).

Thus, there are reasons to accept that dream and REMS are two separate phenomena; however, they may be expressed simultaneously, which needs to be understood accordingly. It is important to find neural substrate(s) for the regulation of those two phenomena. Although we have made significant progress on the neural mechanism of generation and regulation of REMS (Lu *et al.*, 2006; Mallick *et al.*, 1999; Pal and Mallick, 2007; Stickgold and Walker, 2009), we know very little on the neural mechanism of generation and regulation of dreams. The role of neurotransmitters and metabolites may be of immense significance in finding such a structure–function correlation. However, it is important that we must exercise restraint and caution not to oversimplify the two phenomena as identical unless evidence is provided to the contrary. It may be supported by the fact that there is evidence that various drugs, chemicals, neurotransmitters and their agonist/antagonists affect dream/hallucination and REMS, or their associated components, in differential manners in normal or pathological conditions (Chokroverty, 2009; Davis *et al.*, 2002; Mallick and Inoue, 1999; Pillar *et al.*, 2000; Ukai *et al.*, 2007; Yorston and Gray, 2000). In studying in this way, although the ancient literature may not provide definite answers, it may certainly give us some clues and revelations for realization and lead our future steps in a logical direction.

Necessity of REMS with or without associated dream

Since REMS may or may not be associated with dream, they may have independent and overlapping functions. Nature has created a state of REMS with or without

associated dreams and that is preserved through evolution. Several hypotheses with reasonable experimental data have been collected to explain the functional role of REMS (Mallick *et al.*, 1999; Stickgold and Walker, 2009; readers are also encouraged to go through the various chapters devoted to these topics in this volume). The fundamental difference of the neuronal cell as compared to other somatic cells is that neurons have excitability. Mallick combined all the proposed functions of REMS into a unified hypothesis and proposed that "*REMS maintains brain excitability*" (Mallick *et al.*, 1994, 1999) and thus serves "house keeping function of the brain" (Mallick & Singh, 2011). His group further showed that REMS achieves this by maintaining the Na-K ATPase activity in the brain (Madan & Mallick in this volume). Thus, we expect REMS or its analogue in all species, even with a rudimentary brain; however, the criteria to classify REMS need to be redefined.

There is still a deeper question! In terms of expressions of the brain, the states have been defined by appreciation of the brain itself. The question that follows is, can the same brain understand itself or its own expressions? For example, a brain per se does not feel its pain, the eyes cannot see their own color and shape, and one cannot know an object, say a house, by residing inside it only. Thus in order to understand an item or object in its totality, one must study it from within as well as from outside, and by remaining unattached as well as keeping oneself dissociated from it, which in modern language one may term as objective assessment. Further, if the subject/object for study is oneself/itself, it needs to be replicated or the observer must dissociate herself to keep herself at a distance and evaluate. Although we may find these statements logical, we do not have experimental support based on the so-called modern experimental scientific evidence; however, we may find some wisdom from the ancient literatures, the *Vedas* and the *Upanishads*.

During dreaming it is as if one replicates one's self although remaining unattached and, therefore, although one apparently is happy or sad, or expects seeing color, or experience of being killed, one does not usually feel the same sensation as if such things happened during other states. As expressed in *Chandogya Upanishad*, "*the waking individual and the dreaming individual act differently.*" During dream state the *self* can get "*detached*" from the brain and therefore, the *self* can look objectively at what is happening in the brain. The *being* in the state of dreaming is considered to behave as an autonomous creator. The process of dreaming connects between apparently irreconcilable domains leading to resolution of deep conflict and creation of a new reality often with a new Worldview. The phenomenon reaches the level of awareness more frequently when the person remains conscious during dream (dreaming while awake). Thus, in the absence of better justification, we think unlike REMS, which is likely to be present (at least partial REMS associated symptom) through evolution even in those possessing rudimentary brain, dream probably is characteristic of most advanced species in evolution; however, from which species it has started remains to be studied. This potential of dreaming is being harnessed for the creative resolution of complex problems, and has been recognized by scientists such as Otto Loewi, Thomas Edison, and Elias Howe (perfecting the sewing machine) and poets such as William Wordsworth. However, establishing the structure–function correlation, as is demanded by experimental science, is the need of the day. The fallout of this concept is that nature has provided us REMS and dreaming whose understanding in totality probably is very important, and may hold the key to find an objective explanation of consciousness and meditation, self, and non-self, and several such related phenomena in the light of, and explainable by, so-called modern scientific experimental objective criteria.

We conclude by saying that the ancient *Vedic* and *Upanishadic* literatures offer us information based on profound human experience and understanding; however, it has very limited information on physiological and physico-chemico-structural correlates, while present-day science gives us the latter with very limited knowledge on the former. The time has come, or perhaps is fast approaching, to cause them to meet and resonate, rather than reinventing the existing wheel to understand the association between REMS and dreaming. It appears that REMS and dreaming are independent expressions of either physical or mental/conscious states or both, which may or may not be expressed simultaneously in an associated manner. Finally, it is very likely that the answer possibly lies on better segregation and mixing of the structural and anatomical substrates along with those of the chemical substrates, both neurotransmitters as well as receptors, in relation to the expressions by the brain along with the subjective experience of the experiencer, the self. Hence there is a definite need to correlate and connect the present criteria used in modern-day experimental science with those found in the ancient literatures, such as the *Vedas* and the *Upanishads*. Finally, based on the discussions presented in this chapter, at least three directions emerge which need to be looked into, described, and defined for future studies. (1) REMS and dreams are independent phenomenon, which may often overlap; however, the neurobiological substrates and conditions for such overlap/non-overlap are yet unknown. (2) Could the *non-local Turiya* or the "*T*" state be the arbiter of all other states of consciousness; if yes, how? (3) What could be the missing link between neuroscience and the *non-local* existence of expressions? How can we correlate the geometry and mechanism of information with that of behavioral expressions of the person in general and, with neural correlates, constituents or correspondence, for consciousness in particular?

Acknowledgments

Research funding from DST, DBT, and UGC (Networking and Capacity Building) to BNM is acknowledged.

References

Antrobus, J. S. & Wamsley, E. J. (2009) REM/NREM differences in dream content. In *The Neuroscience of Sleep*, eds. R. Stickgold & M. P. Walker. Amsterdam: Academic Press, pp. 310–15.

Aspect, A., Dailibard, J. & Roger, G. (1982) Experimental test of Bell's inequalities using time-varying analyzers. *Phys Rev Lett* **49**: 1804–7.

Barbera, J. (2008) Sleep and dreaming in Greek and Roman philosophy. *Sleep Med* **9**: 906–10.

Beauchamp, H. K. (2007) *Hindu Manners, Customs and Ceremonies*. Trans. A. J. A. Dubois. New Delhi: Rupa & Co., pp. 1–842.

Chokroverty, S. (2009) *Sleep Disorders Medicine: Basic Science, Technical Considerations, and Clinical Aspects*. Philadelphia: Saunders Elsevier, p. 676.

Crick, F. & Mitchison, G. (1983) The function of dream sleep. *Nature* **304** :111–14.

Davis, K. L., Charney, D., Coyle, J. T. & Nemeroff, C. (2002) *Neuropharmacology, the Fifth Generation of Progress*. Lippincott Williams & Wilkins, p. 2010.

Fellin, T., Halassa, M. M., Terunuma, M., *et al.* (2009) Endogenous nonneuronal modulators of synaptic transmission control cortical slow oscillations in vivo. *Proc Natl Acad Sci* **106**: 15,037–42.

Grinberg-Zylberbaum, J., Delaflor, M., Attie, L. & Goswami, A. (1994) The Einstein–Podolsky–Rosen Paradox in the brain: the transferred potential. *Physics Essays* 7(4): 422–8.

Hobson, J. A. (2009) REM sleep and dreaming : towards a theory of protoconsciousness. *Nat Rev Neurosci*, **10**: 803–13.

Kuiken, D. (2009) Theories of dream function. In: *The Neuroscience of Sleep*, eds. R. Stickgold & M. P. Walker. Amsterdam: Academic Press, pp. 295–301.

Lörincz, M. L., Geall, F., Bao, Y., Crunelli, V. & Hughes, S. W. (2009) ATP-dependent infra-slow (<0.1 Hz) oscillations in thalamic networks. *PLoS One* **4**(2): e4447.

Lokeswarananda, S. (1995a) In *Manduyka Upanishad*. Gol Park, Kolkata, India: Ramkrishna Institute of Culture, pp. 27–40.

Lokeswarananda, S. (1995b). In *Prasna Upanishad*. Gol Park, Kolkata, India: Ramkrishna Institute of Culture, pp. 72–98.

Lokeswarananda, S. (1998). In *Chandogya Upanishad*. Gol Park, Kolkata, India: Ramkrishna Institute of Culture, pp. 523–30.

Lu, J., Sherman, D., Devor, M. & Saper, C. B. (2006) A putative flip-flop switch for control of REM sleep. *Nature* **441**: 589–94.

MacLean, P. (1990) *The Triune Brain in Evolution: Role in Paleocerebral Functions*. New York: Plenum Press.

Mallick, B. N. & Inoue, S. (1999) *Rapid Eye Movement Sleep*. Marcel Dekker, pp. 1–419.

Mallick, B. N., Kaur, S., Jha, S. K. & Siegel, J. M. (1999) Possible role of GABA in regulation of REM sleep with special reference to REM-off neurons. In *Rapid Eye Movement Sleep*, eds. B. N. Mallick & S. Inoue. Marcel Dekker, pp. 153–66.

Mallick, B. N. & Singh, A. (2011) REM sleep loss increases brain excitability: role of noradrenalin and its mechanism of action. *Sleep Med. Rev.* (in press).

Mallick, B. N., Thakkar, M. & Gulyani, S. (1994) Rapid eye movement sleep deprivation induced alteration in neuronal excitability: possible role of norepinephrine. In *Environment and Physiology*, eds. B. N. Mallick & R. Singh. Narosa Publishing House, pp. 196–203.

Manni, R. (2005) Rapid eye movement sleep, non-rapid eye movement sleep, dreams, and hallucinations. *Curr Psychiat Rep* **7**(3): 196–200.

McNamara, P., McLaren, D., Smith D., Brown, A. & Stickgold, R. (2005). A "Jekyll and Hyde" within: aggressive versus friendly interactions in REM and Non-REM dreams. *Psychol Sci* **16**(2), 130–6.

Moruzzi, G. (1972) The sleep-waking cycle. *Ergeb der Physiol* **64**: 1–164.

Mukhopadhyay, A. K (1985) States of consciousness: a holistic hypothesis. Supracortical consciousness: an existing reality. In *Frontiers of Research for Human Biologists. Next Hundred Years*. New Delhi: Conscious Publications, pp. 1–6.

Mukhopadhyay, A. K. (2006) Supracortical consciousness. An opening to multiple new doors of Science. In *The Enworlded Subjectivity. Its Three Worlds and Beyond*. Project History of Indian Science, Philosophy and Culture (PHISPC). Vol. XI, Part 4. ed. R. Balasubramanian. New Delhi: Center for Studies in Civilization, pp. 380–446.

Mukhopadhyay, A. K. (2008) A radical view of information. On its nature and science. *Frontier Perspectives* **16**(2): 19–29.

Pal, D. & Mallick, B. N. (2007) Neural mechanism of rapid eye movement sleep generation: with reference to REM-OFF neurons in locus coeruleus. *Ind J Med Res* **125**: 721–39.

Parthasarathy, A. (2007) *Vedanta Treatise: the Eternities*, 14th edn. A. Parthasarathy, www.vedanta-edu.org.

Pillar, G., Malhotra A. & Lavie, P. (2000) Post-traumatic stress disorder and sleep: what a nightmare. *Sleep Med Rev* **4**: 183–200.

Radhakrishnan, S. (2006) *The Principal Upanishads* (translation and edited; 17th impression). India: Harper Collins Publishers, p. 958.

Siegel, J. M. (2001) The REM sleep–memory consolidation hypothesis. *Science* **294**: 1058–63.

Siegel, J. M. (2009) Sleep viewed as a state of adaptive inactivity. *Nat Rev Neurosci* **10**: 747–53.

Smith, M. R., Antrobus, J. S., Gordon, E., *et al.* (2004) Motivation and affect in REM sleep and the mentation reporting process. *Conscious Cogn* **13**(3): 501–11.

Sri Aurobindo (1972) *The Upanishads*, Vol 12 of Sri Aurobindo. Pondicherry, India: Sri Aurobindo Ashrama.

Steriade, M., Contreras, D., Curró Dossi, R. & Nuñez, A. (1993) The slow (< 1 Hz) oscillation in reticular thalamic and thalamocortical neurons: scenario of sleep rhythm generation in interacting thalamic and neocortical networks. *J Neurosci* **13**(8): 3284–99.

Stickgold, R. & Walker, M. P. (2009) *The Neuroscience of Sleep*. Amsterdam: Academic Press, p. 360.

Ukai, S., Yamamoto, M., Tanaka, M., Shinosaki, K. & Takeda, M. (2007) Donepezil in the treatment of musical hallucinations. *Psychiat Clin Neurosci* **61**: 190–2.

Yorston, G. A. & Gray, R. (2000) Hypnopompic hallucinations with donepezil. *J Psychopharmacol* **14** 303–4.

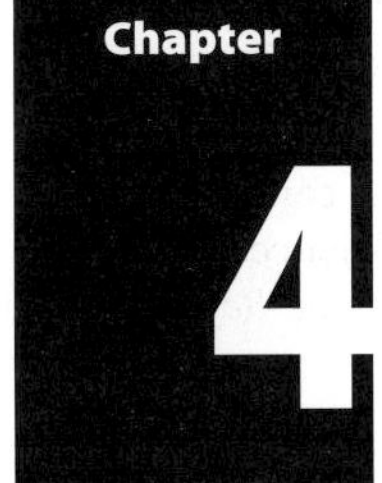

The discovery of REM sleep: the death knell of the passive theory of sleep

Adrian R. Morrison

Summary

Withdrawal from the influence of the outside world seemed a reasonable explanation for the onset of sleep for many years. This view, the passive theory of sleep, held sway despite some evidence to the contrary from lesion and stimulation studies as well as the effects of natural disease of the hypothalamus. Discovery of the ascending reticular activating system did not demolish this idea; for this system was considered merely to transmit the effects of sensory withdrawal, a role previously assigned to long ascending pathways. Even the 1953 discovery of REM sleep, which presented features different from "classical" sleep, could not convince some to abandon the passive theory. By the end of the decade, though, so much evidence for complexity in the organization of sleep and wakefulness had accumulated, including the demonstration of REM sleep in decerebrate cats, that the active theory of sleep finally prevailed.

Early intimations of REM sleep

Eugene Aserinsky, a graduate student of Nathaniel Kleitman at the University of Chicago's sleep research laboratory, first observed and recorded what we now call REM sleep. We regard his 1953 report with Kleitman in *Science* (Aserinsky and Kleitman, 1953) as the starting point for modern sleep research although they did not use the descriptor, "REM," in that paper. In addition to rapid, conjugate eye movements, they observed body movements and significantly increased respiration and heart rates associated with a low-voltage, high-frequency wave pattern in the EEG. And dreams were reported in 20 of the 27 interrogations during the ocular motility episodes.

Aserinsky began his career in sleep research observing eyelid movements in babies and abandoned this approach to observe their eye movements. Only when he attached his balky brain-wave monitors to his sleeping eight-year-old son, Armond, did he observe regularly occurring periods of high ocular motility during sleep. The immediate trigger for this discovery was the decision to use continuous recording with an electroencephalograph (EEG) (Aserinsky, 1996). Perhaps all other researchers had not considered sleep interesting enough to spend reams of paper on continuous recording. If so, they missed one of the great events in biology.

The world of sleep research owes much to Eugene Aserinsky. It seems clear that his was a lonely task, and we remain indebted to his perseverance, ingenuity, and intelligence. Aserinsky later commented on his difficulties in winning Kleitman's attention to his REM sleep observations, since Kleitman – like most scientists of his time – had theorized that sleep was a completely passive phenomenon. The rigorous Kleitman insisted on repeating Aserinsky's experiments on his own daughter. After further long hours of study, Kleitman was willing to acknowledge that the episodes of rapid eye movements were associated with a specific stage of sleep and that they appeared to accompany dreaming. In September 1953, the world received their momentous report (Aserinsky and Kleitman, 1953).

A young medical student, William Dement, aided in the early studies and ultimately published extensive reports on dreams and REM sleep with Kleitman (Dement and Kleitman, 1957a, b). As a budding psychiatrist, Dement was entranced by the possibility of identifying when dreams would appear. Aserinsky, on the other hand, had no interest in the "ephemeral," only hard science.

Of course, REM sleep was always there, only no one's eyes (or more accurately, brain) had had more than a glimpse of it earlier. And there certainly were glimpses, as Claude Gottesmann has dug out of the ancient literature (Gottesmann, 2001). In the nearly 70 pages of

---

REM Sleep: Regulation and Function, eds. Birendra N. Mallick, S. R. Pandi-Perumal, Robert W. McCarley, and Adrian R. Morrison. Published by Cambridge University Press. © Cambridge University Press 2011.

his review from antiquity to 1964 he has provided an amazing array that I only sample here. It is poignant to read brief mention by Derbyshire *et al.* (1936) of what is obviously unrecognized REM sleep intermixed with the large-wave sleep. They were primarily interested in the effects of several anesthetics on the electrical activity of the cerebral cortex, both spontaneous activity and that following sensory stimulation, so that the following words did not merit mention in their discussion or summary. They had REM sleep in their hands, and let it go. (Of course, recording the EEG in humans was a technique that had appeared on the scene only six years earlier; Berger 1930):

> In two of the three cats which we were able to observe without anesthesia, we found during sleep occasional groups of large waves, larger than those recorded in the waking state. At other times when sleep was apparently less tranquil, judging by the twitching of the vibrissae, there were only small rapid waves, as in the alert waking state
>
> *(Derbyshire et al. 1936, p. 582)*

Others in the mid-1930s were interested in recording brain activity in human subjects during sleep. Indeed, Loomis *et al.* (1937), distinguished five different wave patterns (A–E) occurring to varying degrees through a night's sleep. Their figures are "eerily" similar to those graphed in more recent times after the recognition of REM sleep. They summarize their study by saying: "During sleep there is a continual shift in states upward and downward [distinguished by ease of arousing with stimuli] sometimes with recognized stimuli but probably as a result of internal stimuli." Most interesting was this concluding observation: "Dreams in two instances have occurred in the B state" (Loomis *et al.* 1937, p 143). *Low voltage activity characterized the B state.* REM sleep was there, but no one was yet ready to greet it.

Even the animal literature of the time could have introduced us to REM sleep had we been ready to accept it. Klaue (1937, p. 514, as quoted by Gottesmann 2001, p. 215) distinguished something he called deep sleep from other stages this way: "Berhingung in Strombilde" [quiet electrical current], i.e., low amplitude EEG, "eine vollige Entspannung der Muskulatur… und haufige Zunkungen in einzelne Extremitaten" [complete muscular relaxation…and numerous jerks of single extremities]. A figure demonstrates the EEG pattern of REM sleep in the cat that is so familiar to sleep researchers, and of course the description of behavior was the same as that given by Dement (1958) in his study of cats.

There were certainly very early intimations that sleep was not a unitary phenomenon. For example, thanks to Datta and Maclean's recent thorough review (Datta and MacLean, 2007) we have a view extending beyond the Western world to the Hindu or Indus Valley civilization of the centuries 16 to 11 BC that reveals an awareness of some complexity in sleep. Philosophers there divided the states of consciousness into four, sleep comprising two called "Prajna" and "Taijasa," which seem to correspond to NREM sleep and REM sleep as we recognize them today. In this ancient formulation, *Prajna*, meaning dreamless sleep, was a state of consciousness "characterized by abounding bliss in which a veil of apparent unconsciousness envelops our thought and knowledge, and the subtle impressions of our mind seem to vanish." *Taijasa*, on the other hand, "is associated with an internal consciousness equivalent to modern day REM sleep … Characterized by a consciousness only of our dreams, we enjoy the mind's subtle impressions of the deeds we have done in the past." The ancient writings also said that to enter either wakefulness or *Taijasa* one had to pass through *Prajna*.

Then there was the Roman poet, Lucretius, writing more than 2000 years ago, who said: "And hunters' dogs often in their soft sleep yet suddenly toss their legs, and all at once give tongue, and again and again snuff the air with their nostrils, as if they had found and were following the tracks of wild beasts" (Gottesmann, 2001, p. 212). This observation has probably been made by humans closely associated with dogs since time immemorial. Producers of Walt Disney movies even illustrated REM sleep behavior in a dog in the movie *Cinderella*, which was released in 1950, three years before the Aserinsky and Kleitman paper. Bruno, a dog that typically battles with Lucifer, a cat, is found by Cinderella sleeping but "barking, moving his body and paws, beating on the carpet and also biting it." She then asks him if he were dreaming again of chasing Lucifer (Iranzo *et al.*, 2007, p. 532).

Yet, the same Lucretius, in his poetry, described the cessation of waking activity that allowed us to fall asleep, the embodiment of the passive theory of sleep (Moruzzi, 1964). The modern world of sleep researchers and the world in general saw sleep as simply a falling away of the "cares" of the world in the form of all the sensory input impinging upon the brain during wakefulness. With this understanding of sleep, it is no wonder that REM sleep remained beyond the ken of scientists. Who would think that a state so dramatically different from passivity could exist hidden within a so-called passive brain, with many neurons firing just as they do during wakefulness, indeed, with the brain being very much in a state akin to orienting during wakefulness (Morrison, 1983)?

The passive theory of sleep

Actually, there were two competing theories in the nineteenth century, the passive and the hypnotoxin theory. The latter reached its apogee in the latter nineteeth century with the Frenchman Piéron's demonstration of the induction of sleep in a dog transfused with blood from a dog made sleepy by walking it through the streets of Paris. Kleitman, however, rejected the hypnotoxin theory, although he certainly acknowledged Piéron's (1913) contribution to knowledge of sleep up to the early twentieth century in a review of the field that was published ten years before his monumental book, *Sleep and Wakefulness* (Kleitman, 1939).

Dement (2005, p. 2) explained Kleitman's reasoning that put him in opposition to Piéron's theory:

> In the 1920s, the University of Chicago physiologist Nathaniel Kleitman carried out a series of sleep deprivation studies and made the simple but brilliant observation that individuals who stayed up all night were generally less sleepy and less impaired the next morning than in the middle of their sleepless night. Kleitman argued that this observation was incompatible with the notion of a continual buildup of a hypnotoxin in the brain or blood.

Kleitman was a firm believer, though, in the passive theory of sleep and reasoned this way:

> Is it not just as correct to say that a person felt the oncoming of an irresistible attack of sleep as to say it was utterly impossible for him to remain awake? Superficially the two expressions would seem to be equivalent, but their implications are entirely different. The first implies an *active* onset, while the other implies a *cessation* of an active condition of wakefulness.
>
> *(Kleitman, 1939, p. 520)*

Thus, he argued, "from the evolutionary point of view, it is perhaps not sleep that needs to be explained but wakefulness, and indeed there may be different kinds of wakefulness at the different stages of phylogenetic and ontogenetic development" (Kleitman, 1939, p. 502). This proposal he called the evolutionary theory of sleep and wakefulness, proposing two kinds of

wakefulness: "Wakefulness of necessity is a subcortical, probably hypothalamic, function, whereas supplementary wakefulness of choice, as well as the diurnal sleep–wakefulness cycle, is a cortical function" (Kleitman, 1939, p. 504). Consequently, phylogenetically older life forms and new-born humans (and other evolved infants) would of necessity have to be awake to perform various bodily functions, but more complicated wakefulness of choice appears when an organism develops a more sophisticated lifestyle with a discriminating cerebral cortex.

Kleitman laid out his theory of the passive onset of sleep quite nicely in his 1929 review (Kleitman, 1929):

1. Sleep is an easily reversible inactivity of the highest functional centers.
2. The inactivity is due to a functional break between the cerebral cortex and the other parts of the nervous system.
3. The functional break results from a marked decrease in the number of afferent impulses from the sensorium, especially proprioceptive impulses which depend upon the degree of muscle tonus maintained.
4. Sleep is due to fatigue of the neuromuscular mechanism concerned in the maintenance of muscle tonus.
5. In the absence of such fatigue, sleep may result from complete muscular relaxation [as on a warm summer day], intentional or unintentional.
6. Diurnal alternation of wakefulness and sleep is a "conditioned" phenomenon.

The cortex, then, was all-important as an organizer of wakefulness to Kleitman as it was for many others at the time. The first five of his principles are rather self-explanatory, but the sixth requires a bit more explanation. Kleitman noted that, "we are born into a social organization where diurnal sleep is the universally accepted mode of sleeping," but that "The newborn baby is a truly polyphasic creature…" (Kleitman, 1929, p. 658). The development of the mature pattern evolves because night, resulting in poor vision and less movement, encourages relaxation and sleep, leaving the light phase to wakefulness in diurnal beings. He cites Pavlov's view that this is a "natural" conditioned reflex. He then presents an interesting hypothesis: "I feel certain that under conditions of artificial illumination and 24-hour activity of a group, children brought up by that group could be trained into a 12-or 36-hour cycle of existence, instead of the present 24" (Kleitman, 1929, p. 659)" – shades of B. F. Skinner!

The earliest neurophysiological studies

Returning to the nineteenth century, Moruzzi (1964) leads us into the age of the beginnings of attempts to explain the mechanisms of sleep and wakefulness in modern neurophysiological terms with the work of Rolando and Flourens on birds in the early years of that century. Both removed the cerebral hemispheres (such as they are) in birds and found that they induced what they interpreted as constant sleep. Later workers demonstrated that it was not a permanent condition if the diencephalon were not damaged. To Moruzzi, these results pointed to the probability that Rolando and Flourens had induced a cerebral shock analogous to spinal shock. He noted that physiologists in the 1950s demonstrated that stimulation of the mammalian cerebral neocortex would elicit EEG and behavioral signs of arousal via a cortical-reticulo-cortical loop provided that the midbrain is intact. Nevertheless, Moruzzi found it surprising that monographs on sleep neglected mention of Flourens and Rolando because he saw their work as the "beginning of the experimental era of neurophysiology" (Moruzzi, 1964, p. 21).

The great mid-nineteenth century physiologist Purkinje was quite taken by the findings of Flourens and constructed a hypothesis around them. Moruzzi (1964) says, "The concept of sleep as a passive phenomenon – absence of wakefulness – is developed here for the first time as a sheer theoretical development of Flouren's experiments" (p. 22). Purkinje reasoned that the block of sensory inflow that keeps us awake (according to the passive theory) occurred by mechanical blockage at the internal capsule. In a generously sympathetic and poetic comment on this great man's thinking, Moruzzi said, "Purkinje's naïve conception of sleep as a consequence of a mechanical block in the conduction along the internal capsule [between the cerebrum and brain stem] is the tribute that even a great mind had to pay to the limitations of knowledge existing in his times" (p. 22). Moruzzi spoke for even the least of us who have to project our thinking into the unknown.

Bremer's (1935) demonstration that transection through the midbrain caudal to the oculomotor nucleus, the famous cerveau isolé led to an EEG pattern consistent with sleep as it was recognized then – spindles and inter-spindle lulls of low-voltage fast activity – solidified the belief that sleep was a passive phenomenon. The cat remained in a continual state of "sleep." Bremer interpreted the sleep syndrome as:

> The result of the suppression, by the interruption of the corticopetal paths, of the steady flow of excitatory impulses, mainly cutaneous and proprioceptive in origin, which are essential for the maintenance of the waking state of the telencephalon, a condition which the olfactory and visual systems are seemingly unable to maintain."

(Translation by Moruzzi, 1964, p. 23)

Bremer's was an acute syndrome, however, for later studies on the dog and cat revealed that alternation between sleep and wakefulness returned after allowing the brain to recover for a few days (Batsel, 1960, 1961; Genovesi *et al.*, 1956). Nevertheless, Bizzi and Spencer (1962) revealed in a clever way that even in the acute condition the isolated cerebrum that included all of the midbrain had activation mechanisms that were overshadowed by the strong tendency for synchronization following the shock of removal of sensory inflow to the cerebrum. By causing reversible retinal ischemia by means of pressure on the eyeball they were able to increase the amount of synchronization by reducing the inter-spindle lulls that exhibit low-amplitude, high-frequency activity. The conclusion from Bremer's work was that the "sleep" resulting from isolation of the cerebrum stemmed from removal of almost all of the sensory input, that arriving at the thalamus from the major ascending pathways.

The ascending reticular activating system

In 1949, though, a new organ of wakefulness emerged: the ascending reticular activating system. Moruzzi and Magoun (1949) demonstrated that electrical stimulation within the core of the brain stem elicited a change in the EEG from the high-amplitude activity associated with most of natural sleep at the time to the low-voltage rhythm typical of the waking brain. Most importantly, the intensity required was lower than that required to induce the same change when the lateral main sensory paths were stimulated. They concluded that collaterals from the ascending sensory pathways at various levels would influence the activity of the reticular formation. Damaging the central core acutely induced an EEG typical of sleep, but interruption of the lateral pathways did not (Lindsley *et al.*,

1949). In a chronic study, Lindsley *et al.* (1950) created a stuporous condition by placing a lesion in the central core, leaving the lateral pathways intact. Damage to the latter bilaterally did not produce this effect.

Moruzzi and Magoun saw that phasic activity in the reticular formation must underlie the arousal reaction and further proposed that "the presence of a steady background of less intense activity within this cephalically directed brain-stem system, contributed to either by liminal inflows from peripheral receptors or preserved intrinsically, may be an important factor contributing to the maintenance of the waking state, and that absence of such activity in it may predispose to sleep." They concluded their landmark paper this way: "The conception of sleep as a functional deafferentation of the cerebrum is not opposed by this evidence if the term 'deafferentation' is broadened to include interruption of the ascending influence of the brain-stem reticular activating system, the contribution of which to wakefulness now seems more important than that conducted to the cortex over classical sensory paths" (Moruzzi and Magoun, 1949, pp. 470–1).

Thus, we were left with a new organ of wakefulness that passively diminished its activating influence: the ascending reticular activating system. Moruzzi carefully observed, though, that Lindsley *et al.*'s (1949) demonstration that acute interruption of the ascending reticular formation system was responsible for the coma produced by Bremer's complete transections could only suggest that "*physiological sleep* – which is characterized by its spontaneous reversibility and by the intense and prolonged arousal produced by sensory stimulation – *was related with functional decrease of tone of the activating reticular system*". He wanted direct proof that "*integrated* discharge of the ascending reticular system actually decreases during sleep," but admitted it would be difficult to isolate the reticular formation for this task (Moruzzi, 1963, pp. 236–7).

A couple of decades later several workers provided that proof requested by Moruzzi although the results were obtained by recording from isolated, identified units rather than an integrated discharge (Kasamatsu, 1970; Manohar *et al.*, 1972; Steriade *et al.*, 1982). They found units in the rostral region of the reticular formation that increased their firing rates with the appearance of both wakefulness and REM sleep following NREM sleep. The increase in discharge led to the onset of wakefulness and REM sleep from NREM sleep. These neurons projected to midline and intralaminar nuclei (Steriade and Glenn, 1982), and neurons projecting to the cortex from intralaminar nuclei were excited monosynaptically from the rostral reticular formation, providing a disynaptic route for activating the cerebral cortex (Steriade, 1981). Of course, several additional neuronal groups that activate the cerebral cortex have since been identified, but we will encounter these in later chapters.

Berlucchi (1997, p. 12) has reviewed the evolution of Moruzzi's thoughts regarding the role of a unified reticular activating system, reminding us that he very early on questioned that the organization of arousal could be so simple. He summarizes that doubt as follows: "Soon after the birth of the hypothesis of the ascending brainstem activating system, Giuseppe Moruzzi considered the possibility that a fractionated and differentiated arousing action of the reticular formation is required for effective behavior and cognition." In 1954, Moruzzi (1954, p. 48) considered the possibility that "for the lower intensity of sensory stimulation only some districts of the ascending reticular system might be activated, and therefore a more localized (or less diffuse) ascending discharge would contribute to the process of attention for the sensory modality involved." Others made related observations. Olszewski (1954) saw the reticular formation as likely to subserve different functions because it consisted of various groups of neurons of different structure. And Hebb (1955) thought that different drives could not fit into a monolithic arousal system. As Berlucchi (1997, p. 6) summarizes, "Moruzzi felt that the fusion of several reticular functions into one whole might occur solely in association with extreme emotional states during which the power of attention, discrimination and analysis is greatly diminished or lost altogether."

Berlucchi observed that we now know of at least five chemically identified ascending systems projecting diffusely to the diencephalon and telencephalon, particularly to the cerebral cortex: (1) the noradrenergic system from the locus coeruleus; (2) the cholinergic system projecting from the brain stem to the thalamus; (3) the dopaminergic system with two divisions projecting from the midbrain to the striatum and the limbic system and prefrontal cortex; (4) the serotonergic dorsal and median raphé nuclei projecting widely to the telencephalon; and (5) the histaminergic system arising from the tubero-mammillary nucleus with terminals found in most cortical layers. "The designation of these systems as 'arousal systems' is justified by the fact that activation of each of them induces desynchronization of the EEG; all of them cooperate in some form to desynchronize the EEG during waking, while only the cholinergic system is responsible for EEG desynchronization during the phase of sleep with rapid eye movements (REM sleep)" (Berlucchi, 1997, p. 7).

The beginning of the end of the passive theory

The recognition of somewhat more complexity in the regulation of arousal – from withdrawal of input from the main sensory pathways to the more complicated arrangement with the reticular formation – and, even more so, the realization that part of sleep had an EEG pattern quite different from the "lazy" waves always associated with sleep in the past were the beginning of the end for the passive theory of sleep in the middle of the last century. Clear acceptance of the idea that sleep and wakefulness depended upon active processes in the brain had to wait a few more years. What is interesting, though, is that evidence for active processes was clearly there before the recognition of REM sleep, but the world of sleep research was not ready to accept it. Two avenues to understanding were provided by von Economo's analysis of the effects of brain damage that resulted from the influenza pandemic of 1916–17 (von Economo, 1930) and Hess's brain stimulation experiments (Hess, 1944).

Von Economo, based on the various symptoms that his patients with "encephalitis lethargica" exhibited, reasoned that there was a sleep-regulating "center," not overly localized extending from "immediately in front of the nuclei of the eye muscles in the grey junction of interbrain and thalamus where the aqueduct of Sylvius opens into the third ventricle" frontally to "the grey walls of the third ventricle near the caput of the corpus caudatum." He established these boundaries because "inflammation in cases associated with insomnia, is localized anteriorly in the lateral wall of the third ventricle, near the corpus striatum while it is localized in cases showing disturbances of ocular muscles with stupor in the posterior wall of the third ventricle near the nuclei of the oculomotorius in the cap of the interbrain." Patients could exhibit other symptoms we commonly associate with some problem of sleep regulation, such as insomnia and reversal of the normal circadian distribution of sleep and wakefulness. He envisioned the stimuli engaging the sleep center to be essentially hypnotoxins.

Von Economo hastened to add that, "the center of sleep regulation cannot be classified within a narrow definition of this term. It is not considered a narrowly circumscribed seat of sleep function but as a center in a wider sense, i.e., as an accumulation of grey matter the function of which is of primary importance for the normal course of sleep." Further, he emphasized that, "The action of that sleep regulating center consists in a coordination of the different changes which occur in sleep in our vegetative animal and psychic system." This statement hardly supports the concept of a passive arrangement for falling asleep (von Economo, 1930, pp. 255–8).

Von Economo was clearly impressed by the results of Hess's stimulation experiments, which gave a clear indication that the brain was capable of initiating sleep "on its own," not waiting for the environment to stop its barrage. Also, Hess's work was in line with von Economo's desire to prove "the correctness of our conception of a center for the supervision of sleep situated at the junction of the thalamus and the interbrain from which sleep is actively initiated" (von Economo, 1930, p. 258). This statement followed Hess's demonstration (Hess, 1929a, b) that he could induce normal appearing sleep by electrical stimulation in the area of the massa intermedia of the thalamus. Hess certainly did not ascribe to the passive theory of sleep it is clear.

At a famous symposium held in 1953, "Brain Mechanisms and Consciousness," attended by other luminaries of the time, such as Bremer, Jasper, Magoun, and Moruzzi, Hess (actually his son in his absence) introduced his chapter with a brief review of the characteristics of normal sleep: "reduction and eventually loss of psychomotor activity and of the ability to act in a coordinated way … decreased awareness of external and internal stimuli … Vegetative functions are also depressed … Closer observation, however, shows that not all functions are depressed … The orbicular muscles of the eye are more active in sleep than in the waking state … The pupils also are contracted during sleep, even in the dark … Other sphincter muscles at least maintain their tone. With regard to internal organs, their activity is not only decreased but altered in other ways ." He concluded his description with the following prescient analysis, which looked at more than 50 years later, seems so modern. "This demonstrates, that sleep is not simply a passive over-all reduction of activity, such as coma for example, but is a complex and co-ordinated state. A functional organization has therefore to be assumed, which must have a central representation" (Hess,1954, pp. 117–18).

Others were not as impressed. Although Hess had demonstrated to the satisfaction of other scientists that a number of organized behaviors could be elicited by brain stimulation in the hypothalamus, his induction of normally appearing sleep by the stimulation of the midline thalamus presented a problem: the former behaviors, such as defense–aggression, appeared within seconds; but sleep behavior appeared usually after several trains of low-frequency stimulations that occurred over many seconds and even minutes (Moruzzi, 1972). Also, the period of induced sleep lasted far longer than a natural episode although the cat could be aroused. It is interesting that much later study of the effects of the cholinergic agonist, carbachol, in the pons created long-lasting episodes of REM. "Both results suggest that the effects obtained may be the result of a sometimes excessive release into a critical area of appropriate neurotransmitters that succeed in biasing the CNS toward a sleep state" (Parmeggiani *et al.*, 1985, p. 16).

At the same symposium, held in 1953 when REM sleep had yet to dominate the field of sleep research and others (Batsel, 1960, 1961) were yet to show that the chronic cerveau isolé preparation alternated between sleep and wakefulness, Bremer reiterated his skepticism that a center inhibiting sleep functioned in an active way in the paper that followed Hess's: "But in recent years it has become increasingly evident that the neurophysiological problem of sleep is rather that of the mechanism of the waking state." This, of course, echoed Kleitman's earlier statement that wakefulness not sleep was the state in need of explanation. The recognition that the "interruption of the classical sensory (lemniscal) ascending channels plays only a subsidiary part in determining the profound modification in cerebral functioning of the hypnic type following mesencephalic transection … has not invalidated the fundamental notion that a sleep-like functional depression of the telencephalon and diencephalon is linked with the suppression of the continuous flood of ascending dynamogenic impulses which, by maintaining a state of subliminal excitation of their networks, is the waking state." The cerebral cortex, Bremer hastened to add, played an active role: "An exclusively reticular theory of sleep regulation does not explain the facts of common observation which indicate the intervention of the cerebral cortex in the determination of its own awakening" (Bremer, 1954, pp. 137–8; 141–2). He reminded the group that cortical stimulation induced action potentials in the reticular formation just as did

sensory volleys; corticofugal and sensory volleys summated on the same reticular cells; cortical stimulation would awaken the sleeping animal; and removal of cortical auditory areas prevented arousal of the sleeping animal to sounds while cutaneous stimulation continued to do so.

The leading scientists at the symposium were trapped by the dominant thinking of the era: sleep was a passive phenomenon. Other evidence was not yet strong enough apparently to switch thinking. For example, in addition to Hess's tactic of stimulating specific areas to induce various behaviors, including sleep, Nauta had experimentally replicated in rats the clinical phenomena described by von Economo by placing hypothalamic lesions. He concluded that, "There is reason to accept a structure in the preoptic region, which is of specific importance for the capacity of sleeping ('sleep centre')…Evidence is offered that sleep is caused by an inhibitory action of the sleep centre on the [more caudal] waking centre" (Nauta, 1946, p. 314). Yet, it would take the second half of the decade of the 50s to convince the world that active processes determine when we sleep. Without doubt the emerging understanding of REM sleep sounded the death knell of the passive theory.

Rhombencephalic sleep

A very significant contribution to this understanding was the demonstration of the Jouvet laboratory that the peripheral expressions of REM sleep – atonia, muscle twitches, and eye movements – were expressed in cats with brain stems transected at the ponto-mesencephalic border (Jouvet and Michel, 1959; Jouvet *et al.*, 1959). This important observation was the fortunate chance observation that decerebrate rigidity melted periodically into atonia with twitches and pontine spikes because electrodes had been planted there to look for EEG signals. The EMG had been recorded from nuchal muscles as a way to detect the startle reflex and to study its habituation.

At the famous Ciba "Symposium on the Nature of Sleep," Jouvet (1960) announced his conclusion that REM sleep emerged from activity in the caudal brain stem and separated the now clearly different stages of sleep into telencephalic and rhombencephalic sleep, using terminology derived from embryology: the rhombencephalon is the precursor of the pons and medulla oblongata. He then adopted the term, paradoxical sleep, which many of us used until the emergence of clinical sleep medicine. The idea that REM sleep was the purview of the caudal brain stem led to a tremendous amount of work unraveling the mechanisms generating REM sleep that, nevertheless, ignored the fact that entrance into REM sleep required communication with the forebrain in intact animals (Morrison and Reiner, 1985; Parmeggiani, 1968). However, a number of the following chapters demonstrate that the course has been corrected.

Writing in 1964, 10 years after the symposium on "Brain Mechanisms and Consciousness," Moruzzi concluded his paper on the history of the development of the deafferentation hypothesis of sleep with these words: "The results of the last ten years of experimental work have not shaken the foundations of the reticular hypothesis of sleep. They have definitely shown, however, that active processes are at work in the brain stem at the onset and during the different stages of sleep. Sleep can no longer be explained as a purely passive phenomenon" (Moruzzi, 1964, p. 27). In the words of Kuhn (1962) there had been a paradigm shift.

Acknowledgments

Supported by USPH grant MH072897. This review was greatly aided by the tremendous historical efforts of Claude Gottesmann (2001, 2004).

References

Aserinsky, E. (1996) The discovery of REM sleep. *J Hist Neurosci* **5**: 213–27.

Aserinsky, E. & Kleitman, N. (1953) Regularly occurring periods of eye motility, and concomitant phenomena during sleep. *Science* **118**: 273–4.

Batsel, H. L. (1960) Electroencephalographic synchronization and desynchronization in the chronic "cerveau isolé". *Electroenceph Clin Neurophysiol* **12**: 421–30.

Batsel, H. L. (1961) Spontaneous synchronization and desynchronization in the chronic cat cerveau isolé. US Army Medical Research and Development Command Report N: 512.

Berger, H. (1930) Ueber das Elektroenkephalogramm des Menschen. *J Psychol Neurol* **40**: 160–79.

Berlucchi, G. (1997) One or many arousal systems? Reflections on some of Giuseppe Moruzzi's foresights and insights about the intrinsic regulation of brain activity. *Arch Ital Biol* **135**: 5–14.

Bizzi, E. & Spencer, W. A. (1962) Enhancement of EEG synchrony in the acute "cerveau isolé". *Arch Ital Biol* **100**: 234–47.

Bremer, F. (1935) Cerveau "isole" et physiologie du sommeil. *C R Soc Biol* **118**: 1235–41.

Bremer, F. (1954) The neurophysiological problem of sleep. In *Brain Mechanisms and Consciousness*, eds. E. D. Adrian, F. Bremer & H. H. Jasper. Springfield, IL: Charles C. Thomas, pp. 137–58.

Datta, S. & MacLean, R. R. (2007) Neurobiological mechanisms for the regulation of mammalian sleep–wake behavior: reinterpretation of historical evidence and inclusion of contemporary cellular and molecular evidence. *Neurosci Biobehav Rev* **31**: 775–824.

Dement, W. C. (1958) The occurrence of low voltage, fast electroencephalogram patterns during behavioral sleep in the cat. *Electroenceph Clin Neurophysiol* **10**: 291–6.

Dement, W. C. (2005) History of sleep physiology and medicine. In *Principles and Practice of Sleep Medicine*, eds. M. H. Kryger, T. Roth & W. C. Dement. Philadelphia: WB Saunders, pp. 1–12.

Dement, W.C. & Kleitman, N. (1957a) The relation of eye movements during sleep to dream activity: an objective method for the study of dreaming. *J Exp Psychol* **53**: 339–46.

Dement, W. C. & Kleitman, N. (1957b) Cyclic variations of EEG during sleep and their relation to eye movements, body motility, and dreaming. *Electroenceph Clin Neurophysiol* **9**: 673–90.

Derbyshire, A. J., Rempel, B., Forbes, A. *et al.* (1936) The effects of anesthetics on action potentials in the cerebral cortex of the cat. *Amer J Physiol* **116**: 577–96.

Genovesi, U., Moruzzi, G., Palestini, M. *et al.* (1956) EEG and behavioral patterns following lesions of the mesencephalic reticular formation in chronic cats with implanted electrodes. *Abtr Comm 20th Int Physiol Congress Bruxelles*: 335–6.

Gottesmann, C. (2001) The golden age of rapid eye movement sleep discoveries: 1. Lucretius – 1964. *Prog Neurobiol* **65**: 211–87.

Gottesmann, C. (2004) Brain inhibitory mechanisms involved in basic and higher integrated sleep processes. *Brain Res Rev* **45**: 230–49.

Hebb, D. O. (1955) Drives and the C.N.S. (conceptual nervous system). *Psychol Rev* **62**: 243–54.

Hess, E. R. (1954) The diencephalic sleep center. In *Brain Mechanisms and Consciousness*, eds. E. D. Adrian, F. Bremer & H. H. Jasper. Oxford: Blackwell, pp. 117–36.

Hess, W. R. (1929a) Hirnreizversuche uber den Mechanismus des Schlafes. *Arch Psychiat Nervenkr* **86**: 287–92.

Hess, W. R. (1929b) Lokalisatorische Ergebnisse der Hirnreizversuche mit Schlafeffekt. *Arch Psychiat Nervenkr* **88**: 813–16.

Hess, W. R. (1944) Das Schlafsyndrom als Folge dienzephaler Reizung. *Helv Physiol & Pharm Acta* **2**: 305–44.

Iranzo, A. Schenck, C. H. & Fonte, J. (2007) REM sleep behavior disorder and other sleep disturbances in Disney animated films. *Sleep Med* **8**: 531–6.

Jouvet, M. (1960) Telencephalic and rhombencephalic sleep in the cat (with discussion). In *The Nature of Sleep*, eds. G. E. W. Wolstenholme & C. M. O 'Connor. Boston: Little, Brown, pp. 188–208.

Jouvet, M. (1999) Around the discovery of REM sleep in cats. In *Rapid Eye Movement Sleep*, eds. B. N. Mallick & S. Inoué. New Delhi: Narosa, pp. v–ix.

Jouvet, M. & Michel, F. (1959) Corrélations électromyographique du sommeil chez le chat décortiqué et mésencéphalique chronique. *C R Soc Biol* **153**: 422–5.

Jouvet, M., Michel, F. & Courjon, J. (1959) Sur un stade d'activité électrique rapide au cours du sommeil physiologique chez le chat. *C R Soc Biol* **153**: 1024–8.

Kasamatsu, T. (1970) Maintained and evoked unit activity in the mesencephalic reticular formation of the freely behaving cat. *Exp Neurol* **28**: 450–70.

Klaue, R. (1937) Die bioelektrische Tatigkeit der Grosshirnrinde im normalen Schlaf und in der Narkose durch Schlafmittel. *J Psychol Neurol* **47**: 510–31.

Kleitman, N. (1929) Sleep. *Physiol Rev* **9**: 624–65.

Kleitman, N. (1939) *Sleep and Wakefulness.* Chicago: University of Chicago Press.

Kuhn, T. S. (1962) *The Structure of Scientific Revolution.* Chicago: University of Chicago Press.

Lindsley, D. B., Bowden, J. & Magoun, H. W. (1949) Effect upon the EEG of acute injury to the brain stem activating system. *Electroenceph Clin Neurophysiol* **1**: 475–86.

Lindsley, D. B., Schreiner, L. H., Knowles, W. B. *et al.* (1950) Behavioral and EEG changes following chronic brain stem lesions in the cat. *Electroenceph Clin Neurophysiol* **10**: 483–98.

Loomis, A. I., Harvey, E. N. & Hobart, G. A. I. (1937) Cerebral states during sleep, as studied by human brain potentials. *J Exp Psychol* **21**: 127–44.

Manohar, S., Noda, H. & Adey, W. R. (1972) Behavior of mesencephalic reticular neurons in sleep and wakefulness. *Exp Neurol* **34**: 140–57.

Morrison, A. R. (1983) Paradoxical sleep and alert wakefulness: variations on a theme. In *Sleep Disorders, Basic and Clinical Research*, eds. Chase, M. M. & Weitzman, E. D. New York: Spectrum, pp. 95–127.

Morrison, A. R. & Reiner, P. B. (1985) A dissection of paradoxical sleep. In *Brain Mechanisms of Sleep*, eds. D. J. McGinty, R. Drucker-Colin, A. R. Morrison & P. L. Parmeggiani. New York: Raven Press, pp. 97–110.

Moruzzi, G. (1954) The physiological properties of the brain stem reticular system. In *Brain Mechanisms and Consciousness*, eds. E. D. Adrian, F. Bremer & H. H. Jasper. Springfield, IL: Charles C. Thomas, pp. 21–48.

Moruzzi, G. (1963) Active processes in the brainstem during sleep. *Harvey Lect* **58**: 233–97.

Moruzzi, G. (1964) The historical development of the deafferentation hypothesis of sleep. *Proc Am Phil Soc* **108**: 19–28.

Moruzzi, G. (1972) The sleep–waking cycle. In *Neurophysiology and Neurochemistry of Sleep and Wakefulness*. Berlin: Springer-Verlag, pp. 1–165.

Moruzzi, G. & Magoun, H. W. (1949) Brainstem reticular formation and activation of the EEG. *Electroenceph Clin Neurophysiol* **1**: 455–73.

Nauta, W. J. H. (1946) Hypothalamic regulation of sleep in rats: experimental study. *J Neurophysiol* **9**: 285–316.

Olzewski, J. (1954) The cytoarchitecture of the human reticular formation. In: *Brain Mechanisms and Consciousness*, eds. E. D. Adrian, F. Bremer & H. H. Jasper. Springfield, IL: Charles C. Thomas, pp. 54–76.

Parmeggiani, P. L. (1968) Telencephalo-diencephalic aspects of sleep mechanisms. *Brain Res* **7**: 350–9.

Parmeggiani, P. L., Morrison, A. R., Drucker-Colin, R. & McGinty, D. J. (1985) Brain mechanisms of sleep: an overview of methodological issues. In *Brain Mechanisms of Sleep*, eds. McGinty, D.J., Drucker-Colin, R., Morrison, A. R. & Parmeggiani, P. L. New York: Raven Press, pp. 1–34.

Piéron, H. T. (1913) *Le problème physiologique du sommeil.* Masson, Paris.

Steriade, M. (1981) Mechanisms underlying cortical activation: neuronal organization and properties of the midbrain reticular core and intralaminar thalamic nuclei. In *Brain Mechanisms and Perceptual Awareness*, eds. O. Pompeiano & C. A. Marsan. New York: Raven Press, pp. 327–77.

Steriade, M. & Glenn, L. L. (1982) Neocortical and caudate projections of intralaminar neurons and their synaptic excitation from midbrain reticular core. *J Neurophysiol* **48**: 352–71.

Steriade, M., Oakson, G. & Ropert, N. (1982) Firing rates and patterns of midbrain reticular neurons during steady and transitional states of the sleep–waking cycle. *Exp Brain Res* **46**: 37–51.

von Economo, C. (1930) Sleep as a problem of localization. *J Nerv Ment Dis* **71**: 249–59.

Chapter

5

REM sleep and dreaming: the nature of the relationship

Milton Kramer

Summary

The need to study dreaming is the promise that it will unlock the mystery of psychosis and perhaps contribute to resolving the mind–body problem. A number of questions arise in the study of dreams. Can dreams be reliably measured? Do dreams reflect differences where we know psychological differences exist? Do dreams change when there is a change in the state of the dreamer? Do dreams change across the night and across the REM period? Are the dreams of individuals different from one another? And are dreams of an individual different from night to night? Are dreams related to the waking life of the dreamer? Are dreams random or orderly? These are the questions this chapter undertakes to address.

Introduction

The excitement that accompanied the discovery of REM sleep was related to the assumption that the biological basis for psychosis had been discovered. We had been "promised" by many of the great minds in philosophy, psychiatry, and neurology that if we understood dreaming, the sane man's psychosis, we would have clues to unlock the mystery of psychosis (Freud, 1955a). In the early 1950s when Aserinsky and Kleitman (1953, 1955) described the relationship between REM sleep and dreaming, about one hospital bed in ten in the United States was occupied by a mentally ill patient (Lamb and Weinberger, 2005). We thought that a door had been opened to begin dealing more effectively with this enormous public health problem.

A related and intellectually more profound problem, that of the relationship between mind and body (Descartes, 1912), was touched on by having what was thought to be a strong relationship between a mental state, dreaming, and a biological state in the brain,

REM sleep. The conviction developed that, as dreaming was a conscious state, the mind–body divide might be bridged through an examination of this relationship. The use of the term mind–brain is an effort to express a monistic commitment whether evidence for a unity exists or not. McGuinn (1999) has argued that we do not have the tools to explain the transduction from the physiology of brain activity to the conscious activity of mind. Certainly no one would argue at this point that mental function is not dependent on brain function. The question remains what is the nature of the relationship? Hobson (1988; Hobson *et al.*, 2000) has argued that the dreaming state is best analogized to a waking delirium and that the biology of REM sleep determines the nature of the conscious experience, dreaming, that accompanies that state. He explicitly states that his position is one of a biological reduction of the mental to the physical. Solms (2003) has voiced a most compelling critique of Hobson's position pointing out particularly that the relationship between dreaming and REM sleep is doubly dissociated, not all REM periods yield dream reports and not all dreaming occurs during REM sleep.

The description of dreaming that follows is based to a large extent but not exclusively on awakening subjects in a dream/sleep laboratory from REM sleep and asking them what had been going through their minds before they were awakened. The dream reports are tape recorded and transcribed for later "blind" measurement usually by two or more judges using a dream content rating scale, primarily the one described by Hall and Van de Castle (1966). These scales are based on 1000 dreams from college students, 500 from men, and 500 from women, written out as part of a class exercise. We have utilized this scale on the transcripts of dreams collected in the laboratory and found essentially the same content frequencies that they reported in their

REM Sleep: Regulation and Function, eds. Birendra N. Mallick, S. R. Pandi-Perumal, Robert W. McCarley, and Adrian R. Morrison. Published by Cambridge University Press. © Cambridge University Press 2011.

book *The Content Analysis of Dreams* (Reichers *et al.*, 1970; Sandler *et al.*, 1969, 1970).

It is essential to put to rest any residual doubt that the dream experience can be studied scientifically. The basis for any scientific undertaking is to be able to reliably and validly measure the object of study. "When you cannot measure it, when you cannot express it in numbers…you have scarcely in your thoughts advanced to the stage of science…" (Lord Kelvin in Strauss, 1968, 482b). "Vital distinctions are always quantitative" (Fisher in Strauss, 1968, 482b).

The renewed interest in the study of dreams was stimulated by the observation that a particular portion of sleep, REM sleep, was highly correlated with the report on waking of a dream experience. It seemed reasonable to compare the reliability of measuring the content of dreams to the reliability of measuring the stages of sleep. We did two studies to establish the reliability and stability of the physiology of sleep, sleep stages; and that of the psychology of sleep, dream reports (Kramer and Roth, 1979; Roth *et al.*, 1977). The questions we were asking were: (1) Does the reproducibility of measuring dreams approach that of measuring sleep? and (2) Does the stability of dream content approach that of sleep?

We had 11 college-age men sleep for 15 consecutive nights in the sleep laboratory and had their sleep recorded. We then selected two sleep records from each of the subjects and had them scored "blindly" by two judges. The averaged reliability (i.e., agreement) scoring each 30-second period of the eight-hour sleep record for seven sleep parameters for the 30 records was 92.5%. To establish sleep stability, we then correlated actual time and percentage time of each of the seven sleep parameters for each successive night pair then averaged across them for the first and second week. The mean correlation for the time data over two weeks was 0.28 and for the percentage data was 0.44, explaining 8% to 19% of the variance of the sleep physiological parameters.

To establish the reliability and stability of dream content measurement, we had 14 college-age men sleep for 20 consecutive nights in the sleep laboratory and collected dream reports from awakenings from the first four REM periods of each night (Kramer and Roth, 1979). Two scorers using the characters, activities, and descriptive elements scales of the Hall–Van de Castle dream scoring system (1966) rated the transcribed reports "blindly" and independently. The overall exact percentage agreement across the three content scales was 91%. A score for each scale for each night for each subject was established and successive nights were correlated and averaged. The mean overall night-to-night dream content correlation for the two weeks is 0.46, which explains 21% of the night-to-night variability in dream content.

The scoring reliability and night-to-night stability of sleep physiology, 92.5%, 0.28 to 0.44, and sleep psychology, 91%, 0.46, are strikingly similar using the more liberal figure for the physiology. This similarity argues that quantifying dreaming is as reliable an undertaking as quantifying various aspects of sleep physiology. We will test the validity of dream content quantification by studies, which examine whether dream content is different in circumstances where we know that psychological differences exist.

We have reason to believe that at the group level there are meaningful psychological differences related to the various demographic variables such as sex, age, and social class.

Group differences

Demographic variables

Sex

In reviewing the early literature (Winget and Kramer, 1979), it became apparent that the major organizer of dream content was the sex of the dreamer. We found 34 non-lab studies that showed a male/female difference e.g., boys have more mutilation themes while girls have more intimacy themes. Similarly Hall–Van de Castle (1966) in their non-lab normative study of college students showed a systematic and large number of male/female content differences. For example, women have more characters in their dreams, but men have twice as many men as women in their dreams while women have an equal number of men and women in theirs. Sexual interactions are relatively rare in these dreams but are three times as frequent in the dreams of men as women. Men have more physical aggressions while women have more friendly interactions. Men's dreams are more often set outdoors but women's are more likely indoors. Emotions are more frequent in women's dreams. In our stratified random sample of the home dreams of adults in Cincinnati (Kramer *et al.*, 1971; Winget *et al.*, 1972) we found nine content differences related to the sex of the dreamer. Women had more dreams with characters, friendly social interactions, emotions, indoor settings, and home and family references. Men had more aggression, achievement striving with success, castration anxiety, and overt hostility. We compared the laboratory collected dreams of 11 college-age women to 11 college-age men collected over 20 nights for each, 596 dreams from women and 594 from men (Kramer *et al.*, 1983). We found 11 content differences related to the sex of the dreamer. Women had more cognitive activity, and more intensity references. Men had more male characters, single characters, strangers, auditory activity, achromatic colors, old-age references, large sizes, full containers, and crooked or curved references.

The four studies cited clearly support the idea that where we know there are sex differences, systematic and often-replicable differences appear in dream reports. This supports the validity of the study of dreams and points toward looking at the content of dreams as reflecting the dreamer.

Age

We found 20 studies (Winget and Kramer, 1979) that show dream content over the age range of 2 to 95. Unpleasant dreams decrease from ages 1–4 to 9–12. Children's dreams are lower in aggression than adults. Anxiety decreases with age while sex differences in aggression increase with age. Adolescents had more destructive themes and castration threats and concern with self-safety than adults. Dream content changes between age 3 and 15 mirroring waking changes in cognitive development. Older adults, over 65, had more dreams of lost resources, helplessness, or weakness. In a population survey (Winget *et al.*, 1972) we found that references to death and death anxiety were directly correlated with age. Guilt anxiety was highest in young adults, aged 21 to 34. Aggression had a complex relationship to age in the population sample. The young adult is concerned with right and wrong while the elderly are concerned with decline and dying.

In a more recent review of the literature on dreams in the aged (Kramer, 2010), it was found that dream recall and characters decrease with age and that the dreamer is less central to the dream action. Aggressive and friendly interactions decrease with age, but changes in the frequency of sexual interactions are uncertain. Older dreamers are less often the central character in their dreams, report fewer affects that are less intense and less negative. Regression in time occurs in their dreams. The style of dreaming changes with age, with men becoming more passive and women becoming more motorically active. In some degenerative diseases there are concomitant dream content changes.

Important changes occur to dreams as the dreamer ages, although fewer than we see related to the sex of the dreamer. A more extensive systematic study of dreams in relationship to age across the life cycle is necessary. The view (Domhoff, 1996) that "age is not a major factor in shaping dream content once Americans have reached young adulthood" is not tenable.

Socioeconomic class

There has been very little if any (Bastide, 1966) study of the relationship between social class and dreams. In our population study (Winget *et al.*, 1972), we compared the dream content of three social classes; lower, lower middle, and upper middle. There were six content-related class differences. The upper middle class had fewer characters, less death anxiety, and fewer premonitions in their dreams. Misfortune was more common in the two lower social classes. For white dreamers in the upper middle class there was less total anxiety and fewer dreams with home and family themes. Lower class adolescents have more aggression in their dreams than middle class adolescents (Buckley, 1970).

The lower classes have a relatively more troubled dream life than the upper middle class. The conceptualization of the world that the lower classes have in their dreams is a world in which negative events occur over which they have no control in a world crowded with people, and for poor whites focused on home and family. They feel threatened by death and believe that dreams predict the future.

Ullman (1969a, b) has urged that the social aspects of dreaming be more carefully examined and that a sociology of dreams be developed, which should be focused on (1) the ways institutions are experienced in dreams, and (2) how dreaming experience relates to the social ambience and social structure. In our population study (Kramer *et al.*, 1971) we found that 51% of our 182 dream reports contained an institutional reference of which 79% were to the family, 59% to the family by marriage, and 41% to the family of origin. Work references made up 11% of the institutional references, but only 5.6% of our dream reports had a direct work reference. It is not the occupational world of the dreamer that is being manifestly conceptualized, but rather some aspect of the family as it is represented in 40% of the total dream reports.

Race and marital status

Our population study (Winget *et al.*, 1972) revealed very few dream content differences related to the race, only 3 out of 30 variables, or the marital status of the dreamer and those that were found were confounded by small sample size, gender, age, and social class. Blacks had more castration anxiety and penis envy, and whites more covert hostility directed outward. Widows had the most death anxiety. The formerly married dreamed more of family members from their family of marriage than of origin (Cartwright *et al.*, 1984). Cartwright (1991) has pointed out the adaptational significance of who is dreamed about at the time of a divorce.

Psychiatric illness

We expected to find differences in the dream life of patients with major psychiatric illnesses, as this would support the concept of the regularity/stability of dreaming and the validity of dreaming. We asked hospitalized male patients who were diagnosed with either paranoid schizophrenia, psychotic depression, or a medical illness, 40 in each group, to tell us their last dream (Kramer *et al.*, 1969). The dreams were characterized for plausibility, hostility direction, and major character type. The typical dream report of a paranoid schizophrenic patient finds him in an implausible situation in which he is the victim of a hostile attack by a stranger. The psychotically depressed patient is with a family member in the dream, usually in a plausible situation with hostility present about half the time, which is as likely to be directed at others as at the dreamer. The non-psychotic medical patient in his dreams is with a friend in a plausible situation that is rarely hostile, and if it is the dreamer is as likely to be expressing the hostility as receiving it. The dreams of hospitalized women patients with paranoid schizophrenia and psychotic depression patients are similar to what we described for our hospitalized psychotic male patients (Langs, 1966). The dreams of the depressed have family members while family members are essentially absent from the dreams of schizophrenic patients whose dreams are most implausible and filled with conflict.

The dreams of depressed patients (Kramer *et al.*, 1966, 1968) and schizophrenic patients (Kramer *et al*, 1969, 1972, 1973; Kramer and Roth, 1973) show systematic changes concomitant with improvement in their waking condition. The depressed patient with improvement shows a decrease in hostility and anxiety, and an increase in heterosexuality and motility. The schizophrenic patient when improved showed more concise and better organized dreams with proportionately fewer aggressive interactions compared with friendly ones, fewer emotions, and more success and good fortune.

In our laboratory studies of REM dreaming in hospitalized patients with schizophrenia or depression, we found that the schizophrenics had had strangers as their most frequent character type while depressed patients had family members as theirs. The schizophrenics had more groups of people than the depressed. Both patient groups showed changes in their dream life concomitant with their improving clinically.

We compared the dream content laboratory collected REM dreams of mildly brain-damaged men to those who were severely damaged (Kramer and Roth, 1975). The only statistically significant finding was that the severely damaged had more characters in their dreams. We also looked at dream recall rates in the severely damaged. Age and severity of damage contributed to a decreased dream recall rate as recall was lowest in the older, brain-damaged patient. Compared to the Hall–Van de Castle norms (1966) the combined middle-aged brain-damaged group had more family members, friendly social interactions, fewer aggressions, and no scoreable emotions. Age and brain damage result in a significant change in dream content.

Applying a verifiability standard to the dream reports of psychiatric illness (Kramer, 1970; Kramer and Roth, 1979; Kramer and Nuhic, 2007), namely that the findings had to be reported and independently replicated in published studies, both of which were scientifically adequate, significantly reduces our knowledge of the dream life of patients with psychiatric illness. The verified content of the dreams of schizophrenics would be that they are more hostile, more affective, with strangers as a frequent character, and contain more evidence of the schizophrenic thought disorder e.g., more unrealistic, and more bizarre, than non-schizophrenics. For depressed patients the verified findings are that they have shorter dreams and have more family members in their dreams than the non-depressed.

Nevertheless, the orderly and systematic differences in dream content between psychotic patients, in and out of the laboratory, and the differences found in relationship to demographic variables, as well as their dream life changing when their condition improves, makes the suggestion that in producing dreams the brain is making the best of a bad job increasingly implausible. Langs (1966) offers as an example the dream of a paranoid schizophrenic woman, "Dreamed I was going over Niagara Falls in a barrel with a fat roly-poly man made of rubber. I think I had intercourse with the man." And for a psychotically depressed woman, "Dreamed I was with the whole family in former times." The dreams may be implausible but hardly chaotic or resembling the confused verbalization of the delirious (Hobson, 1988). Heynick (1993) makes the point that speech in dreams is well organized and generally grammatically correct.

Individual differences

Between individuals, and between and across nights of the same individual

We have already reviewed the evidence from our work that at the group level dream reports can be reliably quantified at a level equal to if not superior to the quantification of electroencephalographically recorded sleep. Dreams at the group level are regular, orderly, and non-random, showing psychological differences where we would expect content differences to exist; confirming the validity of the content analysis of dreams. Dreams therefore have the characteristics necessary to have meaning. The dream content changes with changes in the dreamer's waking state supports the concept that dreams are meaningful, i.e., related to the waking condition of the dreamer as well.

The question arises whether the orderliness found in the dreams of groups could be extended to individuals, both the normal and the psychiatrically ill (Kramer *et al.*, 1976).

To examine whether the dreams of individuals, normal and schizophrenic, could be distinguished one from the other we did the following study. We gave three judges, of varying experience working with dreams, 75 REM dreams from 5 different male college students, 15 dreams per subject, and 65 dreams from 5 hospitalized schizophrenic patients, 13 dreams per patient. The judges' task was to sort the dreams into 5 groups of 15 dreams each for the normal subjects, and 5 groups of 13 dreams each for the patients. These tasks and the subsequent ones to be described were all done without the judges having any information about the dreamer to increase the likelihood that the judges were basing their decisions primarily on the dream report. All three judges were able to sort the dreams into the correct group for both the normal and schizophrenic subjects. This achievement supports the conclusion that dreams of individuals are distinguishable one from the other at the trait level, i.e., they reflect enduring aspects of the personality.

Freud (1955b) had suggested that the dreams of the same night were related. This is the view reflected as well in the Torah "And Jacob had proclaimed that the dreams of Pharoh are one." (O.T., Genesis: 41:25).

We then gave our judges 15 REM dreams from each of 10 college students and each of 5 schizophrenic patients and they were asked to sort each group of 15 REM dreams into 5 sets of 3 dreams each. Each set of 3 dreams was from the same night. Again, all three judges were able to do the sorting task for the normal and patient group at a statistically significant level.

Not only were dreams distinguishable among people but they were distinguishable by nights for an individual. This systematic result supported the view that dream reports were distinguishable one night from the other at the state level, i.e., day to day. For the individual, it underlines the reactive nature of the dream and opens up the possibility the dream is relatable to the previous day's activity, to the day residue.

We are not denying that the dreams of an individual are not linked to one another across nights. To test this night-to-night dream relationship, we correlated the characters, activities, and descriptive elements, utilizing the Hall–Van de Castle scales (1966), in REM dreams from night to night for 20 consecutive nights (Kramer and Roth, 1976) and found that the overall correlation was a statistically significant 0.46.

Our three judges next were asked to place, in their order of appearance in the night, 50 sets of 3 REM dreams each from the college students, and 34 sets of 3 REM dreams each from the patient group. None of the judges was able to do this at a statistically significant level for the dream sets from the normal subjects, one judge was able to do it for the patients' dreams and one judge showed a trend for ordering the sets of the patients' dreams. It is fair to say that overall the judges were unable to sort the dreams by position of occurrence in the night.

Dreams across a night

We had been unable to demonstrate that the regularity of dreaming extends to the position of the night using judges to determine the dream's position. We pursued the matter further by examining the dream content from REM periods across subjects (Kramer *et al.*, 1981). We collected dreams from the first 4 REM periods of the night from 22 subjects for 20 consecutive nights. We found that the word count for REM I was shorter than for REM II, and that REM III was shorter than for REM IV, but that REM II and REM III were not different from each other. These results could be the consequence of the REM periods being longer across the nights with more dream experience and therefore more to describe and more words per dream being reported. We found nine statistically significant content differences across the night, with word length held constant: four were between REM I and REM II, and five between REM II and REM III, and none between REM III and REM IV. These included total, single and female characters; and total, physical and verbal activities and size minus and total scored content. The ninth was word length. For no single content variable was there a statistically significant change across the four REM periods. There is generally a linear increase in contents across the four REM periods. For the three significant character variables a non-significant decrease occurred in the fourth REM period following the inverted U-shaped function one might hypothesize for a problem-solving function for dreaming across the night. It is the character variables that we have found to be discriminating in other of our studies (Kramer and Roth, 1973; Kramer *et al.*, 1969). The findings are suggestive of a positional difference for a dream within the night related to the content of the dream but only at a group level, and of a possible problem-solving function for the dream across the night. These findings alter any notion that the position of the dream in the night is independent and free of any constraints.

We pursued the question of whether there was a pattern to the dreams of the night both clinically and in laboratory collected REM dreams from across the night. We described two basic patterns (Kramer *et al.*, 1964). One pattern is of a progressive–sequential nature in which a problem is stated thematically, worked on figuratively, and resolved subjectively. The other pattern is a traumatic–repetitive one in which a problem is experienced and reiterated figuratively in each dream of the night with little or no progress. Dreamers have both patterns, probably depending on the immediate current concern they have before going to sleep and their emotional resources at the time.

A progressive–sequential pattern is illustrated by this dream series reported by a 27-year-old married woman to her psychoanalyst in her 497th hour:

> Dream 1: "A man kept knocking at the back door. He said he wanted a knife. I said not to come in. I put the knife behind the washing machine. Finally he got in and got the knife. He was not threatening once he got inside."

> Dream 2: "I was going to an old camp where there was a deep lake. Somebody drowned there and they were finding out the depth of the water by letting down a chain."

> Dream 3: "There was some blood on my breast and I found out that it was partly cut but did not hurt at all."

The sequential progression thematically was from Dream 1: a threat by a male to enter with something penetrating, but when he was inside it was not so threatening. Dream 2: someone died and it was caused by being in too deep? And Dream 3: you may be damaged, but it is not too serious, it doesn't hurt. Without adding the history of the dreamer and her associations to the dream and that much could be made out of possible meanings for the dream, thematically there is a progression from a threat that decreased but could be dangerous – even if there is a cut it is okay as it didn't hurt as anticipated.

A traumatic–repetitive pattern is illustrated by the dream series reported by a 24-year-old single woman to her psychoanalyst in the 54th hour:

> Dream 1: "I went to a beauty shop without an appointment. It was against the rules not to have an appointment. I was afraid that the beautician taking care of me would get fired and I therefore started sobbing dreadfully."

> Dream 2: "I was in the ladies room in the elevated station. I was looking for you at the usual time of our appointment and you were not there. I broke down and began to cry."

> Dream 3: "I was lost in a building like a maze. Couldn't find my way. A girl behind the bar in a taproom talked about going away. I was envious of the fun she was going to have and wished I could go."

> Dream 4: " I was at a bus stop. My friends Helen and Mary were there and were going somewhere. I was seeing them off."

The traumatic–repetitive theme pattern starts with Dream 1: seeking to be made better, but by not following the rules, running the risk of losing the person who can help and being upset. Dream 2: looking for a helping person but they are not there and upset again. Dream 3: a lost person who provides is going away, envious. Dream 4: friends and potential helpers are going, but she isn't. People who could help her (beautician, analyst, bar girl, and friends) are, or could be, leaving in all four dreams – a highly repetitious theme. The affective tone appears to improve from tears to envy to neutral. Nevertheless, the theme remains essentially the same, loss of a helping person. Again much more could be made out of these dreams but the point is to highlight the thematic similarity in all of the dreams.

There has been some work that has suggested that the dream experience is different early as compared to later in the night (Foulkes, 1966; Verdone, 1965). Unfortunately, these studies compared only two points in time across the night and could describe only a linear relationship.

Dream content across an REM period

We examined the content recovered from a series of six time points across the REM period (Kramer *et al.*, 1974, 1975). The content was rated for 12 factors on a Dream Inventory Questionnaire on awakening by the dreamer and later by a judge, and was content analyzed as well using the Hall–Van de Castle (1966) dream content scoring system. There was a statistically significant effect across time for recall, emotionality, anxiety, and pleasantness. The change was linear for all four statistically significant changes, with emotionality also showing a quadratic curve. Each approach to quantifying the dream experience showed the same result and was similarly statistically significant. The rating, judgment, and content-based curves for emotionality rose steeply in intensity from 2.5 minutes into the REM period to 10 minutes then was flat to 20 minutes, then rose a little less steeply to 30 minutes, the last point sampled. This result supports the central role for emotions in guiding the dream experience.

There is a clear regularity to content development across the REM period. The curve, at least for emotions, seems to parallel the ebb and flow of eye movements across the REM period that Aserinsky (1971) described and that we replicated (Johnson *et al.*, 1980). This may be an important point of psycho-physiological parallelism. It further supports the fact that dream content is not randomly displayed across the REM period.

Conclusion

I have reviewed the evidence that dream content could be as reliably measured as the various electrophysiological aspects of sleep. The first step is a scientific (i.e., quantitative) study of dreams. Having established the reliability (i.e., reproducibility), and stability (i.e., night-to-night correlation) of dream measurement, I then explored the validity of the measurement of dreams by showing that where there are known psychological differences among people there are dream content differences. I described studies of the various demographic variables, which have known psychological differences such as sex, age, socioeconomic status, race, and marital status – all of which show statistically significant differences in dream content most prominently for sex and age, and most interestingly for social class. Similarly we were able to show dream content differences between patients with major psychiatric illnesses (i.e., schizophrenia and depression) and dream recall and content differences associated with the degree of brain damage. Dreams are orderly and non-random and therefore have the characteristic necessary for them to have meaning. The dream content changes with changes in the waking state opens the possibility that they are related to the waking state of the dreamer, and to the affective change from night to morning (Kramer and Roth, 1973).

At the individual level we were able to show that dreams of each individual are different from each other, and that for an individual that the dreams of a night are different from each other as well as that dreams night-to-night are connected, correlated to each other. Dreams of a night of an individual cannot be placed in their order of occurrence across the night. However, for groups of subjects there are nine categories that are different across the night: word length, three character categories, three activities, one size minus and one total content scored. No single category changes across all REM periods. Characters show a pattern, an inverted U-shape, consistent with a problem-solving function. Clinically we were able to describe two patterns of dreams across the night: one was of a progressive–sequential nature, in which a problem was stated figuratively, worked on and resolved; and the other of a traumatic–repetitive nature in which the problem was stated figuratively in each dream with no progression. Across an REM period, there was a clear pattern of increased recall, emotion, anxiety, and pleasantness. The change in emotion had a pattern similar to the eye movements of a REM period, a striking psycho-physiologic parallelism.

The impressive discriminatory characteristics of dreaming have not been duplicated by studies of the physiology of REM sleep.

References

Aserinsky, E. (1971) Rapid eye movement density and pattern in the sleep of normal young adults. *Psychophysiology* **8**: 361–76.

Aserinsky, E. & Kleitman, N. (1953) Regularly occurring periods of eye motility, and concomitant phenomena, during sleep. *Science*, **118**(3062): 273–4.

Aserinsky, E. & Kleitman, N. (1955) Two types of ocular motility occurring in sleep. *J Appl Physiol*, **8**(1): 1–10.

Bastide, R. (1966) The sociology of dreams. In *The Dream and Human Societies*, eds. G. Von Gruenbaum & R. Caillois. Berkeley, CA: University of California Press, pp. 199–221.

Buckley, J. J. (1970) The dreams of young adults; a sociological anaysis of 1133 dreams of black and white students. PhD thesis. Wayne State, Detroit.

Cartwright, R. D., Lloyd, S., Knight, S., & Trenholme, I. (1984) Broken dreams: a study of the effects of divorce and depression on dream content. *Psychiatry* **47**(3): 251–9.

Cartwright, R. (1991) The relationship of dream incorporation to adaptation to stressful events. *Dreaming* **1**(1), 3–9.

Descartes, R. (1912) *Philosophical Works of Descartes* (E. Haldane, G. Ross, Trans. Vol. I). Cambridge, UK: Cambridge University Press.

Domhoff, B. (1996) *Finding Meaning in Dreams*. New York: Plenum Press.

Foulkes, D. (1966) *The Psychology of Sleep*. New York: Scribner.

Freud, S. (1955a) *The Interpretation of Dreams*. New York: Basic Books.

Freud, S. (1955b) *Beyond the Pleasure Principle*, vol. XVIII. London: Hogarth Press.

Hall, C. S. & Van de Castle, R. L. (1966) *The Content Analysis of Dreams*. New York: Appleton-Century-Crofts.

Heynick, F. (1993) *Language and its Disturbances in Dreams: the Pioneering Work of Freud and Kraepelin Updated*. New York: Wiley.

Hobson, J. A. (1988) *The Dreaming Brain*. New York: Basic Books.

Hobson, J. A., Pace-Schott, E. F. & Stickgold, R. (2000) Dreaming and the brain: toward a cognitive neuroscience of conscious states. *Behav Brain Sci* **23**(6): 793–842; discussion 904–1121.

Johnson, B., Kramer, M., Bonnet, M., Roth, T. & Jansen, T. (1980) The effect of Ketazolam on ocular motility during sleep. *Curr Ther Res* **28**(5): 792–9.

Kramer, M. (1970) Manifest dream content in normal and psychopathologic states. *Arch Gen Psychiatry* **22**(2): 149–59.

Kramer, M. (2010) Dreaming and dreaming disorders in the elderly. In *Principles and Practice of Geriatric Sleep Medicine*, eds. S. R. Pandi-Perumal, J. M. Monti & A. A. Monjan. Cambridge: Cambridge University Press, pp. 307–18.

Kramer, M., Baldridge, B. J., Whitman, R. M., Ornstein, P. H. & Smith, P. C. (1969) An exploration of the manifest dream in schizophrenic and depressed patients. *Dis Nerv Syst* **30**(2): Suppl 126–30.

Kramer, M., Clark, J. & Day, N. (1973) Dreaming in schizophrenia. In *The Occulomotor System and Brain Function*, ed. V. Zikmund. London: Butterworths, pp. 439–52.

Kramer, M., Czaya, J., Arand, D. & Roth, T. (1974) The development of psychological content across the REM period. *Sleep Res* **3**: 121.

Kramer, M., Hlasny, R., Jacobs, G. & Roth, T. (1976) Do dreams have meaning? An empirical inquiry. *Am J Psychiatry* **133**(7): 778–81.

Kramer, M., Kinney, L. & Scharf, M. (1983) Dream incorporation and dream function. In *Sleep 1982*, ed. W. Koella. Basel: S. Karger, pp. 369–71.

Kramer, M., McQuarrie, E. & Bonnet, M. (1981) Problem solving in dreaming: an empirical test. In *Sleep 1980*, ed. W. Koella. Basel: S.Karger, pp. 357–60.

Kramer, M., & Nuhic, Z. (2007) A review of dreaming by psychiatric patients. In *Sleep and Psychosomatic Medicine*, eds. S.R. Pandi-Perumal & M. Kramer. Boca Raton, Florida: Taylor and Francis, pp. 137–55.

Kramer, M. & Roth, T. (1973) The mood-regulating function of sleep. In *Sleep 1972*, eds. W. Koella & P. Levin. Basel: S. Karger, pp.563–71.

Kramer, M. & Roth, T. (1975) Dreams and dementia: a laboratory exploration of dream recall and dream content in chronic brain syndrome patients. *Int J Aging Hum Dev* **6**(2): 179–82.

Kramer, M. & Roth, T. (1979) The stability and variability of dreaming. *Sleep* **1**(3): 319–25.

Kramer, M., Roth, T. & Czaya, J. (1975) Dream development within an REM period. In *Sleep 1974*, eds. W. Koella & P. Levin. Basel: S. Karger, pp. 406–8.

Kramer, M., Trinder, J. & Roth, T. (1972) Dream content analysis of male schizophrenic patients. *Can Psychiatr Assoc J*, **17**(2): ss251.

Kramer, M., Whitman, R. M., Baldridge, B. J. & Lansky, L. M. (1964) Patterns of dreaming: the interrelationship of the dreams of a night. *J Nerv Ment Dis* **139**: 426–39.

Kramer, M., Whitman, R. M., Baldridge, W. & Lansky, L. (1966) Dreaming in the depressed. *Can Psychiatr Assoc J* **11** Suppl: 178–92.

Kramer, M., Whitman, R. M., Baldridge, B. & Ornstein, P. H. (1968) Drugs and dreams III. The effects of imipramine on the dreams of depressed patients. *Am J Psychiatry* **124**(10): 1385–92.

Kramer, M., Winget, C. & Whitman, R. M. (1971) A city dreams: a survey approach to normative dream content. *Am J Psychiatry* **127**(10): 1350–6.

Lamb, H. R. & Weinberger, L. E. (2005) The shift of psychiatric inpatient care from hospitals to jails and prisons. *J Am Acad Psychiatry Law* **33**(4): 529–34.

Langs, R. J. (1966) Manifest dreams from three clinical groups. *Arch Gen Psychiatry* **14**(6): 634–43.

McGuinn, C. (1999) *The Mysterious Flame.* New York: Basic Books.

Riechers, M., Kramer, M. & Trinder, J. (1970) A replication of the Hall–Van de Castle character scale norms. *Psychophysiology* **7**: 328.

Roth, T., Kramer, M. & Roehrs, T. (1977) The consistency of sleep measures. In *Sleep 1976*, eds. W. Koella & P. Levin. Basel: S. Karger, pp. 286–8.

Sandler, L., Kramer, M., Fishbein, H. & Trinder, J. (1969) Interlaboratory reliability of the Hall–Van de Castle character scale. *Psychophysiology* **6**: 248.

Sandler, L., Kramer, M., Trinder, J. & Fishbein, H. (1970) Interlaboratory reliability of the Hall–Van de Castle characters, social interactions, activities, and emotions scales. *Psychophysiology* **7**: 333.

Solms, M. (2003) Dreaming and REM sleep are controlled by different mechanisms. In *Sleep and Dreaming: Scientific Advances and Reconsiderations,* eds. E. F. Pace-Schott, M. Blagrove & M. Harnad. Cambridge: Cambridge University Press, pp. 51–8.

Strauss, M. B. (1968) *Familiar Medical Quotations*, 1st edn. Boston: Little.

Ullman, M. (1969a) Discussion of Bonime, W. A culturist view. In *Dream Psychology and the New Biology of Dreaming*, ed. M. Kramer. Springfield, IL: Charles C. Thomas, pp. 199–211.

Ullman, M. (1969b) Dreaming as metaphor in motion. *Arch Gen Psychiatry* **21**(6): 696–703.

Verdone, P. (1965) Temporal reference of manifest dream content. *Percept Mot Skills* **20**: suppl:1253–68.

Winget, C., Kramer, M. & Whitman, R. M. (1972) Dreams and demography. *Can Psychiatr Assoc J*, **17**(2): suppl 2: SS203.

Winget, C. & Kramer, M. (1979) *Dimensions of Dreams.* Gainesville: University Presses of Florida.

The ontogeny and function(s) of REM sleep

Marcos G. Frank

Summary

In the decade immediately following the discovery of REM sleep (Aserinsky and Kleitman, 1953), scientists in the United States and in Europe made a second, striking observation (Jouvet-Mounier *et al.*, 1970; Roffwarg *et al.*, 1966; Valatx *et al.*, 1964). In several mammalian species, including humans, REM sleep amounts were two to three times higher in infancy than in adulthood, and then declined dramatically across development. This basic ontogenetic pattern has now been observed in a wide variety of mammals (Davis *et al.*, 1999; Thurber *et al.*, 2008; Walker and Berger, 1980) and suggests that REM sleep may play a crucial role in brain development. In this chapter, I review the evidence in support of this general hypothesis. I begin with an overview of several landmark events in the ontogenesis of sleep and sleep regulation to provide context to the more function-based discussions that follow. I then discuss the results of several studies that provide indirect or suggestive evidence of a role for REM sleep in general brain maturation. This is followed by a review of findings in the developing visual system that more specifically address a possible role for REM sleep in brain development and plasticity.

Ontogenesis of mammalian sleep and sleep regulation

The ontogenesis of mammalian sleep can be broadly divided into three general stages, here referred to as the "dissociation", "concordance," and "maturation" stages (reviewed in Davis *et al.*, 1999). The dissociation stage of sleep ontogeny is characterized by the absence of clear polysomnographic features of REM and non-REM (NREM) sleep. The concordance stage represents the period of time when distinct, immature forms of REM and NREM sleep are first detected. The further

maturation of these immature sleep states and the emergence of regulatory sleep mechanisms occurs in the third developmental stage (Davis *et al.*, 1999).

Dissociation

Recordings of electrographic and autonomic activities in very young, developing mammals do not reveal clear signs of REM and NREM sleep, reflecting the extreme immaturity of the nervous system at this time (reviewed in Davis *et al.*, 1999; Frank and Heller, 2003). Although distinct couplings of autonomic and brain activities typical of adult sleep are not observed, independent oscillations in these systems can occur. In precocial species, such as the guinea pig, dissociation is present in the fetal period. In altricial species, which complete a larger portion of their neural development ex utero, this stage appears to extend into the postnatal period (Davis *et al.*, 1999; Frank and Heller, 2003).

Concordance

During the concordance stage of sleep ontogeny, independent oscillations in autonomic function and brain activity begin to coalesce into discrete episodes that appear to be immature forms of REM and NREM sleep. In precocial species and humans, this concordance begins in utero, whereas in altricial species this begins ex utero. The precise timing of this event in altricial species is not known, with some investigators reporting the presence of pre-EEG "precursor" states several days before the appearance of EEG-defined vigilance states, which in the rat typically occurs near or at the beginning of the second postnatal week (Frank and Heller, 2003).

The nature of these putative precursor states is controversial (Blumberg *et al.*, 2005; Frank and Heller, 2005). As discussed by Frank and Heller (2003), this

REM Sleep: Regulation and Function, eds. Birendra N. Mallick, S. R. Pandi-Perumal, Robert W. McCarley, and Adrian R. Morrison. Published by Cambridge University Press. © Cambridge University Press 2011.

"pre-EEG" sleep condition may be closely related to the spontaneous cyclic activity typical of the immature nervous system. Adult forms of REM and NREM sleep appear approximately at ages when distinct EEG states are first detected (or roughly in the second postnatal week for altricial species like rodents). This position is supported by numerous findings from studies that span the last forty years (Frank and Heller, 2003). According to others, however, the precursor states known as "active sleep" and "quiet sleep" *are* adult forms of REM and NREM sleep that merely lack state-specific EEGs (Blumberg *et al.*, 2005).

While a detailed treatment of this controversy is beyond the scope of this chapter, a few points should be made. Many of the recent studies cited by the proponents of this latter theory are difficult to interpret. For example, behavioral and electrophysiological measurements in neonatal rats are typically performed *within one to four hours* of invasive and painful surgical procedures, including incisions of the skin and underlying fascia, craniotomies, electrolytic lesioning or gross transections of the brain, implantation of screw electrodes into the skull, and insertion of hooks into the orbital and nuchal muscles (Blumberg and Lucas, 1994; Karlsson and Blumberg, 2002, 2005; Karlsson *et al.*, 2005b, 2004). In contrast, four to seven days of post-operative recovery with analgesia is typical for adult animals, and a minimum of 24 hours has been used in other studies of neonatal rats (Frank and Heller, 1997a).

An additional difficulty in interpreting these studies is the use of non-standard analytical techniques such as "state" scoring on millisecond scales. By definition, a behavioral state is a stable constellation of physiological and neurological processes over time. Although the duration of time necessary to score the presence of a state (i.e., epoch length) is somewhat arbitrary, most scientists do not consider that mammalian sleep "states" occur on scales of one second or less. This peculiar method of assigning states can give the appearance of "sleep cycles" that resemble patterns in adults, but it is debatable whether they reflect an actual biological process.

Despite these caveats, the best evidence for a "precursor" REM sleep state from these investigators comes from rats in the second postnatal week (Karlsson *et al.*, 2005a), which is in good agreement with the position of Frank and Heller (2003). It is also interesting that recent lesion studies from this group (Karlsson *et al.*, 2004) confirm earlier reports that destruction of brain-stem areas important in adult REM sleep (reviewed in Frank and Heller, 2003), have no significant effects on pre-EEG REM sleep in the first week of life. This is also consistent with the hypothesis that pre-EEG "sleep" states are not homologous to adult sleep states.

Maturation

In the third stage of sleep ontogeny, the now polysomnographically identified states of REM and NREM sleep rapidly develop and begin to more closely resemble adult forms of sleep. There are rapid increases in the amplitude of the EEG in both NREM and REM sleep, and stereotyped patterns of neuronal activity, such as pontine-geniculate-occipital (PGO) waves in REM sleep are first observed (Davis *et al.*, 1999). In addition, distinct ultradian, homeostatic, and circadian regulatory mechanisms begin to organize sleep into patterns similar to those found in adult mammals. In the rat, homeostatic regulation of NREM sleep is present soon after the appearance of EEG defined states. Sleep deprivation in pre-weanling neonatal rats results in robust compensatory changes in NREM sleep amounts and consolidation, followed, in the fourth postnatal week, by increases in NREM slow-wave activity (Frank *et al.*, 1998).

As is true regarding the appearance of REM sleep in early life, there is some controversy concerning the appearance of REM sleep brain activity and regulation. REM sleep homeostasis – or REM "rebounds" – refers to compensatory increases in REM sleep amounts following total or selective REM sleep deprivation. Blumberg *et al.* (2004) reported that 60-minute sleep deprivation by increasingly intense electric shocks in five-day-old rat pups, resulted in a transient increase in myoclonic twitching (used as an index of putative REM sleep in pre-EEG rats) during the first 30 minutes of recovery. No increases in the amounts of the state itself, however, were reported. On the other hand, two independent laboratories report that REM rebounds are absent in the neonatal rat until approximately the third postnatal week following more gentle forms of selective REM sleep or total sleep deprivation, (Feng *et al.*, 2001; Frank *et al.*, 1998). A similar discrepancy exists for reports of hippocampal theta during neonatal REM sleep, with most investigators finding little to no evidence of theta until approximately the second postnatal week (Frank and Heller, 2003, 2005). Karlsson and Blumberg (2003), however, report adult forms of REM sleep theta in newborn rats; results not replicated by a contemporaneous study (Leinekugel *et al.*, 2002). It is quite difficult to reconcile these conflicting reports, but it seems unlikely that these aspects of REM sleep, if truly present in newborn rats, would subsequently disappear, only to reappear in the third postnatal week.

In addition to the initial absence of regulatory mechanisms and the presence of rudimentary forms of neurophysiologic activity, neonatal sleep during this stage differs from adult sleep in several important ways. Latencies to REM sleep are shortened, and sleep-onset REM periods (SOREMs) are quite frequent (Gramsbergen, 1976; Jouvet-Mounier *et al.*, 1970; McGinty *et al.*, 1977). Sleep is generally more fragmented, possibly reflecting the absence of strong circadian and ultradian mechanisms at these ages (Davis *et al.*, 1999). However, as stated above, the most striking observation is the abundance of REM sleep in early life (Frank and Heller, 1997a; Jouvet-Mounier *et al.*, 1970; Roffwarg *et al.*, 1966). This appears to be a general feature of mammalian development, as it is observed in precocial and altricial placental mammals, marsupials, and phylogenetically "primitive" placental species like the ferret (Frank and Heller, 2003; Thurber *et al.*, 2008). The precise mechanisms governing the initial over-expression and subsequent decline of this state are unknown, but may involve increasing maturation of inhibitory circuits (Garcia-Rill *et al.*, 2008).

REM sleep function in early life

In this section, I review findings from three classes of experiments that provide evidence that REM sleep facilitates brain development. The first are experiments that show associations or correlations between the amount of sleep, or sleep phasic activity, and certain indices of brain development. Mirmiran and colleagues reported that placing juvenile rats in enriched environments resulted in increased brain weight and increased amounts of REM sleep (Mirmiran *et al.*, 1982). Similar enhancements of REM sleep are also reported in adult animals during learning tasks, and may be necessary for the consolidation of the learned material (reviewed in Benington and Frank, 2003). Associations were also reported between the frequency of REM sleep and subsequent eye-opening in the rat, suggesting that the former events represent "preparatory" activation of visual motor circuits (Van Someren *et al.*, 1990).

A second class of experiments employs REM sleep deprivation (RSD) in the postnatal period followed

by behavioral/neurological/biochemical assessments in adulthood. Because sleep pressure is very high in developing animals, the majority of these experiments have used pharmacological means of RSD (antidepressant medications, or related REM sleep-inhibiting compounds). Pharmacological RSD in neonatal rats is reported to induce a number of neurochemical and behavioral changes in adult rats, including changes in REM sleep architecture (Corner *et al.*, 1980; Mirmiran *et al.*, 1981, 1983b; Vogel *et al.*, 1990b) circadian rhythms (Dwyer and Rosenwasser, 1998; Klemfuss and Gillin, 1997; Yannielli *et al.*, 1998), anxiety and sexual behavior (Hilakivi and Hilakivi, 1987; Hilakivi and Sinclair, 1986; Hilakivi *et al.*, 1987; Vogel *et al.*, 1990a), alterations in neurotransmission in cholinergic and monoaminergic systems (Henderson *et al.*, 1991; Hilakivi *et al.*, 1987; Prathiba *et al.*, 1998, 2000), and neuronal survival (Morrissey *et al.*, 2004). However, many of the behavioral effects are not uniform across studies (even within the same laboratory) and vary depending on the drug used in a given experiment (File and Tucker, 1983; Frank and Heller, 1997b). The interpretation of these results is further complicated by the fact that the observed deficits may be caused by non-specific teratogenetic effects of these compounds.

There are additional reasons to doubt that REM sleep loss is an important factor in the results following pharmacological RSD. Gentle forms of mechanical RSD do not produce the suite of deficits reported after neonatal clomipramine exposure (Mirmiran *et al.*, 1983a). More vigorous mechanical RSD is reported to produce some effects similar to drug-induced behavioral changes (Feng, 2001), but the technique employed (periodic shaking of the rat pup) replaces one confounding variable (non-specific teratogenicity) with another (neonatal stress). In addition, many deficits reported after neonatal REM sleep deprivation are more easily explained by chronic alterations in monoaminergic function. For example, changes in adult sleep architecture ascribed to pharmacological RSD are only observed following neonatal treatments with agents that alter serotonergic neurotransmission. Postnatal treatment with REM sleep-inhibiting compounds that target different monoamines has no effect on subsequent adult sleep patterns (Frank and Heller, 1997b). Similarly, changes in anxiety and sexual behavior reported after neonatal REM sleep deprivation are more likely due to changes in serotonergic neurotransmission than pharmacological RSD. Agents that reduce serotonin and REM sleep in neonatal rats decrease anxiety and increase sexual behavior in adulthood; effects that are precisely opposite to those reported after neonatal clomipramine administration (Adlard and Smart, 1974; Farabollini *et al.*, 1988; Wilson *et al.*, 1986). Since both compounds decrease REM sleep, but have opposite effects on serotonin levels, it is unlikely that RSD contributes in a significant way to the behavioral changes noted in adult rats following neonatal antidepressant treatment.

More compelling evidence for a role for REM sleep in neural development comes from a study by Lopez *et al.*, who showed that selective REM sleep deprivation in the third postnatal week (in the rat) destabilizes hippocampal long-term potentiation (LTP) and reduces the expression of several markers of synaptic potentiation, including N-methyl-D-aspartic acid (NMDA) receptor subunits and calcium/calmodulin-dependent protein kinase II (CaMKII). In this particular study, REM sleep deprivation was achieved through mechanical means and was not associated with significant elevations in stress hormones (relative to controls) (Lopez *et al.*, 2008).

The third class of experiments uses manipulations of REM sleep or REM sleep phasic activity followed by measurements of the developing visual system. Endogenous activity in retinal and thalamocortical circuits helps establish initial patterns of synaptic circuitry that are elaborated and sculpted by experience during subsequent critical periods of postnatal development (Shatz, 1996; Sur and Leamey, 2001). The initial development of the central visual pathways and their subsequent sculpting by experience occur at ages when sleep amounts are very high, or during dramatic changes in sleep expression (Davis *et al.*, 1999). A role for REM sleep has been examined in the development of two important components of the central visual pathway, the lateral geniculate nucleus (LGN) and primary visual cortex (V1).

REM sleep and LGN development

The role of REM sleep in subcortical development has been examined by studying the effects of RSD (using mechanical techniques), or the elimination of REM sleep PGO waves, on subsequent visual system development. Davenne and Adrien (1984) examined changes in neuronal morphology in the LGN in kittens after lesioning PGO generating centers in the brain stem. Bilateral electrolytic lesions in the rostral pontine tegmentum abolished PGO waves in the neonatal cat, resulting in smaller LGN volumes and reduced LGN soma sizes. These findings were extended in a second study, which showed that PGO wave elimination in kittens produced much slower LGN responses to stimulation of the optic chiasm (compared to sham or unilaterally lesioned control cats), and also more LGN cells with "mixed" ON–OFF responses (as opposed to pure "ON" or "OFF" responses to an annulus of light centered in the receptive field), and fewer X cell responses (relative to ON–OFF responses) (Davenne *et al.*, 1989). These morphological and functional changes in LGN cells are consistent with delayed development in the LGN (Daniels *et al.*, 1978; Williams and Jeffery, 2001) and suggest that REM sleep neuronal activity may be necessary for normal LGN development.

REM sleep and the critical period for visual development: LGN

REM sleep may also be important for the later occurring, critical periods of visual development. The critical period has been traditionally investigated by surgically closing an eye (monocular deprivation, MD), which rapidly alters responsiveness and morphology in both subcortical and cortical neurons (reviewed in Sengpiel *et al.*, 1998; Singer, 1979). Oksenberg *et al.* found that one week of RSD in kittens (using mechanical means) augmented the effects of MD on cell morphology in the binocular segment of the LGN (Oksenberg *et al.*, 1996). Lateral geniculate nucleus cells innervated by the occluded eye were smaller in kittens deprived of REM sleep and vision in one eye, resulting in a greater difference in the size of LGN cells activated by the open and deprived eyes. A comparable increase in LGN cell size disparity was found when MD was combined with brain-stem lesions that remove PGO waves. In this case, LGN cells receiving input from the open eye appeared to increase in size (Shaffery *et al.*, 1999). An additional, somewhat unusual, finding is that RSD combined with MD also reduces cell sizes in the monocular segment of the LGN, which does not depend upon competitive interactions between the two eyes (Shaffery *et al.*, 1998). Work from this laboratory has also shown that RSD for one week reduces immunoreactivity for the calcium binding protein parvalbumin in GABAergic interneurons in the developing LGN (Hogan *et al.*, 2001). These latter findings are particularly interesting since parvalbumin may play a role in certain forms of synaptic plasticity (Caillard *et al.*, 2000). In sum, these results suggest that REM sleep may influence LGN maturation during critical periods of visual system development.

REM sleep and developmentally regulated cortical plasticity

REM sleep has also been reported to play an important role in a developmentally regulated form of long-term potentiation (LTP) (Shaffery *et al.*, 2002). In this type of LTP, high-frequency white-matter stimulation in cortical slices prepared from postnatal (P) day 28 to 30 rats produces synaptic potentiation in cortical layers II/III. This form of LTP decreases with age (P35+), and is not observed in cortical slices from adult rats (Kirkwood *et al.*, 1995). Using a less stressful version of the pedestal technique of RSD ("multiple small-platform"), Shaffery *et al.* (2002) measured the effects of one week of RSD on this form of LTP in rat visual cortex. The authors reported that one week of RSD prolonged the critical period for the developmentally regulated form of LTP (LTP was evoked from slices of visual cortex from RSD rats at ages when this type of LTP is not normally observed, P34–P40). A similar extension of the critical period was not seen in cortical slices from control rats that were left in their nests, or from rats placed on larger platforms (large-platform control) that presumably permitted REM sleep. Conversely, RSD had no effect on a non-developmentally regulated form of LTP evoked by layer IV stimulation. The extension of the critical period by RSD was similar to effects produced by dark rearing, which also prolongs the period of induction of this form of LTP (Shaffery *et al.*, 2002). These findings suggest a maturational delay in visual cortex, and are in general agreement with previous findings from the same group suggesting that RSD impairs normal brain maturation.

On the other hand, the role of REM sleep in developmental cortical plasticity in vivo is unclear. Following MD, visual cortical neurons rapidly shift their response in favor of the open eye. This type of plasticity (known as ocular dominance plasticity) is enhanced by sleep, but this appears to require NREM sleep (Frank *et al.*, 2001). NREM sleep time is positively correlated with cortical plasticity (Frank *et al.*, 2001), while pharmacological suppression of REM sleep by hypnotic agents or via targeted awakenings does not prevent the normal shift in responses towards the open eye (Aton *et al.*, 2009; Seibt *et al.*, 2008). However, these latter studies were not specifically designed to address the role of REM sleep in these

phenomena. Therefore more detailed investigations are needed before any strong conclusions can be made concerning the role of REM sleep in ocular dominance plasticity.

Theories of sleep function in developing animals: the ontogenetic hypothesis

In their now classic study in human infants, Roffwarg and colleagues hypothesized that REM sleep in early infancy provides an important source of endogenous neural activity necessary for brain maturation (Roffwarg *et al.*, 1966). In the more recent formulations of the ontogenetic hypothesis, it is suggested that REM sleep not only promotes normal brain development, but also insulates the brain from "excessive" experience-dependent plasticity (Oksenberg *et al.*, 1996; Roffwarg and Shaffery, 1999). Both functions are thought to be mediated by the PGO waves, or heightened release of acetylcholine during REM sleep.

The ontogenetic hypothesis and its variants (Marks *et al.*, 1995; Mirmiran and Maas, 1999) is intuitively appealing since REM sleep amounts are unusually high in infants, and decrease as the brain develops. It is supported by findings that indicate that REM sleep deprivation (or inhibition of REM sleep phasic activity) can modify morphological and electrophysiological development of the LGN, and developmentally regulated cortical synaptic plasticity *in situ* (see above discussion). The theory that REM sleep offsets waking experience in infants has less direct support, but is suggested by three findings. Firstly, REM sleep PGO waves in adult cats activate all LGN lamina simultaneously, indicating that this activity, in contrast to visual experience, is not eye specific (Marks *et al.*, 1999). If present in developing animals, this could counterbalance the more specific, experience-dependent activation of neural circuitry present in wake. Secondly, in contrast to normal adult mammals, latencies to REM sleep in infants are very short, and sleep-onset REMs (SOREMs) frequently occur (Jouvet-Mounier *et al.*, 1970; McGinty *et al.*, 1977). Thus it is possible that the more frequent entries into REM sleep and SOREMs in neonates interfere with the consolidation of experience-dependent changes in neural circuitry.

Despite the appeal of the ontogenetic hypothesis, several issues remain to be resolved. Prolonged RSD can lead to fragmentation of NREM sleep and reductions in NREM sleep slow-wave activity (Endo *et al.*,

1997); thus, it is not entirely clear if REM sleep loss alone is responsible for the observed effects of RSD. As discussed above, it is possible that sleep in newborns may not be identical or homologous to adult REM sleep (Frank and Heller, 2003), and even when unambiguous periods of REM sleep are observed, the neurophysiological phenomena typical of adult REM sleep (e.g., PGO waves) are not always present. For example, REM sleep PGO waves in the kitten are not reported at ages when REM sleep is maximally expressed (Bowe-Anders *et al.*, 1974). It is also unclear if other aspects of REM sleep, like heightened cholinergic activity, are present in newborn animals. Considering the slow maturation of cholinergic systems (Coyle and Yamamura, 1976; Lee *et al.*, 1990; Ninomiya *et al.*, 2001), and the late appearance of other REM sleep phenomena (Chase, 1971), this seems rather unlikely. Indeed, the majority of studies suggesting a developmental role for REM sleep have been performed at ages when REM sleep has already declined to near adult levels (Hogan *et al.*, 2001; Oksenberg *et al.*, 1996; Shaffery *et al.*, 1998, 1999, 2002). In summary, while there are data to support predictions of the ontogenetic hypothesis, they are presently limited to a narrow developmental period and rely heavily on prolonged periods of RSD.

Conclusion

The abundance of REM sleep during early life raises a number of interesting questions. Are pre-EEG "sleep" states truly homologous to adult forms of REM sleep? The traditional view, recently revived by some investigators (Blumberg *et al.*, 2005), is that REM sleep is largely intact at birth in animals such as the rat. However, if REM sleep is not present at birth, then its ontogenetic pattern of expression may be quite different than what it is commonly believed. Once REM sleep appears, what are the neurobiological mechanisms governing the expression of this state and its subsequent decline across development? Very importantly, is the abundance of REM sleep and its subsequent decline indicative of an important biological function, or are these changes merely epiphenomena? Although the ontogenetic changes in REM sleep coincide with periods of rapid brain maturation and synaptic plasticity – only a handful of studies have attempted direct investigations of the role of REM sleep in these processes. The best experimental support for this view has come from studies in the visual system, where it appears that REM sleep influences developmental processes in the LGN and in the primary visual cortex. In particular, REM sleep deprivation triggers several morphological and electrophysiological changes in the LGN, and modifies cortical plasticity *in situ*. However, despite the forty years since the initial studies of Rofwarg, Jouvet-Mounier, and Valatx, scientists have made only modest progress in answering these fascinating questions.

Acknowledgments

This research was supported by a grant from the National Institutes of Health (NIH EY019022–01).

References

Adlard, B. P. F. & Smart, J. L. (1974) Some aspects of the behavior of young and adult rats treated with p-chlorophenylalanine in infancy. *Dev Psychobiol* 7: 135–44.

Aserinsky, E. & Kleitman, N. (1953) Regularly occurring periods of eye motility and concomitant phenomena during sleep. *Science* **118**: 273–4.

Aton, S. J., Seibt, J., Dumoulin, M. *et al.* (2009) Mechanisms of sleep-dependent consolidation of cortical plasticity. *Neuron* **61**: 454–66.

Benington, J. H. & Frank, M. G. (2003) Cellular and molecular connections between sleep and synaptic plasticity. *Prog Neurobiol* **69**: 77–101.

Blumberg, M. S., Karlsson, K. A., Seelke, A. M. H. *et al.* (2005) The ontogeny of mammalian sleep: a response to Frank and Heller (2003). *J Sleep Res* **14**: 91–8.

Blumberg, M. S. & Lucas, D. E. (1994) Dual mechanisms of twitching during sleep in neonatal rats. *Behav Neurosci* **108**: 1196–202.

Blumberg, M. S., Middlemis-Brown, J. E. & Johnson, E. D. (2004) Sleep homeostasis in infant rats. *Behav Neurosci* **118**: 1253–61.

Bowe-Anders, C., Adrien, J. & Roffwarg, H. P. (1974) Ontogenesis of ponto-geniculo-occipital activity in the lateral geniculate nucleus of the kitten. *Exp Neurology* **43**: 242–60.

Caillard, O., Moreno, H., Schwaller, B. *et al.* (2000) Role of the calcium-binding protein parvalbumin in short-term synaptic plasticity. *PNAS* **97**: 13,372–7.

Chase, M. H. (1971) Brain stem somatic reflex activity in neonatal kittens during sleep and wakefulness. *Physiol Behav* 7: 165–72.

Corner, M. A., Mirmiran, M., Bour, H. L. *et al.* (1980) Does rapid-eye-movement sleep play a role in brain development? *Prog Brain Res* **53**: 347–56.

Coyle, J. T. & Yamamura, H. I. (1976) Neurochemical aspects of the ontogenesis of cholinergic neurons in the rat brain. *Brain Res* **118**: 429–40.

Daniels, J. D., Pettigrew, J. D. & Norman, J. L. (1978) Development of single-neuron responses in kitten's lateral geniculate nucleus. *J Neurophysiol* **41**: 1373–93.

Davenne, D. & Adrien, J. (1984) Suppression of PGO waves in the kitten: anatomical effects on the lateral geniculate nucleus. *Neurosci Lett* **45**: 33–8.

Davenne, D., Fregnac, Y., Imbert, M. *et al.* (1989) Lesion of the PGO pathways in the kitten. II. Impairment of physiological and morphological maturation of the lateral geniculate nucleus. *Brain Res* **485**: 267–77.

Davis, F. C., Frank, M. G. & Heller, H. C. (1999) Ontogeny of sleep and circadian rhythms. In *Regulation of Sleep and Circadian Rhythms*, eds. P. C Zee & F W Turek. New York: Marcel Dekker, Inc., pp. 19–80.

Dwyer, S. M. & Rosenwasser, A. M. (1998) Neonatal clomipramine treatment, alcohol intake and circadian rhythms in rats. *Psychopharmacol* **138**: 176–83.

Endo, T., Schwierin, B., Borbely, A. A. *et al.* (1997) Selective and total sleep deprivation: effect on the sleep EEG in the rat. *Psychiatry Res* **66**: 97–110.

Farabollini, F., Hole, D. R. & Wilson, C. A. (1988) Behavioral effects in adulthood of serotonin depletion by p-chorophenylalanine given neonatally to male rats. *Int J Neurosci* **41**: 187–99.

Feng, P. (2001) Postnatal REM sleep deprivation and depression: new findings and hypothesis. *Actas de Fisiologica* **7**: 141.

Feng, P., Ma, Y. & Vogel, G. W. (2001) Ontogeny of REM rebound in postnatal rats. *Sleep* **24**: 645–53.

File, S. E. & Tucker, J. C. (1983) Neonatal clomipramine treatment in the rat does not affect social, sexual and exploratory behaviors in adulthood. *Neurobehav Toxicol Teratol* **5**: 3–8.

Frank, M. G. & Heller, H. C. (1997a) Development of REM and slow wave sleep in the rat. *Am J Physiol* **272**: R1792–9.

Frank, M. G. & Heller, H. C. (1997b) Neonatal treatments with the serotonin uptake inhibitors clomipramine and zimelidine, but not the noradrenaline uptake inhibitor desipramine, disrupt sleep patterns in adult rats. *Brain Res* **768**: 287–93.

Frank, M. G. & Heller, H. C. (2003) The ontogeny of mammalian sleep: a reappraisal of alternative hypotheses. *J Sleep Res* **12**: 25–34.

Frank, M. G. & Heller, H. (2005) Unresolved issues in sleep ontogeny: a response to Blumberg *et al. J Sleep Res* **14**: 98–101.

Frank, M. G., Issa, N. P. & Stryker, M. P. (2001) Sleep enhances plasticity in the developing visual cortex. *Neuron* **30**: 275–87.

Frank, M. G., Morrissette, R. & Heller, H. C. (1998) Effects of sleep deprivation in neonatal rats. *Am J Physiol* **275**: R148–57.

Garcia-Rill, E., Charlesworth, A., Heister, D. *et al.* (2008) The developmental decrease in REM sleep: the role of transmitters and electrical coupling. *Sleep* **31**: 673–90.

Gramsbergen, A. (1976) The development of the EEG in the rat. *Dev Psychobiol* **9**: 501–15.

Henderson, M. G., McConnaughey, M. M. & McMillen, B. A. (1991) Long-term consequences of prenatal exposure to cocaine or related drugs: effects on rat brain monoaminergic receptors. *Brain Res Bull* **26**: 941–5.

Hilakivi, L. A. & Hilakivi, I. (1987) Increased adult behavioral 'despair' in rats neonatally exposed to desipramine or zimeldine: an animal model of depression? *Pharmacol Biochem Behav* **28**: 367–9.

Hilakivi, L. A., Hilakivi, I., Ahtee, L. *et al.* (1987) Effect of neonatal nomifensine exposure on adult behavior and brain monoamines in rats. *J Neural Transm* **70**: 99–116.

Hilakivi, L. & Sinclair, J. D. (1986) Effect of neonatal clomipramine treatment on adult alcohol drinking in the AA and ANA rat lines. *Pharmacol Biochem Behav* **24**: 1451–5.

Hogan, D., Roffwarg, H. P. & Shaffery, J. P. (2001) The effects of 1 week of REM sleep deprivation on parvalbumin and calbindin immunoreactive neurons in central visual pathways of kittens. *J Sleep Res* **10**: 285–96.

Jouvet-Mounier, D., Astic, L. & Lacote, D. (1970) Ontogenesis of the states of sleep in rat, cat and guinea pig during the first postnatal month. *Dev Psychobiol* **2**: 216–39.

Karlsson, K. A. & Blumberg, M. S. (2002) The union of the state: myoclonic twitching is coupled with nuchal muscle atonia in infant rats. *Behav Neurosci* **116**: 912–17.

Karlsson, K. A. & Blumberg, M. S. (2003) Hippocampal theta in the newborn rat is revealed under conditions that promote REM sleep. *J Neurosci* **23**: 1114–18.

Karlsson, K. A. & Blumberg, M. S. (2005) Active medullary control of atonia in week-old rats. *Neuroscience* **130**: 275–83.

Karlsson, K., Elig, A., Gall, A. J. *et al.* (2005a) The neural substrates of infant sleep in rats. *PLoS Biology* **3**: e143.

Karlsson, K. A., Gall, A. J., Mohns, E. J. *et al.* (2005b) The neural substrates of infant sleep in rats. *PLoS Biol* **3**: e143.

Karlsson, K. A., Kreider, J. C. & Blumberg, M. S. (2004) Hypothalamic contribution to sleep–wake cycle development. *Neuroscience* **123**: 575–82.

Kirkwood, A., Lee, H. K. & Bear, M. F. (1995) Co-regulation of long-term potentiation and experience-dependent synaptic plasticity in visual cortex. *Nature* **375**: 328–31.

Klemfuss, H. & Gillin, C. J. (1997) Neonatal scopolamine or antidepressant treatment: effect on development of hamster circadian rhythms. *Pharmacol Biochem Behav* **59**: 369–73.

Lee, W., Nicklaus, K. J., Manning, D. R. *et al.* (1990) Ontogeny of cortical muscarinic receptor subtypes and muscarinic receptor-mediated responses in rat. *J Pharmacol Exp Ther* **252**: 284–490.

Leinekugel, X., Khazipov, R., Cannon, R. *et al.* (2002) Correlated bursts of activity in the neonatal hippocampus in vivo. *Science* **296**: 2049–52.

Lopez, J., Roffwarg, H. P., Dreher, A. *et al.* (2008) Rapid eye movement sleep deprivation decreases long-term potentiation stability and affects some glutamatergic signaling proteins during hippocampal development. *Neuroscience* **153**: 44–53.

Marks, G. A., Roffwarg, H. P. & Shaffery, J. P. (1999) Neuronal activity in the lateral geniculate nucleus associated with ponto-geniculate-occipital waves lacks lamina specificity. *Brain Res* **815**: 21–8.

Marks, G. A., Shaffery, J. P., Oksenberg, A. *et al.* (1995) A functional role for REM sleep in brain maturation. *Behav Brain Res* **69**: 1–11.

McGinty, R. J., Stevenson, M., Hoppenbrouwers, T. *et al.* (1977) Polygraphic studies of kitten development: sleep state patterns. *Dev Psychobiol* **10**: 455–69.

Mirmiran, M. & Maas, Y. G. H. (1999) The function of fetal/neonatal REM sleep. In *Rapid Eye Movement Sleep*, eds. B. N. Mallick & S. Inoue. New Delhi: Narosa Publishing House, pp. 326–35.

Mirmiran, M., Scholtens, J., van de Poll, N. E. *et al.* (1983a) Effects of experimental suppression of active (REM) sleep during early development upon adult brain and behavior in the rat. *Brain Res* **283**: 277–86.

Mirmiran, M., Uylings, H. B. & Corner, M. A. (1983b) Pharmacological suppression of REM sleep prior to weaning counteracts the effectiveness of subsequent environmental enrichment on cortical growth in rats. *Brain Res* **283**: 102–5.

Mirmiran, M., van de Poll, N. E., Corner, M. A. *et al.* (1981) Suppression of active sleep by chronic treatment with chlorimipramine during early postnatal development: effects upon adult sleep and behavior in the rat. *Brain Res* **204**: 129–46.

Mirmiran, M., van den Dungen, H. & Uylings, H. B. (1982) Sleep patterns during rearing under different environmental conditions in juvenile rats. *Brain Res* **233**: 287–98.

Morrissey, M. J., Duntley, S. P., Anch, A. M. *et al.* (2004) Active sleep and its role in the prevention of apoptosis in the developing brain. *Med Hypotheses* **62**: 876–9.

Ninomiya, Y., Koyama, Y. & Kayama, Y. (2001) Postnatal development of choline acetyltransferase activity in the rat laterodorsal tegmental nucleus. *Neurosci Lett* **308**: 138–40.

Oksenberg, A., Shaffery, J. P., Marks, G. A. *et al.* (1996) Rapid eye movement sleep deprivation in kittens amplifies LGN cell-size disparity induced by monocular deprivation. *Dev Brain Res* **97**: 51–61.

Prathiba, J., Kumar, K. B. & Karanth, K. S. (1998) Hyperactivity of hypothalamic pituitary axis in neonatal clomipramine model of depression. *J Neural Transm* **105**: 1335–9.

Prathiba, J., Kumar, K. B. & Karanth, K. S. (2000) Effects of REM sleep deprivation on cholinergic receptor sensitivity and passive avoidance behavior in clomipramine model of depression. *Brain Res* **867**: 243–5.

Roffwarg, H. P., Muzio, J. N. & Dement, W. C. (1966) Ontogenetic development of the human sleep–dream cycle. *Science* **152**: 604–19.

Roffwarg, H. P. & Shaffery, J. P. (1999) The ontogenetic hypothesis of REM sleep function: its history, current status and prospects for confirmation. *Sleep Research Online* **2**: 714–15.

Seibt, J., Aton, S., Jha, S. K. *et al.* (2008) The non-benzodiazepine hypnotic Zolpidem impairs sleep-dependent cortical plasticity. *Sleep* **31**: 1381–92.

Sengpiel, F., Godecke, I., Stawinski, P. *et al.* (1998) Intrinsic and environmental factors in the development of functional maps in cat visual cortex. *Neuropharmacology* **37**: 607–21.

Shaffery, J. P., Oksenberg, A., Marks, G. A. *et al.* (1998) REM sleep deprivation in monocularly occluded kittens reduces the size of cells in LGN monocular segment. *Sleep* **21**: 837–945.

Shaffery, J. P., Roffwarg, H. P., Speciale, S. G. *et al.* (1999) Ponto-geniculo-occipital wave suppression amplifies lateral geniculate nucleus cell-size changes in monocularly deprived kittens. *Dev Brain Res* **114**: 109–19.

Shaffery, J. P., Sinton, C. M., Bissette, G. *et al.* (2002) Rapid eye movement sleep deprivation modifies expression of long-term potentiation in visual cortex of immature rats. *Neuroscience* **110**: 431–43.

Shatz, C. J. (1996) Emergence of order in visual system development. *PNAS* **93**: 602–8.

Singer. W. (1979) Neuronal mechanisms in experience dependent modification of visual cortex function. In *Development and Chemical Sensitivity of Neurons*, vol. 31. eds. M. Cuenod, G. W. Kreutzberg & F. E. Bloom.

Amsterdam: Elsevier/North-Holland Biomedical Press, pp. 457–77.

Sur, M. & Leamey, C. A. (2001) Development and plasticity of cortical areas and networks. *Nat Rev Neurosci* **2**: 251–62.

Thurber, A., Jha, S. K., Coleman, T. *et al.* (2008) A preliminary study of sleep ontogenesis in the ferret (*Mustela putorius furo*) *Behav Brain Res* **189**: 41–51.

Valatx, J. L., Jouvet, D. & Jouvet, M. (1964) Evolution Electroencephalographique des differents etats de sommeil chez le chaton. *Electroencephalogr Clin Neurophysiol* **17**: 218–33.

Van Someren, E. J., Mirmiran, M., Bos, N. P. *et al.* (1990) Quantitative analysis of eye movements during REM-sleep in developing rats. *Dev Psychobiol* **23**: 55–61.

Vogel, G., Neill, D., Hagler, M. *et al.* (1990a) A new animal model of endogenous depression: a summary of present findings. *Neurosci Biobehav Rev* **14**: 85–91.

Vogel, G., Neill, D., Kors, D. *et al.* (1990b) REM sleep abnormalities in a new animal model of endogenous depression. *Neurosci Biobehav Rev* **14**: 77–83.

Walker, J. M. & Berger, R J. (1980) The ontogenesis of sleep states, thermogenesis, and thermoregulation in the Virginia opossum. *Dev Psychobiol* **13**: 443–54.

Williams, A. L. & Jeffery, G. (2001) Growth dynamics of the developing lateral geniculate nucleus. *J Comp Neurol* **430**: 332–42.

Wilson, C. A., Pearson, J. R., Hunter, A. J. *et al.* (1986) The effect of neonatal manipulation of hypothalamic serotonin levels on sexual activity in the adult rat. *Pharmacol Biochem Behav* **24**: 1175–83.

Yannielli, P. C., Cutrera, R. A., Cardinali, D. P. *et al.* (1998) Neonatal clomipramine treatment of Syrian hamsters: effect on the circadian system. *Eur J Pharmacol* **349**: 143–50.

Chapter 7

Evolutionary perspectives on the function of REM sleep

Niels C. Rattenborg, John A. Lesku, and Dolores Martinez-Gonzalez

Summary

In most mammals, sleep is composed of two distinct states, rapid eye movement (REM) sleep and slow-wave sleep (SWS). The differentiated nature of mammalian sleep suggests that each state performs a different function, or perhaps different, but complementary components of a unified function. Despite extensive research, the function(s) provided by sleep and its respective sub-states remains the subject of debate (Cirelli and Tononi, 2008; Mignot, 2008; Siegel, 2009; Stickgold and Walker, 2007). One approach to unraveling the function of each sleep state is to trace its evolution. Through identifying the type(s) of animals in which each state evolved, we may reveal biological traits that coevolved with a particular sleep state. Cases of convergent evolution may be particularly informative because they provide the opportunity to isolate traits shared by only those animals that evolved a particular sleep state. The independent coevolution of certain sleep states and traits may be functionally linked. Conversely, the subsequent coevolutionary loss of a particular sleep state and certain traits may also reveal traits that benefit from a particular sleep state. Moreover, assuming that sleep serves an important function, determining how such animals compensate for the loss of a particular sleep state may yield clues to its purpose. Finally, another approach is to identify biological traits that account for the variation in time spent in, and presumably need for, each state. Traits that influence the allocation of time to a particular state may suggest a function for that state. The following chapter summarizes insights into the function of REM sleep gleaned from these comparative approaches.

Phenomenology and evolutionary history of REM sleep

Therian mammals (marsupials and eutherians)

The class Mammalia is composed of three extant groups, monotremes, marsupials, and eutherians (placentals). The electrophysiological and physiological traits that occur during REM sleep, as we know it in therian (marsupial and eutherian) mammals, are typically used as criteria for determining whether other animals exhibit a similar state. Traditional measures of sleep, such as the electroencephalogram (EEG), electromyogram (EMG), and electrooculogram (EOG), have been studied in a diverse range of mammalian species, whereas traits that require more invasive methods, such as deep brain recordings, have only been examined in a few species (Siegel, 2011). In therian mammals, perhaps the defining feature of REM sleep is cortical activation (low-amplitude, high-frequency EEG activity similar to that occurring during wakefulness) occurring in an animal with elevated arousal thresholds (i.e., the paradox that gave REM sleep its other name, paradoxical sleep). In addition to cortical activation, skeletomuscle tone is greatly reduced or absent throughout most REM sleep, although such periods of tonic REM sleep are briefly interrupted by periods of phasic REM sleep characterized by rapid eye movements, twitching of the limbs and whiskers, chewing motions, and irregularities in respiratory and heart rates. In eutherian mammals, rapid eye movements occur in response to spikes of neuronal activity that propagate from the pons through the lateral

REM Sleep: Regulation and Function, eds. Birendra N. Mallick, S. R. Pandi-Perumal, Robert W. McCarley, and Adrian R. Morrison. Published by Cambridge University Press. © Cambridge University Press 2011.

geniculate nucleus of the thalamus to the occipital cortex (i.e., ponto-geniculo-occipital (PGO) spikes). The phasic events occurring during REM sleep are also associated with bursts of fast, irregular neuronal activity in the brain stem. In addition to these electrophysiological events, a hippocampal theta rhythm, similar to that occurring during ambulation while awake, also occurs during REM sleep. REM sleep is associated with penile erections in most eutherian mammals, but not armadillos (*Chaetophractus villosus*), where erections occur during SWS, a difference that apparently reflects alternative erectile mechanisms (vascular vs. muscular in eutherians and armadillos, respectively), rather than differences in REM sleep, per se (Affanni *et al.*, 2001). During REM sleep, brain temperature increases and thermoregulation is suppressed or depressed (Parmeggiani, 2003). The duration of REM sleep episodes and total amount of REM sleep increases across the major sleep period. The time spent in REM sleep increases following sleep deprivation, indicating that as with SWS, REM sleep is homeostatically regulated (Tobler, 2011). Although some studies have found large amounts of REM sleep in South American marsupials, preliminary data from Australasian marsupials suggest that REM sleep is not prevalent in all marsupials (Lesku *et al.*, 2006). Consequently, it is unclear whether the common ancestor to therian mammals engaged in disproportionately large amounts of REM sleep.

Monotremes

The presence of REM sleep with cortical activation in most therian mammals studied (see section on Evolutionary loss of REM sleep, below), suggested that it evolved before the appearance of marsupial and eutherian mammals. To further clarify the origin of REM sleep, Allison *et al.* (1972) examined sleep in the short-beaked echidna (*Tachyglossus aculeatus*), one of the few remaining species of monotremes. Monotremes are the extant representatives of Prototheria, a group of egg-laying mammals that diverged early from the mammalian lineage, before the therian lineage diverged into marsupial and eutherian mammals. If REM sleep, as we know it in therian mammals, was present in the ancestor to all mammals, then monotremes should show a similar state. Interestingly, while Allison *et al.* identified clear EEG signs of SWS, no unequivocal signs of REM sleep could be found despite using a combination of epidurally seated EEG electrodes over the frontal, parietal, and occipital cortex; depth electrodes

in the pyriform cortex and dorsal hippocampus; and EOG, EMG, and EKG, as well as brain temperature measured from the frontal cortex. Allison *et al.* carefully examined a state that bore some gross resemblance to REM sleep (i.e., quiescent periods with EEG activation), but concluded that it reflected quiet wakefulness instead; skeletomuscular twitches, eye movements, hippocampal theta rhythm, increased arousal thresholds, elevated brain temperature, and variability in cardiorespiratory rates were not present during the REM sleep-like state, as would be expected if the state reflected therian mammal-like REM sleep. Moreover, selective deprivation of this state in one echidna for 48 hours failed to induce a compensatory increase in this state during recovery, as expected if it reflected a homeostatically regulated state comparable to REM sleep in eutherian mammals. Collectively, these results indicated that the REM sleep-like state was more akin to quiet wakefulness than to REM sleep. Albeit limited to a single species, the absence of REM sleep in the echidna tentatively suggested that REM sleep evolved only after the appearance of the therian lineage.

A subsequent investigation into the evolution of REM sleep reexamined EEG-defined sleep in the echidna (Siegel *et al.*, 1996). Importantly, however, in addition to epidurally seated cortical electrodes, Siegel *et al.* recorded neuronal unit activity from the pontine tegmentum – an area involved in the initiation of REM sleep in eutherian mammals – and the midbrain reticular formation. Consistent with the findings of Allison *et al.* (1972), Siegel *et al.* found only EEG signs of SWS in sleeping echidnas. However, concurrent with cortical SWS, brain-stem neurons fired in an irregular REM sleep-like pattern with a rate intermediate between the slow, regular rate observed in SWS and the fast, irregular rate observed during REM sleep with cortical activation in cats and dogs (Figure 7.1*a, b*). Sleep data from another species of monotreme – the duck-billed platypus (*Ornithorhynchus anatinus*) – yielded consistent results. As in the echidna, the cortex of sleeping platypuses only showed EEG activity indicative of SWS (Siegel *et al.*, 1999). Cortical SWS was frequently accompanied by bursts of rapid eye movements and twitching of the bill and head, similar to the phasic skeletomuscular activity observed in therian mammals during REM sleep (see www.semel.ucla.edu/ sleepresearch). Although brain-stem neuronal activity was not examined directly, this behavior suggests that the platypus brain stem was in an REM sleep-like state. Thus, as in the echidna, the platypus apparently

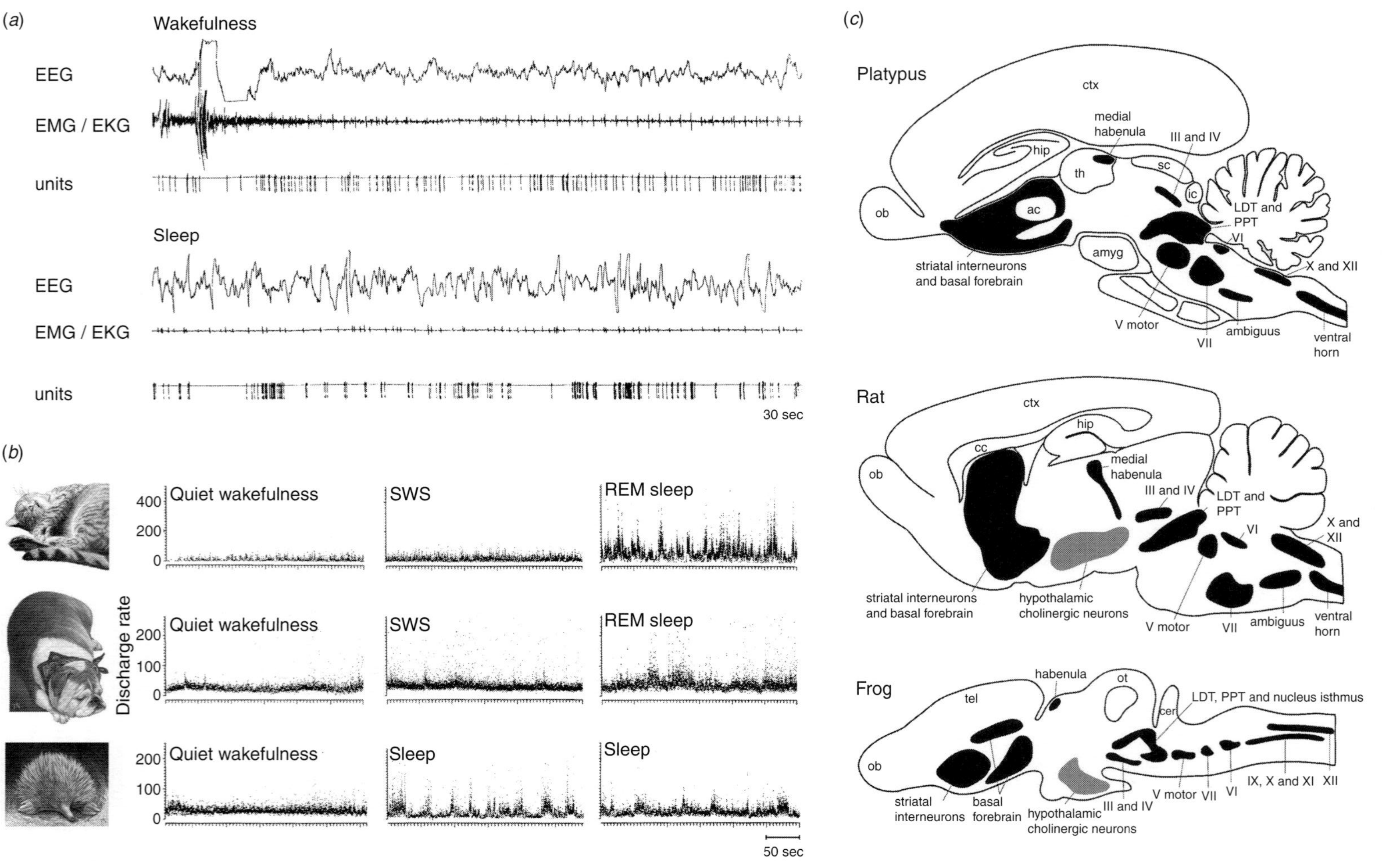

Figure 7.1 The electrophysiological and neuroanatomical correlates of sleep in monotremes. (*a*) Sleep in the echidna is associated with electroencephalogram (EEG) activity characteristic of slow-wave sleep (SWS) occurring concurrently with irregular brain-stem unit activity. (*b*) The rate of brain-stem unit activity observed in sleeping echidnas (bottom) is intermediate between the slow, regular rate observed during SWS and the fast, irregular rate observed during rapid eye movement (REM) sleep in dogs (middle) and cats (top). (*a*) and (*b*) From Siegel *et al.* (1996). (*c*) Cholinergic neuronal groups (shaded in black and gray) in the platypus, rat, and frog. The presence of cortical SWS occurring concurrently with REM sleep-like brain-stem activity in the echidna, and a similar state in the platypus, may reflect the absence of a cholinergic neuronal group in the hypothalamus of monotremes. The presence of this neuronal group in all other tetrapods examined (e.g., depicted in gray for the rat and frog), suggests that monotremes lost this trait, in which case the unique features of sleep in monotremes may reflect a derived trait, rather than the sleep state present in the common ancestor to all mammals. Abbreviations: ac (anterior commissure), amyg (amygdala), cc (corpus callosum), cer (cerebellum), ctx (cortex), EKG (electrocardiogram), EMG (electromyogram), hip (hippocampus), ic (inferior colliculus), LDT (lateral dorsal tegmental nucleus), ob (olfactory bulb), ot (optic tectum), PPT (pedunculopontine tegmentum), sc (superior colliculus), tel (telencephalon), th (thalamus). Cranial nerve nuclei are denoted with their respective Roman numerals. (*c*) From Manger *et al.* (2002). Images of the cat, dog, and echidna are courtesy of Grass-Telefactor, An Astro-Med, Inc. Product Group.

exhibits a heterogeneous sleep state with cortical correlates of SWS occurring concurrently with REM sleep-related brain-stem activity. Moreover, albeit limited by the small number of extant species, the available data suggests that temporally distinct SWS and REM sleep, as seen in therian mammals, evolved from a single, heterogeneous monotreme-like sleep state.

Interestingly, the platypus, or at least its brain stem, may spend a large amount of time in REM sleep. By defining REM sleep as a sleep period with at least one eye movement per minute occurring concurrently with cortical SWS-related EEG activity, Siegel *et al.* (1999) estimated that platypuses spend up to eight hours in REM sleep a day, more than any other animal studied. However, the utility of comparing the time spent in REM sleep based on cortical activation, as seen in therian mammals, to REM sleep estimates derived only from the temporal pattern of twitching in the platypus is unclear. Certainly, based on EEG activity, those same eight hours could be interpreted as SWS. Given that REM sleep-related phasic events are associated with irregular brain-stem activity in placental mammals, perhaps the most accurate way to describe these eight hours is to say that the brain stem (although not recorded directly in platypuses) was in REM sleep, while the cortex was in SWS. Finally, given the absence of direct measures of brain-stem activity, it is conceivable that some of the intervening time between phasic events reflected a SWS state both in the cortex and the brain stem. Indeed, precedent for aspects of REM sleep occurring in short bursts lasting less than ten seconds can be found in birds (see section on Avian reptiles, below). Nonetheless, the results from the echidna and platypus suggest that REM sleep is present, at least at the level of the brain stem, and may have been present in the ancestor to all mammals.

In contrast to the earlier studies (Allison *et al.*, 1972; Siegel *et al.*, 1996), a more recent study of sleep in the echidna reportedly identified REM sleep *with* cortical activation, as seen in therian mammals (Nicol *et al.*, 2000). Because such REM sleep only occurred at temperatures within the thermoneutral zone of echidnas, Nicol *et al.* (2000) argued that unnatural recording temperatures employed in the earlier studies prevented the expression of REM sleep. However, because eye state and arousal thresholds were not determined, it is unclear if the putative REM sleep state reported in Nicol *et al.* (2000) reflected REM sleep or an animal sitting quietly awake, as determined by Allison *et al.* (1972). Furthermore, the notion that REM sleep

with cortical activation was missed in the earlier studies due to the echidnas being housed in temperatures outside their thermoneutral zone is challenged by the absence of REM sleep with cortical activation in platypuses housed in a naturalistic burrow system exposed to natural ambient temperatures (Siegel *et al.*, 1999). Finally, as next discussed, the results from Allison *et al.* and Siegel *et al.* are consistent with recently described neuroanatomical differences between monotreme and therian mammals.

The absence of cortical activation during REM sleep in monotremes suggests that this trait was first acquired in therian mammals. However, an alternative explanation that warrants consideration is the possibility that REM sleep-related cortical activation was present in the common ancestor to all mammals, but monotremes subsequently lost this trait. Although such a scenario may seem speculative, the adaptive loss of genes and associated functions has been a driving force in the evolution of vertebrates, including monotremes (Ordoñez *et al.*, 2008). With regard to sleep, neuroanatomical evidence suggests that monotremes lost a neuronal group involved in REM sleep-related cortical activation in therian mammals. Although the catecholaminergic and serotonergic systems are largely similar in monotreme and eutherian mammals, echidnas and platypuses lack a cholinergic cell group in the hypothalamus (Figure 7.1*c*; Manger *et al.*, 2002). The absence of this neuronal group may create a hiatus in cholinergic transmission between the brain stem and cortex, and thereby explain the unusual phenomenology of sleep in monotremes (Manger *et al.*, 2002). Indeed, a monotreme-like heterogeneous sleep state with REM sleep-like activity in the brain stem occurring concurrently with cortical SWS occurs in cats following lesions in this area (Jouvet, 1962; Siegel, 2011). Interestingly, the absence of this cholinergic group appears to reflect an evolutionary loss in the ancestors to monotremes, because it is present in all other vertebrates examined, including fish, amphibians, reptiles, birds, and eutherian mammals (Manger *et al.*, 2002). Note that this does not necessarily indicate that REM sleep, as we know it in therian mammals, is present in all vertebrate groups; indeed, evidence for REM sleep in fish, amphibians, and non-avian reptiles is equivocal or absent (see section on Fish, amphibians, and non-avian reptiles, below). Rather, the cholinergic hypothalamic group may be necessary, but not sufficient, for generating REM sleep with cortical activation. Fish, amphibians, and non-avian reptiles presumably lack other traits necessary for generating REM sleep. Regardless of whether monotremes lost or never acquired REM sleep-related cortical activation, its apparent absence poses a challenge for functional theories that posit a role for cortical activation in the function of REM sleep.

Fish, amphibians, and non-avian reptiles

Research on sleep in monotremes suggests that aspects of REM sleep evolved prior to the divergence of proto-therian and therian mammals. The following section reviews our current understanding of the evolution of REM sleep (and SWS) in vertebrates through examining sleep in non-avian reptiles, amphibians, and fish. Historically, reptiles were thought to represent the ancestors to mammals. However, Reptilia and Mammalia are actually sister groups forming Amniota that descended from sauropsids and synapsids, respectively (Figure 7.3). Reptilia is composed of Archosauria (crocodilians and birds) and Lepidosauria (lizards and snakes, and tuataras). The relationship between turtles and the rest of Reptilia remains debated, with molecular data supporting their placement as the sister group to Archosauria, and morphological data placing them as either the sister group to Lepidosauria or the sister group to all other reptiles, as historically thought (Lyson and Gilbert, 2009).

The electrophysiological correlates of sleep have been investigated in all reptilian groups with the exception of tuataras. In contrast, few amphibians and fish have been studied (Hartse, 1994). Although REM sleep has been reported in some fish based on the occurrence of eye movements during sleep, it is unclear whether this behavior reflects REM sleep or an unrelated phenomenon. Similarly, while some studies report REM sleep in non-avian reptiles, based on the occurrence of eye and limb movements during sleep, it remains unclear whether such behaviors reflect REM sleep-related twitching similar to that observed in mammals or brief arousals from sleep. Moreover, other researchers failed to detect such behaviors in sleeping reptiles. Notably, Eiland *et al.* (2001) did not observe movements in sleeping turtles or neuronal activity in the brain stem comparable to that observed during sleep in the echidna or REM sleep in eutherian mammals. Perhaps the only electrophysiological feature of sleep in reptiles that bears some gross similarity to mammalian sleep is the intermittent, high-amplitude, sharp-wave often recorded in the EEG of sleeping reptiles (Hartse, 1994).

Rather than reflecting REM sleep-related PGO waves, however, these sharp waves appear to be homologous with the hippocampal sharp waves observed during mammalian SWS (Hartse, 1994; Rattenborg, 2007). Consequently, given the available data, unequivocal evidence for REM sleep in non-avian reptiles is missing. Furthermore, the available evidence suggests that brain-stem correlates of REM sleep evolved in the mammalian lineage prior to the divergence of the prototherian and therian mammals.

Avian reptiles

Although historically considered their own taxonomic group, birds are actually a derived type of reptile that evolved from theropod dinosaurs (Sereno, 1999). Along with their closest living relatives, the crocodilians, birds are the only living members of Archosauria. Interestingly, although birds are clearly perched on a branch of the reptilian phylogenetic tree, avian sleep patterns are more similar to those of their distant therian mammal relatives, than they are to crocodilians or any other group of reptiles. The electrophysiological correlates of sleep have been examined in 12 avian orders including struthioniformes (i.e., ostriches; unpublished data), representatives of the earliest branch of living birds. Although birds lack a truly laminar structure comparable to the mammalian neocortex, the avian pallium – the developmental and functional homologue of the (pallial) neocortex (Jarvis *et al.*, 2005; Medina and Abellán, 2009) – generates EEG activity remarkably similar to that observed in mammals during both wakefulness and sleep (Rattenborg, 2006). As in therian mammals, all birds examined exhibit unequivocal SWS and REM sleep (Figure 7.2), suggesting that both states were present in the common ancestor to modern birds. When compared to wakefulness, the EEG during avian SWS is characterized by high-amplitude, low-frequency activity similar to that observed during mammalian SWS. This pattern is in marked contrast to the EEG pattern observed during sleep in reptiles, which is usually characterized by the absence of high-amplitude, low-frequency EEG activity, and the presence of intermittent, high-amplitude hippocampal sharp waves (Hartse, 1994; Rattenborg, 2007). In addition to the gross similarities in SWS-related EEG activity, recent studies demonstrated that, as in eutherian mammals (Tobler, 2011), SWS is homeostatically regulated in birds (Martinez-Gonzalez *et al.*, 2008), indicating that

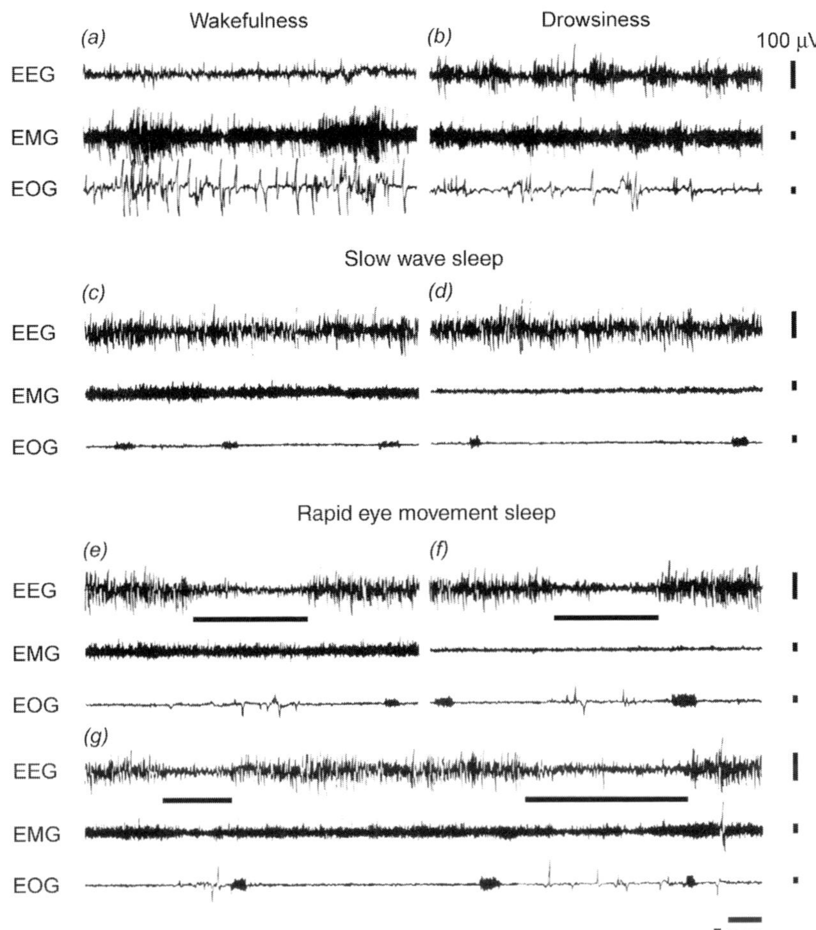

Figure 7.2 Electroencephalogram (EEG), electromyogram (EMG), and electrooculogram (EOG) recordings of wakefulness (*a*), drowsiness (*b*), slow-wave sleep (SWS) (*c–d*), and rapid eye movement (REM) sleep (*e–g*) in an emperor penguin (*Aptenodytes forsteri*). During drowsiness, the EEG alternates rapidly between a pattern typical of wakefulness and that typical of SWS. Slow-wave sleep can occur with high (*c*) or low (*d*) tonic EMG activity. The intermittent increases in EOG amplitude occurring during SWS reflect brief, rapid oscillations of the eyes. Transitions between SWS and REM sleep are shown in (*e–g*); the horizontal black bars mark REM sleep. As with SWS, REM sleep can occur with high (*e*) or low (*f*) tonic EMG activity. In rare cases, however, EMG activity may decrease during episodes of REM sleep (*g*). The states depicted in the penguin are typical of those reported in other bird species. Modified from Buchet *et al.* (1986).

SWS may perform similar functions in homeotherms (Rattenborg *et al.*, 2009).

As in therian mammals, avian REM sleep is characterized by low-amplitude, high-frequency EEG activity similar to that occurring during wakefulness (Figure 7.2). Unlike mammals, however, a hippocampal theta rhythm has not been recorded during avian REM sleep (van Twyver and Allison, 1972). Recordings of brain-stem neuronal activity similar to those performed in the eutherian mammals, echidnas, and turtles, have not been performed in birds. Nonetheless, rapid eye movements and occasional twitching occur during avian REM sleep. The possible equivalent of PGO waves have been reported in the optic tectum in association with rapid eye movements (Sugihara and Gotoh, 1973), although this feature of mammalian REM sleep has not been studied extensively in birds. Although nuchal EMG recordings rarely show reduced amplitude during REM sleep, behavioral signs of reduced tone, including head drooping, are often observed. Interestingly, nuchal hypotonia and atonia are observed in geese only when they support the head on their back (Dewasmes *et al.*, 1985). This suggests that birds actively maintain partial nuchal muscle tone during REM sleep in an attempt to support the head. As in mammals, thermoregulatory responses, such as shivering and feather raising, are reduced during REM sleep when compared to SWS and wakefulness (Heller *et al.*, 1983). Unlike mammals, episodes of REM sleep are short, typically lasting less than ten seconds (e.g., Martinez-Gonzalez *et al.*, 2008). The short duration does not appear to be an adaptation to prevent falling from a perch, because REM sleep episodes are also short in birds that sleep on the ground (Dewasmes *et al.*, 1985). In pigeons (*Columba livia*), the duration of REM sleep episodes and overall time spent in REM sleep increases across the night (Martinez-Gonzalez *et al.*, 2008), a pattern similar to that observed in some mammals. The overall amount of time spent in REM sleep appears to be lower in birds, when compared to mammals (Lesku *et al.*, 2009), although recent studies suggest that songbirds may have more REM sleep than previously recognized (Low *et al.*, 2008; Rattenborg *et al.*, 2004). The time spent in REM sleep increases following 8 and 24 hours of sleep deprivation enforced via gentle handling (Martinez-Gonzalez *et al.*, 2008; Tobler and Borbély, 1988, respectively), and after long-term sleep restriction enforced via the disk-over-water method (Newman *et al.*, 2008). Although pigeons failed to develop the sleep deprivation syndrome observed in rats sleep deprived via the disk-over-water method (Rechtschaffen and Bergmann, 2002), this method was less effective in reducing sleep, particularly REM sleep, in pigeons (Newman *et al.*, 2008). Consequently, it remains unclear whether birds respond to long-term sleep loss in the same manner as rats. Collectively, comparative work in birds indicates that they exhibit sleep states remarkably similar to those in therian mammals. Nonetheless, potentially informative differences include the absence of a hippocampal theta rhythm and the short duration of REM sleep episodes. Functional theories for the evolution of REM sleep that account for these differences between birds and mammals are more likely to explain the core purpose of this state, rather than mammal-specific aspects of REM sleep.

Convergent evolution of REM sleep in mammals and birds

Given the presence of unequivocal REM sleep in birds, and its apparent absence in non-avian reptiles, amphibians, and fish, the most parsimonious evolutionary explanation for the taxonomic distribution of REM sleep is that it evolved independently in birds and mammals (Figure 7.3). Interestingly, SWS also seems to have evolved independently in mammals and birds, although sleep in reptiles, and possibly other vertebrates, may reflect a precursor state that lacks the high-amplitude, low-frequency EEG activity characteristic of SWS (Rattenborg, 2006, 2007). This convergence in sleep states may be interrelated with other trait(s) that among vertebrates are only shared by mammals and birds. Interestingly, in addition to evolving similar sleep states, mammals and birds also independently evolved

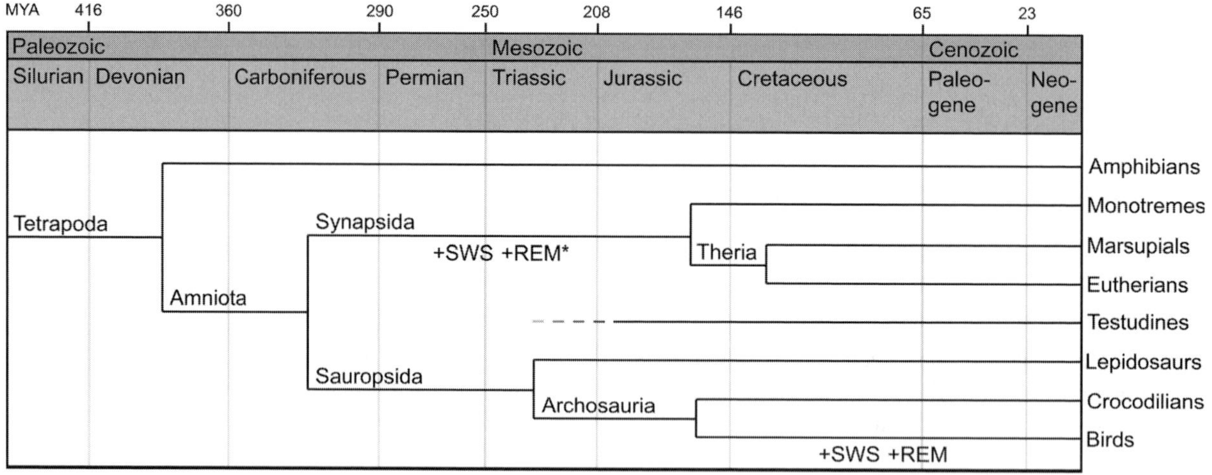

Figure 7.3 A cladogram for tetrapods showing the convergent evolution of rapid eye movement (REM) sleep and slow-wave sleep (SWS) in mammals and birds. The origin of REM sleep and SWS are depicted as +REM and +SWS, respectively. The asterisk after +REM in the mammalian lineage indicates uncertainty over when REM sleep-related cortical activation evolved. Based on evidence for REM sleep-related brain-stem activity in monotremes, this component of REM sleep was probably present in the common ancestor to all mammals. However, the absence of REM sleep-related cortical activation in monotremes suggests that this trait evolved after Prototheria diverged from the mammalian lineage. Alternatively, neuroanatomical data suggest that monotremes may have lost REM sleep-related cortical activation. Based on the presence of high-amplitude, slow waves in the EEG, SWS apparently also originated independently (+SWS) in mammals and birds. Time (millions of years ago, MYA) is given at the top of the plot above geological era (dark gray) and period (light gray). The phylogenetic relationships are well established for all groups except testudines (turtles). As a result, the root of this lineage is not depicted. Lepidosaurs include lizards and snakes, and the tuatara. Estimates of divergence times are from Warren *et al.* (2008).

large (relative to body size), heavily interconnected brains capable of performing complex cognitive processes (Jarvis *et al.*, 2005; Medina and Abellán, 2009). The known taxonomic distribution of REM sleep and SWS is consistent with the notion that both states are involved in maintaining brain function in animals with such brains (Rattenborg, 2006; Rattenborg *et al.*, 2009), although other examples of the coevolution of large, heavily interconnected brains and mammalian-like sleep states would certainly strengthen this argument. Alternatively, REM sleep and SWS might perform conserved sleep functions, but mammals and birds simply differ in the manner in which such states manifest electrophysiologically. The EEG correlates of sleep in mammals and birds could either reflect functionless epiphenomena resulting from large, heavily interconnected brains, or different mechanisms for performing a conserved sleep function. Indeed, genetic work in *Drosophila melanogaster*, suggests that some sleep mechanisms and functions may be highly conserved (Mignot, 2008; Cirelli and Bushey, 2008). Nonetheless, despite the conserved nature of genetic correlates of sleep, the EEG traits, and underlying neurophysiology that characterize sleep and its sub-states in mammals and birds may perform secondarily evolved sleep functions not found in animals lacking REM sleep and SWS (Rattenborg *et al.*, 2009).

Evolutionary loss of REM sleep

Identifying the type of animals in which REM sleep evolved may yield clues to the function of this state through revealing associated traits, such as heavily interconnected brains in mammals and birds. Conversely, the evolutionary loss of REM sleep may also be informative if it occurs concurrent with the loss of other traits. Traits that disappear along with REM sleep may be functionally related to REM sleep, especially if they also coevolved with REM sleep in mammals and birds in the first place. It is also conceivable that animals that lose REM sleep retain traits that depend on REM sleep, but evolve novel mechanisms to compensate for this loss. In this case, revealing the nature of such mechanisms may inform our understanding of REM sleep. Although the evidence remains somewhat equivocal, odontocete cetaceans (dolphins and porpoises) may have lost REM sleep-related cortical activation, a trait thought to be involved in the function of REM sleep in other therian mammals.

Life in an aquatic environment apparently contributed to the evolution of modified forms of SWS and REM sleep in cetaceans (Lyamin *et al.*, 2008). Unlike terrestrial mammals, where SWS occurs simultaneously in both hemispheres, cetaceans primarily engage in unihemispheric SWS (USWS), an unusual state in which one cerebral hemisphere shows EEG activity indicative of SWS while the other shows a waking pattern. During USWS, the eye contralateral to the awake hemisphere is usually open, whereas the eye contralateral to the sleeping hemisphere is usually closed. Cetaceans swim and surface to breathe during USWS, and seem to visually monitor their environment with the open eye during this state. In addition to this specialized form of SWS, REM sleep also seems to have been modified to suit life in an aquatic environment. Most electrophysiological studies of sleep in odontocetes failed to detect unequivocal signs of REM sleep. Although an early study reported a single episode of REM sleep with cortical EEG activation in a pilot whale (*Globicephala scammoni*, an odontocete), subsequent studies were unable to replicate this finding in four other species. Efforts to detect REM sleep were most intense in the bottlenose dolphin, where recordings from both lateral geniculate bodies and hippocampi failed to reveal PGO spikes or a hippocampal theta rhythm, respectively, during wakefulness or sleep. The absence of traditional REM sleep-related traits does not necessarily indicate that cetaceans are completely devoid of an REM sleep-like state. Interestingly, in contrast to studies employing electrophysiological recordings of tethered animals, behavioral studies of untethered captive animals revealed rare head, body, and eye-lid twitching while the animal rested on the bottom of the pool or swam slowly, in both odontocetes and a single young mysticete (balleen) gray whale (*Eschrichtius robustus*). Penile erections have also been observed in sleeping cetaceans. In the Commerson's dolphin (*Cephalorhynchus commersonii*), erections and twitching were temporally associated. Although suggestive of a brief REM sleep-like state, the diagnostic utility of these phenomena is limited by the finding that twitches and penile erections also occur during wakefulness, and twitching can occur during sleep onset and in SWS in terrestrial mammals (Lyamin *et al.*, 2008). Collectively, the electrophysiological and behavioral studies of captive cetaceans suggest that if REM sleep exists in this group, it is greatly reduced when compared to other therian mammals and may occur in a modified manner that does not necessarily include cortical activation.

Manger and colleagues have proposed that these modifications to REM sleep and the almost exclusive reliance on USWS both reflect adaptations aimed at reducing heat loss in an aquatic environment, a significant problem for "warm-blooded" mammals. Unihemispheric SWS allows cetaceans to generate heat via swimming, and the marked reduction or absence of REM sleep prevents the loss of heat that would occur as a result of the immobility and reduced thermoregulation that accompanies REM sleep in terrestrial therian mammals (Lyamin *et al.*, 2008; Manger, 2006). The finding that cetaceans evolved USWS, rather than dispensing with SWS altogether (a more thermogenic alternative than USWS), indicates that SWS must perform an important function, presumably for the cortex itself.

The absence of REM sleep-related cortical activation, or REM sleep altogether, in cetaceans appears to be a derived loss of this trait, because REM sleep has been detected in all other therian mammals studied. Although the potential loss of REM sleep-related cortical activation in cetaceans suggests that it is evolutionarily possible to dispense with this trait under certain ecological circumstances, it does not necessarily challenge the importance of REM sleep in the lives of other mammals. Indeed, the evolutionary preservation of REM sleep with cortical activation in all other therian mammals, despite comparative evidence indicating that REM sleep may be a particularly dangerous state (see below), indicates that it must perform an important function. Otherwise, one would expect the loss of REM sleep to be more common.

Evolutionary determinants of REM sleep duration

A potentially revealing approach to unraveling the functions of REM sleep is to explain why some species spend a great deal of time in REM sleep and others only very little. If we assume that such across-species (or interspecific) variation reflects underlying differences in the need for REM sleep, then identifying the factors responsible for maintaining that variation should provide clues to the function of REM sleep. Although such comparative analyses typically address both REM sleep and SWS, here we only review the more relevant relationships bearing on the functions of REM sleep (see Lesku *et al.*, 2009 for a complete review). Furthermore, our discussion is restricted to recent studies that employed modern phylogenetic comparative methods

to control for pseudoreplication resulting from the inclusion of closely related species with similar sleep traits, a standard in evolutionary biology that only recently has been applied to sleep research (Lesku *et al.*, 2009).

The degree of maturity at birth has consistently been the strongest predictor of the time spent in REM sleep and the allocation of time asleep to REM sleep (or percentage of REM sleep). Altricial species, those that are born largely immobile and rely entirely on their parents for nourishment, warmth, and protection have more REM sleep as adults than more precocial species. This relationship is in agreement with early EEG work by Jouvet-Mounier *et al.* (1970), which shows that the rat and cat, as altricial species, have more REM sleep throughout their life than the precocial guinea pig (Figure 7.4). These findings collectively suggest that REM sleep is important for the early development of the central nervous system (Shaffery *et al.*, 2002), although it is unclear why this difference persists into adulthood (Siegel, 2011).

Increasing evidence indicates that sleep, REM sleep included, is important for memory processing and plasticity (Stickgold and Walker, 2007). What comparative evidence exists to support this hypothesis? If enhancing cognitive performance is a general function of REM sleep across mammals, then one might expect species possessing greater cognitive abilities

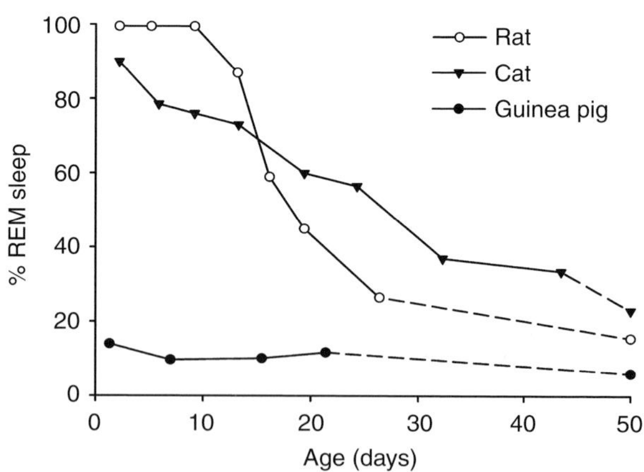

Figure 7.4 Changes in the percentage of total sleep time devoted to rapid eye movement (% REM) sleep across early development in the rat, cat, and guinea pig. In the altricial rat and cat, REM sleep constitutes most of total sleep time and decreases to levels close to that of adults approximately one month after birth. Conversely, % REM sleep in the precocial guinea pig is relatively stable over early ontogeny and into adulthood. Note, however, that even as adults, altricial species have higher %REM sleep than more precocial species. Reprinted Jouvet-Mounier *et al.* (1970).

to engage in more REM sleep. Encephalization is a possible measure of interspecific intelligence as it estimates the degree to which a species' brain is bigger or smaller than that expected for its body size. Encephalization may not be the most precise variable with which to assess interspecific support for sleep-dependent memory consolidation, it is nevertheless readily obtainable for the species for which EEG-based sleep data are available. Although encephalization is not a strong predictor of the time spent in REM sleep, species with greater encephalization allocate a higher percentage of time asleep to REM sleep (Lesku *et al.*, 2006, 2009), as expected if REM sleep is involved in memory processing.

Not all mammals studied were included in the above analyses. Monotremes were excluded because it is unclear how to quantify REM sleep time in animals that exhibit a heterogeneous sleep state with aspects of REM sleep and SWS occurring concurrently (see section on Monotremes, above). Cetaceans were also excluded from these phylogenetic analyses, because it is not clear how to express the time spent asleep in these unihemispherically sleeping animals (see section on Evolutionary loss of REM sleep, above). Nonetheless, they may have bearing on the relationship between encephalization and percentage REM sleep reported above. In addition to engaging primarily in USWS, these animals also apparently lack cortical signs of REM sleep (Lyamin *et al.*, 2008). This apparent loss of REM sleep is surprising as some cetaceans reach a level of encephalization shared by some anthropoid primates (Marino *et al.*, 2008). Thus, if REM sleep is important for information processing, then cetaceans have either found a mechanism other than REM sleep to support their advanced cognition or, as suggested by Manger (2006), cetaceans are not as intelligent as previously thought (but see Marino *et al.*, 2008).

Given the marked reduction or absence of REM sleep in cetaceans, the time spent in REM sleep may be constrained by additional ecological factors, such as the risk of predation. Indeed, species sleeping in more open locations, and more herbivorous species, engage in less REM sleep (both total time and as a percentage of sleep time) relative to their more secure-sleeping and carnivorous counterparts (Lesku *et al.*, 2006), suggesting that REM sleep is a particularly vulnerable sleep state that is selectively reduced when risk is elevated. This comparative result is mirrored in laboratory studies where REM sleep is disproportionately reduced following simulated predatory encounters (Lesku *et al.*, 2008).

Presumably, a trade-off exists between the biological need for REM sleep and ecological factors selecting against REM sleep that accounts for this relationship, as well as the preservation of at least some REM sleep in most mammals.

Although common in other biological disciplines, trade-offs of this sort have not been taken into consideration by sleep researchers. Indeed, much of the variability in sleep times observed in mammals may reflect a combination of species-specific differences in the need for sleep and trade-offs between the benefit and costs of engaging in a particular state. For instance, although two species may have the same biological need for sleep, the cost–benefit ratio of sleeping may differ between the two, resulting in differences in sleep time. Such trade-offs could occur under both evolutionary and ecological time scales, and may vary seasonally within a species in response to changing ecological demands (Rattenborg *et al.*, 2004). Ultimately, it would be informative to determine the short-term costs (e.g., energy expenditure, memory, vigilance, etc.) and potential long-term costs (e.g., longevity, fecundity, etc.) of engaging in more or less of a particular sleep state. The manner in which such trade-offs occur, and their influence on brain function and behavior, may provide insight into the function of sleep. Finally, trade-offs may be best examined in animals living in their natural environment, rather than the laboratory environment (Horne, 2009; Siegel, 2009), a promising approach recently made feasible by the development of techniques for recording sleep in animals living in the ecological context in which sleep evolved (Rattenborg *et al.*, 2008).

Conclusion

Our interpretation of the available research bearing on the evolution of REM sleep is subject to several caveats, and therefore remains tentative. A fundamental caveat of all comparative studies that attempt to trace the evolution of traits that do not fossilize, such as sleep, is that extant representatives of a taxonomic group have undergone millions of years of evolution since their group first appeared, and therefore might not represent the sleep patterns of their ancestors. Other caveats relate to the limited scope of the available data. Many critical points in our understanding are based only on a few species, either because certain taxonomic groups have been poorly studied, or because only a few species are available for study, as is the case in monotremes.

Moreover, certain potentially important defining traits of REM sleep, such as brain-stem activity, have only been examined in a small number of species. As a result, it remains unclear whether these results generalize to an entire taxonomic group. In some cases, the results from the same taxonomic group, or even species, reveal different results, or different interpretations of comparable results. This has been particularly true in fish, amphibians, and non-avian reptiles (Hartse, 1994; Rattenborg, 2007), as well as monotremes. Historically, comparative studies have been based on data obtained from animals sleeping in an unnatural laboratory environment. Given that REM sleep in therian mammals is particularly sensitive to changes in temperature, predation risk, etc., the laboratory environment may influence the amount of time spent in this state, or could even account for reports of its absence in certain taxonomic groups, such as reptiles. Our confidence in concluding that a particular taxonomic group exhibits REM sleep diminishes as fewer therian mammal REM sleep-related traits are identified. This may reflect the simple fact that not all traits exist in a particular taxonomic group and/or that they do not manifest in the same manner, perhaps due to differences in neuroanatomy. Moreover, some traits may exist, but evade detection, either because we are unsure where to look for them or because recording them is technically challenging, as is the case in insects. Some traits that typically occur during REM sleep in therian mammals, such as twitching, may also occur during other sleep states, and therefore are not diagnostic of REM sleep. Conversely, the absence of twitching does not necessarily indicate an absence of REM sleep-related brain-stem activity, as demonstrated in the echidna, where REM sleep-like brain-stem activity occurred in the absence of twitching (Siegel *et al.*, 1996). Finally, our understanding of the evolution of REM sleep also depends on whether a sleep trait is viewed as ancestral or a derived modification of a pre-existing sleep trait. This is particularly problematic in groups thought to represent a pivotal point in evolution. For instance, the lack of cortical activation in monotremes may reflect the sleep state present in the common ancestor to all mammals or a derived modification of REM sleep, as suggested by neuroanatomical data.

Keeping in mind each caveat, the available evidence suggests the following evolutionary scenario for REM sleep. Given the lack of unequivocal evidence for REM sleep in fish, amphibians, and non-avian reptiles, signs of REM sleep first appeared in the common ancestor to monotreme, marsupial, and eutherian mammals. If we assume that the sleep patterns exhibited by extant monotremes have changed little since the monotreme lineage diverged from therian mammals, then the ancestor to all mammals presumably exhibited a heterogeneous sleep state characterized by REM sleep-related activity in the brain stem occurring concurrently with cortical SWS. Alternatively, neuroanatomical data raises the possibility that REM sleep-related cortical activation was present in the common ancestor to all mammals, but monotremes subsequently lost this trait prior to diverging into echidnas and platypuses. Regardless of when REM sleep-related cortical activation evolved, REM sleep-like brain-stem activity was apparently present in the ancestors to all mammals. Furthermore, the absence of REM sleep-like brain-stem activity in a single study of sleeping turtles suggests that this trait evolved after amniotes split into synapsids (the ancestors to mammals) and sauropsids (the ancestors to reptiles, including birds), although more species clearly need to be studied to resolve the evolution of this trait.

The diversification of Mammalia was associated with the evolution of marked interspecific variation in the time spent in REM sleep. Comparative studies have shown that REM sleep in adult mammals is higher in species altricial at birth and those with greater encephalization as adults, both suggesting a neurologically based role for this state. Ecological factors such as the risk of predation during sleep also influenced the amount of REM sleep, with mammals experiencing greater risk engaging in less REM sleep. Nonetheless, despite the inherent risk of predation associated with REM sleep, this state was retained in all, except perhaps one group of, mammals, testament to the biological importance of this state. Only in cetaceans was REM sleep greatly reduced or completely lost, a modification in sleep that along with USWS may be specialized adaptations for life in the sea (Lyamin *et al.*, 2008).

In addition to mammals, REM sleep with EEG activation also evolved in the common ancestor to extant birds. Given the absence of REM sleep in crocodilians, the closest living relatives to birds, as well as other reptiles and amphibians, REM sleep apparently evolved independently in the respective ancestors of birds and mammals. The convergent evolution of REM sleep (and SWS) in mammals and birds suggests that the efficacy of certain biological traits unique to these taxonomic groups depends on these sleep states. For instance, the convergent evolution of similar sleep states may be mechanistically and functionally linked to the associated convergent evolution of large, heavily interconnected brains capable of complex cognition in mammals and birds, although the role of other interrelated traits, such as homeothermy, can not be ruled out (Rattenborg *et al.*, 2009).

Sleep, in general, appears to be a highly conserved trait present in all animals investigated. This suggests that sleep likely serves a basic, perhaps cellular, function in all animals. However, it is also likely that once sleep evolved, other functions became dependent on sleep. The relative importance of such secondarily evolved functions may vary across taxonomic groups. Consequently, our understanding of sleep in humans will be incomplete until we determine both the initial cellular function of sleep and potential secondarily evolved functions associated with the changes in brain activity that characterize SWS and REM sleep. Here, additional comparative work on sleep in vertebrates may be particularly informative. Notably, efforts to determine why only mammals and birds exhibit SWS and REM sleep may reveal overriding principles that might otherwise remain obscure through a strictly mammal-focused research approach.

References

Affanni, J. M., Cervino, C. O. & Marcos, H. J. (2001) Absence of penile erections during paradoxical sleep. Peculiar penile events during wakefulness and slow wave sleep in the armadillo. *J Sleep Res* **10**: 219–28.

Allison, T., van Twyver, H. & Goff, W. R. (1972) Electrophysiological studies of the echidna, *Tachyglossus aculeatus*. I. Waking and sleep. *Arch Ital Biol*, **110**: 145–84.

Buchet, C., Dewasmes, G. & Le Maho, Y. (1986) An electrophysiological and behavioral study of sleep in emperor penguins under natural ambient conditions. *Physiol Behav* **38**: 331–5.

Cirelli, C. & Bushey, D. (2008) Sleep and wakefulness in *Drosophila melanogaster*. *Ann N Y Acad Sci* **1129**: 323–9.

Cirelli, C. & Tononi, G. (2008) Is sleep essential? *PLoS Biology* **6**: e216.

Dewasmes, G., Cohen-Adad, F., Koubi, H. & Le Maho, Y. (1985) Polygraphic and behavioral study of sleep in geese: existence of nuchal atonia during paradoxical sleep. *Physiol Behav* **35**: 67–73.

Eiland, M. M., Lyamin, O. I. & Siegel, J. M. (2001) State-related discharge of neurons in the brainstem of freely moving box turtles, *Terrapene carolina major*. *Arch Ital Biol* **139**: 23–36.

Hartse, K. M. (1994) Sleep in insects and nonmammalian vertebrates. In *Principles and Practice of Sleep Medicine*, 2nd edn. eds. M. H. Kryger, T. Roth & W. C. Dement. Philadelphia: W. B. Saunders, pp. 95–104.

Heller, H. C., Graf, R. & Rautenberg, W. (1983) Circadian and arousal state influences on thermoregulation in the pigeon. *Am J Physiol* **245**: R321–8.

Horne, J. (2009) REM sleep, energy balance and 'optimal foraging'. *Neurosci Biobehav Rev* **33**: 466–74.

Jarvis, E. D., Güntürkün, O., Bruce, L. *et al.* (2005) Avian brains and a new understanding of vertebrate brain evolution. *Nat Rev Neurosci* **6**: 151–9.

Jouvet, M. (1962) Recherches sur les structures nerveuses et les mechanismes responsables des differentes phases du sommeil physiologique. *Arch Ital Biol* **100**: 125–206.

Jouvet-Mounier, D., Astic, L. & Lacote, D. (1970) Ontogenesis of the states of sleep in rat, cat, and guinea pig during the first postnatal month. *Dev Psychobiol* **2**: 216–39.

Lesku, J. A., Roth, T. C., 2nd, Amlaner, C. J. & Lima, S. L. (2006) A phylogenetic analysis of sleep architecture in mammals: the integration of anatomy, physiology, and ecology. *Amer Nat* **168**: 441–53.

Lesku, J. A., Bark, R. J., Martinez-Gonzalez, D. *et al.* (2008) Predator-induced plasticity in sleep architecture in wild-caught Norway rats (*Rattus norvegicus*). *Behavi Brain Res* **189**: 298–305.

Lesku, J. A., Roth, T. C., Rattenborg, N. C., Amlaner, C. J. & Lima, S. L. (2009) History and future of comparative analyses in sleep research. *Neurosci Biobehavi Rev* **33**: 1024–36.

Low, P. S., Shank, S. S., Sejnowski, T. J. & Margoliash, D. (2008) Mammalian-like features of sleep structure in zebra finches. *Proc Nat Acad Sci USA* **105**: 9081–6.

Lyamin, O. I., Manger, P. R., Ridgway, S. H., Mukhametov, L. M. & Siegel, J. M. (2008) Cetacean sleep: an unusual form of mammalian sleep. *Neurosci Biobeh Rev* **32**: 1451–84.

Lyson, T. & Gilbert, S. F. (2009) Turtles all the way down: loggerheads at the root of the chelonian tree. *Evol Dev* **11**:133–5.

Manger, P. R. (2006) An examination of cetacean brain structure with a novel hypothesis correlating thermogenesis to the evolution of a big brain. *Biol Rev* **81**: 293–338.

Manger, P. R., Fahringer, H. M., Pettigrew, J. D. & Siegel, J. M. (2002) The distribution and morphological characteristics of cholinergic cells in the brain of monotremes as revealed by ChAT immunohistochemistry. *Brain Behav Evol* **60**: 275–97.

Marino, L., Butti, C., Connor, R. C. *et al.* (2008) A claim in search of evidence: reply to Manger's thermogenesis hypothesis of cetacean brain structure. *Biol Rev* **83**: 417–40.

Martinez-Gonzalez, D., Lesku, J. A. & Rattenborg, N. C. (2008) Increased EEG spectral power density during sleep following short-term sleep deprivation in pigeons (*Columba livia*): evidence for avian sleep homeostasis. *J Sleep Res* **17**: 140–53.

Medina, L. & Abellán, A. (2009) Development and evolution of the pallium. *Semin Cell Dev Biol* **20**: 698–711.

Mignot, E. (2008) Why we sleep: the temporal organization of recovery. *PLoS Biology* **6**: e106.

Newman, S. M., Paletz, E. M., Rattenborg, N. C., Obermeyer, W. H. & Benca, R. M. (2008) Sleep deprivation in the pigeon (*Columba livia*) using the disk-over-water method. *Physiol Behav* **93**: 50–8.

Nicol, S. C., Andersen, N. A., Phillips, N. H. & Berger, R. J. (2000) The echidna manifests typical characteristics of rapid eye movement sleep. *Neurosci Lett* **283**: 49–52.

Ordoñez, G. R., Hillier, L. W., Warren, W. C. (2008) Loss of genes implicated in gastric function during platypus evolution. *Genome Biol* **9**: R81.

Parmeggiani, P. L. (2003) Thermoregulation and sleep. *Front Biosci* **8**: s557–67.

Rattenborg, N. C. (2006) Evolution of slow-wave sleep and palliopallial connectivity in mammals and birds: a hypothesis. *Brain Res Bull* **69**: 20–9.

Rattenborg, N. C. (2007) Response to commentary on evolution of slow-wave sleep and palliopallial connectivity in mammals and birds: a hypothesis. *Brain Res Bull* **72**: 187–93.

Rattenborg, N. C., Mandt, B. H., Obermeyer, W. H. *et al.* (2004) Migratory sleeplessness in the white-crowned sparrow (*Zonotrichia leucophrys gambelii*). *PLoS Biology* **2**: 924–36.

Rattenborg, N. C., Martinez-Gonzalez, D. & Lesku, J. A. (2009) Avian sleep homeostasis: convergent evolution of complex brains, cognition and sleep functions in mammals and birds. *Neurosci Biobehav Rev* **33**: 253–70.

Rattenborg, N. C., Voirin, B., Vyssotski, A. L. *et al.* (2008) Sleeping outside the box: electroencephalographic measures of sleep in sloths inhabiting a rainforest. *Biol Lett* **4**: 402–5.

Rechtschaffen, A. & Bergmann, B. M. (2002) Sleep deprivation in the rat: an update of the 1989 paper. *Sleep* **25**: 18–24.

Sereno, P. C. (1999) The evolution of dinosaurs. *Science* **284**: 2137–47.

Shaffery, J. P., Sinton, C. M., Bissette, G., Roffwarg, H. P. & Marks, G. A. (2002) Rapid eye movement sleep deprivation modifies expression of long-term potentiation in visual cortex of immature rats. *Neuroscience* **110**:431–43.

Siegel, J. M. (2009) Sleep viewed as a state of adaptive inactivity. *Nat Rev Neurosci*, **10**: 747–53.

Siegel, J. M. (2011) REM sleep. In *Principles and Practice of Sleep Medicine*, 5th edn. eds. M. H. Kryger, T. Roth & W. C. Dement. Philadelphia: W. B. Saunders, pp. 92–111.

Siegel, J. M., Manger, P. R., Nienhuis, R., Fahringer, H. M. & Pettigrew, J. D. (1996) The echidna *Tachyglossus aculeatus* combines REM and non-REM aspects in a single sleep state: implications for the evolution of sleep. *J Neurosci* **16**: 3500–6.

Siegel, J. M., Manger, P. R., Nienhuis, R. *et al.* (1999) Sleep in the platypus. *Neuroscience* **91**:391–400.

Stickgold, R. & Walker, M. P. (2007) Sleep-dependent memory consolidation and reconsolidation. *Sleep Med* **8**: 331–43.

Sugihara, K. & Gotoh, J. (1973) Depth-electroencephalograms of chickens in wakefulness and sleep. *Jpn J Physiol* **23**:371–9.

Tobler, I. (2011) Phylogeny of sleep regulation. In *Principles and Practice of Sleep Medicine*, 5th edn. eds. M. H. Kryger, T. Roth & W.C. Dement. Philadelphia: W. B. Saunders, pp. 112–25.

Tobler, I. & Borbély, A. A. (1988) Sleep and EEG spectra in the pigeon (*Columba livia*) under baseline conditions and after sleep-deprivation. *J Comp Physiol, A* **163**: 729–38.

van Twyver, H. & Allison, T. (1972) A polygraphic and behavioral study of sleep in the pigeon (*Columba livia*). *Exp Neurol* **35**: 138–53.

Warren, W. C., Hillier, L. W., Marshall Graves, J. A., Birney, E., Ponting, C. P. *et al.* (2008) Genome analysis of the platypus reveals unique signatures of evolution. *Nature* **453**: 175–83.

A systems-level approach to human REM sleep

Luca Matarazzo, Ariane Foret, Laura Mascetti, Vincenzo Muto, Anahita Shaffii, and Pierre Maquet

Summary

The organization of regional brain function during human rapid eye movement sleep (REMS) can be characterized at the macroscopic systems level by functional neuroimaging techniques. Several aspects of REMS have been investigated. During REMS, forebrain activation pattern is characterized by a hyperactivity in posterior cortical areas and regions of the limbic and paralimbic system, contrasting with a relative quiescence of the polymodal associative cortices of the lateral frontal and parietal cortices. This activity pattern has been related to the main characteristic of dreams. The activity associated with rapid eye movements has been identified in the thalamus and primary visual cortex, suggesting the existence of ponto-geniculo-occipital (PGO) waves in humans. The variability of heart rate during REMS is associated with the activity in the extended amygdala, suggesting a specific organization of autonomic regulation during REMS. The distribution of regional brain activity during REMS was shown to depend on experience acquired during previous wakefulness. Training on a serial reaction time task induces an increase in activity in the brain stem, thalamus, occipital, and premotor areas during subsequent REMS. These data suggest that REMS is implicated in offline memory processing. With the advent of multimodal functional imaging (electroencephalography/functional magnetic resonance imaging (EEG/fMRI), transcranial magnetic stimulation/electroencephalography (TMS/EEG), and multichannel electroencephalography (MEEG)), a finer grain characterization of human REMS will lead to a better understanding of this intriguing state of vigilance.

Introduction

Rapid eye movement sleep (REMS) represents a state of consciousness distinct from wakefulness and non-REMS (NREMS), characterized by relatively fast-frequency, low-amplitude oscillations on EEG recordings, bursts of rapid eye movements (REMs) on electrooculogram (EOG) channels, and muscular atonia interrupted by muscle twitches on electromyogram (EMG) derivations (Rechtschaffen and Kales, 1968). In addition, dreams occur preferentially, although not exclusively, during REMS (Hobson *et al.*, 2000). All these features suggest that relative to other states of consciousness, REMS is associated with profound modifications in brain function, which might also account for the changes in autonomic regulation (temperature control, variability in heart and respiratory rates) that are typically observed during REMS.

Since its discovery about fifty years ago, the neural mechanisms that regulate, initiate, and maintain REMS are worked out in increasing detail in animals (Fuller *et al.*, 2007; Luppi *et al.*, 2006; Steriade and McCarley, 2005). In contrast, still little is known about the organization of brain function during REMS in humans. The study of neural activity during REMS in humans is necessarily hindered by technical and ethical reasons. Intracranial recordings are restricted to patients in presurgical evaluation: the number of recorded brain regions is limited and their topography imposed by clinical requirements (Cantero *et al.*, 2004; Fell *et al.*, 2003; Magnin *et al.*, 2004). A number of non-traumatic techniques are now available, which all have their own advantages and drawbacks in terms of spatial and temporal resolutions, safety, and cost. Multichannel EEG and magnetoencephalography (MEG) can provide a hint on the topography of electric or magnetic sources that underpin the signal recorded on the surface, based on forward and inverse models that necessarily imply various sets of constraints. Direct measures of brain activity mainly rely on hemodynamic or metabolic measures, provided by emission tomography (positron

REM Sleep: Regulation and Function, eds. Birendra N. Mallick, S. R. Pandi-Perumal, Robert W. McCarley, and Adrian R. Morrison. Published by Cambridge University Press. © Cambridge University Press 2011.

emission tomography – PET, or single photon emission computed tomography – SPECT), fMRI, or optical imaging. These techniques provide a direct measure of local metabolic or hemodynamic signals with a good spatial resolution (millimeter range). However, the time course of the brain processes being assessed is usually slow (seconds to minutes).

Distribution of regional brain activity during REMS

Cerebral neurons typically adopt a tonic firing pattern during REMS, which on average is deemed as intense as during wakefulness (Steriade and McCarley, 2005). Accordingly, cerebral energy metabolism (Maquet *et al.*, 1990) and blood flow (Madsen *et al.*, 1991) reach similar levels during REMS as during wakefulness. However, the distribution of regional brain activity considerably differs between REMS and wakefulness and, in humans, is characterized by three main features. Firstly, in agreement with neurophysiological studies in animals, functional imaging studies reported a high activity in the brain stem and thalamic nuclei (Figure 8.1*a*). Secondly, confirming earlier measures of brain energy metabolism in animals (Ramm and Frost, 1983, 1986; Lydic *et al.*, 1991), they observed a high activity in limbic and paralimbic areas (Figure 8.1*a*). Thirdly, they further highlighted the contrast between this limbic activation and the relative quiescence of the associative frontal and parietal cortices (Figure 8.1*b*).

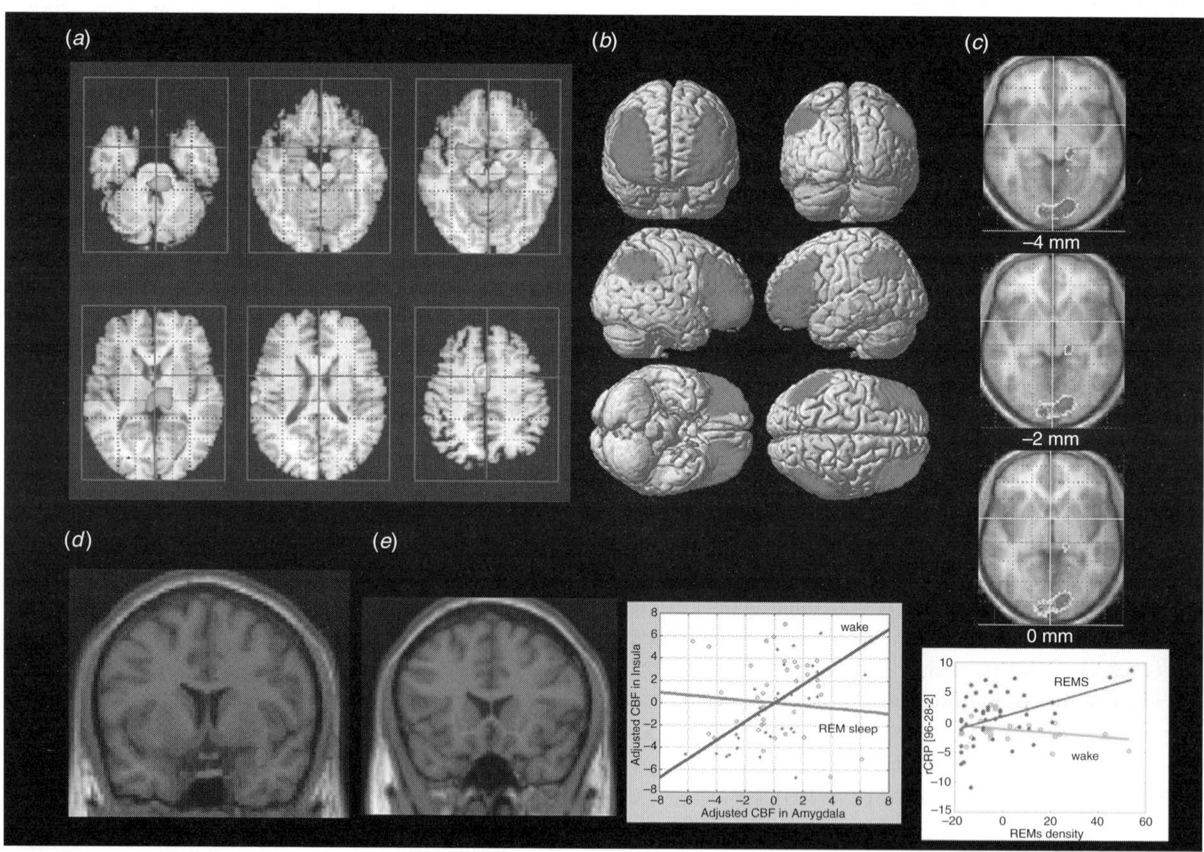

Figure 8.1 (*a*) Brain areas where regional cerebral blood flow is significantly larger during REMS than during wakefulness or slow-wave sleep: mesopontine tegmentum, thalamic nuclei, amygdala, anterior cingulate cortex. Reproduced from Maquet *et al.*, 1996. (*b*) Brain areas where regional cerebral blood flow is significantly decreased relative to wakefulness: ventral prefrontal regions, inferior parietal areas. Reproduced from Maquet *et al.*, 2005. (*c*) Brain areas where the regional cerebral blood flow increases in proportion with the density of eye movements during REMS more than in wakefulness: right medial geniculate nucleus and striate cortex. Reproduced from Peigneux *et al.*, 2001. (*d*) The amygdala is the only brain area where the blood flow is proportional to the variability in heart rate in REMS, relative to wakefulness. Reproduced from Desseilles *et al.*, 2006. (*e*) The interaction that prevails between the insula and the amygdala is involved in the regulation of heart rate during wakefulness, but not during REMS. Reproduced from Desseilles *et al.*, 2006. (See plate section for color version.)

In humans, the activation of the mesopontine tegmentum and thalamic nuclei has been systematically reported during REMS (Braun *et al.*, 1997; Maquet *et al.*, 1996; Nofzinger *et al.*, 1997). This pattern of activity is easily explained by the known neurophysiological mechanisms that generate REMS in animals. During REMS, neuronal populations in the mesopontine tegmentum are the source of a major activating input to the thalamic nuclei (Steriade and McCarley, 1990, 2005), which in turn forward this activation to the entire forebrain.

In the forebrain, REMS is characterized by high activity levels in the amygdala, the hippocampal formation, and the anterior cingulate, orbito-frontal and insular cortices (Braun *et al.*, 1997; Maquet *et al.*, 1996; Nofzinger *et al.*, 1997). In addition to these limbic and paralimbic areas, temporal and occipital cortices were also shown to be very active (Braun *et al.*, 1997), although this result was less systematically reported (Maquet *et al.*, 1996). Finally, the motor and premotor cortices were also very active during REMS (Maquet *et al.*, 2000).

In contrast, the prefrontal and parietal areas were relatively quiescent during REMS, relative to wakefulness (Braun *et al.*, 1997; Maquet *et al.*, 1996). More precisely, the hypoactive areas were located bilaterally in the inferior and middle frontal gyrus as well as the posterior part of the inferior parietal lobule (Maquet *et al.*, 2005). Interestingly, the superior frontal gyrus, the medial frontal areas, the intraparietal sulcus, and the superior parietal cortex were not less active in REMS than during wakefulness (Maquet *et al.*, 2005). It was argued that this peculiar distribution of regional brain activity during REMS might correlate with some features of cognition, as reflected in dream reports (see below).

Not only the distribution of brain activity, but also its functional connectivity, is modified during human REMS. The functional relationship between striate and extrastriate cortices – excitatory during wakefulness – was shown to be inverted during REMS (Braun *et al.*, 1998a, b). Likewise, the functional relationship between the amygdala and the temporal and occipital cortices was different during REMS than during wakefulness or NREMS (Maquet and Phillips, 1998).

The reasons that explain these peculiar functional segregations and integrations remain unclear. It is usually assumed that changes in neuromodulation might participate to a modification of forebrain activity and responsiveness during REMS because REMS is characterized by a prominent cholinergic tone and a decrease in noradrenergic and serotonergic modulation (Steriade and McCarley, 2005). However, objective evidence supporting this hypothesis is still lacking. Another hypothesis assumes that the regional distribution during REMS is partly driven by phasic events concomitant to REMs (see the section below on Neural correlates of rapid eye movements).

The particular pattern of cerebral activity observed during REMS is usually assumed to correlate with, and possibly influence, the main characteristics of dreaming activity (Hobson *et al.*, 2000; Maquet, 2000; Maquet *et al.*, 1996; Maquet and Franck, 1997). The prominent visual and auditory perceptual features of dreams might be related to the activation of posterior (occipital and temporal) cortices. In keeping with this hypothesis, visual imagery in dreams is absent in some patients with occipito-temporal lesions (Solms, 1997). On the other hand, emotions, which are often reported in dreams, would be related to the activation of the amygdala, orbito-frontal cortex, and anterior cingulate cortex (Hobson *et al.*, 2000; Maquet, 2000; Maquet *et al.*, 1996; Maquet and Franck, 1997). The activation of mesio-temporal areas would account for the memory content commonly found in dreams. However this mesio-temporal activity occurs in the context of a relatively low activity of ventral prefrontal cortex, which is deemed participating in memory retrieval (Rugg *et al.*, 2002). This pattern of regional brain activity would explain the peculiar aspects of episodic memory in dreams. Usually, "snips" of recent waking activity are frequently observed in dream reports (65%). In contrast, complete waking life episodes, characterized by the association between specific locations, characters, objects and actions, are seldom described as such in dream reports (1.7%) (Fosse *et al.*, 2003). The relative quiescence of the anterior and ventral prefrontal areas would explain that although the dreamer has access to "day residues," probably spontaneously generated by the coordinated activity of the mesio-temporal areas and the posterior cortices, the successful retrieval of the various details of a specific past episode is hindered. Low frontal activity would also account for the deficits in working memory, and executive functions, that manifest themselves in dream reports from REMS awakenings (Hobson *et al.*, 2000; Maquet, 2000; Maquet *et al.*, 1996; Maquet and Franck, 1997).

None of these hypotheses about the neural correlates of dreaming is yet supported by objective experimental evidence. However, they are based on the implicit assumption that regional brain specialization is identical during REMS and wakefulness, whereas functional integration is profoundly modified. This basic hypothesis is a useful and testable hypothesis, which should ground future research on dreaming in REMS.

Neural correlates of rapid eye movements

One of the main characteristics of REMS in animals consists of prominent phasic bioelectrical potentials, which occur in isolation or in bursts during the transition from slow-wave sleep (SWS) to REMS or during REMS itself (for a review see Callaway *et al.*, 1987). These waves can be observed from many parts of the animal brain (Hobson, 1964), but are most easily recorded in the pons, the lateral geniculate bodies, and the occipital cortex (Mouret *et al.*, 1963) and were therefore called ponto-geniculo-occipital (PGO) waves in cats (Mouret *et al.*, 1963) or pontine waves in rats (Datta, 1997). Typically, bursts of pontine waves are associated with REMs, a prominent feature of phasic REMS.

Several observations suggest that PGO waves also occur during human sleep. In epileptic patients, direct intracerebral recordings in the striate cortex showed monophasic or diphasic potentials during REMS, isolated or in bursts (Salzarulo *et al.*, 1975). Likewise, a recording of the pedunculopontine nucleus in a patient with Parkinson's disease revealed phasic potentials from the human pons occurring during and before REMS with a morphology, temporal distribution, and localization similar to those of PGO waves (Lim *et al.*, 2007). In normal subjects, surface EEG detected transient occipital and/or parietal potentials time-locked to REMs (McCarley *et al.*, 1983). Sources of MEG signals were localized in the brain stem, thalamus, hippocampus, and occipital cortex during REMS (Inoué *et al.*, 1999). The sequence of activation of these magnetic sources suggested that the activation of the frontal eye field and the pons precedes the recruitment of limbic and paralimbic areas (orbitofrontal cortex, amygdala, and parahippocampal gyrus) (Ioannides *et al.*, 2004). Using PET and cerebral blood flow measurements, it was shown that the activity in the right geniculate body and the primary occipital cortex increases in proportion to the density of eye movements to a larger extent during REMS than during wakefulness (Peigneux *et al.*, 2001; Figure 8.1*c*). Similar results were eventually obtained with fMRI (Hong *et al.*, 2009; Miyauchi *et al.*, 2009; Wehrle *et al.*, 2005). Collectively, these results supported the hypothesis of the existence of processes similar to PGO waves in humans, responsible for REMs generation.

The presence of PGO wave mechanisms in humans might have an important functional significance. Indeed, over the years, pontine waves have been implicated in various processes such as dream generation (Hobson and McCarley, 1977), alerting reaction to external stimuli or internal signals (Bowker and Morrison, 1976), sensorimotor integration (Callaway *et al.*, 1987), or memory processing (Datta, 2000; Datta *et al.*, 2004, 2005, 2008).

Neural correlates of the variability in heart rate during REMS

An important feature of REMS is the instability in autonomic function. Usually, during wakefulness or NREMS, physiological control variables are maintained within a narrow range through feedback control loops (Parmeggiani, 1985). In contrast, during REMS, autonomic functions do not rely on such a homeostatic control as strictly as during wakefulness or NREMS, but would resort to an "open-loop" mode of regulation (Parmeggiani, 1985). Indeed, respiratory and heart rates are known to be much more variable during REMS than during NREMS or wakefulness (Orem and Barnes, 1980). The neural mechanisms underpinning the variability in heart rate during REMS have not been described in detail, especially in humans. During wakefulness, the right insula appears as a crucial cortical region involved in cardiovascular regulation (Oppenheimer *et al.*, 1992; Williamson *et al.*, 1997, 1999, 2003, 2009). In contrast, during REMS, the activity in the right amygdala was found to covary more tightly than during wakefulness with the variability in heart rate (Desseilles *et al.*, 2006; Figure 8.1*d*). In addition, the functional relationships between the amygdala and the insula were much weaker during REMS than during wakefulness in relation to the variability of heart rate (Desseilles *et al.*, 2006; Figure 8.1*e*). As the amygdala is one of the most active forebrain areas during REMS, and given its direct projections to critical regions for the cardiovascular regulation (Hopkins and Holstege, 1978) such as the hypothalamus and parabrachial complex, the amygdala is in a good position to influence cardiac rhythm during REMS. These results suggest that during REMS, relative to wakefulness, the insula is less likely to modulate cardiovascular regulation whereas the amygdala seems to take a prominent role in cardiovascular regulation. The participation of the amygdala in cardiovascular regulation during REMS might account for a change in the mode of regulation following an open-loop mode.

Dependence on previous waking experience

The distribution of regional brain activity during REMS is not immutable but in contrast, can be modified by previous waking experience (Figure 8.2). These modifications were demonstrated in PET experiments comparing different groups of subjects. A first group of participants were trained on a probabilistic serial reaction time (SRT) task in the afternoon (Maquet *et al.*, 2000). In this task, six permanent position markers are displayed on a computer screen above six spatially compatible response keys. On each trial, a black circle appears below one of the position markers, and the task consists of pressing as fast and as accurately as possible the corresponding key. The next stimulus is displayed at another location after a 200 ms response–stimulus interval. Unbeknown to the subjects, the sequence of stimulus positions is generated by a probabilistic finite-state grammar that defines legal transitions between successive trials (Cleeremans and McClelland, 1991). To assess learning of the probabilistic rules of the grammar, there is a 15% chance, on each trial, that the stimulus generated based on the grammar (grammatical stimuli, G) is replaced by a non-grammatical (NG), random stimulus. Assuming that response preparation is facilitated by high predictability, predictable G stimuli should thus elicit faster responses than NG stimuli, but only if the context in which stimuli may occur has been encoded by participants. In this task, contextual sensitivity emerges through practice as a gradually increasing difference between the reaction times (RTs) elicited by G and NG stimuli occurring in specific contexts set by two to three previous trials at most (Cleeremans and McClelland, 1991). In this group, the participants were scanned during the post-training night, both during waking and in various sleep stages

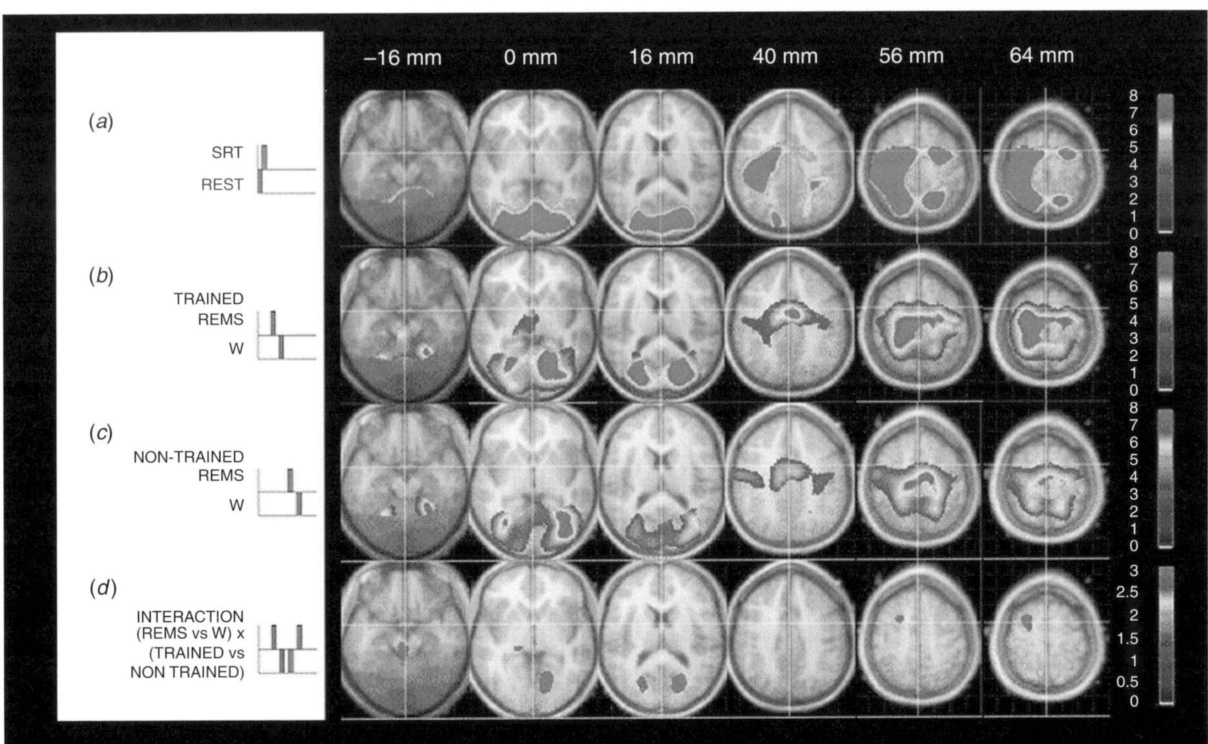

Figure 8.2 Regional brain activity during REMS is modified by previous waking experience (Maquet *et al.*, 2000). (*a*) Brain regions activated during performance of the SRT task during wakefulness (SRT–rest). (*b*) Brain regions activated during REM sleep in trained subjects (REM sleep–wakefulness). (*c*) Brain regions activated during REM sleep in non-trained subjects (REM sleep–wakefulness). (*d*) Brain regions activated more in trained subjects than in non-trained subjects during REM sleep. (See plate section for color version.)

(i.e., slow-wave sleep, stage 2, and REMS). A post-sleep training session again assessed performance to the task. A second group of subjects was not trained to the task but similarly scanned at night, both awake and during sleep. Data showed that the activity of bilateral occipital areas, mesencephalon, and left premotor cortex was larger during post-training REMS, relative to wakefulness, in subjects previously trained on the task, as compared to control subjects without prior training. These findings showed that previous training to the SRT modified the distribution of regional brain activity during subsequent REMS (Maquet *et al.*, 2000). In addition, functional integration during REMS was also modified by prior training. The activity in the left premotor cortex was significantly more correlated with the activity of the pre-supplementary area and posterior parietal cortex in trained participants than in control subjects (Laureys *et al.*, 2001).

However, in this first experiment, it could not be specified whether the experience-dependent changes in regional brain activity during post-training REMS were related to the simple optimization of a visuomotor skill, to the high-order acquisition of the probabilistic structure of the learned material, or to both. A third group of subjects was scanned during sleep after practice on another version of the SRT task, where the sequence of stimulus positions was completely random (Peigneux *et al.*, 2003). In these conditions, any difference in regional cerebral blood flow during post-training REMS between the subjects trained to the probabilistic SRT or to its random version should be specifically related to the acquisition of high-order sequential information. Again, during post-training REMS, activity in the bilateral occipital areas was larger, relative to waking activity, in subjects previously trained to the probabilistic sequence of stimuli than to a random one. These data demonstrated that in the experimental group, changes in regional brain activity during post-training REMS corresponded to the reprocessing of elaborated information about the sequential contingencies contained in the learned material. In contrast, no change in regional brain activity was observed in the subjects trained to the random SRT task. These results are reminiscent of animal experiments. At the behavioral level, an increase in REMS duration was observed in rats following aversive conditioning in which a tone was paired with a footshock, but not after pseudo-conditioning in which the tone and the footshock were not paired (Hennevin *et al.*, 1995). Using a similar procedure at the systems level, tone-evoked responses were obtained in the medial geniculate nucleus during REMS after a conditioning procedure initiated at wake, but not after pseudo-conditioning (Hennevin *et al.*, 1998). Finally, functional integration was shown to be specifically modified by practice of the probabilistic version of the task (Peigneux *et al.*, 2003). During REMS following probabilistic SRT practice, as compared to the practice of the random sequence, the occipital areas established or reinforced functional connections with the ipsilateral caudate nucleus, an area known to play a critical role in implicit sequence learning (Peigneux *et al.*, 2000). The finding that the strength of the functional connections between the occipital cortex and striatum is increased during post-training REMS suggests the involvement of the basal ganglia in the offline reprocessing of implicitly acquired high-order sequential information.

Collectively, these findings show that regional brain activity during REMS is modified when a structured information is acquired during a prior waking period. These data were interpreted as indicating an offline processing of memory traces during post-training REMS.

Conclusions

The distribution of brain activity during REMS substantially differs from wakefulness and depends on previous waking experience. Future research should further address the issue of the function of REMS. For instance, a body of data suggests that REMS participates in offline memory processing. However, the role of REMS in brain plasticity is still unsettled (Rasch *et al.*, 2008; Siegel, 2001). Functional neuroimaging is in a good position to help characterizing the relationship between REMS and memory processes.

Acknowledgments

Personal research reported in this paper was supported by the Belgian Fonds National de la Recherche Scientifique (FNRS), Fondation Médicale Reine Elisabeth (FMRE), Research Fund of the University of Liège and Interuniversity Attraction Programme (Belgian Science Policy).

References

Bowker, R. M. & Morrison, A. R. (1976) The startle reflex and PGO spikes. *Brain Res* **102**: 185–90.

Braun, A. R., Balkin, T. J., Wesenten, N. J. *et al.* (1997) Regional cerebral blood flow throughout the sleep-wake cycle. An H$_2$$^{(15)}$O PET study. *Brain* **120**(Pt 7): 1173–97.

Braun, A. R., Balkin, T. J., Wesensten, N. J. *et al.* (1998a) Dissociated pattern of activity in visual cortices and their projections during human rapid eye movement sleep. *Science* **279**: 91–5.

Braun, A. R., Balkin, T. J., Wesensten, N. J. *et al.* (1998b) Dissociated pattern of activity in visual cortices and their projections during human rapid eye movement sleep. *Science* **279**: 91–5.

Callaway, C. W., Lydic, R., Baghdoyan, H. A. & Hobson, J. A. (1987) Pontogeniculooccipital waves: spontaneous visual system activity during rapid eye movement sleep. *Cell Mol Neurobiol* **7**:105–49.

Cantero, J. L., Atienza, M., Madsen, J. R. & Stickgold, R. (2004) Gamma EEG dynamics in neocortex and hippocampus during human wakefulness and sleep. *Neuroimage* **22**: 1271–80.

Cleeremans, A. & McClelland, J. L. (1991) Learning the structure of event sequences. *J Exp Psychol Gen* **120**: 235–53.

Datta, S. (1997) Cellular basis of pontine ponto-geniculo-occipital wave generation and modulation. *Cell Mol Neurobiol* **17**: 341–65.

Datta, S. (2000) Avoidance task training potentiates phasic pontine-wave density in the rat: a mechanism for sleep-dependent plasticity. *J Neurosci* **20**: 8607–13.

Datta, S., Li, G. & Auerbach, S. (2008) Activation of phasic pontine-wave generator in the rat: a mechanism for expression of plasticity-related genes and proteins in the dorsal hippocampus and amygdala. *Eur J Neurosci* **27**: 1876–92.

Datta, S., Mavanji, V., Ulloor, J. & Patterson, E. H. (2004) Activation of phasic pontine-wave generator prevents rapid eye movement sleep deprivation-induced learning impairment in the rat: a mechanism for sleep-dependent plasticity. *J Neurosci* **24**: 1416–27.

Datta, S., Saha, S., Prutzman, S. L., Mullins, O. J & Mavanji, V. (2005) Pontine-wave generator activation-dependent memory processing of avoidance learning involves the dorsal hippocampus in the rat. *J Neurosci Res* **80**: 727–37.

Desseilles, M., Dang Vu, T., Laureys, S. *et al.* (2006) A prominent role for amygdaloid complexes in the Variability in Heart Rate (VHR) during Rapid Eye Movement (REM) sleep relative to wakefulness. *Neuroimage* **32**: 1008–15.

Fell, J., Staedtgen, M., Burr, W. *et al.* (2003) Rhinal-hippocampal EEG coherence is reduced during human sleep. *Eur J Neurosci* **18**: 1711–16.

Fosse, M. J., Fosse, Rm, Hobson, J. A. & Stickgold, R. J. (2003) Dreaming and episodic memory: a functional dissociation? *J Cogn Neurosci* **15**: 1–9.

Fuller, P. M., Saper, C. B. & Lu, J. (2007) The pontine REM switch: past and present. *J Physiol* **584**: 735–41.

Hennevin, E., Hars, B., Maho, C. & Bloch, V. (1995) Processing of learned information in paradoxical sleep: relevance for memory. *Behav Brain Res* **69**: 125–35.

Hennevin, E., Maho, C. & Hars, B. (1998) Neuronal plasticity induced by fear conditioning is expressed during paradoxical sleep: evidence from simultaneous recordings in the lateral amygdala and the medial geniculate in rats. *Behav Neurosci* **112**: 839–62.

Hobson, J. A. (1964) [The phasic electrical activity of the cortex and thalamus during desychonized sleep in cats.] *C R Seances Soc Biol Fil* **158**: 2131–5.

Hobson, J. A. & McCarley, R. W. (1977) The brain as a dream state generator: an activation-synthesis hypothesis of the dream process. *Am J Psychiatry* **134**: 1335–48.

Hobson, J. A., Pace-Schott, E. F. & Stickgold, R. (2000) Dreaming and the brain: toward a cognitive neuroscience of conscious states. *Behav Brain Sci* **23**: 793–842; discussion 904–1121.

Hong, C. C., Harris, J. C., Pearlson, G. D. *et al.* (2009) fMRI evidence for multisensory recruitment associated with rapid eye movements during sleep. *Hum Brain Mapp* **30**: 1705–22.

Hopkins, D. A. & Holstege, G. (1978) Amygdaloid projections to the mesencephalon, pons and medulla oblongata in the cat. *Exp Brain Res* **32**: 529–47.

Inoué, S., Saha, U. K. & Musha, T. (1999) Spatio-temporal distribution of neuronal activities and REM sleep. *In Rapid Eye Movement Sleep*, eds. B. N. Mallick & S. Inoue. New Dehli: Narosa Publishing, pp. 214–20.

Ioannides, A. A., Corsi-Cabrera, M., Fenwick, P. B. *et al.* (2004) MEG tomography of human cortex and brainstem activity in waking and REM sleep saccades. *Cereb Cortex* **14**: 56–72.

Laureys, S., Peigneux, P., Phillips, C. *et al.* (2001) Experience-dependent changes in cerebral functional connectivity during human rapid eye movement sleep. *Neuroscience* **105**: 521–5.

Lim, A. S., Lozano, A. M., Moro, E. *et al.* (2007) Characterization of REM-sleep associated ponto-geniculo-occipital waves in the human pons. *Sleep* **30**: 823–7.

Luppi, P. H., Gervasoni, D., Verret, L. *et al.* (2006) Paradoxical (REM) sleep genesis: the switch from an aminergic-cholinergic to a GABAergic-glutamatergic hypothesis. *J Physiol Paris* **100**: 271–83.

Lydic, R., Baghdoyan, H. A., Hibbard, L. *et al.* (1991) Regional brain glucose metabolism is altered during rapid eye movement sleep in the cat: a preliminary study. *J Comp Neurol* **304**: 517–29.

Madsen, P. L., Holm, S., Vorstrup, S. *et al.* (1991) Human regional cerebral blood flow during rapid-eye-movement sleep. *J Cereb Blood Flow Metab* **11**: 502–7.

Magnin, M., Bastuji, H., Garcia-Larrea, L. & Mauguiere, F. (2004) Human thalamic medial pulvinar nucleus is not activated during paradoxical sleep. *Cereb Cortex* **14**: 858–62.

Maquet, P. (2000) Functional neuroimaging of normal human sleep by positron emission tomography. *J Sleep Res* **9**: 207–31.

Maquet, P. & Franck, G. (1997) REM sleep and amygdala. *Mol Psychiatry* **2**: 195–6.

Maquet, P. & Phillips, C. (1998) Functional brain imaging of human sleep. *J Sleep Res* **7**: 42–7.

Maquet, P., Dive, D., Salmon, E. *et al.* (1990) Cerebral glucose utilization during sleep-wake cycle in man determined by positron emission tomography and [18F]2-fluoro-2-deoxy-D-glucose method. *Brain Res* **513**: 136–43.

Maquet, P., Peters, J., Aerts, J. *et al.* (1996) Functional neuroanatomy of human rapid-eye-movement sleep and dreaming. *Nature* **383**: 163–6.

Maquet, P., Laureys, S., Peigneux, P. *et al.* (2000) Experience-dependent changes in cerebral activation during human REM sleep. *Nat Neurosci* **3**: 831–6.

Maquet, P., Ruby, P., Maudoux, A. *et al.* (2005) Human cognition during REM sleep and the activity profile within the frontal and parietal cortices: a reappraisal of functional neuroimaging data. In *Progess in Brain Research*, ed. S. Laureys. Elsevier, pp. 219–27.

McCarley, R. W., Winkelman, J. W. & Duffy, F. H. (1983) Human cerebral potentials associated with REM sleep rapid eye movements: links to PGO waves and waking potentials. *Brain Res* **274**: 359–64.

Miyauchi, S., Misaki, M., Kan, S., Fukunaga, T. & Koike, T. (2009) Human brain activity time-locked to rapid eye movements during REM sleep. *Exp Brain Res* **192**: 657–67.

Mouret, J., Jeannerod, M. & Jouvet, M. (1963) [Electrical activity of the visual system during the paradoxical phase of sleep in the cat.] *J Physiol (Paris)* **55**: 305–6.

Nofzinger, E. A., Mintun, M. A., Wiseman, M., Kupfer, D. J. & Moore, R. Y. (1997) Forebrain activation in REM sleep: an FDG PET study. *Brain Res* **770**: 192–201.

Oppenheimer, S. M., Gelb, A., Girvin, J. P. & Hachinski, V. C. (1992) Cardiovascular effects of human insular cortex stimulation. *Neurology* **42**: 1727–32.

Orem, J. & Barnes, C. D. (1980) *Physiology in Sleep*. New York: Academic Press.

Parmeggiani, P. L. (1985) Regulation of circulation and breathing during sleep: experimental aspects. *Ann Clin Res* **17**: 185–9.

Peigneux, P., Maquet, P., Meulemans, T. *et al.* (2000) Striatum forever, despite sequence learning variability: a random effect analysis of PET data. *Hum Brain Mapp* **10**: 179–94.

Peigneux, P., Laureys, S., Fuchs, S. *et al.* (2001) Generation of rapid eye movements during paradoxical sleep in humans. *Neuroimage* **14**: 701–8.

Peigneux, P., Laureys, S., Fuchs, S. *et al.* (2003) Learned material content and acquisition level modulate cerebral reactivation during posttraining rapid-eye-movements sleep. *Neuroimage* **20**: 125–34.

Ramm, P. & Frost, B. J. (1983) Regional metabolic activity in the rat brain during sleep-wake activity. *Sleep* **6**: 196–216.

Ramm, P. & Frost, B. J. (1986) Cerebral and local cerebral metabolism in the cat during slow wave and REM sleep. *Brain Res* **365**: 112–24.

Rasch, B., Pommer, J., Diekelmann, S. & Born, J. (2008) Pharmacological REM sleep suppression paradoxically improves rather than impairs skill memory. *Nat Neurosci* **12**: 396–7.

Rechtschaffen, A. & Kales, A. (1968) *A Manual of Standardized Terminology, Techniques and Scoring System for Sleep Stages of Human Subjects*. University of California, LA: Brain Information Service/Brain Research Institute.

Rugg, M. D., Otten, L. J. & Henson, R. N. (2002) The neural basis of episodic memory: evidence from functional neuroimaging. *Philos Trans R Soc Lond B Biol Sci* **357**: 1097–110.

Salzarulo, P., Lairy, G. C., Bancaud, J. & Munari, C. (1975) Direct depth recording of the striate cortex during REM sleep in man: are there PGO potentials? *EEG Clin Neurophysiol* **38**: 199–202.

Siegel, J. M. (2001) The REM sleep-memory consolidation hypothesis. *Science* **294**: 1058–63.

Solms, M. (1997) *The Neuropsychology of Dreams. A Clinico-anatomical Study*. Mahwah: Lawrence Erlbaum Associates.

Steriade, M. & McCarley, R. W. (1990) *Brainstem Control of Wakefulness and Sleep*. New York: Plenum Press.

Steriade, M. & McCarley, R. W. (2005) *Brain Control of Wakefulness and Sleep*. New York: Kluwer Academic.

Wehrle, R., Czisch, M., Kaufmann, C. *et al.* (2005) Rapid eye movement-related brain activation in human sleep: a functional magnetic resonance imaging study. *Neuroreport* **16**: 853–7.

Williamson, J. W., Nobrega, A. C., McColl, R. *et al.* (1997) Activation of the insular cortex during dynamic exercise in humans. *J Physiol* **503**(2): 277–83.

Williamson, J. W., McColl, R., Mathews, D., Ginsburg, M. & Mitchell, J. H. (1999) Activation of the insular cortex is affected by the intensity of exercise. *J Appl Physiol* **87**: 1213–19.

Williamson, J. W., McColl, R. & Mathews, D. (2003) Evidence for central command activation of the human insular cortex during exercise. *J Appl Physiol* **94**: 1726–34.

Williamson, J. W., Querry, R., McColl, R. & Mathews, D. (2009) Are decreases in insular regional cerebral blood flow sustained during postexercise hypotension? *Med Sci Sports Exerc* **41**: 574–80.

REM-sleep regulation: circadian, homeostatic, and non-REM sleep-dependent determinants

Daniel Aeschbach

Summary

The amount, timing, and structure of REM sleep are regulated. Three major determinants in REM sleep regulation have been identified: (1) the circadian pacemaker in the suprachiasmatic nucleus (SCN) of the hypothalamus, which through its outputs generates daily cycles in REM sleep propensity; (2) a homeostatic (i.e., need-based) drive for REM sleep that increases in the absence of REM sleep and decreases during its presence; (3) the inhibition of REM sleep by non-REM (NREM) sleep. In humans, the circadian modulation of REM sleep shows a maximum shortly after the nadir of the circadian rhythm of core body temperature. A sleep-dependent disinhibition of REM sleep (i.e., a gradual increase of REM sleep in the course of a sleep episode that is distinct from a circadian influence) is also evident and attributed primarily to the decrease in NREM sleep intensity. The circadian rhythm and the sleep-dependent disinhibition of REM sleep are the dominant factors influencing the distribution of REM sleep within a sleep episode. In humans that are normally entrained to the 24-hour day, the interaction of these two factors results in maximal REM sleep propensity in the morning, coinciding with habitual wake time. The homeostatic regulation counteracts deviations from a reference level of REM sleep need such that loss of REM sleep results in increased REM sleep propensity. However, rebounds in REM sleep following selective deprivation often remain partial suggesting that the homeostatic drive is relatively weak. On the other hand, recent studies have emphasized that REM sleep can undergo changes in its quality that may compensate for its loss in duration. In the present chapter, the evidence for circadian and homeostatic regulation of REM sleep will be reviewed, the physiological markers that are indicative of such regulation will be presented, and the interdependence of REM sleep and NREM sleep regulation will be examined.

Circadian regulation of REM sleep

REM sleep propensity

Information on REM sleep propensity can be derived from the duration of REM sleep in a given time interval, or from the REM sleep latency (i.e., the interval between sleep onset and the first occurrence of REM sleep). Healthy adults that are normally entrained to the 24-hour light–dark cycle typically enter sleep through NREM sleep. REM sleep alternates with NREM sleep in a cyclic fashion with a periodicity of approximately 90 to 110 minutes. The proportion of REM sleep to NREM sleep within a sleep cycle exhibits a strong circadian modulation, whereas the duration of the NREM–REM sleep cycle does not appear to be affected by circadian phase (Czeisler et al., 1980). Circadian phase is typically derived from variables with a robust endogenous circadian rhythm such as the plasma melatonin concentration or core body temperature. In humans, the circadian modulation of REM sleep is such that the duration of REM sleep episodes are longest near the end of the interval of endogenous melatonin secretion and shortly after the minimum of the circadian rhythm of core body temperature, which under entrained conditions occurs in the early morning hours (Czeisler et al., 1980; Dijk and Czeisler, 1995; Zulley, 1980; Figure 9.1). The peak in the rhythm of REM sleep propensity measured either as absolute REM sleep duration or as a proportion of total sleep time occurs close to the crest of the sleep propensity rhythm.

The phase relationship between a sleep episode and the endogenous circadian rhythms is an important

REM Sleep: Regulation and Function, eds. Birendra N. Mallick, S. R. Pandi-Perumal, Robert W. McCarley, and Adrian R. Morrison. Published by Cambridge University Press. © Cambridge University Press 2011.

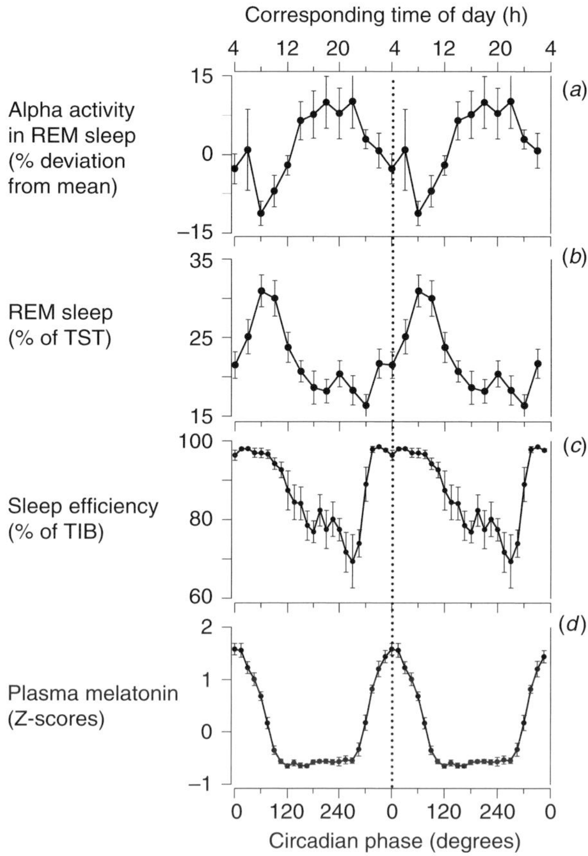

Figure 9.1 Circadian rhythms in EEG alpha activity, REM sleep propensity, and sleep efficiency, and their phase relationship to the endogenous rhythm in plasma melatonin. Data were derived from a one-month long forced desynchrony protocol in seven men. In this protocol the sleep–wake cycle (28 h) was desynchronized from the endogenous circadian rhythm such that the sleep episodes (duration 9.33 h) occurred at all circadian phases over the course of the study. Data are plotted as a function of circadian phase with 0 degrees (bottom *x*-axis) corresponding to the fitted maximum in the melatonin rhythm; for visualization circadian phase is also transformed to corresponding clock time during entrainment to a 24-h day (top *x*-axis). (*a*) EEG alpha activity in REM sleep represents power density in the 8.25 to 10.5 Hz range, expressed as percent deviation from the mean. (*b*) REM sleep is expressed as a percentage of total sleep time (TST). (*c*) Sleep efficiency is TST expressed as percentage of time in bed (TIB). (*d*) Melatonin concentrations are shown as Z-scores. Data are double plotted. (Modified from Dijk *et al.*, 1997 with permission.)

determinant of the REM sleep distribution. This was apparent in studies in which sleep occurred at an unusual circadian phase, such as in long-term studies in time-free environment in which subjects selected their own schedules, in short sleep–wake cycle experiments, in sleep-displacement studies, as well as in the forced desynchrony protocol. In the latter protocol the sleep–wake cycle is uncoupled from the output of the circadian pacemaker such that sleep occurs at all circadian phases over the course of a multiple-week protocol, while the duration of wakefulness prior to sleep is maintained at a similar level (Dijk *et al.*, 1997; Dijk and Czeisler, 1995). It was found that when sleep is initiated at a phase that under entrained conditions typically coincides with the morning hours, the latency to REM sleep is reduced, and the number of sleep-onset REM episodes (SOREMs) is increased compared to normal nighttime sleep. Moreover, REM sleep is more abundant in the early part than in the latter part of the sleep episode, which contrasts with the typical increase in the duration of the REM sleep episodes during normal nighttime sleep. Real-life situations in which the phase relationship between sleep and the output of the circadian pacemaker is altered, and in which changes in the distribution and amount of REM sleep have been observed are shift work (Mignot *et al.*, 2006; Webb, 1983) and jet lag (i.e., the rapid crossing of several time zones; Monk *et al.*, 2000).

There is evidence that aging affects the distribution of REM sleep within a sleep episode and that this may be attributable in part to circadian factors. Shorter REM sleep latencies in older than in young individuals have been observed (Bliwise, 1993). This finding is not necessarily due to a phase advance of the circadian timing system relative to habitual sleep in older individuals. On the contrary, older individuals actually wake up at an earlier circadian phase than young individuals (Duffy *et al.*, 1998). A forced desynchrony protocol revealed that REM sleep latencies were shorter in older than in young individuals at some circadian phases, i.e., in particular during the interval when endogenous plasma melatonin levels were high (Dijk *et al.*, 1999). The authors of this study proposed that aging may be associated with an *internal* phase advance of the REM sleep propensity rhythm.

Electroencephalogram activity

The human electroencephalogram (EEG) during REM sleep is characterized by mixed frequencies of relatively low amplitude. Spectral analysis of the EEG during REM sleep revealed frequency-specific changes as a function of circadian phase. Circadian modulations of power density were found in most frequency bins within the range of 0.75 to 14.0 Hz (Dijk *et al.*, 1997). The magnitude of these modulations is generally modest, particularly in comparison to the prominent circadian modulations within the spindle frequency range (12–15 Hz) during NREM sleep. The largest circadian variation of EEG activity in REM sleep is present within the alpha range (8.25–10.5 Hz). The nadir in this rhythm coincides with the end of the interval of endogenous melatonin secretion, i.e., it occurs close to the maximum of the REM sleep propensity rhythm (Figure 9.1*a*). Interestingly, this rhythm is also similar to the circadian rhythm of EEG activity in the high alpha range during wakefulness (Aeschbach *et al.*, 1999), suggesting that the two rhythms in REM sleep and wakefulness may be functionally related.

REM density

Rapid eye movements are the most prominent phasic events during REM sleep. REM density is a measure of the frequency of rapid eye movements during REM sleep. In contrast to the REM sleep propensity, REM density does not show a substantial circadian modulation. In fact, in a forced desynchrony protocol it was demonstrated that when the data are averaged over the entire sleep episodes there is no significant modulation of REM density with circadian phase (Khalsa *et al.*, 2002). A weak but significant circadian variation of REM density was apparent in the last one-third of the sleep episodes, however. Maximum REM density was observed when the last one-third of sleep coincided with the wake-maintenance zone, a phase during which the circadian wake drive is high, and which typically occurs eight to ten hours prior to the maximum of the REM sleep propensity rhythm. Taken together, the circadian modulation of REM density is minimal and appears to become appreciable only in the latter part of a sleep episode, i.e., at a time when sleep pressure is minimal.

Pathways of circadian control

The suprachiasmatic nucleus (SCN) is the central structure controlling the circadian rhythm of many functions including REM sleep. Lesion studies in animals revealed that the SCN is necessary for the circadian rhythms in total sleep, wakefulness, and REM sleep (Mistlberger *et al.*, 1983; Tobler *et al.*, 1983; Wurts and Edgar, 2000). A recent study pinpointed the origin of the circadian rhythm in REM sleep to a specific subdivision of the SCN, the dorsomedial nucleus (Lee *et al.*, 2009). It is not completely clear how the circadian control of REM sleep is mediated. An SCN lesion study in rats suggested that the circadian pacemaker actively promotes transitions into REM sleep during the animals' resting phase (Wurts and Edgar, 2000). On the other hand, mice with an intact SCN but lacking the orexin (hypocretin) neurons were found to have a blunted circadian rhythm in REM sleep; compared to wildtype mice these animals showed more REM sleep during the active phase but not during the resting phase, suggesting that the excitatory orexin neurons mediate a circadian suppression of REM sleep (Kantor *et al.*, 2009). Orexin neurons are indeed well positioned as they receive direct and indirect input from the SCN, and send projections to various brain regions involved in vigilance-state control and REM sleep inhibition, including the ventrolateral periaqueductal grey, lateral pontine tegmentum, locus coeruleus, and dorsal raphe (Lu *et al.*, 2006). Interestingly, subjects with narcolepsy, a disorder which is characterized by a loss of orexin neurons, showed attenuated circadian variation in several sleep stages including REM sleep, when studied in an ultra-short sleep–wake protocol (Dantz *et al.*, 1994). In addition, these subjects exhibited more REM sleep overall compared to control subjects. In conclusion, it appears that the orexin neurons are critically involved in mediating the SCN signal that shapes the circadian rhythm in REM sleep.

Homeostatic regulation of REM sleep

Origin and concept of sleep homeostasis

The term sleep homeostasis was coined based on observations of compensatory responses in NREM sleep following sleep deprivation. Responses to total sleep deprivation can include an increase in sleep duration in recovery sleep, but always include an intensification of NREM sleep, as reflected in an increase of EEG slow-wave activity (SWA; spectral power density in the range of approximately 0.5–4.5 Hz) (Borbély *et al.*, 1981). Slow-wave activity in NREM sleep increases in proportion to an individual's prior time awake and it decreases in the course of a sleep episode, whereas it is little influenced by circadian phase. Slow-wave activity is thought to be not only a marker of NREM sleep intensity but also an expression of NREM sleep need (i.e., undischarged NREM sleep pressure). The sleep–wake dependent changes of SWA served as the basis of the homeostatic process (Process S) in the two-process model of sleep regulation (Borbély, 1982).

In contrast to NREM sleep, homeostatic regulation of REM sleep has been more difficult to establish, and has rarely been incorporated in models of sleep regulation. The difficulty to delineate homeostatic mechanisms of REM sleep regulation has several reasons. (1) Thus far, an unequivocal physiological marker of REM sleep need and REM sleep intensity has not been identified, although some candidate markers have been proposed (see below). (2) Compensatory responses in REM sleep following total sleep deprivation are not always and immediately evident; this can be due to competing compensatory responses in NREM sleep, or due to confounding circadian influences that can make an interpretation of changes in REM sleep difficult. (3) REM sleep is not a strictly unitary state. In contrast to NREM sleep, the definition of REM sleep uses not only EEG measures but also tonic electromyographic (EMG) activity and phasic electrooculographic activity. The latter two activities can dissociate from a typical REM sleep EEG (Lu *et al.*, 2006) and therefore render the interpretation of changes in response to experimental challenges difficult.

REM sleep propensity and homeostasis

Despite the difficulties mentioned above, compensatory changes in REM sleep in response to its absence or to experimental reduction have been observed. Selective REM sleep deprivation – typically achieved through awakening of a subject at the first signs of REM sleep – is the most direct way to study the homeostatic regulation of REM sleep. It was found that the number of sleep interruptions necessary to minimize the occurrence of REM sleep increased within and across consecutive nights of REM sleep deprivation (Figure 9.2*a*), and that the total duration of REM sleep increased over baseline levels in subsequent recovery sleep (Dement, 1960; Dement *et al.*, 1966; Endo *et al.*, 1998; Kales *et al.*, 1964). Control experiments with interruptions during NREM sleep confirmed that the REM sleep rebound during recovery sleep was indeed caused by the REM sleep deprivation and not by the awakenings. REM sleep rebounds were also apparent in recovery sleep after partial sleep deprivation. In this type of study sleep is restricted to less than eight hours, often for several consecutive nights. Because of the difference in the typical distribution of slow-wave sleep (SWS) and REM sleep – SWS dominating in the early part and REM sleep in the latter part of a normal eight-hour sleep episode – these studies induce primarily a loss of REM sleep, whereas SWS is not or only little affected (e.g., Brunner *et al.*, 1993). Furthermore,

rebounds in REM sleep have not only been observed in recovery nights. An immediate intra-night rebound was found in subjects who were deprived of REM sleep for the first five hours after sleep onset, prior to their being allowed to sleep undisturbed (Beersma *et al.*, 1990). A chronic REM sleep deficit may be manifest in short sleepers (habitual sleep duration < 6 hours); in this group, REM sleep accumulates faster in the course of a sleep episode than in long sleepers (> 9 hours) (Aeschbach *et al.*, 1996).

Evidence for homeostatic control of REM sleep has also been obtained in various animal species (for a review see Franken, 2002). Together with the studies in humans, it appears that a loss of REM sleep is compensated primarily by an increase in REM sleep duration, and that this increase is proportional to the incurred REM sleep deficit. In most studies, however, this compensation remained partial, i.e., the REM sleep rebound was less than the amount of lost REM sleep (e.g., Endo *et al.*, 1998). One interpretation of this discrepancy is that the homeostatic drive is generally weak, and that not all REM sleep during baseline sleep is necessary ("obligate"), but that some portion may be "facultative" (Horne, 2000) and therefore not recovered. Another possibility is that some sub-states of wakefulness or NREM sleep are equivalent to REM sleep and serve as a substitute. Stage 1 may serve such a function given the similarity of its EEG with that in REM sleep, and the fact that stage 1 is greatly increased during REM sleep deprivation (Endo *et al.*, 1998). Finally, there is an additional complexity to REM sleep homeostasis in that at least in humans the individual differences in the REM sleep rebound after selective deprivation are large (Cartwright *et al.*, 1967).

The homeostatic control of REM sleep is independent of its circadian modulation: rats in which the SCN was lesioned still show a REM sleep rebound during recovery after total sleep deprivation or selective REM sleep deprivation (Mistlberger *et al.*, 1983; Tobler *et al.*, 1983; Wurts and Edgar, 2000).

Electroencephalogram activity as a marker of REM sleep need

In humans, EEG alpha activity (~8–11 Hz) in REM sleep was attenuated after selective REM sleep deprivation (Figure 9.2*b*, *c*; Endo *et al.*, 1998). This attenuation even outlasted the REM sleep rebound and was still present in the third recovery night after three nights of REM sleep deprivation. A four-night partial sleep deprivation protocol that resulted in an

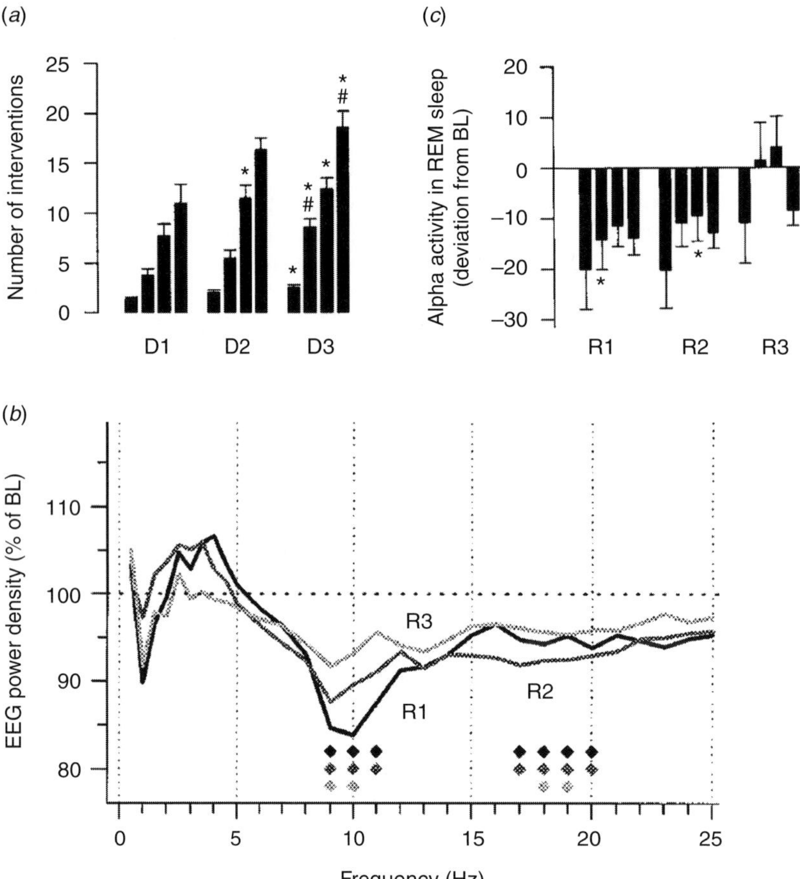

Figure 9.2 Selective REM sleep deprivation during three consecutive nights and its effect on the REM sleep EEG during three recovery nights. Data are from eight men. (*a*) Number of sleep interruptions required during the deprivation nights (D1, D2, D3) to suppress REM sleep. Bars represent means + SEM per two-hour intervals. * Significant difference from corresponding D1 value; # significant difference from corresponding D2 value (P < 0.05, two-tailed paired *t*-test). (*b*) EEG power density spectra during REM sleep in recovery nights (R1, R2, R3) are expressed as percentages of baseline sleep (BL). Diamonds (gray level corresponding to line style) indicate significant differences from baseline (P < 0.05; two-tailed paired *t*-test). (*c*) EEG alpha activity (power density in the range of 8.25–11.0 Hz) in REM sleep during first four NREM–REM sleep cycles in recovery nights. Bars represent percent deviations (mean + SEM) from baseline. * Significant difference between corresponding cycles following REM sleep derivation and control deprivation (i.e., interruptions during NREM sleep, data not shown) (P < 0.05; two-tailed paired *t*-test). The following significant differences from baseline are not indicated: R1 in cycles 1 to 4; R2 in cycles 1, 2, and 4; R3 in cycle 4. (Modified from Endo *et al.*, 1998 with permission.)

accumulating REM sleep deficit was found to induce a gradual attenuation of alpha activity (Brunner *et al.*, 1993). This study also found a reduction of alpha activity in the waking EEG in the presence of an increasing REM sleep deficit. The results indicate that alpha activity in REM sleep and wakefulness is inversely related to REM sleep propensity, and hence may represent a marker of REM sleep homeostasis. In contrast, the typical increase of alpha activity during NREM sleep following total sleep deprivation appears to be functionally distinct and related to NREM sleep pressure (Aeschbach *et al.*, 1996; Borbély *et al.*, 1981).

Muscle atonia during NREM sleep as a marker of REM sleep need

Muscle atonia is one of the hallmarks of REM sleep. Brief episodes of muscle atonia have also been observed in human NREM sleep. Episodes of muscle atonia in NREM sleep (MAN) are most abundant in close proximity to an REM sleep episode indicating that they are functionally related to REM sleep rather than representing an epiphenomenon of NREM sleep (Werth *et al.*, 2002). Particularly high levels of MAN episodes were observed in the initial part of sleep that began in the morning, i.e., at a time when circadian REM sleep propensity was high, and in the initial part of nocturnal recovery sleep that followed selective REM sleep deprivation. It was proposed that episodes of MAN may represent not only a marker of homeostatic and circadian REM sleep propensity, but even be an REM sleep equivalent and contribute to the compensation of an REM sleep deficit. The latter may explain why rebounds in REM sleep were often found to compensate only partially for an REM sleep deficit.

Is REM sleep need related to NREM sleep or waking?

According to one view, the cyclic alternation of NREM and REM sleep episodes is the only relevant process that governs REM sleep homeostasis (Benington and Heller, 1994): REM sleep need would only build up during NREM sleep but not during waking, and it would decrease only during REM sleep. This view was based mainly on the analysis of rat sleep, and in particular on the observation that the number of pre-REM events, i.e., brief, incomplete transitions into REM sleep, increases in the course of an NREM sleep episode prior to a full transition into a sustained REM sleep episode. These pre-REM events were interpreted to be an expression of increasing REM sleep need during NREM sleep. The NREM sleep-related model of REM sleep homeostasis can explain a number of experimental observations, and it is consistent with the concept that the NREM–REM sleep cycle represents a sleep-dependent hourglass process rather than a clock-like oscillator.

There are other observations, however, that cannot convincingly be explained by an NREM sleep-related model of REM sleep homeostasis. They include the large rebounds in REM sleep that were found after extended total sleep deprivation both in humans (> 64 hours; Berger and Oswald, 1962; Kales *et al.*, 1970; Williams *et al.*, 1964) and animals (> 12 hours, e.g., Franken, 2002; Rechtschaffen *et al.*, 1999). In the rat, 24 hours vs. 12 hours of total sleep deprivation induced no measurable difference in NREM sleep rebound during recovery, but the 24-hour sleep deprivation induced a much greater REM sleep rebound than the shorter protocol (Franken, 2002). In humans, it was found that the distribution and total duration of REM sleep during nocturnal sleep was independent of whether or not a sizable amount of NREM sleep was allowed to occur in a preceding daytime bed rest (Whitehead *et al.*, 1969). Together, these data support the view that REM sleep need accumulates during both NREM sleep and wakefulness.

In an effort to resolve the contradictions between the two views of REM sleep homeostasis, it was proposed that the initiation and maintenance of REM sleep are controlled by two separate yet interacting processes (Franken, 2002). According to this model that was based on sleep in the rat, the NREM–REM sleep cycle is controlled by a short-term hourglass process whose level increases during NREM sleep and decreases during REM sleep, whereas the total amount of REM sleep is governed by a long-term process whose level increases during both NREM sleep and waking, and decreases during REM sleep.

Interdependence of REM sleep and NREM sleep

Mutual inhibition of the sleep states

REM sleep and NREM sleep are each homeostatically regulated, but the expression of the two states cannot occur at the same time. The NREM–REM sleep cycle can be viewed as a mechanism that allows for the controlled discharge of both REM sleep need and NREM sleep need. The cycle is thought to arise from the reciprocal interaction and mutual inhibition of several neuron populations in the brain stem (Lu *et al.*, 2006; for a recent review see McCarley, 2007). Inhibition of REM sleep by NREM sleep, in particular when the latter is of high intensity, became apparent also in sleep deprivation studies. In recovery sleep following one night of total sleep deprivation, SWA is greatly increased whereas the amount of REM sleep typically remains unchanged (Borbély *et al.*, 1981). When the bed rest is short such as in short sleepers, a night of total sleep deprivation can even result in reduced REM sleep during the first recovery sleep compared to baseline (Aeschbach *et al.*, 1996). An initial reduction in REM sleep and a delayed rebound over the course of several recovery sleep episodes have been found after extended total sleep deprivation (Berger and Oswald, 1962). The data illustrate that the discharge of NREM sleep pressure takes precedence over the discharge of REM sleep pressure. A sleep-dependent disinhibition of REM sleep, i.e., a gradual increase of the REM sleep fraction in the course of a sleep episode that is independent of a circadian influence, was demonstrated in the forced desynchrony protocol (Dijk and Czeisler, 1995). It is likely that the sleep-dependent decline in SWA contributes to the disinhibition of REM sleep (Borbély, 1982). The shorter REM sleep latencies and higher amounts of REM sleep in the early part of sleep in older people may be a consequence of diminished inhibition due to the age-related decrease in SWA (Bliwise, 1993).

Conversely, increased REM sleep pressure induced by selective REM sleep deprivation was reported to attenuate SWA (Beersma *et al.*, 1990). This finding may explain the small but significant reduction of

SWA at circadian phases during which REM sleep propensity is typically high (Dijk and Czeisler, 1995). Taken together, NREM sleep of increased intensity appears to have a substantial inhibitory influence on REM sleep, whereas the attenuation of NREM sleep intensity by increased REM sleep propensity is more limited.

REM density and homeostatic sleep pressure

Within a sleep episode, REM density increases over consecutive REM sleep episodes; this trend continues when sleep is extended beyond the regular baseline sleep duration (Aserinsky, 1969). This increase is not attributable to a circadian influence since it persisted when sleep occurred at different phases of the circadian cycle (Khalsa *et al.*, 2002; Zimmerman *et al.*, 1980). REM density was found to be inversely related to sleep depth as quantified by the prevalence of slow waves in the NREM sleep EEG (Feinberg *et al.*, 1987). Moreover, recovery sleep after sleep deprivation is associated with a decrease in REM density, and the extent of the decrease is proportional to the lost sleep (Aeschbach *et al.*, 1996; Feinberg *et al.*, 1987). On the other hand, selective REM sleep deprivation seems to have only a limited inhibitory effect on REM density in recovery sleep (Endo *et al.*, 1998). Thus, REM density appears to be related to the changes in homeostatic NREM sleep pressure rather than to changes in REM sleep propensity.

Conclusion

In conclusion, the circadian rhythm and the sleep-dependent disinhibition of REM sleep are the main factors that influence the distribution of REM sleep within a sleep episode. In humans that are normally entrained to the 24-hour day, the interaction of these two factors results in maximal REM sleep propensity in the morning, coinciding with habitual wake time. Studies using an extended bed-rest protocol have shown that spontaneous transitions from sleep to wakefulness occur more frequently out of REM sleep than out of NREM sleep, particularly when REM sleep episodes show high REM densities; this finding may reflect an increased level of a brain arousing process associated with REM sleep (Barbato *et al.*, 1994). Thus, the adequate phase relationship between sleep and the circadian pacemaker is important not only for the consolidation of sleep, but it may also enable the brain's optimal re-arousal by providing a gate to wakefulness (Lavie *et al.*, 1979).

REM sleep homeostasis is the third and least understood factor that influences the expression of REM sleep. Homeostatic responses can be induced by REM sleep deficits. But rebounds in REM sleep duration during recovery often do not match the amount of REM sleep that was lost. The reasons for this discrepancy are still unclear. Possible hypotheses that await further testing are: (1) that the homeostatic drive for REM sleep is weak and that not all REM sleep is necessary; (2) that there are compensatory changes in REM sleep intensity (of which e.g., reduced EEG alpha activity may be a marker); (3) that other components of sleep and wakefulness can serve as substitutes for REM sleep (e.g., stage 1 sleep; NREM sleep with muscle atonia; wakefulness with reduced EEG alpha activity). Advances in the research of REM sleep regulation will require new efforts aimed at understanding the properties of REM sleep homeostasis.

References

Aeschbach, D., Cajochen, C., Landolt, H.-P. & Borbély, A. A. (1996) Homeostatic sleep regulation in habitual short sleepers and long sleepers. *Am J Physiol* **270**: R41–53.

Aeschbach, D., Matthews, J. R., Postolache, T. T. *et al.* (1999) Two circadian rhythms in the human electroencephalogram during wakefulness. *Am J Physiol* **277**: R1771–9.

Aserinsky, E. (1969) The maximal capacity for sleep: rapid eye movement density as an index of sleep satiety. *Biol Psychiatry* **1**: 147–59.

Barbato, G., Barker, C., Bender, C., Giesen, H. A. & Wehr, T. A. (1994) Extended sleep in humans in 14 hour nights (LD 10:14): relationship between REM density and spontaneous awakening. *Electroenceph Clin Neurophysiol* **90**: 291–7.

Beersma, D. G. M., Dijk, D. J., Blok, C. G. H. & Everhardus, I. (1990) REM sleep deprivation during 5 hours leads to an immediate REM sleep rebound and to suppression of non-REM sleep intensity. *Electroenceph Clin Neurophysiol* **76**: 114–22.

Benington, J. H. & Heller, H. C. (1994) Does the function of REM sleep concern non-REM sleep or waking? *Prog Neurobiol* **44**: 433–49.

Berger, R.J. & Oswald, I. (1962) Effects of sleep deprivation on behaviour, subsequent sleep, and dreaming. *J Ment Sci* **108**: 457–65.

Bliwise, D. L. (1993) Sleep in normal aging and dementia. *Sleep* **16**: 40–81.

Borbély, A. A. (1982) A two process model of sleep regulation. *Hum Neurobiol* **1**: 195–204.

Borbély, A. A., Baumann, F., Brandeis, D., Strauch, I. & Lehmann, D. (1981) Sleep deprivation: Effect on sleep stages and EEG power density in man. *Electroenceph Clin Neurophysiol* **51**: 483–93.

Brunner, D. P., Dijk, D. J. & Borbély, A. A. (1993) Repeated partial sleep deprivation progressively changes the EEG during sleep and wakefulness. *Sleep* **16**: 100–13.

Cartwright, R. D., Monroe, L. J. & Palmer, C. (1967) Individual differences in response to REM deprivation. *Arch Gen Psychiatry* **16**: 297–303.

Czeisler, C. A., Zimmerman, J. C., Ronda, J. M., Moore-Ede, M. C. & Weitzman, E. D. (1980) Timing of REM sleep is coupled to the circadian rhythm of body temperature in man. *Sleep* **2**: 329–46.

Dantz, B., Edgar, D. M. & Dement, W. C. (1994) Circadian rhythms in narcolepsy: studies on a 90 minute day. *Electroenceph Clin Neurophysiol* **90**: 24–35.

Dement, W. C. (1960) The effect of dream deprivation. *Science* **131**: 1705–7.

Dement, W. C., Greenberg, S. & Klein, R. (1966) The effect of partial REM sleep deprivation and delayed recovery. *J Psychiatr Res* **4**: 141–52.

Dijk, D. J. & Czeisler, C. A. (1995) Contribution of the circadian pacemaker and the sleep homeostat to sleep propensity, sleep structure, electroencephalographic slow waves, and sleep spindle activity in humans. *J Neurosci* **15**: 3526–38.

Dijk, D. J., Shanahan, T. L., Duffy, J. F., Ronda, J. M. & Czeisler, C. A. (1997) Variation of electroencephalographic activity during non-rapid eye movement and rapid eye movement sleep with phase of circadian melatonin rhythm in humans. *J Physiol (Lond)* **505**(3): 851–8.

Dijk, D. J., Duffy, J. F., Riel, E., Shanahan, T. L. & Czeisler, C. A. (1999) Ageing and the circadian and homeostatic regulation of human sleep during forced desynchrony of rest, melatonin and temperature rhythms. *J Physiol (Lond)* **516**(2): 611–27.

Duffy, J. F., Dijk, D. J., Klerman, E. B. & Czeisler, C. A. (1998) Later endogenous circadian temperature nadir relative to an earlier wake time in older people. *Am J Physiol* **275**: R1478–R87.

Endo, T., Roth, C., Landolt, H. P. *et al.* (1998) Selective REM sleep deprivation in humans: effects on sleep and sleep EEG. *Am J Physiol* **274**: R1186–94.

Feinberg, I., Floyd, T. C. & March, J. D. (1987) Effects of sleep loss on delta (0.3–3Hz) EEG and eye movement density: new observations and hypotheses. *Electroenceph Clin Neurophysiol* **67**: 217–21.

Franken, P. (2002) Long-term vs short-term processes regulating REM sleep. *J Sleep Res* **11**: 17–28.

Horne, J. A. (2000) REM sleep-by default? *Neurosci Biobehav Rev* **24**: 777–97.

Kales, A., Hoedemaker, F. S., Jacobson, A. & Lichtenstein, E. L. (1964) Dream deprivation: an experimental reappraisal. *Nature* **204**: 1337–8.

Kales, A., Tan, T. L., Kollar, E. J. *et al.* (1970) Sleep patterns following 205 hours of sleep deprivation. *Psychosom Med* **32**: 189–200.

Kantor, S., Mochizuki, T., Janisiewicz, A. M. *et al.* (2009) Orexin neurons are necessary for the circadian control of REM sleep. *Sleep* **32**: 1127–34.

Khalsa, S. B., Conroy, D. A., Duffy, J. F., Czeisler, C. A. & Dijk, D. J. (2002) Sleep- and circadian-dependent modulation of REM density. *J Sleep Res* **11**: 53–9.

Lavie, P., Oksenberg, A. and Zomer, J. (1979) It's time, you must wake up now. *Percept Mot Skills* **49**: 447–50.

Lee, M. L., Swanson, B. E., de la Iglesia, H. O. (2009) Circadian timing of REM sleep is coupled to an oscillator within the dorsomedial suprachiasmatic nucleus. *Curr Biol* **19**: 848–52.

Lu, J., Sherman, D., Devor, M. & Saper, C. B. (2006) A putative flip-flop switch for control of REM sleep. *Nature* **441**: 589–94.

McCarley, R. W. (2007) Neurobiology of REM and NREM sleep. *Sleep Med* **8**: 302–30.

Mignot, E., Lin, L., Finn, L. *et al.* (2006) Correlates of sleep-onset REM periods during the Multiple Sleep Latency Test in community adults. *Brain* **129**: 1609–23.

Mistlberger, R. E., Bergmann, B. M., Waldenar, W. & Rechtschaffen, A. (1983) Recovery sleep following sleep deprivation in intact and suprachiasmatic nuclei-lesioned rats. *Sleep* **6**: 217–33.

Monk, T. H., Buysse, D. J., Carrier, J. & Kupfer, D. J. (2000) Inducing jet-lag in older people: directional asymmetry. *J Sleep Res* **9**: 101–16.

Rechtschaffen, A., Bergmann, B. M., Gilliland, M. A. & Bauer, K. (1999) Effects of method, duration, and sleep stage on rebounds from sleep deprivation in the rat. *Sleep* **22**: 11–31.

Tobler, I., Borbély, A. A. & Groos, G. (1983) The effect of sleep deprivation on sleep in rats with suprachiasmatic lesions. *Neurosci Lett* **42**: 49–54.

Webb, W. B. (1983) Are there permanent effects of night shift work on sleep? *Biol Psychol* **16**: 273–83.

Werth, E., Achermann, P., Borbely, A. A. (2002) Selective REM sleep deprivation during daytime. II. Muscle atonia in non-REM sleep. *Am J Physiol* **283**: R527–32.

Whitehead, W. E., Robinson, T. M., Wincor, M. Z. & Rechtschaffen, A. (1969) The accumulation of REM sleep need during sleep and wakefulness. *Commun Behav Biol* **4**: 195–201.

Williams, H. L., Hammack, J. T., Daly, R. L., Dement, W. C. & Lubin, A. (1964) Responses to auditory stimulation, sleep loss and the EEG stages of sleep. *Electroenceph Clin Neurophysiol* **16**: 269–79.

Wurts, S. W. & Edgar, D. M. (2000) Circadian and homeostatic control of rapid eye movement (REM) sleep: promotion of REM tendency by the suprachiasmatic nucleus. *J Neurosci* **20**: 4300–10.

Zimmerman, J. C., Czeisler, C. A., Laxminarayan, S., Knauer, R. S. & Weitzman, E. D. (1980) REM density is dissociated from REM sleep timing during free-running sleep episodes. *Sleep* **2**: 409–15.

Zulley, J. (1980) Distribution of REM sleep in entrained 24 hour and free-running sleep-wake cycles. *Sleep* **2**: 377–89.

Understanding REM sleep: clues from brain lesion studies

Jaime R. Villablanca and Isabel de Andrés

Summary

We have used the brain lesion method and chronically maintained cats to elucidate the contribution of key encephalic structures to the control of REM sleep. The results indicate that the physiological processes that participate in REM sleep generation and maintenance are all located in the pons, with the exception of those involved in REM sleep homeostasis. As we have shown, after a mesencephalic transection, REM sleep-deprived cats show a strong REM sleep pressure, but *rebound* does not occur. This finding indicates that the pontine mechanisms are modulated by a complex forebrain system, which, as we have shown, originates in the neocortex and has a powerful diencephalic stage. Part of this descending influence is a permissive mechanism for REM sleep rebound, which probably originates in the hypothalamus. Therefore the ultimate control of REM sleep *rebound* originates in the forebrain. This makes sense because it allows for a needed tight coupling with NREM sleep, which, as is well known, is also controlled by the forebrain. We have demonstrated that the electrocortical desynchronization induced by REM sleep is stronger that the one seen during waking (W), and this allows for REM sleep to accomplish what, we believe, is perhaps an REM sleep main function, i.e., to maintain the continuity of true sleep (S) given the limited duration of NREM sleep periods (by co-opting W at the end of NREM sleep periods).

Introduction

In this chapter, within the context of the literature, we review and discuss our lifetime work to examine, in the cat, the role of the different levels of the encephalon in the control of REM sleep. Ascending from the lower brain stem to the neocortex, the sections below critically analyze the contribution of each caudo-rostral encephalic level, studied in relative isolation, to the physiology of this fascinating sleep state. REM sleep is defined by using the standard behavioral, electroencephalographic (EEG), oculo-pupillary and electro-oculographic (EOG), electromyographic (EMG, neck muscles), and electrocardiographic (EKG/respiration) patterns that are typical for this state.

The brain stem and the decerebrate animal

In chronic bulbar cats, with a section between the rostral medulla and the lower edge of the pons, and in midpontine cats, with a section just caudal to the nucleus (n.) locus coeruleus (Figure 10.1), Siegel *et al.* (1986) described that, within a fluctuating decerebrate rigidity, quietness dominates, but it is interspersed with brief arousal periods (1–3 min), called phasic activation. Neuronal unitary firing, recorded from the n. gigantocellularis, increases during arousal/motor activation. The authors viewed these periods as a *crude*, primitive waking/arousal behavior alternating with periods of rest akin to drowsiness, but there was an absence of NREM sleep.

A more typical and integrated waking (W) and S behavior is displayed by cats with a section at the mesencephalic level (Figure 10.1c and *d*). Moreover, a high transection just rostral to the 3rd and 4th cranial nerve nuclei (Figure 10.1*d*) allows monitoring of the oculo-pupillary behavior that is typical of REM sleep (Berlucchi *et al.*, 1964).

Jouvet (1962) and ourselves (Villablanca, 1966) were the first to report the presence of REM sleep in cats with a transection in front of the pons. When undisturbed, high mesencephalic cats, in stable conditions and at least 15 days after transection, become quiescent

REM Sleep: Regulation and Function, eds. Birendra N. Mallick, S. R. Pandi-Perumal, Robert W. McCarley, and Adrian R. Morrison. Published by Cambridge University Press. © Cambridge University Press 2011.

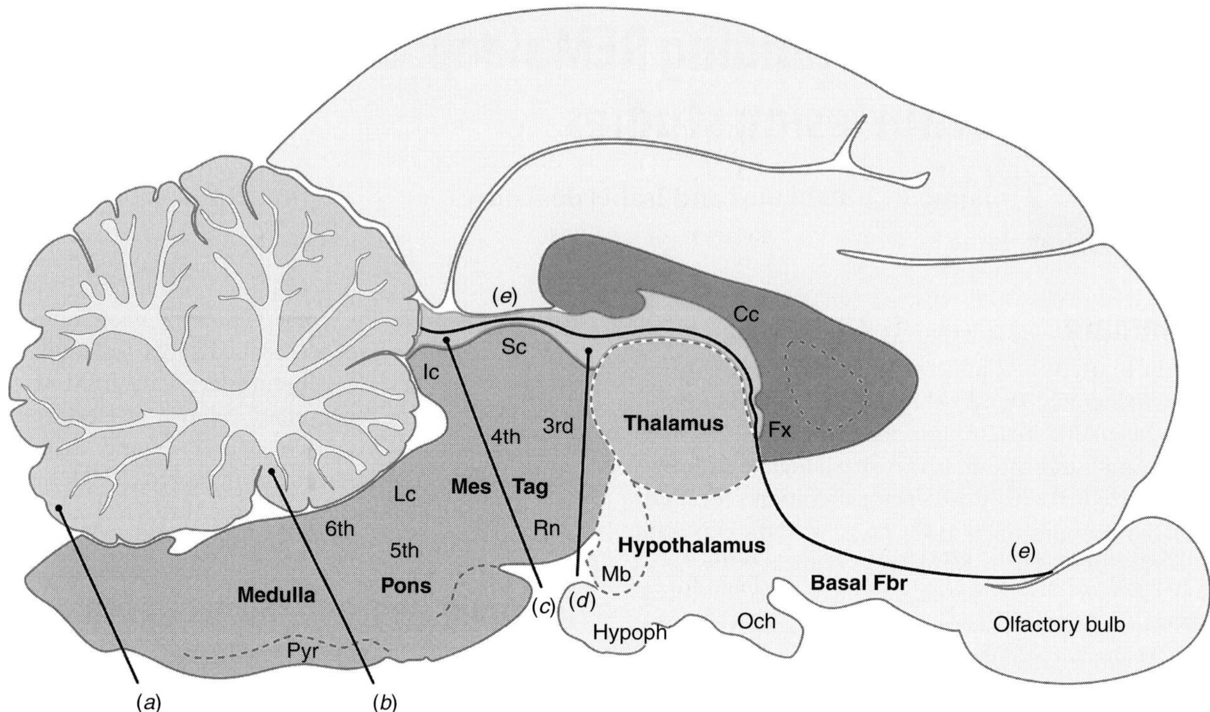

Figure 10.1 Schematic drawing of the midline surface of the cat brain as exposed by a midline sagittal section to illustrate the main transection levels discussed in this chapter. (*a*) spino-medullary: caudally, the spinal cat; rostrally, the isolated encephalon. (*b*) medullary-pontine: caudally, the bulbar or medullary cat. (*c*) mesencephalic inter-collicular (or lower in the midbrain): caudally, the low mesencephalic or pontine decerebrate cat; rostrally, the low isolated forebrain. (*d*) mesencephalic pre-collicular: caudally, the high mesencephalic decerebrate cat; rostrally, the high isolated forebrain. (*e*) telencephalon removed: diencephalic cat. The cerebellum is spared in all cases. In athalamic cats only the thalamus is removed bilaterally. Cc, corpus callosum; Fx, fornix; Hypoph, hypophysis; Ic, inferior colliculus; Lc, nucleus locus coeruleus; Mb, mammillary bodies; Och, optic chiasm; Pyr, pyramid; Rn, red nucleus; Sc, superior colliculus; 3rd, 4th, 5th, and 6th, represent the cranial nerves/ nuclei. The color emphasizes the main brain levels discussed. (See plate section for color version.)

and the pupils decrease in size, but this myosis is variable and fluctuates markedly (Villablanca, 1966). If the cat is undisturbed, the myosis progresses and becomes extreme (slit pupils), the eyeballs rotate downward and inward, the muscle tone decreases with drooping of the head, and quickly reaches total atonia with silence of the neck EMG. Bursts of clonic muscular activity appear over the entire body, but particularly in the face, originating rapid eye movements (as also recorded in the EOG), as well as minute fluctuations in pupil size. Typical ponto-geniculo-occipital (PGO) waves appear in the pontine reticular formation. Altogether, the cat is displaying a full-blown, typical REM sleep episode, which is undistinguishable from those in intact cats. Quantitatively, in our studies, REM sleep occupies 8.9% and 11.4% of the recording time in adult decerebrate cats (Villablanca, 1966) and in developing decerebrate kittens (see Villablanca, 2004), respectively (intact control cats: 11.0%).

If the midbrain is transected in kittens prior to REM sleep maturation (see Villablanca, 2004), i.e., before 40 days of age, all the behavioral and polygraphic REM sleep features develop normally and on a similar developmental timetable to that in intact littermates. Thus, REM sleep appears to be genetically programmed to develop independently from forebrain influences.

In terms of neurological syndromes in humans that may potentially disconnect the forebrain from the brain stem, as in our cats, chances are that midbrain or upper pons lesions very rarely result in a "clean transection" across the entire brain stem. However, it is known that the human brain stem pathologically disconnected from the forebrain, can display REM sleep, such that the typical postural decerebrate rigidity, which is present in many of these cases, dramatically melts away during REM sleep periods (Jouvet *et al.*, 1961).

An important feature in our decerebrate cats is that REM sleep can be triggered as a reflex. In our adult decerebrate cats the introduction of the tube for gastric feeding often induces REM sleep (Villablanca, 1966) and a similar effect is elicited by cutaneous and proprioceptive stimuli. In our mesencephalic kittens, slow, repetitive sounds almost regularly trigger REM sleep (see Villablanca, 2004). Therefore, this S stage has a striking *reflex component*. This phenomenon is reminiscent of cataplexy, a key narcolepsy symptom. Indeed, human cataplexy can be triggered by emotions as well as other stimuli (Guilleminault *et al.*, 1976), and in narcoleptic dogs, by feeding (Mittler *et al.*, 1974). It has been shown (Yamuy *et al.*, 2004) that activation of hypothalamic orexin/hypocretin neurons enhances the excitability and promotes discharges of spinal motoneurons in cats; since these hypothalamic cells are largely lost in human narcolepsy (Siegel, 2004) and since their axons are interrupted in midbrain transected cats, the Yamuy *et al.* (2004) findings may provide the cellular basis for the "reflex component" of REMS in decerebrate animals and in narcolepsy/cataplexy.

After selective, non-stressful, REM sleep deprivation in adult mesencephalic cats, a strong pressure (propensity) to enter REM sleep develops; however, the normal ensuing REM sleep *rebound* of intact cats is absent in these decerebrate cats (Figure 10.2; de Andrés *et al.*, 2003). Moreover, pharmacologically induced (using morphine) REM sleep deprivation in these same animals renders similar results (de Andrés and Corpas, 1991), and yet, the rebound is still present in intact cats after morphine. It is likely that the descending terminals from preoptic and the ventrolateral preoptic areas (VLPOA, see below) are involved in "permitting" the rebound.

The above data is important because it strongly suggests that: (i) pressure and rebound are two different components of the recovery process after REM sleep deprivation; (ii) these components are controlled via different mechanisms, with rebound *requiring* prosencephalic participation, while the brain stem suffices to sustain REM sleep pressure; (iii) since true NREM sleep is not present in decerebrate cats (see Villablanca, 2004), at least the pressure component of REM sleep recovery can not be deemed to depend on the previous occurrence of NREM sleep (Villablanca *et al.*, 2003), as some authors have proposed (Benington and Heller, 1999). The ultimate need for forebrain participation in the full control of REM sleep homeostasis is of particular interest since it suggests that, if there is a physiological need for REM sleep, this need is to benefit the forebrain and not the brain stem.

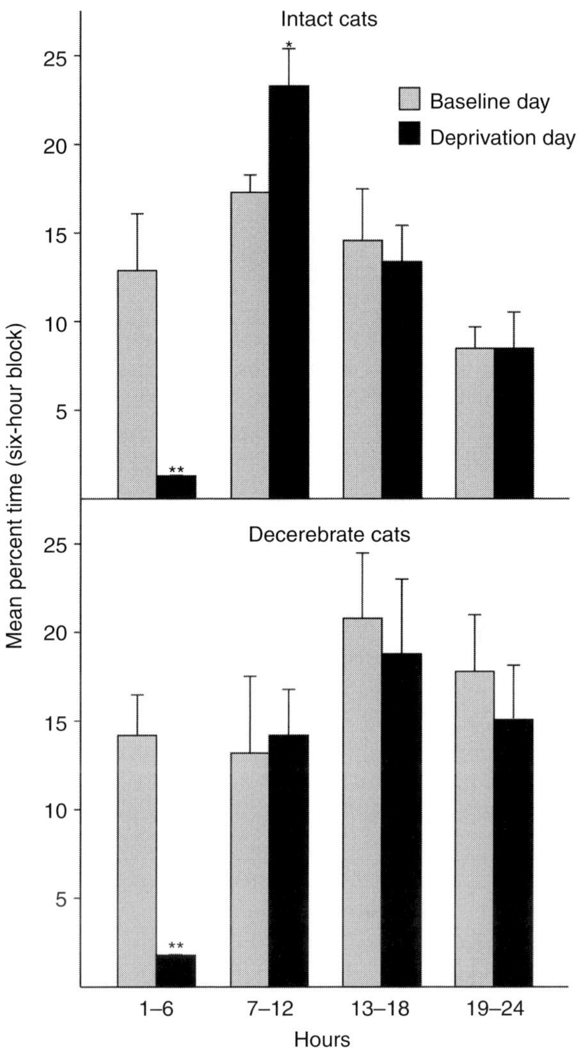

Figure 10.2 Illustrates the absence of rapid eye movement (REM) sleep rebound in decerebrate cats. The bars show that during the six-hour deprivation period (one- to six-hour block) there was a similar large reduction of REM sleep percentage time for both decerebrate and intact cats (**= p < 0.0001). During the six-hour deprivation (seven- to twelve-hour block) there was a significant increase (*= p < 0.05) in REM sleep time (rebound) only in intact but not in decerebrate cats. No other significant differences between the two groups were seen during the two remaining six-hour blocks of the remaining 24-hour recording session. (Reprinted with permission from *Sleep*, 2003, **26**: 419–25, Figure 3).

The diencephalic cat

In this animal model the telencephalon is surgically removed bilaterally, but the thalamus, hypothalamus, and basal forebrain are not damaged (Villablanca and Marcus, 1972). The ablation is followed by partial thalamic degeneration, and this opens a window into the

S–W role of the thalamus as the degeneration *progresses* during the early post-surgical days. In long-term adult cats with only one cerebral hemisphere removed, we reported that the volume of the ipsilateral thalamus decreases by 60%, and that this atrophy is due to widespread neuronal loss (see Villablanca, 2004). In similar hemispherectomized cats, Carreras *et al.* (1969) reported that the actual decrease in neuron counts starts by the tenth day, and a steady state is reached in about 180 days (a 62 to 67% decrease).

Diencephalic cats are usually up and walking by the second day post surgery and, from the start, they are spontaneously insomniac animals (Villablanca and Marcus, 1972). They are extremely active and self-destructive, but placing them in a circular corral with smooth walls and padded floor, precludes damage to the head and paws. Initially, they show obstinate progression and can walk continuously for many hours (a record 17 hours was noted for one cat). Hyperactivity decreases by 20 to 30 days, at least in terms of walking, but they remain restless throughout their survival (5 of our cats lived for 66 to 207 days).

The W behavior of diencephalic cats is certainly more complex than that of decerebrate animals to the point that some hints of awareness can be observed in the former cats. For example, in long-term diencephalic cats, olfactory stimuli elicit intense sniffing and searching, such that the animal can locate a can of fish placed as far as three to four yards away, can walk towards the food, and even initiate, albeit not sustain, eating. During W the electrothalamogram (EThG) shows a low-voltage (< 25 μV), fast (usually > 10 Hz) pattern similar to that seen in intact cats. Spindle waves are present in the EThG but only from four to five days after decortication and they occur in strict parallel with the onset of behavioral drowsiness (D). Beyond this short time period, and having lost its EEG-spindle signature, D is no longer the typical state of intact cats, and its onset and end are hard to determine.

Diencephalic cats exhibit REM sleep with all the typical behavioral and polygraphic features (Villablanca and Marcus, 1972) seen in intact animals. By the end of an episode of NREM sleep and while thalamic S spindles are still present, small amplitude pontine PGO waves and muscle atonia precede the end of spindling by several seconds; thereafter PGO waves become progressively larger and within 15 to 20 seconds they are grouped into complex bursts. By the end of REM sleep, spindles may reappear prior to reactivation of the EMG and cessation of the PGO bursts. By the time spindles are no longer present, REM sleep occurs following NREM sleep and cancels the EThG residual "wavelets" present at the time.

Besides the above qualitative S–W changes, diencephalic cats show impressive quantitative shifts. As already mentioned, throughout their survival these cats are markedly insomniac. We scored the mean amounts of REM and NREM sleep during 12, 24-hour sessions over six months. NREM sleep/24 hr declined progressively from 38% in control cats to 19%, 15%, 8%, and 7% on post-surgery days 5, 10, 20, and 30 respectively; while REM sleep went from 13.8% (controls) to 0.8%, 1.4%, 1.5% and 0.3%, respectively, on the same post-neodecortication days. For the remaining eight sessions the values for NREM sleep ranged between 1.9% and 5%, while the values for REM sleep fluctuated between 0.3% and 0.9% (all with little variability of the standard deviation).

The effects in these cats of a short-acting barbiturate are highly interesting (Villablanca, 1994; Villablanca and Marcus, 1972). Thiopental enhances EThG spindle bursts while they are still present, but fails to elicit them later on (once they have disappeared). In the long-term diencephalic cats a large amount of S is induced by a small thiopental dose (about 20% of that required to induce S in intact cats), a dose level that in control animals *depresses* S (Villablanca and Marcus, 1972). During a four-hour period after thiopental (Figure 10.3) diencephalic cats spend a mean of 51.3% and 33.0 % of the time in NREM and REM sleep, respectively, in sharp contrast with an average of 6.4 % (NREM sleep) and 0.9% (REM sleep) during the four-hour (control) period prior to drug administration (p < 0.005, Student's *t* test). We interpret this effect as a strong S *rebound*, which would indicate that S, and particularly REM sleep, is only spontaneously *suppressed*, but not permanently curtailed, in diencephalic cats.

The effect of opiates administration to diencephalic cats is also highly interesting. A single, low dose of morphine (1.5–2.0 mg/kg i.v.) induces first a brief autonomic stage followed by marked behavioral quietness (de Andrés, 1984) that lasts for about two hours. Thereafter the cats become hyperactive once again for a period of about six hours, and their motor activity becomes so vigorous that recordings must be interrupted. NREM sleep and REM sleep are suppressed for about four hours and seven hours, respectively. However, after this delay, there is a pronounced REM sleep rebound lasting throughout the second, third, and fourth post-morphine days and amounting to

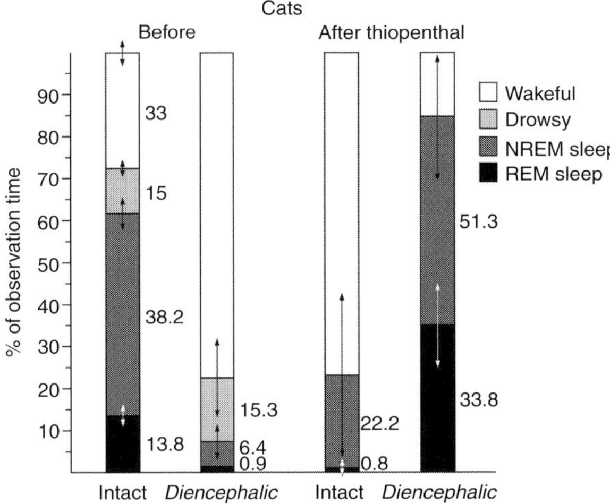

Figure 10.3 Illustrates the effects of thiopenthal in intact and diencephalic cats (8.3 mg/kg, i.p.). Numbers beside the bars indicate the average cumulative percentages for 13 experiments. Note the almost complete suppression of sleep in intact cats, which contrasts with the large REM sleep rebound in diencephalic animals. This shows that the insomnia in diencephalic cats is due to a functional suppression of sleep and it is not permanent. (Reprinted with permission from *Arch. Ital. Biol.* 1972, **110**: 348–82, Figure 11).

23.2%, 24.4%, and 14.9% per 24 hours, respectively). NREM sleep also rebounds, but only through the third day and to a lesser extent than does REM sleep. A similar dose in intact cats (de Andrés and Corpas, 1991; de Andrés *et al.*, 2003) suppresses S for about 12 hours and elicits a rebound that only affects NREM sleep and that lasts for about 12 hours. Therefore, it appears as if morphine pushes the already marked pre-drug REM sleep suppression in these cats to a total blockage. Once the action of morphine fades, the effect ends up in a protracted rebound.

Hyperactivity was a common finding in older studies of neodecorticate cats (e.g., Jouvet, 1962) and dogs (e.g., Kleitman and Camille, 1932). In addition, the nictohemeral periodicity typical of dogs' S was absent after decortication. In the only other study on effects upon NREM sleep *and* REM sleep (Jouvet, 1962), NREM sleep was almost entirely missing, whereas the REM sleep amount was within the normal range. However, it appears that, at difference with our animals, in Jouvet's cats the neostriatum and the limbic cortex were preserved.

The cat without the thalamus

The thalamus was removed bilaterally by pipette aspiration. The midline cortex was first penetrated to expose the corpus callosum, laterally, in order to reach the lateral ventricle via a transcallosal approach (thereby minimizing dorsolateral cortex damage, Villablanca and Salinas-Zeballos, 1972). The thalamus was then exposed and gently aspirated. Six athalamic cats were maintained for a median of 107 days (range 20–189 days). Histologically, thalamectomy was practically complete and additional damage was minimal (Villablanca and Salinas-Zeballos, 1972). Are athalamic cats the mirror image of diencephalic animals? To some extent they are, but not in all aspects.

These animals are also hyperactive and must be kept in a corral. They show pronounced gait ataxia, marked neck hyperextension, and dystonic postures. They are hard to maintain, progressively losing weight and showing increasing motor deterioration. During W the pupils are fully dilated and non-reactive to light (due to damage to the lateral geniculate nuclei). However, during S they show all the pupillary and ocular features seen in intact sleeping cats. Olfactory stimuli induce sniffing, but they can not locate the source of the stimulus. Little indications of awareness can be demonstrated in these animals, and this clearly sets them apart from the much more integrated diencephalic cats. Indeed, the overall behavior and neurological status makes these animals an excellent model for advanced stage fatal familial insomnia cases (e.g., Lugaresi *et al.*, 1986).

From the beginning, there is a pronounced EEG-behavioral dissociation since high-voltage slow waves dominate the electrocorticogram (ECoG). Only by ten days after thalamectomy do epochs of fast activity begin to appear in the ECoG during W, but prolonged periods of W rhythm are not present until 20 to 25 days post lesion. The dissociation decreases progressively, but never fully disappears. These observations indicate that the thalamus has a role in generating fast ECoG activity and the concurrent arousal.

When stopping motor activity athalamic cats lie down either sprawling or in a distorted crouching position. A further postural relaxation and decline in EMG activity together with the corresponding oculo-pupillary behavior, heralds the beginning of NREM sleep. A typical episode of REM sleep may follow indicating that all S stages are possible in these animals. Moreover, REM sleep pressure and rebound readily occur after deprivation showing that these events are not mediated by the thalamus. REM sleep occurs soon after thalamectomy, but as in W, there is also a lasting

REM sleep-ECoG uncoupling. However, it is interesting that ECoG fast activity is consistently seen earlier, by 15 days post thalamectomy, during behavioral REMS than during W, suggesting a stronger influence of REM sleep, compared to W, upon the ECoG. The finding of ECoG fast activity shows that, during REM sleep, the brain stem can activate the neocortex via an extrathalamic route.

Athalamic cats are also insomniac (Villablanca and Salinas-Zeballos, 1972). The mean amount of REM sleep time in the ten, 24-hour recording sessions (the first on day 5 and the last on day 180 post lesion) is markedly reduced ranging from 1.3 % to 3.5 % (controls, 13.8%).

In brief, in terms of REM sleep, changes are mainly quantitative for both diencephalic and athalamic cats. The effects upon NREM sleep, however, include in addition, marked qualitative changes, which render this state atypical for both animal groups, but in very different ways. Importantly, REM sleep (and NREM sleep) pressure and rebound are preserved in both animal groups.

Using the same experimental paradigm as in diencephalic cats, we found that a small dose of thiopental also produces a strong S rebound in these animals (Villablanca and Salinas-Zeballos, 1972). For REM sleep the values were a mean of 2.7% in the four hours prior to administration of the drug vs. 13.5% in the four hours post drug. For NREM sleep the values were 13.4% before and 50.7% after thiopental, respectively. These differences are highly significant (P < 0.005, Student's *t* test).

We know of only one other paper on the S–W effects of *total* thalamectomy (Naquet *et al.*, 1965). The ablation was performed via cortical penetration and the cats survived only two to four days. Spindle waves were absent from the outset. Behaviorally, the cats exhibited periods of "intense agitation", S–W was not quantified, but the authors stated that "the phase of sleep with fast activity was very short or may not exist at all." Perhaps the strongest support for our finding of insomnia in athalamic cats comes from the clinical literature. It is well known that extensive atrophy/degeneration of the thalamus, particularly of the nuclei medialis dorsalis and anterior ventralis, is at the core of the fatal familial insomnia syndrome (e.g., Guilleminault *et al.*, 1994), a disease that also courses with motor, autonomic, and hormonal hyperactivation (Lugaresi *et al.*, 1986). In addition, total insomnia lasting for 72 hours was recorded following bilateral stereotaxic thalamectomy in one patient (Bricolo, 1967).

Insomnia, sleep pressure, and rebound in diencephalic and athalamic cats

The most dramatic finding in diencephalic and athalamic cats was the persistent insomnia followed by the surprising discovery that this was not permanent, since just a small dose of barbiturate could trigger impressive REM sleep and NREM sleep rebounds. However, there is *no insomnia/hyperactivity in decerebrate cats*, and this indicates that, in these cats above, the S–W imbalance is created at ventral forebrain sites. We need, therefore, to very briefly review the role of these latter sites in the control of S–W.

The *S-promoting sites* are located in the ventrolateral preoptic area (VLPO; e.g., Saper *et al.*, 2001) and, more medially, in the anterior preoptic area or POA (e.g., McGinty and Szymusiak, 2001). Within the basal forebrain, the main contributor is the magnocellular nucleus. These cellular groups modulate S–W mainly via projections to the brain stem (e.g., McGinty and Szymusiak, 2003). Data from S deprivation studies in rats (e.g., Gong *et al.*, 2004) suggest that neurons from the median preoptic nucleus might be responsible for "permitting" REM sleep rebound in intact animals, and this would explain the absence of rebound in our decerebate cats (since those axons would have been interrupted).

The W-promoting sites include the (i) histaminergic neurons of the tuberomammillary nucleus, in the posterior hypothalamus, (e.g., McGinty and Szymusiak, 2003); (ii) orexin/hypocretin neurons in the periforniocal/lateral hypothalamus (e.g., Siegel, 2004); and (iii) cholinergic neurons of the basal forebrain (e.g., see Villablanca, 2004). These cellular groups project downstream to mesopontine sites and also, diffusely, to the neocortex.

Based on the above descriptions we would propose that: (i) the hypothalamic–basal forebrain S–W "switch" just described is controlled by telencephalic structures; (ii) this control normally facilitates the VLPO/POA S-promoting, inhibitory components of the "switch"; (iii) removal of the telencephalon disfacilitates this S-promoting process with a resulting disinhibition (or "release") of the posterior hypothalamus-mesopontine reticular formation W-promoting, excitatory side of the switch. The overwhelming consequence of the imbalance would then be behavioral hyperactivity and polygraphic W-arousal dominance with a strong, albeit *functional* suppression, of NREM and REM sleep. That the latter is indeed a functional imbalance is shown by the dramatic S rebound effect of low doses of barbiturate in diencephalic cats. This drug probably acts by depressing the excitability of the above arousal sites (much like the classical barbiturate blockage of the ascending reticular activating system). The probability that dominance of excitatory effects is involved is further supported by our experiments using morphine. It is well known that this opiate has strong excitatory effects in cats (e.g., de Andrés and Corpas, 1991), and we have reported (see Villablanca, 1994) that a single, small dose of morphine produces total and prolonged S suppression as well as behavioral agitation in diencephalic cats.

But why should there be insomnia in athalamic cats with an essentially intact telencephalon? As discussed above, there is no doubt that the thalamus has an important role in the generation of D and NREM sleep, and that spindle waves and delta oscillations, respectively, are most probably involved in this function. Thus, total/partial absence of the thalamus itself most probably underpins the insomnia in athalamic cats and humans with thalamic familial insomnia.

According to the above description, the processes for homeostatic regulation of NREM sleep are all within the forebrain and this is illustrated by the preservation of both sleep pressure *and rebound* after NREM sleep deprivation in diencephalic and athalamic cats. *In contrast*, only REM sleep pressure is seen in decerebrate animals after deprivation, showing that the homoeostatic control of this state is only partially located in the brain stem. Obviously, therefore, a "permissive" descending forebrain influence is needed to elicit a rebound. Because REM sleep rebound can still be elicited in diencephalic cats, we proposed (de Andrés *et al.*, 2003, Villablanca *et al.*, 2003) that this influence descends from the hypothalamus. The thalamus does not appear to play a direct role, since REM sleep rebound can also be elicited in athalamic cats. Therefore, it is likely that the same general S–W interactions that we discussed with regard to the putative hypothalamic S–W "switch," also operate to "permit" or to block the homoeostatic REM sleep rebound. Prime candidates for this descending regulation are pathways from: (i) the lateral hypothalamus orexin/hypocretin cell groups, which are largely lost in human narcolepsy

(e.g., Siegel, 2004); and (ii) the galaninergic neurons in the *extended* VLPO nucleus (Lu *et al.*, 2002). The hypothalamic arcuate (infundibular) nucleus appears to also be involved, at least in REM sleep rebound (Zhang *et al.*, 1987).

We argued that REM sleep pressure is independent of prior occurrence of NREM sleep. The evidence is less strong, but still substantial, for the notion that REM sleep *rebound* is also independent of NREM sleep. We reported (see above) that a *typical* NREM sleep does not exist in diencephalic cats and, regardless, a strong REM sleep rebound can be reliably elicited in these animals. Therefore, we are strongly inclined to believe that the presence of NREM sleep is also *not* required for the occurrence of REM sleep *rebound* (as further documented in Villablanca, 2004; Villablanca *et al.*, 2003), and that therefore, the accumulation of REM sleep pressure *and* its actual expression as a rebound, is the result of the absence of REM sleep *per se* rather than the consequence of an NREM sleep effect on REM sleep homeostasis, as suggested by others (Benington and Heller, 1999).

Specific sites in the telencephalon

The cerebral cortex. A role for this structure was suggested by the finding that low-frequency electrical stimulation of the frontal cortex induces S in cats (e.g., Peñaloza-Rojas *et al.*, 1964). We studied cats with bilateral removal of the frontal pole (Villablanca *et al.*, 1976) in front of stereotaxic plane A22. The S–W and motor activity were evaluated by means of 11, 24-hour polygraphic recording/observation sessions starting on post-surgical day 5 and repeated every 10 to 15 days for the first three months and every 10 to 30 days for three additional months. A significant, albeit moderate, reduction of REM sleep is seen when comparing the grand mean session values for the duration of the study between the afrontal (11.5% of recording time) and control (15.5%) cats. This reduction is coupled with a significant increase in W: afrontal (48.8%; control, 37.9%) and only a tendency to a decrease in NREM sleep. At least two studies on the effects of prefrontal lobotomy in nonpsychotic patients reported either a lasting increase in W time coupled with a decrease in NREM sleep time (Hauri and Hawkins, 1972), or a decrease in REM sleep (Hosokawa *et al.*, 1968).

The caudate nucleus. A number of studies reported induction of S and/or motor relaxation following cholinergic (Hernández-Peón *et al.*, 1967) or electric stimulation of the caudate nucleus in cats (e.g., Lineberry and Siegel, 1971), humans, and monkeys (Heath and Hodes, 1952). We assessed the S–W effects of bilateral caudate nucleus removal in cats. This procedure also alters the S–W pattern of the cats, but not permanently (Villablanca *et al.*, 1976). Comparisons of the partial grand means for the 24-hour sessions of the first post-lesion month show a significant reduction of REM sleep in acaudate cats (10.8%) relative to control animals (15.5%). Wakefulness significantly increases during this period, from 37.9% of the recording time in control cats to 58.2% in acaudate animals. There is only a tendency to a decrease in NREM sleep time.

The suppressing effect of caudate removal upon REM sleep lasts only for a couple of months and, hence, its meaning is hard to evaluate. However, these results complement those on the effects of caudate electrical stimulation cited above, and suggest a positive role of the caudate nucleus in promoting S.

The above results indicate that both the frontal cortex and the caudate are involved in controlling the level of central nervous system (CNS) activation. Thus, caudate ablation resulted in permanent hyperactive cats with a significant decrease in REM sleep time, which lasted for only two months, while the reverse was true for afrontal cats where the impact upon REM sleep was permanent. We have previously postulated the existence of an inhibitory telencephalic system balancing a powerful ventral diencephalic mechanism for W/arousal/motor activity. The above data suggest that the frontal cortex and the neostriatum are a part of this putative inhibitory system.

The hippocampus is another telencephalic structure that has been implicated in S–W control. Electrical stimulation induces S (Passouant and Cadilhac, 1962), or triggers S preparatory behavior in cats. Conversely, bilateral ablation of the hippocampus (Kim *et al.*, 1975) reduces the total time spent in both NREM sleep and REM sleep.

The common denominator in the above results is that ablation of any of the forebrain structures studied tilts the S–W balance towards W, while their electrical stimulation induces S. These observations suggest that the effect of removing telencephalic structures is unspecific and perhaps additive (see de Andrés *et al.*, 1984); i.e., obliteration of most of these sites would have a maximum impact, and this is what we have indeed found in diencephalic cats.

Altogether, the above results lead to the following conclusions:

(i) All the physiological processes involved in REM sleep generation and maintenance are located in the pons, except for the control of REM sleep homeostasis; indeed, following REM sleep deprivation in cats with a mesencephalic transection, there is a strong REM sleep pressure, but rebound does not occur.

(ii) The pontine processes involved in REM sleep control are modulated by a complex forebrain system originating in the neocortex and including a powerful diencephalic stage.

(iii) Part of this descending modulation is a permissive mechanism for REM sleep rebound to occur that probably originates in the hypothalamus.

(iv) Therefore, the ultimate control of REM sleep rebound originates in the forebrain, and this makes sense because it allows the tight coupling with the likewise forebrain-controlled NREM sleep, a coupling that is needed to ensure S continuity.

(v) The electrocortical desynchronization induced by REM sleep is stronger than the one seen during W; this allows for REM sleep to accomplish what we believe is one of REM sleep's main functions, i.e., to maintain the continuity of S given the limited, normal duration of NREM sleep episodes (by co-opting W at the end of NREM sleep periods).

Acknowledgments

This work was supported by USPHS Grants HD-05958 and HD-04612 (USA, J. Villablanca), and Grants MEC BFU006007430/BFI (Spain, I de Andrés). We appreciate D. Crandall's help with the illustrations.

References

Benington, J. H. & Heller, H.C. (1999) Implications of sleep deprivation experiments for our understanding of sleep homeostasis. *Sleep* **22**: 1033–37.

Berlucchi, G. *et al.* (1964) Pupil behavior and ocular movements during synchronized and desynchronized sleep. *Arch Ital Biol* **102**: 230–44.

Bricolo, A. (1967) Insomnia after bilateral stereotactic thalamectomy in man. *J Neurol* **30**: 154–8.

Carreras, M. *et al.* (1969) Residual neurons of the thalamic ventrobasal nuclei: a histological and electrophysiological study in the cat. *Arch Ital Biol* **107**: 570–603.

de Andrés, I. *et al.* (1984) Reassessing morphine effects in cats: II. Protracted effects on sleep-wakefulness and the EEG. *Pharmacol Biochem Behav* **21**: 923–8.

de Andrés, I. & Corpas, I. (1991) Morphine effects in brain stem-transected cats: II. Behavior and sleep of the decerebrate cat. *Behav Brain Res* **44**: 21–6.

de Andrés, I. *et al.* (2003) The disconnected brain stem does not support rapid eye movement sleep rebound after selective deprivation. *Sleep* **26**: 419–25.

Gong, *et al.* (2004) Activation of CABAergic neurons in the preoptic area during sleep and in response to sleep deprivation. *J Physiol* **556**: 935–46.

Guilleminault C., Dement W. C. & Passouant, P. eds. (1976) *Narcolepsy: Advances in Sleep Research.* New York: Spectrum.

Guilleminault, C. *et al.* eds. (1994) *Fatal Familial Insomnia Inherited Prion Disease, Sleep, and the Thalamus.* New York: Raven Press.

Hauri, P. & Hawkins, D. R. (1972) Human sleep after leucotomy. *Arch Gen Psychiat* **26**: 469–73.

Heath, R. G. & Hodes, R. (1952) Induction of sleep by stimulation of the caudate nucleus in macacus rhesus and man. *Trans Amer Neurol Assoc* **77**: 204–10.

Hernández-Peón, R. *et al.* (1967) Sleep and other behavioral effects induced by acetylcholine stimulation of the basal temporal cortex and striate structures. *Brain Res* **4**: 243–67.

Hosokawa, K. J. *et al.* (1968) Follow-up studies on the sleep EEG after frontal lobotomy. *Folia Psychit Neurol Jap* **22**: 233–43.

Jouvet, M. (1962) Recherches sur les structures nerveuses et les méchanismes responsables des différentes phases du sommeil physiologique. *Arch Ital Biol* **100**: 125–206.

Jouvet, M. *et al.* (1961) Etudes polygraphiques des différent phases des sommeil au course des troubles de conscience chronique (commas prolongés). *Rev Neurol* **105**: 181–6.

Kim, C. *et al.* (1975) Effects of hippocampectomy on sleep patterns in cats. *Electroenceph Clin Neurophysiol* **38**: 235–43.

Kleitman, N. & Camille, N. (1932) Studies on the physiology of sleep. VI. The behavior of decorticate dogs. *Am J Physiol* **100**: 474–80.

Lineberry, C. G. & Siegel, J. (1971) EEG synchronization, behavioral inhibition, and mesencephalic unit effects produced by stimulation of the orbital cortex, basal forebrain and caudate nucleus. *Brain Res* **34**: 143–61.

Lu J. *et al.* (2002) Selected activation of the extended ventrolateral preoptic nucleus during rapid eye movement sleep. *J Neurosci* **22**: 4568–76.

Lugaresi, E. *et al.* (1986) Fatal familial insomnia and dysautonomia with selective degeneration of thalamic nuclei. *N Engl J Med* **315**: 997–1003.

McGinty, D. & Szymusiak, R. (2001) Brain structures and mechanisms involved in the generation of NREM sleep: focus on the preoptic hypothalamus. *Sleep Res Rev* **5**: 323–42.

McGinty, D. & Szymusiak, R. (2003) Hypothalamic regulation of sleep and arousal. *Front Biosci* **8**: 1074–83.

Mittler, M. M. *et al.* (1974) Narcolepsy-cataplexy in a female dog. *Exp Neurol* **45**: 332–40.

Naquet, R. *et al.* (1965) Altérations transitoires ou définitives des zones diencéphaliques chez le chat. Leurs effects sur l'activité corticales et le sommeil. In *Aspect Anatomo-fonctionelle de la Physiologie du Sommeil*, ed. M. Jouvet. Paris: Editions de Centre Nationale de la Recherche Scientifique, pp. 107–31.

Passouant, P. & Cadilhac, J. (1962) Les rhythms theta hippocampiques au cours de sommeil. In *Physiologie de l'hippocampe.* ed. P. Passouant. Paris: C. N. R. S., pp. 331–47.

Peñaloza-Rojas *et al.* (1964) Sleep induced by cortical stimulation. *Exp Neurol* **10**: 140–7.

Saper, C. B., Chou, T.C. & Scammel, T. E. (2001) The sleep switch: hypothalamic control of sleep and wakefulness. *Trends Neurosci* **24**: 726–31.

Siegel, J. M. (2004) Hypocretin (Orexin): role in normal behavior and neuropathology. *Ann Rev Psychol* **55**: 125–48.

Siegel, J. M. *et al.* (1986) Behavioral states in the chronic medullary and midpontine cat. *Electroenceph Clin Neurophysiol* **63**: 274–88.

Villablanca, J. (1966) A behavioral and polygraphic study of "sleep" and "wakefulness" in chronic decerebrate cats. *Electroenceph Clin Neurophysiol* **21**: 562–77.

Villablanca, J. R. (1994) Role of the diencephalon in sleep rebound. In *Fatal Familial Insomnia: Inherited Prion Diseases, Sleep, and the Thalamus.* eds. C. Guilleminault *et al.* New York: Raven Press, pp. 143–59.

Villablanca, J. R. (2004) Counterpointing the functional role of the forebrain and of the brain stem in the control of the sleep-waking system. *J Sleep Res* **13**: 178–298.

Villablanca, J. R. *et al.* (1976) Effects of caudate nuclei or frontal cortex ablations in cats. II. Sleep-wakefulness, EEG and motor activity. *Exp Neurol* **53**: 31–50.

Villablanca, J. R. *et al.* (1984) Reassessing morphine effects in cats. I. Specific behavioral responses in intact and unilaterally brain-lesioned animals. *Pharmacol Biochem Behav* **21**: 913–21.

Villablanca, J. R. *et al.* (2003) Debating how rapid eye movement sleep is regulated (and by what). *J Sleep Res* **12**: 259–62.

Villablanca, J. & Marcus, R. J. (1972) Sleep-wakefulness, EEG and behavioral studies of chronic cats without neocortex and striatum: the 201C diencephalic 201D cat. *Arch Ital Biol* **110**: 348–82.

Villablanca, J. & Salinas-Zeballos, M. E. (1972) Sleep-wakefulness, EEG and behavioral studies of chronic cats without the thalamus: the "athalamic" cat. *Arch Ital Biol* **110**: 383–411.

Yamuy, J. *et al.* (2004) Hypocretinergic control of spinal cord motoneurons. *J Neurosci* **24**: 5336–45.

Zhang, J. X. *et al.* (1987) Abscence de rebound de sommeil paradoxale chez de rats hypophysectomisé et prétretés à la naissance par le glutamate de sodioum. *C R Acad Sci* **305**: 605–8.

Chapter 11
Preoptic and basal forebrain modulation of REM sleep

Kazue Semba

Summary

Although the basic mechanisms of REM sleep regulation are thought to reside in the brain stem, considerable evidence suggests that the forebrain, including the preoptic area and the adjacent basal forebrain (BF) as well as the hypothalamus, participates in the regulation of REM sleep. In this review we will first discuss findings that support the role of the preoptic area (POA) in REM sleep, with special focus on the ventrolateral preoptic nucleus (VLPO) and the median preoptic nucleus (MnPO). We will then review evidence for a role of the BF in REM sleep regulation and briefly discuss the role of the suprachiasmatic nucleus (SCN) in the circadian pattern of REM sleep. We will conclude with a view that the POA and BF house a continuum of distinct sleep–wake regulatory neurons with descending and ascending projections that interact with neurons in the posterior hypothalamus, brain stem, and cortex to regulate sleep and wakefulness, including REM sleep.

Since early transection studies, basic neural mechanisms responsible for the occurrence of REM sleep have been thought to reside in the pons, wherein the cyclic occurrence of REM sleep has been postulated to be controlled through the interaction between neurons that execute (REM-on) and those that block (REM-off) REM sleep. The ideas about the identity of these neurons have gone through several revisions. The current reciprocal interaction model focuses on cholinergic REM-on and monoaminergic REM-off neurons (Pace-Schott and Hobson, 2002), whereas the flip-flop model (Lu *et al.*, 2006) and a similar model (Sapin *et al.*, 2009) emphasize GABAergic/glutamatergic REM-on neurons in the sublaterodorsal nucleus and GABAergic REM-off neurons in the ventrolateral periaqueductal gray. Despite this focus on the brain stem for executive mechanisms of REM sleep, there is considerable evidence to suggest that the forebrain, in particular the hypothalamus as well as the POA and the adjacent BF, participates in REM sleep regulation. This review will focus on the role of the POA, including the VLPO and MnPO, and the BF in REM sleep regulation. The role of the SCN of the hypothalamus in the circadian pattern of REM sleep is also discussed briefly. According to the common usage, the BF here refers to those ventral forebrain regions that contain magnocellular cholinergic neurons (Semba, 2000).

The preoptic area

Ever since von Economo's finding in the 1930s of insomnia among patients with viral encephalitis that afflicted rostral ventral forebrain regions (von Economo, 1930), the POA has received much attention as a site that serves to induce sleep by actively inhibiting wake-promoting processes. This notion was corroborated initially by studies using lesions and stimulation (reviewed by Szymusiak *et al.*, 2007). More recently, single-unit recordings were used to demonstrate that the POA contains many neurons that show the highest levels of activity during both NREM and REM sleep, although a small population of neurons is most active during wakefulness (reviewed by Szymusiak *et al.*, 2007; see also Takahashi *et al.*, 2009). In addition, neurons that fire selectively during REM sleep were found throughout the POA in head-restrained rats (Koyama and Hayaishi, 1994), cats (Suntsova and Dergacheva, 2004, and mice (Takahashi *et al.*, 2009) but not in unrestrained rats (Szymusiak *et al.*, 1998). The latter authors speculated that this discrepancy occurs because neurons that are active in both REM sleep and wake could be mistaken for REM sleep-selective neurons if movement is suppressed by head restraint.

REM Sleep: Regulation and Function, eds. Birendra N. Mallick, S. R. Pandi-Perumal, Robert W. McCarley, and Adrian R. Morrison. Published by Cambridge University Press. © Cambridge University Press 2011.

The abundance of sleep-active neurons in the POA supports the notion that sleep is induced by active inhibition and not passively as a result of reduced arousal drive. One wake-promoting area that receives inhibitory input from the POA is the tuberomammillary nucleus; POA stimulation inhibited histaminergic neurons in this nucleus by activating $GABA_A$ receptors (Yang and Hatton, 1997). The POA also sends projections to brain-stem regions that are involved in sleep–wake regulation including REM sleep (Steininger *et al.*, 2001); stimulation of the POA influences the activity of some REM-on and other brain-stem neurons (Mallick *et al.*, 2004).

Sleep regulation and thermoregulation interact, and local warming of the POA increases sleep (reviewed by Szymusiak *et al.*, 2007). About half of the sleep-active neurons in the medial POA (MPOA) and fewer neurons in the lateral POA (LPOA) respond to increases in local temperature (warm sensitivity), whereas wake–active neurons tend to respond to decreases in local temperature (cold sensitivity). Ambient temperatures also modulate the occurrence of REM sleep (Cerri *et al.*, 2005), but the mechanisms underlying this modulation are not well understood.

The POA neurons with different firing patterns across sleep–wake cycles are not segregated anatomically. For example, neurons that fire selectively during REM sleep were mixed with other types of neurons in the MPOA in rats (Koyama and Hayaishi, 1994) and cats (Suntsova and Dergacheva, 2004), and spread throughout the POA and also in the BF in mice (Takahashi *et al.*, 2009).

Perhaps reflecting this anatomical overlap of various types of neurons, the effects of POA lesions are inconsistent, with insomnia occurring consistently only after relatively large lesions (reviewed by Szymusiak *et al.*, 2007). The studies comparing the effects of LPOA and MPOA lesions are also inconsistent. For example, a study using ibotenic acid reported that MPOA lesions had no long-lasting effects on sleep–wake patterns, whereas LPOA lesions resulted in insomnia with a significant decrease in NREM sleep (Schmidt *et al.*, 2000). REM sleep architecture was not significantly affected by either lesion. In contrast, a more recent study using N-methyl-D-aspartic acid (NMDA) reported that lesions of either MPOA or LPOA (encroaching the BF) reduced total sleep, but only MPOA lesions reduced REM sleep (Srividya *et al.*, 2006). Reversible inactivation with microinjection of a local anesthetic in either the MPOA or LPOA increased wakefulness during day, but the effect was greater with the MPOA injection (Alam and Mallick, 1990).

c-Fos immunohistochemistry allows for anatomical mapping of neurons that are activated during a certain behavioral state, and also permits the examination of the neurotransmitter phenotype and projections of activated neurons (Deurveilher and Semba, 2006). Once a region with a high concentration of c-Fos-immunoreactive neurons is identified, single-unit recordings and lesions can be used to characterize the functions of these neurons further. This approach has been taken to identify and study two regions in the POA that play important roles in the regulation of both NREM and REM sleep: the VLPO and the MnPO.

The ventrolateral preoptic nucleus

The VLPO was first identified as a cluster of c-Fos-immunoreactive neurons in a ventrolateral region of the POA in rats that had spent an average of 69% of their time sleeping during the hour before they were killed (Sherin *et al.*, 1996). A retrograde tracer injected into the tuberomammillary nucleus labeled these c-Fos-immunoreactive neurons in the VLPO cluster, as well as c-Fos-immunoreactive neurons that were diffusely distributed in regions dorsal and medial to the cluster (Sherin *et al.*, 1996). These scattered neurons were subsequently called the extended VLPO (Lu *et al.*, 2000). Most (~80%) of the c-Fos-immunoreactive neurons were GABAergic (Gong *et al.*, 2000) and also contained galanin, a neuropeptide with inhibitory action (Sherin *et al.*, 1998). These findings indicate that sleep-active neurons in the VLPO can release GABA and galanin during sleep to inhibit wake-promoting histaminergic neurons in the tuberomammillary nucleus.

The identification of the VLPO as a sleep-active area with c-Fos immunoreactivity was followed by single-unit recording studies. Szymusiak *et al.* (1998) recorded from neurons in the dorsal to ventral extent of the LPOA in rats across sleep–wake cycles and found that the neurons showing higher activity during both NREM and REM sleep compared to wakefulness were concentrated in a ventral region that corresponded to the VLPO cluster. This predominance (>50%) of sleep-active neurons was in contrast to the more dorsal regions of the LPOA, where neurons commonly fired at a higher rate during wakefulness than during NREM sleep. Interestingly, the activity of the ventral neurons increased as NREM sleep progressed from light to deep stages with increasing amounts of electroencephalogram (EEG) delta power. Upon entering REM sleep, the activity of some neurons decreased but this difference was not statistically significant as a group. During recovery sleep after 12 to 14 hours of sleep deprivation, these ventral neurons showed a further increase in firing compared to baseline sleep, but not when the animal was awake during the same recovery period, suggesting that the activity of VLPO neurons is not related to sleep pressure but to the occurrence and the depth of sleep.

Lesion studies investigated the role of the VLPO in sleep regulation further (Lu *et al.*, 2000). Bilateral lesions of the VLPO cluster with ibotenic acid (80–90% cell loss) resulted in a 50 to 60% decrease in NREM sleep and a 60 to 70% decrease in NREM EEG delta power, as well as ~60% decrease in REM sleep; the loss of c-Fos-immunoreactive neurons in the cluster was correlated with NREM sleep time and delta amount but not with REM sleep time. In contrast, lesions of the extended VLPO resulted in smaller decreases in NREM sleep (15–25%) and REM sleep (~35%), but the cell loss was highly correlated with REM sleep amount. These findings suggest that the mechanisms for NREM and REM sleep are anatomically segregated within the VLPO. This conclusion received further support from a study showing a high correlation of c-Fos immunoreactivity in the extended VLPO, but not in the cluster, after REM sleep enhancement with dark-pulse stimulation (Lu *et al.*, 2002).

These lesion and c-Fos studies did not distinguish between REM sleep amount vs. REM sleep pressure. This question was investigated by Gvilia *et al.* (2006a), who examined c-Fos immunoreactivity in rats immediately after REM sleep restriction (two hours; this procedure did not affect NREM sleep amount), and after recovery (one or two hours) following REM sleep restriction. Interestingly, both the VLPO cluster and the extended VLPO showed high levels of c-Fos not only under increased REM sleep amount, but also under increased REM sleep pressure when little REM sleep actually occurred. Furthermore, the c-Fos levels in both VLPO regions showed a stronger correlation with REM sleep pressure (i.e., increased attempts to enter REM sleep) than with REM sleep amount. The results were similar for both GABAergic and non-GABAergic neurons, except that a particularly high responsiveness to REM sleep pressure was seen in GABAergic neurons in the extended VLPO but not those in the cluster. These findings suggest that the VLPO is involved in the homeostatic regulation of REM sleep.

As mentioned above, most VLPO neurons that show c-Fos immunoreactivity during spontaneous or recovery sleep are GABAergic. To determine whether these neurons are responding to sleep pressure or to sleep amount, Gvilia *et al.* (2006b) compared the c-Fos immunoreactivity during spontaneous sleep, immediately after total sleep deprivation (two hours), and during recovery sleep after total sleep deprivation. It was found that GABAergic VLPO neurons were more active during spontaneous or recovery sleep than immediately after the sleep deprivation, suggesting a role of GABAergic VLPO neurons in maintaining and stabilizing sleep.

Various molecules affect the activity of VLPO neurons, including transmitters of wake-promoting neurons in the hypothalamus and brain stem, which likely act to inhibit or disfacilitate the activity of VLPO neurons during wakefulness (reviewed by Szymusiak and McGinty, 2008). In addition, several endogenous sleep-promoting molecules, such as adenosine and prostaglandin D_2, activate VLPO neurons directly or indirectly (reviewed by Szymusiak and McGinty, 2008). However, because these molecules increase both NREM and REM sleep, it is unclear whether the promotion of REM sleep is a direct effect.

The different roles of the VLPO cluster and the extended VLPO in NREM and REM sleep would suggest different projections, and there is some evidence to support this possibility. The VLPO cluster projects heavily to the tuberomammillary nucleus, and less heavily to the lateral hypothalamus (Sherin *et al.*, 1998), which houses neurons containing orexin and melanin-concentrating hormone, two peptides with a role in REM sleep as well as other functions. The VLPO cluster projects further caudally to the midbrain raphe nuclei and the locus coeruleus, which both contain monoaminergic neurons with a permissive role for REM sleep as well as a role in promoting wake (Sherin *et al.*, 1998; Steininger *et al.*, 2001). These projections provide the basis for the flip-flop model of sleep and wake (Saper *et al.*, 2001). Additionally, the VLPO cluster projects to the BF and mesopontine tegmentum, which contain cholinergic neurons that are active during REM sleep or during both REM sleep and wakefulness (Sherin *et al.*, 1998). However, the projections to the sublaterodorsal nucleus or the ventrolateral periaqueductal gray region, two brain-stem sites more recently implicated in REM sleep (see above), appear to be sparse (see Figure 5 in Sherin *et al.*, 1998). In contrast, the extended VLPO projects heavily to the ventrolateral periaqueductal gray region (Lu *et al.*, 2006). The extended VLPO also sends heavier projections than the VLPO cluster to the dorsal raphe nucleus, locus coeruleus, and laterodorsal tegmental nucleus, and about half of these afferent VLPO neurons are GABAergic (Lu *et al.*, 2002).

To summarize, the VLPO contains GABAergic neurons that increase activity in correlation with the depth of NREM sleep and EEG delta power, suggesting their role in the maintenance of sleep. Consistent with this role, lesions of the VLPO cluster decrease sleep and the cell loss is correlated with a decrease in NREM sleep amount. In addition, some VLPO neurons, including both GABAergic and non-GABAergic neurons in the VLPO cluster and GABAergic neurons in the extended VLPO, are responsive to REM sleep pressure, and the loss of neurons in the extended VLPO correlates with a reduction in REM sleep amount, suggesting a role of the VLPO in REM sleep homeostasis. The VLPO is anatomically well positioned to receive various humoural inputs, and to inhibit wake-promoting and REM-off neurons in the hypothalamus and brain stem, thus promoting and consolidating both NREM and REM sleep.

The median preoptic nucleus

Subsequent to the discovery of the VLPO, the MnPO was identified as another site within the POA that contains a high concentration of sleep-responsive neurons in the rat (Gong *et al.*, 2000). Although the nucleus has been implicated in various autonomic regulations, this was the first study to report a role of the MnPO in sleep regulation, a conclusion supported by subsequent studies.

The discharge pattern of MnPO neurons across sleep–wake cycles was investigated using single-unit recording in unrestrained rats (Suntsova *et al.*, 2002). A majority (58%) of all recorded neurons showed increased activity during both NREM and REM sleep relative to wakefulness, whereas 10% and 8% of recorded neurons showed selective activation during NREM and REM sleep, respectively. Thus, as many as 75% of all neurons recorded in the MnPO were sleep active. In addition, 12% of recorded neurons were more active during wake and REM sleep than during NREM sleep.

Interestingly, most of the predominant, NREM/REM-active neurons in the MnPO were more active during REM sleep than during NREM sleep (Suntsova *et al.*, 2002), suggesting a specific role for REM sleep regulation. A small group of NREM/REM-related MnPO neurons, however, were slightly less active during REM compared to NREM sleep, a pattern more typical of VLPO cluster neurons. Most NREM/REM-related neurons also increased firing gradually well before NREM sleep onset. When examined across successive NREM sleep episodes, these neurons showed a gradual decrease in firing rate from the first to the last NREM sleep episode; the activity also gradually decreased, rather than increased as in the case of VLPO neurons, within a single NREM sleep episode, and also during a single REM sleep episode, suggesting a role in promoting NREM and REM sleep under homeostatic pressure. MnPO neurons did not show any change in activity in relation to EEG spindles or delta activity during NREM sleep or theta activity during REM sleep. However, REM sleep-related MnPO neurons showed burst activities in phase with EEG theta waves during REM sleep.

The possibility that MnPO neurons have a specific role in REM sleep regulation was investigated by Gvilia *et al.* (2006a) by comparing c-Fos immunoreactivity during spontaneous sleep, and after REM sleep restriction (two hours) with or without recovery (two hours; the results for the VLPO in the same study were discussed above). The numbers of c-Fos-immunoreactive MnPO neurons were higher both at the end of REM sleep restriction and during the first hour of recovery than during a period of high spontaneous REM sleep. Furthermore, c-Fos immunoreactivity was strongly correlated with the number of attempts to enter REM sleep. Thus, the MnPO is responsive to REM sleep pressure, although the possibility that the c-Fos was correlated with REM sleep onset, rather than REM sleep pressure, cannot be excluded. Interestingly, only 22 to 26% of the c-Fos-immunoreactive neurons in REM sleep-restricted rats were GABAergic, suggesting that glutamatergic MnPO neurons are specifically involved in REM sleep homeostasis. When REM sleep pressure increases, these neurons might activate the REM sleep executive neuronal network in the brain stem.

In a subsequent study, Gvilia *et al.* (2006b) used total sleep deprivation and recovery sleep conditions to distinguish sleep pressure and sleep amount, and found that GABAergic MnPO neurons showed greater c-Fos immunoreactivity in response to increased sleep pressure than to increased sleep amount. In contrast, GABAergic VLPO neurons were, as described above, more responsive to increased sleep amount than to increased sleep pressure. Sleep-related MnPO neurons were separate from non-GABAergic osmosensitive neurons, which are also present in the MnPO (Gvilia *et al.*, 2005). Some interaction, however, is implicated by a selective reduction in REM sleep after intracerebroventricular injection of angiotensin II, which activates osmosensitive glutamatergic neurons in the MnPO (Gvilia *et al.*, 2005). Collectively, these findings suggest that a distinct population of neurons in the MnPO responds to increased sleep pressure, and glutamatergic and GABAergic neurons within this population may respond somewhat differently to increased pressure for REM vs. NREM sleep.

It is noteworthy that the activity pattern of NREM/REM-related neurons in the MnPO described above (Suntsova *et al.*, 2002) was the opposite of the activity pattern of wake-promoting monoaminergic neurons in the brain stem, suggesting that these MnPO neurons, particularly those that are GABAergic, might inhibit these brain-stem regions during sleep (reviewed by Szymusiak and McGinty, 2008). This possibility is supported by the presence of dense anterograde labeling in the perifornical lateral hypothalamus and locus coeruleus from the MnPO (Uschakov *et al.*, 2007). Axon labeling was also present in the dorsal raphe nucleus, extending laterally into the ventrolateral periaqueductal gray region (REM-off), and in the sublaterodorsal nucleus (REM-on; Figures 6 and 7 in Uschakov *et al.*, 2007). MnPO stimulation inhibited wake-active neurons and activated sleep-related neurons in the perifornical lateral hypothalamus (Suntsova *et al.*, 2007). The projections from the MnPO to the BF and the mesopontine tegmentum are relatively sparse, and do not appear to be directed to cholinergic neurons (Uschakov *et al.*, 2006, 2007). Importantly, the MnPO also projects to the VLPO cluster and, less heavily, to the extended VLPO (Chou *et al.*, 2002; Uschakov *et al.*, 2006, 2007). These findings indicate that the MnPO is anatomically well situated to influence sleep/wake regulatory mechanisms in both the forebrain and brain stem.

In summary, like the VLPO, the MnPO contains a large population of both GABAergic and non-GABAergic neurons that are active during sleep. Unlike VLPO neurons, however, MnPO neurons that are GABAergic are more responsive to sleep pressure than to sleep amount. In addition, non-GABAergic neurons in the MnPO are responsive to REM sleep pressure, suggesting a role in REM sleep homeostasis. MnPO neurons project to wake-promoting and REM sleep-regulatory areas in the hypothalamus and brain stem, and through these pathways, they are likely to promote transitions from waking to sleep when sleep pressure is high; once sleep is initiated, the VLPO can act to consolidate and stabilize sleep. Thus, the MnPO and VLPO appear to cooperate in promoting both NREM and REM sleep.

The basal forebrain

The BF consists of a series of nuclei that house a longitudinal column of magnocellular cholinergic neurons (reviewed by Semba, 2000). Most studies on the role of the BF in sleep–wake regulation have focused on middle to caudal levels of the BF, including the magnocellular preoptic nucleus and substantia innominata, which are located just lateral to the POA, and the more caudal magnocellular basal nucleus. These regions contain cholinergic, GABAergic, and putative glutamatergic neurons that project, mostly independently, to the neocortex and various subcortical regions. Many of these targets are involved in sleep–wake regulation, including the perifornical lateral hypothalamus, posterior hypothalamus, and mesopontine tegmentum. The amygdala, another target, plays a role in REM sleep via its descending projections to the dorsolateral tegmentum. Possible BF projections to the recently implicated REM sleep-regulatory areas in the pons (the ventrolateral periaqueductal gray and sublaterodorsal nucleus) remain to be examined.

The predominant pattern of state-dependent activity observed in BF neurons is high levels of activity during both wake and REM sleep compared to during NREM sleep. This pattern is commonly observed in the POA medial to the BF, but uncommon in the VLPO or MnPO. The proportion of neurons showing this pattern, as well as the proportions of other neuronal types, in the BF varies somewhat among studies using different recording conditions and animal species. Szymusiak and McGinty (1986), recording from unrestrained cats, found that about half (48%) of recorded neurons were more active during both wakefulness and REM sleep compared to NREM sleep. In addition, a quarter (24%) of recorded neurons were more active during NREM sleep than during wakefulness and REM sleep; these neurons increased firing prior to transition from wake to NREM sleep and tended to be located ventrally within the BF. Using a test for antidromic activation, some of both types of neurons were found to project to the cortex or midbrain reticular formation (Szymusiak and McGinty, 1989). Somewhat different results were obtained from head-restrained rats (Lee *et al.*, 2004); neurons that were maximally active during REM sleep (49%) or during both REM sleep and wake

(12%) together represented more than half of recorded neurons. These neurons fired in positive correlation with EEG theta and gamma activities, suggesting a role in promoting cortical activation. Some of these neurons also fired in negative correlation with EMG amplitude, suggesting a possible role in postural muscle atonia during REM sleep. REM and REM/wake-active neurons were also commonly found in the BF (as well as in the POA) of head-restrained mice (Takahashi *et al.*, 2009).

The juxtacellular labeling technique allows for identification of the neurotransmitter phenotype of physiologically characterized neurons in vivo. Cholinergic BF neurons were found to be most active during wake and REM sleep and fired in association with EEG theta and gamma activities, consistent with their long-presumed role in cortical activation (Lee *et al.*, 2005). GABAergic BF neurons were heterogeneous: 36% were similar to cholinergic neurons, being most active during wake and REM sleep with a positive correlation with gamma activity, whereas 28% were most active during NREM sleep with a positive correlation with delta activity; 36% fired maximally during REM sleep in negative correlation with EMG (Hassani *et al.*, 2009). In addition to cholinergic and GABAergic neurons, there were putatively glutamatergic neurons, about half (46%) of which were most active during wake and REM sleep, 14% during wake, 17% during NREM sleep, and 17% during REM sleep (Hassani *et al.*, 2009). The GABAergic and glutamatergic REM-active BF neurons may selectively promote REM sleep or its components, such as muscle atonia, through their descending projections to the hypothalamus and brain stem, while activating the cortex via their ascending projections.

Consistent with these neurophysiological results, the c-Fos immunoreactivity in cholinergic neurons was highest during spontaneous or forced wakefulness in rats (McKenna *et al.*, 2009). The c-Fos immunoreactivity during REM sleep was not studied, but acetylcholine released in the cortex, which is derived from the BF, is known to be elevated during both wake and REM sleep, suggesting increased activities of these neurons in these two behavioral states associated with cortical activation. When c-Fos immunoreactivity in the POA and the adjacent BF was examined after three hours of total sleep deprivation, 12% of cholinergic neurons (BF) and 17% of GABAergic neurons (BF and POA) were c-Fos positive; after three hours of recovery, no cholinergic neurons were c-Fos positive, whereas 41% of GABAergic neurons were c-Fos positive; these latter neurons were also immunoreactive for α2-adrenergic

receptors, suggesting that they can be inhibited by noradrenaline during wake (Modirrousta *et al.*, 2004).

Various neurotoxins have been used to study the role of the BF in sleep–wake and cortical activation. Although an early study reported insomnia after kainate lesions of the horizontal limb region, LPOA, and substantia innominata (Szymusiak and McGinty, 1986), subsequent studies using more laterally placed BF lesions with kainate (Stewart *et al.*, 1984), ibotenate (Kaur *et al.*, 2008), or a cholinergic neuron-selective immunotoxin (Kaur *et al.*, 2008) reported no changes in the amount of sleep or wake. Rather, these kainate or ibotenate lesions consistently increased EEG slow waves, an effect demonstrated to be mostly due to loss of non-cholinergic, as opposed to cholinergic, BF neurons (Kaur *et al.*, 2008). Thus, while the BF may not have an exclusive role in modulating the amount of sleep or wake, it has a critical role in cortical activation.

The BF receives various transmitter inputs from the ascending projections originating in wake-modulatory nuclei in the brain stem and hypothalamus (reviewed by Semba, 1991), and attempts have been made to determine the role of these transmitters acting in the BF in modulating cortical EEG and behavioral states. Intra-BF administrations of NMDA, AMPA (Manfridi and Mancia, 1996; Cape and Jones, 2000; Wigren *et al.*, 2007), noradrenaline (Cape and Jones, 1998), orexin (España *et al.*, 2001), and histamine (Ramesh *et al.*, 2004) all increased behavioral arousal, often with increased EEG gamma and EMG activities, and decreased sleep amount and EEG delta power. In contrast, microinjections of GABA$_A$ or GABA$_B$ agonists into the BF increased NREM sleep; the GABA$_A$ agonist additionally decreased REM sleep (Manfridi *et al.*, 2001). These results suggest that wake/REM-related BF neurons are activated by wake-promoting ascending inputs during wake, and inhibited by GABA during NREM sleep. The GABAergic input might originate in the POA, or in putative sleep-active GABAergic interneurons within the BF.

An early study reported induction of REM sleep after injections of acetylcholine or carbachol crystals into the POA-BF region (Hernández-Peón *et al.*, 1963). Interestingly, carbachol injections into the rostral BF triggered cataplexy in narcoleptic dogs (Nishino *et al.*, 1995). Consistent with these findings, acetylcholine release in the BF was highest during REM sleep (Vazquez and Baghdoyan, 2001); the possible sources of acetylcholine released in the BF are the terminals of mesopontine cholinergic neurons, which are known to be REM- or wake/REM-active, and local axon collaterals of cholinergic BF neurons. Incongruently with these previous findings, microinjections of carbachol into middle (Baghdoyan *et al.*, 1993; Nishino *et al.*, 1995), and caudal (Manfridi and Mancia, 1996) levels of the BF in the cat, rat, and dog consistently promoted wakefulness and reduced spontaneous or pharmacologically induced REM sleep. The reason for this discrepancy is not clear.

Neurotensin is an interesting neuropeptide that selectively binds to cholinergic BF neurons and has an excitatory action. Intra-BF microinjection of neurotensin resulted in significant increases in REM sleep and transitional REM sleep, and a decrease in NREM sleep; the EEG was also activated (increased theta and gamma and decreased delta) but there was no change in EMG activity (Cape *et al.*, 2000). Interestingly, REM sleep induced by neurotensin microinjections occurred directly from (usually quiet) wake, and wake and REM sleep often alternated. Thus, neurotensin appears to have a unique ability to promote REM sleep by selectively activating cholinergic neurons in the BF.

There is substantial evidence that the BF is involved not only in promoting behavioral and cortical activation, but also in recovery sleep after prolonged wakefulness; underlying mechanisms appear to involve adenosine, an endogenous somnogen (Basheer *et al.*, 2004; Porkka-Heiskanen *et al.*, 2003). One molecule acting upstream to the adenosine increase is nitric oxide (Kalinchuk *et al.*, 2006c), and nitric oxide production in the BF is required for rebound sleep to occur after total sleep deprivation (Kalinchuk *et al.*, 2006a). Of the three isoforms of nitric oxide synthase (NOS), iNOS is critical for NREM sleep recovery, whereas nNOS is essential for REM sleep recovery (Kalinchuk *et al.*, 2006b). Furthermore, cholinergic BF neurons are required for the increases in nitric oxide and adenosine in the BF during total sleep deprivation (Kalinchuk *et al.*, 2008), and both cholinergic and noncholinergic BF neurons play a role in the recovery of NREM, but not REM, sleep after total sleep deprivation (Kaur *et al.*, 2008).

In summary, unlike in the VLPO and MnPO, the majority of neurons in the BF show activity patterns consistent with a role in the promotion of behavioral and cortical activation during wake, and cortical activation and possibly muscle atonia during REM sleep. The BF receives ascending wake-promoting projections from the hypothalamus and brain stem. Several transmitters of these projections can act in the BF to induce behavioral arousal accompanied by EEG activation. In addition, neurotensin can increase REM sleep presumably by activating cholinergic BF neurons. The promotion of behavioral and cortical activation as well as REM sleep is likely mediated by the BF's multiple, independent output pathways to the sleep/wake-regulatory neurons in the hypothalamus, amygdala, and brain stem.

The suprachiasmatic nucleus

A prominent feature of the organization of sleep and wake is their diurnal rhythms. The amount of REM sleep reaches its maximum during the late rest phase, whereas NREM sleep peaks earlier in the rest phase; increased vigilance occurs during the active phase. This sleep–wake rhythm is thought to be the result of interaction between circadian and homeostatic processes (reviewed by Mistlberger *et al.*, 2000). The circadian process is governed by the principal circadian clock in the SCN in mammals. The circadian clock promotes wakefulness, REM sleep, and some aspects of NREM sleep at specific times of day. The homeostatic process keeps track of prior wakefulness, or sleep need. Consistent with this two-process model, lesions of the SCN abolish circadian sleep–wake patterns but usually have no effects on the amounts of wake, NREM, or REM sleep.

The pathways and mechanisms involved in the circadian regulation of sleep and wake are beginning to be understood. The direct projections from the SCN are largely confined to the hypothalamus and do not reach most of the sleep–wake systems. However, studies using dual tract tracing or transsynaptic tracing have demonstrated that several direct targets of SCN projections, in particular the dorsomedial hypothalamic nucleus, subparaventricular zone, and MPOA may serve as intermediary nuclei to convey the circadian signal indirectly to the VLPO and MnPO, BF, perifornical lateral hypothalamus, tuberomammillary nucleus, and monoaminergic and cholinergic nuclei of the brain stem (reviewed by Saper *et al.*, 2005; see also Deurveilher and Semba, 2005). It is plausible that the SCN also projects indirectly to the ventrolateral periaqueductal gray and sublaterodorsal nucleus. Furthermore, lesions of the dorsomedial hypothalamic nucleus and the subparaventricular zone disrupt the circadian pattern of sleep–wake and the circadian activity of locus coeruleus neurons (reviewed by Saper *et al.*, 2005), consistent with synaptic relay of circadian signals in these nuclei.

One interesting, emerging feature of the output organization of the SCN is that functionally different SCN neurons may be segregated, as shown for the SCN neurons that influence sympathetic vs. parasympathetic functions (Buijs *et al.*, 2003). Thus, SCN neurons that promote REM sleep might be distinct from those that promote wakefulness. Consistent with this possibility, a recent study localized the circadian timing of REM sleep to an oscillator within the dorsomedial region of the rat SCN (Lee *et al.*, 2009). These REM sleep-promoting SCN neurons might use specific indirect output pathways to the hypothalamus and brain stem to inhibit REM-off and activate REM-on neurons at a specific circadian time, i.e., in the late rest phase. This process may also be coordinated by appropriately timed inputs from the REM sleep-regulatory network to these SCN neurons.

Perspectives

The POA and the adjacent BF contain a spectrum of neurons that increase firing during specific behavioral state or states, or specific aspects of a behavioral state, such as EMG activity and cortical activation. The majority of POA and BF neurons appear to be involved in promoting both wake and REM sleep or related cortical and motor activation. However, sleep-active neurons are also present in both the POA and BF, and they are usually mixed with the predominant, wake/REM-active neurons. In addition, sleep-active neurons occur in a high concentration in the VLPO and MnPO, and neurons in these nuclei appear to have different roles. VLPO neurons likely play a role in maintaining and consolidating sleep, whereas MnPO neurons appear to be involved in promoting transitions from wake to sleep in response to sleep pressure. Although the POA and BF neurons with different functions in sleep and wake are largely intermingled, it is possible that those neurons with the same sleep–wake properties and neurochemical phenotype may share similar projections, as well as synaptic inputs, regardless of their anatomical locations.

Neurons that appear to show activity patterns specific to REM sleep or to REM sleep and wakefulness are present in both the POA and BF. In addition, neurons in the extended VLPO (GABAergic), VLPO cluster (GABAergic and glutamatergic), and MnPO (glutamatergic) are likely involved in REM sleep homeostasis. These neurons may promote REM sleep rebound after prolonged wakefulness by inhibiting wake-promoting

and REM-off neurons in the hypothalamus and brain stem. The lack of REM sleep rebound in cats with mesencephalic transection (de Andrés *et al.*, 2003) may be due to the disconnection of the brain stem from these preoptic neurons with a role in REM sleep homeostasis. Various transmitters released in the BF also appear to influence the occurrence of REM sleep. Finally, the timing of REM sleep is strongly controlled by the circadian clock; however, underlying mechanisms and pathways for the circadian control of REM sleep are unclear.

Acknowledgments

Supported by grants from the Canadian Institutes of Health Research (MOP 93673) and the Natural Sciences and Engineering Research Council of Canada (217301–2009). I thank Michelle Black, Samuel Deurveilher, and Doug Rasmusson for a critical reading of an early version of the manuscript.

References

Alam, M. N. & Mallick, B. N. (1990) Differential acute influence of medial and lateral preoptic areas on sleep-wakefulness in freely moving rats. *Brain Res* **525**: 242–8.

Baghdoyan, H. A., Spotts, J. L. & Snyder, S. G. (1993) Simultaneous pontine and basal forebrain microinjections of carbachol suppresses REM sleep. *J Neurosci* **13**: 229–42.

Basheer, R., Strecker, R., Thakkar, M. *et al.* (2004) Adenosine and sleep-wake regulation. *Prog Neurobiol* **73**: 379–96.

Buijs, R. M., la Fleur, S. E., Wortel, J. *et al.* (2003) The suprachiasmatic nucleus balances sympathetic and parasympathetic output to peripheral organs through separate preautonomic neurons. *J Comp Neurol* **464**: 36–48.

Cape, E. G. & Jones, B. E. (1998) Differential modulation of high-frequency gamma-electroencephalogram activity and sleep-wake state by noradrenaline and serotonin microinjections into the region of cholinergic basalis neurons. *J Neurosci* **18**: 2653–66.

Cape, E. G. & Jones, B. E. (2000) Effects of glutamate agonist versus procaine microinjections into the basal forebrain cholinergic cell area upon gamma and theta EEG activity and sleep-wake state. *Eur J Neurosci* **12**: 2166–84.

Cape, E. G., Manns, I. D., Alonso, A. *et al.* (2000) Neurotensin-induced bursting of cholinergic basal forebrain neurons promotes gamma and theta cortical activity together with waking and paradoxical sleep. *J Neurosci* **20**: 8452–61.

Cerri, M., Ocampo-Garces, A., Amici, R. *et al.* (2005) Cold exposure and sleep in the rat: effects on sleep architecture and the electroencephalogram. *Sleep* **28**: 694–705.

Chou, T. C., Bjorkum, A. A., Gaus, S. E. *et al.* (2002) Afferents to the ventrolateral preoptic nucleus. *J Neurosci* **22**: 977–90.

de Andrés, I., Garzón, M. & Villablanca, J. R. (2003) The disconnected brain stem does not support rapid eye movement sleep rebound following selective deprivation. *Sleep* **26**: 419–25.

Deurveilher, S. & Semba, K. (2005) Indirect projections from the suprachiasmatic nucleus to major arousal-promoting cell groups in rat: implications for the circadian control of behavioural state. *Neuroscience* **130**: 165–83.

Deurveilher, S. & Semba, K. (2006) Mapping sleep–wake control with the transcription factor c-Fos. In *Immediate Early Genes in Sensory Processing, Cognitive Performance and Neurological Disorders*, eds. R. Pinaud & L. A. Tremere. New York: Springer, pp. 113–36.

España, R. A., Baldo, B. A., Kelley, A. E. *et al.* (2001) Wake-promoting and sleep-suppressing actions of hypocretin (orexin): basal forebrain sites of action. *Neuroscience* **106**: 699–715.

Gong, H., Szymusiak, R., King, J. *et al.* (2000) Sleep-related c-Fos protein expression in the preoptic hypothalamus: effects of ambient warming. *Am J Physiol* **279**: R2079–88.

Gvilia, I., Angara, C., McGinty, D. *et al.* (2005) Different neuronal populations of the rat median preoptic nucleus express c-fos during sleep and in response to hypertonic saline or angiotensin-II. *J Physiol* **569**: 587–99.

Gvilia, I., Xu, F., McGinty, D. *et al.* (2006a) Preoptic area neurons and the homeostatic regulation of rapid eye movement sleep. *J Neurosci* **26**: 3037–44.

Gvilia, I., Xu, F., McGinty, D. *et al.* (2006b) Homeostatic regulation of sleep: a role for preoptic area neurons. *J Neurosci* **26**: 9426–33.

Hassani, O., Lee, M., Henny, P. *et al.* (2009) Discharge profiles of identified GABAergic in comparison to cholinerigc and putative glutamatergic basal forebrain neurons across the sleep-wake cycle. *J Neurosci* **29**: 11,828–40.

Hernández-Peón, R., Chávez-Ibarra, G., Morgane, P. *et al.* (1963) Limbic cholinergic pathways involved in sleep and emotional behavior. *Exp Neurol* **8**: 93–111.

Kalinchuk, A., Porkka-Heiskanen, T. & McCarley, R. (2006a) Basal forebrain and saporin cholinergic lesions: the devil dwells in delivery details. *Sleep* **29**:1385–7.

Kalinchuk, A., Stenberg, D., Rosenberg, P. *et al.* (2006b) Inducible and neuronal nitric oxide synthases (NOS) have complementary roles in recovery sleep induction. *Eur J Neurosci* **24**: 1443–56.

Kalinchuk, A., Lu, Y., Stenberg, D. *et al.* (2006c) Nitric oxide production in the basal forebrain is required for recovery sleep. *J Neurochem* **99**: 483–98.

Kalinchuk, A., McCarley, R. D. S. *et al.* (2008) The role of cholinergic basal forebrain neurons in adenosine-mediated homeostatic control of sleep: lessons from 192 IgG-saporin lesions. *Neuroscience* **157**: 238–53.

Kaur, S., Junek, A., Black, M. A. *et al.* (2008) Effects of ibotenate and 192IgG-saporin lesions of the nucleus basalis magnocellularis/substantia innominata on spontaneous sleep and wake states and on recovery sleep after sleep deprivation in rats. *J Neurosci* **28**: 491–504.

Koyama, Y. & Hayaishi, O. (1994) Firing of neurons in the preoptic/anterior hypothalamic areas in rat: its possible involvement in slow wave sleep and paradoxical sleep. *Neurosci Res* **19**: 31–8.

Lee, M., Manns, I. D., Alonso, A. *et al.* (2004) Sleep–wake related discharge properties of basal forebrain neurons recorded with micropipettes in head-fixed rats. *J Neurophysiol* **92**: 1182–98.

Lee, M., Hassani, O., Alonso, A. *et al.* (2005) Cholinergic basal forebrain neurons burst with theta during waking and paradoxical sleep. *J Neurosci* **25**: 4365–9.

Lee, M., Swanson, B. & de la Iglesia, H. (2009) Circadian timing of REM sleep is coupled to an oscillator within the dorsomedial suprachiasmatic nucleus. *Curr Biol* **19**: 848–52.

Lu, J., Greco, M. N., Shiromani, P. *et al.* (2000) Effect of lesions of the ventrolateral preoptic nucleus on NREM and REM sleep. *J Neurosci* **20**: 3830–42.

Lu, J., Bjorkum, A., Xu, M. *et al.* (2002) Selective activation of the extended ventrolateral preoptic nucleus during rapid eye movement sleep. *J Neurosci* **22**: 4568–76.

Lu, J., Sherman, D., Devor, M. *et al.* (2006) A putative flip-flop switch for control of REM sleep. *Nature* **441**: 589–94.

Mallick, B. N., Thankachan, S. & Islam, F. (2004) Influence of hypnogenic brain areas on wakefulness- and rapid-eye-movement sleep-related neurons in the brainstem of freely moving cats. *J Neurosci Res* **75**: 133–42.

Manfridi, A. & Mancia, M. (1996) Desynchronized (REM) sleep inhibition induced by carbachol microinjections into the nucleus basalis of Meynert is mediated by the glutamatergic system. *Exp Brain Res* **109**: 174–8.

Manfridi, A., Brambilla, D. & Mancia, M. (2001) Sleep is differently modulated by basal forebrain GABA(A) and GABA(B) receptors. *Am J Physiol Regul Integr Comp Physiol* **281**: R170–5.

McKenna, J., Cordeira, J., Jeffrey, B. *et al.* (2009) c-Fos protein expression is increased in cholinergic neurons of the rodent basal forebrain during spontaneous and induced wakefulness. *Brain Res Bull* 80: 382–8.

Mistlberger, R. E., Antle, M. C., Glass, J. D. *et al.* (2000) Behavioral and serotonergic regulation of circadian rhythms. *Biol Rhythm Res* 31: 240–83.

Modirrousta, M., Mainville, L. & Jones, B. (2004) GABAergic neurons with alpha2-adrenergic receptors in basal forebrain and preoptic area express c-Fos during sleep. *Neuroscience* 129: 803–10.

Nishino, S., Tafti, M., Reid, M. S. *et al.* (1995) Muscle atonia is triggered by cholinergic stimulation of the basal forebrain: implication for the pathophysiology of canine narcolepsy. *J Neurosci* 15: 4806–14.

Pace-Schott, E. & Hobson, J. (2002) The neurobiology of sleep: genetics, cellular physiology and subcortical networks. *Nat Rev Neurosci* 3: 591–605.

Porkka-Heiskanen, T., Kalinchuk, A., Alanko, L. *et al.* (2003) Adenosine, energy metabolism, and sleep. *Scientific World Journal* 3: 790–8.

Ramesh, V., Thakkar, M., Strecker, R. *et al.* (2004) Wakefulness-inducing effects of histamine in the basal forebrain of freely moving rats. *Behav Brain Res* 152: 271–8.

Saper, C. B., Chou, T. C. & Scammell, T. E. (2001) The sleep switch: hypothalamic control of sleep and wakefulness. *Trends Neurosci* 24: 726–31.

Saper, C. B., Lu, J., Chou, T. C. *et al.* (2005) The hypothalamic integration for circadian rhythms. *Trends Neurosci* 28: 152–7.

Sapin, E., Lapray, D., Bérod, A. *et al.* (2009) Localization of the brainstem GABAergic neurons controlling paradoxical (REM) sleep. *PLoS One* 4: e4272.

Schmidt, M. H., Valatx, J.-L., Sakai, K. *et al.* (2000) Role of the lateral preoptic area in sleep-related erectile mechanisms and sleep generation in the rat. *J Neurosci* 20: 6640–7.

Semba, K. (1991) The cholinergic basal forebrain: a critical role in cortical arousal. In *The Basal Forebrain. Anatomy and Function*, eds. T.C. Napier, P. W. Kalivas & I. Hanin. New York: Plenum, pp. 197–218.

Semba, K. (2000) Multiple output pathways of the basal forebrain: organization, chemical heterogeneity, and roles in vigilance. *Behav Brain Res* 115: 117–41.

Sherin, J. E., Shiromani, P. J., McCarley, R. W. *et al.* (1996) Activation of ventrolateral preoptic neurons during sleep. *Science* 271: 216–19.

Sherin, J. E., Elmquist, J. K., Torrealba, F. *et al.* (1998) Innervation of histaminergic tuberomammillary neurons by GABAergic and galaninergic neurons in the ventrolateral preoptic nucleus of the rat. *J Neurosci* 18: 4705–21.

Srividya, R., Mallick, H. & Kumar, V (2006) Differences in the effects of medial and lateral preoptic lesions on thermoregulation and sleep in rats. *Neuroscience* 139: 853–64.

Steininger, T. L., Gong, H., McGinty, D. *et al.* (2001) Subregional organization of preoptic area/anterior hypothalamic projections to arousal related monoaminergic cell groups. *J Comp Neurol* 429: 638–53.

Stewart, D. J., MacFabe, D. F. & Vanderwolf, C. H. (1984) Cholinergic activation of the electrocorticogram: role of the substantia innominata and effects of atropine and quinuclidinyl benzilate. *Brain Res* 322: 219–32.

Suntsova, N. & Dergacheva, O. (2004) The role of the medial preoptic area of the hypothalamus in organizing the paradoxical phase of sleep. *Neurosci Behav Physiol* 34: 29–35.

Suntsova, N., Szymusiak, R., Alam, M. *et al.* (2002) Sleep–waking discharge patterns of median preoptic nucleus neurons in rats. *J Physiol* 543: 665–77.

Suntsova, N., Guzman-Marin, R., Kumar, S. *et al.* (2007) The median preoptic nucleus reciprocally modulates activity of arousal-related and sleep-related neurons in the perifornical lateral hypothalamus. *J Neurosci* 27: 1616–30.

Szymusiak, R. & McGinty, D. (1986) Sleep suppression following kainic acid-induced lesions of the basal forebrain. *Exp Neurol* 94: 598–614.

Szymusiak, R. & McGinty, D. (1989) Sleep–waking discharge of basal forebrain projection neurons in cats. *Brain Res Bull* 22: 423–30.

Szymusiak, R., McGinty, D. (2008) Hypothalamic regulation of sleep and arousal. *Ann N Y Acad Sci* 1129: 275–86.

Szymusiak, R., Alam, N., Steiniger, T. L. *et al.* (1998) Sleep–waking discharge patterns of ventrolateral preoptic/anterior hypothalamic neurons in rats. *Brain Res* 803: 178–88.

Szymusiak, R., Gvilia, I., McGinty, D. (2007) Hypothalamic control of sleep. *Sleep Med* 8: 291–301.

Takahashi, K., Lin, J. & Sakai, K. (2009) Characterization and mapping of sleep–waking specific neurons in the basal forebrain and preoptic hypothalamus in mice. *Neuroscience* 161: 269–92.

Uschakov, A., Gong, H., McGinty, D. *et al.* (2006) Sleep-active neurons in the preoptic area project to the hypothalamic paraventricular nucleus and perifornical lateral hypothalamus. *Eur J Neurosci* 23: 3284–96.

Uschakov, A., Gong, H., McGinty, D. *et al.* (2007) Efferent projections from the median preoptic nucleus to sleep- and arousal-regulatory nuclei in the rat brain. *Neuroscience* 150: 104–20.

Vazquez, J. & Baghdoyan, H. (2001) Basal forebrain acetylcholine release during REM sleep is significantly greater than during waking. *Am J Physiol Regul Integr Comp Physiol* **280**: R598–601.

von Economo, C. (1930) Sleep as a problem of localization. *J Nerv Ment Dis* **71**: 249–59.

Wigren, H., Schepens, M., Matto, V. *et al.* (2007) Glutamatergic stimulation of the basal forebrain elevates extracellular adenosine and increases the subsequent sleep. *Neuroscience* **147**: 811–23.

Yang, Q. Z. & Hatton, G. I. (1997) Electrophysiology of excitatory and inhibitory afferents to rat histaminergic tuberomammillary nucleus neurons from hypothalamic and forebrain sites. *Brain Res* **773**: 162–72.

Chapter 12

Amygdalar regulation of REM sleep

Larry D. Sanford and Richard J. Ross

Summary

The amygdala has a long-recognized role in emotion, and a growing body of work demonstrates that it plays an important part in the regulation of arousal state. Primary findings are that the amygdala, especially its central nucleus, is a strong regulator of rapid eye movement sleep (REMS) and related phenomena, though a smaller body of research indicates a role for the amygdala in regulating non-REM (NREM). Considering its vital place in the limbic circuitry that controls emotion, it is likely that the amygdala mediates fear- and stress-induced alterations in sleep, and investigations in animals have begun to provide confirmatory evidence. In particular, GABAergic regulation of the central nucleus of the amygdala appears to play a significant role in stress-induced reductions in REM. In humans, neuroimaging studies suggest that the pathophysiological mechanisms of narcolepsy and post-traumatic stress disorder (PTSD), two central nervous system disorders with a prominent emotional component and a demonstrated abnormality of REM, involve an amygdalar-mediated reorganization of fundamental REM systems.

Introduction

The amygdala has generally been seen as the center of emotion in the limbic system. It appears to have a pivotal role on the influence emotion has in memory formation and it plays a critical role in conditioned fear, and probably anxiety as well (Davis and Whalen, 2001). The amygdala responds to a variety of positive as well as negative emotional stimuli; it also is important in the regulation of behavioral, physiological, and neuroendocrine responses to stress (reviewed in Davis and Whalen, 2001). Work over the last several years has demonstrated that the amygdala plays an important role in the regulation of REM, a state that appears to be particularly susceptible to stressful influences. The purpose of this chapter is to review the current research demonstrating a role for the amygdala in the regulation of REM and REM-related phenomena including ponto-geniculo-occipital (PGO) waves. We will also place this evidence in the context of the amygdala's established functions in emotion, fear, memory, and stress and their significance for neuropsychiatric disorders, including primary insomnia, depression, narcolepsy, and PTSD.

Anatomical substrate for amygdalar modulation of REM

The basolateral amygdala (BLA) is composed of the basal (BA) and lateral (LA) amygdaloid nuclei. The BA projects to the central nucleus of the amygdala (CNA), through the CNA on to the bed nucleus of the stria terminalis (BNST), considered extended amygdala (Davis and Whalen, 2001), and to other regions such as the hypothalamus and the basal forebrain (Amaral et al., 1992). The CNA projects to brain stem regions considered essential to the control of REM and its related phenomena. Efferents from the CNA are split between two major amygdaloid output tracts, the stria terminalis and the ventral amygdalofugal pathway, the caudal part of which enters the brain stem. Projections from the CNA also go to the pedunculopontine tegmental (PPT) and laterodorsal tegmental (LDT) nuclei, the locus coeruleus (LC), the subcoeruleus, and to the dorsal raphe nuclei (DRN). Each of these regions is implicated in REM and in the control of PGO wave generation, a cardinal sign of REM. In addition, a major pathway originating in the CNA projects to the lateral peribrachial region of the pontomesencephalic

---

REM Sleep: Regulation and Function, eds. Birendra N. Mallick, S. R. Pandi-Perumal, Robert W. McCarley, and Adrian R. Morrison. Published by Cambridge University Press. © Cambridge University Press 2011.

tegmentum. This region also has been demonstrated to have an important role in the generation of REM and PGO waves. There are reciprocal projections from many of these pontine regions back to the CNA (reviewed in Morrison *et al.*, 2000).

These descending projections provide anatomical connections by which the amygdala can influence REM and other arousal states, and studies using a variety of techniques have demonstrated that the CNA is a significant regulator of REM. The amygdala may also influence REM via the BNST, which has descending projections similar to those of the CNA (reviewed in Amaral *et al.*, 1992). Unfortunately, at present, there is minimal information regarding the potential role of the BNST in regulating REM.

Cellular activity in the amygdala correlated with arousal

There have been relatively few studies examining unit activity in the amygdala of freely moving animals in relation to changes in behavioral state. In cats, Jacobs and McGinty (1971) reported that most cells in the BLA were more active in NREM than in quiet wakefulness (W) or REM. A second class of cells fired in bursts and showed more activity in REM and/or W. Also in cats, some projection neurons in the LA are quiet throughout the sleep–wake cycle, but can be activated by stimuli that may be specific for each neuron (Gaudreau and Pare, 1996). By comparison, in rats, approximately 50% of neurons recorded in the LA increased activity during sleep, and some cells had greater firing during REM than NREM (Bordi *et al.*, 1993). In cats, CNA neurons had a higher spontaneous discharge rate in both REM and W compared to NREM (Frysinger *et al.*, 1988). Recently, Jha *et al.* (2005) studied the state-related activity of CNA neurons in chronically implanted rats and found that half had firing patterns related to sleep–wake state. As in cats, a significant population of neurons fired at the highest frequency during W or both W and REM whereas other CNA neurons fired in relation to REM or NREM.

A relationship between amygdala activation and REM generation is also suggested by functional brain imaging findings that the amygdala is spontaneously activated during REM in healthy humans (Maquet *et al.*, 1996). Animal work indicates that regions of the amygdala may be differentially involved in modulating different sleep states. For example, training with inescapable shock, which reduced REM, produced increased Fos activation in several regions of the amygdala (e.g., medial amygdala, cortical amygdala, basal amygdala, lateral amygdala, and amygdalostriatal transition region), but not in the CNA (Liu *et al.*, 2003). This suggests that the probable role of the amygdala in influencing post-stress sleep may involve differential activation and inactivation of various nuclei, and that multiple regions or cell populations of the amygdala can be activated at the same time that REM is reduced.

Amygdala and ponto-geniculo-occipital waves

Ponto-geniculo-occipital waves, so named because they can be recorded from the pons, lateral geniculate body (LGB), and occipital cortex, occur with a high frequency immediately prior to, and during, REM episodes. This relationship to REM has led to suggestions that the neural activity underlying PGO wave generation is causal for the triggering and regulation of REM (Steriade and McCarley, 1990), although it is clear that PGO waves also can be dissociated from REM. For example, depletion of brain serotonin, such as with systemically administered parachlorophenylalanine (PCPA) and reserpine, can release PGO waves into other states (Steriade and McCarley, 1990). Spontaneously occurring PGO or PGO-like waves can be recorded in all states and an elicited analog of the PGO wave (PGO_E) also can be obtained in all states in response to external stimuli (Morrison *et al.*, 2000).

Early work in cats by Calvo *et al.* (1987) demonstrated a linkage between PGO waves and the amygdala. In cats PGO waves can be recorded from the BLA temporally later than PGO waves recorded from the LGB during REM (Calvo and Fernandez-Guardiola, 1984). Calvo *et al.* (1987) found that electrical stimulation of the CNA in cats increased PGO wave frequency by 30% during REM; they did not report on the effects in other states. Electrical stimulation of the CNA in rats did not affect pontine PGO wave frequency, but it did significantly increase PGO wave amplitude during REM; interestingly, PGO wave amplitude was not affected in either W or NREM, but the frequency was actually somewhat reduced in W and significantly reduced in NREM (Morrison *et al.*, 2000). Such electrical stimulation also increased the amplitude of PGO_E waves after the response to auditory stimuli had habituated.

The amygdala is involved in setting emotional tone and is critical for fear conditioning, a classical conditioning paradigm that involves making an association between a neutral stimulus (light or tone) or situational context and an aversive stimulus (usually footshock) (Davis, 1992). Compared to the amplitudes of habituated PGO_E responses and to the amplitudes on test trials where white noise was presented alone, PGO_E amplitudes in rats were greater when white noise was presented in the presence of fear-conditioned light, but were not greater than the amplitudes of PGO_E recorded prior to habituation (Morrison *et al.*, 2000). These results demonstrate that the presence of a fear-inducing stimulus enhances the amplitude of PGO_E responses, an effect likely mediated by the amygdala.

Amygdala and the regulation of REM

Several lines of evidence indicate that inhibition of the CNA suppresses REM and that, under some conditions, activation of the CNA can promote REM and/or REM-related phenomena such as PGO waves. The clearest evidence that inhibition of the CNA decreases REM comes from studies in which the CNA was functionally inactivated with microinjections of the $GABA_A$ agonist muscimol or tetrodotoxin (TTX). Muscimol, which temporarily inactivates cell bodies, administered into the CNA of rats produced a relatively selective decrease in REM without significant alterations in other arousal states, whereas TTX, which inactivates both cell bodies and fibers of passage, decreased REM but enhanced NREM. For example, in addition to the effects on REM, TTX microinjections into the CNA during the light period decreased NREM latency while injections prior to the dark period increased NREM amount (reviewed in Sanford *et al.*, 2006a).

As the effects of muscimol were specific to REM, the alterations in NREM produced by TTX inactivation likely are mediated by blockage of fibers of passage originating in the BLA (Davis and Whalen, 2001). This suggestion is supported by findings that bilateral electrolytic and chemical lesions of the BLA increased NREM and total sleep time without altering REM in rats and that bilateral chemical lesions of the amygdala in chair-restrained Rhesus monkeys produced more consolidated sleep (reviewed in Sanford *et al.*, 2006a). In contrast, electrical and chemical stimulation of the BLA increased low-voltage, high-frequency activity in the cortical EEG and decreased NREM and total sleep time, respectively (reviewed in Sanford *et al.*, 2006a). However, an early study reported that

electrical stimulation of the dorsal and ventral regions of the BLA desynchronized and synchronized the EEG, respectively (Kreindler and Steriade, 1964).

In general, the evidence suggests that the CNA is more involved in the regulation of REM than of NREM and that, by comparison, the BLA has a greater role in the regulation of NREM and general arousal. However, it is important to note that the BLA regulates CNA output and therefore likely controls its influences on REM. Indeed, ongoing studies in our lab (LDS) have found that microinjections into the BLA of the group II metabotropic glutamate (mGlu) receptor agonist LY379268 selectively reduced REM without significantly altering wakefulness or NREM. This suggests that group II mGlu receptors may influence specific cells in the BLA that control descending outputs (possibly via the CNA or BNST) that in turn regulate REM generator regions in the brain stem.

Another drug intervention that likely inhibits the CNA also reduced REM. Serotonin terminated ongoing episodes when microinjected into the CNA during REM but did not alter episode continuity when microinjected during NREM (Morrison *et al.*, 2000). Supporting the specificity of a modulation by CNA of REM, Jha *et al.* (2005) reported that all neurons that fired selectively during REM (REM-on neurons) in the CNA were inhibited by electrical stimulation of the serotonergic DRN whereas firing of other types of cells was not altered. They suggested that REM-on neurons in the CNA could serve as "sentinels," informing REM maintenance systems that serotonergic "tone" was high, and incompatible with REM continuance.

The origin of most cholinergic input into the amygdala is the basal forebrain (Amaral *et al.*, 1992), which also projects to the cerebral cortex (Lehmann *et al.*, 1980). By comparison, brain-stem cholinergic regions implicated in promoting REM generation (the LDT and PPT nuclei) provide only a minor cholinergic projection to the amygdala (Morrison *et al.*, 2000). Activation of forebrain cholinergic neurons resulted in EEG desynchronization that was associated with either W or REM (Cape *et al.*, 2000). In rats, the cholinergic agonist carbachol and the acetylcholinesterase inhibitor neostigmine microinjected into the CNA decreased REM (see Table 12.1) without significantly altering the amounts of NREM and W (Sanford *et al.*, 2006b). However, high dosages of carbachol could induce seizures. In vitro studies of amygdala neurons in rats indicate that carbachol blocks glutamate-mediated

Table 12.1 Time spent (min) in REM and NREM (means ± SEM) during two four-hour blocks and total eight-hour recording period after microinjections into the CNA of saline (SAL), carbachol (low: 0.3 µg; high: 3.0 µg) and neostigmine (low: 0.3 µg; high: 3.0 µg) or scopolamine (low: 0.3 µg; high: 1.0 µg) and mecamylamine (low: 0.3 µg; high: 1.0 µg). Comparisons were conducted with Tukey tests (significant differences relative to SAL: *, p < 0.05; **, p < 0.01; significant difference compared to low dose: #, p < 0.05). Modified from Sanford *et al.* 2006b

	SAL	Carbachol		Neostigmine		SAL	Scopolamine		Mecamylamine	
	0.2 µl	low	high	low	high	0.2 µl	low	high	low	high
REM										
First four-hour	21.2 (1.7)	15.0 (1.7)*	15.3 (2.1)*	19.0 (1.7)	15.3 (1.4)*	18.7 (1.5)	16.8 (1.7)	21.4 (2.9)	20.4 (2.4)	16.6 (1.7)
Second four-hour	29.5 (1.7)	20.7 (1.8)**	22.1 (2.1)*	22.3 (1.2)**	23.4 (1.0)*	27.5 (1.9)	27.4 (1.1)	21.2 (1.7)*#	27.6 (2.1)	27.6 (1.9)
Total eight-hour	50.6 (2.8)	35.6 (3.4)**	37.4 (3.9)*	41.3 (1.3)*	38.6 (2.1)**	46.2 (2.8)	44.2 (2.2)	42.6 (4.4)	48.0 (4.2)	44.2 (2.5)
NREM										
First four-hour	140.3 (3.4)	140.8 (4.9)	140.3 (3.6)	153.5 (5.6)	141.9 (5.0)	128.3 (5.9)	142.5 (6.2)*	152.4 (3.9)***	139.0 (3.7)	125.0 (7.7)
Second four-hour	145.7 (4.6)	144.3 (3.3)	144.3 (4.3)	142.2 (8.1)	148.5 (4.4)	146.2 (3.8)	146.0 (5.8)	149.7 (6.0)	146.3 (4.6)	152.5 (3.8)
Total eight-hour	286.0 (6.8)	285.1 (6.1)	284.6 (6.9)	295.7 (12.9)	290.4 (6.6)	274.5 (8.4)	288.5 (8.5)	302.1 (8.7)**	285.3 (6.4)	277.4 (8.0)

excitation (reviewed in Sanford *et al.*, 2006b), a finding consistent with an inhibitory effect on amygdalar activity.

The CNA contains both muscarinic and nicotinic cholinergic receptor immunoreactive neurons, and muscarinic receptors are generally associated with GABAergic neurons (Van der Zee *et al.*, 1997). Microinjections of the muscarinic cholinergic antagonist scopolamine (see Table 12.1) significantly enhanced NREM whereas a high dosage of scopolamine (1.0 μg) also produced an initial increase in REM (only in the second hour of recording) followed by a significant decrease in the second four-hour period of recording (Sanford *et al.*, 2006b). By comparison, the nicotinic antagonist mecamylamine did not significantly alter sleep, thus suggesting that nicotinic receptors in the CNA have a minor role in the regulation of sleep.

Enhancement of REM or other sleep states has also been found with other experimental manipulations of the CNA. Electrical stimulation of the CNA enhanced REM in rats (reviewed in Sanford *et al.*, 2006a). In cats, microinjections of vasoactive intestinal peptide into either the CNA or BA increased amounts of REM, PGO waves, and NREM with PGO waves for up to five days, with the injections into CNA producing greater effects. Microinjections of carbachol into the CNA, but not the BA, LA, or BLA of cats also have been reported to increase REM and NREM episodes with PGO waves for up to five days post-injection (Calvo *et al.*, 1996). We have never observed prolonged enhancements of REM with any treatments of the amygdala in rats, and the mechanism that accounts for the difference between the REM-suppressing effects of carbachol in rats and REM-enhancing effects in cats is not known. However, in rats, enhancements of REM were observed after blocking GABAergic inhibition in the CNA with the GABA$_A$ antagonist bicuculline (reviewed in Sanford *et al.*, 2006a), and blocking serotonergic inhibition increased the generation of PGO waves outside of REM as well as the amount of NREM (Morrison *et al.*, 2000).

While decreasing overall REM amount, inactivation of the CNA may also be incompatible with the generation of a number of electrophysiological features shared by REM and alert W, including an activated EEG, hippocampal theta, and PGO waves (Morrison *et al.*, 2000). In W, these features are associated with enhanced vigilance or orienting in response to external stimuli, whereas in REM they spontaneously occur in the absence of external stimuli and without behavioral arousal. Prominent in both REM and orienting during W are high-amplitude PGO waves, which we have argued are central correlates of overt behavioral orienting responses. Electrical stimulation of the CNA during W produced "alerting" behaviors along with EEG desynchronization (Kreindler and Steriade, 1964). Electrical stimulation of the CNA also enhanced the amplitude of auditory-elicited PGO waves during W and increased the amplitude (rats) (Morrison *et al.*, 2000) and frequency (cats) (Calvo *et al.*, 1987) of PGO waves during REM. Together, these studies suggest that the amygdala regulates a variety of electrophysiological features common to REM and alert W. They also suggest that interfering with normal activation of the CNA may impede the neural processes underlying the spontaneous generation of the alerting-like phenomena that characterize REM, and that may be necessary for REM to occur.

Amygdala and stress-induced alterations in sleep

Studies in animals have repeatedly demonstrated that stressful experiences during W can significantly influence subsequent sleep and that REM appears to be particularly susceptible to the effects of stress. The extent of the changes in arousal and sleep appears to vary with the type and intensity of the stressor, and a subsequent increase in REM and changes in other sleep parameters have been reported for a great number of stressors, including avoidable footshock, restraint, water maze, exposure to novel objects, open field, ether exposure, cage change, and social stress (reviewed in Pawlyk *et al.*, 2008).

Our recent work has focused on the potential role of the amygdala in regulating stress-induced alterations in arousal and sleep. We have employed extensive fear-conditioning paradigms with multiple shock presentations, recording sleep before and after training. Brief, intense stressful events such as the inescapable footshocks typically used in fear conditioning can produce behavioral and physiological outcomes that resemble the symptoms of anxiety disorders in humans. Conditioned cue and contextual stimuli associated with footshock, i.e., "reminders" of the fearful event, can later produce physiological responses and alterations in behavior similar to those seen directly after training. Our work has demonstrated that both the initial stress and subsequent reminders of the shock can produce significant reductions in the amount of REM; the sleep rebound observed with virtually all other stressors often does not occur. A similar reduction in REM, without recovery, has been reported in rats trained in an intense learned-helplessness paradigm that used inescapable footshock stress (Adrien *et al.*, 1991). There may also be a significant increase in light NREM (Adrien *et al.*, 1991).

By comparison, animals trained with footshock that they could learn to avoid with an appropriate behavior in response to a signal that predicts shock onset showed post-stress increases in sleep, particularly REM (reviewed in Pawlyk *et al.*, 2008). Recently, we (LDS) have demonstrated that mice trained in a paradigm in which they always receive shock, but can terminate it with a simple escape behavior, also show significant increases in post-stress REM compared to both baseline recordings and to yoked control mice trained with inescapable footshock. Contextual reminders of escapable and inescapable footshock also produced significant increases and decreases in REM, respectively, thereby demonstrating that both increases and decreases in REM can occur in response to memories of stressful events.

The role of the amygdala in mediating the physiological and behavioral signs of conditioned fear and its demonstrated role in the regulation of REM and other behavioral states suggest that it may play a central role in regulating stress- and fear-induced alterations in sleep. In a recent study (Liu *et al.*, 2009), we (LDS) microinjected muscimol, bicuculline, or saline vehicle into the CNA prior to training rats with inescapable footshock (Figure 12.1). After saline vehicle, training with inescapable footshock selectively reduced electrographically defined REM, and Fos expression in the LC was increased compared to that in rats that received a microinjection of vehicle alone. Rats treated with muscimol, which inactivates neurons in the CNA, also showed reduced REM and increased Fos expression in the LC. By comparison, microinjection of bicuculline into the CNA prior to training attenuated the reduction in REM and also attenuated Fos expression in the LC. This work suggests the potential involvement of the LC in footshock-induced reductions in REM and its regulation by the amygdala.

Stress-induced alterations in amygdalar neurotransmission that persist after the stressor is removed may be involved in changes in arousal and sleep (Liu *et al.*, 2007). In mice, we (LDS) measured the release of [³H]-norepinephrine ([³H]-NE]) and [¹⁴C]-γ-amino-butyric

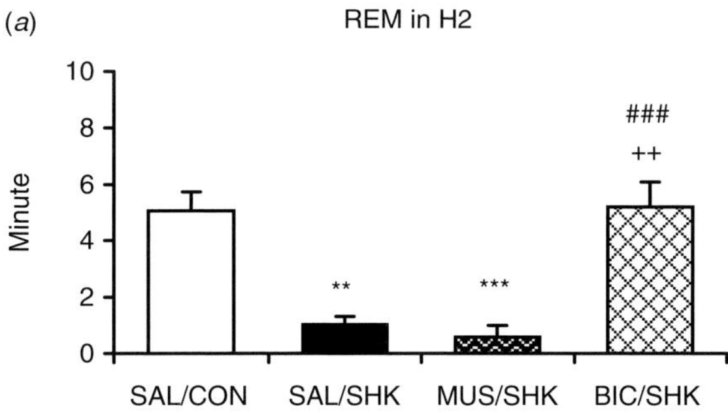

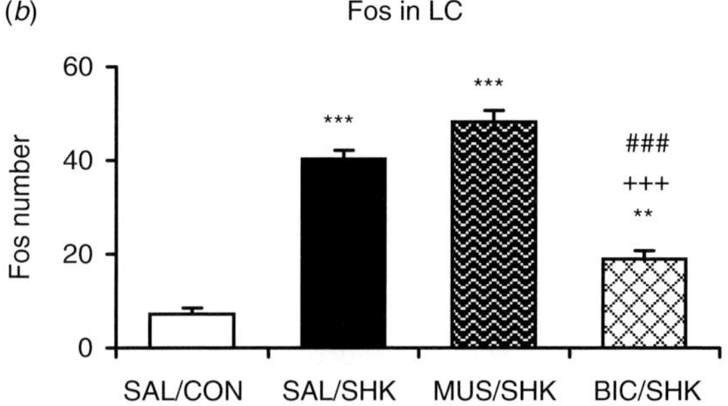

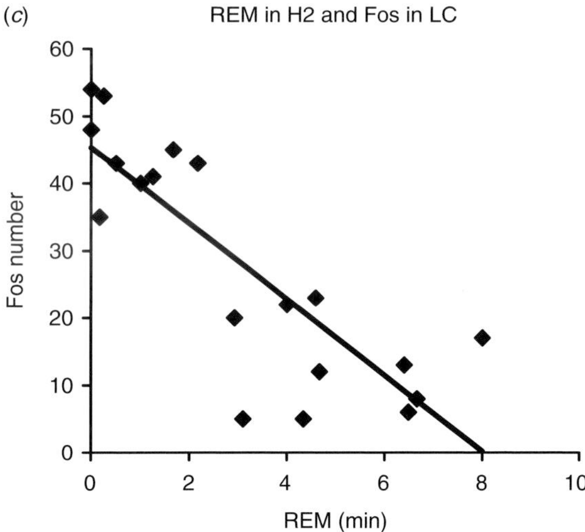

Figure 12.1 Minutes of REM in the second recording hour (H2, *a*) after a footshock stressor and number of Fos granules counted in the LC examined at the end of H2 (*b*) plotted for each treatment condition. The correlation between REM in H2 and Fos counts in the LC is shown in scatterplot form (*c*). Rats in the saline control (SAL/CON, n = 5) condition received only a microinjection of saline into the CNA prior to recording. Rats in the saline shock (SAL/SHK, n = 4) condition received a microinjection of saline prior to footshock. Rats in the muscimol shock (MUS/SHK, n = 5) condition received a microinjection of muscimol (1.0 μM/0.2 μl) prior to shock and rats in the bicuculline shock (BIC/SHK, n = 5) condition received a microinjection of bicuculline (333 pM/0.2 μl). Bicuculline attenuated the stress-induced reduction in REM and Fos expression in the LC whereas muscimol did not. **, $P < 0.01$; ***, 0.001 compared to SAL/CON; ++, $P < 0.01$; +++, 0.001 compared to SAL/SHK, ###, $P < 0.001$ compared to MUS/SHK. Comparisons were conducted with Tukey tests. Modified from (Liu *et al.*, 2009).

acid ([^{14}C]-GABA) from brain regions known to regulate arousal states and REM. Comparing mice that had been fear-conditioned with mice that had received neutral cues only, depolarization-evoked release of [^{3}H]-NE in amygdalar slices was suppressed at two to three hours after cue presentation in the former group. In addition, depolarization-evoked release of [^{14}C]-GABA was significantly increased in the amygdala, and tended to be enhanced in the hippocampus, nucleus pontis oralis, and the DRN at two to three hours after fearful cue presentation. The changes in [^{3}H]-NE and [^{14}C]-GABA release were transient, such that four to five hours after the mice had experienced the cue, no significant differences were detected between the two groups. Thus, fear-induced changes in neurotransmitter release in the amygdala have a time course similar to that of fear-induced reductions in REM (Liu *et al.*, 2003).

The activity of the noradrenergic LC increases during stress (Liu *et al.*, 2003) and there is increased release and turnover of NE in projection regions. Thus, the reduction in evoked [^{3}H]-NE release in the amygdala may reflect a rundown of release machinery in the aftermath of increased activation associated with fear. However, the lack of significant fear-induced alterations in [^{3}H]-NE release in other regions (e.g., the hippocampus, nucleus pontis oralis, and DRN) we (LDS) examined suggests that the effect we saw in the amygdala was not simply due to an effect of fearful cues on the LC causing rundown, but that there were regulatory changes in release specific to noradrenergic projections of the LC to the amygdala.

Together, these studies suggest that the CNA plays a significant role in regulating REM in the aftermath of stress. The results also suggest that the reduction in REM in the aftermath of inescapable footshock may involve local GABAergic inhibitory mechanisms in the CNA and activation of the LC. By comparison, the relative lack of effect on NREM amount suggests that GABAergic regulation of the CNA is minimally involved in stress-induced changes in NREM.

Amygdalar modulation of REM: clinical translation

Sleep is significantly disturbed in a range of neuropsychiatric disorders, and, in several cases, there is evidence for amygdalar involvement in the underlying neurocircuitry. Here we focus on central nervous system disorders with both a prominent emotional component and a demonstrated abnormality of REM. For narcolepsy and PTSD, a strong case can be made that the amygdala participates in a reorganization of fundamental REM-generating mechanisms. The evidence is less clear for major depression and primary insomnia (PI). With all four disorders, considerably more work is required to elucidate the precise neurophysiological disturbances and their neuropharmacological substrates.

REM in primary insomnia

Given the prevailing view that PI often is precipitated by a psychological stressor (Perlis *et al.*, 2005) and the evidence that the pathophysiology of PI involves an entry of the arousal mechanisms usually associated with W into sleep (Perlis *et al.*, 2005), it could be predicted that abnormal amygdalar modulation of REM mechanisms would be evident in PI. In the past decade neuroimaging strategies have been used to elucidate the nature of the sleep disturbances in humans with various mental disorders; however, positron emission tomography (PET) and single photon emission computed tomography (SPECT) studies in PI have focused on the NREM state, and have not, to our knowledge, included scanning during REM. This limited focus can be understood in the context of earlier polysomnographic findings in PI of elevated high-frequency activity in the beta range during NREM (reviewed in Buysse *et al.*, 2008); thus, neuroimaging has been carried out during a phase of sleep that has seemed, by polysomnographic criteria, to be disturbed. It has been suggested that technical difficulties, in the form of electrooculographic (EOG) and electromyographic (EMG) artifacts in the REM EEG, also may have contributed to a de-emphasis of REM mechanisms (Buysse *et al.*, 2008). Therefore, the conclusion drawn by some that there is little reason to implicate a disturbance of REM mechanisms in PI is based more on an absence of appropriate investigations than on experimental results. Neuroimaging may yet be used to identify neurocircuitry incorporating the amygdala that functions abnormally during REM in PI.

Amygdalar modulation of tonic and phasic REM in depression

Abnormalities of REM have been observed in patients with depression since the 1970s, and they were among the first biological measures to be suggested as "markers" of a mental disorder (Reynolds *et al.*, 1987). There is general agreement that a shortened REM latency (time from sleep onset to the beginning of the first REM period of the night) and an increase in REM density (number of rapid eye movements during REM/REM time), particularly in the first REM period (Reynolds *et al.*, 1987), often occur in depressed patients. On the other hand, some investigators have emphasized the reduction of slow-wave sleep and delta wave production in the early part of the sleep period (Reynolds *et al.*, 1987). Polysomnographic studies in patients with mental disorders other than depression, including schizophrenia, have shown that increased pressure to enter REM is by no means specific to depression, and there is as yet no consensus about whether heightened REM pressure is a trait or state sign of depression (Reynolds *et al.*, 1987).

Neuroimaging has been employed to identify brain mechanisms that might underlie REM changes in depression. Noting that "depressed patients demonstrate increases in electroencephalographic sleep measures of REM," and that the normal progression from NREM to REM involves an increase in regional cerebral glucose metabolism in limbic and paralimbic structures (Lydic *et al.*, 1991, Maquet *et al.*, 1996), Nofzinger *et al.* (2004) hypothesized that depressed patients, compared to healthy subjects, would exhibit a greater activation of limbic and paralimbic regions, including the amygdala and the anterior cingulate cortex, in REM vs. W. They found that, consistent with earlier studies in cats and healthy humans (Lydic *et al.*, 1991, Maquet *et al.*, 1996), relative metabolism increased from W to REM in a wide array of anterior limbic and paralimbic structures, including the amygdala, and that the spatial extent of this state-related activation was considerably broader in a group of depressed patients (Nofzinger *et al.*, 2004).

It has been reported that elevated REM density in depressed humans correlates with severity of depression and clinical outcome (Buysse *et al.*, 1999). Although the functional significance of any increase in REM phasic activity in depression remains unknown, some have hypothesized that it indicates hyperarousal during REM, and neuroimaging has been used to identify brain regions that could be implicated in such a highly activated REM state. In an [18]FDG PET study of unmedicated depressed patients, Germain *et al.* (2004) found that regional cerebral glucose metabolism in medial and ventrolateral prefrontal cortices correlated positively with an automated measure of rapid eye movement activity. Interestingly, there was a negative correlation between rapid eye movement activity and glucose metabolism in paralimbic structures including the uncus and parahippocampal gyrus. The authors suggested that, in depressed patients, REM density might be an inverse correlate of occipitotemporal glucose metabolism during REM. They cautioned that any relationship might not be specific to depression, and also observed that previous studies in healthy subjects had found a positive correlation between REM density and regional cerebral blood flow in temporal and lateral occipital cortices during REM (Braun *et al.*, 1998). It can neither be concluded that the amygdala was among the paralimbic structures showing decreased activation during REM in depressed subjects nor that any such decrease was specific to depression. Furthermore, as the authors acknowledged, their imaging was carried out during tonic REM, while rapid eye movements occur phasically during REM, thereby limiting any conclusions that can be drawn about the anatomical substrates of an REM density change in depression.

Amygdalar modulation of REM mechanisms in narcolepsy: cataplexy and REM

Narcolepsy is a neuropsychiatric disorder characterized by excessive sleepiness during W as well as associated features including cataplexy (abrupt loss of muscle tone), hypnagogic and hypnopompic hallucinations, and sleep paralysis. Patients with narcolepsy show a shortened latency to the first REM episode of the night, and narcolepsy has often been viewed as a disorder of REM systems. The atonia of a cataplectic attack may have a mechanism similar to that of the generalized atonia of REM (reviewed in Schwartz *et al.*, 2008). Recently it has been recognized that the pathophysiology of narcolepsy involves a loss or dysfunction of hypocretinergic neurons with cell bodies in the perifornical region of the hypothalamus (reviewed in Schwartz *et al.*, 2008). Because cataplectic attacks typically are triggered by emotional stimuli, it is reasonable to suspect that an abnormality of hypothalamo-amygdalar function has a role in producing the symptoms of narcolepsy (Schwartz *et al.*, 2008).

To our knowledge there have not yet been neuroimaging studies of sleep states in patients with narcolepsy. This gap in our understanding of the pathophysiology of narcolepsy is likely to be filled in the near future, especially as it has been recognized that elucidating fundamental sleep mechanisms in narcolepsy may provide important insights into the ways in which emotion influences REM generally (Fosse *et al.*, 2002). In the study of Fosse *et al.* (2002), patients with narcolepsy and healthy control subjects were awakened from REM and dream mentation reports were elicited. Particularly following sleep-onset REM periods, the narcoleptic group described intensified emotion, especially anxiety/fear and joy/elation, though not anger and surprise. The investigators hypothesized that cholinergic and dopaminergic abnormalities in the "extended amygdala–forebrain region" could be involved in producing the altered emotional intensity of the REM dreams of patients with narcolepsy.

Although the REM state itself has not been imaged in narcolepsy, cataplectic attacks during W have been investigated with functional MRI. Schwartz *et al.* (2008) had subjects with narcolepsy with cataplexy and healthy control subjects watch sequences of humorous pictures. These stimuli produced an enhanced amygdalar response, coupled with a reduced hypothalamic response, in the narcolepsy with cataplexy group. The authors suggested that positive emotions might trigger aberrant patterns of hypothalamo-amygdalar activity that could in turn recruit ponto-medullary neurocircuitry involved in the muscle atonia of REM. On the other hand, as noted by Schwartz *et al.* (2008), there is not a consensus that cataplexy during W partakes of the same forebrain mechanisms as those underlying normal REM atonia. With single-cell recordings in the hypocretin knock-out mouse, Thankachan *et al.* (2009) recently found additional evidence that, at least in the mouse, cataplexy and REM are distinct behavioral states, with only partially overlapping neural control mechanisms. Therefore, a definitive answer to the question of what role the amygdala plays in the REM of narcoleptic patients must await the further application of functional neuroimaging to this population.

Evidence for amygdalar modulation of REM in PTSD

Post-traumatic stress disorder occurs in a substantial minority of people who have been exposed to a psychologically traumatic event. The diagnostic criteria include: reexperiencing the traumatic event as memories or flashbacks during W or nightmares during sleep, or having intense psychological distress from or physiological reactivity to reminders of the event; avoidance of stimuli reminiscent of the traumatic

event and general numbing of responsiveness to the environment; and symptoms of hyperarousal, including insomnia, irritability, hypervigilance, exaggerated startle, and difficulty concentrating. Thus PTSD is unique among mental disorders in that a disturbance of sleep is included twice among the diagnostic criteria. On the basis of evidence that repetitive, stereotypical anxiety dreams are highly prevalent in people with PTSD and are relatively specific to PTSD among the range of mental disorders, as well as the suggestion that dysfunctional REM neurocircuitry likely participates in the pathogenesis of both the post-traumatic anxiety dream and symptoms of PTSD manifested during W, exaggerated startle in particular, we (RJR) originally hypothesized that PTSD may be fundamentally a disorder of REM mechanisms (Ross *et al.*, 1989).

While there is as yet no consensus on the nature of the polysomnographic abnormalities that mark PTSD, there is considerable evidence for various REM disturbances. Two proposed REM abnormalities warrant particular attention. Firstly, REM episodes appear to be more easily interrupted in PTSD patients compared to normal control subjects (reviewed in Mellman, 2006). The authors further suggested that a decreased average REM episode duration in the early aftermath of a traumatic exposure could predict the development of PTSD. The second polysomnographic measure that has seemed, from several studies, to differentiate PTSD from normal sleep is an elevation of the density of REM phasic activity, in the form of both rapid eye movements and leg muscle twitch bursts (reviewed in Mellman, 2006). Given that most disturbing dreams in the general population seem to emerge from REM, this synthesis of the polysomnographic literature, with its emphasis on various REM abnormalities, has considerable face validity.

The likelihood that amygdalar modulation of REM plays a role in producing the sleep disturbance characteristic of PTSD gains strength from earlier observations of amygdalar activation during REM in healthy humans (Lydic *et al.*, 1991, Maquet *et al.*, 1996). Proposing that, with functional neuroimaging techniques, cognitive processes during REM can be mapped onto anatomically segregated brain regions, Schwartz and Maquet (2002) offered as a specific example the likely relationship of "common fear experience in dreams to the activation of the limbic system, in particular the amygdala." As a disorder that can be construed as, in part, one of intrusive reexperiencing in the form of repetitive, stereotypical anxiety dreams, PTSD, we would argue, almost certainly involves a dysfunction of the amygdalo-hypothalamo-brain stem circuitry controlling REM. Our laboratories' use of fear conditioning procedures in rats and mice to model the sleep disturbance of PTSD and to understand the role of the amygdala in fear-conditioned sleep changes should eventually promote the translation of findings in animals to the design of superior treatments for what can often be an intractable clinical problem. Achieving this long-range goal will be facilitated by the more ready application in humans of functional neuroimaging techniques to sleep states including REM. During W, and using various provocation techniques, increased amygdalar activation has been demonstrated in some studies of PTSD (Liberzon and Garfinkel, 2009), but the full extent and significance of amygdalar activation in PTSD will only be appreciated when neuroimaging encompasses the entire sleep–wake cycle.

Acknowledgments

Supported by grants MH61716, MH62483, MH072897, and the Department of Veterans Affairs.

References

Adrien, J., Dugovic, C. & Martin, P. (1991) Sleep-wakefulness patterns in the helpless rat. *Physiol Behav* **49**: 257–62.

Amaral, D., Price, J., Pitkanen, A. & Carmichael, S. (1992) Anatomical organization of the primate amydaloid complex. In *The Amygdala: Neurobiological Aspects of Emotion, Memory, and Mental Dysfunction*, ed. J. Aggleton. New York: Wiley-Liss, Inc.

Bordi, F., Ledoux, J., Clugnet, M. C. & Pavlides, C. (1993) Single-unit activity in the lateral nucleus of the amygdala and overlying areas of the striatum in freely behaving rats: rates, discharge patterns, and responses to acoustic stimuli. *Behav Neurosci* **107**: 757–69.

Braun, A. R., Balkin, T. J., Wesensten, N. J. *et al.* (1998) Dissociated pattern of activity in visual cortices and their projections during human rapid eye movement sleep. *Science* **279**: 91–5.

Buysse, D. J., Germain, A., Hall, M. L. *et al.* (2008) EEG spectral analysis in primary insomnia: NREM period effects and sex differences. *Sleep* **31**: 1673–82.

Buysse, D. J., Tu, X. M., Cherry, C. R. *et al.* (1999) Pretreatment REM sleep and subjective sleep quality distinguish depressed psychotherapy remitters and nonremitters. *Biol Psychiatry* **45**: 205–13.

Calvo, J., Simón-Arceo, K. & Fernández-Mas, R. (1996) Prolonged enhancement of REM sleep produced by carbachol microinjection into the amygdala. *NeuroRep* **7**: 577–80.

Calvo, J. M., Badillo, S., Morales-Ramirez, M. & Palacios-Salas, P. (1987) The role of the temporal lobe amygdala in ponto-geniculo-occipital activity and sleep organization in cats. *Brain Res* **403**: 22–30.

Calvo, J. M. & Fernandez-Guardiola, A. (1984) Phasic activity of the basolateral amygdala, cingulate gyrus, and hippocampus during REM sleep in the cat. *Sleep* **7**: 202–10.

Cape, E. G., Manns, I. D., Alonso, A., Beaudet, A. & Jones, B. E. (2000) Neurotensin-induced bursting of cholinergic basal forebrain neurons promotes gamma and theta cortical activity together with waking and paradoxical sleep. *J Neurosci* **20**: 8452–61.

Davis, M. (1992) The role of the amygdala in fear and anxiety. *Ann Rev Neurosci* **15**: 353–75.

Davis, M. & Whalen, P. J. (2001) The amygdala: vigilance and emotion. *Mol Psychiatry* **6**: 13–34.

Fosse, R., Stickgold, R. & Hobson, J. A. (2002) Emotional experience during rapid-eye-movement sleep in narcolepsy. *Sleep* **25**: 724–32.

Frysinger, R., Zhang, J. & Harper, R. (1988) Cardiovascular and respiratory relationships with neuronal discharge in the central nucleus of the amygdala during sleep–waking states. *Sleep* **11**: 317–32.

Gaudreau, H. & Pare, D. (1996) Projection neurons of the lateral amygdaloid nucleus are virtually silent throughout the sleep–waking cycle. *J Neurophysiol* **75**: 1301–5.

Germain, A., Buysse, D. J., Wood, A. & Nofzinger, E. (2004) Functional neuroanatomical correlates of eye movements during rapid eye movement sleep in depressed patients. *Psychiatry Res* **130**: 259–68.

Jacobs, B. L. & McGinty, D. J. (1971) Amygdala unit activity during sleep and waking. *Exp Neurol* **33**: 1–15.

Jha, S. K., Ross, R. J. & Morrison, A. R. (2005) Sleep-related neurons in the central nucleus of the amygdala of rats and their modulation by the dorsal raphe nucleus. *Physiol Behav* **86**: 415–26.

Kreindler, A. & Steriade, M. (1964) EEG patterns of arousal and sleep induced by stimulating various amygdaloid levels in the cat. *Arch Ital Biol* **102**: 576–86.

Lehmann, J., Nagy, J. I., Atmadia, S. & Fibiger, H. C. (1980) The nucleus basalis magnocellularis: the origin of a cholinergic projection to the neocortex of the rat. *Neuroscience* **5**: 1161–74.

Liberzon, I. & Garfinkel, S. N. (2009) Functional neuroimaging in post-traumatic stress disorder. In *Post-Traumatic Stress Disorder: Basic Science and Clinical Practice*, eds. P. J. Shiromani, T. M. Keane & J. E. LeDoux. New York: Humana Press, pp. 297–318.

Liu, X., Lonart, G. & Sanford, L. D. (2007) Transient fear-induced alterations in evoked release of norepinephrine and GABA in amygdala slices. *Brain Res* **1142**: 46–53.

Liu, X., Tang, X. & Sanford, L. D. (2003) Fear-conditioned suppression of REM sleep: relationship to Fos expression patterns in limbic and brainstem regions in BALB/cJ mice. *Brain Res* **991**: 1–17.

Liu, X., Yang, L., Wellman, L. L., Tang, X. & Sanford, L. D. (2009) GABAergic antagonism of the central nucleus of the amygdala attenuates reductions in rapid eye movement sleep after inescapable footshock stress. *Sleep* **32**: 888–96.

Lydic, R., Baghdoyan, H. A., Hibbard, L. *et al.* (1991) Regional brain glucose metabolism is altered during rapid eye movement sleep in the cat: a preliminary study. *J Comp Neurol* **304**: 517–29.

Maquet, P., Peters, J., Aerts, J. *et al.* (1996) Functional neuroanatomy of human rapid-eye-movement sleep and dreaming. *Nature* **383**: 163–6.

Mellman, T. A. (2006) Sleep and anxiety disorders. *Psychiatr Clin North Am* **29**: 1047–58.

Morrison, A. R., Sanford, L. D. & Ross, R. J. (2000) The amygdala: a critical modulator of sensory influence on sleep. *Biol Signals Recept* **9**: 283–96.

Nofzinger, E. A., Buysse, D. J., Germain, A. *et al.* (2004) Increased activation of anterior paralimbic and executive cortex from waking to rapid eye movement sleep in depression. *Arch Gen Psychiatry* **61**: 695–702.

Pawlyk, A. C., Morrison, A. R., Ross, R. J. & Brennan, F. X. (2008) Stress-induced changes in sleep in rodents: Models and mechanisms. *Neurosci Biobehav Rev* **32**: 99–117.

Perlis, M. L., Smith, M. T. & Pigeon, W. R. (2005) Etiology and pathophysiology of insomnia. In *Principles and Practice of Sleep Medicine*, 4th edn. eds. M. H. Kryger,

T. Roth & W. C. Dement. Philadelphia: Elsevier Saunders.

Reynolds, C. F., Gillin, J. C. & Kupfer, D. J. (1987) Sleep and affective disorders. In *Psychopharmacology: The Third Generation of Progress*. ed. H. Y. Meltzer. New York: Raven Press.

Ross, R. J., Ball, W. A., Sullivan, K. A. & Caroff, S. N. (1989) Sleep disturbance as the hallmark of posttraumatic stress disorder. *Am J Psychiatry* **146**: 697–707.

Sanford, L. D., Yang, L., Liu, X. & Tang, X. (2006a) Effects of tetrodotoxin (TTX) inactivation of the central nucleus of the amygdala (CNA) on dark period sleep and activity. *Brain Res* **1084**: 80–8.

Sanford, L. D., Yang, L., Tang, X. *et al.* (2006b) Cholinergic regulation of the central nucleus of the amygdala in rats: effects of local microinjections of cholinomimetics and cholinergic antagonists on arousal and sleep. *Neuroscience*, **141**, 2167–76.

Schwartz, S. & Maquet, P. (2002) Sleep imaging and the neuro-psychological assessment of dreams. *Trends Cogn Sci* **6**: 23–30.

Schwartz, S., Ponz, A., Poryazova, R. *et al.* (2008) Abnormal activity in hypothalamus and amygdala during humour processing in human narcolepsy with cataplexy. *Brain* **131**: 514–22.

Steriade, M. & McCarley, R. (1990) *Brainstem Control of Wakefulness and Sleep*. New York: Plenum Press.

Thankachan, S., Kaur, S. & Shiromani, P. J. (2009) Activity of pontine neurons during sleep and cataplexy in hypocretin knock-out mice. *J Neurosci* **29**: 1580–5.

van der Zee, E., Roozendaal, B., Bohus, B., Koolhaas, J. & Luiten, P. (1997) Muscarinic acetylcholine receptor immunoreactivity in the amygdala – I Cellular distribution correlated with fear-induced behavior *Neurosci* **76**: 63–73.

Pontomedullary mediated REM-sleep atonia

Yuan-Yang Lai and Jerome M. Siegel

Summary

The medial pontomedullary reticular formation has been implicated in the control of motor activity in REM sleep. Electrical stimulation of points within this area elicits global inhibition of skeletal motor activity in decerebrate animals. This area can be segregated into four distinct subregions based on the response to chemical stimulation. Injection of glutamate, acetylcholine, and corticotropin-releasing factor into the medial pons, the pontine inhibitory area, induces muscle atonia. In the medial medulla, the nucleus magnocellularis (NMC) of the rostroventral medulla responds to glutamate and corticotropin-releasing factor and the nucleus paramedianus of the caudomedial medulla responds to acetylcholine injection, with suppression of muscle tone being induced by these chemicals. In contrast, the transmitter involved in elicitation of atonia by electrical stimulation of the nucleus gigantocellularis of the dorsomedial medulla is unclear. Lesions in this area increase phasic and tonic muscle activity in REM sleep in the chronic animal. Our recent study found that an area rostral to the pons, located at the ventral portion of the junction of the midbrain and pons, the ventral mesopontine junction (VMPJ), is also involved in the control of muscle activity in sleep. Neurotoxic lesions of the VMPJ produce periodic leg movements in slow-wave sleep and increase phasic and tonic muscle activity in REM sleep in the cat, symptoms resembling the human REM sleep behavior disorder (RBD). The anatomical proximity of the VMPJ and the substantia nigra may thus provide a link between RBD and Parkinsonism.

Introduction

The loss of muscle tone in the postural muscles is a characteristic of REM sleep. The pontomedullary reticular formation has been hypothesized to play an important role in this regulation. Activation of a portion of the medial pontomedullary reticular formation suppresses motor activity, whereas, inactivation or damage to this region causes REM sleep without atonia and/or RBD, in which patients appear to act out of their dreams. REM sleep without atonia and RBD are at increased incidence in patients with neurodegenerative diseases, Parkinsonism, Alzheimer's disease and spinocerebellar ataxia type 2.

Electrophysiology studies

Acute animals

Magoun and Rhines (1946) were the first to report that electrical stimulation in the medial medulla completely suppresses reflex activities including the blink, flexor, and patellar reflexes in the chlorolosane anesthetized and decerebrated cats. This bulbar stimulation also suppresses muscle rigidity induced by decerebration and motor responses elicited by motor cortex stimulation. The inhibitory area identified by Magoun and Rhines is mainly located in the ventral portion of the medial medulla, equivalent to the NMC in the cat and nuclei gigantocellularis alpha and ventralis in the rat. However, stimulation in the dorsal part of the medial medulla, the nucleus gigantocellularis (NGC), and the caudal portion of the medial medulla, the nucleus paramedianus (NPM), has also been shown to suppress muscle tone (Hajnik *et al.*, 2000; Kohyama *et al.*, 1998; Lai *et al.*, 1987). The medullary inhibitory system is located in the medial reticular formation. Almost 90% of sites activated within 1.5 mm and 0.8 mm from the midline elicit inhibition of muscle tone in the cat and rat, respectively (Hajnik *et al.*, 2000; Lai *et al.*, 1987). Less than 30% of sites between 1.5 mm to 2.5 mm in the cat and 0.8 mm to 1.5 mm in the rat suppress muscle tone. The latency of suppression of hindlimb muscle tone induced by medial medullary stimulation can be distinguished into early (20.1–22.1 msec) and late (41.3–44.4 msec) phase indicating that two groups of neurons are involved (Kohyama *et al.*, 1998). The conduction velocity of neurons responsible for the early and late phase is about 73 m/sec and 20 m/sec, respectively (Engberg *et al.*, 1968; Kohyama *et al.*, 1998). The suppressive effect of medullary reticulospinal neurons on muscle activity may be mediated through both monosynaptic terminal contact on the motoneuron and polysynaptic action via interneurons. Activation of the medial medulla elicits inhibitory postsynaptic potentials (IPSPs) in spinal motoneurons and interneurons in chloralose anesthetized and decerebrated cats (Engberg *et al.*, 1968; Takakusaki *et al.*, 2001).

Changes in the firing rate of neurons in the pontine inhibitory area (PIA) including nuclei reticular pontis oralis and caudalis have been reported to correlate with the changes in muscle tone. Hoshino and Pompeiano (1976) demonstrated that an increase in PIA neuronal activity correlates with muscle atonia induced by systemic injection of eserine sulfate in the decerebrate animal. They hypothesized that the loss of decerebrate rigidity (muscle atonia) induced by activation of the PIA is mediated through the bulbospinal inhibitory system. Indeed, electrical stimulation of the PIA activates the medial medullary reticulospinal neurons (Kohyama *et al.*, 1998), which in turn project to the spinal cord and suppress postural muscle activity in the decerebrate animal (Hajnik *et al.*, 2000; Kohyama *et al.*, 1998; Lai *et al.*, 1987; Mileykovskiy *et al.*, 2000). The latency of suppression of hindlimb muscle tone induced by pontine stimulation can also be distinguished into the early (21.1–23.0 msec) and late (42.8–46.4 msec) phases (Kohyama *et al.*, 1998). The early and late phases of muscle tone suppression have been hypothesized to be the result of activation of the two groups of the medullary reticulospinal neurons, described above (Kohyama *et al.*, 1998). However, the possibility that pontine reticulospinal neurons exert a direct inhibitory action on spinal motoneurons cannot be ruled out. Anatomical studies have demonstrated that PIA neurons project to the spinal cord (Matsuyama *et al.*, 1999; Figure 13.1).

Muscle-tone suppression has been hypothesized to result from a combination of the release of inhibitory amino acids and cessation of release of the monoaminergic neurons. Electrical stimulation of the PIA produces muscle atonia and simultaneously increases GABA and glycine release and decreases norepinephrine and serotonin release onto motor nuclei in the decerebrate animal (Lai *et al.*, 2001; Kodama *et al.*, 2003; Figure 13.1). The decrease in norepinephrine and serotonin release onto motor neuron pools induced by PIA activation has been suggested to result from an inactivation of the locus coeruleus (LC) and medullary raphe nuclei. Activation of the LC increases motor activity (Lai *et al.*, 1989). In contrast, lesions in the LC or injection of clonidine, an α_2 adrenoreceptor agonist that inhibits noradrenergic neuronal activity, into the LC induces muscle atonia in the decerebrate cat (D'Ascanio *et al.*, 1989). Serotonin has also been shown to play a role in the regulation of motor activity. Electrical stimulation of the raphe pallidus elicits EPSPs in spinal motoneurons (Fung and Barnes, 1989). Activation of the PIA has been shown to exert an inhibitory effect on LC neuronal activity via GABAergic and glycinergic mechanisms (Mileykovskiy *et al.*, 2000; Figure 13.1). Neurons in the PIA also project to the medullary raphe nucleus (Gallager and Pert, 1978), although the phenotypes of the projection neurons have not been identified (Figure 13.1). The increase in inhibitory amino acid release into motor neuron pools induced by the PIA stimulation may result from an activation of medullary GABAergic and glycinergic neurons, which project to the spinal cord (Holstege, 1991; Figure 13.1).

Chronic animals

The phenomenon of generalized loss of muscle tone seen in the decerebrate animals has been identified in REM sleep in the cat, rat, and in humans. The medial pontomedullary reticular formation, whose activation suppresses muscle tone, has been hypothesized to be responsible for the generation and maintenance of REM sleep atonia. Indeed, REM-on cells, whose firing rate increased immediately before and during REM sleep, have been recorded in the pons and medulla (Kanamori *et al.*, 1980). In the medial medulla, REM-on cells have been found in the NGC, NMC, raphe magnus, nucleus parvocellularis, and nucleus paragigantocellularis lateralis (Kanamori *et al.*, 1980), all areas are located within 1.5 mm from the midline in the cat. The REM-on neurons in the pons are located in nuclei reticularis pontis oralis and caudalis, the rostral part of the locus coeruleus alpha (LCα) and peri-LCα, area

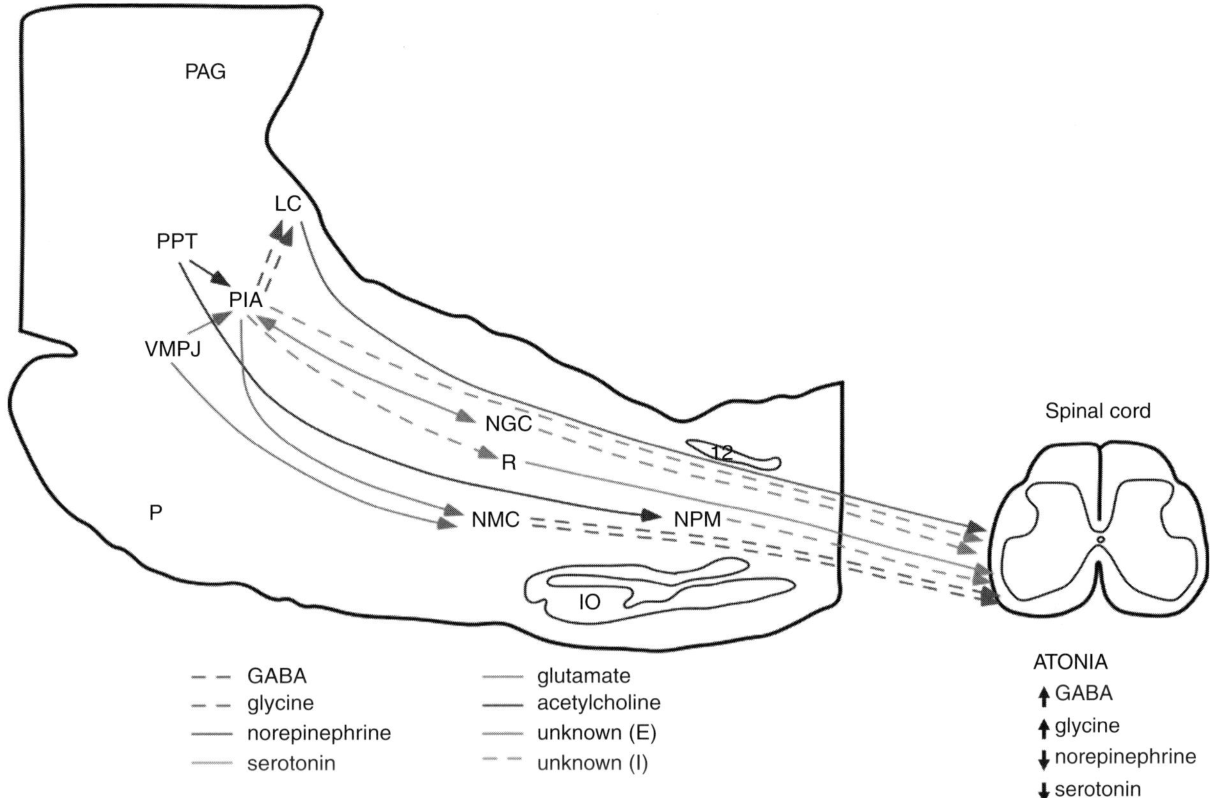

Figure 13.1 Hypothetical neural circuit and transmitters involved in the control of REM sleep atonia. Solid and dashed lines represent excitatory and inhibitory effects on the target site respectively. Glutamatergic and cholinergic activation of the pontine inhibitory area (PIA) elicits muscle atonia, which results from a combination of activation of GABAergic and glycinergic neurons in the medial medulla and inactivation of noradrenergic neurons in the locus coeruleus and serotonergic neurons in the medullary raphe nuclei. The pontine glutamatergic and cholinergic innervations originate from the ventral mesopontine junction (VMPJ) and pedunculopontine nucleus (PPT). Neurons in the VMPJ and PPT also project to the nuclei magnocellularis (NMC) and paramedianus (NPM) in the medial medulla, respectively. IO: inferior olivary nucleus; LC: locus coeruleus; NGC: nucleus gigantocellularis; P: pyramidal tract; PAG: periaqueductal gray; R: medullary raphe nucleus; unknown (E) and unknown (I): transmitter that exerts excitatory and inhibitory effect on the target site; 12: hypoglossal nucleus. (See plate section for color version.)

medial-ventral to the LCα. Extracellular recording combined with antidromic stimulation demonstrated that the REM-on cells in the pons project to the NMC, which in turn project to the spinal cord (Kanamori *et al.*, 1980). Anatomical studies also showed that neurons in the medial pons project to the NGC and NMC, which in turn project to the spinal cord (Kanamori *et al.*, 1980; Kausz, 1991; Lai *et al.*, 1993). As in the findings in the acute animal, activation of the PIA and medial medulla hyperpolarizes motoneurons (Chase *et al.*, 1986). The hyperpolarizing effect of pontomedullary stimulation on spinal motoneurons is state dependent. Medullary stimulation-elicited IPSPs can be seen in all recorded motoneurons during REM sleep, while induced IPSPs are generated in some motoneurons when the stimulation is applied during wakefulness and SWS. The amplitude and latency of the IPSP induced by medullary stimulation during wakefulness and SWS and REM sleep are different, with smaller amplitude and longer latency in wakefulness and SWS (Chase *et al.*, 1986).

The clearest evidence for pontomedullary reticular formation involvement in the control of REM sleep atonia is from studies using lesion technique. In 1960, Jouvet and Mounier showed that electrical coagulation of the dorsolateral pons eliminates REM sleep in the cat. It was later found that small electrolytic lesions in the dorsolateral pons do not eliminate REM sleep but elicit REM sleep without atonia (Hendricks *et al.*, 1982; Shouse and Siegel, 1992). Animals with dorsal pontine electrolytic lesions not only show absence of atonia but also generate orienting, head-raising, walking, and attacking behaviors during REM sleep (Hendricks *et al.*, 1982). However, the neural substrates of the muscle atonia and behavior produced by such lesions in REM sleep are not clear because electrolytic lesion damages both cells and passing fibers. Thus, chemical lesions were used to evaluate the role of pontomedullary reticular formation in the control of muscle activity in REM sleep. Gall *et al.* (2007) showed that neurotoxic ibotenic lesions of the PIA generate REM sleep without atonia. However, exploratory activities seen in the dorsal pontine electrolytic lesioned animals are not found in animals with neurotoxic lesions. In contrast, neurotoxic lesions in the medial medulla generate REM sleep without atonia either with or without change in phasic motor activity in the cat (Holmes and Jones, 1994; Schenkel and Siegel, 1989). Limb and tail movements and head orienting and tracking in REM sleep are observed in animals with large lesions in the medial medulla (Holmes and Jones, 1994). Thus, it is clear that the PIA and medial medulla are important in the generation and maintenance of muscle atonia in REM sleep.

Pharmacological studies

Acute animals

Transmitters in the pons and medulla involved in the control of motor activity can be studied by using microinjection and reverse microdialysis perfusion techniques. Based on motor response to chemical applications, the inhibitory area of the medial medulla can be segregated into three distinct groups, the glutamate responsive area of the NMC, the cholinergic responsive area of the NPM, and the NGC region, which is not responsive to either glutamate or cholinergic agonists (Lai and Siegel, 1988; Figure 13.1). Cholinergic but not glutamatergic agonists injected into the NPM induced muscle atonia. On the other hand, glutamatergic but not cholinergic agonists injected into the NMC suppress muscle tone (Hajnik *et al.*, 2000; Lai and Siegel, 1988). In contrast, the transmitters in the NGC involved in the regulation of muscle tone remain unclear. Neither cholinergic nor glutamatergic agonists injected into the NGC suppresses muscle tone. In the PIA, injection of both cholinergic and glutamatergic agonists has been found to induce muscle atonia (Hajnik *et al.*, 2000; Lai and Siegel, 1988; Figure 13.1). The latency of muscle atonia after glutamate (PIA and NMC) and cholinergic (PIA and NPM) agonist

injections into the pontomedullary reticular formation is 18 to 24 sec and 25 to 34 sec, respectively, with the duration ranging from 4 min to 13 min (Lai and Siegel, 1988). In contrast, carbachol injected into the PIA produces a long-lasting (> 40 min) muscle atonia. Thus, pontine carbachol-induced muscle atonia can be used to determine the neural circuitry involved in the pharmacological control of muscle tone. We have found that unilateral injection of glutamate antagonist, γ-D-glutamyglycine, into the NMC reverses the atonia induced by PIA carbachol injection (Lai and Siegel, 1988) indicating that the descending motor inhibitory system requires an activation of glutamatergic neurons in the PIA, which projects to the NMC (Figure 13.1).

The suppressive effect on motor activity induced by glutamate injections into the PIA and NMC have been shown to be mediated through non-NMDA receptor mechanisms (Hajnik *et al.*, 2000; Lai and Siegel, 1991). Microinjection of non-NMDA receptor agonists, kainate and ibotenic acid, into the PIA and NMC generate muscle atonia, and this effect can be blocked by prior injection of non-NMDA receptor antagonists, 6-cyano-7-nitroquinoxaline-2,3-dione and 6,7-dinitroquinoxaline-2,3-dione, into the PIA and NMC. In contrast, NMDA receptor agonists injected into the same site of the PIA and NMC elicit an opposite effect on motor activity, increased muscle tone and/or rhythmic locomotor activity. The NMDA effect on motor activity can be blocked by local injection of the specific NMDA antagonist, DL-2-amino-5-phosphonovaleric acid (Hajnik *et al.*, 2000; Lai and Siegel, 1991). It has been shown that activation of muscarinic receptors in the PIA and NPM participates in the modulation of motor activity. Atropine, a muscarinic receptor antagonist, blocks muscle atonia induced by acetylcholine injection into the PIA and NPM (Lai and Siegel, 1988). In addition to glutamatergic and cholinergic mechanisms, corticotropin-releasing factor and serotonin also play a role in the control of muscle activity in the PIA and medial medulla. Corticotropin-releasing factor injected into the PIA and NMC suppresses muscle tone. In contrast, injection of serotonin into the PIA increases muscle tone.

Tracing combined with immunohistochemical studies showed that glutamatergic and cholinergic neurons projecting to the PIA originate from the ventral mesopontine junction (VMPJ) and the pedunculopontine/dorsolateral tegmental nuclei, respectively (Lai *et al.*, 1993; Figure 13.1). Cholinergic neurons in the pedunculopontine and dorsolateral tegmental nuclei, that participate in the regulation of muscle tone, also project to the NPM (Shiromani *et al.*, 1990; Figure 13.1). The NMC of the medulla receives glutamatergic projections from the rostroventral pons and caudal ventral midbrain, the VMPJ, and the PIA (Lai *et al.*, 1999; Figure 13.1).

Chronic animals

George *et al.* (1964) first reported that cholinergic agonists, carbachol and oxotremorine, injected into the dorsal part of the PIA produced REM sleep. Van Dongen *et al.* (1978) concluded that the dorsal PIA carbachol injection generates muscle atonia; however, the animal is awake. Further studies by Reinoso-Suarez *et al.* (1994) showed that carbachol injections into the dorsal PIA fail to generate PGO spikes, rapid eye movement, and miosis, despite of muscle atonia. In contrast, REM sleep signs are elicited by carbachol injection into the ventral part of the PIA in the cat. They concluded that carbachol injection into the dorsal and ventral PIA induces wake/atonia and REM sleep/atonia, respectively. As with the dorsal PIA, unilateral injection of acetylcholine into the medullary NPM also suppresses muscle tone without showing any other signs of REM sleep (Lai *et al.*, 1988).

Consistent with the study in acute animals, excitatory amino acid microinjection into the NMC and pons elicits muscle atonia in chronic animals. Glutamate injected into the NMC reduces muscle tone, though the animal remains awake (Lai and Siegel, 1988). Onoe and Sakai (1995) reported that injection of the non-NMDA receptor agonist, kainic acid, into the dorsal PIA suppresses muscle tone. At the motor nucleus level, strychnine, a glycine receptor antagonist, has been shown to reverse medial pontomedullary stimulation induced IPSPs in motoneurons in REM sleep indicating that a glycinergic mechanism is involved in REM sleep atonia (Soja *et al.*, 1987). However, recent studies, using the reverse microdialysis perfusion technique to infuse strychnine into motoneuron pools in naturally sleeping animals have questioned whether REM sleep atonia is solely induced and maintained by glycine. Brooks and Peever (2008) demonstrated that strychnine applied to the trigeminal motor nuclei fails to reverse muscle atonia but increases phasic motor activity in REM sleep. Similarly, bicuculline, a $GABA_A$ receptor antagonist, and strychnine mixed with bicuculline infused into the motoneuron nucleus also fail to eliminate muscle

atonia in REM sleep (Brooks and Peever, 2008). On the other hand, Jelev *et al.* (2001) demonstrated that infusion of 5-tryptamine, a serotonin precursor, into the hypoglossal nucleus partially restores tonic muscle activity in the tongue in REM sleep. Based on our studies in the decerebrate animal, we have hypothesized that muscle atonia may be attributed to the combination of activation of inhibitory amino acid and inactivation of monoamine systems (Kodama *et al.*, 2003; Lai *et al.*, 2001). Further studies are needed to evaluate the hypothesis.

REM sleep behavior disorder and the ventral mesopontine junction

REM sleep behavior disorder (RBD) is characterized by violent behavior that appears to correlate with subsequent dream reports. The dream-related behaviors include talking, yelling, kicking, and jumping (Schenck and Mahowald, 1990). Patients with RBD may cause injury to themselves and to their bed partners. Atonia in REM sleep can prevent such motor behaviors and has obvious adaptive value. In addition to behavior responses, an increase in percentage of REM sleep without atonia and an increase in phasic motor activity in SWS and REM sleep have also been reported in RBD (Schenck and Mahowald, 1990). It has been hypothesized that dorsal pontine lesions may cause RBD. However, the dorsal pontine area appears normal in most RBD patients (Mazza *et al.*, 2006; Schenck and Mahowald, 1990).

We have reported that electrical stimulation in the rostral ventral pons elicits muscle atonia during stimulation, whereas, rhythmic activities are elicited during interstimulation periods (Lai and Siegel, 1990). We further found that neurotoxic lesions in this area and the caudal ventral midbrain, the VMPJ, induces spontaneous or sensory (touching, puffing) induced locomotor-like activity and/or phasic motor activity in the decerebrate cat. Ventral mesopontine junction lesion-induced motor hyperactivity can be attenuated or blocked by the injection of non-NMDA agonists, kainate and ibotenic acid, and NMDA antagonist, DL-2-amino-5-phosphonovaleric acid into the NMC. We hypothesized that the VMPJ may be involved in the regulation of motor activity in sleep. To evaluate our hypothesis, we performed neurotoxic NMDA lesions in the VMPJ in the chronic cat (Lai *et al.*, 2008). After VMPJ lesion (Figure 13.2), cats develop motor hyperactivity in

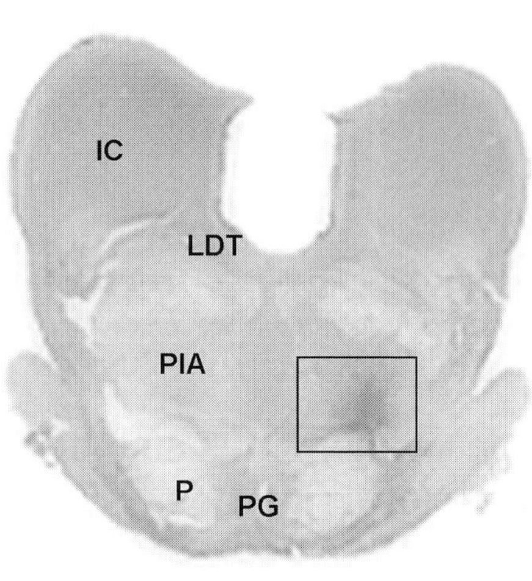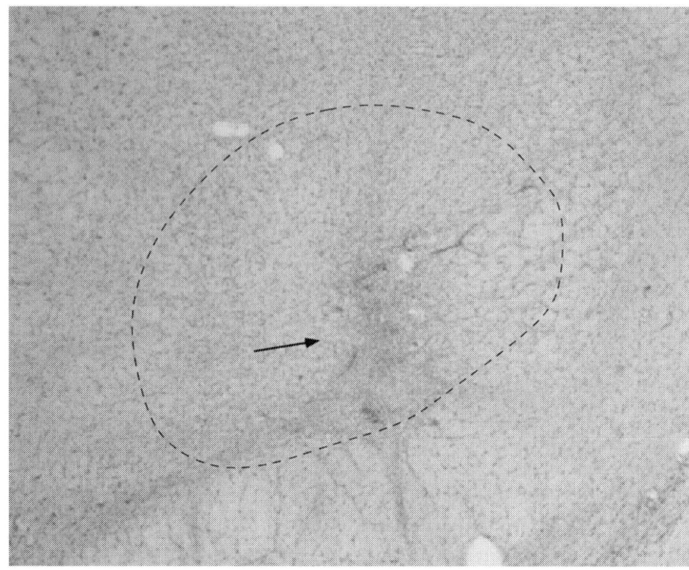

Figure 13.2 Photomicrograph showing the NMDA lesion site in the ventral mesopontine junction (VMPJ). Unilateral lesion in the caudal VMPJ was performed in this cat, which developed RBD-like activity after lesion. Tissue section was processed with neutral red. The circled area shown on the right was taken from the rectangular area shown on the left. Arrow shown on the right represents the tip of NMDA injection. IC: inferior colliculus; LDT: laterodorsal tegmental nucleus; P: pyramidal tract; PG: pontine gray; PIA: pontine inhibitory area.

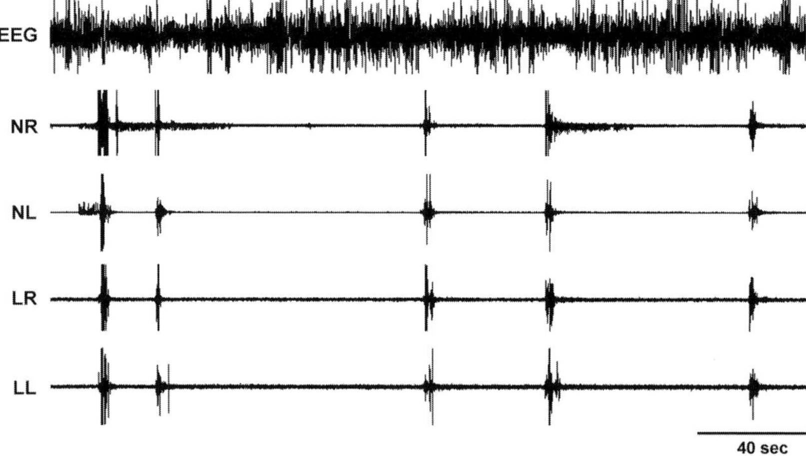

Figure 13.3 Polygraphic recording showing periodic leg movements in slow-wave sleep in the cat after VMPJ lesion. NL and NR: left and right neck EMG; LL and LR: left and right limb EMG.

sleep. The VMPJ-lesioned cat shows periodic leg movements in SWS (Figure 13.3) and an increase in phasic and tonic muscle activity in REM sleep (Figure 13.4). Leg twitching, head raising, and moving in REM sleep (Figure 13.5) were also seen in the VMPJ-lesioned cat. However, motor activity and behavior responses in wake are normal. Behavioral responses in wake and motor hyperactivity in sleep seen in our VMPJ-lesioned animal resemble that in human RBD. Indeed, recent studies have shown dysfunction of the ventral pons in human RBD (Mazza *et al.*, 2006; Schenck and Mahowald, 1990).

In conclusion, postural skeletal muscle tone is absent in REM sleep and is associated with brief intrusions of phasic motor activity. The pontomedullary reticular formation has been suggested to play a key role in the generation and maintenance of muscle atonia. Activation of the PIA not only excites the inhibitory amino acid system in the medullary NGC and NMC but also inhibits monoaminergic neuronal

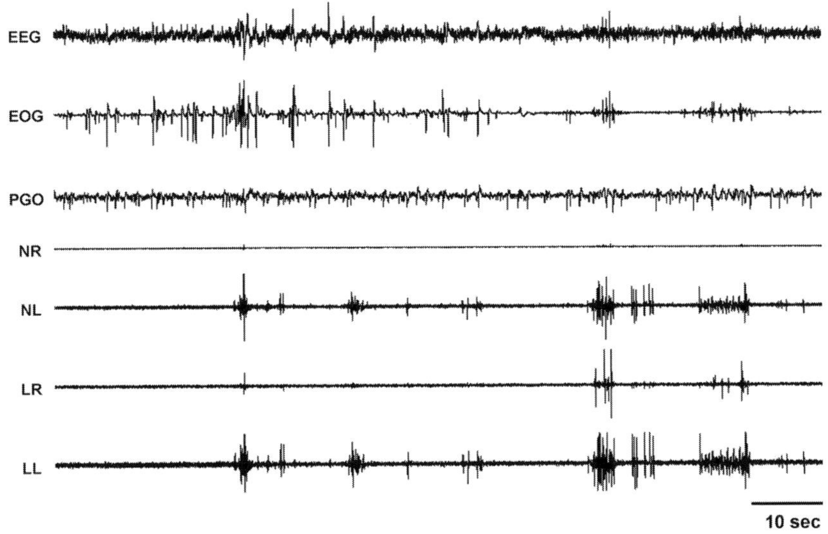

Figure 13.4 Polygraphic recording showing abnormal motor activity in REM sleep after VMPJ lesion. The cat showed an increase in basal muscle tone and phasic motor activity in REM sleep. EOG: electrooculogram; PGO: pontogeniculooccipital.

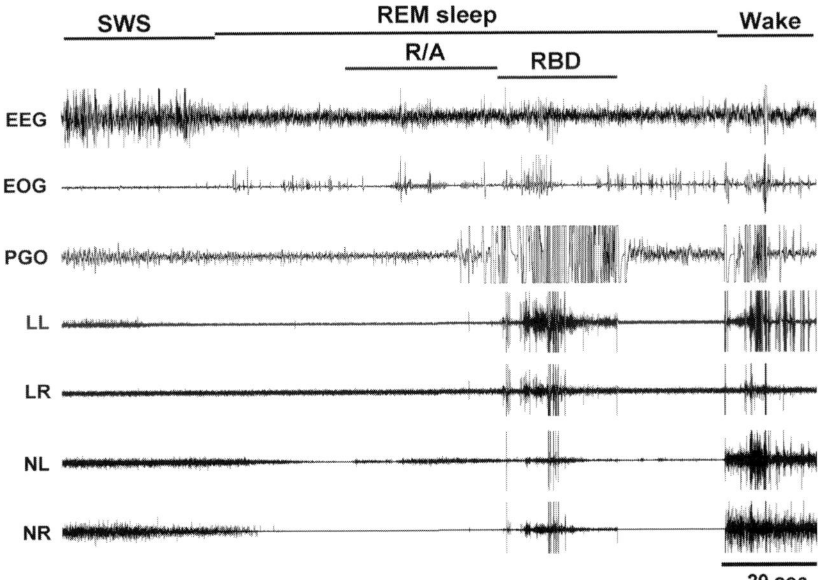

Figure 13.5 REM sleep behavior disorder-like activity in a cat after VMPJ lesion. The RBD-like activity was preceded with an increase in muscle tone. Leg twitching and head raising were seen to be accompanied with polygraphic recording of RBD-like activity. R/A: REM sleep without atonia.

activity in the LC and medullary raphe nuclei. As a consequence, an increase in glycine and GABA release and a simultaneous decrease in norepinephrine and serotonin release into motoneuron pools may be required in the inducing and maintaining of muscle atonia in REM sleep. Dysfunction of the medial pontomedullary reticular formation may result in an imbalance of these transmitters' release into the motoneuron pools thus causing REM sleep without atonia and RBD.

References

Brooks, P. L. & Peever, J. H. (2008) Glycinergic and GABAA-mediated inhibition of somatic motoneurons does not mediate rapid eye movement sleep motor atonia. *J Neurosci* **28**: 3535–45.

Chase, M. H., Morales, F. R., Boxer, P. A., Fung, S. J. & Soja, P. (1986) Effect of stimulation of the nucleus reticularis gigantocellularis on the membrane potential of cat lumbar motoneurons during sleep and wakefulness. *Brain Res* **386**: 237–44.

D'Ascanio, P., Pompeiano, O. & Tononi, G. (1989) Inhibition of vestibulospinal reflexes during the episodes of postural atonia induced by unilateral lesion of the locus coeruleus in the decerebrate cat. *Arch Ital Biol* **127**: 81–97.

Engberg, I., Lundberg, A. & Ryall, R. W. (1968) Reticulospinal inhibition of transmission in reflex pathways. *J Physiol* **194**: 201–23.

Fung, S. J. & Barnes, C. D. (1989) Raphe-produced excitation of spinal cord motoneurons in the cat. *Neurosci Lett* **103**: 185–90.

Gall, A. J., Poremba, A. & Blumberg, M. S. (2007) Brainstem cholinergic modulation of muscle tone in infant rats. *Eur J Neurosci* **253**: 367–75.

Gallager, D. W. & Pert, A. (1978) Afferents to brain stem nuclei (brain stem raphe, nucleus reticularis pontis caudalis and nucleus gigantocellularis) in the rat as demonstrated by microiontophoretically applied horseradish peroxidase. *Brain Res* **144**: 257–75.

George, R., Haslett, W. L. & Jenden, D. J. (1964). A cholinergic mechanism in the brainstem reticular formation: induction of paradoxical sleep. *Int J Neuropharmacol* **3**: 541–52.

Hajnik, T., Lai, Y. Y. & Siegel, J. M. (2000). Atonia-related regions in the rodent pons and medulla. *J Neurophysiol* **84**: 1942–8.

Hendricks, J. C., Morrison, A. R. & Mann, G. L. (1982) Different behaviors during paradoxical sleep without atonia depend on pontine lesion site. *Brain Res* **239**: 81–105.

Holmes, C. J. & Jones, B. E. (1994) Importance of cholinergic, GABAergic, serotonergic and other neurons in the medial medullary reticular formation for sleep–wake states studied by cytotoxic lesions in the cat. *Neuroscience* **62**: 1179–200.

Holstege, J. C. (1991) Ultrastructure evidence for GABAergic brain stem projections to spinal motoneurons in the rat. *J Neurosci* **11**: 159–67.

Hoshino, K. & Pompeiano, O. (1976) Selective discharge of pontine neurons during the postural atonia produced by an anticholinesterase in the decerebrate cat. *Arch Ital Biol* **114**: 244–7.

Jelev, A., Sood, S., Liu, H., Nolan, P. & Horner, R. L. (2001) Microdialysis perfusion of 5-HT into hypoglossal motor nucleus differentially modulates genioglossus activity across natural sleep-wake states in rats. *J Physiol* **532**: 467–81.

Jouvet, M. & Mounier, D. (1960) Effects des lesions de la formation reticule pontique sur le sommeil du chat. *C R Soc. de Biol* **154**: 2301–5.

Kanamori, N., Sakai, K. & Jouvet, M. (1980) Neuronal activity specific to paradoxical sleep in the ventromedial medullary reticular formation of unrestrained cats. *Brain Res* **189**: 251–5.

Kausz, M. (1991) Arrangement of neurons in the medullary reticular formation and raphe nuclei projecting to thoracic, lumbar and sacral segments of the spinal cord in the cat. *Anat Embryol* **183**: 151–63.

Kodama, T., Lai, Y. Y. & Siegel, J. M. (2003) Changes in inhibitory amino acid release linked to pontine-induced atonia: an *in vivo* microdialysis study. *J Neurosci* **23**: 1548–54.

Kohyama, J., Lai, Y. Y. & Siegel, J. M. (1998) Reticulospinal systems mediate atonia with short and long latencies. *J Neurophysiol* **80**: 1839–51.

Lai, Y. Y. & Siegel, J. M. (1988) Medullary regions regulating atonia. *J Neurosci* **8**: 4790–6.

Lai, Y. Y. & Siegel, J. M. (1990) Muscle tone suppression and stepping produced by stimulation of the midbrain and rostral pontine reticular formation. *J Neurosci* **10**: 2727–38.

Lai, Y. Y. & Siegel, J. M. (1991) Pontomedullary glutamate receptors mediating locomotion and muscle tone suppression. *J Neurosci* **11**: 2931–7.

Lai, Y. Y., Siegel, J. M. & Wilson, W. J. (1987) Effect of blood pressure on medial medulla-induced muscle atonia. *Am J Physiol* **252**, H1249–57.

Lai, Y. Y., Strahlendorf, H. K., Fung, S. J. & Barnes, C. D. (1989) The actions of two monoamines on spinal motoneurons from stimulation of the locus coeruleus. *Brain Res* **484**: 268–72.

Lai, Y. Y., Clements, J. R. & Siegel, J. M. (1993) Glutamatergic and cholinergic projections to the pontine inhibitory area identified with horseradish peroxidase retrograde transport and immunohistochemistry. *J Comp Neurol* **336**: 321–30.

Lai, Y. Y., Clements, J. R., Wu, X. Y. *et al.* (1999) Brainstem projections to the ventromedial medulla in cat: retrograde transport horseradish peroxidase and immunohistochemical studies. *J Comp Neurol* **408**: 419–36.

Lai, Y. Y., Kodama, T. & Siegel, J. M. (2001) Changes in monoamine release in the ventral horn and hypoglossal nucleus linked to pontine inhibition of muscle tone: an *in vivo* microdialysis study. *J Neurosci* **21**: 7384–91.

Lai, Y. Y., Hsieh, K. C., Nguyen, D., Peever, J. & Siegel, J. M. (2008) Neurotoxic lesions at the ventral mesopontine junction change sleep time and muscle activity during sleep: an animal model of motor disorders in sleep. *Neuroscience* **154**: 431–43.

Magoun, H. W. & Rhines, R. (1946) An inhibitory mechanism in the bulbar reticular formation. *J Neurophysiol* **9**: 165–71.

Matsuyama, K., Mori, F., Kuze, B. & Mori, S. (1999). Morphology of single pontine reticulospinal axons in the lumbar enlargement of the cat: a study using anterograde tracer PHA-L. *J Comp Neurol* **410**: 413–30.

Mazza, S., Soucy, J., Gravel, P. *et al.* (2006) Assessing whole brain perfusion changes in patients with REM sleep behavior disorder. *Neurology* **67**: 1618–22.

Mileykovskiy, B. Y., Kiyashchenko, L. I., Kodama, T., Lai, Y. Y. & Siegel, J. M. (2000) Activation of pontine and medullary motor inhibitory regions reduces discharge in neurons located in the locus coeruleus and the anatomical equivalent of the midbrain locomotor region. *J Neurosci* **20**: 8551–8.

Onoe, H. & Sakai, K. (1995) Kainate receptors: a novel mechanism in paradoxical (REM) sleep generation. *NeuroReport* **6**: 353–6.

Pompeiano, O., D'Ascanio, P., Horn, E. & Stampacchia. G. (1987) Effects of local injection of the α2-adrenergic agonist clonidine into the locus coeruleus complex on the gain of vestibulospinal and cervicospinal reflexes in decerebrate cats. *Arch Ital Biol* **125**: 225–89.

Reinoso-Suarez, F., De Andres, I., Rodrigo-Angulo, M. L. & Rodriguez-Veiga, E. (1994) Location and anatomical connections of a paradoxical sleep induction site in the cat ventral pontine tegmentum. *Eur J Neurosci* **6**: 1829–36.

Schenck, C. H. & Mahowald, M. W. (1990) Polysomnographic, neurologic, psychiatric, and clinical outcome report on 70 consecutive cases with REM sleep behavior disorder (RBD): sustained clonazepam efficacy in 89.5% of 57 treated patients. *Cleveland Clin J Med* **37**: Suppl, S9–23.

Schenkel, E., & Siegel, J. M. (1989) REM sleep without atonia after lesions of the medial medulla. *Neurosci Lett* **98**: 159–65.

Shiromani, P. J., Lai, Y. Y. & Siegel, J. M. (1990) Descending projections from the dorsolateral pontine tegmentum to the paramedian reticular nucleus of the caudal medulla in the cat. *Brain Res* **517**: 224–8.

Shouse, M. N. & Siegel, J. M. (1992) Pontine regulation of REM sleep components in cats: integrity of the pedunculopontine tegmentum (PPT) is important for phasic events but unnecessary for atonia during REM sleep. *Brain Res* **571**: 50–63.

Soja, P. J., Morales, F. R., Baranyi, A. & Chase, M. H. (1987) Effect of inhibitory amino acid antagonists on IPSPs induced in lumbar motoneurons upon stimulation of the nucleus reticularis gigantocellularis during active sleep. *Brain Res* **423**: 353–8.

Takakusaki, K., Kohyama, J. & Matsuyama, K. (2001) Medullary reticulospinal tract mediating the generalized motor inhibition in cats: parallel inhibitory mechanisms acting on motoneurons and on interneuronal transmission in reflex pathways. *Neuroscience* **103**: 511–27.

Van Dongen, P. A. M., Broekkamp, C. L. E. & Cools, A. R. (1978) Atonia after carbachol microinjections near the locus coeruleus in cats. *Pharmacol Biochem Behav* **8**: 527–32.

Phenomenology and function of myoclonic twitching in developing rats

Mark S. Blumberg

Summary

The development of adult sleep is a complex process comprising the emergence and coalescence of sleep components and the consolidation of sleep into progressively longer bouts. Achieving adequate descriptions of infant sleep and its development requires the use of methods that are scaled to the structural and temporal properties of sleep at early ages. This chapter reviews work demonstrating in infant rats how measures of sleep–wake behavior (e.g., myoclonic twitching during REM sleep, high-amplitude movements during wakefulness) coupled with electromyography of skeletal muscle (e.g., nuchal muscle) reveal sleep–wake cycles that are highly structured in space and time. Consideration of other measures – for example, extraocular muscle and cortical activity – provides further support for the notion that adult sleep is constructed in an orderly fashion through the addition of components (e.g., delta waves) and alterations in the statistical structure of sleep and wake bouts. Neurophysiological recordings and lesions in the medulla, mesopontine region, hypothalamus, and forebrain indicate that the brain critically contributes to sleep–wake processes as early as the first postnatal week. Finally, sensory feedback produced by twitches of the limbs is transmitted to the contralateral somatosensory cortex (where cortical activity is also modulated by the corpus callosum) before being transmitted to the hippocampus. Thus, we are moving closer to a full description of sleep–wake processes in the newborn as well as an understanding of the contributions of sleep-related spontaneous activity to the self-organization of the nervous system.

Introduction

The earliest behavior of invertebrate and vertebrate animals comprises spontaneous movements of the head, limbs, and tail (Corner, 1977). In mammalian and avian embryos, this spontaneous motor activity (SMA) is a ubiquitous feature of behavioral expression and has been a major focus of investigation for behavioral embryologists (Hamburger, 1973). In considering these various embryonic and infant movements, Corner (1977) proposed that they exhibit continuity across the lifespan. Indeed, he maintained that "sleep motility in its entirety… is nothing less than the continued postnatal expression of primordial nervous functional processes" (p. 292).

The SMA of fetal and infant rats exhibits organization in both spatial and temporal dimensions. One particular form of spatiotemporal organization comprises limb movements occurring in close temporal proximity. Although synchronous, these movements do not typically occur simultaneously and certainly do not resemble the whole-body *startles* – comprising sudden, spontaneous, and simultaneous contraction of multiple skeletal muscle groups – that have long been recognized (Gramsbergen *et al.*, 1970; Karlsson *et al.*, 2006). Furthermore, movement synchrony reflects more than simply a temporal dependence among pairs of limbs; rather, patterns of movements among two or more limbs are organized into discrete *bouts*. Using this bout-analytic approach in rats (Robinson *et al.*, 2000), similarities in bout structure between fetuses (embryonic day [E]17–21) and infants (postnatal day [P]1–9) become readily apparent, thus providing additional empirical support for Corner's continuity hypothesis. Interestingly, the movements that qualify as SMA in perinatal rats – and especially those that are expressed in postnatal rats – are also properly designated as myoclonic twitching, that is, the form of twitching that is most closely associated with the phasic movements of REM sleep (hereafter designated as active sleep, or AS) in infants and adults.

REM Sleep: Regulation and Function, eds. Birendra N. Mallick, S. R. Pandi-Perumal, Robert W. McCarley, and Adrian R. Morrison. Published by Cambridge University Press. © Cambridge University Press 2011.

Notwithstanding such behavioral observations, some have remained skeptical about the phenomenological link between perinatal behavior (such as twitching) and sleep. There are several reasons for this skepticism. Firstly, some remain convinced that infant sleep – to be "true" sleep – should conform to the conventional criteria used to define sleep in adults (Rechtschaffen and Kales, 1968), especially including the presence of state-dependent EEG activity in the form of delta waves (Frank and Heller, 2003).

Secondly, although the conventional use of 30-second (or shorter) epochs can safely be used to quantify durations of sleep and wakefulness in human adults, the application of such epochs to animals that cycle more rapidly between states effectively filters out valuable high-frequency information (Blumberg *et al.*, 2005; Seelke and Blumberg, 2008). Similarly, the application of a 30-second criterion for defining QS in early infancy appears to have contributed to the mistaken notion that QS emerges suddenly in rats after P10 (Jouvet-Mounier *et al.*, 1970, Seelke and Blumberg, 2008).

Thirdly, the successful integration of sleep research with neuroscience has engendered the expectation that sleep processes must be accompanied by state-dependent neural activity (Hendricks *et al.*, 2000). Despite some early studies reporting state-dependent brainstem activity in infant rats (for review, see Blumberg and Seelke, 2010), some continued to believe that infant sleep is produced by "a very primitive system of diffuse activation within the whole central nervous system" (Adrien and Lanfumey, 1984). More recently, continuing doubts concerning the control of infant sleep by "executive sleep mechanisms" buttressed the view that infant sleep is not really sleep at all, but rather should be designated as "presleep," a protostate that only outwardly resembles the state of sleep expressed in older animals (Frank and Heller, 2003).

It should be noted that the "presleep hypothesis" was presented as an alternative to the traditional view, which holds that sleep – especially AS – predominates in early infancy before decreasing to adult levels. This traditional view emerged from the influential papers of Roffwarg and his colleagues on human infants (Roffwarg *et al.*, 1966) and of Jouvet-Mounier and her colleagues on sleep in the infants of several mammalian species, including rats (Jouvet-Mounier *et al.*, 1970). Of particular relevance to this chapter, Roffwarg's paper established the view that the activational state of AS serves a functional role in early brain development. Although this hypothesis has been extended and elaborated over the intervening decades (Blumberg and Lucas, 1996; Corner *et al.*, 1980; Mirmiran, 1995; Shaffery *et al.*, 2002), we have not yet achieved a final theory that effectively and comprehensively explains the predominance of sleep in early infancy and its precise functional roles in the development of the infant nervous system.

The present chapter reviews recent advances in our understanding of infant sleep and, in particular, the role that AS-related myoclonic twitches play in the development of the nervous system. To make this recent research more comprehensible – and to place it in proper context – it is useful to also review our current understanding of the phenomenology and neural control of infant sleep.

From behavioral to electrographic measures of infant sleep and wakefulness

When an infant rat is placed in a thermoneutral and humidified environment, it is readily observed to cycle rapidly between behavioral states. When actively awake, the pup exhibits high-amplitude movements including locomotion, head-lifting, kicking, stretching, and yawning. When this activity ceases, there ensues a period of behavioral quiescence as muscles in the body visibly relax. After this period of quiescence, myoclonic twitching commences, characterized by phasic bursts of activity in the fore and hind limbs, head, and tail. Waves of twitching with interposed periods of quiescence continue until the pup suddenly reawakens and resumes high-amplitude movements. A typical cycle exhibits this basic order of expression – wakefulness followed by quiet sleep (QS) and AS – with the duration of each bout of sleep and wakefulness varying significantly within and between individuals, as well as across age (Gramsbergen *et al.*, 1970; Seelke and Blumberg, 2008).

Although behavioral analysis alone can effectively identify behavioral states, it was clear that the demonstration of a stable relationship between sleep–wake behaviors and a second measure would be useful. Figure 14.1 depicts a segment of electromyographic (EMG) data, recorded from the nuchal muscle, for an infant rat. A cycle from high muscle tone to atonia and back to high muscle tone is presented; myoclonic twitches in the EMG record are indicated, as are behaviorally scored limb twitches. This representative example also illustrates how twitching – whether

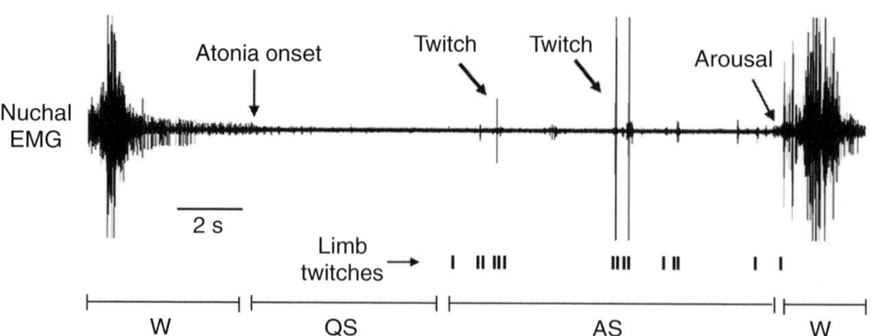

Figure 14.1 Representative cycle of high nuchal muscle tone and atonia in a P8 rat at 35°C. Nuchal muscle twitches against a background of atonia are indicated, as are instances of visually scored limb twitches. This cycle has been divided into periods of wakefulness (W), quiet sleep (QS) and active sleep (AS). (Adapted from Seelke *et al.*, 2005.)

recorded behaviorally or from the EMG record – occurs only against a background of nuchal atonia. In addition, wake behaviors (e.g., kicking, yawning) occur only during periods of high muscle tone. Thus, sleep and wakefulness in infant rats are reliably defined using these two components – nuchal EMG and behavior – and these components are highly concordant at a very early age in this altricial species.

We next reexamined the development of rapid eye movements (REMs) during sleep. Although work in rats had addressed the development of REMs using electrooculography (EOG) (Jouvet-Mounier *et al.*, 1970; Van Someren *et al.*, 1990), the EOG does not yield useful information in very young animals. Thus, we developed a method to record EMG activity directly from the extraocular muscles as soon after birth as possible (Seelke *et al.*, 2005). We reasoned that if REMs are produced by twitches of the extraocular muscles, as had been suggested (Chase and Morales, 1983), and if these extraocular muscle twitches are similar to the twitches produced by skeletal muscles in the limbs, then extraocular muscle activity should exhibit patterns of activity similar to those found in other skeletal muscle groups.

Consistent with these expectations, as early as P3, extraocular muscle tone waxes and wanes similarly to nuchal muscle tone. Secondly, even before eye movements are detected, twitches of the extraocular muscles are detectible in the EMG record and these twitches are tightly coupled with similar activity recorded from the nuchal muscle and limbs. Thus, the extraocular EMG provides information about muscle tone that is qualitatively and quantitatively similar to that provided by the nuchal EMG. Accordingly, the extraocular and nuchal muscles control their associated "limbs" – that is, the eyes and head, respectively – and provide redundant information concerning behavioral state (Seelke *et al.*, 2005).

The neural substrates of infant sleep–wake states and myoclonic twitching

The demonstrated linkage between sleep–wake behaviors and nuchal EMG afforded opportunities for exploring the neural bases of behavioral state organization in early infancy. It was first necessary, however, to overcome the technical challenges posed by these small, fragile subjects. Accordingly, a novel method was developed for stimulating and recording from the brain of unanesthetized, head-fixed infants as nuchal EMG activity and behavior are also monitored (Karlsson and Blumberg, 2005).

Using this method, it was demonstrated that atonia in P8 rats results when neurons in the ventromedial medulla become activated (Karlsson and Blumberg, 2005), as is the case in adults (Siegel, 2005). Moreover, lesions within this area reduced or eliminated atonia to produce a condition reminiscent of "REM without atonia" (Morrison, 1988).

We next sought to delineate other medullary and mesopontine components of the neural circuit mediating behavioral states in week-old rats (Karlsson *et al.*, 2005). As expected, a diversity of state-dependent neurons was found, including "atonia-on neurons" (indicative of sleep), "EMG-on" neurons (indicative of wakefulness), and neurons associated with periods of AS ("AS-on"). Also, consistent with the recording data, atonia durations decreased after lesions of the nucleus subcoeruleus or nucleus pontis oralis and myoclonic twitching decreased after lesions within the dorsolateral pontine tegmentum, an area that includes the laterodorsal tegmental nucleus (LDT).

The LDT was notable in that EMG-on neurons were highly concentrated within it. In addition, some LDT neurons exhibited a burst of activity in anticipation of myoclonic twitches (see Figure 14.2). The

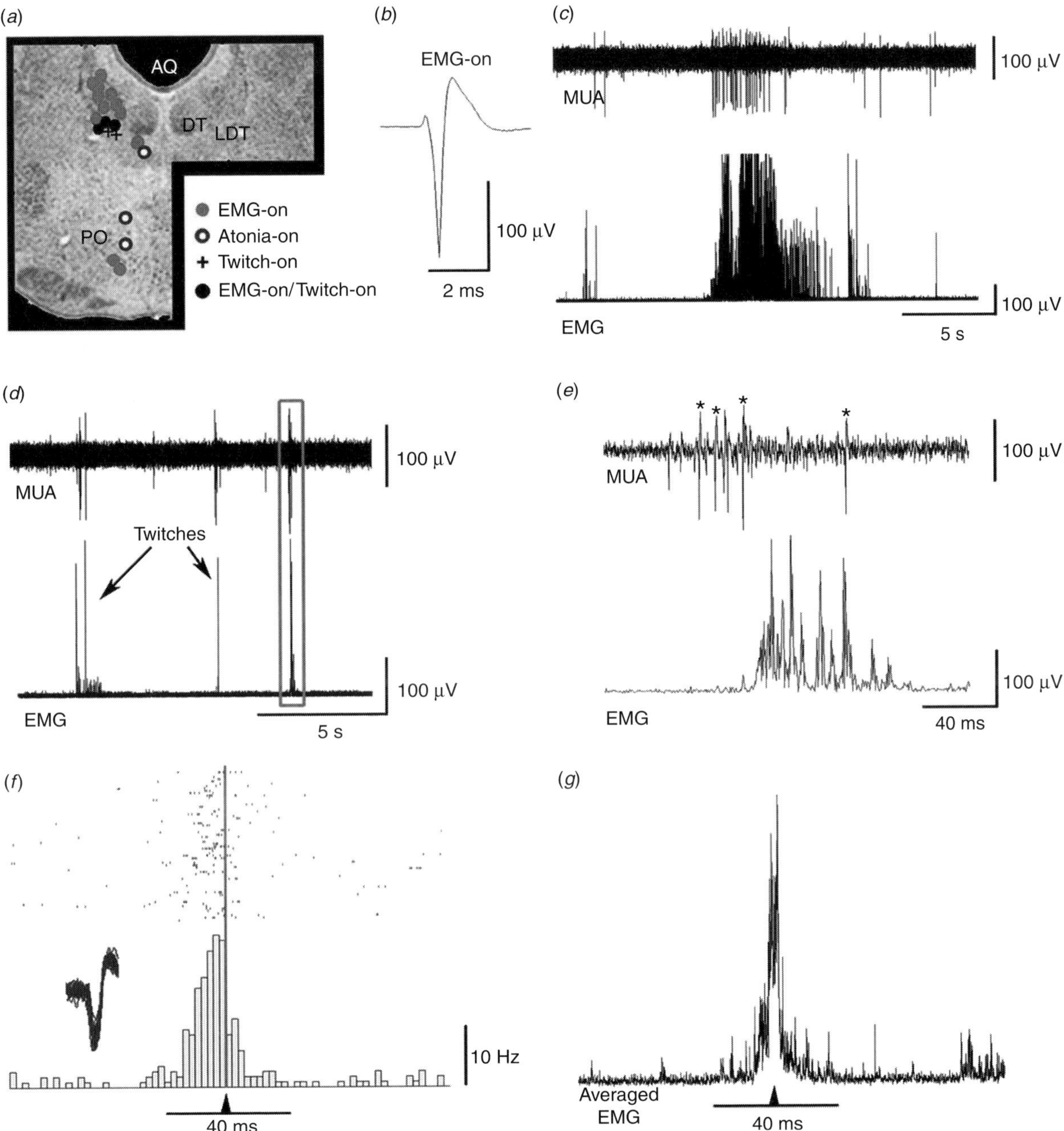

Figure 14.2 State-dependent neuronal discharges within the pontine tegmentum. (*a*) Recording sites of state-dependent neurons reconstructed on a coronal section of the brain stem. Note the predominance of EMG-on neurons. (*b*) Averaged waveform of a representative EMG-on neuron. (*c*) Upper trace: multiunit activity. Lower trace: concurrently recorded nuchal EMG. One EMG-on neuron was isolated from the multiunit record; note its tonic discharge during the period of high muscle tone. (*d*) Upper trace: multiunit activity. Lower trace: concurrently recorded nuchal EMG. (*e*) Expanded view of the boxed area from (*d*). Note how multiunit activity precedes the twitch. Asterisks identify a single isolated unit. (*f*) Peristimulus histogram and raster plot for the twitch-on neuron identified in (*e*) during a ten-minute recording session in a P7 rat (83 total twitches). Inset depicts 55 superimposed action potential waveforms for this unit. This unit's mean discharge rate peaks 5 to 10 ms before the twitch (red line). (*g*) Averaged nuchal EMG for all 83 twitches. AQ: cerebral aqueduct; DT: dorsal tegmental nucleus; LDT: laterodorsal tegmental nucleus; PO: nucleus pontis oralis. (From Karlsson *et al.*, 2005.) (See plate section for color version.)

discovery of these "twitch-on" neurons provided substantial support for an inference, based on an earlier study (Kreider and Blumberg, 2000), that there must exist neurons within the mesopontine region of week-old rats that contribute to twitching.

Thus, the infant brain stem is intimately involved in the generation of cyclic changes in muscle tone and the production of the phasic activity that defines AS. Still, we have much to learn about the neural circuit involved in infant sleep and how it changes across development.

Sleep-state organization upon the developmental emergence of delta activity

Despite having established the value of the EMG as a reliable measure of infant behavioral state, the question remained as to whether and how EMG activity is modified upon the emergence of state-dependent EEG differentiation, especially delta (or slow-wave) activity, at P11 (Gramsbergen, 1976). An initial examination of this issue revealed that at P14 (i.e., just several days after delta's emergence), delta activity occupies the "location" designated as quiet sleep (QS) in younger subjects using EMG data alone (see Figure 14.1) (Seelke et al., 2005). More recently, we assessed the microstructure of sleep bouts in P9, P11, and P13 subjects – that is, before, during, and after the emergence of delta activity (Seelke and Blumberg, 2008). Again, all evidence pointed to delta activity merging seamlessly with the organizational structure that had already developed. Thus, the emergence of delta activity may help to refine estimates of QS duration, but it does not reflect or produce a significant alteration of sleep-state organization.

Thus, using methods and criteria outlined above, very soon after birth we can identify sleep periods comprising periods of quiescence interspersed with bursts of phasic activity, including twitches of the limbs and tail as well as nuchal and extraocular muscles. These bursts of activity, comprising synchronized activity in multiple muscle groups throughout the body, begin shortly after the onset of atonia and continue throughout the duration of the sleep period. The periods of quiescence are initially very brief – during the first postnatal week, they may last less than two seconds. With age, the duration of these periods of quiescence increase and, by P11, are often accompanied by delta activity (Seelke and Blumberg, 2008).

Myoclonic twitching and its effect on infant neocortical activity

As discussed above, the single most influential developmental hypothesis regarding the function of AS remains that of Roffwarg and his colleagues (Roffwarg et al., 1966) who, noting the developmental relation between sleep and brain development in newborns, suggested that the two processes are related. In light of subsequent research detailing the role of spontaneous activity in, for example, the development of the visual system (Wong, 1999), some have raised the possibility that sleep – and, in particular, AS-related twitching – presents an opportunity for spontaneous activity to contribute to the self-organization of the nervous system (Blumberg and Lucas, 1996; Blumberg and Seelke, 2010; Khazipov et al., 2004; Petersson et al., 2003).

To address the possible functional role of twitching, first recall that myoclonic twitches are expressed as phasic, bursts of activity in skeletal muscle groups throughout the body, a pattern of activity that suggests they are generated by a highly connected network of neurons. These neurons are located in the mesopontine region, including the LDT (Karlsson et al., 2005; Kreider and Blumberg, 2000). As has been shown in the adult trigeminal system, twitch-on neurons appear to use glutamate to drive motoneuron activity (Burgess et al., 2008). Then, when a muscle twitch is produced, the associated movement produces a flexion at a joint – thereby triggering proprioceptive feedback – and may also result in physical contact between the limb and a nearby surface – thereby triggering tactile feedback. Might this sensory feedback, associated as it is with discrete motor output in the form of a twitch, contribute to the self-organization of the nervous system?

Recent work supports a role for myoclonic twitching in the development of somatotopic maps in the spinal cord (Petersson et al., 2003; Schouenborg, 2010). Schouenborg and colleagues set out to explore the development of spinal withdrawal reflex circuits. The specific problem that they addressed concerns the fact that somatosensory information is multisensory and each developing animal is confronted with the difficult task of associating specific sensory inputs with appropriate motor outputs as bodies (and limbs) grow in size and change in shape. Their proposed solution is that these complex relations arise from a self-organizational process in which self-generated motor outputs – that is, sleep-related twitches – help to sculpt and refine spinal reflex circuits to produce the somatotopy that is readily observed in adults.

Beyond the spinal cord (and even more surprising in light of conventional views of cortical activity before the developmental onset of delta) was the discovery of brief bursts of spatially confined oscillatory activity – so called spindle-bursts (SBs) – in primary somatosensory cortex (S1) in P1 to P6 rats (Khazipov *et al.*, 2004). Because SBs occurred in a topographic fashion during periods of limb twitching, it was suggested that they reflect a self-organizational process underlying sensorimotor development (Khazipov *et al.*, 2004). In subsequent work, SBs have been detected in S1 barrel cortex and primary visual cortex (V1) in association with whisker activity (Minlebaev *et al.*, 2007) and retinal waves (Hanganu *et al.*, 2006, 2007), respectively. In the visual cortex, SBs are modulated by the cholinergic basal forebrain acting on cortical muscarinic receptors (Hanganu *et al.*, 2007).

The existence of topographically organized events in S1 offered the opportunity to assess interhemispheric communication during the early postnatal period when callosal projections are undergoing rapid developmental change (Marcano-Reik and Blumberg, 2008). Specifically, many commissural fibers have crossed the midline by the day of birth in rats and, during the first postnatal week, callosal fibers grow into the maturing cortex and topographic relations are established (Innocenti and Price, 2005). Accordingly, if sleep-related SBs reflect the activity of a developing, self-organizing cortical system, it was hypothesized that surgically disrupting transcallosal communication (i.e., with callosotomy) would alter SB activity in S1. To test this hypothesis, we modified existing methods to visualize limb activity in unanesthetized pups during sleep (as well as to deliver precise tactile and proprioceptive stimulation to the forepaw), all while monitoring activity in the forepaw regions of the left and right S1s (see Figure 14.3*a*).

As illustrated in Figure 14.3*b*, spontaneous SBs are closely associated with AS-related twitching of the distal limbs. Moreover, consistent with previous findings (Khazipov *et al.*, 2004), SBs result from peripheral stimulation, as they are evoked with >95% reliability by stimulation of the contralateral forepaw. In fact, proprioceptive stimulation in the form of dorsiflexion of the contralateral wrist – but not tactile stimulation of the palmar surface of the forepaw – produces a discrete SB in S1.

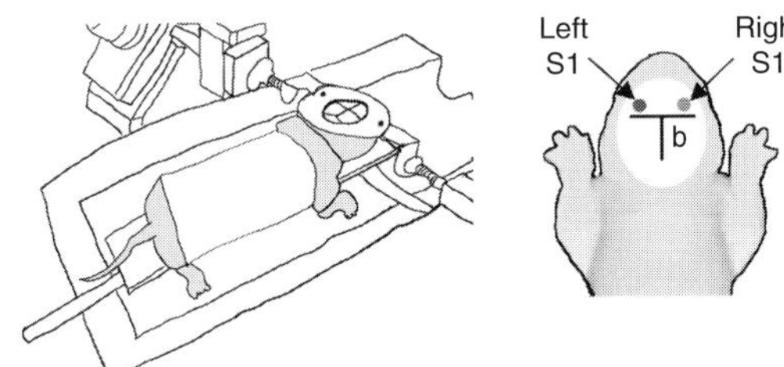

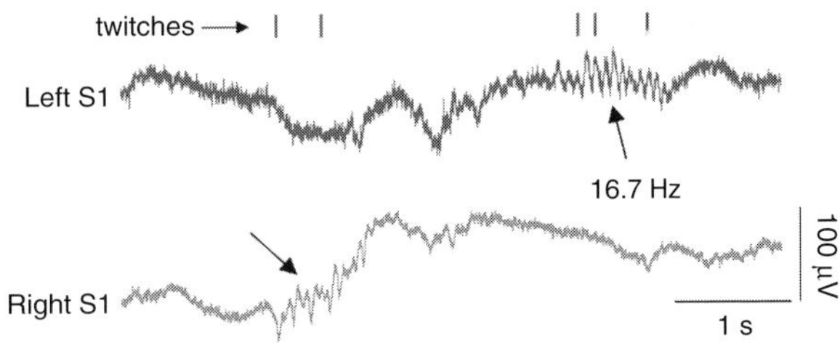

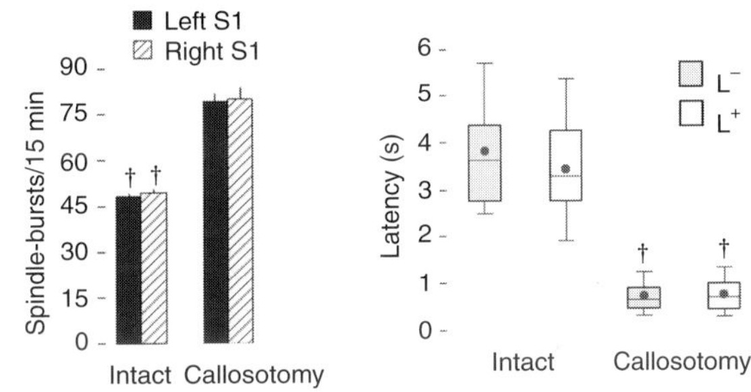

Figure 14.3 Spontaneous spindle-bursts (SBs) in a P5 rat. (*a*) Left: Experimental procedure for recording SBs. The infant rat was head-fixed in a stereotaxic apparatus, placed on a narrow platform, lightly wrapped in gauze, and suspended over a temperature-controlled glass chamber. A heating lamp was also used to maintain brain temperature at 37 °C. Right: View of skull showing approximate location of electrodes in relation to bregma (b). Pairs of Ag/AgCl electrodes were placed in left and right somatosensory cortex (S1) and SB responses to contralateral forepaw plantar surface stimulation were confirmed. (*b*) Spontaneous SBs (denoted by arrows) in left and right S1 in relation to active sleep-related myoclonic twitches of the limbs (vertical ticks) assessed through behavioral observation. The oscillation frequencies of one spontaneous SB is also shown. (*c*) Mean number of spontaneous SBs in left (solid) and right (hatched) S1 during 15-minute recording periods in intact and callosotomized P1 to P6 rats. $n = 6$ per group. † $P < 0.001$ in relation to the callosotomy group. Mean + s.e. (*d*) Box plots depicting distributions of SB latencies for intact and callosotomized subjects ($n = 6$ per group). For this analysis, 20 "anchor" SBs in the left S1 recording were selected at random for each subject and its duration determined. Then, for each of these SBs, the latency between it and the prior (L⁻) and subsequent (L⁺) SBs in the right S1 recording was determined. The top, middle, and bottom horizontal lines of the box represent the 75th, 50th (median), and 25th percentiles, respectively. The thin vertical lines above and below the box represent the 90th and 10th percentiles, respectively. Dots are means. † $P < 0.0001$ in relation to the intact group. (Adapted from Marcano-Reik and Blumberg, 2008.) (See plate section for color version.)

As shown in Figure 14.3*c*, callosotomy resulted in an immediate doubling of the number of spontaneous, AS-related SBs in both S1s. This callosotomy-induced increase in the occurrence of spontaneous SBs could have resulted from generalized functional disinhibition of these cortical oscillations, perhaps allowing them to occur independently of behavioral state. However, even in callosotomized pups the close association between periods of myoclonic twitching and SBs was retained. Thus, we hypothesized that callosotomy exerts its effects on SBs by reducing mutually inhibitory interactions between homotopic areas in left and right S1s. Indeed, as shown in Figure 14.3*d*, the interval between SBs in the two hemispheres was dramatically reduced in callosotomized pups. Thus, in intact pups, the triggering of an SB in one hemisphere results in the inhibition of SBs in the homotopic region of the contralateral hemisphere. With callosotomy, this mutual inhibition disappears, thereby increasing the probability that an SB will occur in response to twitch-related sensory feedback.

We have posited the existence of homologous activational states of the forebrain (EEG) and skeletal muscle (EMG) during sleep–wake states (Seelke *et al.*, 2005). Viewed in this way, we can think of sleep as a body-wide process that links muscle and brain into a single system that establishes, refines, and maintains topographic relations and, thereby, coordinative functioning. The need to flexibly integrate relations between muscle and brain forms the basis for the notion that infant sleep states, including myoclonic twitching, contribute to neural and neuromuscular development. The discrete nature of a twitch, especially when performed against a background of muscle atonia, may provide an enhanced signal-to-noise ratio for accurately processing relationships between outgoing motor signals and sensory feedback.

Myoclonic twitching and its effect on infant hippocampal activity

In the first study describing the firing patterns of neonatal hippocampal neurons in vivo (Leinekugel *et al.*, 2002), regularly recurring waves of synchronized activity were observed; such waves are thought to facilitate activity-dependent development. Because behavioral state was not quantitatively assessed in that earlier study, it remained unclear whether this hippocampal activity is state dependent. We hypothesized that this activity is state dependent and, moreover, predicted

that hippocampal neural activity would increase specifically during periods of twitching (Mohns and Blumberg, 2008). Indeed, using unanesthetized P1 to P12 rats, we found that the majority of neurons in CA1 and the dentate gyrus are significantly more active during AS than during either quiet sleep or wakefulness. All AS-active neurons increased their firing rates during periods of twitching, and a subset of these AS-active neurons fired preferentially within several hundred milliseconds after a twitch, thus suggesting that twitching during the early postnatal period provides sensory feedback that modulates activity not only within the spinal cord and neocortex, but within the hippocampus as well.

We also found an interesting developmental progression in the twitch-related events and oscillations in the infant hippocampus (Mohns and Blumberg, 2008). Specifically, at P1, twitching was accompanied by bursts of unit activity; at P5, this unit activity was also accompanied by gamma-frequency oscillatory activity; at P8, theta activity was first detected and it occurred together with gamma and unit activity; finally, by P11, high-amplitude theta and gamma activity extended beyond periods of twitching, but continued to show amplitude and frequency increases during periods of twitching. Thus, hippocampal oscillations appear to develop on a foundation comprising neuronal activity produced in response to twitch-related feedback.

Given the newly established relations between AS-related twitching and neocortical SBs, we further hypothesized a direct connection between twitch-related neocortical activity and hippocampal activity (Mohns and Blumberg, 2010). In support of this hypothesis, we found a clear temporal progression from muscle twitch to cortical SB to hippocampal activity. Critically, when we surgically disconnected the neocortex from the hippocampus, SBs were unaffected but hippocampal activity was no longer tightly coupled with twitching.

These findings suggest that the phasic motor events of AS provide the developing hippocampus with discrete sensory stimulation that contributes to the development and refinement of hippocampal circuits as well as the development of synchronized interactions between hippocampus and neocortex. Such synchronized activity between neocortex and hippocampus may underlie the integrative interactions that are central to the learning and memory functions of these forebrain structures.

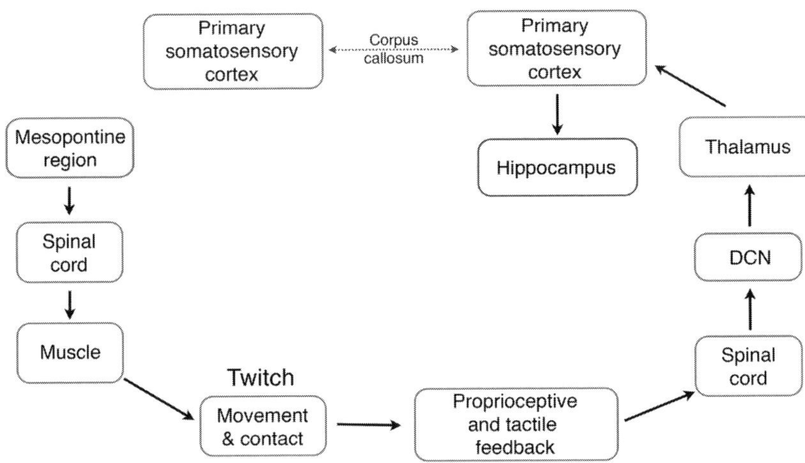

Figure 14.4 Schematic representation of our current understanding of the "life of a twitch." A twitch is produced in the mesopontine area (including the laterodorsal tegmental nucleus), from which a signal is sent through the spinal cord to skeletal muscle in a distal limb to produce a twitch. The resulting limb movement produces proprioceptive and (if a surface is touched) tactile feedback that ascends through the spinal cord and dorsal column nuclei (DCN) to the thalamus and primary somatosensory cortex (S1). When a twitch-related spindle-burst is produced in S1, it is followed by neuronal activation in the hippocampus. In addition, the corpus callosum mediates reciprocal interactions between homotopic regions of S1.

The life of a twitch

Our current understanding of the "life of a twitch" – from its initiation within the mesopontine region, to the movement of a limb, to the sensory feedback that modulates activity within the neocortex and hippocampus – is summarized in Figure 14.4. Of course, sensory feedback likely influences the activity of other structures that have not yet been examined. A complete understanding of the causes and consequences of a twitch will be necessary for refining and testing hypotheses regarding the functions of twitching for the developing animal.

Although current evidence seems to support the notion that the sensory feedback produced by a twitch during AS constitutes a unique or special condition for the establishment, refinement, and maintenance of neocortical and hippocampal circuits, this issue has not yet been resolved. One intriguing direction for future investigation that may address this issue concerns the possible co-generation during twitching of an efference copy – perhaps projecting to the cholinergic basal forebrain – that could "prepare" the cortex for the ensuing arrival of twitch-related sensory information (Kilgard and Merzenich, 1998). These and other possible mechanisms will need to be explored if we are to fully understand the functional significance of sleep for the developing animal.

Acknowledgments

Preparation of this chapter was supported by a grant (MH50701) and a Research Scientist Award (MH66424) from the National Institute of Mental Health to M.S.B.

References

Adrien, J. & Lanfumey, L. (1984) Neuronal activity of the developing raphe dorsalis: its relation with the states of vigilance. *Exp Brain Res*, Suppl. **8**: 67–78.

Blumberg, M. S., Karlsson, K. Æ., Seelke, A. M. H. & Mohns, E. J. (2005). The ontogeny of mammalian sleep: A response to Frank and Heller (2003). *J Sleep Res* **14**: 91–101.

Blumberg, M. S. & Lucas, D. E. (1996) A developmental and component analysis of active sleep. *Dev Psychobiol* **29**: 1–22.

Blumberg, M. S. & Seelke, A. M. (2010) The form and function of infant sleep: from muscle to neocortex. In *The Oxford Handbook of Developmental Behavioral Neuroscience*, eds. M. S. Blumberg, J. H. Freeman & S. R. Robinson. New York: Oxford University Press, pp. 391–423.

Burgess, C., Lai, D., Siegel, J. & Peever, J. (2008) An endogenous glutamatergic drive onto somatic motoneurons contributes to the stereotypical pattern of muscle tone across the sleep-wake cycle. *J Neurosci* **28**: 4649–60.

Chase, M. H. & Morales, F. R. (1983) Subthreshold excitatory activity and motoneuron discharge during REM periods of active sleep. *Science* **221**: 1195–8.

Corner, M. A. (1977) Sleep and the beginnings of behavior in the animal kingdom: studies of ultradian motility cycles in early life. *Prog Neurobiol* **8**: 279–95.

Corner, M. A., Mirmiran, M., Bour, H. L. *et al.* (1980) Does rapid-eye-movement sleep play a role in brain development? *Prog Brain Res* **53**: 347–56.

Frank, M. G. & Heller, H. C. (2003) The ontogeny of mammalian sleep: a reappraisal of alternative hypotheses. *J Sleep Res* **12**: 25–34.

Gramsbergen, A. (1976) The development of the EEG in the rat. *Dev Psychobiol* **9**: 501–15.

Gramsbergen, A., Schwartze, P. & Prechtl, H. F. R. (1970) The postnatal development of behavioral states in the rat. *Dev Psychobiol* **3**: 267–80.

Hamburger, V. (1973) Anatomical and physiological bases of embryonic motility in birds and mammals. In *Studies on the Development of Behavior and the Nervous System, Behavioral Embryology, Volume 1.* ed. G. Gottlieb. New York: Academic Press, pp. 51–76.

Hanganu, I. L., Ben-Ari, Y. & Khazipov, R. (2006) Retinal waves trigger spindle bursts in the neonatal rat visual cortex. *J Neurosci* **26**: 6728–36.

Hanganu, I. L., Staiger, J. F., Ben-Ari, Y. & Khazipov, R. (2007) Cholinergic modulation of spindle bursts in the neonatal rat visual cortex in vivo. *J Neurosci* **27**: 5694–705.

Hendricks, J. C., Sehgal, A. & Pack, A. (2000) The need for a simple animal model to understand sleep. *Prog Neurobiol* **61**: 339–51.

Innocenti, G. M. & Price, D. J. (2005) Exuberance in the development of cortical networks. *Nat Rev Neurosci* **6**: 955–65.

Jouvet-Mounier, D., Astic, L. & Lacote, D. (1970) Ontogenesis of the states of sleep in rat, cat, and guinea pig during the first postnatal month. *Dev Psychobiol* **2**: 216–39.

Karlsson, K. Æ. & Blumberg, M. S. (2005) Active medullary control of atonia in week-old rats. *Neuroscience* **130**: 275–83.

Karlsson, K. Æ., Gall, A. J., Mohns, E. J., Seelke, A. M. H. & Blumberg, M. S. (2005) The neural substrates of infant sleep in rats. *PLoS Biol* **3**: 891–901.

Karlsson, K. Æ., Mohns, E. J., Vianna di Prisco, G. & Blumberg, M. S. (2006) On the co-occurrence of startles and hippocampal sharp waves in newborn rats. *Hippocampus* **16**: 959–65.

Khazipov, R., Sirota, A., Leinekugel, X., *et al.* (2004) Early motor activity drives spindle-bursts in the developing somatosensory cortex. *Nature* **432**: 758–61.

Kilgard, M. P. & Merzenich, M. M. (1998) Cortical map reorganization enabled by nucleus basalis activity. *Science* **279**: 1714–18.

Kreider, J. C. & Blumberg, M. S. (2000) Mesopontine contribution to the expression of active 'twitch' sleep in decerebrate week-old rats. *Brain Res* **872**: 149–59.

Leinekugel, X., Khazipov, R., Cannon, R. *et al.* (2002) Correlated bursts of activity in neonatal hippocampus in vivo. *Science* **296**: 2049–52.

Marcano-Reik, A. J. & Blumberg, M. S. (2008) The corpus callosum modulates spindle-burst activity within homotopic regions of somatosensory cortex in newborn rats. *Eur J Neurosci* **28**: 1457–66.

Minlebaev, M., Ben-Ari, Y. & Khazipov, R. (2007) Network mechanisms of spindle-burst oscillations in the neonatal rat barrel cortex in vivo. *J Neurophysiol* **97**: 692–700.

Mirmiran, M. (1995) The function of fetal/neonatal rapid eye movement sleep. *Behav Brain Res* **69**: 13–22.

Mohns, E. J. & Blumberg, M. S. (2008) Synchronous bursts of neuronal activity in the developing hippocampus: modulation by active sleep and association with emerging gamma and theta rhythms. *J Neurosci* **28**: 10,134–44.

Mohns, E. J. & Blumberg, M. S. (2010) Neocortical activation of the hippocampus during sleep in newborn rats. *J Neurosci* **30**(9): 3438–49.

Morrison, A. R. (1988) Paradoxical sleep without atonia. *Arch Ital Biol* **126**: 275–89.

Petersson, P., Waldenström, A., Fåhraeus, C. & Schouenborg, J. (2003) Spontaneous muscle twitches during sleep guide spinal self-organization. *Nature* **424**: 72–5.

Rechtschaffen, A. & Kales, A. eds. (1968) *A Manual of Standardized Terminology, Techniques, and Scoring System for Sleep Stages of Human Subjects.* Los Angeles: UCLA Brain Information Service/Brain Research Institute.

Robinson, S. R., Blumberg, M. S., Lane, M. S. & Kreber, L. A. (2000) Spontaneous motor activity in fetal and infant rats is organized into discrete multilimb bouts. *Behav Neurosci* **14**: 328–36.

Roffwarg, H. P., Muzio, J. N. & Dement, W. C. (1966) Ontogenetic development of the human sleep–dream cycle. *Science* **152**: 604–19.

Schouenborg, J. (2010) Role of spontaneous movements in imprinting an action-based body representation in the spinal cord. In *The Oxford Handbook of Developmental Behavioral Neuroscience,* eds. M. S. Blumberg, J. H. Freeman & S. R. Robinson. New York: Oxford University Press, pp. 254–61.

Seelke, A. M. H. & Blumberg, M. S. (2008) The microstructure of active and quiet sleep as cortical delta activity emerges in infant rats. *Sleep* **31**: 691–9.

Seelke, A. M. H., Karlsson, K. Æ., Gall, A. J. & Blumberg, M. S. (2005) Extraocular muscle activity, rapid eye movements, and the development of active and quiet sleep. *Eur J Neurosci* **22**: 911–20.

Shaffery, J. P., Sinton, C. M., Bissette, G., Roffwarg, H. P. & Marks, G. A. (2002) Rapid eye movement sleep deprivation modifies expression of long-term potentiation in visual cortex of immature rats. *Neuroscience* **110**: 431–43.

Siegel, J. M. (2005) REM sleep. In: *Principles and Practice of Sleep Medicine*. eds. M. H. Kryger, T. Roth & W. C. Dement. Philadelphia: W. B. Saunders Company, pp. 120–35.

van Someren, E. J. W., Mirmiran, M., Bos, N. P. A. *et al.* (1990) Quantitative analysis of eye movements during REM-sleep in developing rats. *Dev Psychobiol* **23**: 55–61.

Wong, R. O. (1999) Retinal waves and visual system development. *Ann Rev Neurosci* **22**: 29–47.

Chapter

15

Pontine-wave generator: a key player in REM sleep-dependent memory consolidation

Subimal Datta

Summary

The data outlined in this chapter provides evidence to support a concept that the activation of pontine-wave (P-wave) generating neurons plays a critical role in long-term memory formation. The P-wave, generated by the phasic activation of glutamatergic neurons in the pons, is one of the most prominent phasic events of REM sleep. These P-wave generating neurons project to the hippocampus, amygdala, entorhinal cortex and many other regions of the brain known to be involved in cognitive processing. These P-wave generating glutamatergic neurons remain silent during wakefulness and slow-wave sleep (SWS), but during the transition from SWS to REM sleep and throughout REM sleep these neurons discharge high-frequency spike bursts in the background of tonically increased firing rates. Activation of these P-wave generating neurons increases glutamate release and activates postsynaptic N-methyl-D-aspartic acid (NMDA) receptors in the dorsal hippocampus. Activation of P-wave generating neurons increases phosphorylation of transcription factor cAMP response element binding protein (CREB) in the dorsal hippocampus and amygdala by activating intracellular protein kinase A (PKA). The P-wave generating neurons activation-dependent PKA-CREB phosphorylation increases the expression of activity-regulated cytoskeletal-associated protein (Arc), brain-derived neurotrophic factor (BDNF), and early growth response-1 (Egr-1) genes in the dorsal hippocampus and amygdala. The P-wave generator activation-induced increased activation of PKA and expression of pCREB, Arc, BDNF, and Egr-1 in the dorsal hippocampus is shown to be necessary for REM sleep-dependent memory processing. Continued research on P-wave generation and its functions may provide new advances in understanding memory and treating its disorders.

Introduction

Sleep, especially REM sleep, provides an exceptional opportunity to study the brain-based physical and physiological foundation of cognitive processes (Datta, 2006). As one proceeds from wake (W) into non-REM (SWS) and then REM sleep, a series of dramatic and well defined changes occur in the neurophysiology and neurochemistry of the brain. REM sleep is a constellation of multiple events with specific cellular and molecular mechanisms. Each of these REM sleep events may provide some specific, as well as some common, beneficial effects to a species that possesses this state of sleep. The goal of this chapter is to describe mechanisms and cognitive functions of one of the most prominent physiological signs of REM sleep, the P-wave. The focus of this chapter is on the P-wave, which normally occurs only during REM sleep; thus, I will provide a brief description on polygraphic signs of REM sleep and mechanisms for the generation of those signs. I will then describe the characteristics of both the P-wave and the generator of this wave. Finally, I will describe the role of the P-wave generator in memory processing.

Mechanisms of REM sleep sign generation

REM sleep is characterized by a constellation of events including the following: (1) an activated pattern of cortical EEG activity; (2) marked atonia of the postural muscles; (3) rapid eye movements; (4) a theta rhythm within the hippocampus; (5) field potentials in the pons (P-wave), lateral geniculate nucleus, and occipital cortex (ponto-geniculo-occipital [PGO]) spikes; (6) myoclonic twitches, most apparent in the facial and distal limb musculature; (7) pronounced fluctuations in cardiorespiratory rhythms and core body temperature;

REM Sleep: Regulation and Function, eds. Birendra N. Mallick, S. R. Pandi-Perumal, Robert W. McCarley, and Adrian R. Morrison. Published by Cambridge University Press. © Cambridge University Press 2011.

and (8) penile erection and clitoral tumescence (Datta and MacLean, 2007).

During the past decade, evidence from both rat and cat studies have suggested that each of the events of REM sleep is executed by distinct cell groups located in the brain stem (reviewed in Datta, 1995; Datta and McLean, 2007). These cell groups are discrete components of a widely distributed network, rather than a single REM sleep "center." For example, muscle atonia is executed by the activation of neurons in the locus coeruleus alpha (LCα), rapid eye movements result from the activation of neurons in the peri-abducens reticular formation (PAb), PGO waves emerge from activation of neurons in the caudo-lateral peribrachial area (C-PBL) of predator mammals and in the dorsal part of the nucleus subcoeruleus (SubCD) of prey mammals, hippocampal theta rhythm is produced via the activation of neurons in the pontis oralis (PO), muscle twitches appear with the activation of neurons in the nucleus gigantocellularis (especially the caudal part), and increased brain temperature and cardiorespiratory fluctuations result from the activation of neurons in the parabrachial nucleus (PBN). The cortical EEG activation sign of REM sleep, however, is executed jointly by the activation of neurons in the mesencephalic reticular formation (MRF) and rostrally projecting bulbar reticular formation (also called medullary magnocellular nucleus, MN).

It should be emphasized here that these particular cell groups simply represent the executive neurons for the individual signs. For the final expression of each distinct sign, the relevant executive neurons employ a specific neuronal circuit unique to that REM sleep sign. In essence, each of these REM sleep signs has a separate, specialized network. Thus, each of these REM sleep signs could be modulated by multiple neurotransmitters at multiple sites of their circuit. For detailed mechanisms of REM sleep generation, readers are referred to one of the more comprehensive reviews elsewhere (Datta and Maclean, 2007).

Turn-on or turn-off conditions of REM sleep-generating executive neurons are regulated by the ratios of available aminergic and cholinergic neurotransmitters within those cell groups. The source of aminergic neurotransmitters is the locus coeruleus (LC) and raphe nucleus (RN), while cholinergic neurotransmitters originate from the pedunculopontine tegmentum (PPT). The activity of both aminergic and cholinergic cells is approximately equal during wakefulness, and the onset of SWS results in an equal reduction in

activity. Therefore, the ratio of aminergic to cholinergic neurotransmitters in REM sleep generators is proportionate during wakefulness and through SWS. During REM sleep, however, aminergic cell activities are markedly reduced or absent and cholinergic cell activities are comparatively high (Datta et al., 2009b). The level of cholinergic cell activity during REM sleep is roughly 35% less than that of wakefulness. Thus, when a hypothetical ratio of aminergic and cholinergic neurotransmitters is 1:1, the REM sleep sign-generator remains in turned-off condition; however, when this ratio is 0:0.65, the generator is turned-on to express REM sleep signs (Datta and Siwek, 2002).

Description of PGO/P-waves

Prominent phasic events of REM sleep are field potentials in the pontine tegmentum, which begin just prior to the onset of REM sleep and continue through its duration (Brooks and Bizzi, 1963; Datta and Hobson, 1994, 1995; Datta et al., 1998; Jouvet et al., 1959). These field potentials have been recorded both in the lateral geniculate body (LGB) and in the occipital cortex of the cat (Mikiten et al., 1961; Mouret et al., 1963). Since, in the cat, these field potentials originate in the pons (P) and then propagate to the geniculate (G) and occipital cortex (O), they are called PGO waves (Bizzi and Brooks, 1963; Brooks and Bizzi, 1963). Subsequent studies found that PGO waves in the cat could also be recorded from points throughout the extent of the thalamus and cortex. However, such PGO waves reach their highest amplitude in the LGB, primary visual cortex, and association visual cortex (reviewed in Datta, 1997). In addition to the pons, thalamus, and cortex, phasic potentials have been recorded in the oculomotor nuclei (Brooks and Bizzi, 1963) and the cerebellum of the cat (Jouvet et al., 1965). Phasic potentials of pontine origin have also been recorded from the amygdala, cingulate gyrus, and hippocampus, suggesting that the PGO waves also occur in the limbic system (Calvo and Fernandez-Guardiola, 1984). More importantly all of these studies, mapping PGO waves in the cat, have demonstrated that the pons is the primary site of origin for PGO wave activity (reviewed in Datta, 1995, 1997).

Ponto-geniculo-occipital waves have also been documented and studied in other mammalian species including humans, non-human primates, and rodents. In non-human primates, PGO wave-like phasic field potentials have been recorded from the LGB and pons of macaques (Cohen and Feldman, 1968; Feldman and

Cohen, 1968) and in the LGB of baboons (Vuillon-Cacciuttolo and Seri, 1978). Phasic potentials have been recorded in the striate cortex of humans during REM sleep (Salzarulo *et al.*, 1975). Such striate field potentials are probably cortical components of state-specific phasic potentials of pontine origin. The observation of phasic scalp potentials associated with eye movements during REM sleep has suggested that PGO wave-like activity may also be present in humans (McCarley *et al.*, 1983; Miyauchi *et al.*, 1987). Indeed, PGO waves have recently been recorded in the human pons occurring during and immediately before REM sleep (Lim *et al.*, 2007).

Based on recordings of PGO waves in the cat, initial attempts to record similar potentials from the LGB of the rat were unsuccessful (Gottesman, 1969; Stern *et al.*, 1974). Subsequent studies have recorded PGO-like waves in the pons of the rat that are equivalent to those in the pons of the cat (Datta *et al.*, 1998, 1999; Farber *et al.*, 1980; Gottesman, 1969; Sanford *et al.*, 1995). The initial failures indicated that state-specific pontine phasic waves in rats do not excite LGB neurons in a way that could produce geniculate components of PGO waves (Datta, 1995). More recently, the absence of PGO wave-like activity in the rat LGB has been shown to be due to the lack of afferent inputs from P-wave generating cells to the LGB (Datta *et al.*, 1998). This field potential in the rat is therefore called a pontine-wave (P-wave), since it does not activate the geniculate nucleus (Datta *et al.*, 1999, Datta, 2000).

The waveform, amplitude, and frequency characteristics of PGO waves recorded from the pons, geniculate, and occipital cortex have been most intensively examined in the cat (reviewed in Datta, 1997). Ponto-geniculo-occipital waves are biphasic in shape with a duration of 60 to 120 ms and an amplitude between 200 to 300 μV (Datta and Hobson, 1994). The P-wave in the rat is equivalent to the pontine component of the PGO wave in the cat (Datta and Hobson, 1994; Datta *et al.*, 1998, 1999), with similar duration (75 to 100 msec) and amplitude (100–150 μV) (Datta *et al.*, 1998). The PGO/P-waves can occur as singlets or as clusters containing a variable number of waves (3–5 waves/burst) at a density range of 30 to 60 spikes/min during REM sleep (Datta and Hobson, 2000). Singlet PGO/P-waves, known as Type I waves, occur commonly in non-REM sleep and are independent of eye movement; conversely, clusters of PGO waves (Type II waves) are associated with eye movement bursts and are typically indicative of REM sleep (Morrison and Pompeiano, 1966). Type II PGO

wave activity accounts for 55 to 65% of the total number of PGO waves recorded during REM sleep (Datta *et al.*, 1992; Datta and Hobson, 2000).

Description of the PGO/P-wave generator

Early transection and PGO-wave recording studies indicated that the PGO-wave generator is located within the pons (Bizzi and Brooks, 1963; Datta, 1997; Gottesman, 1969; Jouvet *et al.*, 1965). Subsequently, a number of single-cell activity recordings in and around the PPT and laterodorsal tegmentum (LDT) observed a small population of neurons (about 3–5%) that discharged in bursts (of 3–5 spikes/burst) immediately preceding individual LGB PGO waves (McCarley *et al.*, 1978; Steriade *et al.*, 1990a, b). Based on this observation, these cells were originally believed to be PGO-wave generating neurons (McCarley *et al.*, 1978; Steriade *et al.*, 1990a). Recent studies, however, clearly indicate that the burst cells in the PPT/LDT are not PGO-wave generating neurons (reviewed in Datta, 1995). Instead these cells, called transferring neurons, are responsible for conveying information from the pontine PGO-wave generator to the forebrain in the cat (Datta, 1997). Because P-wave generating cells transmit P-wave information directly to the forebrain of rats, (Datta *et al.*, 1998), these transferring neurons are absent in the rat (Datta and Siwek, 2002).

Utilizing chemical microstimulation, cell-specific lesions, and single-cell recording techniques, the P-wave generator in the cat was localized within the C-PBL area (Datta *et al.*, 1992; Datta and Hobson, 1994, 1995). Subsequently, using similar experimental techniques to those used in the cat, the P-wave generator in the rat was localized within the SubCD (Datta *et al.*, 1998, 1999). In humans, as in the cat, the PGO-wave generator is located in the C-PBL (Lim *et al.*, 2007). Immunohistochemical identification of cholinergic and glutamatergic types of cells in the brain stem indicates that PGO-wave generating cells in the cat are capable of synthesizing both acetylcholine and glutamate (Quattrochi *et al.*, 1998), thus these cells could be labeled as both cholinergic and glutamatergic; whereas in the rat, P-wave generating cells have been identified by specific monoclonal antibodies as glutamatergic, but not cholinergic (Datta, 2006).

Since the P-wave generator is also involved in sensorimotor integration (Morrison and Bowker, 1975), the differences in anatomical location and in neurotransmitter identity of the P-wave generator between the rat and cat may provide a species-specific advantage. Specifically, in prey animals (i.e., the rat), the P-wave generator is anatomically closer to the LC. This shorter distance is advantageous during REM sleep (when animals are naturally paralyzed due to muscle atonia), because it permits quick communication with the LC for flight response, and facilitates escape from predators. This rapid flight response is vital for the survival of prey animals. In contrast, the predatory mammalian (such as the cat) PGO-wave generator is further from the LC and close to the PPT. Since predators rarely face the threat of predation, there is no advantage to having a quick arousal response to any non-threatening type of noise during REM sleep. On the contrary, frequent interruptions could actually harm a predatory animal by preventing necessary regenerative functions of REM sleep. Thus, for these types of noises, the P-wave generator signals the cholinergic PPT to intensify REM sleep rather than to wake the animal up by activating the LC.

Single-cell recording studies have shown that P-wave generating neurons discharge high-frequency spike bursts (>500 Hz, 3–5 spikes/burst) on the background of tonically increased firing rates (30–40 Hz) during the P-wave related transitional state between SWS and REM sleep (tS-R) and REM sleep (Datta and Hobson, 1994; Datta, 1997). Normally, the glutamatergic P-wave generating cells remain silent during W and SWS (Datta and Hobson, 1994). A neuroanatomical pathway tracing study has demonstrated that functionally identified P-wave generator cells in the rat project to the dorsal hippocampus (DH), amygdala, entorhinal cortex, visual cortex, as well as many other regions of the brain involved in cognitive functions (Datta et al., 1998). Similar studies have also demonstrated that the P-wave generator in both the cat and rat receives afferent projections from the RN and LC (Datta et al., 1999; Quattrochi et al., 1998). It has been demonstrated that the cholinergic activation of the P-wave generator increases glutamate release in the DH (Datta, 2006). In addition, the P-wave activity has been shown to have a positive influence on hippocampal theta-wave activity in the DH (Karashima et al., 2002, 2005). Most recently, we have demonstrated that the activation of the P-wave generator increases: (1) phosphorylation of cAMP response element-binding protein (CREB); (2) activity-regulated cytoskeletal-associated protein (Arc); and (3) brain-derived neurotrophic factor (BDNF), as well as the messenger ribonucleic acid (mRNAs) of Arc, BDNF, and early growth response-1 (Egr-1) in the DH and amygdala (Datta et al., 2008, 2009; Saha and Datta, 2005; Ulloor and Datta, 2005).

REM sleep and memory consolidation

Since the formal discovery of REM sleep, many animal and human studies of sleep and learning have focused on the role of REM sleep in memory consolidation (for reviews see Datta and Patterson, 2003; Smith, 2003; Stickgold and Walker, 2007; Walker and Stickgold, 2006). Using a variety of protocols and test paradigms, sleep and learning studies in both humans and animals have produced two different types of correlative evidence: (1) learning training trials increase SWS and/or REM sleep during the subsequent sleep period; (2) post learning-training REM sleep deprivation impairs learning performance by impairing memory formation. These correlative evidences suggest that memory consolidation following task training requires processes selectively active during REM sleep and that the organism homeostatically adjusts its SWS and/or REM sleep in response to memory consolidation demands.

The current views of memory consolidation have their roots in the perseveration–consolidation hypothesis originally proposed in 1900. The perseveration–consolidation hypothesis suggests that the neural processes underlying memory perseverate in a labile form following an experience and subsequently become fixed or consolidated with time. More than fifty years of sleep and memory research have revealed that for memories to successfully consolidate, not only the passage of time, but also an adequate amount of sleep during that time is required (for reviews and individual references, please see Datta, 2006; Datta and Patterson, 2003; Stickgold and Walker, 2007). At the end of the consolidation stage, a memory becomes stable and resistant to even extreme disruptions, such as electroconvulsive shock or the application of neuronal gene and protein activation inhibitors. Following consolidation, a memory can be retained for any range of days to years, during which time it can be recalled from long-term memory storage.

Memory consolidation is not a single step, but rather is a multistep process. All of these processes occur over time, automatically, outside of awareness and without intent. Thus, they are specifically different from changes that result from conscious reminiscing or from intentional rehearsal. Operationally, the cascade of memory consolidation processes can be divided into four stages: (1) search and readout of the intermediate form of memory; (2) elimination of unnecessary or redundant memory; (3) strengthening of a cognitively relevant memory; and (4) transfer of stable memory to long-term storage. It is likely that separate sleep states are differentially involved in the separate steps of memory consolidation (Datta, 2010). Based on the wake–sleep stage-specific neurochemical and physiological status of the brain and neurochemical and physiological environment that are conducive for these specific consolidation stages, it is suggested that the first stage of consolidation occurs during NREM II (humans)/SWS-1 (animals) and the second stage of consolidation occurs during NREM III–IV/SWS-2. It has been demonstrated that the third and fourth stages of memory consolidation occur during tS-R and REM sleep (Datta, 2010).

Evidence to link P-wave generator with memory consolidation

Physiological evidence

Long-term potentiation (LTP) of synaptic transmission is widely considered to be a model of activity-dependent synaptic plasticity that could be involved in certain forms of learning and memory (Bliss and Collingridge, 1993; Datta, 2006). It has been shown that REM sleep increases following learning trials and that deprivation of REM sleep soon after learning trials causes a subsequent decrease in performance of a learned task (Datta *et al.*, 2004; Datta and Patterson, 2003; Karni *et al.*, 1994;). Associated with these changes in REM sleep are changes in the efficacy of synaptic transmission in the brain, manifested as long-term potentiation (LTP) (for references see Datta, 2006). Long-term potentiation is significant in that it is thought to be the physiological substrate of learning and memory at the level of the hippocampus and the amygdala (Bliss and Collingridge, 1993). The standard protocols used by most researchers to induce LTP in the hippocampus, amygdala, neocortex, and many other areas of the brain are: (1) high-frequency stimulation in which several hundred pulses at frequencies of 250 to 400 Hz are given; and (2) short high-frequency (>200 Hz) bursts of stimuli with an interburst interval of ~200 msec, called theta-patterned stimulation (for references see Datta and Patterson, 2003; Datta, 2006). In an experimental situation, the high-frequency electrical stimulation of an

afferent pathway is key for induction of LTP. However, during REM sleep, the physiological source of that presynaptic high-frequency stimulation is unclear. Therefore, the identification of the source of this presynaptic high-frequency stimulus for LTP during REM sleep would be a significant contribution to the current body of knowledge about the physiological substrates of learning and memory.

For REM sleep-dependent memory processing and learning, the source of the LTP-inducing high-frequency stimulus must come from the REM sleep sign generating structures of the brain stem. Over the past 25 years, a number of laboratories have recorded the single-cell activity patterns of the different REM sleep sign generating structures in rats, cats, and non-human primates (for reviews see Datta, 1995, 1997; Datta and MacLean, 2007). Depending on the specific REM sleep sign generating structure, neuronal activity patterns of those generating cells are classified as tonic single-spike type, bursting type, or both tonic and bursting type. The only type of cell within the REM sleep sign generating structures that fires as a high-frequency burst, similar to the high-frequency stimulus required for the generation of LTP, is located within the P-wave generator (Datta, 1997). These P-wave generating neurons discharge high-frequency (>500 Hz) spike bursts (3–5 spikes/burst) on the background of tonically increased firing rates (30–40 Hz) during the P-wave related states of tS-R and REM sleep (Datta and Hobson, 1994; Datta, 1997). High-frequency bursting patterns of these P-wave generating cells support the idea that the P-wave generator may be the source of electrical stimulus for the induction of physiological LTP. Indeed, there is now experimental evidence that the activation of P-wave generating cells is capable of inducing LTP. Microinjection of the cholinergic agonist carbachol into the P-wave generator activates P-wave generating cells (Datta *et al.*, 1991, 1998). The cholinergic activation of the P-wave generator in the cat markedly increases P-wave activity and REM sleep (Datta *et al.*, 1991, 1992). This cholinergic stimulation-induced potentiation of P-wave density and REM sleep in the cat lasts for about seven to ten days. This long-lasting increase in P-wave density and REM sleep is a physiological sign of synaptic, as well as intracellular, plasticity. Activation of the P-wave generator facilitates hippocampal theta activity (Datta, 2006; Karashima *et al.*, 2002, 2005). Physiological evidence suggests that the hippocampal theta rhythm favors induction of LTP in the hippocampus as well as in many different parts of the cerebral cortex (for references see Booth and Poe, 2006; Pavlides and Ribeiro, 2003; Poe *et al.*, 2000). Thus, the collection of P-wave generating cells is not only capable of inducing physiological LTP, but also represents the only group of cells in the REM sleep generating network that are capable of inducing this type of physiological plasticity.

Anatomical evidence

If the P-wave generator is the presynaptic input for the induction of synaptic plasticity, a prerequisite for learning and memory processing, it is expected that the P-wave generating cells will send anatomical connections to the forebrain structures known to be involved in memory processing. To test this hypothesis, the anterograde tracer biotinylated dextran amine (BDA) was microinjected into the physiologically identified cholinoceptive pontine P-wave generating site of rats to identify brain structures receiving efferent projections from those P-wave generating sites (Datta *et al.*, 1998). In all cases, small volume injections of BDA in the cholinoceptive P-wave generating sites resulted in anterograde labeling of fibers and terminals in many regions of the brain. The most important output structures of those P-wave generating cells were the occipital cortex, entorhinal cortex, piriform cortex, amygdala, hippocampus, and many other thalamic, hypothalamic, and brain-stem nuclei that participate in the generation of REM sleep (Datta, 1995, 1997; Datta *et al.*, 1998). All of these forebrain structures are already known to be involved in memory processing (for references see Datta and Patterson, 2003). More recently, it has been demonstrated that those functionally identified P-wave generating cells are glutamatergic and stimulation of those cells releases glutamate in the DH (Datta, 2006). These monosynaptic axonal connections between P-wave generating glutamatergic cells and forebrain structures provide anatomical evidence that P-wave generating cells have the necessary anatomical substrate to be the presynaptic input for the induction of synaptic plasticity, a required process for learning and memory processing.

Behavioral evidence

Several studies indicate that rapid eye movements may represent the element of REM sleep that is crucial for memory consolidation (Mandai *et al.*, 1989; Smith and Lapp, 1991; Smith and Weeden, 1990; Verschoor and Holdstock, 1984). For example, when a background clicking noise was presented during acquisition of a learned skill, presentation of the same auditory stimulus during subsequent eye movements during REM sleep (cueing), was correlated with a 23% improvement on retest performance one week later. The same cueing applied during non-eye movement REM sleep episodes correlated with only an 8.8% retest improvement. It has been hypothesized, therefore, that the eye movements (or at least that segment of REM sleep in which they occur) are selectively important in REM sleep-dependent memory consolidation (Smith and Weeden, 1990). Visual learning tests in human volunteers showed that in addition to increases in percentage of REM sleep, the percentage of eye bursts during post-training REM sleep increased (Verschoor and Holdstock, 1984). Researchers hypothesize that these augmented eye bursts represent the scanning of visual stimuli encountered during the learning task, as part of the process of sorting, organizing, and consolidating daily input (Verschoor and Holdstock, 1984). A study of Morse language learning in humans provides further evidence for an eye movement role in learning and memory processing during REM sleep. After a 90-minute Morse language learning session immediately prior to bedtime, subjects who had the greatest success had the densest rapid eye movements (Mandai *et al.*, 1989). It is well established that the occurrence and direction of rapid eye movements during REM sleep depends exclusively on the excitation of P-wave generating cells (Datta and Hobson, 1994). Therefore, the studies described above indirectly suggest that the excitation of pontine P-wave generating cells may be involved in REM sleep-dependent memory consolidation. The following paragraph describes some of the behavioral studies that have tested directly the relationship between P-wave generator activity and memory consolidation.

Using two different types of learning paradigms – two-way active avoidance (TWAA) and spatial learning in the Morris water maze – studies have shown that learning training increases REM sleep and P-wave activity (Datta, 2000, 2006). More importantly, the results of those studies have shown that the increase in P-wave density during the post-training REM sleep episodes is positively correlated with the effective consolidation, retention, and recall of the learning task. Together the results of those studies indicate that P-wave generator activation may have a positive influence in the REM sleep-dependent memory processing of TWAA and spatial navigational learning behavior.

In another behavioral study, we have demonstrated that the supplemental activation of the P-wave generator above the normal post-training increase in P-wave activity boosts retention of TWAA learning in the test trials (Mavanji and Datta, 2003). The results of this study provided experimental evidence to suggest that P-wave generator activation during REM sleep may enhance consolidation and integration of memories, resulting in improved performance on a recently learned task. Subsequently, another study using selective REM sleep deprivation and activation of P-wave generator methods, has shown that activation of the P-wave generator prevents the memory-impairing effects of post-training REM sleep deprivation (Datta et al., 2004). The results of this study further substantiated the idea that activation of the P-wave generator during REM sleep enhances the physiological process of memory processing that naturally occurs during post-training REM sleep. Finally, another study has shown that selective elimination of cell bodies from the P-wave generator prevents retention of TWAA learning memory (Mavanji et al., 2004). The results of this study also show that lesions in the P-wave generator eliminated P-waves during REM sleep without changing the amount of time spent in W, SWS, or REM sleep. These findings provided direct evidence that P-wave generating cells are crucial for normal REM sleep-dependent memory processing.

Biochemical/molecular evidence

A number of studies have shown that the afferent path for DH reactivation-dependent LTP and/or memory formation is glutamatergic, and transmission at these synapses involves NMDA receptors in the postsynaptic side (Morris et al., 1986; Packard and Teather, 1997; Steward and Worley, 2001; Zanatta et al., 1996). Interestingly, we have shown that the P-wave generator directly projects to the DH, amygdala, and many other forebrain structures that are known to be involved in memory processing (Datta et al., 1998). More importantly, we have shown that P-wave generating cells are glutamatergic and activation of P-wave generating cells increases glutamate release in the DH (Datta, 2006). Additionally, our behavioral studies have shown that learning training increases P-wave activity and that the activation of the P-wave generator during a post-training period improves memory (Datta, 2000, 2006; Datta et al., 2004; Mavanji and Datta, 2003). We have also demonstrated that the elimination of

P-wave generating cells prevents retention of memory (Mavanji et al., 2004). Collectively, the results of these studies suggest that P-wave generating cells are one of the major sources of glutamate for the postsynaptic NMDA receptor activation mediated memory processing in the DH.

A number of studies have suggested that neuronal activation-induced stimulation of the cAMP and/or Ca^{++}-PKA-CREB pathway is involved in the induction of a variety of gene expressions and ultimately in the protein synthesis of long-term memory formation (Abel et al., 1997; Datta et al., 2009a: Kandel and Schwartz, 1982). Using molecular and cellular techniques, we have shown that TWAA learning training causes P-wave generator activation and spatio-temporal phosphorylation of CREB (pCREB) in the DH and amygdala (Saha and Datta, 2005). Similarly, we have also demonstrated that TWAA learning training increases pCREB, BDNF, and Arc proteins in the DH and amygdala (Ulloor and Datta, 2005). The results of this study showed that the increase in P-wave activity during the post-training three-hour recording session is positively correlated with the increased levels of pCREB, BDNF, and Arc in the DH. These results suggest that memory processing of TWAA learning involves excitation of P-wave generating cells and increased expression of pCREB, Arc, and BDNF proteins in the DH and amygdala. Finally, using a combination of cell-specific localized lesions and molecular techniques, we have shown that elimination of P-wave generating cells abolished P-wave activity and TWAA learning training trials-induced expression of pCREB and Arc proteins and Arc, BDNF, Egr-1 mRNAs in the DH and amygdala (Datta et al., 2008). More recently, we have demonstrated that the P-wave generator activation-dependent TWAA memory processing involved intracellular PKA signaling system in the DH (Datta et al., 2009a). This study also showed that this P-wave generator activation-mediated PKA activation is necessary for the expression of TWAA learning training-induced BDNF gene expression in the DH. Collectively, these cellular and molecular studies have shown that TWAA memory processing-specific gene activation and protein synthesis in the DH and amygdala are initiated by the activation of the P-wave generator. These studies also suggest that the P-wave generator activation is the primary mechanism for the REM sleep-dependent memory consolidation process.

Here, I discuss some of the compelling evidence that I believe to be significant for our understanding of the mechanisms for REM sleep-dependent memory processing. These findings are the following: (1) Both TWAA and Morris water maze spatial navigation learning training increase REM sleep and P-wave activity during the subsequent sleep period. Improvement in TWAA and spatial navigation learning performance in the Morris water maze test trials session is proportional to the increase in P-wave density during the REM sleep episodes following training trials (Datta, 2000, 2006). (2) After TWAA training trials, immediate supplemental activation of the P-wave generator above the normal post-training increase in P-wave activity significantly increases retention of learning in the test trials (Mavanji and Datta, 2003). (3) Activation of the P-wave generator prevents the TWAA memory-impairing effects of post-training REM sleep deprivation (Datta *et al.*, 2004). (4) Elimination of P-waves by selective elimination of P-wave generating cells prevents retention of TWAA learning in the test trials (Mavanji *et al.*, 2004). (5) We have shown that the P-wave generating cells are glutamatergic, which project directly to a number of forebrain regions, including the DH and amygdala (Datta *et al.*, 1998; Datta, 2006). P-wave generating cell target areas are directly involved in learning and memory processing. Activation of the P-wave generator increases glutamate release and frequency of theta waves in the DH; both of these conditions have a positive influence on memory processing (Datta, 2006). (6) REM sleep-dependent TWAA memory processing depends on P-wave generator activation-mediated interaction with the DH-CA3 region (Datta *et al.*, 2005). (7) Chemical activation of P-wave generator and/or TWAA learning training increases the phosphorylation of transcription factor CREB and expression of immediate early genes Arc, BDNF, and Egr-1 in the DH, amygdala, and cerebral cortex (Datta *et al.*, 2008; Saha and Datta, 2005; Ulloor and Datta, 2005). (8) P-wave generator activation-mediated TWAA memory processing involves PKA activation and PKA activation-mediated BDNF expression in the DH-CA3 (Datta *et al.*, 2009a). These findings are significant because they provide the most direct evidence to substantiate the idea that P-wave generator activation during post-training REM sleep is critical for REM sleep-dependent memory processing of two-way active avoidance and spatial learning.

At present, our understanding of REM sleep-dependent memory processing mechanisms remains incomplete. Nevertheless, based on the existing findings, I suggest that learning training causes an increased homeostatic demand for the activation of P-wave generating cells in the brain stem that ultimately increases the total duration of the P-wave related states, tS-R, and REM sleep. Activation of P-wave generating cells during post-learning-training tS-R and REM sleep provides a glutamatergic-activating stimulus to the hippocampus and amygdala, leading to the physiological reactivation and neuronal activation-dependent gene expression and protein synthesis necessary for long-term neuronal plasticity and memory formation.

Acknowledgments

This work was supported by National Institutes of Health (USA) Research Grants: NS 34004 and MH 59839. The author thanks Mr. Brian W. Macone for his assistance in the production of this manuscript.

References

Abel, T., Nguyen, P. V., Barad, M. *et al.* (1997) Genetic demonstration of a role for PKA in the late phase of LTP and in hippocampus-based long-term memory. *Cell* **88**: 615–26.

Bizzi, E. & Brooks, D. C. (1963) Functional connections between pontine reticular formation and lateral geniculate nucleus during deep sleep. *Arch Ital Biol* **101**: 666–80.

Bliss, T. V. & Collingridge, G. L. (1993) A synaptic model of memory: long-term potentiation in the hippocampus. *Nature* **361**: 31–9.

Booth, V. & Poe, G. R. (2006) Input source and strength influences overall firing phase of model hippocampal CA1 pyramidal cells during theta: relevance to REM sleep reactivation and memory consolidation. *Hippocampus* **16**: 161–73.

Brooks, D. C. & Bizzi, E. (1963) Brain stem electrical activity during deep sleep. *Arch Ital Biol* **101**: 648–65.

Calvo, J. M. & Fernandez- Guardiola, A. (1984) Phasic activity of the basolateral amygdala, cingulate gyrus and hippocampus during REM sleep in the cat. *Sleep* **7**: 202–10.

Cohen, J. M. & Feldman, M. (1968) Relationship to electrical activity in the pontine reticular formation and lateral geniculate body to rapid eye movements. *J Neurophysiol* **31**: 807–17.

Datta, S. (1995) Neuronal activity in the peribrachial area: relationship to behavioral state control. *Neurosci Biobehav Rev* **19**: 67–84.

Datta, S. (1997). Cellular basis of pontine ponto-geniculo-occipital wave generation and modulation. *Cell Molec Neurobiol* **17**: 341–65.

Datta, S. (2000) Avoidance task training potentiates phasic pontine-wave density in the rat: a mechanism for sleep-dependent plasticity. *J Neurosci* **20**: 8607–13.

Datta, S. (2006) Activation of phasic pontine-wave generator: a mechanism for sleep-dependent memory processing. *Sleep Biol Rhythms* **4**: 16–26.

Datta, S. (2010) Sleep: learning and memory. In *Encyclopedia of Behavioral Neuroscience*, eds. G. F. Koob, M. Le Moal & R. F. Thompson. Oxford: Academic Press, pp. 218–226.

Datta, S. & Hobson, J. A. (1994) Neuronal activity in the caudo-lateral peribrachial pons: Relationship to PGO waves and rapid eye movements. *J Neurophysiol* **71**: 95–109.

Datta, S. & Hobson, J. A. (1995) Suppression of ponto-geniculo-occipital waves by neurotoxic lesions of pontine caudo-lateral peribrachial cells. *Neurosci* **67**: 703–12.

Datta, S. & Hobson, J. A. (2000) The rat as an experimental model for sleep neurophysiology. *Behav Neurosci* **114**: 1239–44.

Datta, S. & Maclean, R. R. (2007) Neurobiological mechanisms for the regulation of mammalian sleep-wake behavior: reinterpretation of historical evidence and inclusion of contemporary cellular and molecular evidence. *Neurosci Biobehav Rev* **31**: 775–824.

Datta, S. & Patterson, E. H. (2003) Activation of phasic pontine wave (P-wave): a mechanism of learning and memory processing. In *Sleep and Brain Plasticity*, eds. J. Maquet, R. Stickgold & C. Smith. Oxford: Oxford University Press, pp. 135–56

Datta, S. & Siwek, D. F. (2002) Single cell activity patterns of pedunculopontine tegmentum neurons across the sleep-wake cycle in the freely moving rats. *J Neurosci Res* **70**: 611–21.

Datta, S., Calvo, J. M., Quattrochi, J. J. & Hobson, J. A. (1991) Long-term enhancement of REM sleep following cholinergic stimulation. *Neuroreport* **2**: 619–22.

Datta, S., Calvo, J. M. & Quatrochi, J. (1992) Cholinergic microstimulation of the peribrachial nucleus in the cat. I. immediate and prolonged increases in ponto-geniculo-occipital waves. *Arch Ital Biol* **130**: 263–84.

Datta, S., Siwek, D. F., Patterson, E. H. & Cipolloni, P. B. (1998) Localization of pontine PGO wave generation sites and their anatomical projctions in the rat. *Synapse* **30**: 409–23.

Datta, S., Patterson, E. H. & Siwek, D. F. (1999) Brainstem afferents of the cholinoceptive pontine wave generation sites in the rat. *Sleep Res Online* **2**: 79–82.

Datta, S., Mavanji, V., Ulloor, J. & Patterson, E. H. (2004) Activation of phasic pontine-wave generator prevents rapid eye movement sleep deprivation-induced learning impairment in the rat: a mechanism for sleep-dependent plasticity. *J Neurosci* **24**: 1416–27.

Datta, S., Saha, S., Prutzman, S. L., Mullins, O. J. & Mavanji, V. (2005) Pontine-wave generator activation-dependent memory processing of avoidance learning involves the dorsal hippocampus in the rat. *J Neurosci Res* **80**: 727–37.

Datta, S., Li, G. & Auerbach, S. (2008) Activation of phasic pontine-wave generator in the rat: a mechanism for expression of plasticity-related genes and proteins in the dorsal hippocampus and amygdala. *Eur J Neurosci* **27**: 1876–92.

Datta, S., Siwek, D. F. & Huang, M. P. (2009a) Improvement of two-way active avoidance memory requires protein kinase a activation and brain-derived neurotrophic factor expression in the dorsal hippocampus. *J Mol Neurosci* **38**: 257–64.

Datta, S., Siwek, D. F. & Stack, E. C. (2009b) Identification of cholinergic and non-cholinergic neurons in the pons expressing phosphorylated cyclic AMP response element-binding protein as a function of rapid eye movement sleep. *Neuroscience* doi: **10**.1016/j. neuroscience. 2009.06.035.

Farber, J., Marks, G. A. & Roffwarg, H. P. (1980) Rapid eye movement sleep PGO-type waves are present in the dorsal pons of the albino rat. *Science* **209**: 615–17.

Feldman, M. & Cohen, B. (1968). Electrical activity in the lateral geniculate body of the alert monkey associated with eye movements. *J Neurophysiol* **31**: 455–66.

Gottesmann, C. (1969) Etude sur les activites electrophysiologiques phasiques chez la rat. *Physiol Behav* **4**: 495–504.

Jouvet, M., Jeannerod, M. & Delorme, F. (1965) Organization of the system responsible for phase activity during paradoxal sleep. *C R Seances Soc Biol Fil* **159**: 1599–604.

Jouvet, M., Michel, F. & Courjon, J. (1959) L'activite electrique du rhinencephale au cours du sommeil chez le chat. *C R Soc Biol* **153**: 101–5.

Kandel, E. R. & Schwartz, J. H. (1982) Molecular biology of learning: modulation of transmitter release. *Science* **218**: 433–43.

Karashima, A., Nakamura, K., Sato, N. *et al.* (2002) Phase-locking of spontaneous and elicited ponto-geniculo-occipital waves is associated with acceleration of hippocampal theta waves during rapid eye movement sleep in cats. *Brain Res* **958**: 347–58.

Karashima, A., Nakao, M., Katayama, N. & Honda, K. (2005) Instantaneous acceleration and amplification of hippocampal theta wave coincident with phasic pontine activities during REM sleep. *Brain Res* **1051**: 50–6.

Karni, A., Tanne, D., Rubenstein, B. S., Askenasy, J. J. & Sagi, D. (1994) Dependence on REM sleep of overnight improvement of a perceptual skill. *Science* **265**: 679–82.

Lim, Y. G., Kim, K. K. & Park, K. S. (2007) ECG recording on a bed during sleep without direct skin-contact. *IEEE Trans Biomed Eng* **54**: 718–25.

Mandai, O., Guerrien, A., Sockeel, P., Dujardin, K. & Leconte, P. (1989) REM sleep modifications following a Morse code learning session in humans. *Physiol Behav* **46**: 639–42.

Mavanji, V. & Datta, S. (2003) Activation of the phasic pontine-wave generator enhances improvement of learning performance: a mechanism for sleep-dependent plasticity. *Eur J Neurosci* **17**: 359–70.

Mavanji, V., Ulloor, J., Saha, S. & Datta, S. (2004) Neurotoxic lesions of phasic pontine-wave generator cells impair retention of 2-way active avoidance memory. *Sleep* **27**: 1282–92.

McCarley, R. W., Nelson, J. P. & Hobson, J. A. (1978). Ponto-geniculo-occipital (PGO) burst neurons: correlative evidence for neuronal generators of PGO waves. *Science* **201**: 269–72.

McCarley, R. W., Winkelman, J. W. & Duffy, F. H. (1983) Human cerebral potentials associated with REM sleep rapid eye movements: links to PGO waves and waking potentials. *Brain Res* **274**: 359–64.

Mikiten, T. M., Niebyl, P. H. & Hendley, C. D. (1961) EEG desynchronization during behavioral sleep associated with spike discharges from the thalamus of the cat. *Fed Proc.* **20**: 327.

Miyauchi, S., Takino, R., Fukuda, H. & Torii, S. (1987) Electrophysiological evidence for dreaming: human cerebral potentials associated with rapid eye movement during REM sleep. *Electroencephalogr Clin Neurophysiol* **66**: 383–90.

Morris, R. G., Anderson, E., Lynch, G. S. & Baudry, M. (1986) Selective impairment of learning and blockade of long-term potentiation by an N-methyl-D-aspartate receptor antagonist, AP5. *Nature* **319**: 774–6.

Morrison, A. R. & Bowker, R. M. (1975) The biological significance of PGO spikes in the sleeping cat. *Acta Neurobiol Exp (Wars)* **35**: 821–40.

Morrison, A. R. & Pompeiano, O. (1966) Vestibular influences during sleep. IV. Functional relations between vestibular nuclei and lateral geniculate nucleus during desynchronized sleep. *Arch Ital Biol* **104**: 425–58.

Mouret, J., Jeannerod, M. & Jouvet, M. (1963) L'active electrique du systeme visuel au cours de la phase paradoxale du sommeil chez le chat. *J Physiol (Paris)* **55**: 305–6.

Packard, M. G. & Teather, L. A. (1997) Posttraining injections of MK-801 produce a time-dependent impairment of memory in two water maze tasks. *Neurobiol Learn Mem* **68**: 42–50.

Pavlides, C. & Ribeiro, S. (2003) Recent evidence of memory processing in sleep. In *Sleep and Brain Plasticity*, eds, J. Maquet, R. Stickgold & C. Smith. Oxford: Oxford University Press, pp. 327–62.

Poe, G. R., Nitz, D. A., McNaughton, B. L. & Barnes, C. A. (2000) Experience-dependent phase-reversal of hippocampal neuron firing during REM sleep. *Brain Res* **855**: 176–80.

Quattrochi, J., Datta, S. & Hobson, J. A. (1998) Cholinergic and non-cholinergic afferents of the caudolateral parabrachial nucleus: a role in the long-term enhancement of rapid eye movement sleep. *Neuroscience* **83**: 1123–36.

Saha, S. & Datta, S. (2005) Two-way active avoidance training-specific increases in phosphorylated cAMP response element-binding protein in the dorsal hippocampus, amygdala, and hypothalamus. *Eur J Neurosci* **21**: 3403–14.

Salzarulo, P., Pelloni, G. & Lairy, G. C. (1975) [Electrophysiologic semiology of daytime sleep in 7 to 9-year-old children]. *Electroencephalogr Clin Neurophysiol* **38**: 473–94.

Sanford, L. D., Tejani-Butt, S. M., Ross, R. J. & Morrison, A. R. (1995) Amygdaloid control of alerting and behavioral arousal in rats: involvement of serotonergic mechanisms. *Arch Ital Biol* **134**: 81–99.

Smith, C. (2003) The REM sleep window and memory processing. In *Sleep and Brain Plasticity*, eds. J. Maquet, R. Stickgold & C. Smith. Oxford: Oxford University Press, pp. 117–33.

Smith, C. & Lapp, L. (1991) Increases in number of REMS and REM density in humans following an intensive learning period. *Sleep* **14**: 325–30.

Smith, C. & Weeden, K. (1990) Post training REMs coincident auditory stimulation enhances memory in humans. *Psychiatr J Univ Ott* **15**: 85–90.

Steriade, M., Datta, S., Pare, D., Oakson, G. & Curro Dossi, R. C. (1990a) Neuronal activities in brain-stem cholinergic nuclei related to tonic activation processes in thalamocortical systems. *J Neurosci* **10**: 2541–59.

Steriade, M., Pare, D., Datta, S., Oakson, G. & Curro Dossi, R. (1990b) Different cellular types in mesopontine cholinergic nuclei related to ponto-geniculo-occipital waves. *J Neurosci* **10**: 2560–79.

Stern, W. C., Forbes, W. B. & Morgane, P. J. (1974) Absence of ponto-geniculo-occipital (PGO) spikes in rats. *Physiol Behav* **12**: 293–5.

Steward, O. & Worley, P. F. (2001) Selective targeting of newly synthesized Arc mRNA to active synapses requires NMDA receptor activation. *Neuron* **30**: 227–40.

Stickgold, R. & Walker, M. P. (2007) Sleep-dependent memory consolidation. *Sleep Med* **8**: 331–43.

Ulloor, J. & Datta, S. (2005). Spatio-temporal activation of cyclic AMP response element-binding protein, activity-regulated cytoskeletal-associated protein and brain-derived nerve growth factor: a mechanism for pontine-wave generator activation-dependent two-way active-avoidance memory processing in the rat. *J Neurochem* **95**: 418–28.

Verschoor, G. J. & Holdstock, T. L. (1984) REM bursts and REM sleep following visual and auditory learning. *S Afr J Psychol* **14**: 69–74.

Vuillon-Cacciuttolo, G. & Seri, B. (1978) Effects of optic nerve section in baboons on the geniculate and cortical spike activity during various states of vigilance. *Electroencephalogr Clin Neurophysiol* **44**: 754–68.

Walker, M. P. & Stickgold, R. (2006) Sleep, memory, and plasticity. *Annu Rev Psychol* **57**: 139–66.

Zanatta, M. S., Schaeffer, E., Schmitz, P. K. *et al.* (1996) Sequential involvement of NMDA receptor-dependent processes in hippocampus, amygdala, entorhinal cortex and parietal cortex in memory processing. *Behav Pharmacol* **7**: 341–5.

Chapter 16

Hippocampal theta rhythm of REM sleep

Robert P. Vertes

Summary

The theta rhythm of the hippocampus is a large-amplitude (1–2 mV), nearly sinusoidal oscillation of 5 to 12 Hz. Theta is present in the hippocampus of the rat during the exploratory movements of waking and continuously throughout REM sleep. In early reports, we identified neurons of the nucleus pontis oralis (RPO) of the pons that discharged in association with the theta of waking and REM sleep, and subsequently showed that electrical stimulation or carbachol injections into the RPO very effectively elicited theta. These findings indicated that RPO was the brain-stem source for the generation of theta. In related studies, we described an ascending RPO to septohippocampal system routed through the hypothalamic supramammillary nucleus controlling theta, and further demonstrated that the serotonin-containing median raphe (MR) nucleus desynchronized the hippocampal EEG – or blocked theta. The latter indicates that theta, like other events of REM sleep, is subject to aminergic modulation; that is, the suppression of MR activity during REM releases theta in that state. Theta serves a well recognized role in memory processing in waking. We suggest that theta does not serve the same function in REM sleep (memory processing), but rather theta (of REM) is a by-product of the intense forebrain activation of REM sleep, which serves the important function of maintaining the minimum requisite levels of activity periodically throughout sleep to ensure and promote recovery from sleep.

Introduction

The theta rhythm of the hippocampus is a large-amplitude (1–2 mV), nearly sinusoidal oscillation of 5 to 12 Hz in the rat (Bland, 1986; Vertes and Kocsis, 1997; Vertes *et al.*, 2004). It is the largest extracellular synchronous signal that can be recorded in the mammalian brain. Theta is present in the hippocampus during the exploratory movements of waking and continuously throughout REM sleep. As documented in this volume, REM sleep is composed of a constellation of events, which include: (1) a desynchronized pattern of cortical electroencephalographic (EEG) activity; (2) theta rhythm in the hippocampus; (3) marked atonia of the postural muscles; (4) ponto-geniculo-occipital (PGO) spikes; (5) rapid eye movements; (6) myoclonic twitches; and (7) pronounced cardiorespiratory fluctuations (Datta and MacLean, 2007; Vertes, 1984). Although theta is a prominent event of REM sleep, it has not received the same degree of attention as other indices of REM. This may be a consequence of the fact that most of the early examinations of REM sleep in cats did not record theta, possibly because theta is not as robust in cats as in rats.

Our initial interest in theta developed from early unit recording studies in behaving rats designed to examine the role of the pontine reticular formation (PRF) in REM sleep control (Vertes, 1977, 1979). In the early 1970s, Hobson, McCarley, and associates published a series of papers describing the discharge properties of cells of the PRF (or their terminology, the gigantocellular tegmental field or FTG) during sleep–wake states in cats (Hobson *et al.*, 1974; McCarley and Hobson, 1971). They reported in awake, restrained cats that FTG cells fired "selectively" during REM sleep; that is, at very low rates during waking (without movements) and slow-wave (or non-REM) sleep and at very high rates during REM sleep. These results, in part, formed the basis of their reciprocal interaction model of sleep–wake control (Hobson *et al.*, 1975).

In accord with Hobson and McCarley, we found that PRF neurons in behaving rats fired at significantly greater rates during REM sleep than during either

REM Sleep: Regulation and Function, eds. Birendra N. Mallick, S. R. Pandi-Perumal, Robert W. McCarley, and Adrian R. Morrison. Published by Cambridge University Press. © Cambridge University Press 2011.

SWS or quiet waking, but unlike them, further showed that PRF cells maintained the same high rates of discharge during waking with movements as observed in REM. Siegel *et al.* (1977) similarly described a population of PRF cells in the behaving cat that fired at enhanced rates during waking mobility and REM, and also failed to identify cells that discharged selectively in REM sleep. These findings suggested, then, that PRF cells do not serve to generate the state of REM sleep, but rather perform some function(s) common to waking motor behavior and REM sleep.

Following our initial examination of PRF cells (Vertes, 1977), we recorded from a larger population of these neurons and found that 83% of them discharged at high rates during both waking with movements and REM sleep (Vertes, 1979). We termed these cells MOV-REM neurons, and found they could be subdivided into phasically and tonically firing MOV-REM neurons. The phasic MOV-REM cells fired in association with specific and readily identifiable types of movements during waking, such as facial or head movements, and phasically occurring replicas of these movements (twitches) during REM sleep. By contrast, the discharge of the tonic MOV-REM cells during waking (with movements), unlike that of the phasic MOV-REM neurons, did not appear to be associated with specific motor acts. Instead, the "tonic cells" tended to fire during various, seemingly unrelated, motor acts of waking, and in a sense, their discharge appeared to signal a transition from non-movement (still) to movement conditions. As such, their activity appeared to be correlated with the theta rhythm of waking; that is, both unit discharge and theta were present during active motor behavior but not with quiescent states of the rat. In addition, tonic MOV-REM cells fired at high tonic rates throughout REM sleep and showed fluctuations in rates of discharge that directly varied with changes in the degree to which theta was regular or sinusoidal in REM (Vertes, 1979). These observations led us to suggest that PRF cells, or more specifically the tonic MOV-REM neurons, served a direct role in the generation of theta of waking and REM sleep.

Recording in rabbits, Green and Arduini (1954) were among the first to describe the theta rhythm of the hippocampus, and in their original report showed that theta was associated with a desynchronized cortical EEG, and further that theta could be elicited with an array of natural sensory stimuli as well as by activation of the brain-stem reticular formation (RF). Accordingly, they viewed theta as an "arousal reaction"

of the hippocampus and stated that this interpretation was "strengthened by the observation that excitation of the reticular activating system of the brain stem evokes an identical pattern of hippocampal activity" (Green and Arduini, 1954). Although Green and Arduini (1954), as well as others that followed, showed that stimulation of the brain-stem RF generated theta, no attempt was made to specifically identify the reticular sites responsible for this effect (for a review see Vertes, 1982). At best, it was stated that stimulation was delivered to the midbrain RF. Our unit recording studies identifying PRF neurons with "theta-related" discharge properties suggested that the PRF region containing these cells was the principal brain-stem site for the generation of theta. Tonic MOV-REM cells were predominantly localized to the nucleus pontis oralis (RPO) of the rostral PRF.

In a series of follow-up studies, then, we demonstrated that: (1) stimulation of, or carbachol injections into, the RPO, but not in adjacent regions of the brain stem, generated theta; (2) stimulation of the serotonin-containing MR nucleus desynchronized the hippocampal EEG (or blocked theta); and (3) theta is controlled by an ascending system of connections from the RPO to the supramammillary nucleus (of the hypothalamus) and to the septum/hippocampus (for reviews see Vertes and Kocsis, 1997; Vertes *et al.*, 2004).

Nucleus pontis oralis – brain-stem source for the generation of the theta: recording and stimulation studies

As discussed, in early reports we identified cells of the RPO that exhibited "theta-like" properties; that is, they fired at high tonic rates selectively during the two states in which theta is present in the rat (voluntary movements of waking and REM sleep) and displayed changes in patterns of discharge directly correlated with fluctuations of theta of waking and REM. In accord with these findings, Nūñez *et al.* (1991) demonstrated in urethane-anesthetized rats that approximately 64% (46/72) of RPO neurons discharged at significantly greater rates during theta elicited with sensory stimulation or carbachol injections in the (contralateral) RPO. In addition, RPO cells fired tonically with theta; that is, none were identified that discharged rhythmically in bursts with theta. More recently, Takano and Hanada (2009), recording from several regions of the brain stem in anesthetized rats, reported that 14 of 22

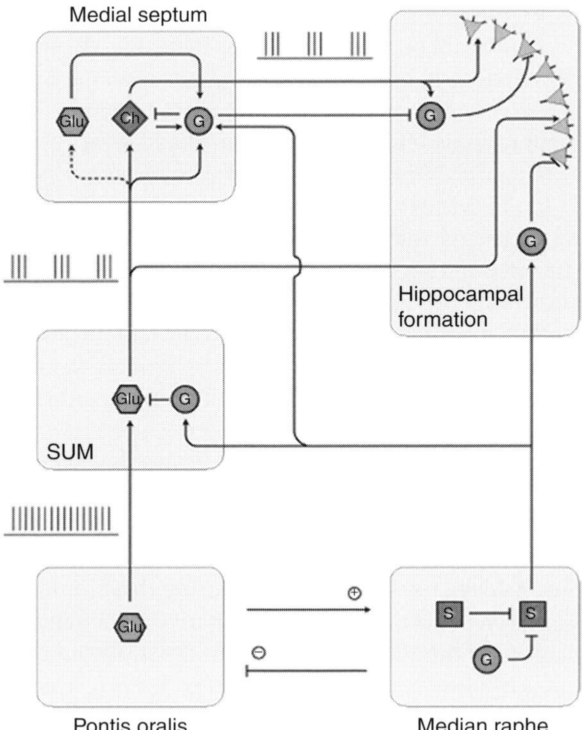

Figure 16.1 Schematic diagram showing the major interconnections of ascending systems controlling theta and non-theta (desynchronization) states of the hippocampal EEG. During theta, tonically firing cells of the nucleus pontis oralis activate putative glutamatergic neurons of the supramammillary nucleus, which, in turn, convert this steady barrage into a rhythmical pattern of discharge that is relayed to cholinergic and GABAergic pacemaking cells of the medial septum. Medial septal GABAergic neurons connect with and inhibit GABAergic cells of the hippocampus thereby exerting a disinhibitory action on the pyramidal cells of the hippocampus. Medial septal GABAergic cells receive intraseptal excitatory input from both septal cholinergic and glutamatergic neurons. Cholinergic septohippocampal pacemaking cells terminate on both interneurons and principal cells of the hippocampus. During states of hippocampal desynchronization (non-theta), a subset of serotonergic septal-projecting cells of the median raphe nucleus discharge at enhanced rates, activate GABAergic cells of the medial septum, which, in turn, inhibit GABAergic/cholinergic pacemaking cells of the medial septum in the desynchronization of the hippocampal EEG. Serotonergic neurons of the median raphe nucleus also project directly to the supramammillary nucleus and to the hippocampus and could also exert desynchronizing actions on the hippocampal EEG through these connections. Dashed line signifies presently undetermined SUM glutamatergic projections to glutamatergic cells of the septum. Arrows (at the end of lines) indicate excitatory connections; straight lines, indicate inhibitory connections. Abbreviations: Ch, acetylcholine; G, GABA; Glu, glutamate; S, serotonin; SUM, supramammillary nucleus.

cells of the RPO showed changes in firing rates with the onset of theta, and further RPO neurons exhibited the earliest changes with respect to theta onset, indicating that they were the brain-stem trigger for theta.

As initially demonstrated by Petsche, Stumpf, and colleagues (Petsche *et al.*, 1965), and subsequently by several others (for review see Vertes *et al.*, 2004), the medial septum and vertical limb of the diagonal band nucleus (MS/DBv): (1) contains populations of cells (cholinergic, GABAergic, and glutamatergic) that fire rhythmically in bursts with theta to pace the rhythm; and (2) MS/DBv cells are driven by input arising from lower levels of the brain (brain stem and diencephalon) in the generation of theta (Figure 16.1). Lesions of the MS/DBv abolish theta in the hippocampus.

In early reports, we mapped the PRF (as well as the midbrain and medullary RF) with stimulation in anesthetized rats to determine its effect on the hippocampal EEG, and found that RPO of the rostral pons was the most effective brain-stem site for stimulation-elicited theta (Vertes, 1981). Stimulation of brain-stem regions adjacent to RPO were either ineffective in producing theta or marginally effective at significantly higher levels of stimulation. We further demonstrated that injections of carbachol into this same region (RPO) produced theta at short latencies (mean: 38.5 sec) and for long durations (mean: 12.9 min) (Vertes *et al.*, 1993). In most instances, carbachol injections into the RPO gave rise to theta almost instantaneously; that is, before the completion of the injection. Finally, working with Brian Bland and colleagues at the University of Calgary, we demonstrated that stimulation of, or carbachol injections into, the RPO activated theta rhythmically bursting neurons (pacemaking cells) of the MS/DBv and generated theta, but had no effect on non-theta related cells of the MS/DBv (Bland *et al.*, 1994). The foregoing findings indicate, then, that the nucleus pontis oralis (RPO) of the rostral pons is the primary (or sole) brain-stem source for the generation of theta, and like other indices of REM (see below), theta is a cholinergically mediated event.

Ascending brain stem-diencephalo-septohippocampal systems controlling the hippocampal theta rhythm

As discussed, the pacemaking neurons of the MS/DBv that directly drive theta are activated by input arising from lower levels of the brain. Although it was originally thought that the reticular formation exerted direct actions on the MS/DBv in the generation of theta (see Vertes and Kocsis, 1997), it has subsequently been shown that the supramammillary nucleus (SUM) of the hypothalamus represents a critical link between the brain stem (RPO) and septum/hippocampus in the control of theta. For instance, in an early anatomical study (Vertes, 1988), examining putative brain-stem sources of input to the MS/DBv subserving theta, we unexpectedly found that injections of retrograde tracers in the MS/DBv gave rise to very few labeled cells in the pontine RF. This suggested that RPO actions on the MS/DBv were indirect or mediated by an intervening cell group(s) between RPO and MS/DBv. Interestingly, in that same report, we showed that MS/DBv injections produced massive cell labeling in the SUM, dorsal to the mammillary bodies, indicating that SUM may be a link between RPO and the septum in the control of theta.

As developed below, this was confirmed by the following lines of evidence: (1) the SUM receives projections from the RPO and, in turn, projects heavily to the septum and hippocampus (Figure 16.1); (2) SUM cells fire rhythmically with theta; (3) electrically or chemically elicited activation of the SUM drives theta; and (4) suppression of the SUM disrupts the bursting discharge of septal pacemaking cells and eliminates theta in the hippocampus.

Using anterograde tracing techniques, we demonstrated that: (1) the RPO projects to the SUM (Vertes and Martin, 1988); and (2) the SUM distributes densely to the medial (MS/DBv) and lateral septum as well as to the hippocampus (Vertes, 1992). Within the hippocampus, SUM fibers selectively target the dentate gyrus and CA2/CA3a of Ammon's horn (Vertes, 1992). There are essentially no SUM projections to the CA1 region of Ammon's horn.

Recording multi-unit activity in anesthetized rats, Kirk and McNaughton (1991) initially identified a population of cells of the SUM that fired rhythmically with the hippocampal theta rhythm. They further showed that this activity was not dependent on "downstream" actions of the MS/DBv on the SUM; that is, procaine injections in the MS/DBv that abolished hippocampal theta did not alter the rhythmical firing of supramammillary neurons. In a subsequent examination of the activity of SUM cells as well as those in surrounding regions of the caudal diencephalon, we found that 29 of 170 neurons discharged rhythmically, synchronous with theta (Kocsis and Vertes, 1994). All 29 theta-related cells were localized to the SUM or to the mammillary bodies (MB), ventral to the SUM; none of 141 neurons located outside of the SUM/MB fired synchronously with theta. Bland et al. (1995) similarly demonstrated that 16 of 16 SUM cells and 19 of 23 MB cells discharged rhythmically with theta – their phasic theta-on cells.

Finally, the activation or suppression of SUM drives or blocks theta, respectively. Specifically, electrical stimulation of, or carbachol injections into, the SUM activate theta-bursting neurons of the septum and hippocampus and produce theta (Bland et al., 1994; Vertes et al., 2004), while the reversible suppression of the SUM with procaine injections in anesthetized rats disrupts the spontaneous as well as the RPO-elicited bursting discharge of septal pacemaking cells and eliminates theta (Bland et al., 1994; Vertes et al., 2004). Procaine injections into the SUM in awake (non-anesthetized) rats significantly reduces the frequency of theta but does not totally eliminate it (Pan and McNaughton, 2004).

In summary, the foregoing indicates that theta is controlled by a network of cells extending from the brain stem to the forebrain; that is, from the RPO to the supramammillary nucleus to the septum/hippocampus. As depicted in Figure 16.1, during theta tonically firing cells of the RPO activate putative glutamatergic neurons of the SUM, which convert the steady barrage into a rhythmical pattern of discharge that is relayed to cholinergic and GABAergic "pacemaking" cells of the MS/DBv that rhythmically drive large populations of hippocampal neurons to produce theta.

Ascending systems controlling non-theta states of the hippocampal EEG (hippocampal EEG desynchronization): role of the median raphe nucleus (MR) nucleus

The MR nucleus is a major serotonin-containing cell group of the midbrain with extensive projections to the forebrain (Morin and Meyer-Bernstein, 1999; Vertes and Martin, 1988; Vertes et al., 1999). A large body of evidence indicates that the MR serves a direct role in controlling non-theta (or desynchronized) states of the hippocampal EEG. Early reports showed that MR stimulation desynchronized the hippocampal EEG (Assaf and Miller, 1978; Vertes, 1981; Yamamoto et al. 1979), and that MR lesions produced continuous, uninterrupted theta, independent of behavior (Maru et al. 1979; Yamamoto et al., 1979). It was further demonstrated that the desynchronizing effects of the MR on the hippocampal EEG were mediated by serotonergic MR neurons. Specifically, Assaf and Miller (1978) demonstrated that the disruptive effect of MR stimulation on septal pacemaking cells and the hippocampal EEG was blocked by pre-treatment with the 5-hydroxytryptamine (5-HT) synthesis inhibitor, p-chlorophenylalanine (PCPA), which produced a 60 to 80% depletion of forebrain serotonin, while Yamamoto *et al.* (1979) reported that ongoing theta produced by MR lesions could be temporarily disrupted by injections of the serotonin precursor L-5-hydroxytryptophan (L-5-HTP). More recently, we demonstrated that injections of various substances into the MR that either suppressed 5-HT MR neurons (5-HT$_{1A}$ autoreceptor agonists or GABA agonists) or reduced excitatory drive to them (excitatory amino acid antagonists) produced theta at short latencies (1–2 min) and for long durations (20–80 min) (Kinney *et al.*, 1994, 1995, 1996; Vertes *et al.*, 1994). In a similar manner, Varga *et al.* (2002) identified GABA$_B$ receptors on serotonergic MR neurons, and further reported that infusions of the GABA$_B$ agonist, baclofen, into the MR produced long-lasting theta. They concluded that the effects of baclofen on theta "resulted from suppression of the serotonergic output from the median raphe" (Varga *et al.*, 2002).

In examinations of the effects of manipulations of the MR on the hippocampal EEG in awake rabbits, Vinogradova and colleagues (Kitchigina *et al.*, 1999; Vinogradova *et al.*, 1999) showed that low-amplitude MR stimulation disrupted the bursting discharge of medial septal cells and abolished theta in the hippocampus, and that the reversible suppression of the MR with local injections of lidocaine increased the frequency and regularity of discharge of theta-bursting neurons of the septum and hippocampus and produced continuous theta in the hippocampus. Kitchigina *et al.* (1999) concluded that: "the median raphe nucleus can be regarded as a functional antagonist of the reticular formation, powerfully suppressing theta bursts of the medial septal area neurons and the hippocampal theta rhythm." More recently, Kudina *et al.* (2004) demonstrated that injections of the serotonin reuptake inhibitor, fluoxetine, into the lateral ventricles produced a greater than 50% reduction in the amplitude of theta that persisted for 60 to 90 minutes.

Median raphe stimulation-induced hippocampal desynchronization: large-amplitude irregular activity, small-amplitude irregular activity, or neither?

Until fairly recently, it was thought that the hippocampal EEG essentially consisted of two states: large-amplitude irregular activity (LIA) and theta rhythm (Bland, 1986; Vertes and Kocsis, 1997). In effect, theta was present during voluntary movements of waking and REM sleep (see above), and LIA during "automatic" behaviors of waking and SWS. Although a few early reports identified a third state of the hippocampal EEG, termed small-amplitude irregular activity (SIA) (Vanderwolf, 1971), SIA has only recently received detailed attention (Jarosiewicz and Skaggs, 2004). Small-amplitude irregular activity is a less common form of hippocampal EEG activity than LIA. For instance, according to a recent report (Jarosiewicz and Skaggs, 2004), SIA is mainly present in the hippocampus during transitions between stages of sleep, transitions from sleep to waking, or with the presentation of novel or unexpected stimuli during waking that are not accompanied by orienting movements. Jarosiewicz and Skaggs (2004) have suggested that SIA represents a level of arousal intermediate between that of sleep and waking.

Early studies that examined the effects of MR stimulation on the hippocampal EEG (Assaf and Miller, 1978; Vertes, 1981; Yamamoto *et al.* 1979) generally failed to describe specific properties of the EEG produced by the stimulation, referring to it as hippocampal desynchronization, non-theta, or perhaps LIA. By contrast, Bland and colleagues (Jackson *et al.*, 2008) recently reported that MR stimulation produces SIA. Specifically, they showed that high-intensity MR stimulation gave rise to very low-amplitude (~ 25–50 µV) hippocampal EEG activity, or according to them "a near flattening of the electroencephalogram." They stated that MR stimulation "does not elicit hippocampal field activity typical of non-theta (LIA, sharp wave, slow oscillation) but rather produces an activated neocortex and small amplitude irregular hippocampal activity" (Jackson *et al.*, 2008). Although this remains possible, it may be the case that the very low-amplitude EEG (flattening) produced by MR stimulation represents a nearly complete suppression of hippocampal EEG activity (SIA, LIA, and theta) – as apposed to the generation of a third pattern of activity or SIA.

Consistent with a near-total MR suppression of the hippocampal EEG, Jackson *et al.* (2008) further reported that MR stimulation inhibited the activity of several types of hippocampal cells including phasic theta-on, tonic theta-on, theta-off, and non-theta related cells. For instance, MR stimulation was shown to completely suppress the discharge of 40% (16/40) of hippocampal phasic theta-on cells, and inhibit the firing with a loss of rhythmicity of an additional 53% of them. It is evident, then, that MR stimulation produces a profound reduction in the amplitude of the hippocampal EEG (a near flattening) that may, at least in part, result from the marked suppression of the activity of various types of hippocampal neurons.

Unit activity in the MR nucleus in relation to the hippocampal EEG: serotonergic and non-serotonergic neurons

In an initial examination of the discharge properties of neurons of the dorsal (DR) and median raphe (MR) nuclei in urethane anesthetized rats, we showed that a relatively large percentage of DR/MR cells fired synchronously with the hippocampal theta rhythm (Kocsis and Vertes, 1996). For instance, 5 of 10 MR cells displayed theta rhythmical patterns of discharge and high unit-EEG coherence values (0.47 to 0.89), indicating strong theta rhythmicity. Interestingly, the "theta-rhythmic" MR cells fired at high mean rates (21–42 Hz), suggesting that they were not serotonergic neurons – or the classically defined population of 5-hydroxytryptamine (5-HT) raphe cells with slow (1–4 Hz), regular rates of discharge (Jacobs and Azmitia, 1992). Accordingly, it was tentatively suggested that these MR cells were GABAergic neurons.

In a follow-up analysis of the firing characteristics of MR neurons with respect to theta, we demonstrated that 145 of 181 MR cells (or ~80%) showed theta-related changes in activity; that is, they fired at significantly higher (theta-on cells) or lower (theta-off cells) rates of activity during theta compared to non-theta states (Viana Di Prisco *et al.*, 2002). The theta-on (68%) and theta-off (32%) MR neurons were further divided into slow (~1–3 Hz), moderate (5–11 Hz), and fast-firing (>12 Hz) cells. Unlike the previous report (which involved a much smaller population of MR neurons) (Kocsis and Vertes, 1996), approximately one-third (49/145) of MR cells discharged at slow regular rates of activity similar to "classic" serotonin-containing neurons of the raphe and were presumed to be 5-HT cells. About 30% of the slow-firing (SF) neurons were theta-off cells, while the remaining (or the majority) were theta-on cells.

Several recent reports, using various methods to identity 5-HT raphe neurons (mainly of DR) have shown that serotonergic cells are not a homogeneous population of neurons as originally described (Jacobs and Azmitia, 1992), but rather discharge over a range of frequencies up to >20 Hz (Kocsis *et al.*, 2006; Urbain

et al., 2006). In this regard, we identified a second population of MR neurons, termed moderately firing (MF) cells, that discharged at mean baseline rates of ~7 Hz (range 5–11 Hz) (Viana Di Prisco *et al.*, 2002). These cells constituted about 37% (53/145) of MR neurons, and unlike SF neurons, more were theta-off (60%) than theta-on (40%) cells. The theta-off MF cells showed a dramatic decrease in firing rate from non-theta to theta states; that is, from mean rates about 7.0 Hz to rates of 2.0 Hz. An interesting subset of theta-off MF cells discharged at very regular rates similar to classic slow-firing MR neurons – the main difference being their rates of discharge during baseline conditions: SF cells ~1 to 3 Hz and MF cells ~5 to 7 Hz.

The discharge profile of a moderately firing, putative serotonergic, theta-off cell is shown in Figure 16.2. As depicted, the cell discharged at very regular rates during control (non-theta) conditions (Figure 16.2*a*), and abruptly ceased firing with the onset, and essentially for the duration, of theta elicited with tail pinch (TP) (Figure 16.2*a*) or by electrical stimulation of the tail (Figure 16.2*b*). Although not systematically examined, a few regular firing MF theta-off cells were strongly inhibited by systemic injections of the 5-HT1$_A$ agonist, 8-hydroxy-2(di-*n*-propylamino)tetralin (8-OH-DPAT), indicating that they were serotonergic neurons.

A third population of MR neurons (37/145) discharged at high baseline rates (12–22 Hz) and exhibited further increases in discharge from non-theta to theta states. All fast-firing (FF) MR neurons had narrow action potentials, were theta-on cells (no theta-off FF neurons), and could be subdivided into tonic and phasically discharging cells. The phasic FF neurons not only showed pronounced increases in rates of discharge with theta (from mean rates of 12.0 to 20.7 Hz), but fired rhythmically, synchronous with theta. Based on high rates of activity and other factors including narrow action potentials (APs), the FF MR neurons (phasic and tonic) were considered to be GABAergic cells.

It is well established that in addition to 5-HT cells, the MR contains significant numbers of GABAergic neurons (Jacobs and Azmitia, 1992; Maloney *et al.*, 1999), which contact and inhibit 5-HT MR cells (Forchetti and Meek, 1981). As discussed, injections of GABA$_A$ (Kinney *et al.*, 1995) or GABA$_B$ agonists (Varga *et al.*, 2002) into the MR generate persistent theta. This suggests a GABAergic MR influence on 5-HT cells of the MR in the modulation of the hippocampal EEG.

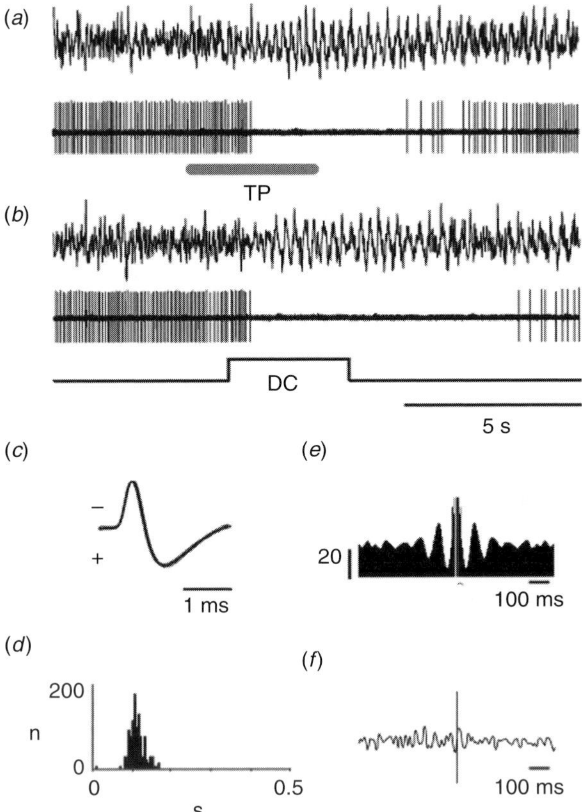

Figure 16.2 (*a,b*) The discharge characteristics of a moderately firing "theta-off" neuron of the median raphe nucleus. The cell showed an abrupt cessation of firing at the onset and for the duration of hippocampal theta elicited with either tail pinch (TP) (*a*) or with electrical stimulation of the tail (DC) (*b*). (*c*) Superimposed action potentials of the cell showing a wide spike of ~2 msec. (*d*) ISI histogram of the cell demonstrating a sharp peak at 110 ms indicating that the cell fired at very regular rates during control (non-theta) conditions. (*e*) Autocorrelogram depicting the steady rate of discharge of the cell at ~9 Hz (peaks in *e*). (*f*) Crosscorrelogram (spike triggered averaging) showing that the cell did not discharge rhythmically synchronous with theta as indicated by the flat unit-EEG crosscorrelogram.

Based on the foregoing, then, we suggested the following interactions for the various types of MR cells (Viana Di Prisco *et al.*, 2002) in the modulation of the hippocampal EEG: (1) the slow-firing cells (theta-on and theta-off) and a subset of the moderately discharging cells are serotonergic neurons, and the phasic and tonic fast-firing cells are mainly GABAergic neurons; (2) the 5-HT theta-off (or desynchronization-on) cells are projection neurons, and the 5-HT theta-on and GABAergic cells are primarily interneurons; and (3) these populations of cells mutually interact in the modulation of the hippocampal EEG. In effect, the activation of local 5-HT theta-on cells as well as the GABAergic theta-on cells would inhibit 5-HT theta-off projection cells to release or generate theta, whereas suppression of 5-HT theta-on and/or GABAergic theta-on activity would disinhibit 5-HT theta-off (desynchronization-on) cells resulting in a blockade of theta or a desynchronization of the hippocampal EEG.

Site(s) of action of MR desynchronizing effects on the hippocampal EEG

As discussed above, it is now well established that the theta rhythm is generated by a network of structures extending from the brain stem to the hippocampus, including the RPO, SUM, MS/DBv, and the hippocampus. The MR projects to each of these sites (Morin and Meyer-Bernstein, 1999; Vertes and Martin, 1988; Vertes *et al.*, 1999) and as such could influence some or all of them in the desynchronization of the hippocampal EEG – or blockade of theta of waking and REM sleep. Since MS/DBv pacemaking cells directly drive theta, the medial septum would appear to be the primary MR target for effects on the hippocampal EEG. In this regard, MR stimulation disrupts the rhythmical discharge of septal pacemaking cells and eliminates theta (Assaf and Miller, 1978; Kitchigina *et al.*, 1999), while the suppression of MR with either lidocaine (Kitchigina *et al.*, 1999) or 8-OH-DPAT (Kinney *et al.*, 1996) increases the frequency and regularity of discharge of septal bursting neurons and produces continuous theta. As discussed, Jackson *et al.* (2008) demonstrated that MR stimulation desynchronized the hippocampal EEG and suppressed the activity of a large percentage of theta-related hippocampal neurons. While the authors acknowledged that it is difficult to determine whether MR-elicited effects are routed through the septum or directly affect the hippocampus, their findings seem to favor direct actions on the hippocampus. Finally, it is very possible that MR could directly influence the adjacent RPO in the modulation of the hippocampal EEG. Vinogradova *et al.* (1999) raised this possibility, stating that a suppression of MR activity could result in the "elimination of MR inhibitory influences on the reticular formation" and thereby "stimulate the generation of theta rhythm and increase of its frequency in the septo-hippocampal system."

This latter possibility wherein a suppression of 5-HT MR neurons disinhibits RPO cells to produce theta is very comparable to the situation shown for other events of REM sleep, notably PGO waves. Specifically, the dorsal raphe (DR) nucleus projects to the two acetylcholine-containing nuclei of the brain stem, the laterodorsal (LDT) and pedunculopontine tegmental (PPT) nuclei, that have been implicated in the control PGO waves of REM sleep. Similar to the putative actions of the MR on the RPO in the elicitation of theta, DR reportedly serves a permissive role in PGO spike generation. For instance, it has been shown that: (1) the discharge of DR neurons is inversely correlated with the occurrence of PGO spikes; (2) serotonergic agonists suppress PGO spikes, while 5-HT antagonists enhance them; and (3) electrical DR stimulation inhibits PGO spikes (for review see Vertes and Linley, 2007). Median raphe 5-HT cells, like those of the DR (and other monoaminergic groups) fire at highest rates in waking, slow in non-REM sleep, and are virtually silent in REM sleep (Jacobs and Azmitia, 1992). In effect, then, a suppression of 5-HT MR activity in REM could disinhibit RPO cells in the generation of theta of REM sleep.

Distinct brain-stem "modules" for the control of individual events of REM sleep

While the "Holy Grail" of REM research seems to be the search for *the* REM sleep control "center" of the brain stem, in an early review (Vertes, 1984) we essentially avoided the "big issue" and instead focused on putative brain-stem structures that control the individual indices of REM sleep. This was not to deny, however, the existence of a central command region (probably in the brain stem), which coordinated the activity of the various subregions to produce the unified state of REM sleep.

In effect, then, using information available at the time, which in some instances was incomplete, we described distinct nuclei of the brain stem responsible for the control of the separate events of REM sleep. We further noted that each of the events of REM involve analogous or identical types of activity during wakefulness; that is, none of the signs of REM are specific to that state. For example, as described here, RPO is a source for the generation of theta of waking and REM sleep.

Although some of the following has been updated, particularly in this volume, we initially reviewed evidence showing that major indices of REM are controlled by the following cell groups of the brain stem: cortical EEG desynchronization – the mesencephalic reticular formation; hippocampal theta rhythm – nucleus pontis oralis; muscle atonia – the locus coeruleus, pars alpha area (LCα); PGO spikes – primarily the X area; rapid eye movements – the peri-abducens region; muscle twitches – caudal parts of nucleus pontis caudalis and nucleus gigantocellularis; and cardiorespiratory fluctuations – the parabrachial complex (Vertes, 1984).

With respect to the (older) nomenclature for some of these structures, the LC, pars alpha area, responsible for atonia, is located ventral and slightly medial to the LC, proper; the X area of Sakai and Jouvet (Sakai and Jouvet, 1980), generating PGO spikes, is located on the dorsolateral border of the brachium conjunctivum and extends rostrally from the lateral parabrachial nucleus to the ventrolateral edge of the nucleus cuneiformis and is the region now identified as the PPT; and the peri-abducens region, controlling rapid eye movements, is located in the dorsomedial pons, just rostral to the abducens nucleus (Vertes, 1984).

Finally, although the aminergic–cholinergic hypothesis for REM sleep genesis is constantly under siege (Luppi *et al.*, 2007), it is worth noting that the major events of REM sleep including cortical EEG desynchronization, theta rhythm, atonia, PGO waves, and rapid eye movements can be elicited either independently or as a constellation with acetylcholine (ACh) agonists (Datta and MacLean, 2007; Vertes, 1990). This would indicate a cholinergic drive for REM, likely originating from the brain-stem ACh cells of the LDT and PPT (see also below).

Recent analysis of brain-stem substrates controlling the indices and state of REM sleep: the cellular-molecular-network model of Datta and MacLean for REM sleep regulation

In a recent overview of substrates for the regulation of the events and state of REM, Datta and MacLean (2007) updated and significantly refined the "distributed network theory" of REM (Vertes, 1984) wherein each of the indices of REM are controlled by separate "REM sleep sign generators" – and they, in turn, are driven by ACh systems of the LDT/PPT.

Datta and MacLean (2007) marshaled solid support for the position that the brain stem contains a discrete set of nuclei that generate the individual signs of REM sleep (see their Figure 5, p. 794.) In particular, they reviewed a wealth of evidence showing that the various signs of REM are controlled by the following structures of the brain stem: (1) cortical EEG activation – jointly, by the mesencephalic reticular formation (MRF) and the rostral part of the magnocellular reticular nucleus of the medulla; (2) hippocampal theta rhythm – by RPO; muscle atonia – by the LCα; PGO/P waves – by the dorsal part of the subcoeruleus nucleus in rats and by the caudolateral peribrachial area in cats; rapid eye movements – by the peri-abducens RF; and autonomic functions – by the parabrachial nucleus.

Important updates to earlier descriptions include their demonstration that cortical EEG activation involves both the MRF and the medullary magnocellular reticular nucleus and that PGO waves (or P-waves in the rat) are generated by nucleus subcoeruleus (in rats) and by the peribrachial area (in cats). Regarding the latter, Datta and MacLean (2007) indicated that previous claims that the PPT (or the X area of Sakai and Jouvet) was the source for the generation of PGO waves was largely based on the identification of "PGO burst neurons" in the PPT, but that these cells are not true PGO "generators" but rather serve to transfer PGO signals (generated in the pons) to the forebrain.

In a strong reaffirmation of the aminergic–cholinergic hypothesis for REM sleep genesis, Datta and MacLean (2007) showed that each of the REM sleep sign generators receives both aminergic (from the LC and/or raphe nuclei) and cholinergic (from the LDT and PPT) inputs, which exert dual actions on the individual events of REM. In effect, REM signs (and hence REM) are triggered by a combined reduction of aminergic tone and an increase in cholinergic tone. They state: "The net result of aminergic tone withdrawal and increased cholinergic tone is the activation of each individual REM sleep sign-generator to express specific REM sleep signs" – and by extension the REM sleep state. The model applies to the theta rhythm of REM, for as discussed, theta involves an inhibition of 5-HT neurons of the MR and an ACh-mediated activation of cells of the RPO.

Function of the hippocampal theta rhythm of wakefulness

Although the theta rhythm has been implicated in a host of functions, the prevailing view is that theta is directly involved in mnemonic processes of the hippocampus (Buzsaki, 2002; Vertes, 2005; Vertes *et al.*, 2004; Vertes and Kocsis, 1997). This is supported by the following lines of evidence: (1) reversible or irreversible lesions of the MS/DBv that abolish theta produce severe learning/memory deficits; (2) long-term potentiation (LTP) is optimally elicited in the hippocampus with stimulation at theta frequency (i.e., theta burst or primed burst stimulation) and this mode of stimulation (theta) is now commonly used to induce LTP at sites throughout the forebrain; (3) stimulation delivered in the presence of theta, and on its positive phase, significantly potentiates population responses in the hippocampus; (4) the loss of LTP with primed burst stimulation in mutant mice is accompanied by a pronounced disruption of place cell activity and spatial memory; and (5) several reports in humans have described task-dependent theta activity in the cortex with a range of behavioral tasks (for reviews see Vertes *et al.*, 2004; Vertes, 2005). Regarding the latter, Anderson *et al.* (2009) recently described a marked coherence of theta oscillations between the prefrontal cortex and medial temporal lobe with the successful recall of words in a free recall task.

Although the precise nature of the involvement of theta in memory processing remains to be fully determined (Buzsaki, 2002), we recently proposed that theta serves as a "tag" for the short-term encoding of information in the hippocampus (Vertes, 2005). In brief, we proposed that the hippocampus receives two main types of input, theta from ascending brainstem-diencephalo-septal systems, and "information bearing" mainly from thalamocortical and cortical systems. The temporal convergence of activity of these two systems results in the encoding of information in the hippocampus, primarily reaching it via cortical routes. By analogy to processes associated with LTP, we suggest that theta represents a strong depolarizing influence on NMDA receptor-containing cells of the hippocampus. The temporal coupling of a theta-induced depolarization and the release of glutamate to these cells from intra- and extra-hippocampal sources activates them. This, in turn, initiates processes leading to a (short-term) strengthening of connections between presynaptic ("information bearing") and postsynaptic neurons of the hippocampus.

As described, theta is present in rats during active exploratory movements of waking. During exploration, a rat continually gathers and updates information about its environment. If this information is temporally coupled to theta (as is the case with locomotion), it becomes temporarily stored in the hippocampus by mechanisms similar to the early phase of LTP (E-LTP). If the exploratory behavior of the rat goes unreinforced, these relatively short-lasting traces (1–3 hours) gradually weaken and eventually fade – to be re-updated. On the other hand, if the explorations of the rat lead to rewards (or punishments), additional modulatory inputs to the hippocampus become activated (amygdala, monoaminergic systems) and convert the short-term, theta-dependent memory, into long-term stores. In sum, events associated with exploratory behaviors of rats would be temporarily held in the hippocampus and, depending on the consequences of those behaviors, would either be erased or stored in long-term memory.

Function of the hippocampal theta rhythm in REM sleep

As discussed, theta serves a well recognized role in the mnemonic functions of waking and it might be expected that theta would serve this same function in REM sleep: encoding/consolidation of memories. This notion gains additional support from the (seemingly) widely held view that memories are processed/consolidated in sleep/REM sleep. Although it might seem reasonable to attribute the same function to theta during waking and REM (memory processing), we would contend that theta serves very different functions in waking and REM. Or specifically, theta is not involved in the encoding (or consolidation) of information during REM, mainly because information is not processed in REM sleep (Siegel, 2001; Vertes, 2004; Vertes and Eastman, 2000; Vertes and Siegel, 2005).

Although the sleep-memory consolidation hypothesis continues to be a dominant theory in the field (Diekelmann *et al.*, 2009; Walker and Stickgold, 2004), several recent studies have failed to demonstrate a relationship between sleep and memory consolidation (Rasch *et al.*, 2009; Rickard *et al.*, 2008; Song *et al.*, 2007). Perhaps one of the strongest arguments refuting a role for REM sleep in memory processing, is the demonstration that the pronounced suppression (or virtual elimination) of REM sleep resulting from either brainstem damage or the use of antidepressants, is largely without effect on cognitive functions (see Siegel, 2001; Vertes, 2004 ; Vertes and Eastman, 2000). In this regard, Born and colleagues (Rasch *et al.*, 2009), proponents of the sleep-memory consolidation hypothesis, recently showed that the marked suppression of REM sleep in healthy adults with serotonin or norepinephrine reuptake inhibitors failed to disrupt performance on procedural (mirror tracing and finger tapping) or declarative (word paired associate) memory tasks. In fact, somewhat surprisingly, they described gains in performance on the finger-tapping tasks following pronounced REM suppression. These findings are consistent with early descriptions from clinical populations on antidepressants showing little or no disruption of skill or cognitive functions with long-term REM suppression.

If, as argued, theta does not serve to encode information in REM, what is its function in REM sleep? We suggest that theta is a reflection (or by-product) of the large-scale, brain stem-elicited activation of REM sleep and that the widespread hippocampal (and cortical) EEG activation of REM does not serve the same higher order processes associated with these patterns of EEG activity of waking (e.g., sensory, motor, cognition, or consciousness). We nonetheless suggest that the intense forebrain activation of REM is a defining feature of the state and alternatively serves to promote recovery from sleep and prepare the brain for wakefulness. In an early theoretical article (Vertes, 1986) and subsequent minor modifications (Vertes and Eastman, 2000; Vertes, 2004), we proposed that the primary function of REM sleep is to provide periodic endogenous stimulation to the brain/forebrain, which serves to maintain minimum requisite levels of CNS activity throughout sleep. REM is the mechanism used by the brain to ensure and promote recovery from sleep. We suggest that the brain is strongly depressed in non-REM sleep, particularly in delta sleep, and is incapable of tolerating long continuous periods of relative suppression. REM serves the critical function of periodically activating the brain during sleep without awakening the subject or disturbing the continuity of sleep. The progressively increasing length of the REM periods throughout sleep serve to prime the brain for a return to consciousness as waking approaches. Consistent with this scheme, the periodic excitation of large populations of hippocampal neurons during theta of REM (Vertes and Kocsis, 1997; Vertes, 2005) would offset their relative quiescence in non-REM, maintaining their viability throughout sleep and promoting readiness for wakefulness.

Acknowledgments

This work was supported by National Science Foundation Grant, IOS-082639.

References

Anderson, K. L., Rajagovindan, R., Ghacibeh, G. A., Meador, K. J. & Ding, M. (2009) Theta oscillations mediate interaction between prefrontal cortex and medial temporal lobe in human memory. *Cereb Cortex*, Epub 2009 Oct 27.

Assaf, S. Y. & Miller, J. J. (1978) Role of a raphe serotonin system in control of septal unit-activity and hippocampal desynchronization. *Neuroscience* **3**: 539–50.

Bland, B. H. (1986) The physiology and pharmacology of hippocampal formation theta rhythms. *Prog Neurobiol* **26**: 1–54.

Bland, B. H., Oddie, S. D., Colom, L. V. & Vertes, R. P. (1994) The extrinsic modulation of medial septal cell discharges by the ascending brainstem hippocampal synchronizing pathway. *Hippocampus* **4**: 649–60.

Bland, B. H., Konopacki, J., Kirk, I. J., Oddie, S. D. & Dickson, C. T. (1995) Discharge patterns of hippocampal theta-related cells in the caudal diencephalon of the urethane-anesthetized rat. *J Neurophysiol* **74**: 322–33.

Buzsaki, G. (2002) Theta oscillations in the hippocampus. *Neuron* **33**: 325–40.

Datta, S. & Maclean, R. R. (2007) Neurobiological mechanisms for the regulation of mammalian sleep-wake behavior: reinterpretation of historical evidence and inclusion of contemporary cellular and molecular evidence. *Neurosci Biobehav Rev* **31**: 775–824.

Diekelmann, S., Wilhelm, I. & Born, J. (2009) The whats and whens of sleep-dependent memory consolidation. *Sleep Med Rev* **13**: 309–21.

Forchetti, C. M. & Meek, J. L. (1981) Evidence for a tonic GABAergic control of serotonin neurons in the median raphe nucleus. *Brain Res* **206**: 208–12.

Green, J. D. & Arduini, A. A. (1954) Hippocampal electrical activity in arousal. *J Neurophysiol* **17**: 533–57.

Hobson, J. A., McCarley, R. W., Pivik, R. T. & Freedman, R. (1974) Selective firing by cat pontine brain stem neurons in desynchronized sleep. *J Neurophysiol* **37**: 497–511.

Hobson, J. A., McCarley, R. W., Wyzinski, P. W. (1975) Sleep cycle oscillation: reciprocal discharge by two brainstem neuronal groups. *Science* **189**: 55–8.

Jackson, J., Dickson, C.T. & Bland, B. H. (2008) Median raphe stimulation disrupts hippocampal theta via rapid inhibition and state-dependent phase reset of theta-related neural circuitry. *J Neurophysiol* **99**: 3009–26.

Jacobs, B. L. & Azmitia, E. C. (1992) Structure and function of the brain serotonin system. *Physiol Rev* **72**: 165–229.

Jarosiewicz, B. & Skaggs, W. E. (2004) Level of arousal during the small irregular activity state in the rat hippocampal EEG. *J Neurophysiol* **91**: 2649–57.

Kinney, G. G., Kocsis, B. & Vertes, R. P. (1994) Injections of excitatory amino acid antagonists into the median raphe nucleus produce hippocampal theta rhythm in the urethane anesthetized rat. *Brain Res* **654**: 96–104.

Kinney, G. G., Kocsis, B. & Vertes, R. P. (1995) Injections of muscimol into the median raphe nucleus produce hippocampal theta rhythm in the urethane anesthetized rat. *Psychopharmacology* **120**: 244–48.

Kinney, G. G., Kocsis, B. & Vertes, R. P. (1996) Medial septal unit firing characteristics following injections of 8-OH-DPAT into the median raphe nucleus. *Brain Res* **708**: 116–22.

Kirk, I. J. & McNaughton, N. (1991) Supramammillary cell firing and hippocampal rhythmical slow activity. *Neuroreport* **2**: 723–5.

Kitchigina, V. F., Kudina, T. A., Kutyreva, E. V. & Vinogradova, O. S. (1999) Neuronal activity of the septal pacemaker of theta rhythm under the influence of stimulation and blockade of the median raphe nucleus in the awake rabbit. *Neuroscience* **94**: 453–63.

Kocsis, B., Varga, V., Dahan, L. & Sik, A. (2006) Serotonergic neuron diversity: identification of raphe neurons with discharges time-locked to the hippocampal theta rhythm. *Proc Natl Acad Sci USA* **103**: 1059–64.

Kocsis, B. & Vertes, R. P. (1994) Characterization of neurons of the supramammillary nucleus and mammillary body that discharge rhythmically with the hippocampal theta rhythm in the rat. *J Neurosci* **14**: 7040–52.

Kocsis, B. & Vertes, R. P. (1996) Midbrain raphe cell firing and hippocampal theta rhythm in urethane anaesthetized rats. *Neuroreport* **7**: 2867–72.

Kudina, T. A., Sudnitsyn, V. V., Kutyreva, E. V. & Kichigina, V. F. (2004) The serotonin reuptake inhibitor fluoxetine suppresses theta oscillations in the electroencephalogram of the rabbit hippocampus. *Neurosci Behav Physiol* **34**: 929–33.

Luppi, P. H., Gervasoni, D., Verret, L. *et al.* (2007) Paradoxical (REM) sleep genesis: the switch from an aminergic-cholinergic to a GABAergic-glutamatergic hypothesis. *J Physiol (Paris)* **100**: 271–83.

Maloney, K. J., Mainville, L. & Jones, B. E. (1999) Differential c-Fos expression in cholinergic, monoaminergic, and GABAergic cell groups of the pontomesencephalic tegmentum after paradoxical sleep deprivation and recovery. *J Neurosci* **19**: 3057–72.

Maru, E., Takahashi, L. K. & Iwahara, S. (1979) Effects of median raphe nucleus lesions on hippocampal EEG in the freely moving rat. *Brain Res* **163**: 223–34.

McCarley, R. W. & Hobson, J. A. (1971) Single neuron activity in cat gigantocellular tegmental field: selectivity of discharge in desynchronized sleep. *Science* **174**: 1250–2.

Morin, L.P. & Meyer-Bernstein, E. L. (1999) The ascending serotonergic system in the hamster: comparison with projections of the dorsal and median raphe nuclei. *Neuroscience* **91**: 81–105.

Nuñez, A., de Andrés, I. & García-Austt, E. (1991) Relationships of nucleus reticularis pontis oralis neuronal discharge with sensory and carbachol evoked hippocampal theta rhythm. *Exp Brain Res* **87**: 303–8.

Pan, W. X. & McNaughton, N. (2004) The supra-mammillary area: its organization, functions and relationship to the hippocampus. *Prog Neurobiol* **74**: 127–66.

Petsche, H., Gogolak, G. & Vanzwiet, P. A. (1965) Rhythmicity of septal cell discharges at various levels of reticular excitation. *Electroenceph Clin Neurophysiol* **19**: 25–33.

Rasch, B., Pommer, J., Diekelmann, S. & Born, J. (2009) Pharmacological REM sleep suppression paradoxically improves rather than impairs skill memory. *Nat Neurosci* **12**: 396–7.

Rickard, T. C., Cai, D. J., Rieth, C. A., Jones, J. & Ard, M. C. (2008) Sleep does not enhance motor sequence learning. *J Exp Psychol Learn Mem Cogn* **34**: 834–42.

Sakai, K. & Jouvet, M. (1980) Brain stem PGO-on cells projecting directly to the cat dorsal lateral geniculate nucleus. *Brain Res* **194**: 500–5.

Siegel, J. M. (2001) The REM sleep-memory consolidation hypothesis. *Science* **294**: 1058–63.

Siegel, J. M., McGinty, D. J. & Breedlove, S. M. (1977) Sleep and waking activity of pontine gigantocellular field neurons. *Exp Neurol* **56**: 553–73.

Song, S., Howard, J. H. & Howard, D. V. (2007) Sleep does not benefit probabilistic motor sequence learning. *J Neurosci* **27**: 12475–83.

Takano, Y. & Hanada, Y. (2009) The driving system for hippocampal theta in the brainstem: an examination by single neuron recording in urethane-anesthetized rats. *Neurosci Lett* **455**: 65–9.

Urbain, N., Creamer, K. & Debonnel, G. (2006) Electrophysiological diversity of the dorsal raphe cells across the sleep–wake cycle of the rat. *J Physiol* **573**: 679–95.

Vanderwolf, C. H. (1971) Limbic-diencephalic mechanisms of voluntary movement. *Psychol Rev* **78**: 83–113.

Varga, V., Sik, A., Freund, T. F. & Kocsis, B. (2002) GABA(B) receptors in the median raphe nucleus: distribution and role in the serotonergic control of hippocampal activity. *Neuroscience* **109**: 119–32.

Vertes, R. P. (1977) Selective firing of rat pontine gigantocellular neurons during movement and REM sleep. *Brain Res* **128**: 146–52.

Vertes, R. P. (1979) Brain stem gigantocellular neurons: patterns of activity during behavior and sleep in the freely moving rat. *J Neurophysiol* **42**: 214–28.

Vertes, R. P. (1981) An analysis of ascending brain stem systems involved in hippocampal synchronization and desynchronization. *J Neurophysiol* **46**: 1140–59.

Vertes, R. P. (1982) Brain stem generation of the hippocampal EEG. *Prog Neurobiol* **19**: 159–86.

Vertes, R. P. (1984) Brainstem control of the events of REM sleep. *Prog Neurobiol* **22**: 241–88.

Vertes, R. P. (1986) A life-sustaining function for REM sleep: a theory. *Neurosci Biobehav Rev* **10**: 371–6.

Vertes, R. P. (1988) Brainstem afferents to the basal forebrain in the rat. *Neuroscience* **24**: 907–35.

Vertes, R. P. (1990) Brainstem mechanisms of slow wave sleep and REM sleep. In *Brainstem Mechanisms of Behavior*, eds. R. P. Vertes & W. R. Klemm. New York: John Wiley & Sons, pp. 535–83.

Vertes, R. P. (1992) PHA-L analysis of projections from the supramammillary nucleus in the rat. *J Comp Neur* **326**: 595–622.

Vertes, R. P. (2004) Memory consolidation in sleep: dream or reality. *Neuron* **44**: 135–48.

Vertes, R. P. (2005) Hippocampal theta rhythym: a tag for short-term memory. *Hippocampus* **15**: 923–35.

Vertes, R. P. & Martin, G. F. (1988) Autoradiographic analysis of ascending projections from the pontine and mesencephalic reticular formation and the median raphe nucleus in the rat. *J Comp Neurol* **275**: 511–41.

Vertes, R. P. & Kocsis, B. (1997) Brainstem-diencephalo-septohippocampal systems controlling the theta rhythm of the hippocampus. *Neuroscience* **81**: 893–926.

Vertes, R. P. & Eastman, K. E. (2000) The case against memory consolidation in REM sleep. *Behav Brain Sci* **23**: 867–76.

Vertes, R. P. & Siegel, J. M. (2005) Time for the sleep community to take a critical look at the purported role of sleep in memory processing. *Sleep* **28**:1228–9.

Vertes, R. P. & Linley, S. B. (2007) Comparisons of projections of the dorsal and median raphe nuclei, with some functional considerations. In *Interdisciplinary Conference on Tryptophan and Related Substances: Chemistry, Biology, and Medicine*, ed. K. Takai. International Congress Series, 1304, pp. 98–120.

Vertes, R. P., Colom, L. V., Fortin, W. J. & Bland, B. H. (1993) Brainstem sites for the carbachol elicitation of the hippocampal theta rhythm in the rat. *Exp Brain Res* **96**: 419–29.

Vertes, R. P., Kinney, G. G., Kocsis, B. & Fortin, W. J. (1994) Pharmacological suppression of the median raphe nucleus with serotonin1A agonists, 8-OH-DPAT and buspirone, produces hippocampal theta-rhythm in the rat. *Neuroscience* **60**: 441–51.

Vertes, R. P., Fortin, W. J. & Crane, A. M. (1999) Projections of the median raphe nucleus in the rat. *J Comp Neurol* **407**: 555–82.

Vertes, R. P., Hoover, W.B. & Viana Di Prisco, G. (2004) Theta rhythm of the hippocampus: subcortical control and functional significance. *Behav Cogn Neurosci Rev* **3**: 173–200.

Viana Di Prisco, G., Albo, Z., Vertes, R. P. & Kocsis, B. (2002) Discharge properties of neurons of the median raphe nucleus during hippocampal theta rhythm in the rat. *Exp Brain Res* **145**: 383–94.

Vinogradova, O. S., Kitchigina, V. F., Kudina, T. A. & Zenchenko, K. I. (1999) Spontaneous activity and sensory responses of hippocampal neurons during persistent theta-rhythm evoked by median raphe nucleus blockade in rabbit. *Neuroscience* **94**: 745–53.

Walker, M. P. & Stickgold, R. (2004) Sleep-dependent learning and memory consolidation. *Neuron* **44**: 121–33.

Yamamoto, T., Watanabe, S., Oishi, R. & Ueki, S. (1979) Effects of midbrain raphe stimulation and lesion on EEG activity in rats. *Brain Res Bull* **4**: 491–5.

Chapter

17

Respiration during REM sleep and its regulation

Jimmy J. Fraigne and John M. Orem

Summary

There have been many studies of the atonia of REM sleep and of its effects on the respiratory system. In contrast, excitatory processes that affect the respiratory system in REM sleep are poorly understood. Nevertheless, these processes may be the main determinants of respiratory behavior in REM sleep (e.g., the higher rate of breathing). In this chapter, findings relevant to excitation of the respiratory system in REM sleep are presented and discussed.

(1) Most medullary respiratory neurons are more active in REM sleep than in NREM sleep, and both diaphragmatic and hypoglossal motor neurons reportedly have greater overall activity in REM sleep than in NREM sleep.

(2) The source of the excitation of respiratory neurons and motor neurons in REM sleep is internal because excitation is seen even when mechanical and chemical respiratory stimuli are removed or held constant and respiratory drive is eliminated.

(3) Studies under conditions of mechanically induced apnea show that the excitation develops with a delay after the onset of REM sleep, that it is episodic, and that it peaks in the latter half of the REM period. It simultaneously affects inspiratory and expiratory neurons and may either stimulate breathing or disorganize it.

(4) The activity of the genioglossal muscles is greater than that of the nuchal muscles in REM sleep, and there is no evidence suggesting that the two muscle groups are excited in the same way in that state. Therefore motor control of respiratory and non-respiratory muscle groups in REM sleep is apparently different.

(5) The neural structures necessary for the excitation of the respiratory system in REM sleep are unknown. Some but not all of the excitation may be correlated with dreams, which implies a cortical role. Within the medulla, REM-specific neurons in the ventrolateral reticular formation have activity profiles similar to the excitation seen in respiratory neurons and muscles in REM sleep – suggesting that these cells might cause the excitation.

Introduction

Breathing parameters are highly variable in REM sleep. The respiratory pattern varies from hyperpnea with rates greater than 200 min^{-1} (in the cat) to apneas lasting for many seconds. The average rate of breathing is greater than that in NREM sleep, and it may be greater than the rate in wakefulness. And notably end-tidal CO_2 levels decrease in REM sleep in the cat – signifying hyperventilation in that state.

Ventilatory responses to chemical stimuli (hypoxia and hypercapnia) are more variable and often weaker in REM sleep than in NREM sleep or wakefulness (Douglas, 2005), and patients with obstructive sleep apnea fare worse in REM sleep than in NREM sleep, just as patients with chronic obstructive pulmonary disease (COPD) are more hypoxemic in REM than in NREM sleep. Yet, it is in REM sleep when the first respiratory movements are made in utero (Dawes *et al.*, 1972), and it is in REM sleep when patients with congenital hypoventilation syndrome breathe and do not require mechanical ventilation (Fleming *et al.*, 1980). These and other apparent contradictions, e.g., the low arousal threshold of normal subjects to airway occlusion in REM sleep and yet the prolonged obstructive apneas in that state, belie the complexity of the control of breathing in REM sleep.

REM Sleep: Regulation and Function, eds. Birendra N. Mallick, S. R. Pandi-Perumal, Robert W. McCarley, and Adrian R. Morrison. Published by Cambridge University Press. © Cambridge University Press 2011.

The respiratory system is controlled in REM sleep by excitatory and inhibitory processes. The inhibitory processes are relevant to the pathophysiology of obstructive sleep apnea and have been the subject of many studies, particularly neuropharmacological studies of the hypoglossal motor pool that controls the genioglossus muscle (Horner, 2008). However, it is still unclear if the loss of activity of this tongue muscle is due to disfacilitation (decrease in the aminergic excitatory drive) and/or direct inhibition (GABAergic or glycinergic or cholinergic) of the hypoglossal motor neurons. Excitatory processes that affect the respiratory system have been the subject of fewer studies and are poorly understood. Nevertheless, we believe these processes are the main determinants of respiratory behavior in REM sleep, and accordingly they are the primary subjects of this chapter.

Excitatory drive to the respiratory system in REM sleep

Central respiratory neurons

Most medullary respiratory neurons are more active in REM sleep than in NREM sleep (Figure 17.1). The source of the excitation of respiratory neurons in REM sleep is evidently internal because the excitation can still be seen when mechanical and chemical respiratory stimuli are removed or held constant and when respiratory drive is eliminated by mechanical ventilation. In the latter state there are only non-respiratory inputs affecting respiratory neurons, and these inputs in REM sleep excite the neurons to discharge in the absence of breathing at mean rates that are 65% of the discharge rates in REM sleep during breathing (Figure 17.2). Characteristically, the excitation develops with a delay of several seconds after the onset of the REM period. It can induce at times rhythmic breathing out of the background apnea produced by mechanical ventilation – indicating that this drive can stimulate rhythmogenesis with synchronous neuronal and diaphragmatic activity (Figure 17.3*b*1), whereas at other times it excites only the neuron or the diaphragmatic motor neurons (Figure 17.3*b*2, *b*3). Simultaneous recordings of respiratory neurons that discharge during different phases of the respiratory cycle, for example, an inspiratory and expiratory neuron, show that the endogenous drive at times excites them simultaneously and thereby disturbs their normal reciprocal relation (Figure 17.4). From these data it follows that

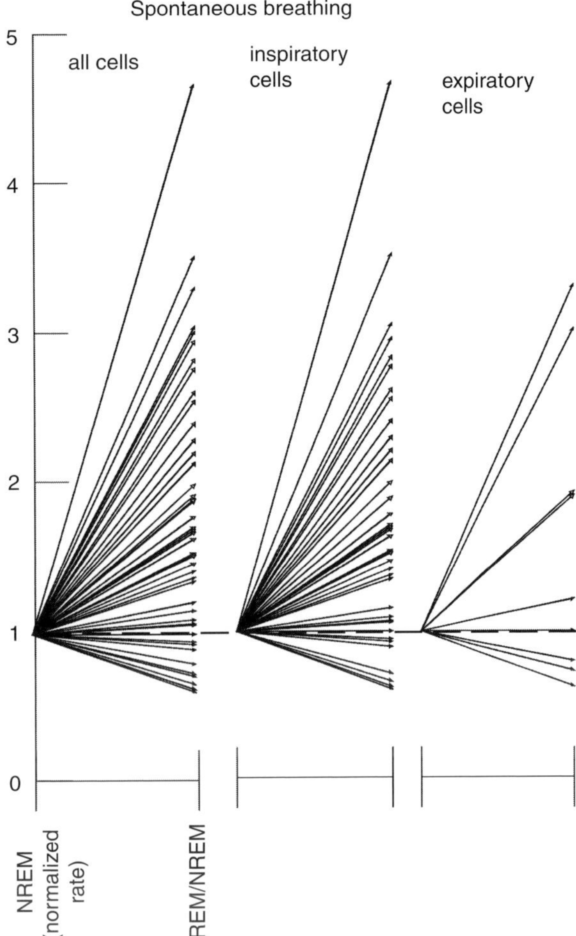

Figure 17.1 Change in activity of respiratory cells from NREM to REM sleep during eupnea. NREM activity is normalized to a value of "1" and REM activity is expressed as the ratio of REM to NREM mean discharge rates. (Reprinted with permission from Orem *et al.*, 2005. Excitation of medullary respiratory neurons in REM sleep. *Sleep,* **28**: 801–7.)

the endogenous drive can either stimulate breathing or disorganize it. These ideas are expressed in Figure 17.5, which shows the possible subsets of excitation of respiratory neurons and motor neurons and the form of the excitation that develops with a delay and then waxes and wanes.

Respiratory motor neurons

The evidence is mixed that the greater central respiratory neuronal activity seen in REM sleep is associated with greater respiratory efforts. Recordings of diaphragmatic activity in the cat in REM sleep show that

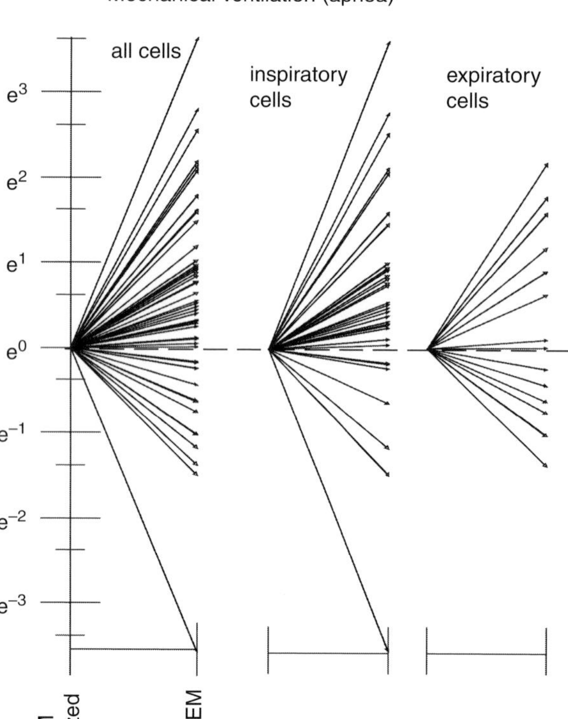

Figure 17.2 Change in activity of respiratory cells from NREM to REM sleep during apnea induced by mechanical hyperventilation. NREM activity is normalized to a value of "1" and REM activity is expressed as the natural log of the ratio of REM to NREM mean discharge rates. The natural log is to the base e where e = 2.718281828… (Reprinted with permission from Orem *et al.*, 2005. Excitation of medullary respiratory neurons in REM sleep. *Sleep*, **28**: 801–7.)

the rate of rise of diaphragmatic activity in REM sleep is greater than in NREM sleep. This is associated with a change in the recruitment pattern of diaphragmatic motor units such that large motor units that discharge late in inspiration during NREM sleep and relaxed wakefulness are active from the onset of inspiration in REM sleep (Orem and Anderson, 1996). Mean diaphragmatic activity is also greater, but peak activity is not greater in REM sleep than in NREM sleep, and indeed some authors have argued that the diaphragm, like many other muscles, is affected by the motor inhibition of the state (Hendricks *et al.*, 1990). Post-inspiratory diaphragmatic activity is notably absent in REM sleep (Lovering *et al.*, 2003). This and the abrupt rate of rise of diaphragmatic activity are associated

with a square-wave-like inspiratory airflow profile that contrasts with the step-ramp profile of inspiratory airflow in NREM sleep.

Many accessory respiratory muscles are atonic in REM sleep, and this atonia may account for REM-related hypoventilation in some cases of lung disease. For example, if the action of the diaphragm is compromised, as can occur because of the high lung volumes in obstructive lung disease, ventilation may be nevertheless adequate in wakefulness and NREM sleep, but not in REM sleep (Johnson and Remmers, 1984), because of reliance on accessory respiratory muscles (sternocleidomastoid, intercostal, and scalene muscles). However, there is evidence that respiratory muscles that are normally inactive in REM sleep can become active in that state to compensate for diaphragmatic paralysis caused by lesions of the phrenic nerves (Bennett *et al.*, 2004; Sherrey and Megirian, 1990). It seems therefore that atonia of accessory respiratory muscles is not inevitable in REM sleep.

Reports on the level of activity of upper airway muscles in REM sleep are also mixed. A recent study comparing normal subjects and patients with obstructive sleep apnea found that both tonic and phasic genioglossal activity declined from NREM sleep to REM sleep and was minimal during phasic REM sleep (Eckert *et al.*, 2009). Yet there are reports to the contrary. For example, Wiegand and colleagues (1991) studied six normal men and found no significant differences in genioglossus or alae nasi electromyograph (EMG) activity between NREM and REM sleep. Activity of these muscles during phasic REM sleep (REM sleep associated with rapid eye movements) was less than activity during NREM sleep, but activity during tonic REM sleep was equivalent to or greater than activity during NREM sleep. Another study in humans showed that phasic cricothyroid muscle activity is greater in REM sleep than in NREM sleep (Kuna *et al.*, 1994). In the intact, unanesthetized cat, Richard and Harper (1991) recorded hypoglossal neurons and found that most respiratory-related cells discharged at rates in REM sleep that were similar to those in wakefulness. In dogs, there is also evidence of excitation, not depression, of the hypoglossal nerve in REM sleep (Sahin *et al.*, 1999). This excitation in REM sleep was observed both during normal breathing and in response to a submental force that caused narrowing of the airway. The excitation appeared to cause both phasic activity associated with the respiratory cycle and irregular and intense activity that

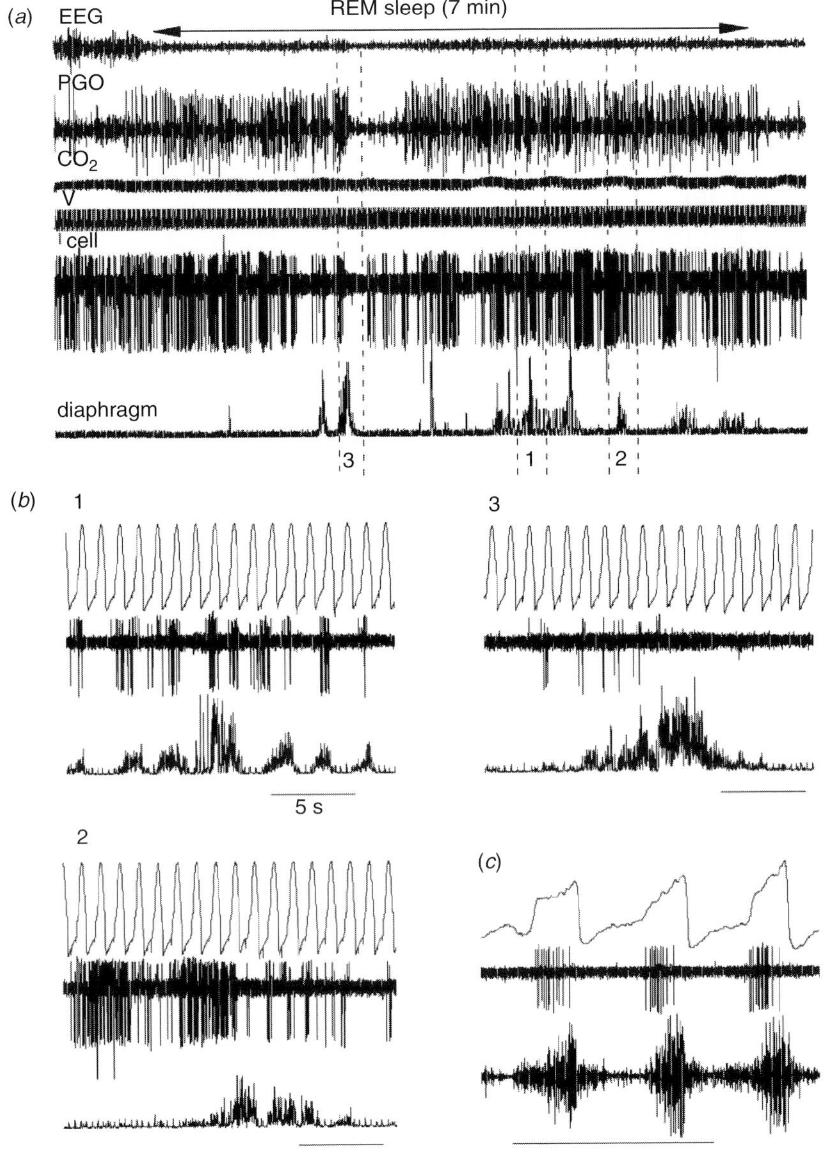

Figure 17.3 Activity of an inspiratory cell and of the diaphragm during mechanical hyperventilation in REM sleep. (*a*) EEG refers to electroencephalogram; PGO, ponto-geniculo-occipital waves; CO_2, tidal CO_2; V, airflow; I cell, action potentials of inspiratory cell; diaphragm, halfwave integrated diaphragmatic electromyogram. (*b*, *c*) Traces are, from top down, airflow, action potentials and the half-wave integrated diaphragmatic electromyogram in (*b*) and raw diaphragmatic activity in (*c*). (*b*) Varying relations between action potentials and diaphragmatic activity shown in (*a*) (designated as 1, 2, and 3) and expanded here. (*c*)Activity of the cell during spontaneous breathing in wakefulness. Inspiratory airflow is upward. Calibration is 5 seconds in (*b*) and (*c*). (Reprinted with permission from Orem *et al.*, 2005. Excitation of medullary respiratory neurons in REM sleep. *Sleep*, **28**: 801–7.)

occurred episodically with no apparent relation to breathing. Also, there are complex tongue movements in REM sleep in humans (Chokroverty, 1980), and phasic bursts in lingual activity progressively increase throughout REM sleep in the rat (Lu *et al.*, 2005). The lingual bursts have a distinctive time course with a delayed onset and then a progressive increase to a peak before a decline preceding the end of the REM period. A similar profile has been demonstrated in the activity of the diaphragm and of respiratory neurons in REM sleep (Orem *et al.*, 2000; 2005) (Figures 17.5 and 17.6). These reports contradict the generally accepted idea that REM sleep is the state in which upper-airway muscle activity is most depressed.

Sources of excitation of the respiratory system in REM sleep

It is not known if the REM-sleep excitation of respiratory neurons and muscles is part of a widespread phenomenon that affects motor systems throughout the body or if it is unique to the respiratory system. In general, little is known about the excitation of motor systems in REM sleep. We know that myoclonic twitches

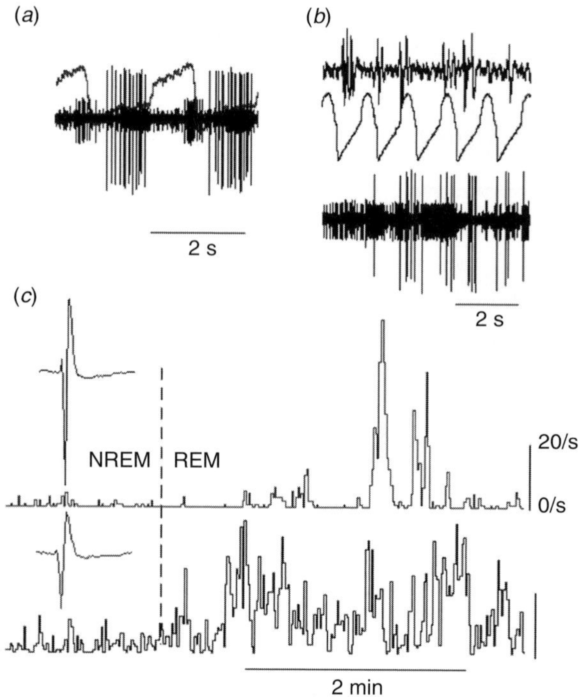

Figure 17.4 An inspiratory–expiratory phase-spanning cell (small action potentials) and a late expiratory cell (large action potentials) recorded simultaneously during normal breathing in NREM (*a*) and in REM sleep during mechanical hyperventilation (*b*, *c*). (*a*) Action potentials and airflow (inspiratory flow indicated by upward deflection of flow trace) during eupnea. (*b*) Ponto-geniculo-occipital (PGO) waves (top trace), airflow (middle trace), and action potentials of neurons shown in (*a*). The airflow trace shows artificial ventilation (50 breaths/minute, 50-mL tidal volumes); presence of PGO waves indicates the state was REM sleep. Action potentials occurred at times simultaneously and at other times independently. (*c*) Discharge rates of cells shown in (*a*) and (*b*) during late NREM sleep and REM sleep. (Reprinted with permission from Orem *et al.*, 2005. Excitation of medullary respiratory neurons in REM sleep. *Sleep*, **28**: 801–7.)

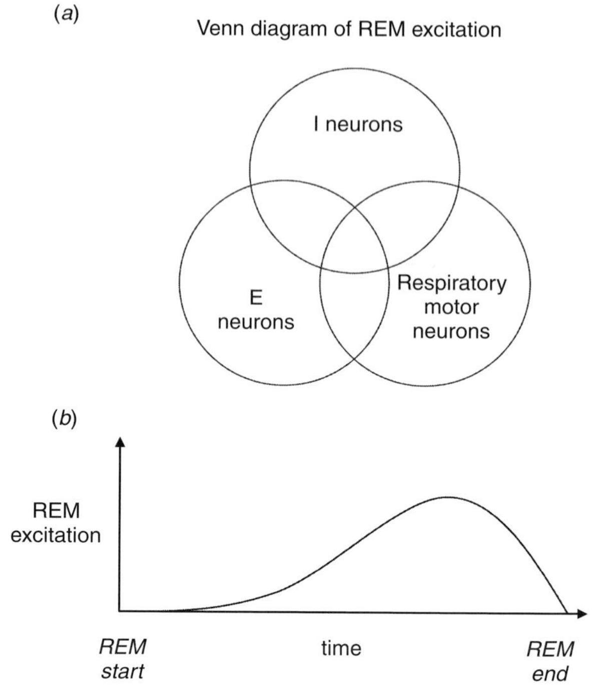

Figure 17.5 REM excitation of the respiratory system. (*a*) Venn diagram showing distribution of excitation to inspiratory and expiratory neurons and to respiratory muscles in REM sleep. The diagram illustrates subsets of excitation during which respiratory neurons and motor neurons are excited separately and collectively. For simplicity, medullary respiratory neurons are denoted as either inspiratory or expiratory, but, as shown in this chapter, respiratory neurons of all types are excited in REM sleep. (*b*) Schematic illustrating the time course of excitation of the respiratory system in REM sleep. The excitation develops after a delay and then waxes and wanes. The profile of the waxing and waning has not been quantified but is shown here as a gradual increase to a maximum and then a decay prior to the end of the REM period. (Reprinted with permission from Orem *et al.*, 2005. Excitation of medullary respiratory neurons in REM sleep. *Sleep*, **28**: 801–7.)

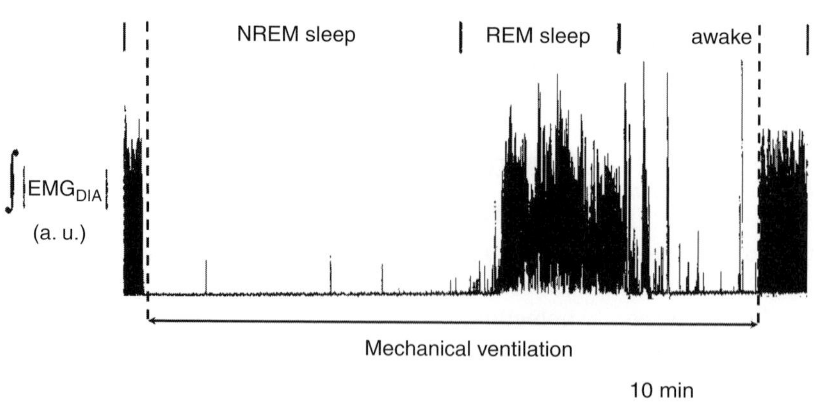

Figure 17.6 Rhythmic diaphragmatic activity during eupnea and during mechanical hyperventilation in NREM and REM sleep and wakefulness. (Reprinted with permission from Orem *et al.*, 2000. Endogenous excitatory drive to the respiratory system in rapid eye movement sleep in cats. *J. Physiol.*, **527**: 365–76.)

in non-respiratory muscles occur in REM sleep in slow twitch as well as fast twitch fibers, more frequently in distal than in proximal muscles, and more in flexors than in extensors (Pompeiano, 1967). Twitching can occur simultaneously in antagonistic muscles and in association with or independently of rapid eye movements. Paradoxically, excitation of muscles in REM sleep is most likely when inhibition is most intense (Pomeiano, 1967). Intracellular recordings of motor neurons show that inhibitory postsynaptic potentials occur simultaneously with the excitatory postsynaptic potentials that give rise to the twitches of somatic muscles (Chase and Morales, 1982). Attempts to define the motor pathways for twitching have produced inconclusive results (Pompeiano, 1967). The descending pathways may be in the dorsolateral columns because lesions there cause a reduction in twitching, but nevertheless twitching is not eliminated by either destruction of corticospinal fibers in the pyramidal tract or by fibers arising from the red nucleus, both of which course in the dorsolateral columns of the spinal cord.

It may be that excitation of muscles in REM sleep arises from a phasic generator that affects both non-respiratory and respiratory muscles. If so, there should be a temporal correlation between them. Only a few studies have compared the activity of respiratory muscles and neurons with the activity in other motor systems in REM sleep. However, there is evidence of phasic inhibition of both non-respiratory and respiratory motor neurons in REM sleep. Inhibitory postsynaptic potentials occur in lumbar motor neurons in association with ponto-geniculo-occipital (PGO) waves (Lopez-Rodriguez et al., 1990), and diaphragmatic EMG activity is depressed with a duration (~80 ms) coinciding with the temporal duration of the PGO wave (Dunin-Barkowski and Orem, 1998). This suggests that they may be affected by a common inhibitory source. There is evidence also that the respiratory system receives an excitatory drive, in addition to the phasic inhibition described above, in association with PGO waves. There is a positive, albeit weak, correlation between PGO-wave activity and emergent diaphragmatic activity in cats ventilated to apnea (Orem et al., 2000) and between PGO-wave activity and respiratory neuronal activity (Orem, 1980). Thus, like other motor pools, respiratory motor neurons may receive simultaneously excitatory and inhibitory drives in REM sleep. However, respiratory muscles may be more intensely activated

than non-respiratory muscles in REM sleep. This has been convincingly demonstrated in a comparison of the activity during REM sleep of the genioglossal and nuchal muscles (Lu et al., 2005).

Generally motor activation in REM sleep is attributed to the dreaming process. And, according to this view, were it not for active motor inhibition the dreamer would act out his dream. This idea is supported by the troublesome motor behavior of patients with REM sleep behavior disorder (Mahowald and Schenck, 2005) when they act out their dream and similarly by the oneiric behavior of experimental animals (Sastre and Jouvet, 1979) having lesions that block motor inhibition in REM sleep. It follows from this that motor excitation in REM sleep arises from voluntary or intended actions or from species-specific action patterns such as flight and attacking and not from random, behaviorally, and physiologically meaningless activations of motor neurons.

Respiratory excitation may occur also in relation to dreaming. Hobson et al., (1965) found that breathing rates were high and variable in association with dreams of physical activity and high emotional content. They found also that specific respiratory content was twice as likely when the subject was awakened following apnea as compared to following other respiratory patterns. Baust and Engel (1971) found that highly variable respiratory rates were associated with reports of the sleeper having little active participation in the dream and of little physical aggression in it. However, large-amplitude breaths were associated with the sleeper having intense active participation in the dream, and variability in amplitude was associated with dreams containing a high degree of physical aggression. These results support the idea that breathing patterns may parallel the content of the dream. However, other data are less convincing. Hauri and Van de Castle (1973) examined heart rate, the galvanic skin response, and breathing in relation to dream emotionality, physical activity in the dream, and dream intensity. Respiration rate was related to emotionality and to dream intensity, but they found that there was no significant relation between physical activity in the dream and the rate of breathing.

Consistent with evidence questioning a relation between breathing pattern and dream content, studies in animals show that respiratory neuronal and muscular activity patterns in REM sleep are generally unrecognizable and cannot be attributable to dream enactment of a behavior involving the respiratory system. Emergent respiratory neuronal and muscular activity in REM sleep in cats ventilated to apnea is generally unrecognizable (Orem *et al.*, 2000, 2005). It consists characteristically of bursts of activity, and, in the case of simultaneously recorded respiratory neurons that are normally active during different phases of the respiratory cycle, the bursts can occur at the same time (Figure 17.3). Rarely rhythmic breathing occurs as a short fragment (Figure 17.3). Recognizable behavioral respiratory acts, such as purring or meowing, are extremely rare. In these rare cases, behavioral drives arising from dreams may excite the respiratory system in REM sleep, but generally the emergent motor activity has no recognizable pattern. Also, lesioned animals that display at times oneiric behaviors in REM sleep and patients with REM sleep behavior disorder have erratic movements in REM sleep that are not components of a dream enactment (Mahowald and Schenck, 2005). Irregular jerking and twitching occur before and after development of the disorder in many patients. Full dream enactments vary from as many as four per night to only one every two weeks. It is interesting that the enactments may occur either with or without the autonomic responses that accompany the same behaviors in wakefulness.

Finally, the neural structures necessary for the excitation of the respiratory system in REM sleep are unknown. Respiratory patterns that are components of dream enactments might arise from mesencephalic or higher nervous structures, but the rapid breathing characteristic of REM sleep persists in pontile and neonatal animals, and in decorticate humans, none of whom presumably have dream content.

Physiological effects of REM-specific endogenous drive

There have been many studies of motor inhibition but few of motor excitation in REM sleep. Yet, most neurons throughout the brain, including most respiratory neurons, are more active in REM sleep than in NREM sleep. This excitation, however, does not prevent or mitigate respiratory disorders that in REM sleep result in blood oxygen levels lower than those occurring in NREM sleep, a state when the brain is much less active. REM atonia may have a role in the worsening hypoxemia. Yet the respiratory system is obviously not paralyzed in REM sleep – the diaphragm contracts, the larynx opens, and even respiratory accessory muscles that are normally atonic in REM sleep can become active to compensate for muscles that

are paralyzed. Furthermore, there is clear evidence of excitation of respiratory neurons and muscles in REM sleep. However, this excitation, evident in the activity of both pump and upper airway muscles, does not necessarily stimulate breathing. Indeed, Douglas (1998) has proposed that excitation of the respiratory generator in REM sleep, because of simultaneous and erratic stimulation of cells of the respiratory network, causes dysrhythmic breathing and worsening of the hypoxemia of patients with COPD – and, we propose, the irregularities characteristic of breathing in REM sleep in normal subjects. However, in other cases excitation may sustain breathing in the absence of chemical stimuli or functioning chemoreceptors (Fleming *et al.*, 1980). The source(s) of the excitation are not known. The excitation may in some cases arise from dreams and have a pattern corresponding to known respiratory behaviors. In other cases it has an unrecognizable pattern.

The cause of the excitation is internal and not the result of afferent information from respiratory chemoreceptors or proprioceptors. In fact, excitation of premotor and motor respiratory neurons may cause, by interference, blunted responses to chemical and mechanical stimuli. Animal experiments show a dose–response relation between ventilation and carbon dioxide level in REM sleep: there is more ventilation in REM periods with higher inspired levels of carbon dioxide (Fraigne *et al.*, 2008) – indicating that the chemoreceptors are functional in that state. Indeed at high levels of carbon dioxide, chemical drive overrides endogenous excitatory drive, and variability of respiratory parameters is decreased. Yet there are reports of blunted ventilatory responses to carbon dioxide particularly during phasic REM sleep. This may indicate either reduced chemosensitivity or altered motor activity. There is no evidence of the former, but ample evidence of the latter, in which case, endogenous drive may override chemical drive.

The pattern of REM-specific endogenous drive

Characteristically, excitation of respiratory neurons and motor neurons develops with a delay after the onset of REM sleep and gradually rises to a peak before declining abruptly before the end of the REM period. The excitation is potent: genioglossal activity in REM sleep in the rat is 25% greater than activity in NREM sleep, and respiratory neuronal activity in REM sleep in the cat under conditions of hypocapnic apnea may be as much as 20 times greater than the activity in NREM sleep. The distinctive late-onset pattern of the excitation is a clue to understanding its source, which must have a similar activity pattern. The activity of the REM sleep-specific neurons described by Netick and colleagues (1977) has this pattern (unpublished observations), but whether these neurons are the source or recipients of the excitation is not known.

References

Baust, W. & Engel, R. (1971) The correlation of heart and respiratory frequency in natural sleep of man and their relation to dream content. *Electroencephalogr Clin Neurophysiol* **30**: 262–3.

Bennett, J. R., Dunroy, H. M. A., Corfield, D. R. *et al.* (2004) Respiratory muscle activity during REM sleep in patients with diaphragm paralysis. *Neurology* **62**: 134–7.

Chase, M. H. & Morales, F. R. (1982) Phasic changes in motoneuron membrane potential during REM periods of active sleep. *Neurosci Lett* **34**: 177–82.

Chokroverty, S. (1980) Phasic tongue movements in human rapid eye-movement sleep. *Neurology* **30**: 665–8.

Dawes, G. S., Fox, H. E., Leduc, B. M., Liggins, G. C. & Richards, R. T. (1972) Respiratory movements and rapid eye movement sleep in the foetal lamb. *J Physiol* **220**: 119–43.

Douglas, N. J. (1998) Sleep in patients with chronic obstructive pulmonary disease. *Clin Chest Med* **19**: 115–25.

Douglas, N. J. (2005) Respiratory physiology: control of ventilation. In *Principles and Practice of Sleep Medicine*, 4th edn. eds. M. H. Kryger, T. Roth & W. C. Dement. Philadelpia, PA: Elsevier Saunders, pp. 224–31.

Dunin-Barkowski, W. L. & Orem, J. M. (1998) Suppression of diaphragmatic activity during spontaneous ponto-geniculo-occipital waves in cat. *Sleep* **21**: 671–5.

Eckert, D. J., Malhotra, A., Lo, Y. L. *et al.* (2009) The influence of obstructive sleep apnea and gender on genioglossus activity during rapid eye movement sleep. *Chest* **135**: 957–64.

Fleming, P. J., Cade, D., Bryan, M. H. & Bryan, A. C. (1980) Congenital central hypoventilation and sleep state. *Pediatrics* **66**: 425–8.

Fraigne, J. J., Dunin-Barkowski, W. L. & Orem, J. M. (2008) Effect of hypercapnia on sleep and breathing in unanesthetized cats. *Sleep* **31**(7): 1025–33.

Goodenough, D. R., Witkin, H. A., Koulack, D. & Cohen, H. (1975) The effects of stress films on dream affect and on respiration and eye-movement activity during rapid-eye-movement sleep. *Psychophysiol* **12**: 313–20.

Hauri, P. & Van de Castle, R. L. (1973) Psychophysiological parallels in dreams. *Psychosom Med* **35**: 297–308.

Hendricks, J. C., Kline, L. R., Davies, R. O. & Pack, A. I. (1990) Effect of dorsolateral pontine lesions on diaphragmatic activity during REMS. *J Appl Physiol* **68**: 1435–42.

Hobson, J. A., Goldfrank, F. & Snyder, F. (1965) Respiration and mental activity in sleep. *J Psychiatr Res* **3**:79–90.

Horner, R. L. (2008) Neuromodulation of hypoglossal motoneurons during sleep. *Respir Physiol Neurobiol* **164**: 179–96.

Johnson, M. W. & Remmers, J. E. (1984) Accessory muscle activity during sleep in chronic obstructive pulmonary disease. *J Appl Physiol* **57**: 1011–17.

Kuna, S. T., Smickley, J. S., Vanoye, C. R. & McMillan, T. H. (1994) Cricothyroid muscle activity during sleep in normal adult humans. *J Appl Physiol* **76**: 2326–32.

Lopez-Rodriguez, F., Morales, F.R., Soja, P. J. *et al.* (1990) Suppression of the PGO-related lumbar motoneuron IPSP by strychnine. *Brain Res* **535**: 331–4.

Lovering, A. T., Dunin-Barkowski, W. L., Vidruk, E. H. & Orem, J. M. (2003) Ventilatory response of the cat to hypoxia in sleep and wakefulness. *J App Physiol* **95**: 545–54.

Lu, J. W., Mann, G. L., Ross, R. J. *et al.* (2005) Differential effect of sleep–wake states on lingual and dorsal neck muscle activity in rats. *Respir Physiol Neurobiol* **147**: 191–203.

Mahowald, M. W. & Schenck, C. H. (2005) REM sleep parasomnias. In *Principles and Practice of Sleep Medicine*, 4th edn. ed. M. H. Kryger, T. Roth & W. C. Dement. Philadelpia, PA: Elsevier Saunders, pp. 897–916.

Netick, A., Orem, J. & Dement, W. (1977) Neuronal activity specific to REM sleep and its relationship to breathing. *Brain Res* **120**: 197–207.

Orem, J. (1980) Medullary respiratory neuron activity: relationship to tonic and phasic REM sleep. *J Appl Physiol* **48**: 54–65.

Orem, J. & Anderson, C. A. (1996) Diaphragmatic activity during REM sleep in the adult cat. *J Appl Physiol* **81**: 751–60.

Orem, J., Lovering, A. T., Dunin-Barkowski, W. & Vidruk, E. H. (2000) Endogenous excitatory drive to the respiratory system in rapid eye movement sleep in cats. *J Physiol* **527**: 365–76.

Orem, J. M., Lovering, A. T. & Vidruk, E. H. (2005) Excitation of medullary respiratory neurons in REM sleep. *Sleep* **28**: 801–7.

Pompeiano, O. (1967) The neurophysiological mechanisms of the postural and motor events during desynchronized sleep. *Proc Assoc Res Nerv Ment Dis* **45**: 351–423.

Richard, C. A. & Harper, R. M. (1991) Respiratory-related activity in hypoglossal neurons across sleep-waking states in cats. *Brain Res* **542**: 167–70.

Sahin, M., Durand, D. M. & Haxhiu, M. A. (1999) Chronic recordings of hypoglossal nerve activity in a dog model of upper airway obstruction. *J Appl Physiol* **87**: 2197–206.

Sastre, J. P. & Jouvet, M. (1979) [Oneiric behavior in cats]. *Physiol Behav* **22**: 979–89.

Sherrey, J. H. & Megirian, D. (1990) After phrenicotomy the rat alters the output of the remaining respiratory muscles without changing its sleep–waking pattern. *Respir Physiol* **81**: 213–25.

Wiegand, L., Zwillich, C. W., Wiegand, D. & White, D. P. (1991) Changes in upper airway muscle activation and ventilation during phasic REM sleep in normal men. *J Appl Physiol* **71**: 488–97.

Modulation of REM sleep by non-REM sleep and waking areas in the brain

Sushil K. Jha and Birendra N. Mallick

Summary

The brain-stem cholinergic neurons, having higher activity during rapid eye movement (REM) sleep, located in several isolated nuclei are known as REM-on neurons. In contrast, the monoaminergic neurons in the brain stem and in the forebrain areas exhibit higher activity during wakefulness, almost completely cease their firing during REM sleep and have been termed as REM-off neurons. The norepinephrin (NE)-ergic neurons located in the locus coeruleus (LC) could be the negative REM sleep-executive neurons and their cessation during REM sleep seems to be obligatory for its occurrence. Our findings that the wakefulness-promoting neurons are inhibitory to REM-on neurons and excitatory to the REM-off neurons led us to suggest that the wakefulness-related neurons do not allow REM sleep to occur and cessation of REM-off neurons is a necessity for the generation of REM sleep. The caudal brain-stem reticular formation (CRF), which induces cortical synchronization, facilitates the activity of REM-on neurons. However, the hypothalamic non-REM sleep-related neurons do not seem to have significant effect on the spontaneous activity of the REM-on neurons, although they may be indirectly modulating REM sleep. Taken together these findings suggest that normally waking neurons do not allow REM sleep to appear; at a certain depth of non-REM sleep the CRF facilitates the onset of REM sleep and re-activation of the wake-active neurons in the brain stem is requisite for its termination.

Introduction

Sleep is a natural and periodic state of rest with decreased contextual consciousness. It is generated by complex but active involvement of specific neuronal circuitry in the brain and heavily influenced by biological rhythms, hormonal changes, and also by environmental factors (for a review see Zepelin *et al.*, 2005). Although apparently by looking at the external behavioral expression sleep appears to be a homogeneous process, based on associated electrophysiological signals, sleep in the birds and mammals has been characterized into two distinct stages; REM sleep and non-REM (NREM) sleep. These stages appear in non-rhythmic cycles of varying durations; five stages in humans and mainly two to three stages in rats, cats, dogs, and other mammals (Zepelin *et al.*, 2005). Consistent efforts across the globe for over more than half a century have made significant advancement to our understanding about the mechanism of neural regulation of sleep–wakefulness which has been covered in several reviews and monographs; however, a lot still remains to be known.

The neuronal components involved in the regulation of wakefulness, NREM, and REM sleep are closely interrelated anatomically as well as functionally and regarded as antagonistic systems, which are under the sway of central as well as peripheral neuronal influences for the recurring appearance of sleep–wakefulness cycles. The classical experiments by W. R. Hess and Frederic Bremer may be considered as the stepping stones of experimental research toward understanding the neurophysiological mechanism of sleep–wakefulness (Bremer, 1935; Hess, 1927). They showed induction of sleep-like behavior by protracted low-rate electrical stimulation of the midline thalamus and by transection of the neuraxis at the midbrain level ("cerveau isole" preparation). The pioneering studies by Moruzzi and Magoun and several others showed the influence of the brain-stem reticular formation on alertness and drowsiness. While the reticular formation of the rostral part of the brain stem (pontine and midbrain) was attributed to alertness and waking,

REM Sleep: Regulation and Function, eds. Birendra N. Mallick, S. R. Pandi-Perumal, Robert W. McCarley, and Adrian R. Morrison. Published by Cambridge University Press. © Cambridge University Press 2011.

electroencephalogram (EEG) and behavioral signs of sleep and drowsiness were associated to activation of other brain sites, such as CRF and the basal forebrain (BF) (Moruzzi, 1972).

The sleep-like EEG pattern of the "cerveau isole" animal was attributed to the withdrawal of influences from the rostral reticular activating system. Thus, the neuronal substrates involved in the induction and maintenance of waking and sleep are located in the rostral brain-stem reticular formation, CRF, and BF, respectively. There is evidence suggesting that neurons located in these areas mutually interact and inhibit each other for smooth regulation of sleep and wakefulness (Moruzzi, 1972). Further, as detailed in other sections of this volume, around the mid-twentieth century a distinct state, REM sleep, was identified within the sleep period. Over the past half a century, significant efforts have been put into understanding its regulation. It is important to know that under normal conditions the REM sleep state does not appear after waking, it appears only after a period of NREM sleep, although the duration of the NREM sleep period varies and every NREM sleep episode is not followed by an REM sleep period; however, REM sleep may continue either into NREM sleep or into wakefulness. It is likely that the neural circuitry for the regulation of REM sleep must have modulating inputs from the NREM sleep and waking areas.

The neural mechanism associated with the specific vigilant state commencement or swapping is still unclear. We do not have complete understanding as to how the neural circuitry responsible for one specific vigilant state gets re-energized to induce the other vigilant state. Also, we are unaware about how the potency and mechanism of one neuronal circuitry associated with a specific vigilant state keeps the other circuitry(ies), responsible for the other vigilant state, suppressed/inhibited. Here, we review the neural regulation of REM sleep, especially the possible role of waking and NREM sleep-regulating areas in the initiation and termination of REM sleep. We have proposed that the cessation of LC NE-ergic neuronal activity is a prerequisite for the genesis and maintenance of REM sleep (Pal *et al.*, 2005).

Brain areas modulating wakefulness

Neurons in the brain-stem ascending reticular activating system (ARAS), BF-cholinergic neurons, hypothalamic histaminergic and orexinergic neurons are the main components for inducing cortical arousal. Based on the histochemical features, functional properties, and anatomical connections, the ARAS is mainly considered to have four discrete nuclei: (1) the classical reticular formation; (2) the monoaminergic area; (3) the cholinergic area; and (4) the autonomic nuclei (Parvizi and Damasio, 2001). In the rostral half of the brain stem (midbrain and upper pons) some of the prominent nuclei are the deep mesencephalic nucleus, the pararubral nucleus, the non-cholinergic portion of the pedunculopontine tegmental (PPT) nucleus, and the pontis oralis nuclei. The nuclei in the lower pons and the medulla are the pontis caudalis (PNC), paragigantocellularis, parvocellularis, and subnucleus reticular dorsalis.

The monoaminergic nucleus of the brain stem encompasses the NE-ergic LC area, the serotonergic dorsal raphe complex, and the dopaminergic substantia nigra and ventral tegmental nucleus. The physiological involvement of the serotonergic and NE-ergic systems in modulating the global activity of the cortex and in supporting increased attentiveness and behavioral responses to environmental stimuli is well documented. The cholinergic nuclei located in the upper brain stem include the laterodorsal tegmental (LDT) neurons and the cholinergic portion of the PPT area (Lydic and Baghdoyan, 2005). The activity of the brainstem cholinergic system blocks the generation of sleep spindles and thereby initiates the wake state (Steriade, 1993). The autonomic nuclei, which include the upper brain-stem parabrachial nucleus and the periaqueductal gray matter, have the anatomical means to modulate the activity of the cerebral cortex either through the thalamus or the basal forebrain, or through the classical reticular monoaminergic and cholinergic nuclei. Hence, these discrete nuclei of the ARAS play a crucial role in the generation and maintenance of wakefulness and alertness (Parvizi and Damasio, 2001).

Besides the neurons of the ARAS, the BF-cholinergic cells also play an important role in cortical arousal as identified by EEG desynchronization. Electrical or chemical stimulation of the BF induces cortical activation and the neurons of this area discharge at higher rates in association with cortical activation during wakefulness and REM sleep. The cholinergic neurons represent only approximately 5% of the total BF cell population, which is both chemically and physiologically heterogeneous, but a very potent system for inducing alertness (Lee *et al.*, 2005).

The tuberomammillary nucleus (TMN), located in the caudolateral portion of the posterior hypothalamus, is the sole source of histaminergic neurons in the mammalian brain and its pharmacological manipulation greatly alters sleep–wakefulness. For example, activation of histaminergic neurons induces arousal and, conversely, blocking the histaminergic receptors or inhibiting its synthesis machinery induces both NREM and REM sleep (Monti *et al.*, 1988). Reversible inactivation or permanent lesion of the TMN neurons induces sleep. Further, the TMN neurons demonstrate maximal firing rate during arousal, decreased firing rate during NREM sleep, and are virtually silent during REM sleep (for a review see Saper *et al.*, 2001). The inhibitory signal presumably is transmitted by NREM sleep-related neurons, which possibly acts like a sentinel for sleep induction and its maintenance; otherwise the activated TMN neurons would promote wakefulness.

In addition, several relatively recent reports suggest that the orexinergic system is involved in sensing the body's external and internal environments and also regulates sleep–wakefulness. Orexin maintains vigilant states by activating the wake-related monoaminergic and cholinergic neurons in the brain stem to maintain long periods of wakefulness. If these neurons in the central nervous system are permanently lost, it leads to a sleep disorder "narcolepsy" (for a review see Szymusiak and McGinty, 2008). Additionally, the orexin neurons receive abundant inputs from the limbic system, which might be important for modulating alertness during emotional situations.

NREM sleep-generating areas

Similar to the wake-inducing areas, some of the hypothalamic nuclei have been implicated in the generation and maintenance of NREM sleep (for a review see Saper *et al.*, 2001). Historically, during the Spanish-flu pandemic that raged after World War I, a Viennese neurologist, Constantin von Economo, observed that some flu patients fell into a state of lethargy or coma before dying, while others went several days without sleeping and then died. The brain autopsies exhibited lesions at two different brain areas in these two types of patients. The patients who were comatosed before their death had lesions in the posterior hypothalamic region, whereas those who experienced sleeplessness before dying had brain lesions in the preoptic area of the anterior hypothalamus (POAH) (von Economo, 1930; Kleitman, 1963) suggesting that anterior and posterior regions of the basal forebrain induce sleep and wakefulness, respectively (Saper *et al.*, 2001). Nauta supported the

existence of a "sleep facilitatory region" in the POAH, which was then confirmed by stimulation and lesion studies by several workers (McGinty and Sterman, 1968; Nauta, 1946; Sterman and Clemente, 1962). Later, in unanesthetized encephale isole cats (Mallick *et al.*, 1983) and subsequently in freely moving cats (Kaitin, 1984) it was shown that indeed a majority of neurons in the POAH are sleep active. Further studies localized the sleep-active neurons in the ventrolateral preoptic area (VLPO) and in the median preoptic nucleus; a significant proportion (50–75%) of these neurons are GABA-ergic (Szymusiak and McGinty, 2008). The number of c-Fos expressive sleep-active GABA-ergic neurons in the VLPO, median preoptic nucleus, and BF was increased during recovery sleep following sleep deprivation. Subsequent studies demonstrated that VLPO neurons may be predominantly involved in promoting sleep during the recovery phase, whereas median preoptic nucleus neurons may be responsive to increased sleep pressure (for review see Szymusiak and McGinty, 2008).

The POAH neurons also serve several other physiological functions including body-temperature regulation. A progressive decrease in body temperature is accompanied with NREM sleep while the thermoregulatory machinery loses its sensitivity during REM sleep (Parmeggiani *et al.*, 1999). The thermal messages are conceivably relayed to the medial POAH (mPOAH) primarily via the NE-ergic cell groups in the ponto-medullary area, a part of the ARAS that also controls alertness (Jha and Mallick, 2009). Further, we have shown that NE, ACh, and GABA neurotransmitters in the mPOAH jointly help regulate body temperature and sleep–wakefulness (Jha and Mallick, 2009; Mallick and Joseph, 1997). Additionally, we have noticed that the brain-stem wakefulness-inducing area tightly modulates the activity of thermosensitive neurons in the mPOAH (Jha and Mallick, 2009), which shows the integration of sleep–wakefulness and thermoregulatory inputs in the POAH and may elucidate the fine tuning of the temporal changes in body temperature along with sleep and wakefulness.

REM sleep-generating areas

Several models have been proposed to explain neural regulation of REM sleep. However, the precise driving force that triggers its cyclic generation, maintenance, and termination is still unknown. The reader's

Effects of CRF and POAH stimulation on an REM-on neuron of the LDT

(*a*) Spontaneous activity of an REM-on neuron of the LDT

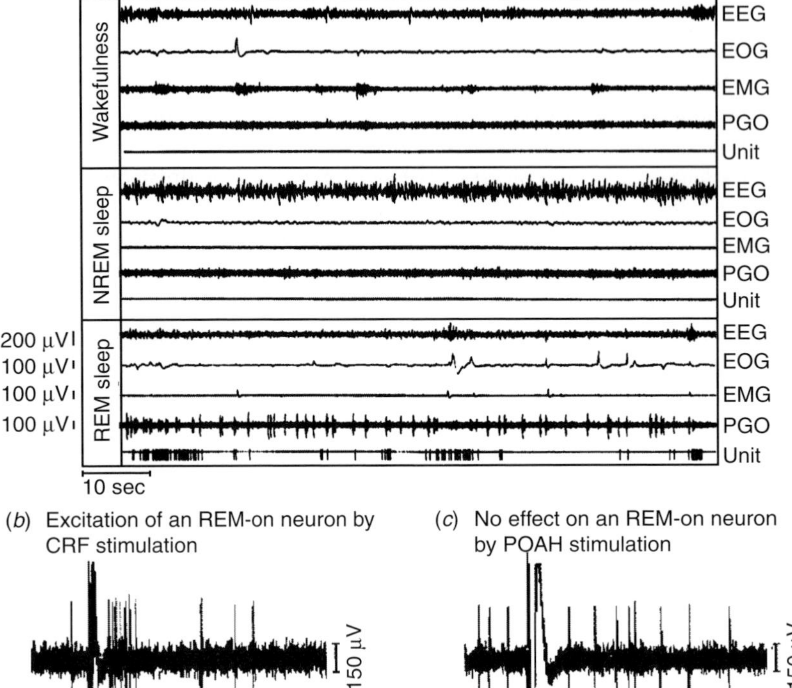

Figure 18.1 Spontaneous activity of an REM-on neuron of the laterodorsal tegmental (LDT) area in the brain stem during different vigilant states and the effect of caudal reticular formation (CRF) and preoptic anterior hypothalamus (POAH) stimulation. (*a*) The neuron was active during REM sleep with no activity during NREM sleep and wakefulness. (*b*) This neuron was excited by CRF stimulation whereas (*c*) POAH stimulation did not induce any change in its activity. (Adapted from Mallick *et al.*, 2004)

attention is drawn to the preface by Jouvet (1999) in an earlier related book (Jouvet, 1999) and to the chapters in this volume by Villablanca and Andrés, and by Morrison, where it has been shown that the pontine region in the brain stem is essential for the generation and regulation of REM sleep.

Brain-stem REM-on neurons

It has been generally accepted that the pontine tegmentum area in the brain stem is necessary for generating REM sleep and its phasic events in particular. Some of the neurons in this part of the brain stem are active or significantly increase their activity almost exclusively during REM sleep; they have been termed as REM-on neurons (Figure 18.1*a*) (Hobson *et al.*, 1975). These neurons have been identified mainly in the LDT and PPT regions in the brain stem and the majority of these neurons are presumably cholinergic (Sakai and Koyama, 1996). There are mainly four sites in the pontine area, where application of the cholinergic

agonist, carbachol, induces REM sleep or REM sleep-like state: (1) the pontine tegmental area corresponding to the most ventral and rostral part of the PNC (Baghdoyan *et al.*, 1987; Lydic and Baghdoyan, 2005); (2) the mediodorsal pontine tegmentum area (Vanni-Mercier *et al.*, 1989); (3) the dorsal part of the rostral pontine tegmentum around the LC (Yamamoto *et al.*, 1990); and (4) the oral pontine reticular nucleus (RPO) (McCarley *et al.*, 1987). Although it is known that the pontine cholinergic group of neurons is the executive machinery for REM sleep, how these neurons interact for REM sleep regulation is not yet clear.

Brain-stem REM-off neurons

In contrast to the REM-on neurons there is another group of neurons, the REM-off neurons. The typical discharge profile of this latter group of neurons is highest in waking, decreases during NREM sleep, and almost stops activity during REM sleep. The REM-off neurons are monoaminergic in nature and are located in the brain stem primarily in the LC, the dorsal raphe nucleus (DRN), and the peribrachial area.

Role of the locus coeruleus in REM sleep regulation

Several reports suggest that the LC and NE play a very important role in REM sleep regulation though mostly as a negative regulator (for a review see Gottesmann, 2008). Jouvet's group had shown that lesion of the LC did not affect REM sleep as such but caused irreversible disappearance of muscle atonia during REM sleep, REM sleep without atonia (Roussel *et al.*, 1976). However, Braun and Pivik, from their lesion study in rabbits, suggested that the LC regions are essential for the integrity of sleep and are especially important for the control of motor mechanisms during sleep (Braun and Pivik, 1981). Further, local cooling of the LC led to an increase in NREM sleep as well as REM sleep (Cespuglio *et al.*, 1982). Injections of a cholinergic agonist mimicking the actions of acetylcholine (ACh) into the RPO, including the LC, triggered REM sleep (Baghdoyan *et al.*, 1987; Mallick *et al.*, 2001). This suggested that ACh is normally released in this area for the initiation of REM sleep.

The LC contains REM-off neurons (Aston-Jones and Bloom, 1981) and these neurons do not cease activity during REM sleep deprivation (Mallick *et al.*, 1990). Hence, it was proposed that keeping these neurons persistently active should prevent REM sleep generation and induce a condition simulating REM sleep deprivation. It was observed in chronically prepared normally behaving rats that when the LC was stimulated bilaterally with mild, low-intensity, and low-frequency electrical pulses (an average frequency at which the LC neurons normally fire) REM sleep was significantly reduced; in those animals the REM sleep was inhibited throughout the period of stimulation (eight hours), which showed a rebound increase after the stimulation was withdrawn before attaining normal level (Singh and Mallick, 1996). Similar to the LC neurons, normally the activity of DRN serotonergic neurons is at its highest during wakefulness, diminishes during NREM sleep, and is virtually suppressed during REM sleep and thus they also have been categorized as REM-off neurons (Trulson and Jacobs, 1979). Activation of serotonergic neurons in the DRN inhibits REM sleep as well as REM-on neurons (Jha *et al.*, 2005; Monti and Monti, 2000). These findings suggest that a condition that keeps the REM-off neurons activated or disinhibited, delays the emergence of REM sleep.

Is inhibition of monoaminergic transmission requisite for REM sleep genesis?

The activated monoaminergic REM-off neurons probably drive down the generation of REM sleep and the effects last until the activation is withdrawn. The first line of evidence in this support primarily comes from our group which found that a mild electrical stimulation of the LC reduced REM sleep significantly (Singh and Mallick, 1996). Further, we observed that the effect of electrical stimulation was annulled in the presence of an NE-ergic antagonist, which suggests the inactivity-dependent role of the LC's NE-ergic neurons in the generation of REM sleep (Mallick *et al.*, 2005). Additionally, we found that the microinjection of picrotoxin, a GABA-A receptor antagonist, in the LC reduced REM sleep genesis (Kaur *et al.*, 1997) and the effects were so pronounced that six bolus of such microinjection of picrotoxin into the LC at an interval of every 6 hours for 36 hours, kept REM sleep inhibited (Kaur *et al.*, 2004). The second line of evidence can be drawn from the DRN REM-off neurons, where similar such phenomenon has been observed. It has been found that the activation of serotonergic autoreceptors in the DRN that induce self-neuronal hyper-polarization, increases REM sleep (Monti and Monti, 2000). This is consistent with electrophysiological studies showing virtually no firing of the serotonergic raphe neurons during REM sleep (Trulson and Jacobs, 1979). Also, perfusion of 8-OH-DPAT (a serotonergic receptor agonist) into the DRN led to a four-fold increase in only REM sleep but NREM sleep or wakefulness did not change (Monti and Monti, 2000). These studies support our view that suppression of the monoaminergic REM-off neurons, a condition that hands-off the circuitry for REM sleep to begin, seems to be prerequisite for REM sleep genesis.

Is activation of the wake center requisite for REM sleep termination?

Sleep–wakefulness normally progresses from wakefulness to NREM sleep to REM sleep except under certain altered neurological conditions. REM sleep terminates into either wakefulness or NREM sleep, but the underlying mechanism of its precise termination into a specific vigilant state is unknown. Although REM sleep appears at a certain depth of NREM sleep, it does not tag along with every NREM sleep episode. Hence, one would expect that (once certain yet unknown conditions are fulfilled) NREM sleep-promoting neural machinery would activate REM sleep-executive neurons, which would in turn induce REM sleep. On the contrary, since normally REM sleep does not appear during waking, the wake-promoting brain areas would inhibit REM sleep-executive neurons to prevent its appearance during waking. Experiments were conducted to study such neuronal phenomenon in the brain and the revelations of our investigations were (1) the midbrain reticular formation (MRF), a wake-inducing area in the brain stem, excited the REM-off neurons, while it inhibited the REM-on neurons (Thankachan *et al.*, 2001); (2) the CRF area, one of the hypnogenic brain-stem neural groups, excited the REM-on neurons (Figure 18.1*b*) (Mallick *et al.*, 2004); (3) the hypothalamic sleep center (mPOAH) did not significantly influence the REM-on cells (Figure 18.1*c*) (Mallick *et al.*, 2004). The REM-on neurons have also been identified in other brain areas such as the central nucleus of the amygdala (Figure 18.2*a*), which were inhibited by the electrical stimulation of raphe nucleus (Figure 18.2*b*) (Jha *et al.*, 2005).

The studies mentioned above suggest that the activated wake area (MRF) is likely to prevent the appearance of REM sleep during arousal. However, for normal sleep progression from NREM sleep to REM sleep, the hypothalamic NREM sleep area does not have a direct switching influence on REM sleep-executive neurons, although they may provide bias to the REM-on neurons. Instead, the slow and recurrent excitation of these neurons by the CRF help the onset of REM sleep. It is noteworthy that activation of the POAH, a sleep center, would strengthen the circuitry associated with NREM sleep and thereby may provide bias to the system and indirectly influence REM sleep. Hence, we reasoned that the CRF hypnogenic area could be the driving force for REM sleep initiation; this is possibly why we observe REM sleep only after a certain depth of NREM sleep. On the other hand, once the downscaled wake-circuitry during REM sleep gets re-energized (maybe through the flip-flop mechanism), it terminates REM sleep into wakefulness by simultaneously inhibiting the REM sleep-executive neurons and exciting the REM-off neurons. However, we still do not know how REM sleep terminates sometimes into NREM sleep. We need to have a better understanding about the progression of sleep–wakefulness, but these studies demonstrate that the activation of wake-promoting areas is possibly obligatory for the termination of REM sleep into wakefulness.

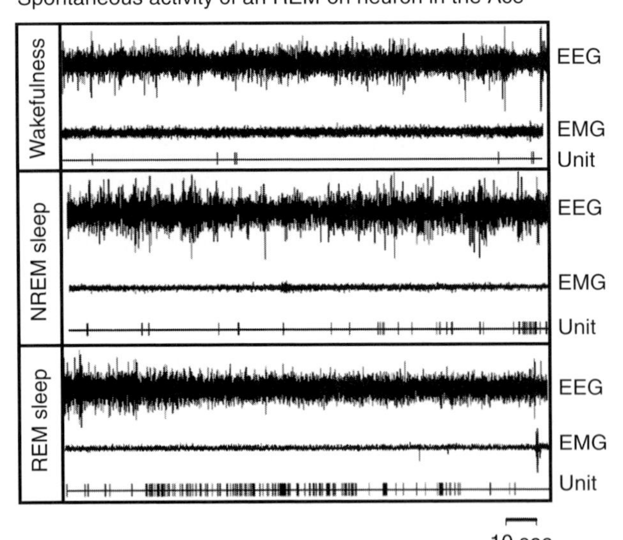
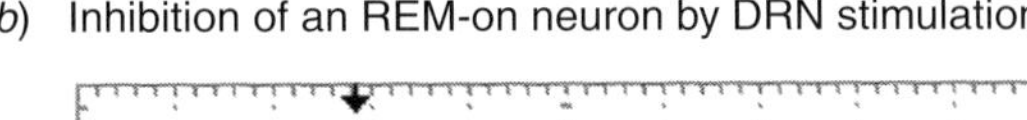
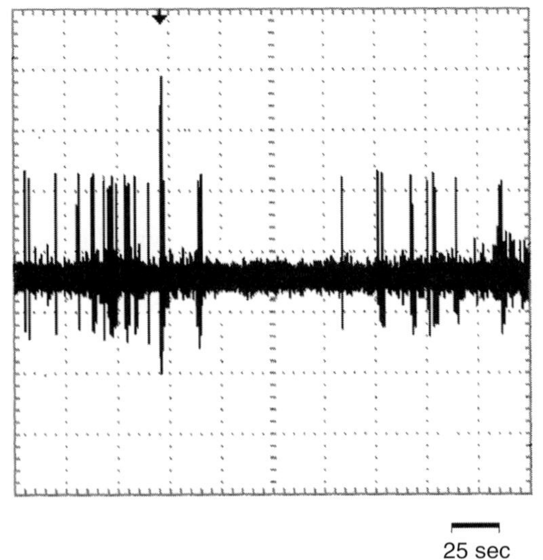

Effect of DRN stimulation on an REM-on neuron of the central nucleus of the amygdala (Ace)

(*a*) Spontaneous activity of an REM-on neuron in the Ace

(*b*) Inhibition of an REM-on neuron by DRN stimulation

Figure 18.2 An REM-on neuron from the central nucleus of the amygdala (Ace) and its modulation by dorsal raphe nucleus (DRN) stimulation. (*a*) Spontaneous activity of an REM-on neuron recorded from Ace during wakefulness, NREM sleep, and REM sleep. (*b*) This neuron was inhibited by electrical stimulation of the DRN. (Adapted from Jha *et al.*, 2005.)

REM sleep generation and termination: regulation solely through the brain-stem cog

An antagonistic interaction between REM-on and REM-off neurons: a GABA-ergic reciprocal-interaction model

REM sleep is generated and terminated through the brain-stem nuclei by its integrated neuronal circuitries. According to the *reciprocal-interaction model*, the REM-off neurons in the LC inhibit the REM-on neurons, while the REM-on neurons exert an excitatory effect on the LC REM-off neurons (Hobson *et al.*, 1975). This model suggested the role of REM-off neurons in REM-sleep termination but was unable to explain the mechanism of activation of REM-on neurons. Later on, Sakai (1988) put forward a *mutual-inhibitory model*, which offered mutual inhibition between REM-on and REM-off neurons for the generation and termination of REM sleep. However, the nature of neurotransmitters involved in the projections on these neuronal groups was not considered at the time of proposition. According to the mutual-inhibitory model, the cessation of REM-off neurons at the onset of REM sleep is the result of active REM sleep-specific inhibitory processes originating from the cholinergic REM-on cells (Sakai, 1988). However, ACh depolarizes the LC NE-ergic neurons (Egan and North, 1986) and is only weakly inhibitory to the serotonergic DRN neurons (Koyama and Kayama, 1993).

We therefore reasoned that the REM-on neurons might use some inhibitory interneurons, such as GABA, for the execution and/or termination of REM sleep. During REM sleep, elevated GABA levels have been observed in the LC (Nitz and Siegel, 1997) and GABA inhibits the LC NE-ergic neurons (Gervasoni *et al.*, 1998). Hence, GABA-ergic interneurons stimulated by the REM-on cholinergic neurons could be involved in the cessation of NE-ergic REM-off neurons at the onset of REM sleep. Also, REM sleep should be decreased after blocking the GABA transmission. Interestingly, we found that blocking GABA receptors in the LC reduced REM sleep (Kaur *et al.*, 1997). Although GABA interneurons could be playing a role in REM sleep, we also observed that GABA-ergic inputs to the LC from the area prepositus hypoglossi also increase REM sleep (Kaur *et al.*, 2001). Thus, the above studies suggest that the activated cholinergic REM-on neurons inhibit the REM-off neurons in the LC through GABA-ergic inputs, which could be either by means of interneurons or projecting neurons.

Further, any condition that keeps the LC neurons activated (for example, during wakefulness or NREM sleep), forbids REM-on neurons to fire. This could be mediated by GABA-ergic inputs to the REM-on neurons; the former being activated directly or indirectly by the NE-ergic REM-off neurons. We reasoned that blocking the GABA-ergic transmission in PPT, the site of REM-on neurons, would increase REM sleep but interestingly we observed an opposite effect. Microinjection of picrotoxin (a GABA-A receptor antagonist) into the PPT significantly decreased REM sleep while muscimol (a GABA-A receptor agonist) increased REM sleep (Pal and Mallick, 2006). The above findings indicated an excitatory role of GABA in the PPT for REM sleep genesis, which is likely to be acting presynaptically on an NE-ergic inhibitory input on the REM-on neurons as we have proposed earlier (Pal and Mallick, 2006).

An antagonistic interaction between the neuronal circuitries of the midbrain and caudal brain-stem reticular area

The interaction between the brain-stem mesencephalic reticular area and the caudal brain-stem reticular area plays an important role for REM sleep genesis and its termination. In general, the wake-active neurons in the brain stem are more active during wakefulness than during sleep. In contrast, the sleep-related neurons exhibit higher firing rates during sleep and low during wakefulness (Moruzzi, 1972). Such behavior of wakefulness and sleep-active neurons during waking facilitate REM-off neurons to be active but inhibit or disfacilitate the firing of REM-on neurons. However, during sleep, the wake-active neurons gradually slow down causing withdrawal of inhibitory and excitatory effects on the REM-on and REM-off neurons, respectively. Subsequently, at a certain depth of NREM sleep when some yet unknown conditions are fulfilled, the CRF-mediated excitation of REM-on neurons stimulates the GABA-ergic interneurons in the LC, which in turn inhibits the REM-off neurons and initiates REM sleep. Although the detailed neurochemical nature of the circuitries are unknown, based on recent studies we propose an antagonistic interaction between the neuronal circuitries of the midbrain and caudal

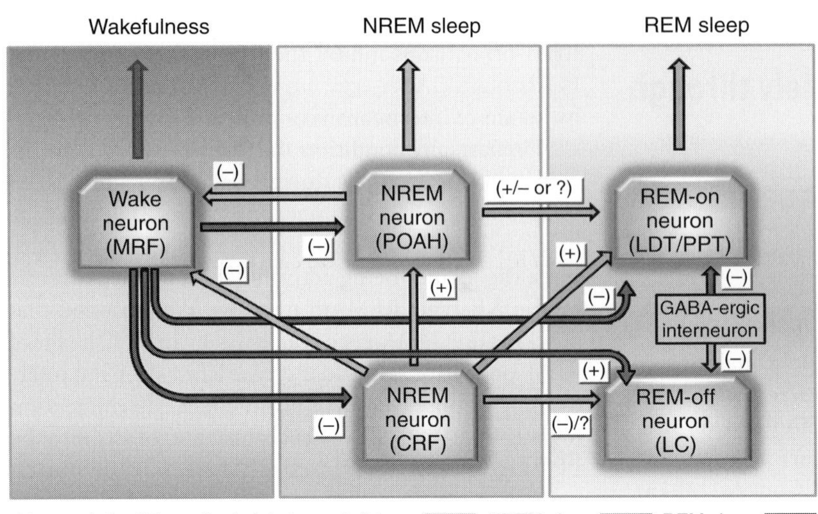

Figure 18.3 Proposed model for the induction of wakefulness, NREM sleep, and REM sleep.

brain-stem reticular areas and their influence on the REM-on and REM-off neurons for non-appearance of REM sleep during waking, progression of REM sleep from NREM sleep, and its termination into wakefulness (Figure 18.3).

The current knowledge persuasively suggests that the reciprocal antagonistic communiqué between brain-stem REM-on and REM-off neurons sets off the neural system for REM sleep genesis or its termination. Although, the precise mechanism of the generation of REM sleep and its phasic activities are yet to be determined, based on some known facts, it seems that until the REM-off neurons are inhibited, the appearance of REM sleep would not occur. Thus, the LC NE-ergic REM-off cells seem to be negative REM sleep-executive neurons and their cessation, mediated by GABA, is a pre-requisite for the regulation of REM sleep. If these neurons do not cease firing it would prevent REM sleep genesis, a condition similar to REM sleep deprivation. Further, the inhibition of REM-on neurons by wake-active areas would help terminate REM sleep into wakefulness.

Acknowledgments

Funding from CSIR and DBT to SKJ and from CSIR, DST, and UGC, India to BNM is highly acknowledged.

References

Aston-Jones, G. & Bloom, F. E. (1981) Activity of norepinephrine-containing locus coeruleus neurons in behaving rats anticipates fluctuations in the sleep–waking cycle. *J Neurosci* **1**: 876–86.

Baghdoyan, H. A., Rodrigo-Angulo, M. L., McCarley, R. W. & Hobson, J. A. (1987) A neuroanatomical gradient in the pontine tegmentum for the cholinoceptive induction of desynchronized sleep signs. *Brain Res* **414**: 245–61.

Braun, C. M. & Pivik, R. T. (1981) Effects of locus coeruleus lesions upon sleeping and waking in the rabbit. *Brain Res* **230**: 133–51.

Bremer, F. (1935) Cerveau 'isolé' et physiologie du sommeil. *C R Soc Biol (Paris)* **118**: 1235–42.

Cespuglio, R., Gomez, M. E., Faradji, H. & Jouvet, M. (1982) Alterations in the sleep-waking cycle induced by cooling of the locus coeruleus area. *Electroencephalogr Clin Neurophysiol* **54**: 570–8.

Egan, T. M. & North, R. A. (1986) Actions of acetylcholine and nicotine on rat locus coeruleus neurons in vitro. *Neuroscience* **19**: 565–71.

Gervasoni, D., Darracq, L., Fort, P. *et al.* (1998) Electrophysiological evidence that noradrenergic neurons of the rat locus coeruleus are tonically inhibited by GABA during sleep. *Eur J Neurosci* **10**: 964–70.

Gottesmann, C. (2008) Noradrenaline involvement in basic and higher integrated REM sleep processes. *Prog Neurobiol* **85**: 237–72.

Hess, W. R. (1927) Stammganglien Reizversuche. *Tagg Dtsch Physiol Frankfurt* 554–5.

Hobson, J. A., McCarley, R. W. & Wyzinski, P. W. (1975) Sleep cycle oscillation: reciprocal discharge by two brainstem neuronal groups. *Science* **189**: 55–8.

Jha, S. K. & Mallick, B. N. (2009) Presence of alpha-1 norepinephrinergic and GABA-A receptors on medial preoptic hypothalamus thermosensitive neurons and their role in integrating brainstem ascending reticular activating system inputs in thermoregulation in rats. *Neuroscience* **158**: 833–44.

Jha, S. K., Ross, R. J. & Morrison, A. R. (2005) Sleep-related neurons in the central nucleus of the amygdala of rats and their modulation by the dorsal raphe nucleus. *Physiol Behav* **86**: 415–26.

Jouvet, M. (1999) Preface. In *Rapid Eye Movement Sleep*, eds. B. N. Mallick & S. Inoue. Marcel-Dekker.

Kaitin, K. I. (1984) Preoptic area unit activity during sleep and wakefulness in the cat. *Exp Neurol* **83**: 347–57.

Kaur, S., Panchal, M., Faisal, M. *et al.* (2004). Long term blocking of GABA-A receptor in locus coeruleus by bilateral microinfusion of picrotoxin reduced rapid eye movement sleep and increased brain Na-K ATPase activity in freely moving normally behaving rats. *Behav Brain Res* **151**: 185–90.

Kaur, S., Saxena, R. N. & Mallick, B. N. (1997) GABA in locus coeruleus regulates spontaneous rapid eye movement sleep by acting on GABAA receptors in freely moving rats. *Neurosci Lett* **223**: 105–8.

Kaur, S., Saxena, R. N. & Mallick, B. N. (2001) GABAergic neurons in prepositus hypoglossi regulate REM sleep by its action on locus coeruleus in freely moving rats. *Synapse* **42**: 141–50.

Kleitman, N. (1963) *Sleep and Wakefulness*, Midway Reprint 1987 edn. The University of Chicago Press.

Koyama, Y. & Kayama, Y. (1993) Mutual interactions among cholinergic, noradrenergic and serotonergic neurons studied by ionophoresis of these transmitters in rat brainstem nuclei. *Neuroscience* **55**: 1117–26.

Lee, M. G., Hassani, O. K., Alonso, A. & Jones, B. E. (2005) Cholinergic basal forebrain neurons burst with theta during waking and paradoxical sleep. *J Neurosci* **25**: 4365–9.

Lydic, R. & Baghdoyan, H. A. (2005) Sleep, anesthesiology, and the neurobiology of arousal state control. *Anesthesiology* **103**: 1268–95.

Mallick, B. N., Chhina, G. S., Sundaram, K. R., Singh, B. & Kumar, V. M. (1983) Activity of preoptic neurons during synchronization and desynchronization. *Exp Neurol* **81**: 586–97.

Mallick, B. N. & Joseph, M. M. (1997) Role of cholinergic inputs to the medial preoptic area in regulation of sleep– wakefulness and body temperature in freely moving rats. *Brain Res* **750**: 311–17.

Mallick, B. N., Kaur, S. & Saxena, R. N. (2001) Interactions between cholinergic and GABAergic neurotransmitters in and around the locus coeruleus for the induction and maintenance of rapid eye movement sleep in rats. *Neuroscience* **104**: 467–85.

Mallick, B. N., Siegel, J. M. & Fahringer, H. (1990) Changes in pontine unit activity with REM sleep deprivation. *Brain Res* **515**: 94–8.

Mallick, B. N., Singh, S. & Pal, D. (2005) Role of alpha and beta adrenoceptors in locus coeruleus stimulation-induced reduction in rapid eye movement sleep in freely moving rats. *Behav Brain Res* **158**: 9–21.

Mallick, B. N., Thankachan, S. & Islam, F. (2004) Influence of hypnogenic brain areas on wakefulness- and rapid-eye-movement sleep-related neurons in the brainstem of freely moving cats. *J Neurosci Res* **75**: 133–42.

McCarley, R. W., Ito, K. & Rodrigo-Angulo, M. L. (1987) Physiological studies of brainstem reticular connectivity. II. Responses of mPRF neurons to stimulation of mesencephalic and contralateral pontine reticular formation. *Brain Res* **409**: 111–27.

McGinty, D. & Sterman, M. B. (1968) Sleep suppression after basal forebrain lesions in the cat. *Science* **160**: 1253–5.

Monti, J. M., D'Angelo, L., Jantos, H. & Pazos, S. (1988). Effects of a-fluoromethylhistidine on sleep and wakefulness in the rat. Short note. *J Neural Transm* **72**: 141–5.

Monti, J. M. & Monti, D. (2000) Role of dorsal raphe nucleus serotonin 5-HT1A receptor in the regulation of REM sleep. *Life Sci* **66**: 1999–2012.

Moruzzi, G. (1972) *The Sleep Waking Cycle*. Ergeb. Physiol. Springer-Verlag.

Nauta, W. J. H. (1946) Hypothalamic regulation of sleep in rats: an experimental study. *J. Neurophysiol* **9**: 285–316.

Nitz, D. & Siegel, J. M. (1997) GABA release in the locus coeruleus as a function of sleep/wake state. *Neuroscience* **78**: 795–801.

Pal, D., Madan, V. & Mallick, B. N. (2005) Neural mechanism of rapid eye movement sleep generation: cessation of locus coeruleus neurons is a necessity. *Sheng Li Xue Bao* **57**: 401–13.

Pal, D. & Mallick, B. N. (2006) Role of noradrenergic and GABA-ergic inputs in pedunculopontine tegmentum for regulation of rapid eye movement sleep in rats. *Neuropharmacology* **51**: 1–11.

Parmeggiani, P. L., Azzaroni, A. & Calasso, M. (1999) Selective brain cooling is impaired in REM sleep. *Arch Ital Biol* **137**: 161–4.

Parvizi, J. & Damasio, A. (2001) Consciousness and the brainstem. *Cognition* **79**: 135–60.

Roussel, B., Pujol, J. F. & Jouvet, M. (1976). [Effects of lesions in the pontine tegmentum on the sleep stages in the rat]. *Arch Ital Biol* **114**: 188–209.

Sakai, K. (1988) Executive mechanisms of paradoxical sleep. *Arch Ital Biol* **126**: 239–57.

Sakai, K. & Koyama, Y. (1996) Are there cholinergic and non-cholinergic paradoxical sleep-on neurones in the pons? *Neuroreport* **7**: 2449–53.

Saper, C. B., Chou, T. C. & Scammell, T. E. (2001) The sleep switch: hypothalamic control of sleep and wakefulness. *Trends Neurosci* **24**: 726–31.

Singh, S. & Mallick, B. N. (1996) Mild electrical stimulation of pontine tegmentum around locus coeruleus reduces rapid eye movement sleep in rats. *Neurosci Res* **24**: 227–35.

Steriade, M. (1993) Cholinergic blockage of network- and intrinsically generated slow oscillations promotes waking and REM sleep activity patterns in thalamic and cortical neurons. *Prog Brain Res* **98**: 345–55.

Sterman, M. B. & Clemente, C. D. (1962) Forebrain inhibitory mechanisms: sleep patterns induced by basal forebrain stimulation in the behaving cat. *Exp Neurol* **6**: 103–17.

Szymusiak, R. & McGinty, D. (2008) Hypothalamic regulation of sleep and arousal. *Ann N Y Acad Sci* **1129**: 275–86.

Thankachan, S., Islam, F. & Mallick, B. N. (2001) Role of wake inducing brain stem area on rapid eye movement sleep regulation in freely moving cats. *Brain Res Bull* **55**: 43–9.

Trulson, M. E. & Jacobs, B. L. (1979) Raphe unit activity in freely moving cats: correlation with level of behavioral arousal. *Brain Res* **163**: 135–50.

Vanni-Mercier, G., Sakai, K., Lin, J. S. & Jouvet, M. (1989) Mapping of cholinoceptive brainstem structures responsible for the generation of paradoxical sleep in the cat. *Arch Ital Biol* **127**: 133–64.

von Economo, C. (1930) Sleep as a problem of localization. *J Nerv Ment Dis* **71**: 249–59.

Yamamoto, K., Mamelak, A. N., Quattrochi, J. J. & Hobson, J. A. (1990) A cholinoceptive desynchronized sleep induction zone in the anterodorsal pontine tegmentum: locus of the sensitive region. *Neuroscience* **39**: 279–93.

Zepelin, H., Siegel, J. M. & Tobler, I. (2005) Mammalian sleep. In *Principles and Practice of Sleep Medicine*, eds. M. H. Kryger, T. Roth & W. C. Dement. W. B. Saunders Company, pp. 91–100.

Aminergic influences in the regulation of basic REM sleep processes

Claude Gottesmann

Summary

Research into the influence of monoamines on REM sleep-generating processes began as early as 1964, 11 years after the discovery of REM sleep. Various studies have now established that noradrenergic neurons of the locus coeruleus must be silent for REM sleep to occur. However, the maintenance of a low level of noradrenaline is still necessary. This phenomenon is linked to the persistence of noradrenaline in the brain resulting from its diffuse release at the varicosity level and the absence of rapid noradrenaline elimination by reuptake and enzymatic destruction. The role of dopamine in the regulation of REM sleep was discovered more recently. The infusion of dopamine agonists into the REM sleep-inducing structure called the peri-locus coeruleus-α inhibits REM sleep. However, this effect can be blocked by the concurrent administration of dopamine antagonists, indicating a basic noradrenergic function. In the same way, lesions of the dopaminergic ventral periaqueductal gray matter increase REM sleep. Serotonergic neurons become silent during REM sleep, and serotonin, which is involved in processes that support waking, also has REM sleep-off influences. Finally, histamine appears to have indirect influences on REM sleep, as histaminergic neurons become silent as soon as sleep onset occurs. This monoamine acts in connection with orexin, a deficit of which favors REM sleep and narcolepsy. The narcoleptic attacks seen in knock-out mice lacking orexin can be prevented by antagonists of the H_3 histamine autoreceptor.

Introduction

It is slightly artificial to focus attention on only one family of neurotransmitters when studying basic and higher integrated rapid eye movement (REM) sleep processes. Although amines are indeed important for the generation of this sleep stage, other transmitters such as acetylcholine (ACh), GABA, and glutamate are also involved, in the brain stem and forebrain. Moreover, the numerous interactions that take place between the different neurotransmitters in the regulation of REM sleep must be taken into account.

Indeed, although monoamines were among the first agents to be identified as being involved in REM sleep (Matsumoto and Jouvet, 1964), cholinergic processes were implicated even earlier, for example by showing that REM sleep increases after agonist administration (physostigmine and eserine) and is inhibited by antagonists like atropine (Jouvet and Michel, 1960). Gamma aminobutyric acid (GABA) derivatives were also shown to increase REM sleep at an early date (Jouvet *et al.*, 1961), curiously, prior to the discovery that barbiturates inhibit REM sleep (Jouvet, 1962) and cause it to be replaced by an intermediate stage (Gottesmann, 1996). Both of these phenomena were later explained with the discovery of their underlying GABAergic processes. However, during decades, the monoamines were the transmitters most often studied.

Catecholamines

The monoamines comprise dopamine, noradrenaline, and adrenaline (by extension), which together constitute the catecholamine chain. Other amines include serotonin, an indolamine, and histamine. All these compounds are directly, indirectly, or potentially involved in basic or integrated processes of REM sleep.

Noradrenaline

The first-identified and most important amine with respect to basic REM sleep processes is noradrenaline. This neuromodulator is primarily released from

REM Sleep: Regulation and Function, eds. Birendra N. Mallick, S. R. Pandi-Perumal, Robert W. McCarley, and Adrian R. Morrison. Published by Cambridge University Press. © Cambridge University Press 2011.

neurons located in the locus coeruleus, the A_6 area. Higher integrated forebrain activities are also supported by neurons with axons originating in the locus coeruleus and with terminals running along the dorsal noradrenergic tract, as well as by neurons originating in the medulla oblongata (areas A_1 and A_2) that particularly innervate the limbic system through the noradrenergic ventral tract. It should be mentioned that noradrenaline is mainly released by varicosities (Descarries *et al.*, 1977; Fuxe *et al.*, 1968) and binds to different brain receptors with differing effects: postsynaptic excitatory α_1 receptors, mostly presynaptic inhibitory α_2 receptors, and postsynaptic mainly excitatory β_1 and inhibitory β_2 receptors (Langer, 2008).

Noradrenergic neuron activity is important during waking, even though they fire at a slow rate; their influence is evidenced by the fact that α_1 agonists promote waking in the initial stages of slow-wave sleep and they become silent during subsequent REM sleep episodes (Aston-Jones and Bloom, 1981; Hobson *et al.*, 1975; Rasmussen *et al.*, 1986).

Today, most researchers seem to agree that the noradrenergic neurons must be silent for REM sleep to occur. This conclusion is mainly based on the observed silence of the neurons and on numerous other consistent results (for this reason, these neurons were called REM-off neurons (Sakai, 1985, 1988). For example, REM sleep occurrence decreases following the administration of monoamine oxidase inhibitors in humans (Toyoda, 1964) and animals (Delorme *et al.*, 1966; Khazan and Sulman, 1966), of uptake inhibitors (blockage of transporters) (Python *et al.*, 1997), and of α_1 agonists (Cirelli *et al.*, 1992; Hilakivi and Leppävuori, 1984). Consistent with this, β-receptor antagonists increase REM sleep (Tononi *et al.*, 1989). Moreover, REM sleep is induced by cooling (Cespuglio *et al.*, 1982) or destruction (Caballero and De Andres, 1986) of the locus coeruleus, and is inhibited by the local infusion of noradrenaline into the locus coeruleus (Masserano and King, 1982) or the peri-locus coeruleus-α (Cirelli *et al.*, 1992; Crochet and Sakai, 1999b). Recent results (Hou *et al.*, 2002) extending older ones (Stevens *et al.*, 1994) strongly suggest that noradrenaline activates α_1-receptors situated on mesopontine neurons and involved in waking processes, and it inhibits α_2-receptors situated on REM sleep-on neurons. Consequently, these results indicate that noradrenergic silence in the locus coeruleus deactivates processes involved in the induction of waking and disinhibits REM sleep-on mechanisms.

Despite these results associating noradrenergic silence in the locus coeruleus with REM sleep, a number of older findings suggested the contrary conclusion, namely that noradrenaline is in fact involved in the induction of REM sleep. The first such result was obtained by Matsumoto and Jouvet (Matsumoto and Jouvet, 1964), who showed that reserpine, which inhibits noradrenaline storage, thus inducing its destruction by monoamine oxidase, decreases REM sleep in cats, and that REM reappears after DOPA administration. Soon afterwards, it was shown that alpha-methyl-*para*-tyrosine (AMPT), which blocks tyrosine hydroxylase, decreases REM sleep in monkeys (Weitzman *et al.*, 1969) and in humans (Wyatt *et al.*, 1971). Similarly, alpha-methyl-DOPA, which inhibits catecholamine synthesis, was shown to decrease REM sleep (Dusan-Peyrethon *et al.*, 1968). The positive influence of noradrenaline (in fact of catecholamines) was also demonstrated by intracerebroventricular (icv) (Laguzzi *et al.*, 1972) or pontine (Zolovick *et al.*, 1973) injection of 6-hydroxy-dopamine (6–0H-DA), which destroyed catecholaminergic neurons and terminals and decreased REM sleep. Further evidence of the rather specific influence of noradrenaline was provided by the demonstration that inhibiting dopamine β-hydroxylase decreases REM sleep in rats (Satoh and Tanaka, 1973).

Subsequent results with AMPT confirmed the role of noradrenaline in inducing REM sleep (Gaillard, 1983), as did results with the α_2-agonist, clonidine, which reduces noradrenaline release by collateral inhibition of locus coeruleus or noradrenergic pontine targets and decreases REM sleep in animals (Kleinlogel *et al.*, 1975; Ma *et al.*, 2003; Mallick *et al.*, 2005; Putkonen *et al.*, 1977; Tononi *et al.*, 1991) and in humans (Autret *et al.*, 1977; Gentili *et al.*, 1996; Spiegel and Devos, 1980). This decrease of REM sleep was confirmed using β_1-receptor blockers administered either icv or intraperitoneally (ip) into animals (Lanfumey *et al.*, 1985) or given orally to humans (Betts and Alford, 1985). The involvement of noradrenaline in REM sleep generation has also been confirmed by experiments using α_2 antagonists (Bier and McCarley, 1994) and agonists (Cirelli *et al.*, 1992). Finally, the above-described results showing that inhibiting dopamine β-hydroxylase decreases REM sleep were confirmed in studies of humans with enzyme deficiencies (Tulen *et al.*, 1990), and further extended using knock-out mice with disruptions of the same enzyme (Ouyang *et al.*, 2004).

How can we reconcile the apparently opposite, and yet necessarily complementary, results regarding the well established necessary silence of noradrenergic locus coeruleus neurons during REM sleep and the decrease in this sleep stage following the central loss of noradrenaline?

A first point we can make is that, although the neurons are silent, a certain level of noradrenaline is still present during REM sleep (Léna *et al.*, 2005). Indeed, as already mentioned, this neuromodulator is released by varicosities, and because of this diffuse dispersal it does not immediately disappear from target neurons due to a lack of rapid reuptake or destruction in the synaptic space. Thus, the low level of noradrenaline that results from the final neuron spikes upon entrance into REM sleep could be maintained for a substantial duration. In animals, noradrenaline is maintained at a level of 24% during REM sleep (Shouse *et al.*, 2000). However, there is a potential problem here for the longest human REM sleep period in the early morning, which lasts for up to 50 minutes; no locus coeruleus has been recorded during sleep in humans to date, however.

Today, a generally accepted conclusion is that noradrenaline indeed seems to be important for REM-sleep occurrence although locus coeruleus neurons have to stop firing. This is a conclusion that has been long and consistently supported by Gaillard (1983). He wrote that "REM sleep preparation would be positively linked to noradrenergic cell activity, but actual REM sleep realization would be negatively related to this activity" (p. 221S). This statement was also recently supported by Mallick *et al.* (2005): "A critical level of noradrenaline in the system (is) required for generation of REM sleep. However, a higher level may be inhibitory" (p. 9). Thus, locus coeruleus neurons have to be silent for REM sleep occurrence (Pal *et al.*, 2005); however, there is maintenance of a low central level of noradrenaline.

One major remaining question is: how do the noradrenergic neurons become silent at the onset of REM sleep? One possibility is that residual noradrenaline previously released through collaterals could induce auto-inhibition (Aghajanian *et al.*, 1977) by α_2 receptors and participate in the progressive deactivation of locus coeruleus neurons. Indeed, infusing clonidine into the locus coeruleus decreases noradrenaline release. Moreover, although it has not been studied during sleep–waking stages, the adrenergic medulla oblongata C_2 neurons, which ascend along the ipsilateral medullary longitudinal bundle, appear to inhibit locus coeruleus neurons: the lesion of C_2 increases locus coeruleus tyrosine hydroxylase activity by 104%

(Astier *et al.*, 1986). These could thus be activated during REM sleep.

In addition, the locus coeruleus is under the powerful inhibitory influence of GABA originating from the medulla oblongata prepositus hypoglossi (Ennis and Aston-Jones, 1989a, b; Kaur *et al.*, 2001) and dorsal paragigantocellular reticular (Verret *et al.*, 2006) nuclei, and GABA release in the locus coeruleus increases during REM sleep (Nitz and Siegel, 1997); this increase also probably partly originates in local interneurons. The function of GABA has been directly demonstrated by the infusion of GABA antagonists into the locus coeruleus, which inhibits REM sleep, and by the local infusion of bicuculine, which activates the firing of locus coeruleus neurons (Gervasoni *et al.*, 1998). Moreover, the silence of the locus coeruleus could also be at least partly due to disfacilitation originating in the medulla (Ennis and Aston-Jones, 1986, 1988) and involving glutamate (Sakai and Crochet, 2004).

Finally, REM-sleep modulation could partly occur through more anterior structures. Indeed, it has been shown that lesions of the anterior hypothalamic preoptic area shorten REM sleep. Neurons of this area are specifically activated during REM sleep (Lu *et al.*, 2002).

To conclude, for several decades the reciprocal cholinergic–noradrenaline model of Hobson's group (Hobson *et al.*, 1975) dominated the history of REM-sleep research. There were numerous arguments in favor of a cholinergic role in REM sleep-on processes and of a correlated noradrenaline silence.

There are now additional arguments that strongly suggest that processes other than those involving noradrenaline are also crucial for the genesis of REM sleep. Firstly, the strongest evidence regarding the role of noradrenaline in inducing REM sleep should come from the inhibition of dopamine β-hydroxylase, which should show whether or not the neuromodulator is necessary for REM sleep to occur. However, β-hydroxylase knock-out mice show either no disturbance of REM sleep (Hunsley and Palmiter, 2003) or only a decrease (Ouyang *et al.*, 2004), while one would predict that the loss of the gene should suppress or increase REM sleep if it has a sleep-on or sleep-off role, respectively. Moreover, although the pharmacological blockade of the enzyme indeed initially suppressed REM sleep (Satoh and Tanaka, 1973), it needs to be explained why a rebound effect was observed if the basic process responsible for REM sleep had been suppressed. These particular experiments thus satisfy neither the noradrenaline REM sleep-off defenders nor the sleep-on defenders (for further discussion see Gottesmann, 2008).

For this reason, researchers are now focusing attention not only on the role of cholinergic and noradrenergic processes in REM-sleep generation, but also on those involving glutamate and GABA. While glutamate infusion in the pedunculopontine nucleus promotes REM sleep, GABA does the same in the locus coeruleus (see above) and in a dorsocaudal central tegmental field located just beneath the ventrolateral periaqueductal gray (Crochet *et al.*, 2006; Luppi *et al.*, 2006). At the same time, in the reticular pontine oralis nucleus area, REM sleep is enhanced when GABA is at its lowest level (McCarley *et al.*, 2005) or after pharmacological GABA blockade (Sanford *et al.*, 2003; Xi *et al.*, 1999), although this only occurs in the presence of locally available acetylcholine (Marks *et al.*, 2008). This highlights the importance of acetylcholine for REM sleep in addition to the required local disinhibition of noradrenaline (Hou *et al.*, 2002).

The above results show that, in spite of intensive research, much remains to be deciphered regarding the interrelated, complex regulation of REM sleep by noradrenaline, acetylcholine, GABA, and glutamate. However, it appears that while noradrenaline and acetylcholine neurons act as REM-sleep modulators, glutamate and GABA seem to be involved in the basic processes of REM-sleep generation (Luppi *et al.*, 2006).

Dopamine

Dopamine is the most abundant amine in the brain. It intervenes through the activity of different nuclei, including: (1) the midbrain A_9 nucleus, which gives rise to the mesostriatal tract but also sends some terminals to the thalamus; (2) the A_{10} nucleus in the ventral tegmental area, which mainly gives rise to the mesocortical and mesolimbic tracts; (3) the ventral periaqueductal gray matter, which sends projections to different diencephalic and forebrain structures; (4) the hypothalamic A_{11} nucleus, which mainly sends descending influences to the brain stem and spinal cord, although there are also terminals in the amygdala, prefrontal cortex, and a small number in the nucleus accumbens; and (5) different hypothalamic areas (A_{12}, A_{13}, A_{14}, A_{15}) with the tuberoinfundibular short tract and some A_{13}-originating brain-stem descending axons.

Dopamine acts on different receptors. Receptors of the D_1 subfamily, which comprise the D_1 and D_5 receptors, activate adenylate cyclase through sodium currents. The D_2 subfamily, which comprises the D_2, D_3, and D_4 receptors, inhibit adenylate cyclase through potassium currents. While D_1 receptors are postsynaptic, D_2 receptors can be either postsynaptic – where they induce hyperpolarization – or at the dendrite, cell body, or axon terminal levels, where they act as autoreceptors. Neurons of the ventral tegmental and nigral areas fire during waking as well as during slow-wave and REM sleep (contrary to all other amines), and a recent study showed that there is firing by bursts during both waking and REM sleep in the ventral tegmental area (Dahan *et al.*, 2007), implying increased dopamine release (Chergui *et al.*, 1994).

Although the influence of dopamine on REM sleep was first studied in the 1980s (see Monti and Monti, 2007), recent research has produced significant results regarding its intervention in REM sleep-regulating processes.

As discussed above, the most important evidence regarding the role of noradrenaline in REM sleep should have come from pharmacological (Satoh and Tanaka, 1973) or genetic (Ouyang *et al.*, 2004) suppression of the specific synthesis enzyme, dopamine β-hydroxylase. This type of approach is impossible for the study of dopamine, however. The nearest possible approach is the deletion of the gene coding the dopamine transporter (knock-out mice), which prevents dopamine reuptake in terminals and thus increases its available amount; these animals show a correlated increase in waking. Another approach is the deletion of dopamine receptors, which has not been characterized in relation to REM-sleep processes (Monti and Monti, 2007). Accordingly, to date the direct infusion of dopamine into structures responsible for the generation of REM sleep remains the most precise and informative method.

Dopamine was infused by reverse microdialysis (Crochet and Sakai, 2003) into the peri-locus coeruleus-α of cats (the sublaterodorsal nucleus in rats), a structure crucial for REM-sleep genesis (Sakai and Crochet, 2003) (REM sleep-on structure). This pontine area is innervated by axon terminals originating in A_{10} and A_{13}. The experiment of Sakai's team (Crochet and Sakai, 2003) showed that, following dopamine infusion, REM sleep was selectively decreased in a dose-dependent manner. Further, at high doses, the remaining REM sleep occurred without atonia. These effects were observed only when the perfusion was performed in the caudal part of the nucleus, and not when it was performed in any other mesopontine structures. The decrease was related to an increased latency of REM-sleep episode occurrence and to a decrease in the mean duration and number of episodes. Consistent with this result, older findings showed that systemic L-DOPA inhibits REM sleep (Wyatt *et al.*, 1970).

Crochet and Sakai (2003) also tried to identify the dopamine receptors involved in this REM-inhibiting effect. While D_1-like agonists injected in the locus coeruleus-α had little influence on REM sleep (although systemic administration reduces REM sleep by increasing waking; Trampus *et al.*, 1991), D_2-like agonists increased REM sleep by raising the number of episodes. D_3-like agonists had the same effect. Similar results with D_2 and D_3 agonists were obtained by systemic administration. Antagonists of the D_4 receptor, a member of the same D_2 family, increased the latency of REM sleep while globally decreasing sleep.

The inhibitory effect of dopamine on REM sleep in the peri-locus coeruleus-α was blocked by simultaneous administration of a selective antagonist of $α_2$ receptors (RX821002) (Crochet and Sakai, 1999a). The conclusion that dopamine inhibits REM sleep through $α_2$ receptor activation was confirmed by infusing the $α_2$ receptor agonist clonidine. This result was in agreement with previous published findings (Bier and McCarley, 1994).

The increased REM sleep that was observed with D_2-like agonists could be consecutive to: (1) the observed increase in the amount of global sleep; (2) the direct postsynaptic $α_2$ inhibition of neighboring noradrenergic neurons of the locus coeruleus or coeruleus-α, which promotes waking; (3) the presynaptic inhibition of glutamate release, and thus to a waking disfacilitation process that promotes REM sleep-inducing processes; or (4) GABAergic disinhibition of REM sleep-on neurons, since bicuculline in the peri-locus coeruleus-α area increases REM sleep (Crochet and Sakai, 2003).

A further decisive finding related to the influence of dopamine on REM sleep-generating processes was provided by the study of the ventral periaqueductal gray matter. Specifically, Lu *et al.* (2006) showed that the dopaminergic neurons of this area, which is anatomically and functionally different from the ventral tegmental area (and is adjacent to the dorsal raphe nucleus), are specifically active during spontaneous or induced waking. Its lesion decreases waking and increases sleep, particularly REM sleep when the lesion is performed using ibotenic acid. It is important that midbrain ventral lesions, including those of the A_{10} area, induce rather opposite effects on waking, sleep, and REM sleep (Rye, 2004), with the dopaminergic neurons of the ventral tegmental area being activated during REM sleep recovery following deprivation (Maloney *et al.*, 2002). It is probable that, just as neurons of the ventrolateral periaqueductal gray inhibit the sleep-inducing neurons of the hypothalamic ventrolateral preoptic nucleus by acting on $α_2$ receptors (Gallopin *et al.*, 2004), its neurons may also activate $α_2$ receptors of the peri-locus coeruleus area to inhibit REM sleep-on neurons. Indeed, the ventrolateral periaqueductal area is reciprocally connected to the locus coeruleus. It is worth mentioning that the increase in REM sleep following lesions to this area is certainly primarily linked to the global sleep increase, as is the case with D_2 agonists (see above); at the same time, the greater increase in REM sleep after ibotenic acid lesions as compared to those induced by 6-hydroxydopamine (Lu *et al.*, 2006) suggests a complementary specific effect on REM sleep-inducing processes.

Sleep disturbances related to dopamine dysfunction have long been noted in human pathology. The first to be described were the decreased REM sleep and persistence in muscle activity in drug-free patients with Parkinson's disease (Mouret, 1975). More recently, it has been shown that the frequently observed REM sleep decrease is accompanied by daily sleepiness and rapid entry into REM sleep (sleep-onset REM sleep: SOREM) during naps, as in narcolepsy. These disturbances are correlated with disturbed night sleep (Rye, 2004). The daytime sleepiness observed in Parkinson's could be explained not only by a decreased level of waking induction by dopamine (dopamine transporter blockers enhance waking), but also by disturbances in night sleep. The SOREM attacks can be explained by Crochet and Sakai's (2003) results in two ways. The first is a possible direct dopamine disinhibition of the peri-locus coeruleus-α, which would thus promote the occurrence of rapid REM sleep during daytime sleep bursts. The second is a decrease or disappearance of dopaminergic activating influences on hypothalamic orexinergic (hypocretin) neurons, which send activating influences to the locus coeruleus; the silence of these neurons also favors idiopathic narcolepsy (Thannickal *et al.*, 2000), again characterized by the same rapid REM-sleep irruption during daytime sleep attacks as well as during nighttime sleep. In support of this, antagonists of orexin-2 receptors promote sleep, including REM sleep (Shelton *et al.*, 2008).

In addition, complex behavior disturbances called REM sleep behavior disorder (RBD) often occur with Parkinson's disease, including "laughing, talking, shouting, kicking, jumping out of bed, walking, and running" (Lai and Siegel, 2003 : p. 138), with generally bilateral motor disturbances. REM sleep behavior disorder appears in 15 to 47% of Parkinson's cases (Gagnon *et al.*, 2002). Interestingly, during RBD, the usual motor symptoms of Parkinson's disease (rigidity, tremor, akinesia) disappear. REM sleep behavior disorder motor disturbances may precede the appearance of Parkinson's disease by several years (Arnulf *et al.*, 2008).

In Parkinson's disease, other motor abnormalities such as periodic leg movements appear in 38% of cases during all of the night sleep stages, thus including REM sleep (Schenck and Mahowald, 2002). During REM sleep, the spinal dopamine level is 28% lower than during waking (Taepavarapruk *et al.*, 2008). This must be related to a decrease in A_{11} area function, although there is a decrease in postsynaptic D_2 receptor binding in the striatum, and a lower concentration of iron, the cofactor of tyrosine hydroxylase, in the substantia nigra and putamen. However, the glutamate-mediated disfacilitation of medulla oblongata-originating GABA and glycine influences on the spinal cord are sufficient to explain the motor disturbances of restless legs syndrome.

Serotonin

Serotonin influence on REM sleep-generating processes has also been considered as early as 1964 (Matsumoto and Jouvet, 1964). The main nuclei involved in serotonin functioning are the mesencephalic dorsal and medial raphe nuclei, both of which innervate the forebrain and also send axons to the neighboring mesencephalon and to the pontine level. However, there are also rhombencephalic serotonergic neurons, which mainly innervate the spinal cord. There are 15 different types of receptors, all of which are metabotropic, except the ionotropic $5-HT_3$ receptor (Monti and Jantos, 2009). Serotonergic neurons are active during waking, decrease their firing rate during slow-wave sleep, and become silent during REM sleep (McGinty and Harper, 1976; Rasmussen *et al.*, 1984); serotonin release follows the same pattern (Portas *et al.*, 1998). This cessation of activity is related to a disfacilitation process (Sakai and Crochet, 2001b).

Table 19.1 Influence of serotonergic agonists on sleep–waking stages.

Compound	W	SWS	REMS
8-OH-DPAT, flesinoxan			
(5-HT$_{1A}$ agonists)			
Somatodendritic			
(Microinjection into the DRN)	n.s.	n.s.	+
Postsynaptic			
(Systemic injection)	+	–	–
Buspirone, ipsapirone, gepirone			
(Partial agonists at postsynaptic sites)			
(Systemic injection)	+	–	–
Fluoxetine			
(Selective serotonin reuptake inhibitor)			
Somatodendritic			
(Microinjection into the DRN)	n.s.	n.s.	+
Postsynaptic			
(Systemic injection)	n.s.	n.s.	–
CGS 12066B; CP-94,253			
(5-HT$_{1B}$ agonists)			
(Systemic injection)	4–	–	–
DOI			
(5-HT$_{2A/2C}$ agonist)			
(Microinjection into the DRN)	n.s.	n.s.	–
(Systemic injection)	+	–	–
m-chlorophenylbiguanide			
(5-HT$_3$ agonist)			
(icv injection)	+	–	–

Abbreviations: DRN: dorsal raphe nucleus; W: waking; SWS: slow-wave sleep; REMS: REM sleep; n.s., non-significant; +: increased; –: decreased.

(Reprinted from *Progress in Brain Research* with permission.)

The first result showing that serotonin does not promote REM sleep came from Matsumoto and Jouvet (1964). They showed that 5-HTP induces the reappearance of slow-wave sleep but not of REM sleep in reserpinized cats, contrarily to l-DOPA. Today it is not useful to analyze the REM sleep influences of serotonergic receptors in detail. Indeed, as extensively studied by Monti and Jantos (2009), and as shown in their table 2 (Table 19.1), direct or indirect agonists of the different serotonin receptors generally inhibit REM sleep except when injected in the raphe nucleus. This latter result is because such agonists activate 5-HT$_{1A}$ receptors, which are autoreceptors, and thus inhibit serotonergic neurons and induce the disinhibition of pontine REM sleep-on neurons. This inhibitory influence of serotonin on REM sleep is supported by experiments on knock-out mice showing that mutants that lack 5-HT$_{1A}$ or 5-HT$_{1B}$ (Adrien, 2005) receptors show increased REM sleep. However, while other results have shown that serotonin does not significantly influence REM sleep generation (Sakai and Crochet, 2001a)– dorsal raphe neurons can fire without suppressing REM sleep (Trulson *et al.*, 1981) – microdialysis studies have shown that it does regulate waking processes (Sakai and Crochet, 2001a).

Histamine

Histamine was first considered as influencing waking processes. The histaminergic neurons are located in the tuberomammillary area of the posterior hypothalamus, and the axon terminals are either local or directed to the brain stem or forebrain, particularly to structures involved in sleep and waking regulation (Lin *et al.*, 1994). There are H$_1$, H$_2$, H$_3$, and H$_4$ receptors, with H$_3$ acting as both auto- and heteroreceptors. Histamine promotes waking: classical antihistamines used as antiallergics have long been shown to induce sleepiness, and inverse H$_3$ receptor agonists increase waking (Sander *et al.*, 2008). Indeed, histaminergic neurons fire during waking and become silent as soon as the first stages of slow-wave sleep appear (Vanni-Mercier *et al.*, 1984). However, histamine only has an indirect connection with REM sleep, since histamine acts in connection with the orexinergic system. This latter system supports waking by increasing histamine release, and deficits in orexin promote REM sleep and narcolepsy (Liu *et al.*, 2008). Consistent with this, knock-out mice lacking the H$_1$ receptor do not show increased waking after orexin administration (Huang *et al.*, 2002). Moreover, the narcoleptic attacks of knock-out mice without orexin can be prevented by H$_3$ receptor antagonists (Guo *et al.*, 2009).

Conclusion

Amines have various distinct influences on REM sleep. Noradrenaline, for a long time, and dopamine, more recently, have been shown to modulate the occurrence and maintenance of this sleep stage. In addition these two neuromodulators have crucial influences for higher integrated activities, as revealed by the mind disturbances observed during dreaming. The maximal release of dopamine during REM sleep and the correlated decrease in noradrenaline in the nucleus accumbens, as well as the decrease in both neuromodulators in the prefrontal cortex as compared to waking (Léna *et al.*, 2005), are also classical indices of schizophrenia; significantly, dreaming because of these neurochemical disturbances mainly shows psychotic-like characteristics (Gottesmann, 1999, 2006).

Acknowledgments

The author thanks Dr. Peter Follette for improving the English of the manuscript.

References

Adrien, J. (2005) REM sleep and the serotonergic system:What we learn from mutant mice. *Sleep Biol Rhyt* **3**: suppl. 1: A.17.

Aghajanian, G. K., Cedarbaum, J. M. & Wang, R. Y. (1977) Evidence for norepinephrine-mediated collateral inhibition of locus coeruleus neurons. *Brain Res* **136**: 570–7.

Arnulf, I., Leu, S. & Oudiette, D. (2008) Abnormal sleep and sleepiness in Parkinson's disease. *Curr Opin Neurol* **21**: 472–7.

Astier, B., Kitahama, K., Denoroy, L., Berod, A. & Jouvet, M. (1986) Biochemical evidence for an interation bertween adrenaline and noradrenaline neurons in the rat brainstem. *Brain Res* **397**: 333–40.

Aston-Jones, G. & Bloom, F. E. (1981) Activity of norepinephrine-containing neurons in behaving rats anticipates fluctuations in the sleep-waking cycle. *J Neurosci* **1**: 876–86.

Autret, A., Minz, M., Beillevaire, T., Cathala, H. P. & Schmitt, H. (1977) Effect of clonidine on sleep patterns in man. *Eur J Clin Pharmacol* **12**: 319–22.

Betts, T. A. & Alford, C. (1985) Beta-blockers and sleep: a controlled trial. *Eur J Clin Pharmacol* **28** suppl: 65–8.

Bier, M. J. & McCarley, R. W. (1994) REM-enhancing effects of the adrenergic antagonist idazoxan infused into the medial pontine reticular formation of the freely moving cat. *Brain Res* **634**: 333–8.

Caballero, A. & De Andres, I. (1986) Unilateral lesions in locus coeruleus area enhance paradoxical sleep. *Electroenceph Clin Neurophysiol* **64**: 339–46.

Cespuglio, R., Gomez, M. E., Faradji, H. & Jouvet, M. (1982) Alterations in the sleep-waking cycle induced by cooling of the locus coeruleus area. *Electroenceph Clin Neurophysiol* **54**: 570–8.

Chergui, K., Suaud-Chagny, M. F. & Gonon, F. (1994) Non-linear relationship between impulse flow. Dopamine release and dopamine elimination in the rat in vivo. *Neuroscience* **62**: 641–5.

Cirelli, C., Tononi, G. M., Pompeiano, O. & Genneri, A. (1992) Modulation of desynchronized sleep through microinjection of alpha1-adrenergic agonists and antagonists in the dorsal pontine tegmentum of the cat. *Pflügers Arch* **422**: 273–9.

Crochet, S. & Sakai, K. (1999a) Alpha-2 adrenoceptor mediated paradoxical (REM) sleep inhibition in the cat. *NeuroReport* **10**: 2199–204.

Crochet, S. & Sakai, K. (1999b) Effects of microdialysis application in monoamines on the EEG and behavioral states in the cat mesopontine tegmentum. *Eur J Neurosci* **11**: 3738–52.

Crochet, S. & Sakai, K. (2003) Dopaminergic modulation of behavioral states in mesopontine tegmentum: a reverse microdialysis study in freely moving cats. *Sleep* **26**: 801–6.

Crochet, S., Onoe, H. & Sakai, K. (2006) A potent non-monoaminergic paradoxical sleep inhibitory system: a reverse microdialysis and single-unit recording study. *Eur J Neurosci* **24**: 1404–12.

Dahan, L., Astier, B., Vautrelle, N. *et al.* (2007) Prominent burst firing of dopaminergic neurons in the ventral tegmental area during paradoxical sleep. *Neuropsychopharmacology* **32**: 1232–41.

Delorme, F., Froment, J. L. & Jouvet, M. (1966) Suppression du sommeil par la p. chlorométhamphetamine et la p. chlorophénylalanine. *C R Soc Biol* **160**: 2347–460.

Descarries, L., Watkins, K.C. & Lapierre, Y. (1977) Noradrenergic axon terminals in the cerebral cortex of rats. III. Topometric ultrastructural analysis. *Brain Res* **133**: 197–222.

Dusan-Peyrethon, D., Peyrethon, J. & Jouvet, M. (1968) Suppression élective du sommeil paradoxal chez le Chat par α méthyl DOPA. *C R Soc Biol* **162**: 116–18.

Ennis, M. & Aston-Jones, G. (1986) A potent excitatory input to the locus coeruleus from the ventrolateral medulla. *Neurosci Lett* **71**: 299–305.

Ennis, M. & Aston-Jones, G. (1988) Activation of locus coeruleus from nucleus paragigantocellularis: a new excitatory amino acid pathway in brain. *J Neurosci* **8**: 3644–57.

Ennis, M. & Aston-Jones, G. (1989a) Potent inhibitory input to the locus coeruleus from the nucleus prepositus hypoglossi. *Brain Res Bull* **22**: 793–803.

Ennis, M. & Aston-Jones, G. (1989b) GABA-mediated inhibition of locus coeruleus from the dorsomedial rostral medulla. *J Neurosci* **9**: 2973–81.

Fuxe, K., Hamberger, B. & Hökfelt, T. (1968) Distribution of noradrenaline nerve terminals in cortical areas in the rat. *Brain Res* **8**: 125–31.

Gagnon, J. F., Bédard, M. A., Fantinin, M. L. *et al.* (2002) REM sleep disorder and REM sleep without atonia in Parkinson's disease. *Neurology* **59**: 585–9.

Gaillard, J. M. (1983) Biochemical pharmacology of paradoxical sleep. *Br J Pharmacol* **16**: S205–30.

Gallopin, T., Luppi, P.-H., Rambert, F. A., Fryman, A. & Fort, P. (2004) Effect of the wake-promoting agent modafinil on sleep-promoting neurons from the ventrolateral preoptic nucleus an in vitro pharmacologic study. *Sleep* **27**: 19–25.

Gentili, A., Godschalk, M. F., Gheorghiu, D. *et al.* (1996) Effect of clonidine and yohimbine on sleep in healthy men: a double-blind, randomized, controlled trial. *Eur J Clin Pharmacol* **50**: 463–5.

Gervasoni, D., Darracq, L., Fort, P. *et al.* (1998) Electrophysiological evidence that noradrenergic neurons of the locus coeruleus are tonically inhibited by GABA during sleep. *Eur J Neurosci* **10**: 964–70.

Gottesmann, C. (1996) The transition from slow wave sleep to paradoxical sleep: evolving facts and concepts of the neurophysiological processes underlying the intermediate stage of sleep. *Neurosci Biobehav Rev* **20**: 367–87.

Gottesmann, C. (1999) Neurophysiological support of consciousness during waking and sleep. *Prog Neurobiol* **59**: 469–508.

Gottesmann, C. (2006) The dreaming sleep stage: a new neurobiological model of schizophrenia? *Neuroscience* **140**: 1105–15.

Gottesmann, C. (2008) Noradrenaline involvement in basic and higher integrated REM sleep processes. *Prog Neurobiol* **82**: 237–72.

Guo, R., Anaclet, C., Roberts, J. C. *et al.* (2009) Differential effects of acute and repeat dosing with the H3 antagonist GSK189254 on the sleep-wake cycle and narcoleptic episodes in Ox–/– mice. *Br J Pharmacol* **157**: 104–17.

Hilakivi, I. & Leppävuori, A. (1984) Effects of methoxamine, an alpha-1 adrenoceptor agonist, and prazosin, an alpha-1 antagonist, on the stages of the sleep-waking cycle in the cat. *Acta Physiol Scand* **120**: 363–72.

Hobson, J. A., McCarley, R. W. & Wyzinski, P. W. (1975) Sleep cycle oscillation: reciprocal discharge by two brainstem neuronal groups. *Science* **189**: 55–8.

Hou, Y. P., Manns, I. D. & Jones, B. E. (2002) Immunostaining of cholinergic pontomesencephalic neurons for alpha1 versus alpha2 adrenergic receptors suggests different sleep-wake state activities and roles. *Neuroscience* **114**: 517–21.

Huang, Z. L., Qu, W. M., Li, W.D. *et al.* (2002) Arousal effect of orexin-A depends on activation of the histaminergic system. *Proc Nat Acad Sci (USA)* **99**: 1098.

Hunsley, M. S. & Palmiter, R. D. (2003) Norepinephrine-deficient mice exhibit normal sleep-wake states but have shorter sleep latency after mild stress and low doses of amphetamine. *Sleep* **26**: 521–6.

Jouvet, M. (1962) Recherches sur les structures nerveuses et les mécanismes responsables des différentes phases du sommeil physiologique. *Arch Ital Biol* **100**: 125–206.

Jouvet, M. & Michel, F. (1960) Nouvelles recherches sur les structures responsables de la "phase paradoxale" du sommeil. *J Physiol Paris* **52**: 130–1.

Jouvet, M., Cier, A., Mounier, D. & Valatx, J. L. (1961) Effets du 4-butyrolactone et du 4-hydroxybutyrate de sodium sur l'E.E.G et le comportement du Chat. *C R Soc Biol* **155**: 1313–16.

Kaur, S., Saxena, R. N. & Mallick, B. N. (2001) GABAergic neurons in prepositus hypoglossi regulate REM sleep by its action on locus coeruleus in freely moving rats. *Synapse* **42**: 141–50.

Khazan, N. & Sulman, F. G. (1966) Effect of imipramine on paradoxical sleep in animals with reference to dreaming and enuresis. *Psychopharmacologia* **10**: 89–95.

Kleinlogel, H., Scholtysik, G. & Sayers, A. C. (1975) Effects of clonidine and BS 100–141 on the EEG sleep pattern in rats. *Eur J Pharmacol* **33**: 159–63.

Laguzzi, R., Petitjean, F., Pujol, J. F. & Jouvet, M. (1972) Effets de l'injection intraventriculaire de 6-hydroxydopamine. II. Sur le cycle veille-sommeil du Chat. *Brain Res* **48**: 295–310.

Lai, Y.Y. & Siegel, J. M. (2003) Physiological and anatomical link between Parkinson-like disease and REM sleep behavior disorder. *Mol Neurobiol* **27**: 137–51.

Lanfumey, L., Dugovic, C. & Adrien, J. (1985) β1 and β2 adrenergic receptors: their role in the regulation of paradoxical sleep in the rat. *Electroenceph Clin Neurophysiol* **60**: 558–67.

Langer, S. Z. (2008) Presynaptic autoreceptors regulating transmitter release. *Neurochemistry International* **52**: 26–30.

Léna, I., Parrot, S., Deschaux, O. *et al.* (2005) Variations in the extracellular levels of dopamine, noradrenaline, glutamate and aspartate across the sleep-wake cycle in the medial prefrontal cortex and nucleus accumbens of freely moving rats. *J Neurosci Res* **81**:891–9.

Lin, J. S., Sakai, K. & Jouvet M. (1994) Hypothalamo-preoptic histaminergic projections in sleep-wake control in the cat. *Eur J Pharmacol* **6**: 618–25.

Liu, M., Thankachan, S., Kaur, S. *et al.* (2008) Orexin (hypocretin) gene transfer improves narcoleptic symptoms in orexin null mice. *J Sleep Res* **17**(Suppl. 1): 26–7.

Lu, J., Bjorkum, A. A., Xu, M. *et al.* (2002) Selective activation of the extended ventrolateral preoptic nucleus during rapid eye movement sleep. *J Neurosci* **22**: 4568–76.

Lu, J., Jhou, T. C. & Saper, C. B. (2006) Identification of wake-active dopaminergic neurons in the ventral periaqueducal grey matter. *J Neurosci* **26**: 193–202.

Luppi, P. H., Gervasoni, D., Verret, L. *et al.* (2006) Paradoxical (REM) sleep genesis: the switch from an aminergic-cholinergic to a GABAergic-glutamatergic hypothesis. *J Physiol Paris* **100**: 271–83.

Ma, J., Ye, N., Lange, N. & Cohen, B. M. (2003) Dynorphynergic GABA neurons are a target of both typical and atypical antipsychotic drugs in the nucleus accumbens shell, central amygdaloid nucleus and thalamic central medial nucleus. *Neuroscience* **121**: 991–8.

Mallick, B. N., Singh, S. & Pal, D. (2005) Role of alpha and beta adrenoceptors in locus coeruleus stimulation-induced reduction in rapid eye movement sleep in freely moving rats. *Behav Brain Res* **158**: 9–21.

Maloney, K. J., Mainville, L. & Jones, B. E. (2002) c-Fos expression in dopaminergic and GABAergic neurons of the ventral mesencephalic tegmentum after paradoxical sleep deprivation and recovery. *Eur J Neurosci* **15**: 774–8.

Marks, G. A., Sachs, O. W. & Birabil, C. G. (2008) Blockade of GABA, typeA, receptors in the rat pontine reticular formation induces rapid eye movement sleep that is dependent upon the cholinergic system. *Neuroscience* **156**: 1–10.

Masserano, J. M. & King, C. (1982) Effects on sleep of phentolamine and epinephrine infused into the locus coeruleus of cats. *Eur J Pharmacol* **84**: 199–204.

Matsumoto, J. & Jouvet, M. (1964) Effets de la réserpine, DOPA et 5 HTP sur les deux états de sommeil. *C R Soc Biol* **158**: 2137–40.

McCarley, R. W., Brown, R. M. & Thakkar, M. (2005) GABA: inhibition and/or disinhibition in REM sleep control? *Sleep Biol Rhyt* **3**(Suppl. 1): A13.

McGinty, D. J. & Harper, R. M. (1976) Dorsal raphe neurons: depression of firing during sleep in cats. *Brain Res* **101**: 569–75.

Monti, J. M. & Jantos, H. (2009) The role of dopamine and serotonin, and of their receptors, in regulating sleep and waking. *Prog Brain Res* **172**: 625–46.

Monti, J. M. & Monti, D. (2007) The involvement of dopamine in the modulation of sleep and waking. *Sleep Med Rev* **11**: 113–33.

Mouret, J. (1975) Differences in sleep with Parkinson's disease. *Elecroenceph Clin Neurophysiol* **38**: 653–7.

Nitz, D. & Siegel, J. (1997) GABA release in the locus coeruleus as a function of sleep–wake state. *Neuroscience* **78**: 795–801.

Ouyang, M., Hellman, K., Abel, T. & Thomas, S. A. (2004) Adrenergic signaling plays a critical role in the maintenance of waking and in the regulation of REM sleep. *J Neurophysiol* **92**: 2071–82.

Pal, D., Madan, V. & Mallick, B. N. (2005) Neural mechanism of rapid eye movement sleep generation: cessation of locus coeruleus neurons is a necessity. *Acta Physiol Sinica* **57**: 401–13.

Portas, C., Bjorvatn, B., Fagerland, S. *et al.* (1998) On-line detection of extracellular levels of serotonin in dorsal raphe nucleus and frontal cortex over the sleep/wake cycle in the freely moving rat. *Neuroscience* **83**: 807–14.

Putkonen, P. T. S., Leppävuori, A. & Stenberg, D. (1977) Paradoxical sleep inhibition by central alpha-adrenoceptor stimulant clonidine antagonized by alpha-receptor blocker yohimbine. *Life Sci* **21**: 1059–66.

Python, A. Y., Charnay, R., Mikolajewski, H. *et al.* (1997) Effects of nisoxetine, a selective noradrenaline transporter blocker, on sleep in rats. *Pharm Bioch Behav* **58**: 369–72.

Rasmussen, K., Heym, J. & Jacobs, B. L. (1984) Activity of serotonin-containing neurons in nucleus centralis superior of freely moving cats. *Exp Neurol* **83**: 302–17.

Rasmussen, K., Morilak, D. A. & Jacobs, B. L. (1986) Single unit activity of locus coeruleus neurons in the freely moving cat. I. Naturalistic behaviors and in response to simple and complex stimuli. *Brain Res* **371**: 324–34.

Rye, D. B. (2004) The two faces of Eve: dopamine's modulation of wakefulness and sleep. *Neurology* **63**: S2–7.

Sakai, K. (1985) Anatomical and physiological basis of paradoxical sleep. In *Brain Mechanisms of Sleep*, eds. R. Drucker-Colin, A. R. Morrison & P. L. Parmeggiani. pp. 111–37.

Sakai, K. (1988) Executive mechanisms of paradoxical sleep. *Arch Ital Biol* **126**: 239–57.

Sakai, K. & Crochet, S. (2001a) Role of dorsal raphe neurons in paradoxical sleep generation in the cat: no evidence for serotonergic mechanisms. *Eur J Neurosci* **13**: 103–12.

Sakai, K. & Crochet, S. (2001b) Increase in antidromic excitability in presumed serotonergic dorsal raphe neurons during paradoxical sleep in the cat. *Brain Res* **98**: 332–41.

Sakai, K. & Crochet, S. (2003) A neural mechanism of sleep and wakefulness. *Sleep Biol Rhyt* **1**: 29–42.

Sakai, K. & Crochet, S. (2004) Role of the locus coeruleus in the control of paradoxical sleep generation in the cat. *Arch Ital Biol* **142**: 421–7.

Sander, K., Kottke, T. & Stark, H. (2008) Histamine H3 receptor antagonists go to clinics. *Biol Pharm Bull* **31**: 2163–81.

Sanford, L. D., Tang, X., Xiao, J., Ross, R. J. & Morrison, A. R. (2003) GABAergic regulation of REM sleep in reticularis pontis oralis and caudalis in rats. *J Neurophysiol* **90**: 938–45.

Satoh, T. & Tanaka, R. (1973) Selective suppression of rapid eye movement sleep (REM) by fusaric acid, an inhibitor of dopamine-β-oxydase. *Experientia* **29**: 177–8.

Schenck, C. H. & Mahowald, M. W. (2002) REM sleep behavior disorder: clinical, developmental, and neuroscience perspectives 16 years after its formal identification in sleep. *Sleep* **25**: 120–30.

Shelton, J., Sutton, S., Yun, S. *et al.* (2008) Sleep-inducing effects mediated by a selective orexin-2 receptor antagonist during the light phase in the rat. *J Sleep Res* **17** (Suppl. 1): 201.

Shouse, M. N., Staba, R. J., Saquib, S. F. & Farber, P. R. (2000) Monoamines and sleep: microdialysis findings in pons and amygdala. *Brain Res* **860**: 181–9.

Spiegel, R. & Devos, J. E. (1980) Central effects of guanfacine and clonidine during wakefulness and sleep in healthy subjects. *Brit J Clin Pharmacol* **10**: S165–8.

Stevens, D. R., McCarley, R. W. & Greene (1994) The mechanism of noradrenergic alpha1 excitatory modulation of pontine reticular formation neurons. *J Neurosci* **14**: 6481–7.

Taepavarapruk, N., Taepavarapruk, P., John, J. *et al.* (2008) State-dependent changes in glutamate, glycine, GABA, and dopamine levels in cat lumbar spinal cord. *J Neurophysiol* **100**: 598–608.

Thannickal, T. C., Moore, R. Y., Nienhuis, R. *et al.* (2000) Reduced number of hypocretin neurons in human narcolepsy. *Neuron* **27**: 464–74.

Tononi, G., Pompeiano, M. & Pompeiano, O. (1989) Modulation of desynchronized sleep through microinjection of beta-adrenergic agonists and antagonists in the dorsal pontine tegmentum of the cat. *Pflügers Arch* **415**: 142–9.

Tononi, G., Pompeiano, M. & Cirelli, C. (1991) Suppression of desynchronized sleep through microinjection of alpha2-adrenergic agonist clonidine in the dorsal pontine tegmentum of the cat. *Pflügers Arch* **418**: 512–18.

Toyoda, J. (1964) The effects of chlorpromazine and imipramine on the human nocturnal sleep electroencephalogram. *Folia Psychiat Neurol* **18**: 198–221.

Trampus, M., Ferri, N., Monopoli, A. & Ongini, E. (1991) The dopamine D1 receptor is involved in the regulation of REM sleep in the rat. *Eur J Pharmacol* **194**: 189–94.

Trulson, M. E., Jacobs, B. L. & Morrison, A. R. (1981) Raphe unit activity during REM sleep in normal cats and in pontine lesioned cats displaying REM sleep without atonia. *Brain Res* **226**: 75–91.

Tulen, J. H., Man in 't Veld, A. J., Mechelse, K. & Boomsma, F. (1990) Sleep patterns in congenital dopamine beta-hydroxylase deficiency. *J Neurol* **237**: 98–102.

Vanni-Mercier, G., Sakai, K. & Jouvet, M. (1984) Neurones spécifiques de l'éveil dans l'hypothalamus postérieur. *C R Acad Sci* **298**: 195–200.

Verret, L., Fort, P., Gervasoni, D., Léger, L. & Luppi, P. H. (2006) Localization of the neurons active during paradoxical (REM) sleep and projecting to the locus coeruleus noradrenergic neurons in the rat. *J Comp Neurol* **495**: 573–86.

Weitzman, E., McGregor, P., Moore, C. & Jacoby, J. (1969) The effect of alpha-methyl-para-tyrosine on sleep patterns of the monkey. *Life Sciences* **8**: 751–7.

Wyatt, R. J., Chase, T. N., Kupfer, D. J., Scott, J. & Snyder, F. (1971) Brain catecholamines and human sleep. *Nature* **133**: 63–5.

Wyatt, R. S., Chase, T. N., Scott, J., Snyder, F. & Engelman, K. (1970) Effect of L-dopa on the sleep of Man. *Nature* **228**: 999–1001.

Xi, M. C., Morales, F. R. & Chase, M. H. (1999) Evidence that wakefulness and REM sleep are controlled by a GABAergic pontine mechanism. *J Neurophysiol* **82**: 2015–19.

Zolovick, A. J., Stern, W. C., Jalowiec, J. E., Panksepp, J. & Morgane, P. J. (1973) Sleep-waking patterns and brain biogenic amine levels in cats after administration of 6-hydroxydopamine into the dorsolateral pontine tegmentum. *Pharm Bioch Behav* **1**: 557–67.

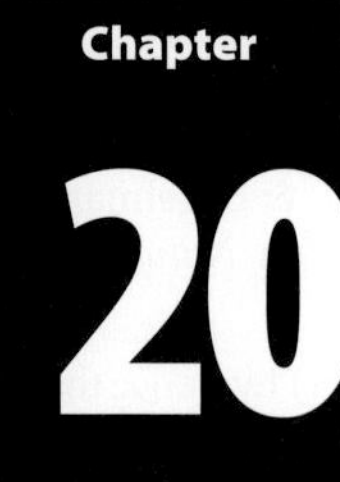

Chapter

20

REM sleep regulation by cholinergic neurons: highlights from 1999 to 2009

Christopher J. Watson, Helen A. Baghdoyan, and Ralph Lydic

Summary

Rapid eye movement (REM) sleep is a behavioral state initiated and maintained by the interaction of multiple neurotransmitters, including acetylcholine. Numerous studies confirm that cholinergic transmission contributes to the regulation of REM sleep. Cholinergic signaling in the basal forebrain modulates the cortical activation that occurs during REM sleep. It is also well documented that cholinergic transmission in the pontine reticular formation plays a role in REM-sleep generation and maintenance. This chapter highlights evidence supporting that acetylcholine regulates REM sleep and focuses on the mechanisms that regulate cholinergic transmission within arousal-regulating brain regions. The chapter also considers how other arousal-regulating neurotransmitters, such as hypocretin, GABA, adenosine, and opioids modulate both cholinergic signaling and REM sleep. A greater understanding of how neurotransmitter interactions regulate REM sleep will further clarify the role of cholinergic transmission in REM-sleep generation. Employing new analytical techniques will facilitate understanding the effects of multiple neurotransmitter interactions on physiologically relevant time scales. Capillary electrophoresis and biosensors, which can quantify neurochemical changes on the order of seconds, will allow insights that could not be achieved with more conventional sampling techniques.

Introduction

Studies investigating the cholinergic regulation of rapid eye movement (REM) sleep date back to the 1960s. A PubMed search in July of 2009 combining the search terms "cholinergic" and "rapid eye movement sleep" revealed 709 publications. Editorial directives for this chapter were to limit citations. Readers are referred to previous reviews (Datta and Maclean, 2007; Jones, 2005; Kubin, 2001; Lydic and Baghdoyan, 2005, 2008; McCarley, 2007; Steriade and McCarley, 2005) for detailed consideration of REM-sleep regulation by cholinergic neurotransmission. This chapter selectively highlights data published from 1999 to 2009 relating to cholinergic regulation of REM sleep. Available evidence supports the view that cholinergic signaling in the pontine reticular formation, basal forebrain, and prefrontal cortex plays a unifying role in the mechanisms by which other neurotransmitters, such as adenosine, GABA, hypocretins, and opioids, modulate REM sleep. Essential findings prior to 1999 are referenced to previous reviews containing the original citation. In cases where multiple reports between 1999 and 2009 have shown similar findings, only the most recent finding is cited. The editorial constraints on citations resulted in exclusion of many remarkable papers and we apologize to our colleagues whose work is not cited here.

Acetylcholine-containing neurons and cholinergic receptors

Cholinergic neurons are phenotypically defined by the presence of choline acetyltransferase (ChAT), the enzyme that synthesizes acetylcholine (ACh), and by the presence of the vesicular ACh transporter (VAChT) (Figure 20.1). Seven major clusters of ChAT-positive neurons have been identified as contributing to sleep neurobiology (reviewed in Steriade and McCarley, 2005). The present selective review focuses on ChAT-positive neurons in the laterodorsal and pedunculopontine tegmental nuclei (LDT/PPT) and the basal forebrain. The LDT/PPT neurons project to numerous brain regions that regulate sleep and wakefulness, including the basal forebrain and pontine reticular formation. Selective lesions of cholinergic neurons within the LDT/PPT causes a decrease in REM sleep that is

REM Sleep: Regulation and Function, eds. Birendra N. Mallick, S. R. Pandi-Perumal, Robert W. McCarley, and Adrian R. Morrison. Published by Cambridge University Press. © Cambridge University Press 2011.

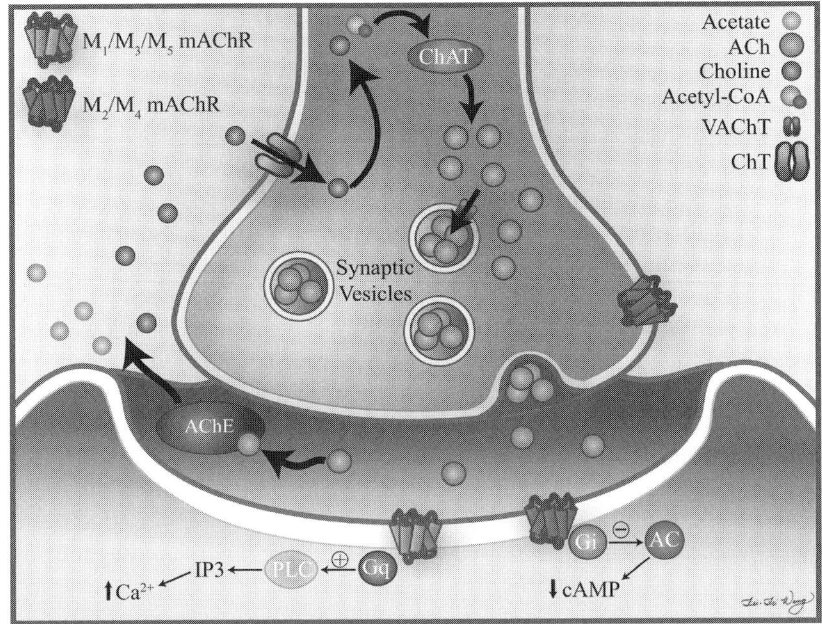

Figure 20.1 Muscarinic cholinergic signaling at the synapse. Acetylcholine (ACh) enters synaptic vesicles via a vesicular acetylcholine transporter (VAChT). Upon exocytosis into the synapse, ACh may bind to pre- or postsynaptic muscarinic cholinergic receptors (mAChR), or ACh may be degraded to acetate and choline by acetylcholinesterase (AChE). Choline is transported back into the presynaptic terminal via a choline transporter (ChT) where choline acetyltransferase (ChAT) synthesizes ACh by catalyzing a reaction between choline and acetyl-coenzyme A (Acetyl-CoA). M1, M3, and M5 muscarinic receptors couple to excitatory (Gq) proteins that activate (+) phospholipase C (PLC). PLC causes a degradation of phosphatidylinositol-4,5-bisphosphate into inositol 1,4,5-triphosphate (IP3) and diacylglycerol (not shown). IP3 mobilizes stores of intracellular calcium (Ca²⁺) and diacylglycerol initiates protein kinase C signaling. M2 and M4 receptors couple to inhibitory (Gi) proteins. Activation of M2 and M4 receptors inhibits (–) adenylyl cyclase (AC) resulting in a decrease of cyclic adenosine mono-phosphate (cAMP). When associated with G protein-gated potassium channels, activated M2 and M4 receptors hyperpolarize neurons (Ishii and Kurachi, 2006). (See plate section for color version.)

proportional to the amount of cholinergic cell loss (Jones, 2005). Cholinergic neurons within the basal forebrain project to the entire cerebral cortex (Datta and Maclean, 2007; McCarley, 2007) and promote cortical activation during REM sleep and wakefulness (Lee *et al.*, 2005). Although the basal forebrain and LDT/PPT are known to contain ChAT-positive neurons, these brain regions are chemically heterogeneous and not exclusively cholinergic (Jones, 2005). To understand how these brain regions regulate REM sleep, it is vital to characterize the functional roles of each neurotransmitter in these brain regions. Furthermore, elucidating the interactions between neurotransmitters is likely to provide new insights into how REM sleep is generated and maintained.

Cholinergic cell discharge and ACh release during REM sleep

The LDT/PPT and the basal forebrain contain subsets of putatively cholinergic neurons that show state-dependent discharge activity. One subset of LDT/PPT neurons, described as REM-on neurons, discharges with the fastest frequency during REM sleep (Datta and Maclean, 2007). The second subset of LDT/PPT neurons, described as Wake-on/REM-on neurons, fires with the fastest frequency during wakefulness and REM sleep (Steriade and McCarley, 2005). A subset of basal forebrain neurons also displays the fastest firing frequency during wakefulness and REM sleep (Lee *et al.*, 2005). The observations that some neurons discharge at their fastest rates during REM sleep are consistent with the view that these neurons may play a role in the regulation of REM sleep.

Cholinergic modulation of REM sleep may also be inferred from measures of ACh release in discrete brain regions across states of sleep and wakefulness. In the PPT of the cat, ACh levels are lowest during NREM sleep and highest during wakefulness and REM sleep (Kodama and Honda, 1999). Acetylcholine release in the basal forebrain of the cat varies as a function of arousal state with ACh levels being lowest during NREM sleep, higher during quiet wakefulness, and highest during REM sleep (Vazquez and Baghdoyan, 2001). Likewise, basal forebrain neurons provide cholinergic input to the cortex, and cortical ACh release is higher during wakefulness and REM sleep than during NREM sleep (reviewed in Datta and Maclean, 2007; Lydic and Baghdoyan, 2005). These data support the view that basal forebrain ACh promotes cortical activation during wakefulness and REM sleep. Acetylcholine release in the pontine reticular formation also shows state dependence in that it is highest during REM sleep compared to wakefulness and NREM sleep (Lydic and Baghdoyan, 2008), consistent with multiple lines of evidence outlined above that cholinergic signaling within the pontine reticular formation promotes REM sleep.

Cholinergic receptors

Cholinergic neurotransmission occurs at two distinct groups of ACh receptors, muscarinic and nicotinic (reviewed in Hogg *et al.*, 2003; Ishii and Kurachi, 2006). Neuronal nicotinic ACh receptors are pentameric, ligand-gated cation channels that can be located pre-, post-, or extrasynaptically (Hogg *et al.*, 2003). Each transmembrane protein subunit comes from a pool of 12 identified subunits designated as α2 to α10 and β2 to β4 (Hogg *et al.*, 2003). Although nicotinic receptors have been shown to play a role in REM-sleep modulation (Salin-Pascual *et al.*, 1999), a majority of research related to cholinergic regulation of REM sleep focuses on the muscarinic receptors. Five subtypes of muscarinic receptors (M1–M5) have been identified (Ishii and Kurachi, 2006). Each muscarinic receptor is composed of seven transmembrane protein domains, coupled to a guanine nucleotide binding (G) protein, and is categorized into one of two subgroups (Figure 20.1). M1, M3, and M5 muscarinic receptors couple to excitatory $G_{q/11}$ proteins, whereas M2 and M4 receptors couple to inhibitory $G_{i/o}$ proteins (Ishii and Kurachi, 2006). As reviewed below, muscarinic receptor agonists delivered into the pontine reticular formation cause large increases in REM sleep. Several studies also have shown that direct administration into the pontine reticular formation of drugs that disrupt M2/M4-activated signal transduction cascades decreases REM sleep (Lydic and Baghdoyan, 2005).

Cholinergic regulation of REM sleep

Increasing endogenous ACh increases REM sleep

Endogenous cholinergic transmission can be enhanced by inhibiting the enzymatic degradation of ACh by acetylcholinesterase or by electrically stimulating cholinergic neurons. Both of these approaches cause significant increases in REM sleep in experimental animals. Consistent with these findings are data showing that inhibiting ACh release or disrupting secondary messenger systems activated by muscarinic cholinergic receptors decreases REM sleep. REM sleep also is decreased by inhibiting the VAChT (Figure 20.1) in the pontine reticular formation. Inhibiting the packaging of ACh into vesicles would be expected to result in decreased local ACh release (Lydic and Baghdoyan, 2005).

Acetylcholinesterase inhibitors also have been used in humans to determine whether increasing endogenous ACh increases REM sleep. Intravenous administration of physostigmine to healthy volunteers during NREM sleep induces REM sleep (reviewed in Lydic and Baghdoyan, 2005; Lydic and Baghdoyan, 2008). Donepezil is an acetylcholinesterase inhibitor used for the treatment of Alzheimer's disease (Kanbayashi *et al.*, 2002). When given to healthy adults (Kanbayashi *et al.*, 2002; Nissen *et al.*, 2006), donepezil causes an increase in REM sleep. Donepezil also decreases REM latency and increases the density of rapid eye movements during REM sleep in elderly healthy volunteers (Schredl *et al.*, 2006). These data are consistent with the pioneering studies of Domino and Gillin (Lydic and Baghdoyan, 2008) showing that enhancing cholinergic transmission promotes REM sleep in humans.

Nicotinic and muscarinic receptors differentially modulate REM sleep

Subcutaneous or intravenous administration of nicotine decreases REM sleep in naïve rats, but increases REM sleep in chronically treated rats (Salin-Pascual *et al.*, 1999). These data indicate that nicotinic receptors act to suppress REM sleep, but also suggest that activation of compensatory mechanisms or receptor desensitization may occur during chronic activation in order to restore REM sleep.

Intravenous administration of arecoline, a selective muscarinic receptor agonist at low doses, to healthy human volunteers decreases REM latency and increases the number of REM episodes (reviewed in Lydic and Baghdoyan, 2005; Lydic and Baghdoyan, 2008). In healthy human volunteers, the muscarinic antagonist scopolamine increases REM sleep latency and also blocks the effects of the cholinergic agonist arecoline (reviewed in Lydic and Baghdoyan, 2005; Lydic and Baghdoyan, 2008). Oral administration of the putatively selective M1 receptor agonist RS-86 to healthy human volunteers shortens REM latency, suggesting that M1 receptors play a role in the onset of REM sleep (Nissen *et al.*, 2006). Taken together, these data show that systemically administered agonists of muscarinic receptors act to increase REM sleep in humans.

Regulation of REM sleep by cholinoceptive neurons of the pontine reticular formation

Cholinergic innervation of the pontine reticular formation originates mainly from the LDT/PPT (Reinoso-Suarez *et al.*, 2001), and medial regions of the pontine reticular formation are known to promote REM sleep (Lydic and Baghdoyan, 2008). Electrical stimulation of the LDT/PPT increases ACh release in the pontine reticular formation and increases REM sleep (reviewed in Lydic and Baghdoyan, 2005; Lydic and Baghdoyan, 2008). Together these data suggest that one mechanism by which the LDT/PPT increases REM sleep is by increasing cholinergic transmission in the pontine reticular formation.

Neostigmine, an acetylcholinesterase inhibitor, microinjected into the pontine reticular formation of the C57BL/6J (B6) mouse increases REM sleep (Coleman *et al.*, 2004; Douglas *et al.*, 2005; Lydic *et al.*, 2002). Figure 20.2 shows that this neostigmine-induced increase in REM sleep is concentration dependent and is blocked by the muscarinic receptor antagonist atropine (Douglas *et al.*, 2005). These data from B6 mice are consistent with evidence from many laboratories indicating that increasing endogenous ACh levels in the pontine reticular formation of the cat and rat increases REM sleep. The atropine blockade of REM-sleep enhancement by neostigmine indicates mediation by muscarinic receptors.

Microinjection of carbachol, a cholinergic agonist, into the pontine reticular formation of the cat, induces a REM sleep-like state with short latency, and carbachol-induced REM sleep is blocked by co-administration of atropine (reviewed in Lydic and Baghdoyan, 2008). The carbachol-evoked REM

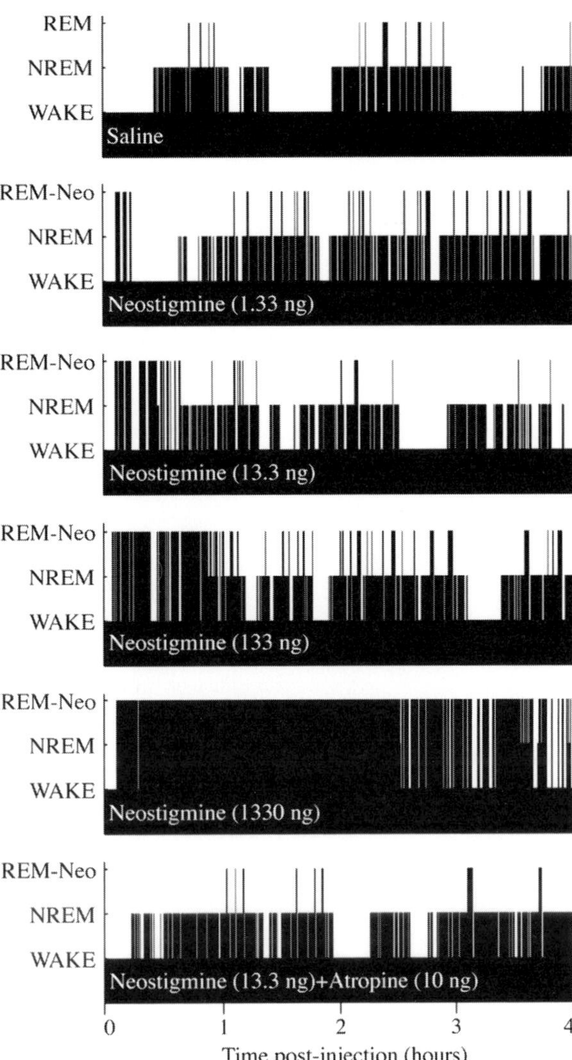

Figure 20.2 Neostigmine causes a concentration dependent increase in REM sleep. Time-course plots of sleep and wakefulness reveal that increasing the amount of neostigmine microinjected into the pontine reticular formation of the C57BL/6J mouse increases the amount of REM sleep. The neostigmine-induced increase in REM sleep was reversed by co-administration of the muscarinic receptor antagonist atropine, indicating a role for pontine reticular formation muscarinic receptors in the generation of REM sleep. (From Douglas, Bowman, Baghdoyan and Lydic, *Journal of Applied Physiology*, 2005. American Physiological Society, with permission.)

sleep-like state is homologous in many ways to spontaneously occurring REM sleep (Table 20.1). The two states are not identical, however, leading some to a diminished enthusiasm for this heuristically valuable cholinergic model. If the strident criterion of orthogonal identity between naturally occurring sleep and

Table 20.1 Similarities and differences between spontaneous (S) and carbachol-induced (C) REM sleep

Dependent measure	Principal finding	Reference
REM sleep	Microinjection of carbachol into the pontine reticular formation (PRF) induces an REM sleep-like state.	*Brain Res* 1974, **68**: 335 *Brain Res* 1984, **306**: 39 *Brain Res* 1986, **384**: 29 *Pharm Biochem Behav* 1986, **25**: 1253 *Brain Res* 1987, **414**: 245 *Arch Ital Biol* 1989, **127**: 133 *Neuropsychopharmacol* 1989, **2**: 67 *Brain Res* 1994, **636**: 68 *Neuroreport* 1995, **6**: 532 *Neuroscience* 1998, **86**: 29 *Brain Res* 2001, **922**: 299 *Eur J Neurosci* 2003, **18**: 2611
EEG frequency	Power spectra of neocortical and hippocampal EEGs recorded during spontaneous and carbachol-induced REM sleep reveal that both states display the same EEG activity. Microinjection of carbachol into the PPT or PRF of urethane-anesthetized rat causes REM sleep-like alterations in the cortical and hippocampal EEG.	*Brain Res* 1997, **766**: 266 (S,C) *Brain Res* 1998, **809**: 307 (C) *Neuroscience* 1999, **93**: 215 (C)
Eye movements and abducens motoneuron activity	Traits (convergence, downward rotations, phasic complex rapid eye movements associated with PGO waves, codified eye velocity) are very similar between spontaneous and carbachol-evoked REM sleep.	*J Physiol* 2008, **586**: 3461 (S) *J Physiol* 2008, **586**: 3479 (S) *Sleep* 2009, **32**: 471 (C)
Motor atonia	REM sleep or carbachol microinjection into the PRF causes genioglossus and laryngeal airway muscle hypotonia.	*Neuroscience* 1999, **93**: 215 (C) *FASEB J* 1989, **3**: 1625 (C) *Sleep* 1978, **1**: 49 (S)
Gene expression	c-fos expression in PRF is increased during REM sleep rebound and carbachol-induced REM sleep. Cat trigeminal premotor interneurons express c-fos during prolonged carbachol-induced REM sleep.	*Eur J Neurosci* 2005, **21**: 2488 (S) *Brain Res* 1992, **580**: 351 (C) *J Neurosci* 1993, **13**: 2703 (C) *J Neurosci* 1995, **15**: 3500 (C) *J Neurosci* 1999, **19**: 9508 (C)
Single neuron activity	In the rat subcoeruleus, carbachol inhibited over 50% of measured neurons (putative PGO neurons) and excited remaining neurons (putative REM-on neurons). Neurons in the cat mPRF increase discharge rate during both natural and carbachol-induced REM sleep.	*Neuroscience* 2006, **143**: 739 (C) *Brain Res* 1986, **386**: 20 (S,C)
Neuronal excitability	PRF neurons depolarize during spontaneous REM sleep and in response to carbachol.	*Brain Res* 1984, **292**: 169 (S) *Brain Res* 1989, **476**: 154 (C)
Respiratory rate	PRF microinjection of carbachol into urethane-anesthetized rat caused alterations in breathing that are similar to those occurring during spontaneous REM sleep. PRF microinjection of carbachol into urethane-anesthetized rat decreased respiratory rate, respiratory minute ventilation, and increased tidal volume, similar to REM sleep.	*Respir Physiol Neurobiol* 2004, **143**: 235 (C) *Neuroscience* 1999, **93**: 215 (C) *J Appl Physiol* 1999, **87**: 1059 (C) *Neurosci Lett* 1989, **102**: 211 (C)

Table 20.1 (*cont.*)

Blood pressure	Blood pressure is decreased during spontaneous and carbachol-induced REM sleep.	*J Appl Physiol* 1999, **87**: 1059 (C) *Exp Neurol* 1986, **120**: 241 (C)
Heart rate	Carbachol microinjection into the rat PRF caused a decrease in heart rate that is associated with spontaneous REM sleep.	*Brain Res* 1998, **797**: 103 (C)
Penile erection	Occurs in spontaneous REM sleep but does not occur in carbachol-induced REM sleep.	*Behav Brain Res* 2004, **154**: 585 (S,C)

drug enhancement of a sleep-like state were imposed on every sleep medication, there would be no pharmacological treatments for insomnia. For example, some benzodiazepine hypnotics disrupt the temporal organization of naturally occurring sleep by decreasing deep NREM sleep and REM sleep while increasing light NREM sleep (Wagner and Wagner, 2000).

The pontine reticular formation contains muscarinic receptors (Brischoux *et al.*, 2008; DeMarco *et al.*, 2003), and the REM sleep-promoting effects of administering cholinergic agonists and acetylcholinesterase inhibitors into the pontine reticular formation occur mainly via M2 muscarinic receptors (Baghdoyan and Lydic, 1999; Coleman *et al.*, 2004). Table 20.1 summarizes some of the physiological and behavioral traits characteristic of REM sleep that are enhanced by carbachol-induced increases in cholinergic neurotransmission in the pontine reticular formation.

Muscarinic receptors localized to the prefrontal cortex modulate EEG activation, which is a trait characteristic of REM sleep and wakefulness. Dialysis administration of relatively subtype-selective muscarinic receptor antagonists to the prefrontal cortex of a halothane-anesthetized mouse revealed that cholinergic signaling via local presynaptic M2 autoreceptors and postsynaptic M1 receptors causes cortical activation (Douglas *et al.*, 2002). One puzzling finding is that microdialysis delivery of carbachol to the pontine reticular formation of the B6 mouse decreases ACh release in the prefrontal cortex (Figure 20.3) (DeMarco *et al.*, 2004). This decrease in prefrontal cortex ACh release may result from activation of M2/M4 muscarinic receptors in the pontine reticular formation, because these receptors activate inhibitory G proteins that in turn inhibit ACh and decrease cAMP (Figure 20.1). Additionally, the effects of pontine reticular formation carbachol on prefrontal cortex ACh release are likely to be mediated by polysynaptic pathways and additional neurotransmitters.

The dorsal subcoeruleus, a region dorsolateral to the pontine reticular formation, is thought to play a role in the regulation of muscle atonia and ponto-geniculo-occipital waves, which are hallmark traits of REM sleep. Whole-cell patch-clamp recordings of neurons in the dorsal subcoeruleus reveal that carbachol inhibits excitatory postsynaptic currents and excites inhibitory postsynaptic currents (Heister *et al.*, 2009). The excitatory postsynaptic currents measured in this study were presumed to be from glutamatergic neurons, and the inhibitory postsynaptic currents were presumed to be from GABAergic or glycinergic neurons. These data suggest that cholinergic signaling in the dorsal subcoeruleus may coordinate the activity of dorsal subcoeruleus projection neurons in order to produce ponto-geniculo-occipital waves (Heister *et al.*, 2009).

Neurotransmitters that modulate ACh release

Gamma aminobutyric acid (GABA) and hypocretin

GABA is the main inhibitory neurotransmitter in the brain and many pharmacological studies of sleep have focused on GABAergic signaling via $GABA_A$ receptors (see Vanini *et al.*, this volume). $GABA_A$ receptors are ligand-gated ion channels that, when activated, allow an influx of chloride ions causing neuronal hyperpolarization. Bicuculline, a $GABA_A$ receptor antagonist, delivered to the pontine reticular formation of the cat, increases local ACh release in a concentration-dependent manner (Vazquez and Baghdoyan, 2004) and increases REM sleep in the cat (Xi *et al.*, 2004) and rat (Marks *et al.*, 2008). Together, these data suggest that $GABA_A$ receptor blockade increases REM sleep by increasing ACh release. In the cat, the REM sleep-enhancing effects of pontine reticular formation

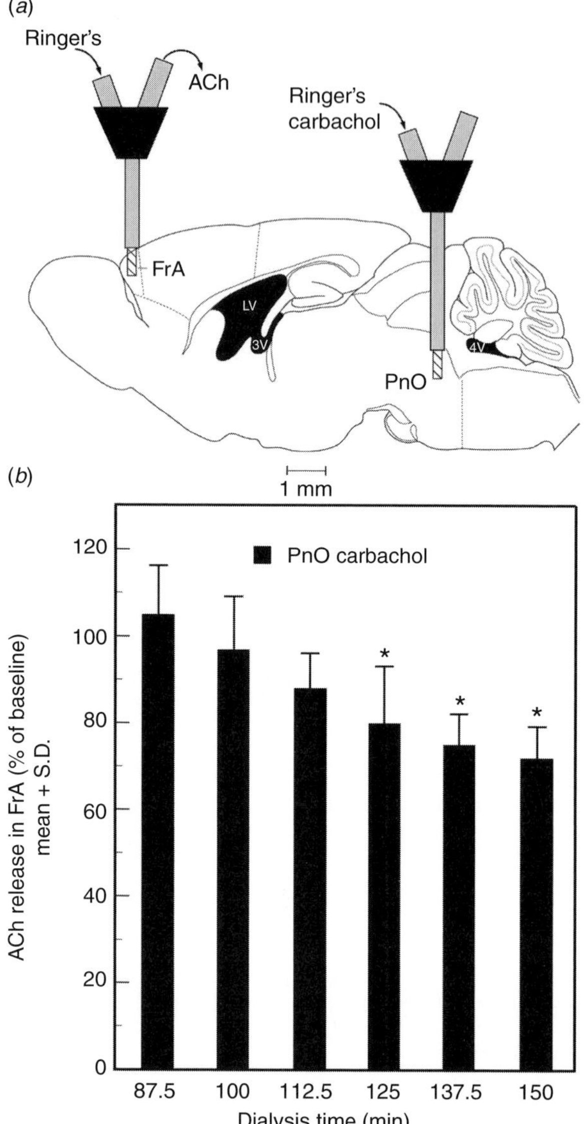

Figure 20.3 Cholinergic signaling within the pontine reticular formation decreases acetylcholine release in the prefrontal cortex. (*a*) Illustrates the placement of one microdialysis probe into the pontine reticular formation (PnO) for delivery of carbachol and a second microdialysis probe in the prefrontal cortex (to measure ACh). (*b*) Shows that administering carbachol into the pontine reticular formation caused a significant decrease in prefrontal cortex (FrA) ACh release. (From DeMarco *et al.*, 2004).

administration of bicuculline were not blocked by pretreatment with scopolamine, a muscarinic receptor antagonist (Xi *et al.*, 2004). However, in the rat pontine reticular formation the REM sleep-enhancing effects of gabazine, another GABA$_A$ receptor antagonist, were blocked by the muscarinic receptor antagonist atropine

(Marks *et al.*, 2008). The contradictory nature of these findings may be attributed to differences in species, muscarinic receptor antagonist, GABAergic receptor antagonist, or brain region of drug administration. These findings warrant further investigation to clarify the effect of muscarinic receptors on GABAergic signaling within the pontine reticular formation.

Microdialysis delivery of the GABA$_A$ receptor antagonist bicuculline to the substantia innominata portion of the basal forebrain in halothane-anesthetized cat causes a concentration-dependent increase in ACh release (Vazquez and Baghdoyan, 2003). Microinjection of the GABA$_A$ receptor agonist muscimol to the nucleus basalis of Meynert, another region of the basal forebrain, increases NREM sleep and decreases REM sleep and wakefulness (Manfridi *et al.*, 2001). Together, these data support the interpretation that GABAergic signaling in the basal forebrain decreases ACh release and also decreases cortical activation.

Delivery of the arousal-promoting peptide hypocretin to the pontine reticular formation increases ACh release (Bernard *et al.*, 2006) and increases GABA levels (Watson *et al.*, 2008) within the pontine reticular formation. Administering hypocretin to the pontine reticular formation increases wakefulness, and decreases both NREM sleep and REM sleep (Watson *et al.*, 2008). Wakefulness can be increased or decreased by pontine reticular formation administration of drugs that, respectively, decrease or increase local GABA levels (Watson *et al.*, 2008). The foregoing data point the way for future studies aiming to clarify the relationship between pontine reticular formation ACh, hypocretin, and GABA (see Vanini *et al.*, this volume).

Adenosine

Adenosinergic signaling plays an important role in sleep-cycle control (Porkka-Heiskanen *et al.*, 2002). Four types of adenosine receptors have been identified and denoted A$_1$, A$_{2A}$, A$_{2B}$, and A$_3$. Each adenosine receptor is a G-protein coupled receptor. A$_1$ and A$_3$ receptors couple to inhibitory G$_{i/o}$ proteins and A$_{2A}$ and A$_{2B}$ receptor subtypes couple to stimulatory G$_s$ proteins (Marks *et al.*, 2003). Dialysis delivery of an A$_1$ receptor agonist (N^6-*p*-sulfophenyladenosine; SPA) to the pontine reticular formation of halothane-anesthetized cat significantly decreases ACh release in the pontine reticular formation and increases anesthesia recovery time (Tanase *et al.*, 2003). The finding that an adenosine A$_1$ receptor agonist delays emergence from anesthesia suggests that A_1 receptors in the pontine reticular formation function to decrease wakefulness. This idea is supported by data showing that microinjection of the adenosine A_1 receptor agonist cyclohexaladenosine (CHA) into the pontine reticular formation of the rat increases REM sleep (Marks *et al.*, 2003). The CHA-induced increase in REM sleep is not blocked by atropine, suggesting that adenosine A_1 receptors do not modulate REM sleep via muscarinic cholinergic receptors in the pontine reticular formation.

Adenosine A_{2A} receptors in the pontine reticular formation may regulate REM sleep via cholinergic mechanisms. Dialysis delivery of an A_{2A} receptor agonist (2-*p*-(2-carboxyethyl)phenethylamino-5′-N-ethylcarboxamidoadenosine; CGS) to the pontine reticular formation of the B6 mouse increases local ACh release, decreases wakefulness, and increases NREM sleep and REM sleep (Coleman *et al.*, 2006). Similarly, microinjection of CGS into the pontine reticular formation of the rat increases REM sleep, and pretreatment with atropine blocks the enhancement of REM sleep induced by CGS (Marks *et al.*, 2003). These findings support the interpretation that adenosine A_{2A} receptors in the pontine reticular formation increase REM sleep by increasing ACh release.

Adenosine in the prefrontal cortex also regulates ACh release in the cortex, ACh release in the pontine reticular formation, cortical EEG activation, recovery time from anesthesia, and sleep (Van Dort *et al.*, 2009). Dialysis delivery of the adenosine A_1 receptor agonist SPA to the prefrontal cortex of the B6 mouse causes a concentration-dependent decrease in prefrontal cortical ACh release, a delayed emergence from anesthesia, and an increase in EEG delta power (Van Dort *et al.*, 2009). This study also showed that dialysis delivery of an A_1 receptor antagonist (8-cyclopentyl-1,3-dipropylxanthine; DPCPX) to the prefrontal cortex causes a concentration-dependent increase in ACh release in the prefrontal cortex, an increase in ACh release in the pontine reticular formation (Figure 20.4), and a decrease in anesthesia recovery time. These findings demonstrate that endogenous adenosine in the prefrontal cortex inhibits waking phenotypes. DPCPX blocks the SPA-evoked decrease in ACh release and increase in anesthesia recovery time. Furthermore, microinjection of DPCPX into the prefrontal cortex causes a significant increase in wakefulness and decrease in NREM sleep. These data suggest that adenosine A_1 receptors in the prefrontal cortex promote sleep by decreasing ACh release, and support the

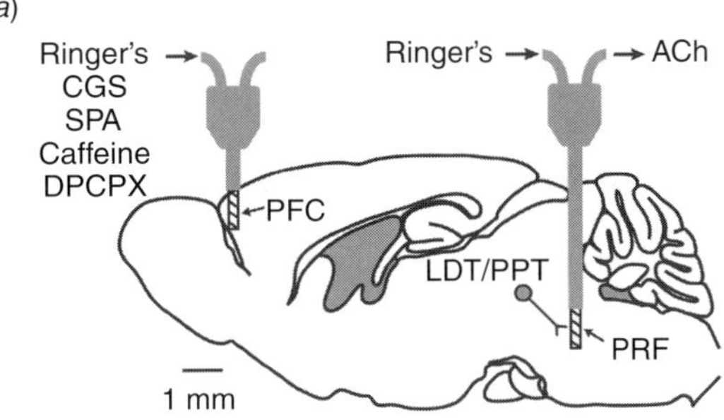

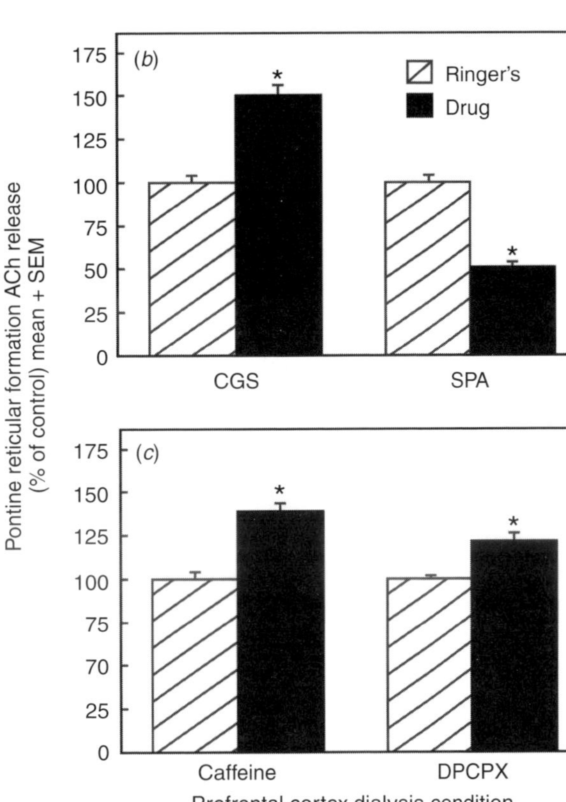

Figure 20.4 Adenosinergic signaling in the prefrontal cortex modulates acetylcholine release in the pontine reticular formation. (*a*) Shows one microdialysis probe inserted into the prefrontal cortex to deliver adenosine agonists and antagonists and a second microdialysis probe inserted into the pontine reticular formation to measure acetylcholine (ACh) release. (*b*) Dialysis delivery of 2-*p*-(2-carboxyethyl)phenethylamino-5′-N-ethylcarboxamidoadenosine (CGS; an adenosine A_{2A} receptor agonist) increases ACh release in the pontine reticular formation whereas dialysis delivery of N^6-*p*-sulfophenyladenosine (SPA; an adenosine A_1 receptor agonist) to the prefrontal cortex decreases pontine reticular formation ACh release. (*c*) Shows that dialysis delivery of an adenosine A_1 (8-cyclopentyl-1,3-dipropylxanthine; DPCPX) or an A_1/A_{2A} mixed antagonist (caffeine) increases pontine reticular formation ACh release. These data indicate that adenosinergic signaling via A_1 and A_{2A} receptors in the prefrontal cortex modulates ACh release within the pontine reticular formation. (From Van Dort *et al.*, 2009.)

interpretation that adenosine A_1 receptors within the prefrontal cortex comprise part of a descending system that inhibits wakefulness (Van Dort *et al.*, 2009). Taken together with the data in Figure 20.3 (DeMarco *et al.*, 2004), these findings demonstrate the existence of a functional network between the prefrontal cortex and the pontine reticular formation.

Opioids

Opioids are widely used for pain management but cause the unwanted side effect of disrupting sleep (Lydic and Baghdoyan, 2007). Morphine administration to the pontine reticular formation decreases pontine reticular formation ACh release (Lydic and Baghdoyan, 2005), increases wakefulness, and decreases NREM sleep and REM sleep (Watson *et al.*, 2007). Morphine also decreases ACh release in the substantia innominata when administered by microdialysis to the substantia innominata and when administered systemically by intravenous injection (Osman *et al.*, 2005). Intravenous administration of morphine causes a significant increase in EEG delta power (Osman *et al.*, 2005; Watson *et al.*, 2007). Direct administration of morphine into the substantia innominata also causes increased EEG delta power (Osman *et al.*, 2005). However, morphine does not increase EEG delta power when administered directly into the pontine reticular formation (Watson *et al.*, 2007). These data suggest that the EEG slowing caused by systemic administration of morphine is mediated at the level of the basal forebrain.

Future directions

Current challenges for neurochemical characterization of a temporally expressed phenomenon such as REM sleep include the limited spatial and temporal resolution of measurement techniques. These limitations can be overcome by the development of analytical methods that enable rapid separation and detection of multiple transmitters in small sample volumes. The most common method for sample collection in neuroscience is in vivo microdialysis (Watson *et al.*, 2006). Typical microdialysis probes have a diameter of 0.24 mm, a membrane length of 1 to 4 mm, and a molecular weight cut-off ranging from 5 to 20 kDaltons. When a microdialysis probe is inserted into a brain region of interest, compounds that have a molecular weight less than the molecular weight cut-off of the probe diffuse into the lumen of the probe along a concentration gradient. Given the correct separation and detection

techniques with the appropriate sensitivity, microdialysis enables the monitoring of almost any endogenous brain molecule of interest. Currently, most methods utilizing in vivo microdialysis are coupled off-line to high performance liquid chromatography (HPLC). Unfortunately, conventional HPLC requires sample volumes in the tens of microliters and is typically optimized to measure a single compound. However, HPLC methods can be optimized to detect multiple compounds in 2 µL sampling volumes (McKenzie *et al.*, 2002). Figure 20.5*a* shows the separation and detection of 11 neuroactive molecules in a single chromatogram. This separation was achieved using capillary liquid chromatography with amperometric detection.

Another capillary-based method that decreases sample volume requirements is capillary electrophoresis (CE). Instead of relying on the partitioning of the analytes between a stationary and mobile phase to achieve a separation (as is done for HPLC), CE utilizes a high voltage to separate analytes based on the charge and size of the molecule. Capillary electrophoresis has been used to monitor state-dependent changes of dopamine, noradrenaline, glutamate, and aspartate in the prefrontal cortex and nucleus accumbens (Lena *et al.*, 2005). According to CE theory, the separation efficiency is independent of capillary length, but the separation time is proportional to the length of the capillary squared. What this means is that if the length of the capillary is cut in half, the separation time is a quarter of the original separation time and the resolution of the peaks remains the same. Optimizing this attribute of CE allows for the separation of eight identified amino acids in 10.5 sec (Figure 20.5*b*) and reduces the sample volume requirements down to the tens of nL range. With this technology it is possible to collect over 240 measurements per hour (Smith *et al.*, 2004), which is a vast improvement over the 4 to 12 measurements typical of HPLC.

Biosensors also address the needs of improving spatial and temporal resolution. Sensor technologies have recently been employed to monitor second-by-second changes in ACh (Bruno *et al.*, 2006). These sensors immobilize choline oxidase and acetylcholinesterase onto platinum electrodes in conjunction with an *m*-polyphenylene diamine coating that acts as a size-exclusion layer. This technology allows for the highly specific detection of ACh on a sub-second time scale. Thus, ongoing advances in chemical sensing technology can be anticipated to further enrich understanding of ACh in REM sleep-generation and maintenance.

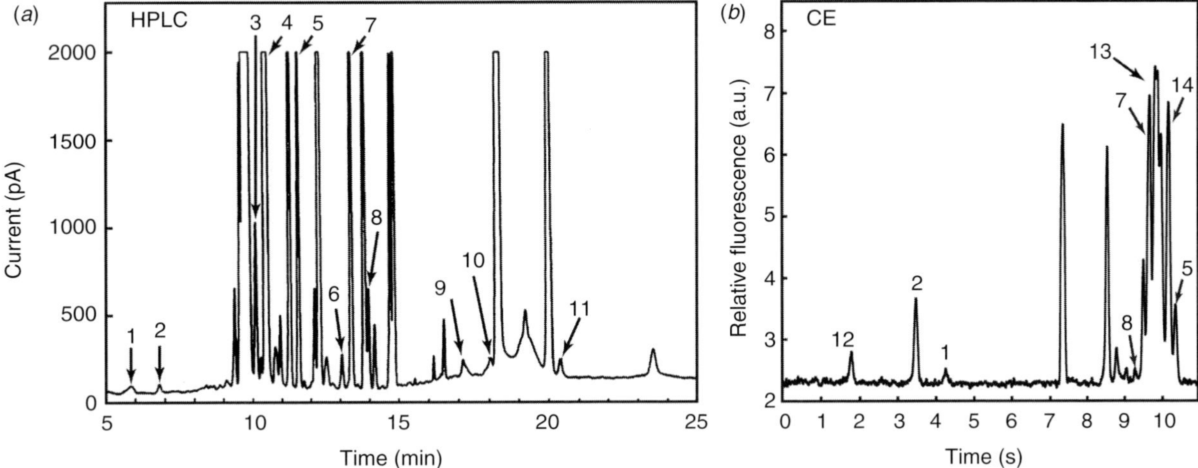

Figure 20.5 Simultaneous detection of multiple neuroactive compounds. (*a*) Shows the HPLC separation and amperometric detection of over 30 compounds (11 of which have been identified) collected via microdialysis from the striatum of the rat. (*b*) Shows that 15 compounds (8 identified) can be separated and detected using capillary electrophoresis with laser-induced fluorescence. Both separations derivatized the analytes using *o*-phthalaldehyde and a thiol (*tert*-butyl thiol for HPLC and β-mercaptoethanol for CE). Notice that the HPLC separation simultaneously measures neuroactive amino acids and monoamines and that the time scale for the CE separation is in seconds. Peak identification key for (*a*) and (*b*): 1, aspartate; 2, glutamate; 3, citrulline; 4, arginine; 5, glycine; 6, β-alanine; 7, taurine; 8, GABA; 9, norepinephrine; 10, histamine; 11, dopamine; 12, *o*-phosphoethanolamine; 13, glutamine; 14, serine. ((*a*) Modified from McKenzie *et al.*, 2002).

Acknowledgments

This work is supported by National Institutes of Health grants HL40881, MH45361, HL57120, HL65272, and the Department of Anesthesiology. This work was not industry-supported and the authors have no financial conflicts of interest.

References

Baghdoyan, H. A. & Lydic, R. (1999) M2 muscarinic receptor subtype in the feline medial pontine reticular formation modulates the amount of rapid eye movement sleep. *Sleep* **22**: 835–47.

Bernard, R., Lydic, R. & Baghdoyan, H. A. (2006) Hypocretin (orexin) receptor subtypes differentially enhance acetylcholine release and activate G protein subtypes in rat pontine reticular formation. *J Pharmacol Exp Ther* **317**: 163–71.

Brischoux, F., Mainville, L. & Jones, B. E. (2008) Muscarinic-2 and orexin-2 receptors on GABAergic and other neurons in the rat mesopontine tegmentum and their potential role in sleep-wake control. *J Comp Neurol* **510**: 607–30.

Bruno, J. P., Gash, C., Martin, B. *et al.* (2006) Second-by-second measurement of acetylcholine release in prefrontal cortex. *Eur J Neurosci* **24**: 2749–57.

Coleman, C. G., Baghdoyan, H. A. & Lydic, R. (2006) Dialysis delivery of an adenosine A$_{2A}$ agonist into the pontine reticular formation of C57BL/6J mouse increases pontine acetylcholine release and sleep. *J Neurochem* **96**:1750–9.

Coleman, C. G., Lydic, R. & Baghdoyan, H. A. (2004) M2 muscarinic receptors in pontine reticular formation of C57BL/6J mouse contribute to rapid eye movement sleep generation. *Neuroscience* **126**: 821–30.

Datta, S. & Maclean, R. R. (2007) Neurobiological mechanisms for the regulation of mammalian sleep-wake behavior: reinterpretation of historical evidence and inclusion of contemporary cellular and molecular evidence. *Neurosci Biobehav Rev* **31**:775–824.

DeMarco, G. J., Baghdoyan, H. A. & Lydic, R. (2003) Differential cholinergic activation of G proteins in rat and mouse brainstem: relevance for sleep and nociception. *J Comp Neurol* **457**: 175–84.

DeMarco, G. J., Baghdoyan, H. A. & Lydic, R. (2004) Carbachol in the pontine reticular formation of C57BL/6J mouse decreases acetylcholine release in prefrontal cortex. *Neuroscience* **123**: 17–29.

Douglas, C. L., Baghdoyan, H. A. & Lydic, R. (2002) Postsynaptic muscarinic M1 receptors activate prefrontal cortical EEG of C57BL/6J mouse. *J Neurophysiol* **88**: 3003–9.

Douglas, C. L., Bowman, G. N., Baghdoyan, H. A. *et al.* (2005) C57BL/6J and B6.V-LEPOB mice differ in the cholinergic modulation of sleep and breathing. *J Appl Physiol* **98**: 918–29.

Heister, D. S., Hayar, A. & Garcia-Rill, E. (2009) Cholinergic modulation of GABAergic and glutamatergic transmission in the dorsal subcoeruleus: mechanisms for REM sleep control. *Sleep* **32**: 1135–47.

Hogg, R. C., Raggenbass, M. & Bertrand, D. (2003) Nicotinic acetylcholine receptors: from structure to function. *Rev Physiol Biochem Pharmacol* **147**: 1–46.

Ishii, M. & Kurachi, Y. (2006) Muscarinic acetylcholine receptors. *Curr Pharm Des* **12**: 3573–81.

Jones, B. E. (2005) From waking to sleeping: neuronal and chemical substrates. *Trends Pharmacol Sci* **26**:578–86

Kanbayashi, T., Sugiyama, T., Aizawa, R. *et al.* (2002) Effects of donepezil (Aricept) on the rapid eye movement sleep of normal subjects. *Psychiatry Clin Neurosci* **56**: 307–8.

Kodama, T. & Honda, Y. (1999) Acetylcholine and glutamate release during sleep-wakefulness in the pedunculopontine tegmental nucleus and norepinephrine changes regulated by nitric oxide. *Psychiatry Clin Neurosci* **53**: 109–11.

Kubin, L. (2001) Carbachol models of REM sleep: recent developments and new directions. *Arch Ital Biol* **139**: 147–68.

Lee, M. G., Hassani, O. K., Alonso, A. *et al.* (2005) Cholinergic basal forebrain neurons burst with theta during waking and paradoxical sleep. *J Neurosci* **25**: 4365–9.

Lena, I., Parrot, S., Deschaux, O. *et al.* (2005) Variations in extracellular levels of dopamine, noradrenaline, glutamate, and aspartate across the sleep–wake cycle in the medial prefrontal cortex and nucleus accumbens of freely moving rats. *J Neurosci Res* **81**: 891–9.

Lydic, R. & Baghdoyan, H. A. (2005) Sleep, anesthesiology, and the neurobiology of arousal state control. *Anesthesiology* **103**: 1268–95.

Lydic, R. & Baghdoyan, H. A. (2007) Neurochemical mechanisms mediating opioid-induced REM sleep disruption. In *Sleep and Pain*, eds. G. Lavigne, B. Sessle, M. Choinière & P. Soja. Seattle: IASP Press, pp. 99–122.

Lydic, R. & Baghdoyan, H. A. (2008) Acetylcholine modulates sleep and wakefulness: a synaptic perspective. In *Neurochemistry of Sleep and Wakefulness*, eds. J. M. Monti, S. R. Pandi-Perumal & C. M. Sinton. New York: Cambridge University Press, pp. 109–43.

Lydic, R., Douglas, C. L. & Baghdoyan, H. A. (2002) Microinjection of neostigmine into the pontine reticular formation of C57BL/6J mouse enhances rapid eye movement sleep and depresses breathing. *Sleep* **25**: 835–41.

Manfridi, A., Brambilla, D. & Mancia, M (2001) Sleep is differently modulated by basal forebrain GABA(A) and GABA(B) receptors. *Am J Physiol Regul Integr Comp Physiol* **281**: R170–5.

Marks, G. A., Sachs, O. W. & Birabil, C. G. (2008) Blockade of GABA, type A, receptors in the rat pontine reticular formation induces rapid eye movement sleep that is dependent upon the cholinergic system. *Neuroscience* **156**:1–10.

Marks, G. A., Shaffery, J. P., Speciale, S. G. *et al.* (2003) Enhancement of rapid eye movement sleep in the rat by actions at A1 and A2a adenosine receptor subtypes with a differential sensitivity to atropine. *Neuroscience* **116**: 913–20.

McCarley, R. W. (2007) Neurobiology of REM and NREM sleep. *Sleep Med* **8**: 302–30.

McKenzie, J.A., Watson, C.J., Rostand, R.D. *et al.* (2002) Automated capillary liquid chromatography for simultaneous determination of neuroactive amines and amino acids. *J Chromatogr A* **962**: 105–15.

Nissen, C., Nofzinger, E.A., Feige, B. *et al.* (2006) Differential effects of the muscarinic M1 receptor agonist RS-86 and the acetylcholine-esterase inhibitor donepezil on REM sleep regulation in healthy volunteers. *Neuropsychopharmacology* **31**:1294–300.

Osman, N. I., Baghdoyan, H. A. & Lydic, R. (2005) Morphine inhibits acetylcholine release in rat prefrontal cortex when delivered systemically or by microdialysis to basal forebrain. *Anesthesiology* **103**: 779–87.

Porkka-Heiskanen, T., Alanko, L., Kalinchuk, A. *et al.* (2002) Adenosine and sleep. *Sleep Med Rev* **6**: 321–32.

Reinoso-Suarez, F., de Andrés, I., Rodrigo-Angulo, M. L. *et al.* (2001) Brain structures and mechanisms involved in the generation of REM sleep. *Sleep Med Rev* **5**: 63–77.

Salin-Pascual, R. J., Moro-Lopez, M. L., Gonzalez-Sanchez, H. *et al.* (1999) Changes in sleep after acute and repeated administration of nicotine in the rat. *Psychopharmacology (Berl)* **145**: 133–8.

Schredl, M., Hornung, O., Regen, F. *et al.* (2006) The effect of donepezil on sleep in elderly, healthy persons: a double-blind placebo-controlled study. *Pharmacopsychiatry* **39**: 205–8.

Smith, A., Watson, C. J., Frantz, K. J. *et al.* (2004) Differential increase in taurine levels by low-dose ethanol in the dorsal and ventral striatum revealed by microdialysis with on-line capillary electrophoresis. *Alcohol Clin Exp Res* **28**: 1028–38.

Steriade, M. M. & McCarley, R. W. (2005) *Brain Control of Wakefulness and Sleep*. New York: Kluwer Academic/ Plenum Publishers.

Tanase, D., Baghdoyan, H.A. & Lydic, R. (2003) Dialysis delivery of an adenosine A_1 receptor agonist to the pontine reticular formation decreases acetylcholine release and increases anesthesia recovery time. *Anesthesiology* **98**: 912–20.

Van Dort, C. J., Baghdoyan, H. A. & Lydic, R. (2009) Adenosine A_1 and A_{2A} receptors in mouse prefrontal cortex modulate acetylcholine release and behavioral arousal. *J Neurosci* **29**: 871–981.

Vazquez. J. & Baghdoyan, H. A. (2001) Basal forebrain acetylcholine release during REM sleep is significantly greater than during waking. *Am J Physiol Regul Integr Comp Physiol* **280**: R598–601.

Vazquez, J. & Baghdoyan, H. A. (2003) Muscarinic and $GABA_A$ receptors modulate acetylcholine release in feline basal forebrain. *Eur J Neurosci* **17**: 249–59.

Vazquez, J. & Baghdoyan, H. A. (2004) $GABA_A$ receptors inhibit acetylcholine release in cat pontine reticular formation: implications for REM sleep regulation. *J Neurophysiol* **92**: 2198–206.

Wagner, J. & Wagner, M. L. (2000) Non-benzodiazepines for the treatment of insomnia. *Sleep Med Rev* **4**: 551–81.

Watson, C. J., Lydic, R. & Baghdoyan, H. A. (2007) Sleep and GABA levels in the oral part of rat pontine reticular formation are decreased by local and systemic administration of morphine. *Neuroscience* **144**: 375–86.

Watson, C. J., Lydic, R. & Baghdoyan, H. A. (2008) Pontine reticular formation (PnO) administration of hypocretin-1 increases PnO GABA levels and wakefulness. *Sleep* **31**: 453–64.

Watson, C.J., Venton, B. J. & Kennedy, R. T. (2006) In vivo measurements of neurotransmitters by microdialysis sampling. *Anal Chem* **78**: 1391–9.

Xi, M. C., Morales, F. R. & Chase, M. H. (2004) Interactions between GABAergic and cholinergic processes in the nucleus pontis oralis: neuronal mechanisms controlling active (rapid eye movement) sleep and wakefulness. *J Neurosci* **24**: 10,670–8.

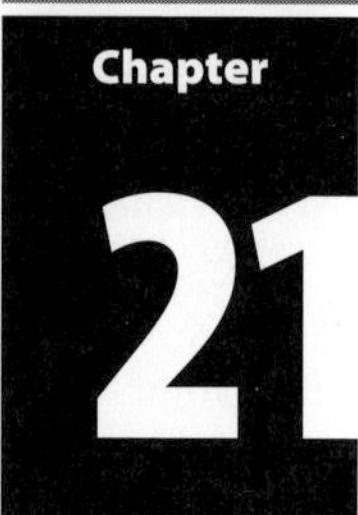

Chapter 21

GABAergic modulation of REM sleep

Giancarlo Vanini, Ralph Lydic, and Helen A. Baghdoyan

Summary

Gamma-aminobutyric acid (GABA) is the main inhibitory neurotransmitter in the adult mammalian brain. GABA receptors are ubiquitous and are highly expressed in many brain areas modulating states of sleep and wakefulness. The consistent finding that drugs that enhance GABAergic transmission also enhance sleep supports the conclusion that endogenous GABA promotes sleep. The effects of GABA on sleep, however, vary as a function of brain region. GABAergic transmission in the pontine reticular formation, the tuberomammillary region of the posterior hypothalamus, and the ventrolateral part of the periaqueductal gray has been shown to promote wakefulness, non-rapid eye movement (NREM) sleep, or rapid eye movement (REM) sleep, respectively. The finding that hypothalamic GABA-containing neurons project to the dorsal raphe nucleus, locus coeruleus, and pontine reticular formation encourages future studies aiming to determine the extent to which these GABAergic neurons play a causal role in the generation and maintenance of REM sleep. Functional neuroanatomical studies have identified neural pathways that contribute to REM-sleep generation. Simultaneous, in vivo single-cell recordings of identified GABAergic neurons combined with direct measures of endogenous GABA offer a productive approach for gaining future insights.

Introduction

Gamma-aminobutyric acid is the major inhibitory neurotransmitter in the adult mammalian brain and is a key element in the central regulation of behavior. The majority of its effects are mediated through the GABA receptor type A ($GABA_A$), which increases chloride conductance causing fast, transient membrane hyperpolarization. GABA-containing neurons, synaptic terminals, and $GABA_A$ receptors are abundant in all brain areas modulating states of sleep and wakefulness (Pirker *et al.*, 2000). The widespread distribution of GABAergic neurons and GABA receptors through diverse brain areas involved in the control of sleep and wakefulness is a challenge for efforts to derive a unifying hypothesis for GABAergic modulation of sleep and wakefulness. Additionally, GABAergic transmission is complex due to the regulation of synaptic and extrasynaptic GABA levels by glia as well as by neurons.

The sleep-promoting effects of GABAmimetic drugs are well known (Charney *et al.*, 2006). Systemic administration of benzodiazepine or non-benzodiazepine hypnotics decreases wakefulness, shortens sleep latency, and increases NREM sleep. Accumulating preclinical evidence aiming to understand the neural substrates regulating states of sleep and wakefulness supports the interpretation that the effects of activating $GABA_A$ receptors on arousal states vary as a function of brain region. In fact, in some brain regions GABAergic transmission promotes wakefulness and inhibits sleep. This chapter highlights the functional and anatomical evidence for the role of GABA in regulating sleep and arousal with an emphasis on the state of REM sleep.

The hypothalamus and REM sleep

The location of the preoptic area (POA) of the anterior hypothalamus (AH) is schematized in Figure 21.1. Not shown in the figure but included in the area of the POA/AH are the median preoptic nucleus (MnPN) and the ventrolateral preoptic area (VLPO) of the hypothalamus. Single-cell recording and *c-fos* expression studies have revealed that the majority of the preoptic neurons display a sleep-active pattern of activity (Szymusiak and McGinty, 2008). Sleep-active preoptic neurons are GABAergic and have reciprocal connections with the tuberomammillary nucleus of the posterior

REM Sleep: Regulation and Function, eds. Birendra N. Mallick, S. R. Pandi-Perumal, Robert W. McCarley, and Adrian R. Morrison. Published by Cambridge University Press. © Cambridge University Press 2011.

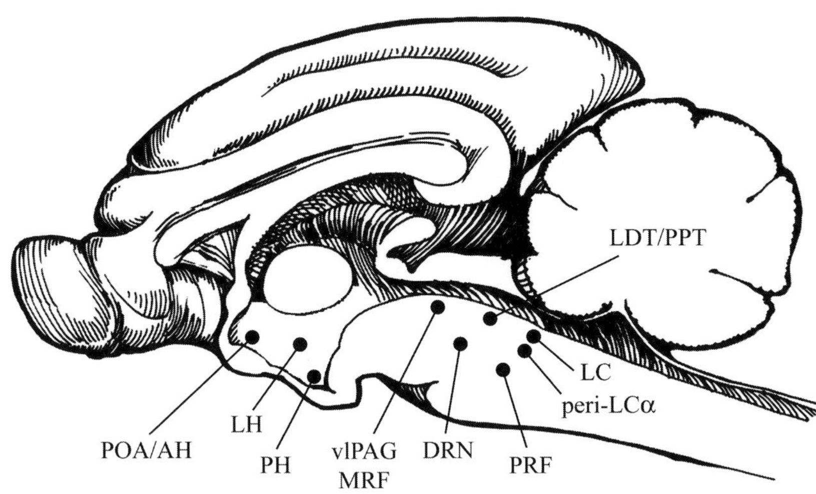

Figure 21.1 Sagittal view of the cat brain illustrating the wakefulness and sleep-promoting areas most studied to date. Localization of each area is indicated by black dots. Abbreviations: DRN, dorsal raphe nucleus; LH, lateral hypothalamus; LC, locus coeruleus; LDT/PPT, laterodorsal/pedunculopontine tegmental nucleus; MRF, mesencephalic reticular formation; peri-LCα, peri-locus coeruleus alpha; PH; posterior hypothalamus; POA/AH, preoptic area/anterior hypothalamus; PRF, pontine reticular formation; vlPAG, ventrolateral periaqueductal gray.

hypothalamus (PH), the lateral hypothalamus (LH), and brain-stem monoaminergic nuclei (dorsal raphe nucleus (DRN) and locus coeruleus (LC); Figure 21.1). Sleep-active preoptic neurons are inhibited by the wakefulness-promoting neurotransmitters serotonin and noradrenaline (reviewed in Szymusiak and McGinty, 2008). These data suggest that MnPN and VLPO GABAergic neurons may mediate the inhibition of wakefulness-promoting systems that is a prerequisite for REM sleep generation. Furthermore, expression of *c-fos* in MnPN and VLPO neurons increases during enhanced homeostatic drive for REM sleep (Gvilia *et al.*, 2006). The presence of anatomical connections between the preoptic area (MnPN and VLPO) and posterior hypothalamic and brain-stem monoaminergic nuclei suggest that the MnPN and VLPO neurons could work to facilitate REM sleep generation by inhibiting posterior hypothalamic and brain-stem arousal circuits. Disinhibition of the medial preoptic area by microinjection of picrotoxin, which functions as a GABA$_A$ receptor antagonist by blocking the chloride ion channel, increases wakefulness and decreases both NREM sleep and REM sleep (Ali *et al.*, 1999). This finding shows that GABA acts via GABA$_A$ receptors within the preoptic hypothalamus to modulate NREM sleep and REM sleep.

Histaminergic neurons in the posterior hypothalamus and hypocretinergic neurons in the lateral hypothalamus (Figure 21.1) are wakefulness promoting and have a wake-on, REM-off discharge profile (Szymusiak and McGinty, 2008). GABAergic neurotransmission in the posterior and lateral hypothalamus is postulated to inhibit the discharge of histaminergic and hypocretinergic neurons, facilitating REM sleep. Microinjection of the GABA$_A$ receptor agonist muscimol into the posterior hypothalamus reverses the insomnia produced by experimental preoptic lesions. The increase in sleep produced by muscimol is comprised of both NREM sleep and REM sleep (Sallanon *et al.*, 1989). GABA levels in the posterior hypothalamus are greatest during NREM sleep, and microinjection of muscimol into the same area increases NREM sleep with no effect on REM sleep (Nitz and Siegel, 1996). GABAergic neurons in the posterior hypothalamus that project directly to the pontine reticular formation (PRF) could modulate REM sleep by inhibiting REM-on cells during wakefulness (Rodrigo-Angulo *et al.*, 2008). Although the majority of data supports a role for the hypothalamus in promoting NREM sleep (Szymusiak and McGinty, 2008), the anatomical and functional evidence reviewed above indicate that future functional studies are needed to determine whether the hypothalamus plays a causal role in the generation and maintenance of REM sleep.

Role of brain-stem GABAergic transmission in sleep and arousal

The reciprocal interaction model provided the first conceptual and mathematical description of the neural mechanisms responsible for the generation of REM sleep (McCarley and Hobson, 1975). This model originally hypothesized functional and anatomical reciprocal connections between REM-on neurons in the pontine reticular formation (PRF) and REM-off monoaminergic neurons of the locus coeruleus and dorsal raphe nucleus. The model has been updated to specify that the cholinergic REM-on neurons are located in the laterodorsal and pedunculopontine tegmental nuclei (LDT/PPT) and promote REM sleep, in part, via activation of "effector" PRF neurons. Updates of the model also include GABAergic input to the PRF REM sleep effector neurons (Steriade and McCarley, 2005). Additional data have identified a role for glutamatergic neurons in the rat sublaterodorsal nucleus (corresponding to the peri-locus coeruleus α in the cat) in REM sleep generation, and it has been hypothesized that these glutamatergic neurons are controlled by discrete groups of brain-stem GABAergic neurons (Luppi *et al.*, 2006). The following subsections review the role of brain-stem GABAergic inhibition in the generation of REM sleep. It should be clear, however, that data from multiple laboratories support a pluralistic control system in which acetylcholine, GABA, glutamate, and monoamines interact to generate all the traits comprising the state of REM sleep.

Ventrolateral periaqueductal gray and adjacent reticular formation

Early lesion studies of the ventrolateral periaqueductal gray (vlPAG) and adjacent mesencephalic reticular formation (MRF) of the cat (Figure 21.1) suggested that these brain-stem regions are involved in modulating pontine structures responsible for REM sleep generation (Petitjean *et al.*, 1975). The finding that a substantial increase in REM sleep caused by delivery of muscimol into the mesencephalic tegmentum suggests that GABA-mediated inhibition is required to deactivate a group of REM-off neurons within the vlPAG-MRF (Crochet *et al.*, 2006; Kaur *et al.*, 2009; Sapin *et al.*, 2009; Sastre *et al.*, 1996; Vanini *et al.*, 2007). These REM-off neurons are likely wakefulness active (wake-on/REM-off), and modulate REM sleep occurrence via descending projections acting on either REM sleep permissive mechanisms or pontine effector neurons. Thus, GABAergic mechanisms within the vlPAG-MRF may promote REM sleep by: (a) inhibition of descending excitatory pathways that project to wakefulness-on neurons, allowing the activation of REM sleep-effector neurons; and/or, (b) inhibition of GABAergic cells that project directly to the PRF, causing disinhibition of REM sleep-effector neurons. Other possible mechanisms may involve the excitation of LDT/PPT cholinergic neurons, or a tonic inhibition during REM sleep of noradrenergic and serotonergic neurons.

Based on the foregoing postulated mechanism, a subgroup of neurons within the vlPAG-MRF must be tonically active during wakefulness, with scarce or absent discharge as the GABAergic system becomes active prior to and during REM sleep. Single-cell activity recorded across the sleep–wake cycle of behaving animals revealed that groups of vlPAG and MRF neurons display state-dependent discharge patterns. However, only the discharge of neurons recorded in the MRF fulfilled the criteria for a tonic descending modulation of REM sleep generation (Crochet *et al.*, 2006; Steriade *et al.*, 1982; Thakkar *et al.*, 2002). Based on *c-fos* expression criteria, Sapin *et al.* (2009) reported two subpopulations of GABAergic neurons in the vlPAG and MRF (dorsal part of the deep mesencephalic reticular nucleus). One group of cells included REM-on neurons that may project to and inhibit the brain-stem monoaminergic nuclei. A second group of neurons displaying a REM-off activity pattern may inhibit REM-on neurons and REM sleep-effector neurons during wakefulness (Sapin *et al.*, 2009). These data suggest that a GABAergic mechanism modulates the activity of neurons within the vlPAG-MRF regions to facilitate REM sleep generation. More studies are needed to identify the chemical phenotype and connections of the neurons that are modulated by GABA. It will also be important to determine whether these neurons have an exclusive role in REM sleep generation or whether they also modulate other state-dependent phenotypes.

Laterodorsal and pedunculopontine tegmental nucleus

Cholinergic LDT/PPT neurons (Figure 21.1) are important for the generation of REM sleep. A large number of GABAergic neurons are codistributed with cholinergic neurons in the pontomesencephalic tegmentum (Ford *et al.*, 1995) and express *c-fos* during carbachol-induced REM sleep (Torterolo *et al.*, 2001). Microinjection of muscimol into the PPT increases REM sleep and decreases wakefulness, whereas microinjection of the GABA$_A$ receptor antagonist bicuculline (Torterolo *et al.*, 2002) or picrotoxin (Pal and Mallick, 2004) increases wakefulness and decreases REM sleep and NREM sleep. These data suggest that GABA-mediated inhibition of wakefulness-promoting neurons, or their projections within the PPT, facilitates REM sleep. In agreement with the foregoing evidence, GABAergic inhibition of noradrenergic projections from the locus coeruleus to the PPT participates in the generation of REM sleep (Pal and Mallick, 2006). In addition to the proposed modulatory actions of GABAergic interneurons, putative GABAergic projections from the substantia nigra to the PPT could be involved in regulating the motor atonia (Takakusaki *et al.*, 2004) and ponto-geniculo-occipital waves (Datta *et al.*, 1991) characteristic of REM sleep.

Dorsal raphe nucleus and locus coeruleus

Serotonergic neurons in the DRN and noradrenergic neurons in the LC are wakefulness promoting and are characterized by a wake-on, REM-off discharge pattern. Thus, both of these monoaminergic cell groups likely play a permissive role in the generation of REM sleep. The subsections below describe anatomical and functional evidence that tonic GABAergic inhibition of these monoaminergic neurons contributes to REM sleep generation.

Dorsal raphe nucleus

GABA levels in the DRN (Figure 21.1) are greater during REM sleep than during NREM sleep and wakefulness, and increasing or blocking GABAergic transmission within the DRN increases or decreases REM sleep, respectively (Nitz and Siegel, 1997a). GABAergic neurons in the DRN express *c-fos* during recovery sleep after REM deprivation (Maloney *et al.*, 1999) and during the REM sleep-like state induced by pontine microinjection of carbachol (Torterolo *et al.*, 2000). Iontophoretic delivery of bicuculline to the DRN increases the discharge rates of serotonergic neurons. Combined retrograde tracing and glutamic acid decarboxylase immunochemistry revealed that neurons in the VLPO and vlPAG are possible sources of GABA-mediated inhibition of DRN neurons (Gervasoni *et al.*, 2000).

Locus coeruleus

Similar to the DRN, endogenous GABA levels in the LC (Figure 21.1) are highest during REM sleep, intermediate during NREM sleep, and lowest during wakefulness (Nitz and Siegel, 1997b). Iontophoretic drug application during extracellular recording of LC neuron discharge from behaving, head-restrained animals showed that bicuculline increases the discharge rates of noradrenergic neurons during wakefulness, and restores tonic firing during NREM sleep and REM sleep (Gervasoni *et al.*, 1998). Furthermore, blockade

of GABA$_A$ receptors in the LC of behaving animals decreases the duration of REM-sleep episodes (Kaur *et al.*, 1997). These data are consistent with the presence of tonic GABAergic inhibition of noradrenergic neurons in the LC during NREM sleep and REM sleep. GABAergic neurons within the LC express *c-fos* in association with recovery sleep after REM-sleep deprivation (Maloney *et al.*, 1999). In addition to these local neurons, combined retrograde labeling and *c-fos* expression during recovery sleep after REM-sleep deprivation suggested that the GABAergic inhibition of neurons in the LC could originate in the vlPAG and in the more caudally located dorsal and lateral paragigantocellular reticular nuclei (Verret *et al.*, 2006). Collectively, the data summarized above provide support for the interpretation that increasing GABAergic inhibition of monoaminergic neurons in the DRN and LC facilitates REM sleep.

Pontine reticular formation

The rostral portion of the cat PRF (Figure 21.1), the pontine reticular nucleus, called the oral part (PnO) in the rat, encompasses the area into which unilateral microinjection of cholinomimetics induces, with short latency, a long-lasting REM sleep-like state (Lydic and Baghdoyan, 2008). Several lines of evidence indicate that GABA in the PRF promotes wakefulness. The PRF contains GABA$_A$ receptors (Pirker *et al.*, 2000), and GABAergic terminals that originate from local interneurons and distant projecting neurons (de la Roza and Reinoso-Suarez, 2006; Liang and Marks, 2009; Rodrigo-Angulo *et al.*, 2008). Extracellular GABA levels in the cat PRF (Figure 21.2) during REM sleep are significantly lower than during wakefulness and NREM sleep (Vanini *et al.*, 2011). Microinjection of GABA$_A$ and GABA$_B$ receptor agonists into the rostral part of the PRF increases wakefulness and suppresses sleep (Camacho-Arroyo *et al.*, 1991; Sanford *et al.*, 2003; Xi *et al.*, 1999, 2001). Conversely, microinjection of GABA$_A$ and GABA$_B$ receptor antagonists into the same area of the PRF decreases wakefulness and increases REM sleep (Sanford *et al.*, 2003; Xi *et al.*, 1999, 2001). Increasing GABA levels by blocking GABA uptake mechanisms or decreasing GABA levels by interfering with the synthesis of GABA in the PRF increases or decreases wakefulness, respectively (Watson *et al.*, 2008). Furthermore, administration of hypocretin-1 to the rat PRF increases GABA levels and increases wakefulness (Watson *et al.*, 2008).

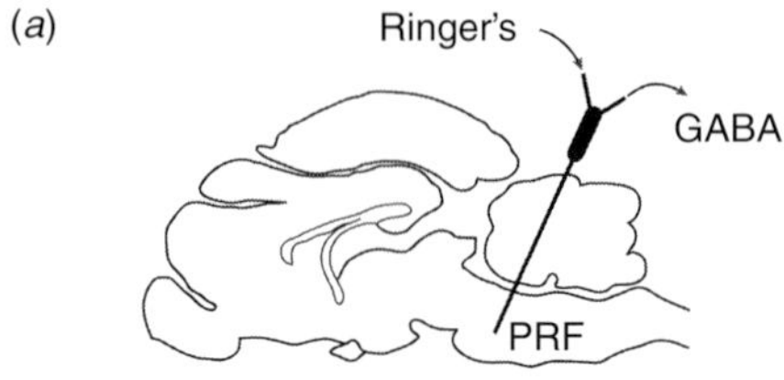

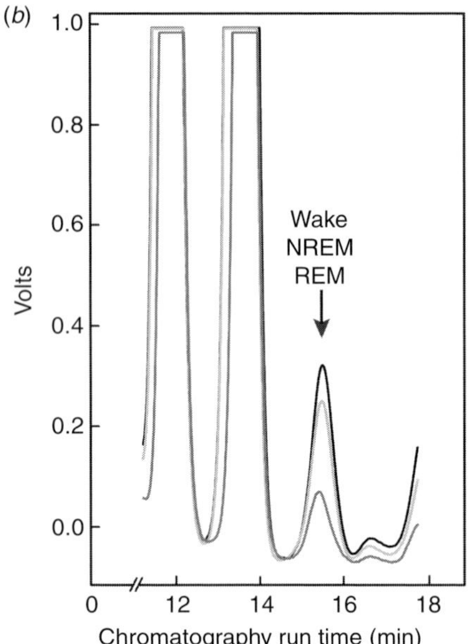

Figure 21.2 Pontine reticular formation GABA levels during states of wakefulness, NREM sleep, and REM sleep. (*a*) Schematic sagittal view of the cat brain showing a microdialysis probe used to collect endogenous GABA from the pontine reticular formation (PRF). (*b*) The graph shows three superimposed GABA peaks (arrow) generated using high performance liquid chromatography with electrochemical detection. Peak area represents the amount of GABA collected from the brain during wakefulness (black), NREM sleep (red), and REM sleep (blue). (See plate section for color version.)

Taken together, the foregoing evidence suggests that endogenous GABA in the PRF promotes wakefulness and inhibits REM sleep.

The mechanisms by which GABA within the PRF promotes wakefulness are unknown. GABA inhibits PRF acetylcholine release (Vazquez and Baghdoyan, 2004) suggesting that GABA exerts a postsynaptic inhibition of the PRF neurons that generate REM sleep (Marks *et al.*, 2008; Xi *et al.*, 2004). In agreement with the concept that decreasing GABAergic neurotransmission in the PRF decreases behavioral arousal, pontine GABA levels are significantly decreased below waking levels during isoflurane anesthesia (Vanini

et al., 2008). The decrease in PRF GABA levels caused by isoflurane is accompanied by an electroencephalographic (EEG) burst-suppression and muscle atonia. Furthermore, decreasing or increasing PRF GABA levels decreases or increases, respectively, the time needed to induce anesthesia with isoflurane. The results suggest that decreasing PRF GABAergic transmission comprises one mechanism by which isoflurane causes loss of consciousness (Vanini *et al.*, 2008).

Subcoeruleus

The area of the rat PRF ventral to the LC and named the dorsal and alpha subcoeruleus (SubC) by Paxinos and Watson (2007) and sublaterodorsal nucleus (SLD) by Swanson (1998) is homologous to the peri-locus coeruleus α in the cat (Figure 21.1), and has been proposed to contain neurons contributing to the generation of REM sleep. Whereas microinjecting cholinomimetics into the PRF or PnO increases REM sleep, iontophoresis delivery of carbachol to the SubC of the head-restrained rat produces wakefulness (Boissard *et al.*, 2002). Iontophoretic application of the GABA$_A$ receptor antagonists bicuculline or gabazine to the SubC causes a dissociated state resembling REM sleep (Boissard *et al.*, 2002). This REM-like state is characterized by unresponsiveness to stimuli, muscle atonia, and EEG activation. However, the REM-like state produced by antagonism of GABA$_A$ receptors within the SubC differs from spontaneous REM sleep by the absence of rapid eye movements and penile erections. These pharmacological data indicate that removal of GABA-mediated inhibition in the rat SubC participates in the generation of hypersomnia with muscle atonia, a hallmark of REM sleep. GABAergic REM-off neurons in the vlPAG and MRF are suggested as probable contributors to the tonic inhibition of SubC neurons during wakefulness and NREM sleep (Lu *et al.*, 2006; Sapin *et al.*, 2009). Whole-cell recordings from knock-in mice expressing green fluorescent protein under the control of the GAD67 promoter showed that carbachol excites GABAergic cells in the SubC and causes either excitation or inhibition of GABAergic cells in the PnO (Brown *et al.*, 2008). This finding led to the postulate that the PnO neurons inhibited by carbachol project to and inhibit REM-on SubC neurons during wakefulness, whereas SubC and PnO neurons that are excited by carbachol project to and inhibit brain-stem REM-off neurons at the onset of and during REM sleep episodes. Carbachol-induced inhibition of

PRF GABAergic neurons is likely to be mediated by M2 muscarinic cholinergic receptors (Baghdoyan and Lydic, 1999; Brischoux *et al.*, 2008).

Conclusion

GABAergic neurotransmission contributes to the generation of sleep and wakefulness. Functional and anatomical mapping studies continue to identify the location, projections, and activity profiles (based on *c-fos* expression) of GABAergic neurons that inhibit wake-on, REM-off neurons and disinhibit REM-on neurons to generate REM sleep. In most cases, these findings are consistent with pharmacologic studies using GABA receptor agonists and antagonists. Additional support comes from direct measures of GABA in specific brain areas known to participate in REM sleep generation (Vanini *et al.*, 2008). An exciting opportunity for continued research includes simultaneous single-cell recording of identified GABAergic neurons combined with measurement of endogenous GABA. The clinical relevance of such studies is emphasized by the fact that sedative-hypnotics and anesthetics achieve their desired effects by altering GABAergic neurotransmission.

Acknowledgments

National Institutes of Health grant numbers: MH45361, HL40881, HL57120, HL65272, and the Department of Anesthesiology.

References

Ali, M., Jha, S. K., Kaur, S. *et al.* (1999) Role of GABA-A receptor in the preoptic area in the regulation of sleep-wakefulness and rapid eye movement sleep. *Neurosci Res* **33**: 245–50.

Baghdoyan, H. A. & Lydic, R. (1999) M2 muscarinic receptor subtype in the feline medial pontine reticular formation modulates the amount of rapid eye movement sleep. *Sleep* **22**: 835–47.

Boissard, R., Gervasoni, D., Schmidt, M. H. *et al.* (2002) The rat ponto-medullary network responsible for paradoxical sleep onset and maintenance: a combined microinjection and functional neuroanatomical study. *Eur J Neurosci* **16**: 1959–73.

Brischoux, F., Mainville, L. & Jones, B. E. (2008) Muscarinic-2 and orexin-2 receptors on GABAergic and other neurons in the rat mesopontine tegmentum and their potential role in sleep-wake state control. *J Comp Neurol* **510**: 607–30.

Brown, R. E., McKenna, J. T., Winston, S. *et al.* (2008) Characterization of GABAergic neurons in rapid-eye-movement sleep controlling regions of the brainstem reticular formation in GAD67-green fluorescent protein knock-in mice. *Eur J Neurosci* **27**: 352–63.

Camacho-Arroyo, I., Alvarado, R., Manjarrez, J. *et al.* (1991) Microinjections of muscimol and bicuculline into the pontine reticular formation modify the sleep-waking cycle in the rat. *Neurosci Lett* **129**: 95–7.

Charney, D. S., Mihic, S. J. & Harris, R. A. (2006) Hypnotics and sedatives. *In the Pharmacological Basis of Therapeutics*, 11th edn, eds. L. L. Brunton, J. S. Lazo and K. L. Parker. McGraw-Hill, pp. 401–27.

Crochet, S., Onoe, H. & Sakai, K. (2006) A potent non-monoaminergic paradoxical sleep inhibitory system: a reverse microdialysis and single-unit recording study. *Eur J Neurosci* **24**: 1404–12.

Datta, S., Curro Dossi, R., Pare, D. *et al.* (1991) Substantia nigra reticulata neurons during sleep-waking states: relation with ponto-geniculo-occipital waves. *Brain Res* **566**: 344–7.

de la Roza, C. & Reinoso-Suarez, F. (2006) GABAergic structures in the ventral part of the oral pontine reticular nucleus: an ultrastructural immunogold analysis. *Neuroscience* **142**: 1183–93.

Ford, B., Holmes, C. J., Mainville, L. *et al.* (1995) GABAergic neurons in the rat pontomesencephalic tegmentum: codistribution with cholinergic and other tegmental neurons projecting to the posterior lateral hypothalamus. *J Comp Neurol* **363**: 177–96.

Gervasoni, D., Darracq, L., Fort, P. *et al.* (1998) Electrophysiological evidence that noradrenergic neurons of the rat locus coeruleus are tonically inhibited by GABA during sleep. *Eur J Neurosci* **10**: 964–70.

Gervasoni, D., Peyron, C., Rampon, C. *et al.* (2000) Role and origin of the GABAergic innervation of dorsal raphe serotonergic neurons. *J Neurosci* **20**: 4217–25.

Gvilia, I., Turner, A., McGinty, D. *et al.* (2006) Preoptic area neurons and the homeostatic regulation of rapid eye movement sleep. *J Neurosci* **26**: 3037–44.

Kaur, S., Saxena, R. N. & Mallick, B. N. (1997) GABA in locus coeruleus regulates spontaneous rapid eye movement sleep by acting on GABAA receptors in freely moving rats. *Neurosci Lett* **223**: 105–8.

Kaur, S., Thankachan, S., Begum, S. *et al.* (2009) Hypocretin-2 saporin lesions of the ventrolateral periaquaductal gray (vlPAG) increase REM sleep in hypocretin knockout mice. *PLoS One* **4**: e6346.

Liang, C. L. & Marks, G. A. (2009) A novel GABAergic afferent input to the pontine reticular formation: the mesopontine GABAergic column. *Brain Res* doi:**10**.1016/j.brainres.2009.08.045.

Lu, J., Sherman, D., Devor, M. *et al.* (2006) A putative flip-flop switch for control of REM sleep. *Nature* **441**: 589–94.

Luppi, P. H., Gervasoni, D., Verret, L. *et al.* (2006) Paradoxical (REM) sleep genesis: the switch from an aminergic-cholinergic to a GABAergic-glutamatergic hypothesis. *J Physiol Paris* **100**: 271–83.

Lydic, R. & Baghdoyan, H. A. (2008) Acetylcholine modulates sleep and wakefulness: a synaptic perspective. In *Sleep and Wakefulness*, eds. J. M. Monti, S. R. Pandi-Perumal & C. M. Sinton. Cambridge University Press, pp. 109–43.

Maloney, K. J., Mainville, L. & Jones, B. E. (1999) Differential c-Fos expression in cholinergic, monoaminergic, and GABAergic cell groups of the pontomesencephalic tegmentum after paradoxical sleep deprivation and recovery. *J Neurosci* **19**: 3057–72.

Marks, G. A., Sachs, O. W. & Birabil, C. G. (2008) Blockade of GABA, type A, receptors in the rat pontine reticular formation induces rapid eye movement sleep that is dependent upon the cholinergic system. *Neuroscience* **156**: 1–10.

McCarley, R. W. & Hobson, J. A. (1975) Neuronal excitability modulation over the sleep cycle: a structural and mathematical model. *Science* **189**: 58–60.

Nitz, D. & Siegel, J. M. (1996) GABA release in posterior hypothalamus across sleep–wake cycle. *Am J Physiol* **271**: R1707–12.

Nitz, D. & Siegel, J. (1997a) GABA release in the dorsal raphe nucleus: role in the control of REM sleep. *Am J Physiol* **273**: R451–5.

Nitz, D. & Siegel, J. M. (1997b) GABA release in the locus coeruleus as a function of sleep/wake state. *Neuroscience* **78**: 795–801.

Pal, D. & Mallick, B. N. (2004) GABA in pedunculo pontine tegmentum regulates spontaneous rapid eye movement sleep by acting on GABAA receptors in freely moving rats. *Neurosci Lett* **365**: 200–4.

Pal, D. & Mallick, B. N. (2006) Role of noradrenergic and GABA-ergic inputs in pedunculopontine tegmentum for regulation of rapid eye movement sleep in rats. *Neuropharmacology* **51**: 1–11.

Paxinos, G. & Watson, C. (2007) *The Rat Brain in Stereotaxic Coordinates*. Burlington, MA: Academic Press.

Petitjean, F., Sakai, K., Blondaux, C. *et al.* (1975) [Hypersomnia by isthmic lesion in cat. II. Neurophysiological and pharmacological study]. *Brain Res* **88**: 439–53.

Pirker, S., Schwarzer, C., Wieselthaler, A. *et al.* (2000) GABAA receptors: immunocytochemical distribution of 13 subunits in the adult rat brain. *Neuroscience* **101**: 815–50.

Rodrigo-Angulo, M. L., Heredero, S., Rodriguez-Veiga, E. *et al.* (2008) GABAergic and non-GABAergic thalamic, hypothalamic and basal forebrain projections to the ventral oral pontine reticular nucleus: their implication in REM sleep modulation. *Brain Res* **1210**: 116–25.

Sallanon, M., Denoyer, M., Kitahama, K. *et al.* (1989) Long-lasting insomnia induced by preoptic neuron lesions and its transient reversal by muscimol injection into the posterior hypothalamus in the cat. *Neuroscience* **32**: 669–83.

Sanford, L. D., Tang, X., Xiao, J. *et al.* (2003) GABAergic regulation of REM sleep in reticularis pontis oralis and caudalis in rats. *J Neurophysiol* **90**: 938–45.

Sapin, E., Lapray, D., Berod, A. *et al.* (2009) Localization of the brainstem GABAergic neurons controlling paradoxical (REM) sleep. *PLoS One* **4**: e4272.

Sastre, J. P., Buda, C., Kitahama, K. *et al.* (1996) Importance of the ventrolateral region of the periaqueductal gray and adjacent tegmentum in the control of paradoxical sleep as studied by muscimol microinjections in the cat. *Neuroscience* **74**: 415–6.

Steriade, M. & McCarley, R. W. (2005) *Brain Control of Wakefulness and Sleep*. New York: Kluwer Academic/Plenum Press.

Steriade, M., Oakson, G. & Ropert, N. (1982) Firing rates and patterns of midbrain reticular neurons during steady and transitional states of the sleep-waking cycle. *Exp Brain Res* **46**: 37–51.

Swanson, L. W. (1998) *Brain Maps: Structure of the Rat Brain: A Laboratory Guide with Printed and Electronic Templates for Data, Models, and Schematics*. New York: Elsevier.

Szymusiak, R. & McGinty, D. (2008) Hypothalamic regulation of sleep and arousal. *Ann N Y Acad Sci* **1129**: 275–86.

Takakusaki, K., Saitoh, K., Harada, H. *et al.* (2004) Evidence for a role of basal ganglia in the regulation of rapid eye movement sleep by electrical and chemical stimulation for the pedunculopontine tegmental nucleus and the substantia nigra pars reticulata in decerebrate cats. *Neuroscience* **124**: 207–20.

Thakkar, M. M., Strecker, R. E. & McCarley, R. W. (2002) Phasic but not tonic REM-selective discharge of periaqueductal gray neurons in freely behaving animals: relevance to postulates of GABAergic inhibition of monoaminergic neurons. *Brain Res* **945**: 276–80.

Torterolo, P., Morales, F. R. & Chase, M. H. (2002) GABAergic mechanisms in the pedunculopontine tegmental nucleus of the cat promote active (REM) sleep. *Brain Res* **944**: 1–9.

Torterolo, P., Yamuy, J., Sampogna, S. *et al.* (2000) GABAergic neurons of the cat dorsal raphe nucleus express c-fos during carbachol-induced active sleep. *Brain Res* **884**: 68–76.

Torterolo, P., Yamuy, J., Sampogna, S. *et al.* (2001) GABAergic neurons of the laterodorsal and pedunculopontine tegmental nuclei of the cat express c-fos during carbachol-induced active sleep. *Brain Res* **892**: 309–19.

Vanini, G., Torterolo, P., McGregor, R. *et al.* (2007) GABAergic processes in the mesencephalic tegmentum modulate the occurrence of active (rapid eye movement) sleep in guinea pigs. *Neuroscience* **145**: 1157–67.

Vanini, G., Wathen, B. L., Lydic, R. *et al.* (2011) Endogenous GABA levels in the pontine reticular formation are greater during wakefulness than during REM sleep. *J Neurosci* **31**: 2649–56.

Vanini, G., Watson, C. J., Lydic, R. *et al.* (2008) Gamma-aminobutyric acid-mediated neurotransmission in the pontine reticular formation modulates hypnosis, immobility, and breathing during isoflurane anesthesia. *Anesthesiology* **109**: 978–88.

Vazquez, J. & Baghdoyan, H. A. (2004) GABAA receptors inhibit acetylcholine release in cat pontine reticular formation: implications for REM sleep regulation. *J Neurophysiol* **92**: 2198–206.

Verret, L., Fort, P., Gervasoni, D. *et al.* (2006) Localization of the neurons active during paradoxical (REM) sleep and projecting to the locus coeruleus noradrenergic neurons in the rat. *J Comp Neurol* **495**: 573–86.

Watson, C. J., Soto-Calderon, H., Lydic, R. *et al.* (2008) Pontine reticular formation (PnO) administration of hypocretin-1 increases PnO GABA levels and wakefulness. *Sleep* **31**: 453–64.

Xi, M. C., Morales, F. R. & Chase, M. H. (1999) Evidence that wakefulness and REM sleep are controlled by a GABAergic pontine mechanism. *J Neurophysiol* **82**: 2015–19.

Xi, M. C., Morales, F. R. & Chase, M. H. (2001) Induction of wakefulness and inhibition of active (REM) sleep by GABAergic processes in the nucleus pontis oralis. *Arch Ital Biol* **139**: 125–45.

Xi, M. C., Morales, F. R. & Chase, M. H. (2004) Interactions between GABAergic and cholinergic processes in the nucleus pontis oralis: neuronal mechanisms controlling active (rapid eye movement) sleep and wakefulness. *J Neurosci* **24**: 10,670–8.

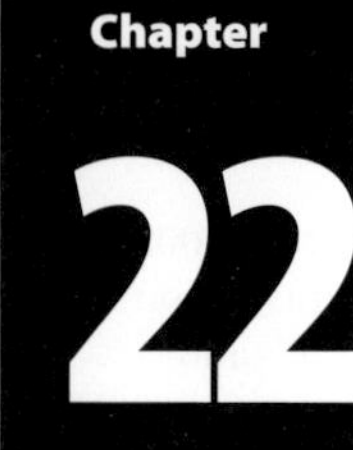

Chapter 22

Glutamatergic regulation of REM sleep

Pierre-Hervé Luppi, Olivier Clement, Emilie Sapin, Damien Gervasoni, Denise Salvert, and Patrice Fort

Summary

Since the discovery of rapid eye movement (REM) sleep (also known as paradoxical sleep, PS), it has been accepted that sleep is an active process. Paradoxical sleep is characterized by electroencephalogram (EEG) rhythmic activity resembling that of waking with a disappearance of muscle tone and the occurrence of REMs in contrast to slow-wave sleep (SWS, also known as non-REM sleep) identified by the presence of delta waves. Here, we review the most recent data indicating that glutamatergic neurons play a key role in the genesis of PS. We propose an updated integrated model of the mechanisms responsible for PS integrating these neurons. We hypothesize that the entrance from SWS to PS is due to the activation of PS-active glutamatergic neurons localized in the pontine sublaterodorsal tegmental nucleus (SLD). We further propose that these neurons are tonically excited across all the sleep–waking cycle by glutamatergic neurons localized in the lateral periaqueductal gray. We finally hypothesize that the onset of activity of the SLD glutamatergic neurons is due to the removal of a GABAergic input from neurons localized in the ventrolateral periaqueductal gray and the adjacent deep mesencephalic reticular nucleus.

Neuronal network responsible for paradoxical (REM) sleep

The discovery of the pontine generator of REM sleep and the cholinergic hypothesis

In 1959, Jouvet and Michel discovered in cats a sleep phase characterized by a complete disappearance of muscle tone, paradoxically associated with a cortical activation and rapid eye movements (REMs) (Jouvet and Michel, 1959; Jouvet et al., 1959). Rapidly, they demonstrated that the brain stem is necessary and sufficient to trigger and maintain PS in cats. By using electrolytic and chemical lesions, it was then evidenced that the dorsal part of pontis oralis (PnO) and caudalis (PnC) nuclei contain the neurons responsible for PS onset (Carli and Zanchetti, 1965; Jouvet, 1962, 1965; Sastre et al., 1981; Webster and Jones, 1988). Furthermore, large bilateral injections of a cholinergic agonist, carbachol, into the PnO and PnC promotes PS in cats (George et al., 1964). It was later shown that PS is induced with shortest latencies when carbachol injections are restricted to the dorsal area of the PnO and PnC, coined the peri-locus coeruleus α (peri-LCα), pontine inhibitory area (PIA), or subcoeruleus nucleus (SubC) (Baghdoyan, 1997; Garzon et al., 1998; Lai and Siegel, 1990; Sakai et al., 1979, 1981; Vanni-Mercier et al., 1989; Yamamoto et al., 1990). An experimental milestone in that field was the discovery by unit recordings in freely moving cats that many peri-LCα neurons show a tonic firing selective to PS (called "PS-on" neurons) (Sakai, 1985; Sakai and Koyama, 1996; Sakai et al., 1981, 2001). Two types of PS-on neurons were segregated. The first ones were inhibited by carbachol, an indication that they might be cholinergic. They were restricted to the rostro-dorsal peri-LCα and projected to rostral brain areas including the intralaminar thalamic nuclei, posterior hypothalamus, and basal forebrain. The second type of PS-on neurons recorded over the whole peri-LCα were excited by carbachol and projected caudally to the nucleus reticularis magnocellularis (Mc) within the ventromedial medullary reticular formation (Sakai et al., 1979, 1981; Sakai and Koyama, 1996).

It has been proposed that (1) the ascending PS-on neurons are cholinergic and are responsible for the cortical activation during PS; and (2) the descending PS-on neurons are not cholinergic and generate muscle

REM Sleep: Regulation and Function, eds. Birendra N. Mallick, S. R. Pandi-Perumal, Robert W. McCarley, and Adrian R. Morrison. Published by Cambridge University Press. © Cambridge University Press 2011.

atonia during PS through excitatory projections to medullary glycinergic pre-motoneurons (Chase *et al.*, 1989; Fort *et al.*, 1990, 1993; Luppi *et al.*, 1988; Sakai and Koyama, 1996; Sakai *et al.*, 2001).

In contrast to the data in cats, carbachol iontophoresis into the rat sublaterodorsal tegmental nucleus (SLD), the equivalent of the cat peri-LCα induces waking (W) with increased muscle activity (Boissard *et al.*, 2002). Other studies using carbachol administration in freely moving rats described either a moderate PS enhancement compared to cats (Bourgin *et al.*, 1995; Gnadt and Pegram, 1986; Shiromani and Fishbein, 1986; Velazquez-Moctezuma *et al.*, 1989;) or no effect (Deurveilher *et al.*, 1997). Finally, the number of pedunculo-pontine and laterodorsal cholinergic neurons expressing c-Fos increases in rats during PS recovery following its selective deprivation by the flower-pot technique (Maloney *et al.*, 1999). However, in our recent study reproducing these experiments, we observed that only occasional cholinergic neurons stained for c-Fos in the same pontine nuclei (Verret *et al.*, 2005). In conclusion, our results in rats are strongly against a role of cholinergic neurons in PS genesis although unit recording combined with juxtacellular labeling is required to draw a more definitive conclusion because c-Fos is not a perfect marker for activated neurons (Kovacs, 1998).

Evidence that SLD neurons triggering PS are glutamatergic

As described above, SLD neurons activated during PS are not cholinergic. We further recently showed that they are not GABAergic. Indeed, the small number of Fos-GAD neurons in the SLD did not increase in rats displaying a PS rebound compared to control or PS-deprived animals (Sapin *et al.*, 2009). It is more likely that the Fos+ neurons observed in the SLD specifically after PS recovery are glutamatergic. Indeed, Lu *et al.* (2006) reported the presence of vGlut2-containing neurons in the SLD. Our recent preliminary results further showed that most of the Fos-labeled neurons localized in the SLD after PS recovery express vGlut2 (Figure 22.1; Clement, 2009). Altogether, these results strongly suggest that the SLD neurons triggering PS are glutamatergic.

Further, it has been shown that the SLD sends direct efferent projections to glycinergic neurons from the ventral and alpha gigantocellular nuclei (corresponding to the cat magnocellular reticular nucleus,

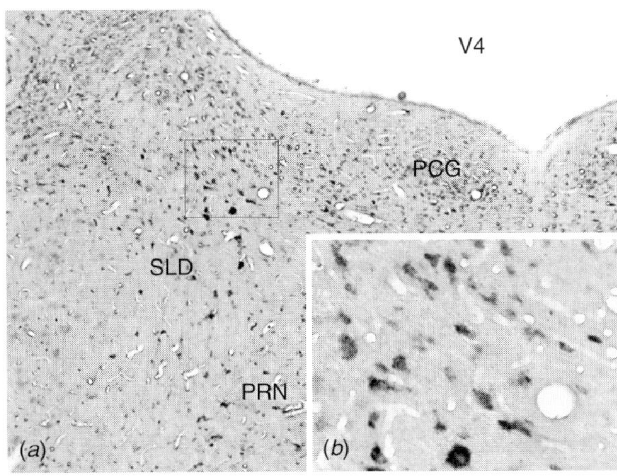

Figure 22.1 Illustration showing a section double-stained with "in situ" hybridization of vGlut2 and immunohistochemistry of c-Fos. Note the large number of double-labeled neurons characterized by a brown nucleus and a blue cytoplasm in the SLD. (See plate section for color version.)

Mc) previously shown in cats to generate atonia during PS by direct projections to cranial and spinal motoneurons. In addition, these glycinergic neurons express Fos after induction of PS by bicuculline injection in the SLD (Boissard *et al.*, 2002), and we have shown that when SLD neurons are disinhibited by Bic, they excite glycinergic neurons of the RMg, GiA, and GiV and also the intralaminar thalamic relay neurons (Boissard *et al.*, 2002). Further, glutamate release in the medullary nuclei containing the glycinergic neurons (namely the ventral and alpha gigantocellular nuclei, GiV and GiA) responsible for muscle atonia during PS increases specifically during PS (Kodama *et al.*, 1998). In addition, injection of non-NMDA glutamate agonists in GiA and GiV suppresses muscle tone while an increased tonus is induced during PS in cats with GiA and GiV cytotoxic lesion (Holmes and Jones, 1994; Lai and Siegel, 1991). It is likely that these neurons are also GABAergic since a large majority of the Fos-labeled neurons localized in these nuclei after 3 hours of PS recovery following 72 hours of PS deprivation express GAD67mRNA (Sapin *et al.*, 2009). The role of these neurons has been recently challenged by results showing that some SLD neurons directly project to the spinal cord and that lesions of the ventral medulla have no effect on PS atonia (Lu *et al.*, 2006). However, it was not determined whether the SLD neurons projecting to the spinal cord express Fos after PS recovery and the lesions were located rostral to the Mc. In addition, it has been shown in cats that SLD PS-on neurons directly project to the medullary level but not the spinal cord, whereas SLD neurons with a firing rate unrelated to PS display spinal cord projections (Sakai *et al.*, 1981). Besides, it has also been recently shown that co-application by microdialysis of bicuculline and strychnine (GABA and glycine agonists) in the trigeminal nucleus during PS induced no effect on atonia (Brooks and Peever, 2008). However, negative results obtained with microdialysis should be interpreted with caution (Chase, 2008).

Sublaterodorsal tegmental nucleus neurons triggering PS are tonically excited by glutamate

In cats, the microdialysis administration of kainic acid, a glutamate agonist in the peri-LCα, induces a PS-like state (Onoe and Sakai, 1995). We reproduced these experiments in rats with iontophoretic application in the SLD of kainic acid and we also observed a firing activation of PS-on neurons reliably associated with the PS-like induction (Figures 22.2 and 22.3) (Boissard *et al.*, 2002). Further, application of kynurenate, a glutamate antagonist, reversed the PS-like state induced by bicuculline (Boissard *et al.*, 2002). These results suggest that PS-on neurons are under a permanent glutamatergic barrage throughout the sleep–waking cycle, unmasked at the onset of PS by the removal of tonic GABAergic inputs. The best candidate structure for containing the glutamatergic neurons permanently activating SLD PS-on neurons is the lateral and ventro-lateral periaqueductal gray (PAG). Indeed, we observed that numerous non-GABAergic neurons in these two structures project to the SLD (Boissard *et al.*, 2003) and they both contain glutamatergic neurons (Beitz, 1990). Although established by Jouvet (1962) that structures responsible for PS are restricted to the brain stem, numerous non-GABAergic neurons projecting to the SLD located in the primary motor area of the frontal cortex, the bed nucleus of the stria terminalis, or the central nucleus of the amygdala could also use glutamate as a neurotransmitter and contribute to the activation of the SLD PS-on neurons during PS (Boissard *et al.*, 2003).

Sublaterodorsal tegmental nucleus glutamatergic neurons are inhibited by GABAergic neurons during W and SWS

By early 2000, we observed that a long-lasting PS-like hypersomnia can be pharmacologically induced with a short latency in head-restrained unanesthetized rats by iontophoretic applications of bicuculline or gabazine, two $GABA_A$ receptor antagonists, specifically into a very small area of the dorso-lateral pontine tegmentum (Boissard *et al.*, 2002). We found that this region exactly corresponds to the SLD defined by Swanson (1998) and not with the dorsal subcoeruleus nucleus of Paxinos and Watson (1997) localized more caudally at the LC level. The SLD also seems to

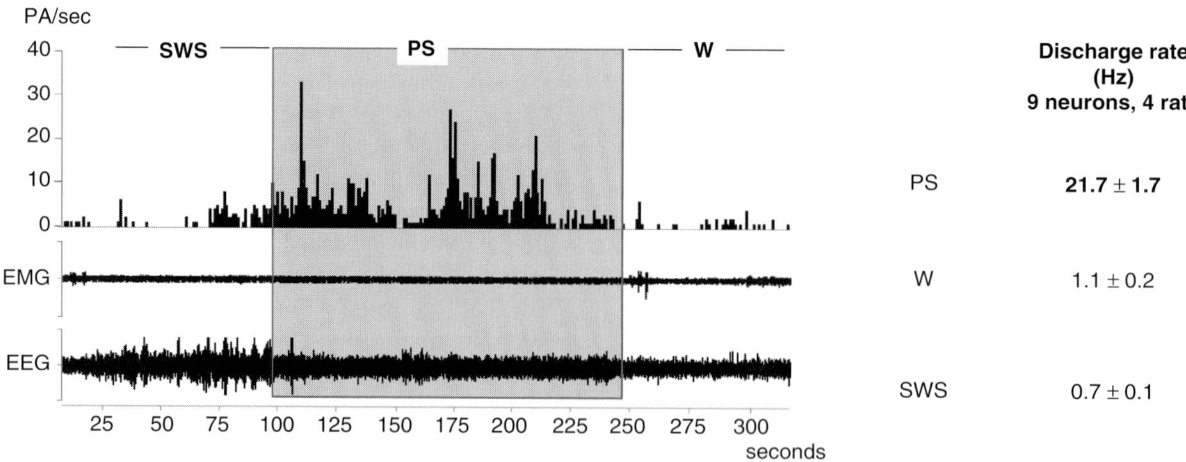

Figure 22.2 Polygraphic recordings displaying the electromyogram (EMG), electroencephalogram (EEG), the unit activity of SLD neurons before, during, and after a PS episode. Note that PS starts slowly from a SWS episode and is abruptly terminated by a microarousal. The SLD unit discharges specifically during PS characterized by the muscle atonia concomitant to EEG activation. The neurons start to fire a few seconds before the onset of PS.

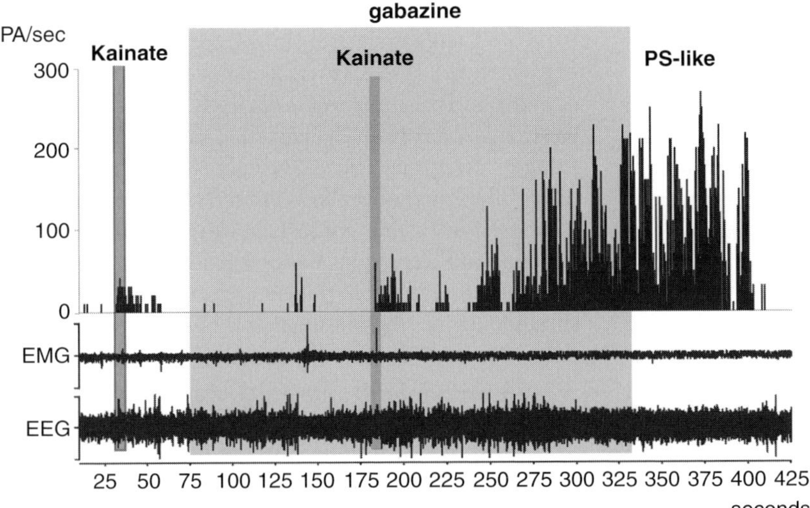

Figure 22.3 Illustration of the effect of iontophoretic application of kainate (a glutamatergic agonist) and gabazine (a GABA$_A$ antagonist) on the activity of an SLD neuron. The ejection of kainate during SWS induces a strong, short-lasting activation of the SLD neurons otherwise nearly silent during W and SWS. The application of gabazine induces after a few minutes a long-lasting increase in firing of the SLD neuron and then an episode of PS.

correspond to the peri-LCα previously identified in the cat. Our results have been reproduced in freely moving rats (Pollock and Mistlberger, 2003; Sanford *et al.*, 2003) and also in cats with pressure injection of bicuculline in the dorsal portion of the nucleus pontis oralis (roughly corresponding to the peri-LCα) (Xi *et al.*, 1999, 2001). In the head-restrained rat, we also recorded neurons within the SLD specifically active during PS (Figure 22.2) and excited following bicuculline or gabazine iontophoresis (Figure 22.3) (Boissard *et al.*, 2000). Taken together, our data indicate that the onset of SLD PS-on neurons is mainly due to the removal during PS of a tonic GABAergic tone present during W and SWS. Combining retrograde tracing with cholera toxin b subunit (CTb) injected in SLD and GAD immunostaining, we thus identified neurons at the origin of these GABAergic inputs. They were localized within the pontine (including the SLD itself) and the dorsal deep mesencephalic reticular nuclei (dDpMe) and to a minor extent in distant areas (Boissard *et al.*, 2003). Supporting the contribution of local GABAergic neurons in the inhibition of PS-on neurons during SWS and W, a significant increase in PS is produced by administration of antisense oligonucleotides against glutamic acid decarboxylase (GAD) mRNA targeted to the cat nucleus pontis oralis including peri-LCα (Xi *et al.*, 1999). In rats, the number of GABAergic neurons expressing c-Fos in the rostral pontine reticular nucleus decreased following PS rebound, suggesting they are active during W and SWS and inactive during PS (Maloney *et al.*,

2000). However, we recently demonstrated that the ventrolateral part of the periaqueductal gray (vlPAG) and the dDpMe are the only ponto-medullary structures containing a large number of Fos-positive neurons expressing GAD67mRNA after 72 hours of PS deprivation (Sapin *et al.*, 2009). Further, injections of muscimol in the vlPAG and/or the dDpMe induce strong increases in PS quantities in cats (Crochet *et al.*, 2006; Sastre *et al.*, 1996, 2000) and rats (Boissard *et al.*, 2000; Sapin *et al.*, 2009). These congruent experimental data led us to propose that GABAergic neurons within the vlPAG and the dDpMe are gating PS by tonically inhibiting PS-on neurons from the SLD during W and SWS.

Role of the monoaminergic neurons in the control of SLD glutamatergic neurons

Another achievement in the research for PS regulatory mechanisms was the finding that serotonergic neurons from the raphe nuclei, and noradrenergic neurons from the locus coeruleus cease firing specifically during PS, i.e, they show a PS-off firing activity, reciprocal to that of PS-on neurons (Aghajanian and Vandermaelen, 1982; Aston-Jones and Bloom, 1981; Hobson *et al.*, 1975; McGinty and Harper, 1976). Later, it has been shown that histaminergic neurons from the tuberomammillary nucleus and hypocretinergic neurons from the perifornical hypothalamic area also depict a PS-off firing activity (Alam *et al.*, 2002; Goutagny *et al.*, 2005; Lee *et al.*, 2005; Mileykovskiy *et al.*, 2005; Takahashi *et al.*,

2006; Vanni-Mercier *et al.*, 1984). These electrophysiological data were the basis for a well accepted hypothesis suggesting that PS onset is gated by reciprocal inhibitory interactions between PS-on and PS-off neurons (Sakai *et al.*, 1981). Supporting this neuronal model, drugs enhancing serotonin and noradrenergic transmission (monoamine oxidase inhibitors, and serotonin and norepinephrine reuptake blockers) specifically suppress PS (Jones, 1991; Jones *et al.*, 1969; Gervasoni *et al.*, 2002). Further, applications of noradrenaline, adrenaline, or benoxathian (an α2 agonist) into the peri-LCα inhibit PS but that of serotonin has no effect (Crochet and Sakai, 1999a, b; Tononi *et al.*, 1991). In addition, noradrenaline via α2-adrenoceptors inhibits the non-cholinergic PS-on neurons but has no effect on the putative cholinergic PS-on neurons from the peri-LCα while serotonin has no effect on both types of neurons (Sakai and Koyama, 1996).

Importantly, our recent data combining TH and Fos staining after PS deprivation and recovery suggest that LC noradrenergic neurons are likely not involved in the inhibition of PS particularly during PS deprivation. Indeed, LC noradrenergic neurons do not display Fos after 72 hours of PS deprivation in contrast to the dDpMe and vlPAG GABAergic neurons. Nevertheless, a substantial number of noradrenergic neurons from A1 and 2 noradrenergic cell groups displayed Fos after PS deprivation indicating that noradrenergic neurons from these cell groups might contribute to PS inhibition (Léger *et al.*, 2009).

A network model for PS onset and maintenance

As described above, the majority of the populations of neurons responsible for PS onset and maintenance was identified, primarily based on Fos labeling evoked by PS deprivation or Fos labeling that is associated with recovery from PS. In the future, it will be important to employ additional experimental approaches to fully determine the role of these neurons, including tract tracing, single-unit recordings, and local neuropharmacological manipulations of these neurons' excitability. Furthermore, several regions that contain a large number of Fos-labeled neurons require extensive study, including the lateral paragigantocellular nucleus, the lateral parabrachial nucleus, and the nucleus raphe obscurus or the dorsal PAG (Verret *et al.*, 2005).

The observation that PS episodes in the rat start from SWS after a relatively long intermediate state during which the EEG displays a mix of spindles and theta activity, and then terminate abruptly, associated with a short microarousal (Gervasoni *et al.*, 2004), deserves further attention. These findings suggest fundamentally different mechanisms underlying the onset and offset of PS. In this context, is worth noting that the duration of PS episodes varies considerably across species. Paradoxical sleep periods generally are shorter in smaller animals suggesting that it might depend on the animal's metabolic rate (Siegel, 2005).

Altogether, these characteristics, as well as our current knowledge of the neuronal network, lead us to propose an updated model of the mechanisms controlling PS onset and maintenance (Figure 22.4). Paradoxical sleep onset is due to the activation of glutamatergic PS-on neurons from the SLD. During W and SWS, the activity of these PS-on neurons would be inhibited by a tonic inhibitory GABAergic tone originating from PS-off neurons localized in the vlPAG and the dDpMe. These neurons would be activated during W by the hypocretin-containing (Hcrt) neurons and the monoaminergic neurons. The onset of PS would be due to the activation by intrinsic mechanisms of PS-on MCH/GABAergic hypothalamic neurons and PS-on GABAergic neurons localized in the DPGi and vlPAG. These neurons would also inactivate the PS-off monoaminergic and Hcrt neurons during PS. The disinhibited ascending SLD PS-on neurons would in turn induce cortical activation via their projections to intralaminar thalamic relay neurons in collaboration with W/PS-on cholinergic and glutamatergic neurons from the LDT and PPT, mesencephalic and pontine reticular nuclei, and the basal forebrain. Descending PS-on SLD neurons would induce muscle atonia and sensory inhibition via their excitatory projections to glycinergic premotoneurons localized in the alpha and ventral gigantocellular reticular nuclei and the nucleus raphe magnus. The exit from PS would be due to the activation of waking systems since PS episodes are almost always terminated by an arousal. The waking systems would inhibit the MCH/GABAergic and GABAergic PS-on neurons localized in the DPGi and vlPAG. Since the duration of PS is negatively coupled with the metabolic rate, we propose that the activity of the waking systems is triggered to end PS to restore competing physiological parameters like thermoregulation.

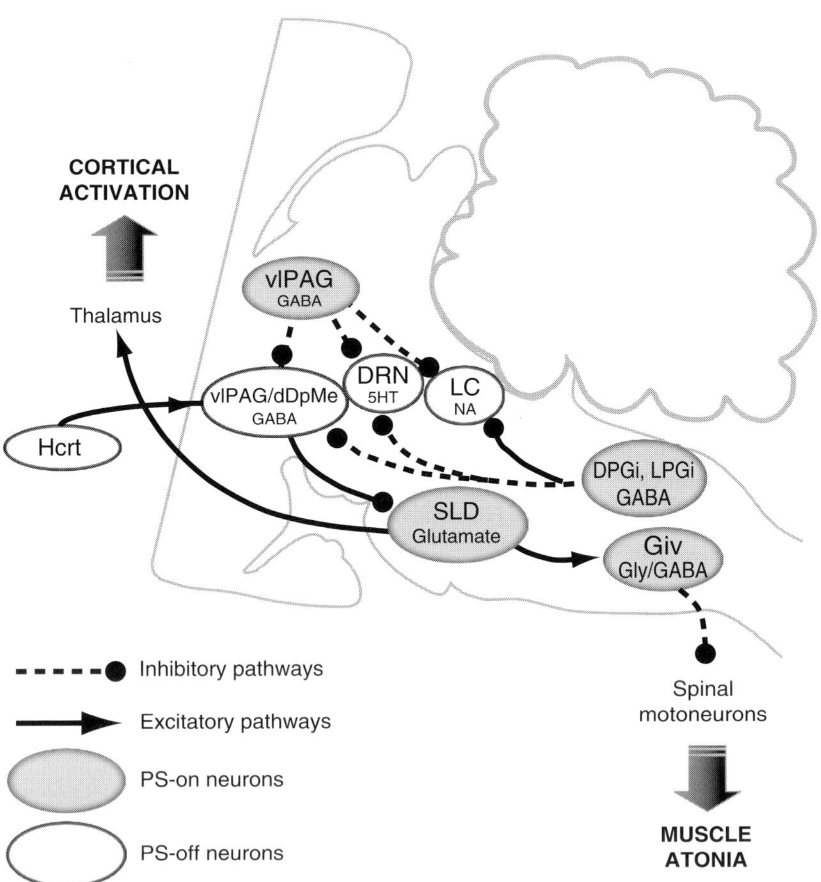

Figure 22.4 Model of the network responsible for paradoxical sleep. (See plate section for color version.) Abbreviations: DPGi, dorsal paragigantocellular reticular nucleus; dDpMe, dorsal deep mesencephalic reticular nucleus; DRN, dorsal raphe nucleus; Giv, ventral gigantocellular reticular nucleus; Gly, glycine; Hcrt, hypocretin- (orexin) containing neurons; LC, locus coeruleus; LPGi, lateral paragigantocellular reticular nucleus, vlPAG, ventrolateral periaqueductal gray; SLD, sublaterodorsal nucleus.

Acknowledgments

This work was supported by CNRS and Université Claude Bernard Lyon.

References

Aghajanian, G. K. & Vandermaelen, C. P. (1982) Intracellular identification of central noradrenergic and serotonergic neurons by a new double labeling procedure. *J Neurosci* **2**: 1786–92.

Alam, M. N., Gong, H., Alam, T. *et al.*, (2002) Sleep-waking discharge patterns of neurons recorded in the rat perifornical lateral hypothalamic area. *J Physiol* **538**: 619–31.

Aston-Jones, G. & Bloom, F. E. (1981) Activity of norepinephrine-containing locus coeruleus neurons in behaving rats anticipates fluctuations in the sleep–waking cycle. *J Neurosci* **1**: 876–86.

Baghdoyan, H. A. (1997) Cholinergic mechanisms regulating REM sleep. In *Sleep Science: Integrating Basic Research and Clinical Practice*, ed. W. J. Schwartz. Basel: S. Karger Publishing, pp. 88–116.

Beitz, A. J. (1990) Relationship of glutamate and aspartate to the periaqueductal gray-raphe magnus projection: analysis using immunocytochemistry and microdialysis. *J Histochem Cytochem* **38**: 1755–65.

Boissard, R., Fort, P., Gervasoni, D., Barbagli, B. & Luppi, P. H. (2003) Localization of the GABAergic and non-GABAergic neurons projecting to the sublaterodorsal nucleus and potentially gating paradoxical sleep onset. *Eur J Neurosci* **18**: 1627–39.

Boissard, R., Gervasoni, D., Fort, P. *et al.* (2000) Neuronal networks responsible for paradoxical sleep onset and maintenance in rats: a new hypothesis. *Sleep,* **23** Suppl: 107.

Boissard, R., Gervasoni, D., Schmidt, M. H. *et al.* (2002) The rat ponto-medullary network responsible for paradoxical sleep onset and maintenance: a combined microinjection and functional neuroanatomical study. *Eur J Neurosci* **16**: 1959–73.

Bourgin, P., Escourrou, P., Gaultier, C. & Adrien, J. (1995) Induction of rapid eye movement sleep by carbachol infusion into the pontine reticular formation in the rat. *Neuroreport* **6**: 532–6.

Brooks, P. L. & Peever, J. H. (2008) Glycinergic and GABA(A)-mediated inhibition of somatic motoneurons does not mediate rapid eye movement sleep motor atonia. *J Neurosci* **28**: 3535–45.

Carli, G. & Zanchetti, A. (1965) A study of pontine lesions suppressing deep sleep in the cat. *Arch Ital Biol* **103**: 751–88.

Chase, M. H. (2008) Confirmation of the consensus that glycinergic postsynaptic inhibition is responsible for the atonia of REM sleep. *Sleep* **31**, 1487–91; discussion 1492–97.

Chase, M. H., Soja, P. J. & Morales, F. R. (1989) Evidence that glycine mediates the postsynaptic potentials that inhibit lumbar motoneurons during the atonia of active sleep. *J Neurosci* **9**: 743–51.

Crochet, S., Onoe, H. & Sakai, K. (2006) A potent non-monoaminergic paradoxical sleep inhibitory system: a reverse microdialysis and single-unit recording study. *Eur J Neurosci* **24**: 1404–12.

Crochet, S. & Sakai, K. (1999a) Alpha-2 adrenoceptor mediated paradoxical (REM) sleep inhibition in the cat. *Neuroreport* **10**: 2199–204.

Crochet, S. & Sakai, K. (1999b) Effects of microdialysis application of monoamines on the EEG and behavioural states in the cat mesopontine tegmentum. *Eur J Neurosci* **11**: 3738–52.

Deurveilher, S., Hars, B. & Hennevin, E. (1997) Pontine microinjection of carbachol does not reliably enhance paradoxical sleep in rats. *Sleep* **20**: 593–607.

Fort, P., Luppi, P. H. & Jouvet, M. (1993) Glycine-immunoreactive neurones in the cat brain stem reticular formation. *Neuroreport* **4**: 1123–6.

Fort, P., Luppi, P. H., Wenthold, R. & Jouvet, M. (1990) [Glycine immunoreactive neurons in the medulla oblongata in cats]. *C R Acad Sci III*, **311**: 205–12.

Garzon, M., De Andres, I. & Reinoso-Suarez, F. (1998) Sleep patterns after carbachol delivery in the ventral oral pontine tegmentum of the cat. *Neuroscience* **83**: 1137–44.

George, R., Haslett, W. L. & Jenden, D. J. (1964) A cholinergic mechanism in the brainstem reticular formation: induction of paradocixal sleep. *Int J Neuropharmacol* **3**: 541–52.

Gervasoni, D., Lin, S. C., Ribeiro, S., *et al.* (2004) Global forebrain dynamics predict rat behavioral states and their transitions. *J Neurosci* **24**: 11,137–47.

Gervasoni, D., Panconi, E., Henninot, V., *et al.* (2002) Effect of chronic treatment with milnacipran on sleep architecture in rats compared with paroxetine and imipramine. *Pharmacol Biochem Behav* **73**: 557–63.

Gnadt, J. W. & Pegram, G. V. (1986) Cholinergic brainstem mechanisms of REM sleep in the rat. *Brain Res* **384**: 29–41.

Goutagny, R., Luppi, P. H., Salvert, D., Gervasoni, D. & Fort, P. (2005) GABAergic control of hypothalamic melanin-concentrating hormone-containing neurons across the sleep-waking cycle. *Neuroreport* **16**: 1069–73.

Hobson, J. A., McCarley, R. W. & Wyzinski, P. W. (1975) Sleep cycle oscillation: reciprocal discharge by two brainstem neuronal groups. *Science* **189**: 55–8.

Holmes, C. J. & Jones, B. E. (1994) Importance of cholinergic, GABAergic, serotonergic and other neurons in the medial medullary reticular formation for sleep-wake states studied by cytotoxic lesions in the cat. *Neuroscience* **62**: 1179–200.

Jones, B. E. (1991) Paradoxical sleep and its chemical/structural substrates in the brain. *Neuroscience* **40**: 637–56.

Jones, B.E., Bobillier, P. & Jouvet, M. (1969) [Effect of destruction of neurons containing catecholamines of the mesencephalon on the wake-sleep cycle in cats]. *C R Seances Soc Biol Fil* **163**; 176–80.

Jouvet, M. (1962) Recherches sur les structures nerveuses et les mécanismes responsables des différentes phases du sommeil physiologique. *Arch Ital Biol* **100**: 125–206.

Jouvet, M. (1965) [The paradoxical phase of sleep]. *Int J Neurol* **5**: 131–50.

Jouvet, M. & Michel, F. (1959) Corrélations électromyographiques du sommeil chez le chat décortiqué et mésencéphalique chronique. *CR Soc Biol* **153**: 422–5.

Jouvet, M., Michel, F. & Courjon, J. (1959) Sur un stade d'activité électrique cérébrale rapide au cours du sommeil physiologique. *CR Seances Soc Biol* **153**: 1024–8.

Kodama, T., Lai, Y. Y. & Siegel, J. M. (1998) Enhanced glutamate release during REM sleep in the rostromedial medulla as measured by in vivo microdialysis. *Brain Res* **780**: 178–81.

Kovacs, K. J. (1998) c-Fos as a transcription factor: a stressful (re)view from a functional map. *Neurochem Int* **33**: 287–97.

Lai, Y. Y. & Siegel, J. M. (1990) Cardiovascular and muscle tone changes produced by microinjection of cholinergic and glutamatergic agonists in dorsolateral pons and medial medulla. *Brain Res* **514**: 27–36.

Lai, Y. Y. & Siegel, J. M. (1991) Pontomedullary glutamate receptors mediating locomotion and muscle tone suppression. *J Neurosci* **11**: 2931–7.

Lee, M. G., Hassani, O. K. & Jones, B. E. (2005) Discharge of identified orexin/hypocretin neurons across the sleep-waking cycle. *J Neurosci* **25**: 6716–20.

Léger, L., Goutagny, R., Sapin, E. *et al.* (2009) Noradrenergic neurons expressing Fos during waking and paradoxical sleep deprivation in the rat. *J Chem Neuroanat* **37**: 149–57.

Lu, J., Sherman, D., Devor, M. & Saper, C. B. (2006) A putative flip-flop switch for control of REM sleep. *Nature* **441**: 589–94.

Luppi, P. H., Sakai, K., Fort, P., Salvert, D. & Jouvet, M. (1988) The nuclei of origin of monoaminergic, peptidergic, and cholinergic afferents to the cat nucleus reticularis magnocellularis: a double-labeling study with cholera toxin as a retrograde tracer. *J Comp Neurol* **277**: 1–20.

Maloney, K. J., Mainville, L. & Jones, B. E. (1999) Differential c-Fos expression in cholinergic, monoaminergic, and GABAergic cell groups of the pontomesencephalic tegmentum after paradoxical sleep deprivation and recovery. *J Neurosci* **19**: 3057–72.

Maloney, K. J., Mainville, L. & Jones, B. E. (2000) c-Fos expression in GABAergic, serotonergic, and other neurons of the pontomedullary reticular formation and raphe after paradoxical sleep deprivation and recovery. *J Neurosci* **20**: 4669–79.

McCarley, R. W. & Hobson, J. A. (1975) Neuronal excitability modulation over the sleep cycle: a structural and mathematical model. *Science* **189**: 58–60.

McGinty, D. J. & Harper, R. M. (1976) Dorsal raphe neurons: depression of firing during sleep in cats. *Brain Res* **101**: 569–75.

Mileykovskiy, B. Y., Kiyashchenko, L. I. & Siegel, J. M. (2005) Behavioral correlates of activity in identified hypocretin/orexin neurons. *Neuron* **46**: 787–98.

Onoe, H. & Sakai, K. (1995) Kainate receptors: a novel mechanism in paradoxical (REM) sleep generation. *Neuroreport* **6**: 353–6.

Paxinos, G. & Watson, C. (1997) *The Rat Brain in Stereotaxic Coordinates*. Orlando: Academic Press, Sydney.

Pollock, M. S. & Mistlberger, R. E. (2003) Rapid eye movement sleep induction by microinjection of the GABA-A antagonist bicuculline into the dorsal subcoeruleus area of the rat. *Brain Res* **962**: 68–77.

Sakai, K. (1985) Neurons responsible for paradoxical sleep. In *Sleep: Neurotransmitters and Neuromodulators*, eds. A. Wauquier & Janssen Research Foundation. New York: Raven Press, pp. 29–42.

Sakai, K., Crochet, S. & Onoe, H. (2001) Pontine structures and mechanisms involved in the generation of paradoxical (REM) sleep. *Arch Ital Biol* **139**: 93–107.

Sakai, K., Kanamori, N. & Jouvet, M. (1979) [Neuronal activity specific to paradoxical sleep in the bulbar reticular formation in the unrestrained cat]. *C R Seances Acad Sci D* **289**: 557–61.

Sakai, K. & Koyama, Y. (1996) Are there cholinergic and non-cholinergic paradoxical sleep-on neurones in the pons? *Neuroreport* **7**: 2449–53.

Sakai, K., Sastre, J. P., Kanamori, N. & Jouvet, M. (1981) State-specific neurones in the ponto-medullary reticular formation with special reference to the postural atonia during paradoxical sleep in the cat. In *Brain Mechanisms of Perceptual Awareness and Purposeful Behavior*, eds. O. Pompeiano & C. Aimone Marsan. New York: Raven Press, pp. 405–29.

Sanford, L. D., Tang, X., Xiao, J., Ross, R. J. & Morrison, A. R. (2003) GABAergic regulation of REM sleep in reticularis pontis oralis and caudalis in rats. *Journal of Neurophysiology* **90**: 938–45.

Sapin, E., Lapray, D., Berod, A. *et al.* (2009) Localization of the brainstem GABAergic neurons controlling paradoxical (REM) sleep. *PLoS ONE* **4**: e4272.

Sastre, J. P., Buda, C., Kitahama, K. & Jouvet, M. (1996) Importance of the ventrolateral region of the periaqueductal gray and adjacent tegmentum in the control of paradoxical sleep as studied by muscimol microinjections in the cat. *Neuroscience* **74**: 415–26.

Sastre, J. P., Buda, C., Lin, J. S. & Jouvet, M. (2000) Differential c-fos expression in the rhinencephalon and striatum after enhanced sleep-wake states in the cat. *Eur J Neurosci* **12**: 1397–410.

Sastre, J. P., Sakai, K. & Jouvet, M. (1981) Are the gigantocellular tegmental field neurons responsible for paradoxical sleep? *Brain Res* **229**: 147–61.

Shiromani, P. J. & Fishbein, W. (1986) Continuous pontine cholinergic microinfusion via mini-pump induces sustained alterations in rapid eye movement (REM) sleep. *Pharmacol Biochem Behav* **25**: 1253–61.

Siegel, J. M. (2005) Clues to the functions of mammalian sleep. *Nature* **437**: 1264–71.

Swanson, L. W. (1998) *Brain Maps: Structure of the Rat Brain: A Laboratory Guide with Printed and Electronic Templates for Data, Models, and Schematics*. New York: Elsevier.

Takahashi, K., Lin, J. S. & Sakai, K. (2006) Neuronal activity of histaminergic tuberomammillary neurons during wake–sleep states in the mouse. *J Neurosci* **26**: 10,292–8.

Tononi, G., Pompeiano, M. & Cirelli, C. (1991) Suppression of desynchronized sleep through microinjection of the alpha 2-adrenergic agonist clonidine in the dorsal pontine tegmentum of the cat. *Pflugers Arch* **418**: 512–18.

Vanni-Mercier, G., Sakai, K. & Jouvet, M. (1984) [Specific neurons for wakefulness in the posterior hypothalamus in the cat]. *C R Acad Sci III* **298**: 195–200.

Vanni-Mercier, G., Sakai, K., Lin, J. S. & Jouvet, M. (1989) Mapping of cholinoceptive brainstem structures responsible for the generation of paradoxical sleep in the cat. *Arch Ital Biol* **127**: 133–64.

Velazquez-Moctezuma, J., Gillin, J. C. & Shiromani, P. J. (1989) Effect of specific M1, M2 muscarinic receptor agonists on REM sleep generation. *Brain Res* **503**: 128–31.

Verret, L., Leger, L., Fort, P. & Luppi, P. H. (2005) Cholinergic and noncholinergic brainstem neurons expressing Fos after paradoxical (REM) sleep deprivation and recovery. *Eur J Neurosci* **21**: 2488–504.

Webster, H. H. & Jones, B. E. (1988) Neurotoxic lesions of the dorsolateral pontomesencephalic tegmentum-cholinergic cell area in the cat. II. Effects upon sleep-waking states. *Brain Res* **458**: 285–302.

Xi, M. C., Morales, F. R. & Chase, M. H. (1999) Evidence that wakefulness and REM sleep are controlled by a GABAergic pontine mechanism. *J Neurophysiol* **82**: 2015–19.

Xi, M. C., Morales, F. R. & Chase, M. H. (2001) The motor inhibitory system operating during active sleep is tonically suppressed by GABAergic mechanisms during other states. *J Neurophysiol* **86**: 1908–15.

Yamamoto, K., Mamelak, A. N., Quattrochi, J. J. & Hobson, J. A. (1990) A cholinoceptive desynchronized sleep induction zone in the anterodorsal pontine tegmentum: locus of the sensitive region. *Neuroscience* **39**: 279–93.

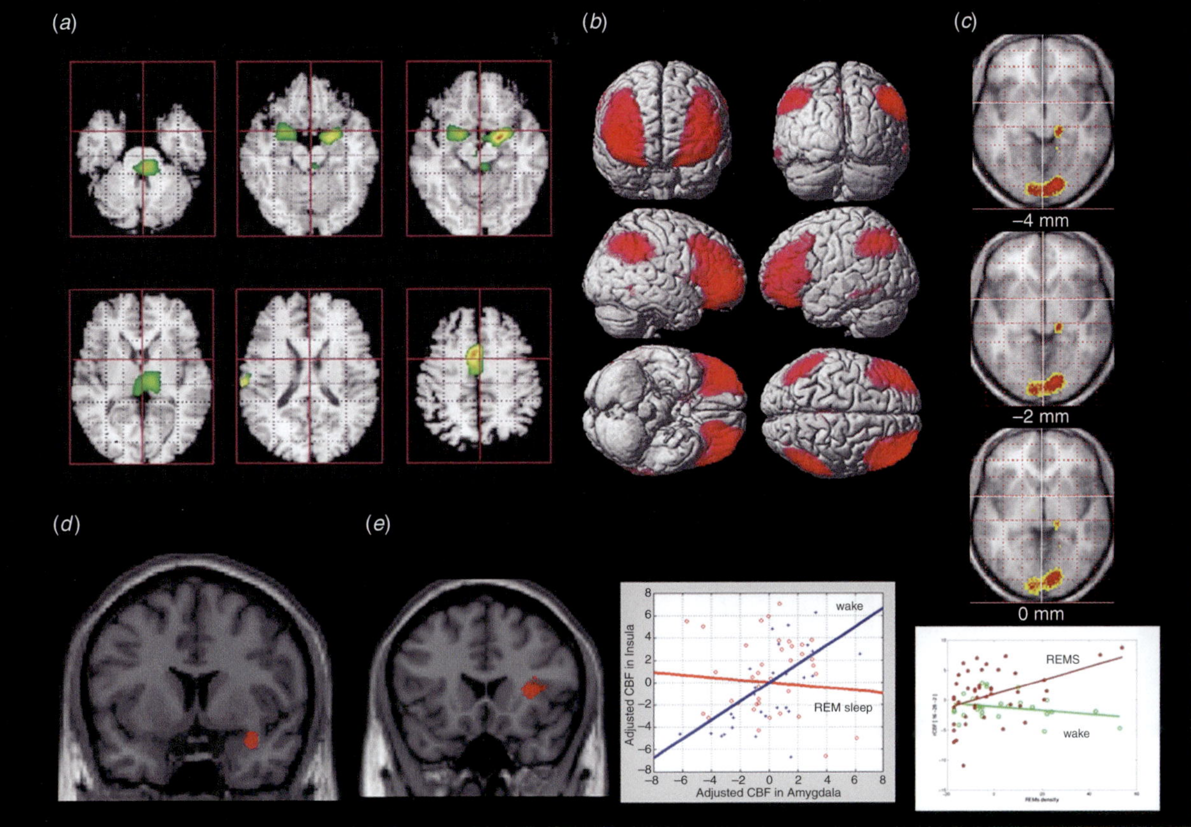

Figure 8.1 (*a*) Brain areas where regional cerebral blood flow is significantly larger during REMS than during wakefulness or slow-wave sleep: mesopontine tegmentum, thalamic nuclei, amygdala, anterior cingulate cortex. Reproduced from Maquet *et al.*, 1996. (*b*) Brain areas where regional cerebral blood flow is significantly decreased relative to wakefulness: ventral prefrontal regions, inferior parietal areas. Reproduced from Maquet *et al.*, 2005. (*c*) Brain areas where the regional cerebral blood flow increases in proportion with the density of eye movements during REMS more than in wakefulness: right medial geniculate nucleus and striate cortex. Reproduced from Peigneux *et al.*, 2001. (*d*) The amygdala is the only brain area where the blood flow is proportional to the variability in heart rate in REMS, relative to wakefulness. Reproduced from Desseilles *et al.*, 2006. (*e*) The interaction that prevails between the insula and the amygdala is involved in the regulation of heart rate during wakefulness, but not during REMS. Reproduced from Desseilles *et al.*, 2006.

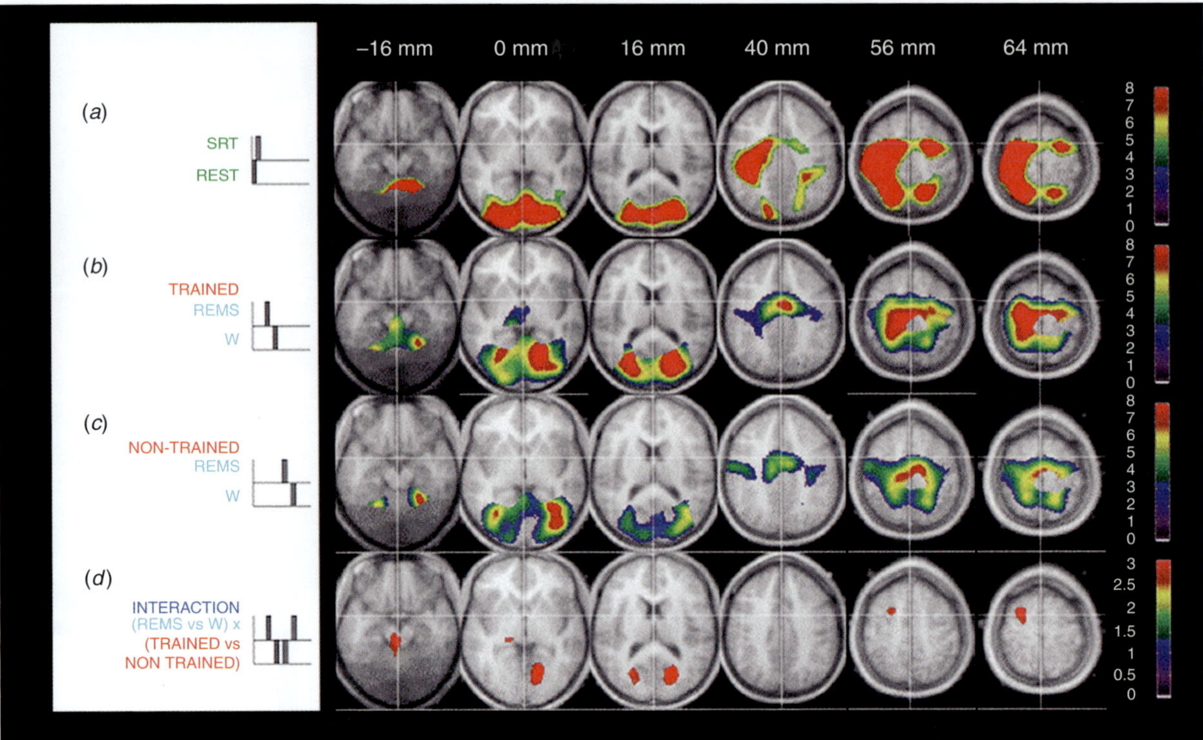

Figure 8.2 Regional brain activity during REMS is modified by previous waking experience (Maquet *et al.*, 2000). (*a*) Brain regions activated during performance of the SRT task during wakefulness (SRT–rest). (*b*) Brain regions activated during REM sleep in trained subjects (REM sleep–wakefulness). (*c*) Brain regions activated during REM sleep in non-trained subjects (REM sleep–wakefulness). (*d*) Brain regions activated more in trained subjects than in non-trained subjects during REM sleep.

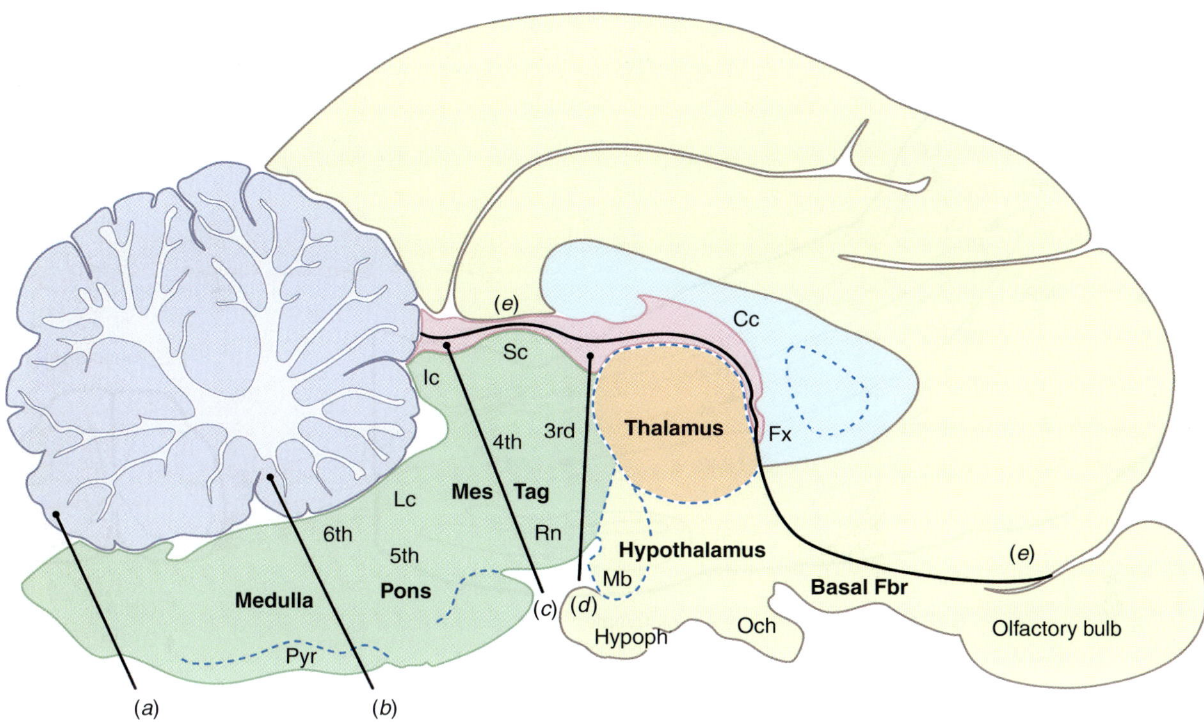

Figure 10.1 Schematic drawing of the midline surface of the cat brain as exposed by a midline sagittal section to illustrate the main transection levels discussed in this chapter. (*a*) spino-medullary: caudally, the spinal cat; rostrally, the isolated encephalon. (*b*) medullary-pontine: caudally, the bulbar or medullary cat. (*c*) mesencephalic inter-collicular (or lower in the midbrain): caudally, the low mesencephalic or pontine decerebrate cat; rostrally, the low isolated forebrain. (*d*) mesencephalic pre-collicular: caudally, the high mesencephalic decerebrate cat; rostrally, the high isolated forebrain. (*e*) telencephalon removed: diencephalic cat. The cerebellum is spared in all cases. In athalamic cats only the thalamus is removed bilaterally. Cc, corpus callosum; Fx, fornix; Hypoph, hypophysis; Ic, inferior colliculus; Lc, nucleus locus coeruleus; Mb, mammillary bodies; Och, optic chiasm; Pyr, pyramid; Rn, red nucleus; Sc, superior colliculus; 3rd, 4th, 5th, and 6th, represent the cranial nerves/nuclei. The color emphasizes the main brain levels discussed.

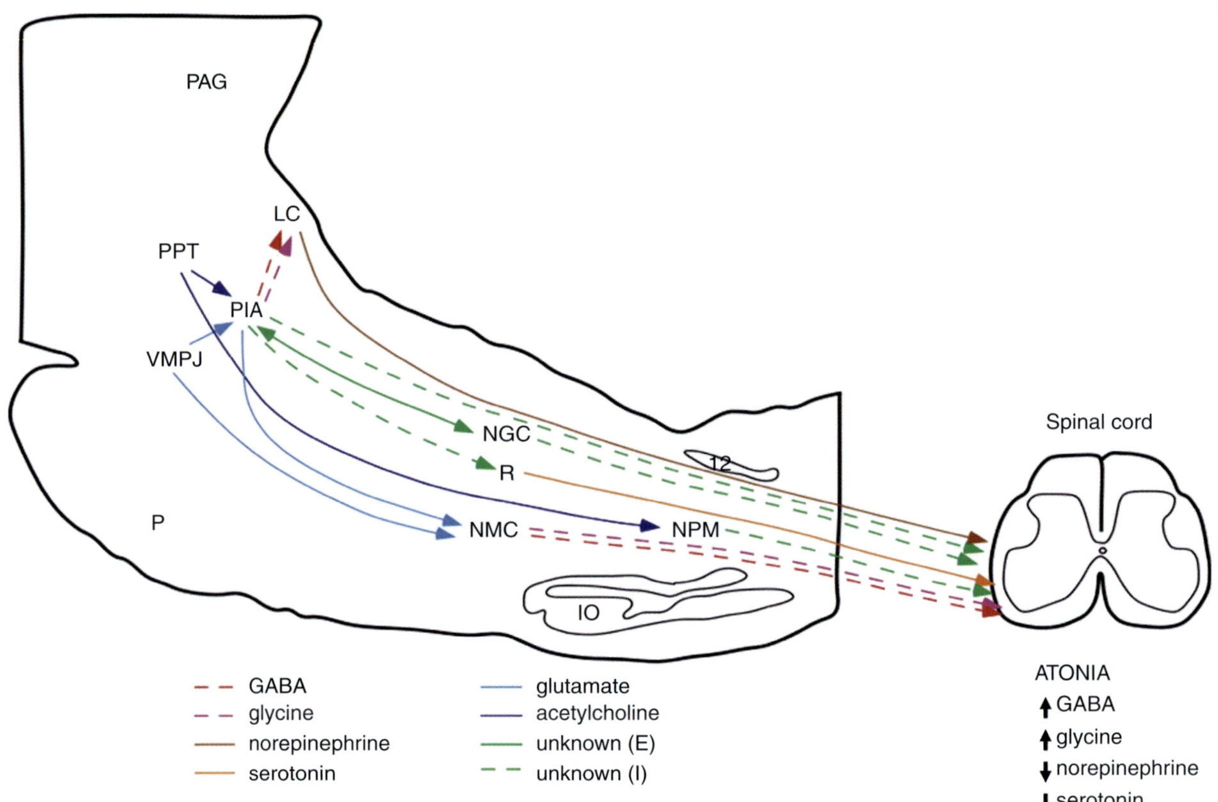

Figure 13.1 Hypothetical neural circuit and transmitters involved in the control of REM sleep atonia. Solid and dashed lines represent excitatory and inhibitory effects on the target site respectively. Glutamatergic and cholinergic activation of the pontine inhibitory area (PIA) elicits muscle atonia, which results from a combination of activation of GABAergic and glycinergic neurons in the medial medulla and inactivation of noradrenergic neurons in the locus coeruleus and serotonergic neurons in the medullary raphe nuclei. The pontine glutamatergic and cholinergic innervations originate from the ventral mesopontine junction (VMPJ) and pedunculopontine nucleus (PPT). Neurons in the VMPJ and PPT also project to the nuclei magnocellularis (NMC) and paramedianus (NPM) in the medial medulla, respectively. IO: inferior olivary nucleus; LC: locus coeruleus; NGC: nucleus gigantocellularis; P: pyramidal tract; PAG: periaqueductal gray; R: medullary raphe nucleus; unknown (E) and unknown (I): transmitter that exerts excitatory and inhibitory effect on the target site; 12: hypoglossal nucleus.

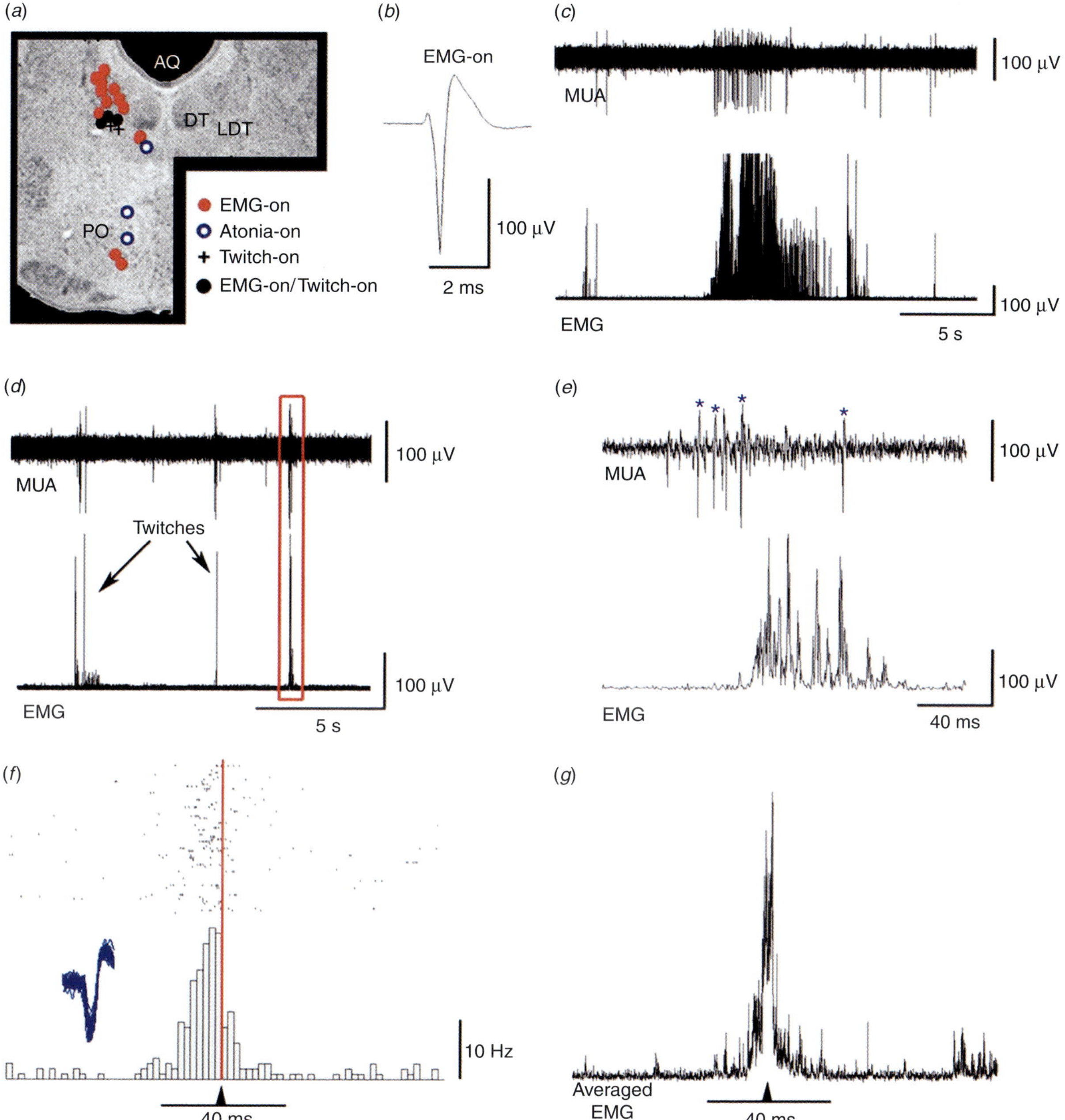

Figure 14.2 State-dependent neuronal discharges within the pontine tegmentum. (*a*) Recording sites of state-dependent neurons reconstructed on a coronal section of the brain stem. Note the predominance of EMG-on neurons. (*b*) Averaged waveform of a representative EMG-on neuron. (*c*) Upper trace: multiunit activity. Lower trace: concurrently recorded nuchal EMG. One EMG-on neuron was isolated from the multiunit record; note its tonic discharge during the period of high muscle tone. (*d*) Upper trace: multiunit activity. Lower trace: concurrently recorded nuchal EMG. (*e*) Expanded view of the boxed area from (*d*). Note how multiunit activity precedes the twitch. Asterisks identify a single isolated unit. (*f*) Peristimulus histogram and raster plot for the twitch-on neuron identified in (*e*) during a ten-minute recording session in a P7 rat (83 total twitches). Inset depicts 55 superimposed action potential waveforms for this unit. This unit's mean discharge rate peaks 5 to 10 ms before the twitch (red line). (*g*) Averaged nuchal EMG for all 83 twitches. AQ: cerebral aqueduct; DT: dorsal tegmental nucleus; LDT: laterodorsal tegmental nucleus; PO: nucleus pontis oralis. (From Karlsson *et al.*, 2005.)

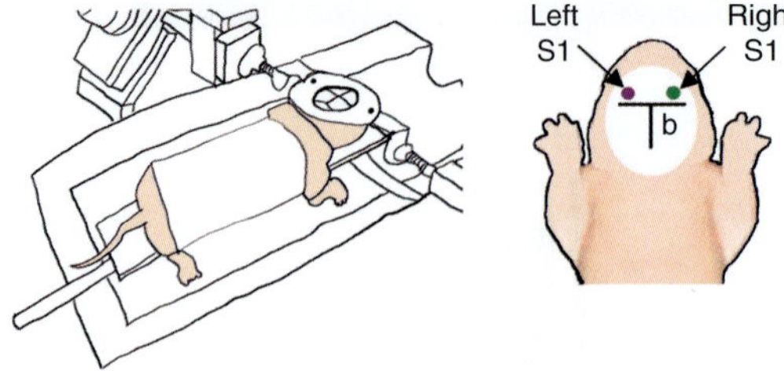

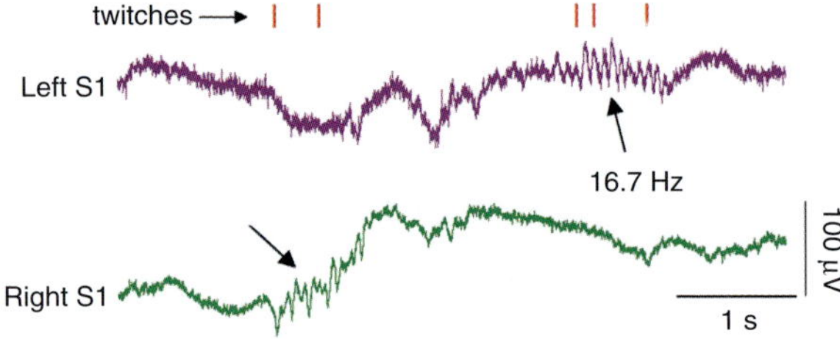

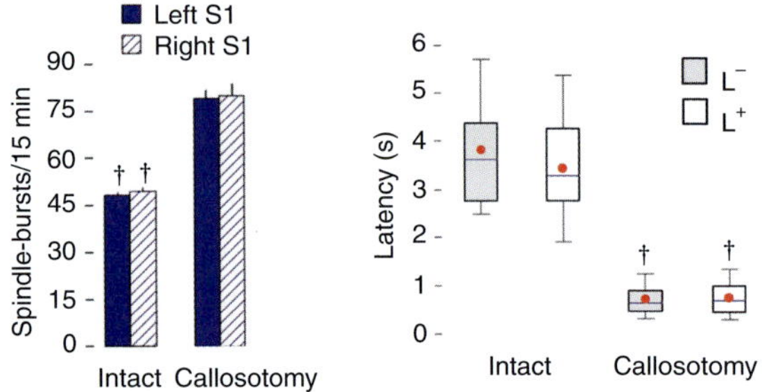

Figure 14.3 Spontaneous spindle-bursts (SBs) in a P5 rat. (*a*) Left: Experimental procedure for recording SBs. The infant rat was head-fixed in a stereotaxic apparatus, placed on a narrow platform, lightly wrapped in gauze, and suspended over a temperature-controlled glass chamber. A heating lamp was also used to maintain brain temperature at 37°C. Right: View of skull showing approximate location of electrodes in relation to bregma (b). Pairs of Ag/AgCl electrodes were placed in left (purple dot) and right (green dot) somatosensory cortex (S1) and SB responses to contralateral forepaw plantar surface stimulation were confirmed. (*b*) Spontaneous SBs (denoted by arrows) in left (purple) and right (green) S1 in relation to active sleep-related myoclonic twitches of the limbs (red ticks) assessed through behavioral observation. The oscillation frequencies of one spontaneous SB is also shown. (*c*) Mean number of spontaneous SBs in left (solid) and right (hatched) S1 during 15-minute recording periods in intact and callosotomized P1 to P6 rats. n 6 per group. † $P < 0.001$ in relation to the callosotomy group. Mean + s.e. (*d*) Box plots depicting distributions of SB latencies for intact and callosotomized subjects ($n = 6$ per group). For this analysis, 20 "anchor" SBs in the left S1 recording were selected at random for each subject and its duration determined. Then, for each of these SBs, the latency between it and the prior (−L) and subsequent (+L) SBs in the right S1 recording was determined. The top, middle, and bottom horizontal lines of the box represent the 75th, 50th (median), and 25th percentiles, respectively. The thin vertical lines above and below the box represent the 90th and 10th percentiles, respectively. Red circles are means. † $P < 0.0001$ in relation to the intact group. (Adapted from Marcano-Reik and Blumberg, 2008.)

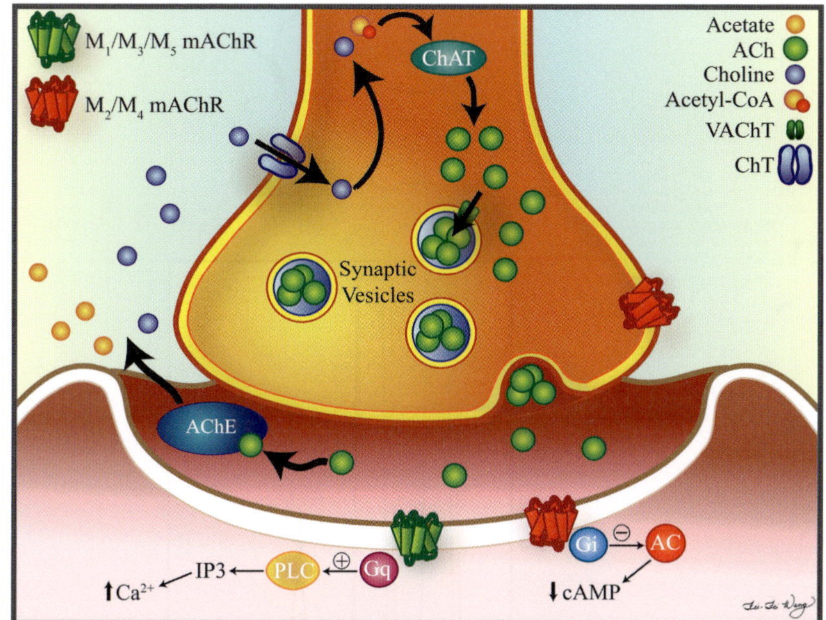

Figure 20.1 Muscarinic cholinergic signaling at the synapse. Acetylcholine (ACh) enters synaptic vesicles via a vesicular acetylcholine transporter (VAChT). Upon exocytosis into the synapse, ACh may bind to pre- or postsynaptic muscarinic cholinergic receptors (mAChR), or ACh may be degraded to acetate and choline by acetylcholinesterase (AChE). Choline is transported back into the presynaptic terminal via a choline transporter (ChT) where choline acetyltransferase (ChAT) synthesizes ACh by catalyzing a reaction between choline and acetyl-coenzyme A (Acetyl-CoA). M1, M3, and M5 muscarinic receptors couple to excitatory (Gq) proteins that activate (+) phospholipase C (PLC). PLC causes a degradation of phosphatidylinositol-4,5-bisphosphate into inositol 1,4,5-triphosphate (IP3) and diacylglycerol (not shown). IP3 mobilizes stores of intracellular calcium (Ca²⁺) and diacylglycerol initiates protein kinase C signaling. M2 and M4 receptors couple to inhibitory (Gi) proteins. Activation of M2 and M4 receptors inhibits (–) adenylyl cyclase (AC) resulting in a decrease of cyclic adenosine mono-phosphate (cAMP). When associated with G protein-gated potassium channels, activated M2 and M4 receptors hyperpolarize neurons (Ishii and Kurachi, 2006).

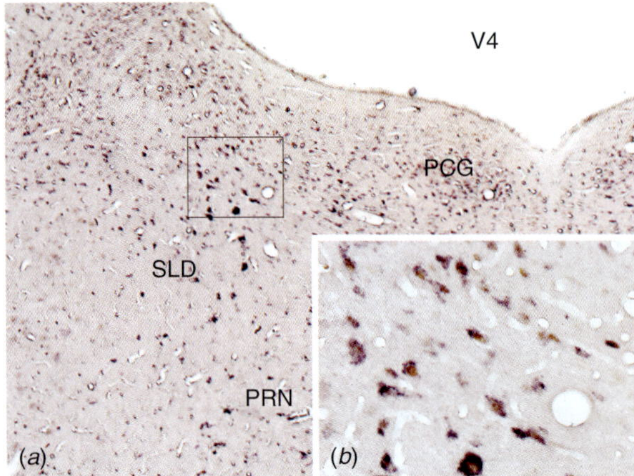

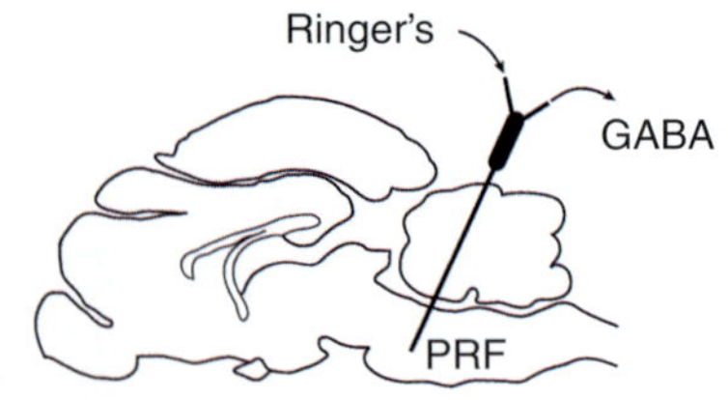

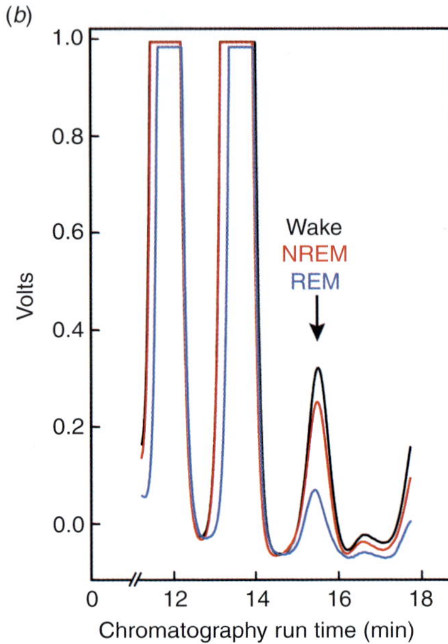

Figure 22.1 Illustration showing a section double-stained with "in situ" hybridization of vGlut2 and immunohistochemistry of c-Fos. Note the large number of double-labeled neurons characterized by a brown nucleus and a blue cytoplasm in the SLD.

Figure 21.2 Pontine reticular formation GABA levels during states of wakefulness, NREM sleep, and REM sleep. (a) Schematic sagittal view of the cat brain showing a microdialysis probe used to collect endogenous GABA from the pontine reticular formation (PRF). (b) The graph shows three superimposed GABA peaks (arrow) generated using high performance liquid chromatography with electrochemical detection. Peak area represents the amount of GABA collected from the brain during wakefulness (black), NREM sleep (red), and REM sleep (blue).

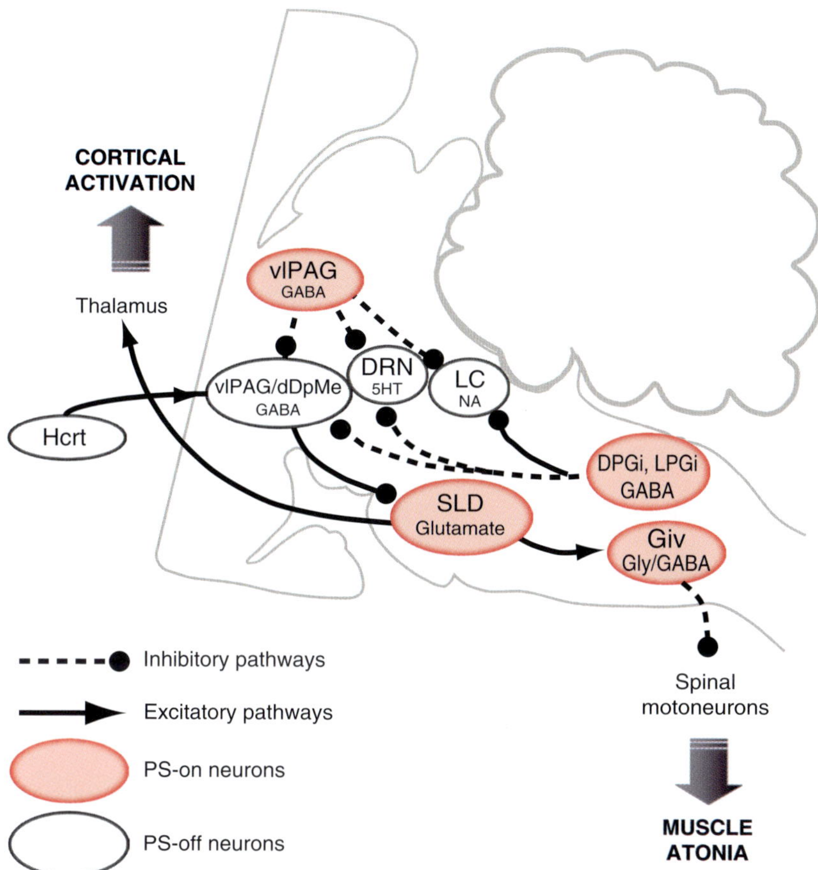

Figure 22.4 Model of the network responsible for paradoxical sleep. Abbreviations: DPGi, dorsal paragigantocellular reticular nucleus; dDpMe, dorsal deep mesencephalic reticular nucleus; DRN, dorsal raphe nucleus; Giv, ventral gigantocellular reticular nucleus; Gly, glycine; Hcrt, hypocretin- (orexin) containing neurons; LC, locus coeruleus; LPGi, lateral paragigantocellular reticular nucleus, vlPAG, ventrolateral periaqueductal gray; SLD, sublaterodorsal nucleus.

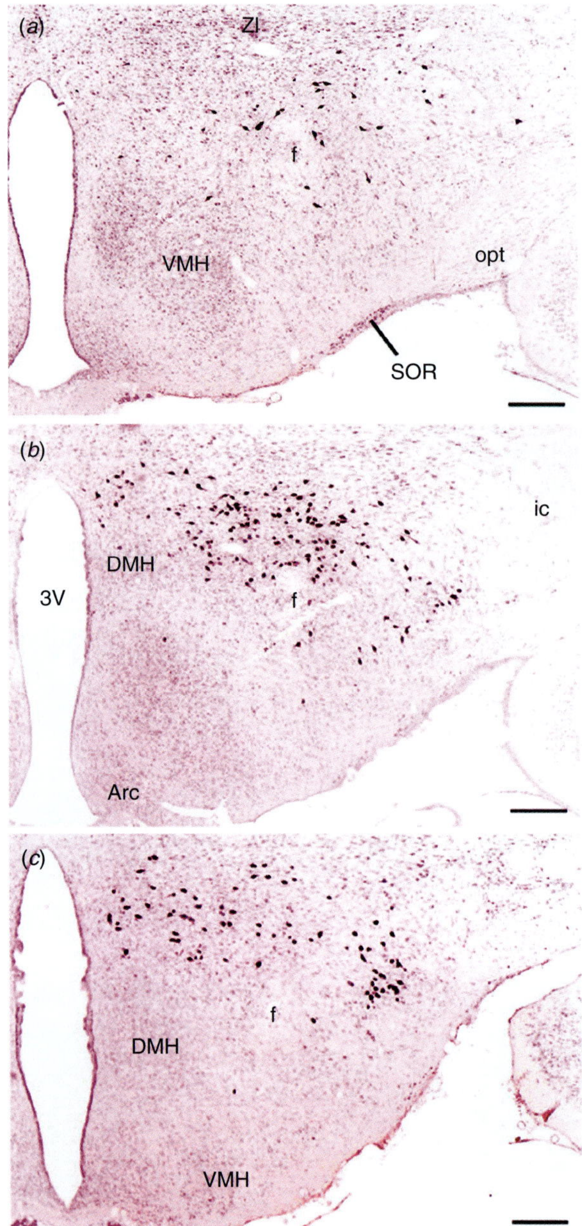

Figure 24.1 Distribution of HCRT neurons at three rostrocaudal levels of the tuberal region of the hypothalamus. 3V, 3rd ventricle; Arc, arcuate nucleus; DMH, dorsomedial hypothalamic nucleus; f, fornix; ic, internal capsule; opt, optic tract; SOR, retrochiasmatic part of the supraoptic nucleus; VMH, ventromedial hypothalamic nucleus; ZI, zona incerta. Scale bars, 275 μm. (Adapted from Peyron *et al.*, 1998, *J. Neuroscience*, with permission.)

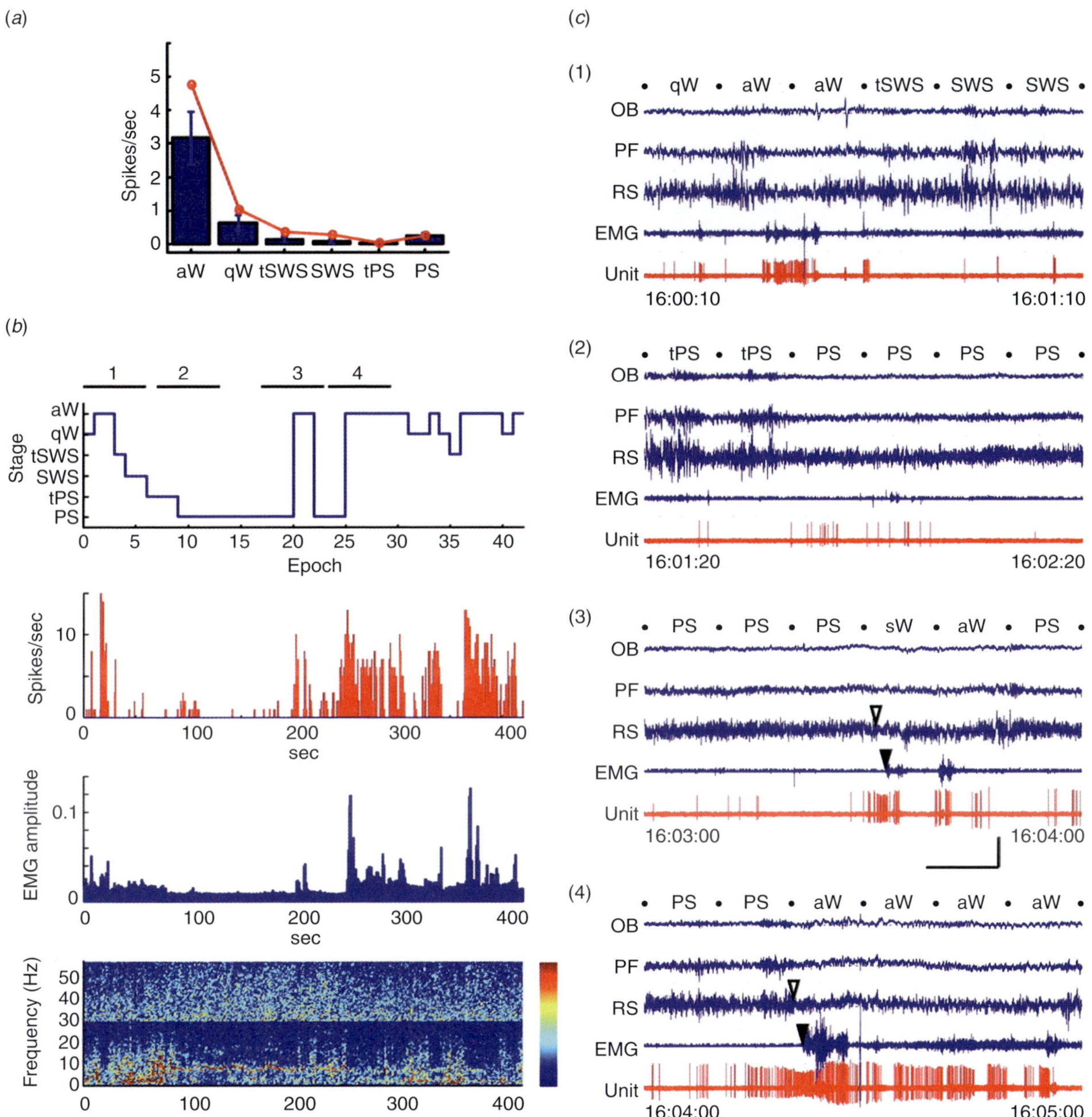

Figure 24.4 Sleep–wake discharge profile of identified HCRT neuron. (*a*) Bar diagram showing mean spike rate. The line drawing shows the discharge rate of an individual HCRT neuron shown in (*b*) and (*c*). (*b*) Hypnogram, spike-rate histogram, and EMG amplitude and EEG frequency spectra over the recording session. (*c*) One-minute segments of unit, EEG, and EMG activity during state transitions. The increase in firing before arousal from REM sleep (in 3 and 4) anticipates the transition from REM to waking judged by EEG (open arrowhead) and also EMG (filled arrowhead). OB, Olfactory bulb; PF, prefrontal cortex; RS, retrosplenial cortex. (Adapted from Lee *et al.*, 2005, *J. Neuroscience*, with permission.)

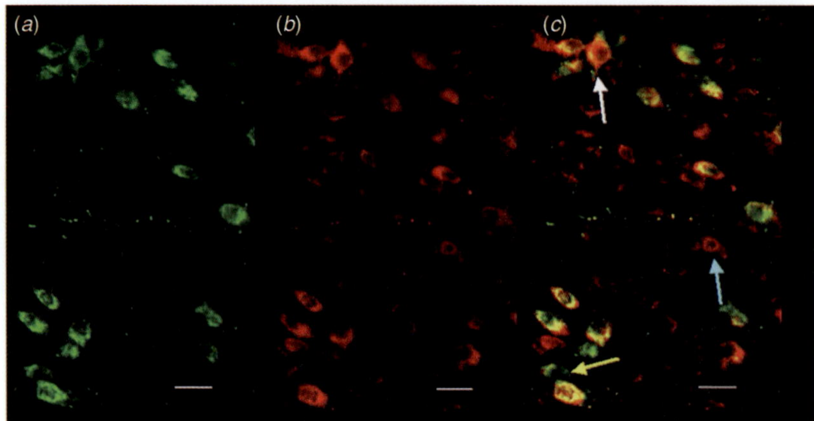

Figure 26.1 (*a*) Orexin-A containing neurons present in the perifornical-lateral hypothalamus region. Orexin-A containing neurons (green) were identified with fluorescence immunohistochemistry using a secondary antibody conjugated to FITC. Numerous cell bodies and fibers containing orexin-A are also visible. Calibration bar = 25 μm. (*b*) Same visual field and section as (*a*), here showing immunoreactivity (red) to the adenosine A_1 receptor in neurons in the perifornical-lateral hypothalamus. The A_1 receptor immunoreactivity is widely distributed and not restricted to orexin-A containing neurons. Calibration bar = 25 μm. (*c*) The same section and visual field, as shown in (*a*) and (*b*) describing double labeling of orexin-A and A_1 receptors. The white arrow indicates a double-labeled neuron, whereas the yellow arrow marks an orexin-A containing neuron without A_1 receptor. The blue arrow indicates a non-orexin containing A_1 receptor-labeled neuron. Calibration bar = 25 μm.

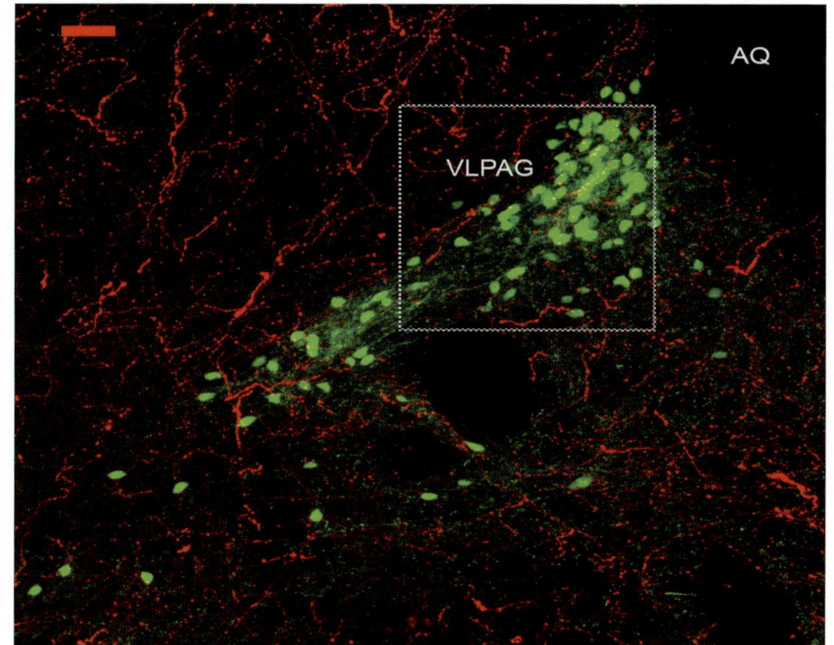

Figure 28.1 GABA neurons (green) in the ventral lateral periaquaductal gray area. These neurons are innervated by hypocretin (red), which activates the GABA neurons thereby inhibiting REM sleep. Lesion of these GABA neurons in the vlPAG releases the inhibition and leads to more REM sleep even in mice that lack hypocretin (Kaur *et al.*, 2009).

Abbreviations: AQ= cerebral aqueduct; VLPAG= ventral lateral periaqueductal gray.

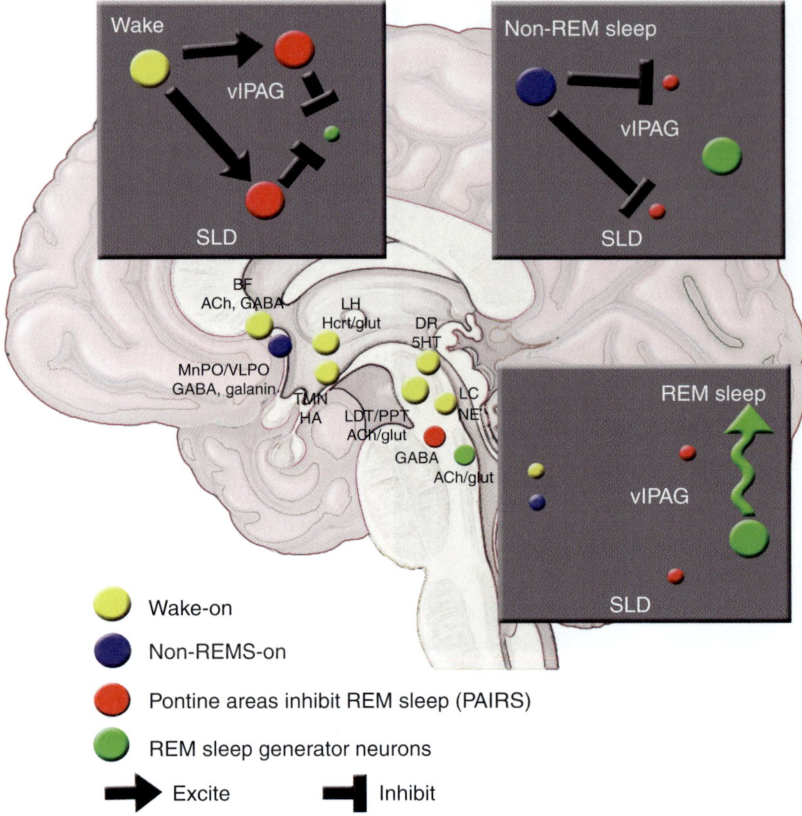

Figure 28.2 Model of neuronal populations that regulate wake, non-REM sleep, and REM sleep (Kaur *et al.*, 2009). This model represents an effort by a number of investigators (for a review see Kaur *et al.*, 2009). There are several neuronal populations that are considered to generate wakefulness and these are identified in yellow. Neurons that are considered to generate non-REM sleep are identified in blue. Both of these neuronal populations act on neurons in the pontine brain stem (red) and influence the generation of rapid-eye movement sleep (REM sleep). Wake-on neurons inhibit REM sleep by activating pontine GABA neurons in the pons. The strength of the excitatory input to the pontine GABA neurons influences REM sleep. A strong input will inhibit REM sleep while a weakened input will facilitate it. This excitatory input to the GABA pontine neurons is from hypocretin and from other sources. The purpose of this excitation is to keep the animal upright and mobile while foraging for food. During non-REM sleep the excitatory input to the pontine GABA neurons is lost and is replaced by a strong inhibitory input. This enables REM-sleep generator neurons (green) to become active and when sufficient numbers of these are activated then REM sleep ensues. The hypothesis that the pontine areas inhibit REM sleep has been tested in two separate studies from our lab (Blanco-Centurion *et al.*, 2004; Kaur *et al.*, 2009). The earlier study tested the hypothesis in rats whereas the second study tested it in mice. In both studies REM sleep increased when the GABA neurons were lesioned with hypocretin-2-saporin thereby supporting the hypothesis of PAIRS.

Abbreviations: Ach = acetylcholine; BF = basal forebrain; DR = dorsal raphe; GABA = gamma-aminobutyric acid; GLUT = glutamic acid; HA = histamine; HCRT = hypocretin; LC = locus coeruleus; LH = lateral hypothalamus; MnPO = median preoptic nucleus; NE = norepinephrine; LDT = lateral dorsal pontine tegmentum; PPT = pedunculopontine tegmentum; SLD = sublateral dorsal nucleus; TMN = tuberomammillary nucleus; vlPAG = ventral lateral periaqueductal gray; VLPO = ventral lateral preoptic nucleus.

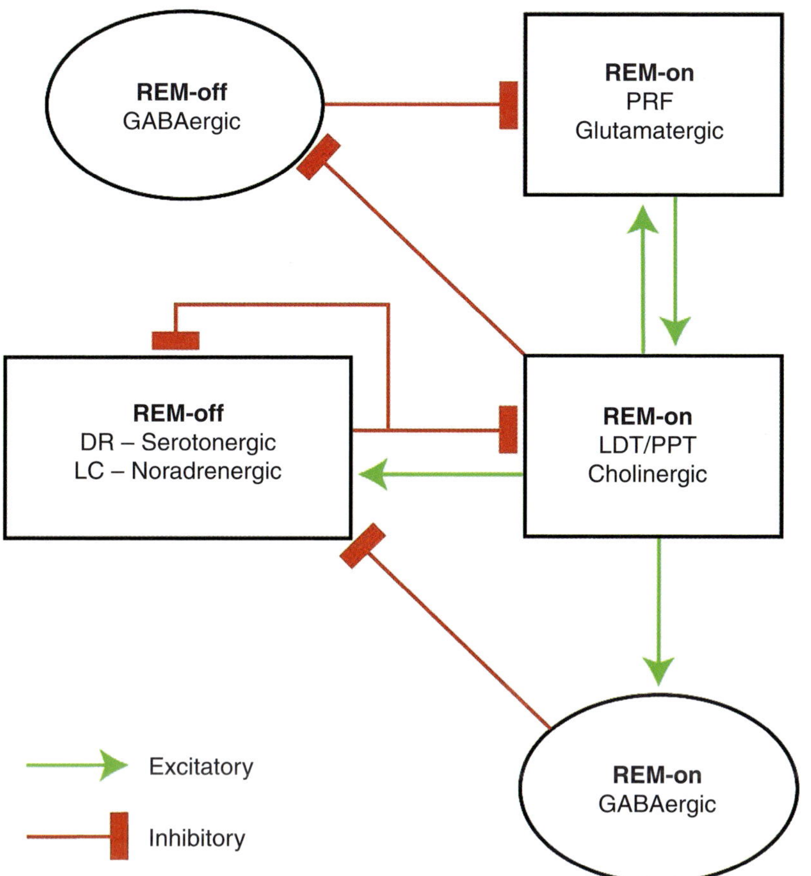

Figure 29.3 Graphic depiction of the modified reciprocal-interaction model of REM-sleep control, originally proposed by McCarley and Hobson (1975a,b), and here modified from McCarley (2007). The dorsal raphe (DR) and locus coeruleus (LC) REM-off neurons inhibit laterodorsal/pedunculopontine tegmental nuclei (LDT/PPT) REM-on neurons during waking and NREM sleep. Self-inhibition of these REM-off neurons leads to disinhibition of REM-on neurons, allowing REM sleep to begin. LDT/PPT REM-on activity excites PRF (pontine reticular formation) glutamatergic REM-on cells that are responsible for muscle atonia, PGO waves, and hippocampal theta rhythmicity during REM sleep. REM-on cells begin to excite the REM-off cells as REM sleep progresses, leading to eventual REM-sleep cessation. REM-on LDT/PPT neurons excite local GABAergic interneurons, in turn inhibiting REM-off neurons. Also, REM-on output inhibits GABAergic REM-off interneurons, which then inhibit REM-on PRF neurons. Red lines denote excitation; blue, inhibition.

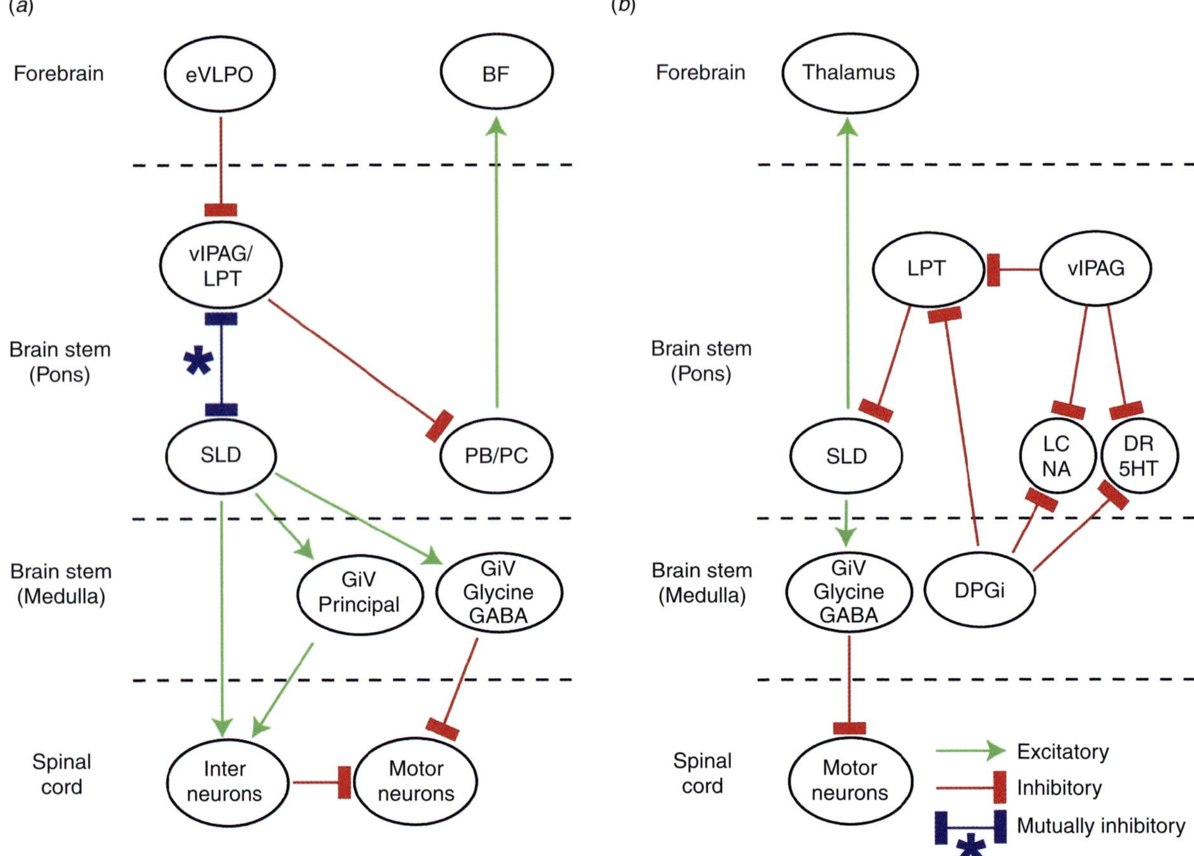

Figure 29.4 Graphic depiction of two suggested models of REM-sleep control. (*a*) The REM-sleep "flip-flop" circuit model of Lu and colleagues (2006b); this REM regulatory model is different from the NREM sleep/wake "flip-flop" switch previously proposed (Saper *et al.*, 2001). During REM sleep, REM-off vlPAG/LPT regions are inhibited by GABAergic/galaninergic eVLPO input, in turn releasing GABAergic and glutamatergic SLD (also known as the subcoeruleus, SubC) and glutamatergic PB/PC neurons. The SLD GABAergic REM-on neurons mutually inhibit vlPAG/LPT GABAergic REM-off neurons, providing a "flip-flop" (asterisk). The PB/PC projects rostrally to the basal forebrain, and plays a crucial role in the expression of LVFA and the hippocampal theta rhythm. The SLD glutamatergic descending output excites GiV principal cells, which in turn excite spinal cord interneurons. These glycinergic/GABAergic interneurons inhibit spinal-cord motoneuronal activity, and muscle atonia results. Also, SLD output excites GiV glycinergic/GABAergic neurons, which directly inhibit the spinal-cord motoneurons. The SLD may also directly excite the inhibitory spinal-cord interneurons, bypassing GiV. (*b*) The revised model of paradoxical sleep control proposed by Luppi and colleagues. During REM sleep, vlPAG and DPGi GABAergic REM-on neurons inhibit DR, LC, and LPT REM-off activity. The SLD glutamatergic output ascends to forebrain regions responsible for LVFA, such as the thalamus, and descends to activate the GiV glycinergic/GABAergic output responsible for muscle atonia. Recent work suggests that GABAergic MCH REM-on hypothalamic neurons may inhibit vlPAG REM-off neurons, thereby promoting REM sleep. We further note that this sketch, adapted from Fort *et al.* (2009, Figure 1), is somewhat less complex than suggested in the Fort *et al.* review's text. Abbreviations: BF, basal forebrain; DPGi, dorsal aspect of the paragigantocellular reticular nucleus; DR, dorsal raphe nucleus; eVLPO, extended region of the ventrolateral preoptic nucleus; GiV, medullary ventral gigantocellular nucleus; LC, locus coeruleus; LPT, lateral pontine tegmentum; PB/PC, parabrachial/precoeruleus nuclei; SLD, sublaterodorsal nucleus, also known as the subcoeruleus SubC; vlPAG, ventrolateral aspect of the periaqueductal gray. Red lines denote excitation; blue, inhibition; and green with asterisk, mutual inhibition.

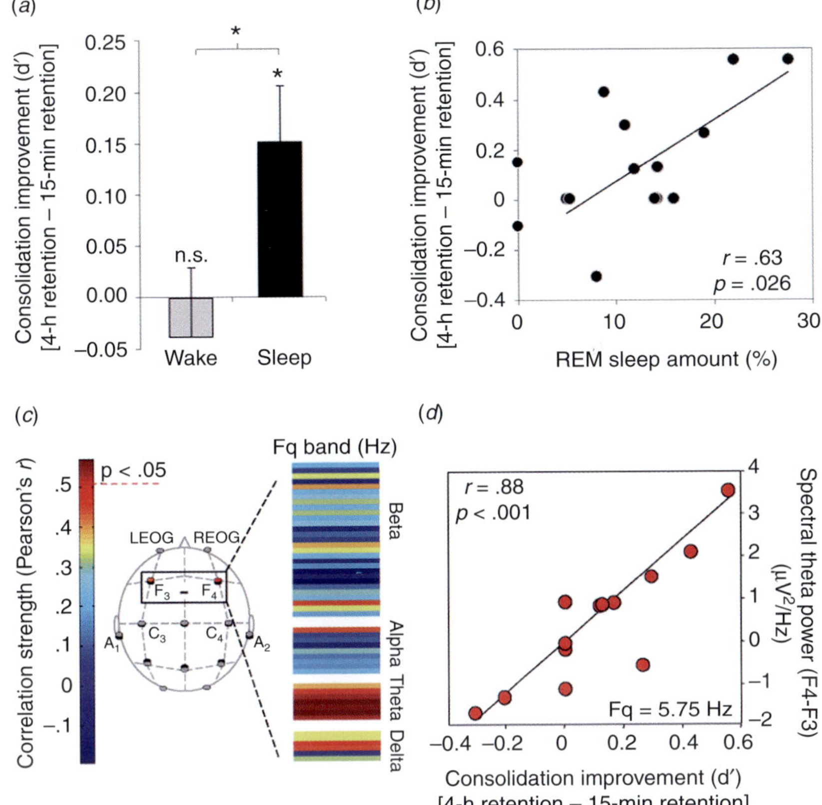

Figure 34.3 REM-sleep enhancement of negative emotional memories. (a) Offline benefit (change in memory recall for 4 hours versus 15 minutes old memories) across the day (wake, grey bar) or following a 90-minute nap (sleep, filled bar). (b) Correlation between the amount of offline emotional memory improvement in the nap group (i.e., the offline benefit expressed in filled bar of figure (a), and the amount of REM sleep obtained within the nap. (c) Correlation strength (Pearson's r-value) between offline benefit for emotional memory in the sleep group (the benefit expressed in filled bar of figure (a)) and the relative right versus left prefrontal spectral-band power (F4–F3) within the delta, alpha, theta, and beta spectral bands, expressed in average 0.5 Hz bin increments. Correlation strength is represented by the color range, demonstrating significant correlations within the theta frequency band (hot colors), and (d) exhibiting a maximum significance at the 5.75 Hz bin. *p < 0.05; error bars indicate s.e.m. (Modified from Nishida et al., 2009).

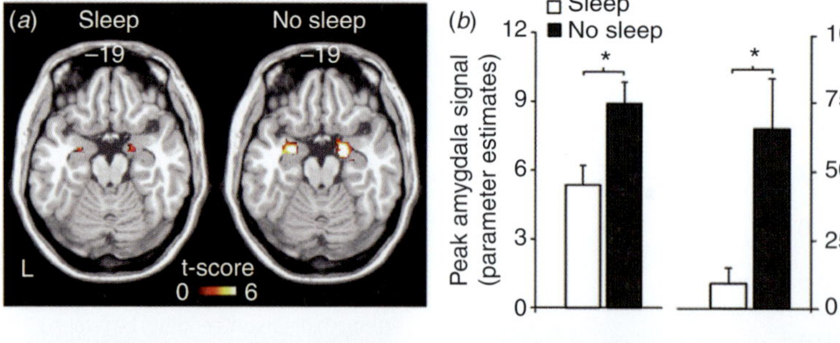
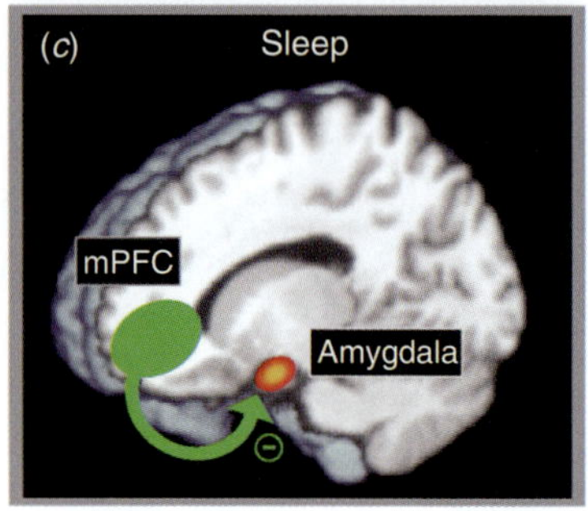
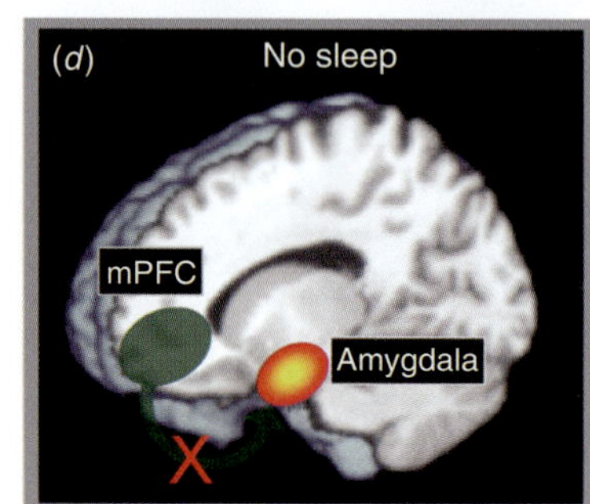

Figure 34.4 The impact of sleep deprivation on emotional-brain reactivity and functional connectivity. (*a*) Amygdala response to increasingly negative emotional stimuli in the sleep-deprivation and sleep-control groups, and (*b*) corresponding differences in intensity and volumetric extent of amygdala activation between the two groups (average ± s.e.m. of left and right amygdala). (*c*) Depiction of associated changes in functional connectivity between the medial prefrontal cortex (mPFC) and the amygdala. With sleep, the prefrontal lobe was strongly connected to the amygdala, regulating and exerting an inhibitory top-down control. (*d*) Without sleep, however, amygdala-mPFC connectivity was decreased, potentially negating top-down control and resulting in an overactive amygdala.

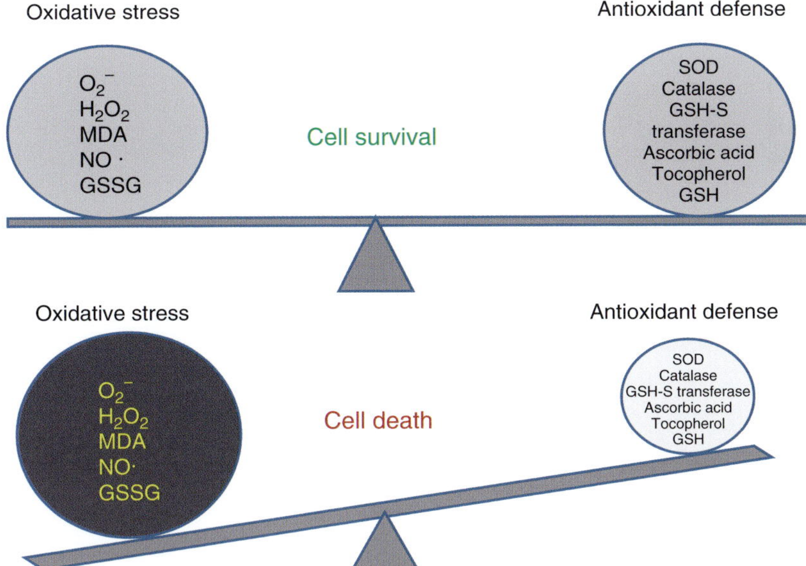

Figure 35.1 Cartoon representation of the oxidative balance in the cell. In a healthy cell, a balance between the oxidant production and antioxidant response is maintained. However, an increase in oxidant production, if uncompensated by an increase in antioxidant response, leads to oxidative damage and cell death.

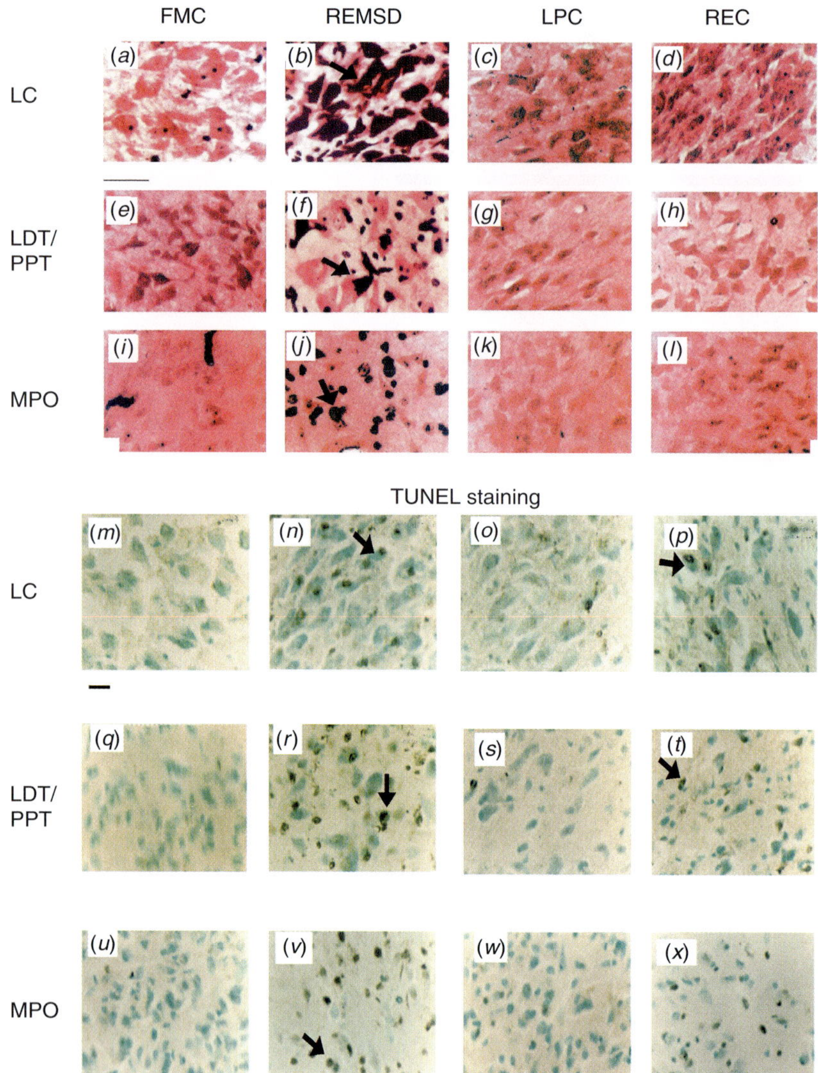

Figure 35.2 Representative photomicrographs of amino-cupric silver stained (*a–l*) and TUNEL stained (*m–x*) sections in the LC, LDT/PPT, and MPO under different conditions.

Top panel (*a–l*): Following amino-cupric silver staining, degenerated neurons seen as black–silver deposited stains (black arrows) were observed after REMSD in the LC (*b*), LDT/PPT (*f*), and MPO (*j*). Scale bar = 40 μm.

Bottom panel (*m–x*): Significant increased number of TUNEL-positive neurons can be observed following REMSD in the LC (*n*), LDT/PPT (*r*), and MPO (*v*) suggesting increased apoptosis in the REM sleep-related areas. Black arrows point to TUNEL-stained apoptotic neurons. Scale bar = 20 μm. (Modified from Biswas *et al.*, 2006.)

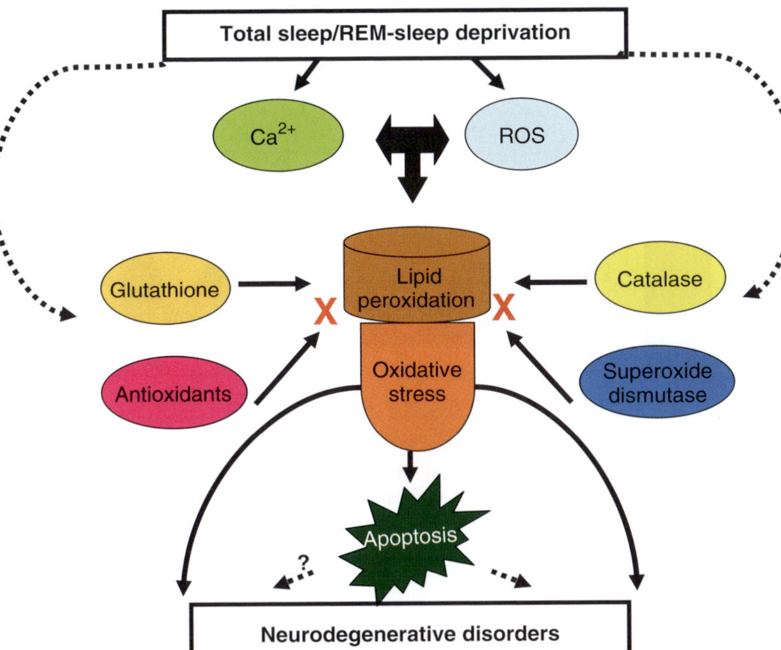

Figure 35.3 Effect of sleep deprivation (TSD and REMSD) on oxidative stress and apoptosis: a working model. Sleep deprivation, including REM-sleep deprivation, may induce lipid peroxidation and oxidative stress leading to apoptosis in some brain regions and may be the underlying cause of several neurodegenerative disorders. In contrast, it may also elevate the levels of protective enzymes such as glutathione, SOD, and antioxidants and prevent lipid peroxidation.

The model was compiled based on the following studies: Singh and Kumar (2008); Ramanathan *et al.* (2002) ; Singh *et al.*(2008); Das *et al.* (2008); Biswas *et al.* (2006); Andersen *et al.* (2009); Lai and Siegel (2003); Coppede and Migliore (2009).

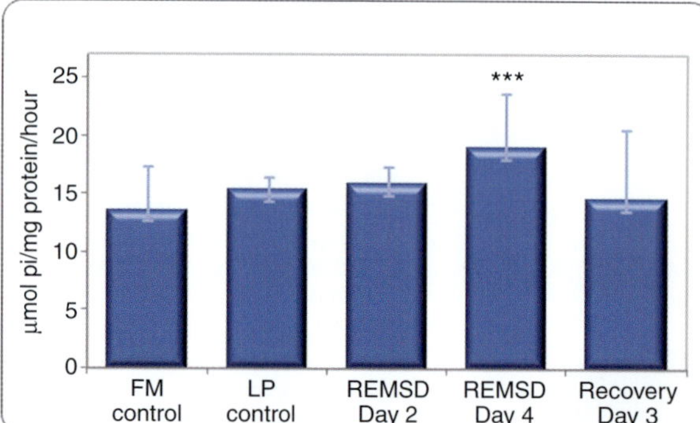

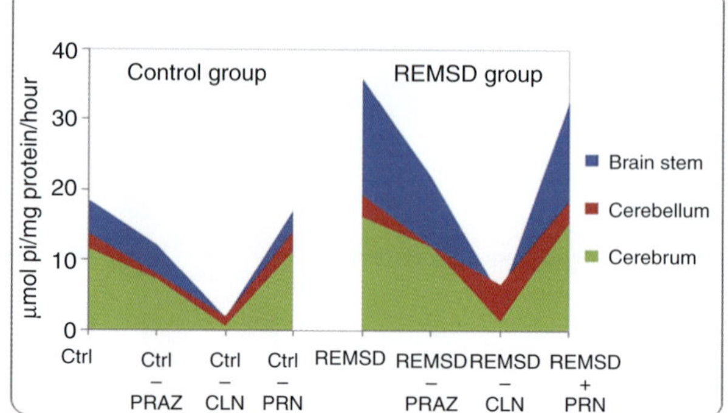

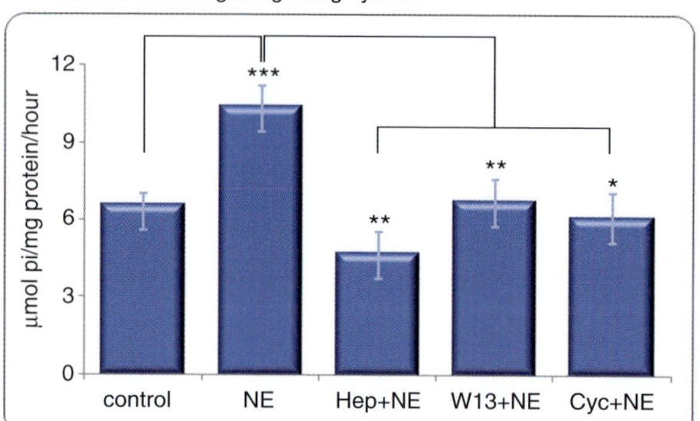

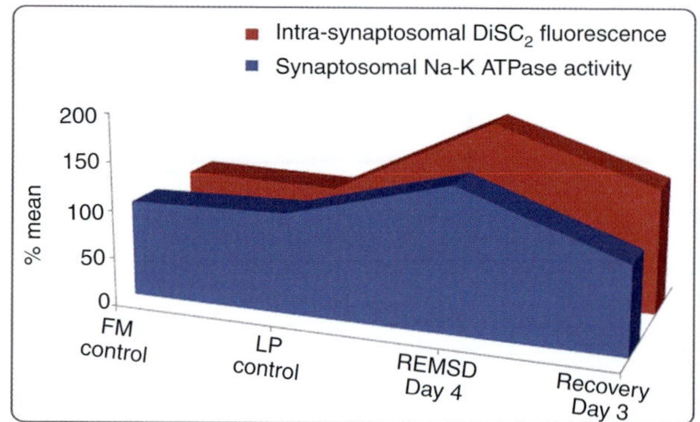

Figure 36.1 REM sleep deprivation-induced increase in the Na-K ATPase activity and intrasynaptosomal potential as a reflection of intracellular potential. (*a*) Four days of REMSD significantly increased the Na-K ATPase activity as compared to the free moving (FM) control. The enzyme activity did not alter significantly after two days of REMSD and in large-platform (LP) control animals. The increased activity returned to its normal level after three days of recovery of REM-sleep loss. (*b*) Significant increase in Na-K ATPase activity after REMSD were observed in all three regions studied, i.e., the cerebrum, cerebellum, and brain stem. However, maximum changes were observed in the brain-stem region. The increase in Na-K ATPase activity was modulated by NE specifically through its action via the alpha-1 NE-ergic receptors in both the control and REM sleep-deprived groups. (Abbreviations: PRAZ, prazosin; CLN, clonidine; PRN, propranolol). (*c*) Na-K ATPase activity was significantly inhibited by heparin (an IP3 antagonist), W13 (a calmodulin antagonist), and Cyc (a calcineurin inhibitor) suggesting that the NE-mediated increase in the enzyme activity involves intracellular calcium for signaling. (Abbreviations: NE, norepinephrine; Hep, heparin; Cyc, cyclosporin A). (*d*) Na-K ATPase activity and intra-synaptosomal positive potential increased significantly after four days of REMSD. Intra-synaptosomal positive potential (as a reflection of intracellular potential) was estimated using the membrane permeable mono-cationic fluorescent dye, 3,3′-diethylthiacarbocyanine iodide ($DiSC_2$). Significance level: * $p<0.05$; ** $p<0.01$; *** $p<0.001$. Figures reconstructed based on previous reports from this lab; Gulyani and Mallick, 1993 (*a*); Gulyani and Mallick, 1995 (*b*); Mallick *et al.*, 2000 (*c*); Das and Mallick, 2008 (*d*).

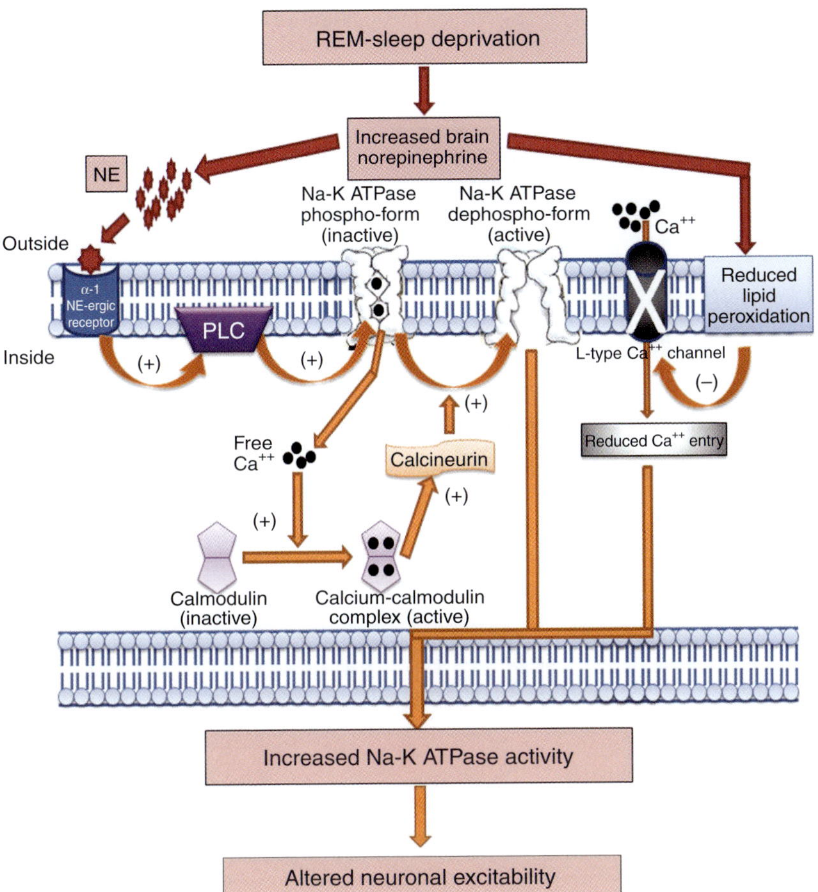

Figure 36.2 Schematic representation of the underlying mechanism of REMSD-induced changes in Na-K ATPase activity. Norepinephrine (NE) concentration increases in the brain after REMSD. The increased NE binds to the alpha-1A adrenoceptor on the neuronal membrane and activates PLC, which then releases membrane-bound calcium that activates calcineurin causing dephosphorylation of the Na-K ATPase, the active form of the enzyme. Additionally, the increased NE in the brain decreases the neuronal membrane lipid peroxidation causing a reduction in Ca++ influx into the neurons possibly by closing the L-type calcium channels, which also activates the Na-K ATPase activity. Figure reconstructed based on several reports cited in the text.

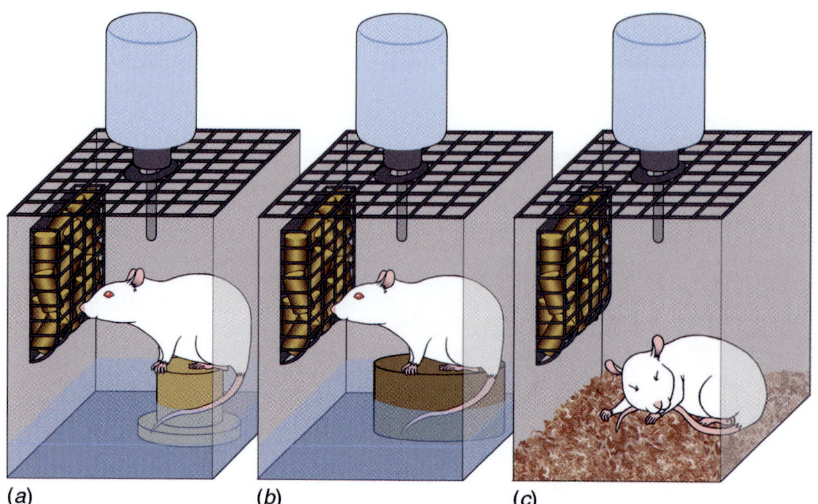

Figure 37.1 The single platform method (SPM), including the narrow platform (*a*), large platform, which has been used as a form of stress control (*b*), and the cage control, in which rats are placed in the same container as REMsd rats, but are allowed to sleep freely, lying down on a bedding made of sawdust (*c*). Water and food are available throughout the entire sleep-deprivation period, and the water inside the chambers is changed once or twice a day, depending on the study.

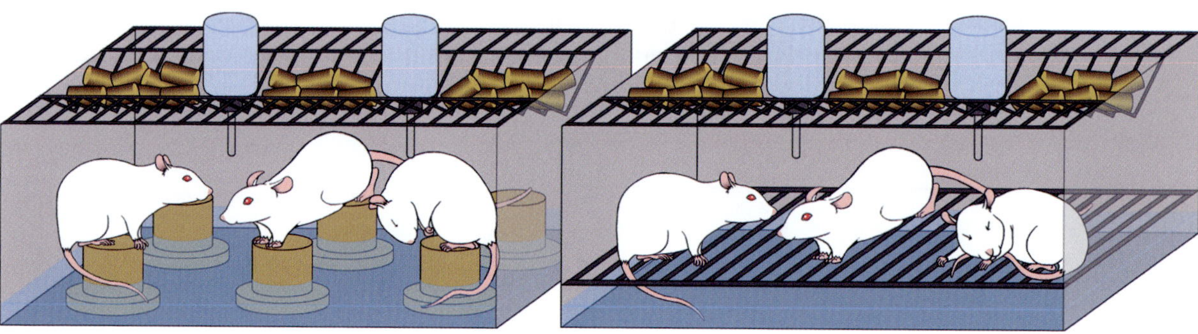

Figure 37.2 The modified multiple platform method (MMPM) was elaborated based on the SPM, but with sufficient platforms so the rats would be allowed to move around the water tank. Rats are placed in the large water tanks as a socially stable group, to prevent additional, non-sleep related stressors. One possible stress-control group consists of placing large platforms, but alternatively, a grid can be placed inside the water tank, so the rats can lay down and sleep freely. Previous results show some loss of sleep in the grid, but far less than that seen in large platforms (Machado *et al.*, 2004).

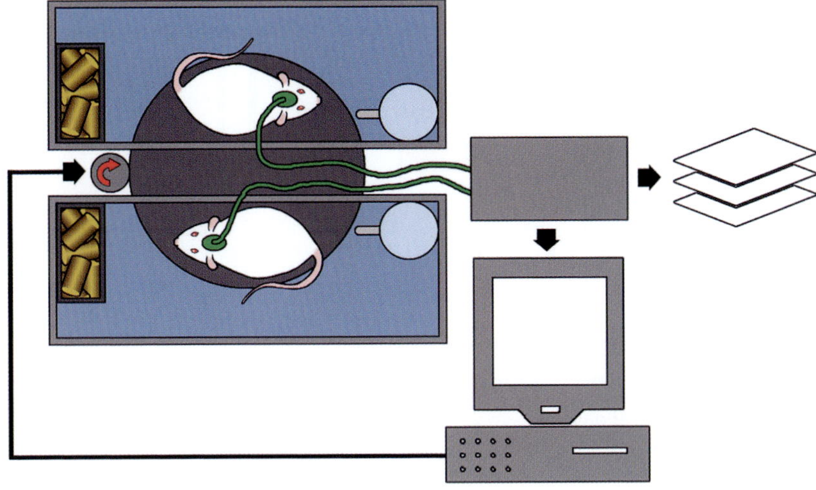

Figure 37.3 The disk-over-water (DOW) method involves the implant of electrodes for sleep monitoring. Because a computer detects the sleep phase, it is possible to deprive rats of specific sleep phases. Therefore, upon sleep (or REM sleep) onset, the disk turns on and the rat walks counterwise to avoid falling in the water. The yoked rat is also obliged to walk regardless of whether it is awake or not.

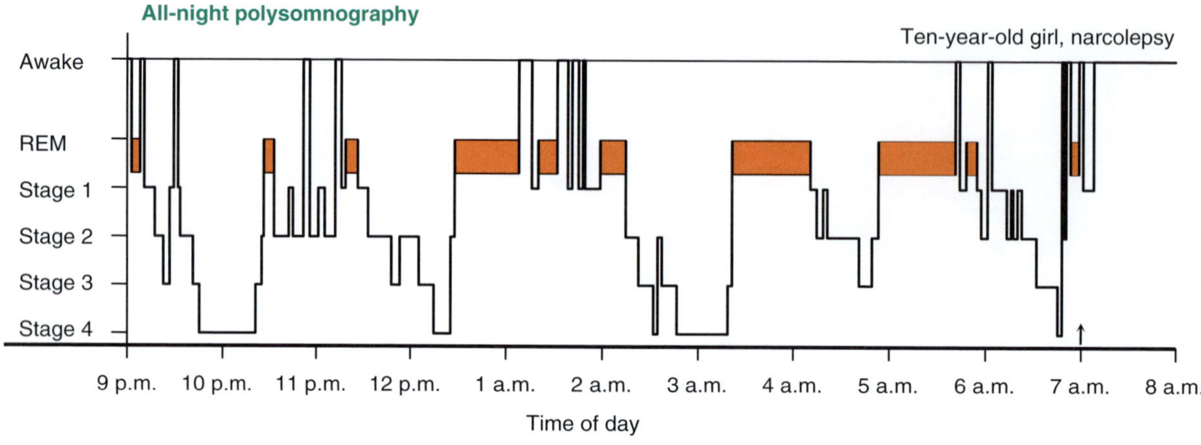

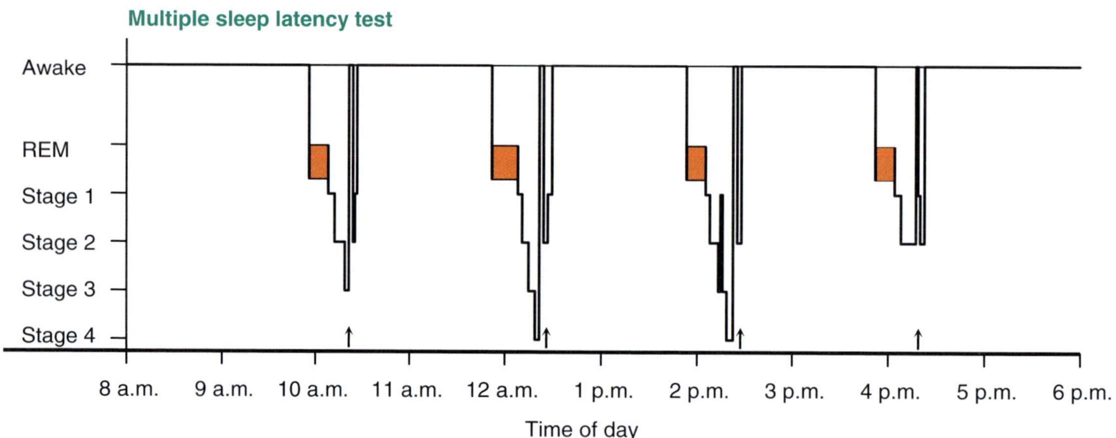

Figure 40.1 All-night polysomnography and MSLT of a narcoleptic patient (adapted from Honda, 1988).

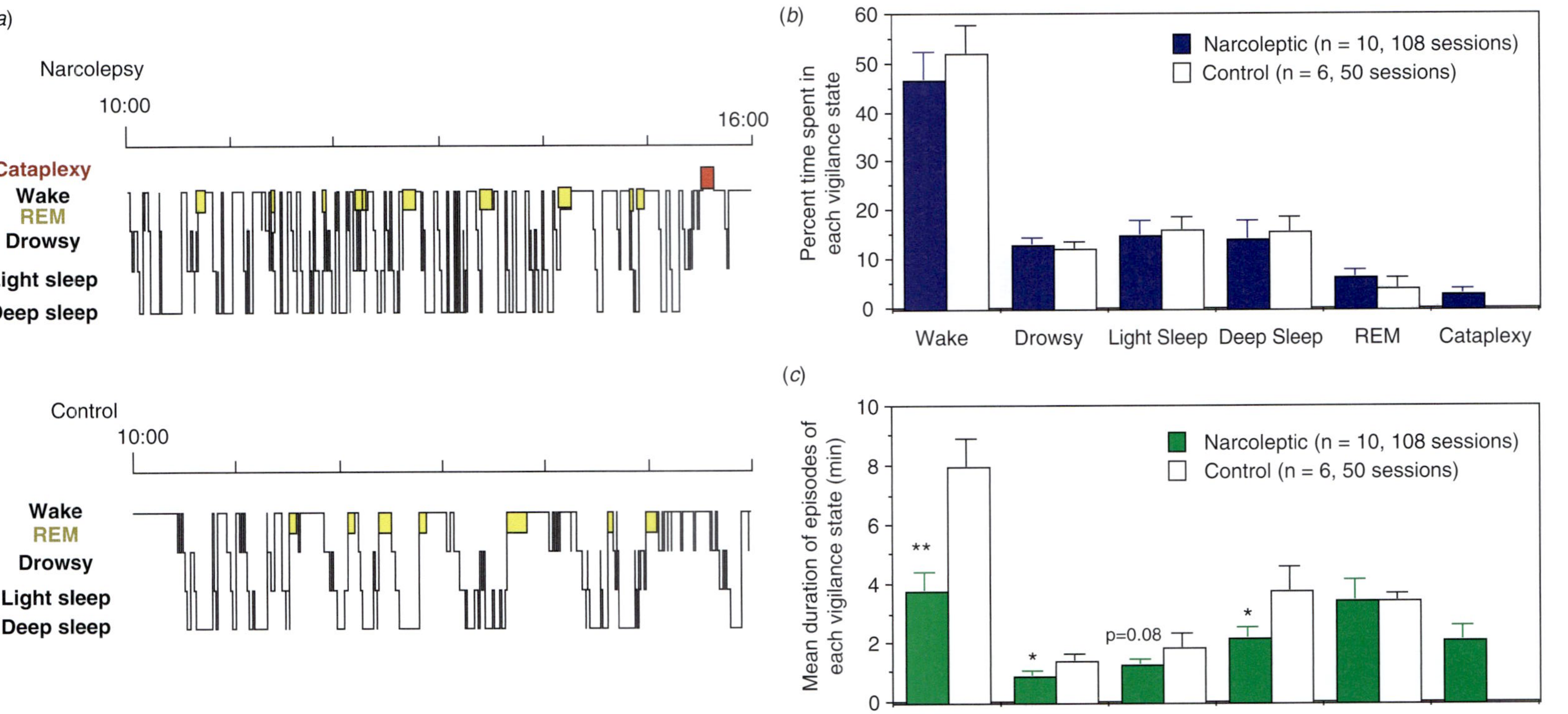

Figure 40.2 (a) Typical hypnograms from a narcoleptic and a control Doberman. (b, c) Percentage of time spent in, mean frequency of, and mean duration for each vigilance state of narcoleptic and control Dobermans during daytime six-hour recordings (10:00 to 16:00). No significant difference was found in the percentage of time spent in each vigilance state between narcoleptic and control dogs. However, the mean duration of wake, drowsy state, and deep-sleep episodes were significantly shorter in the narcoleptics, suggesting a fragmentation of the vigilance states (wake and sleep) in these animals. To compensate for the influence of cataplectic episodes on wake and drowsiness, those episodes interrupted by the occurrence of cataplexy were excluded.

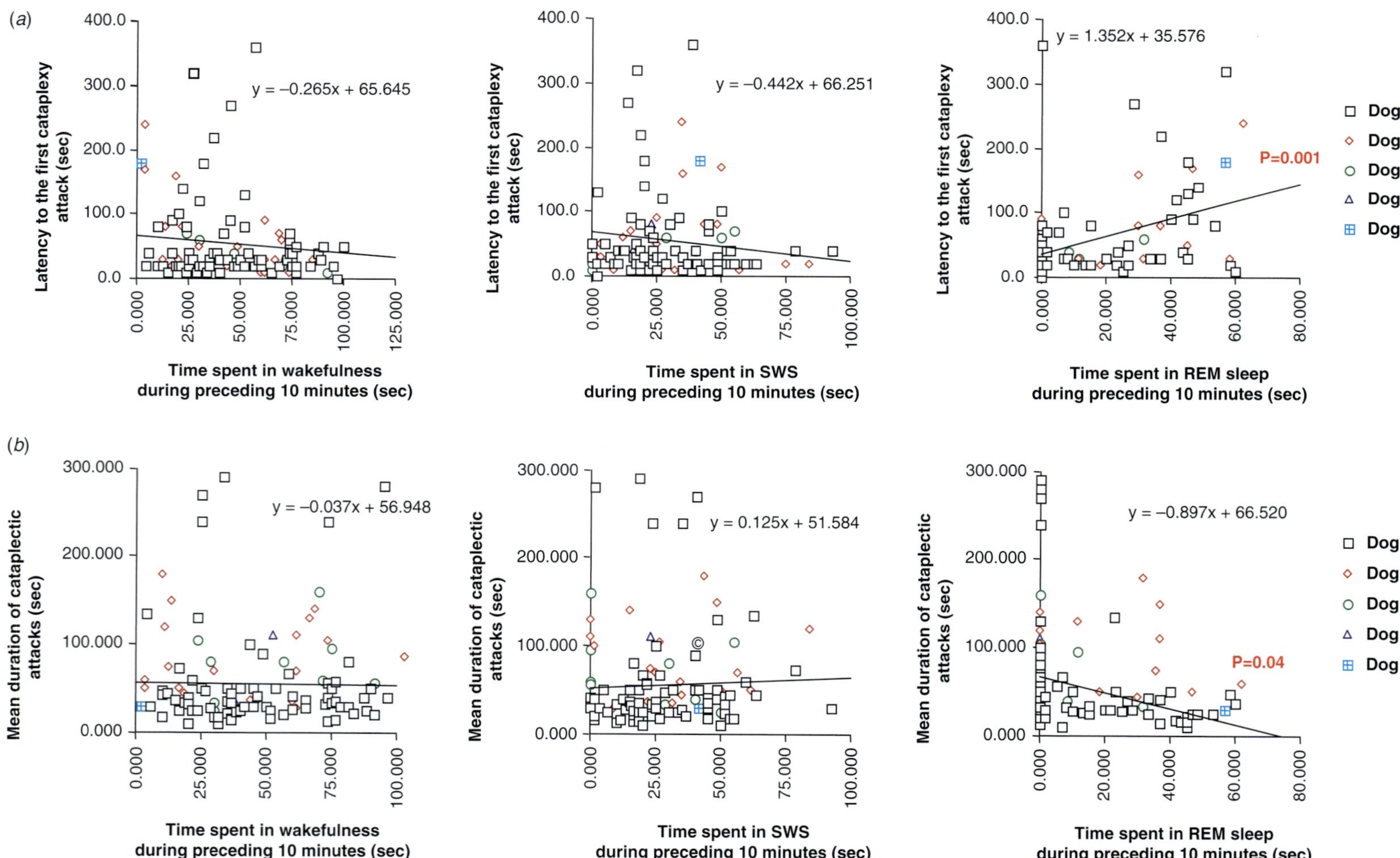

Figure 40.5 (a) Correlation between ten minutes preceding amount of wakefulness, SWS and REM sleep, and latencies to the first cataplectic attacks and (b) mean duration of cataplectic attacks. Preceding REM-sleep amount is positively correlated to the latency to the first cataplectic attack (p = 0.001), and is negatively correlated with the mean duration of cataplectic attacks (p = 0.04). Preceding REM-sleep amount is also negatively correlated with the duration of the first cataplectic attacks and total time spent in cataplexy (TSC) (data not shown). In contrast, preceding wake and SWS amount do not influence these parameters.

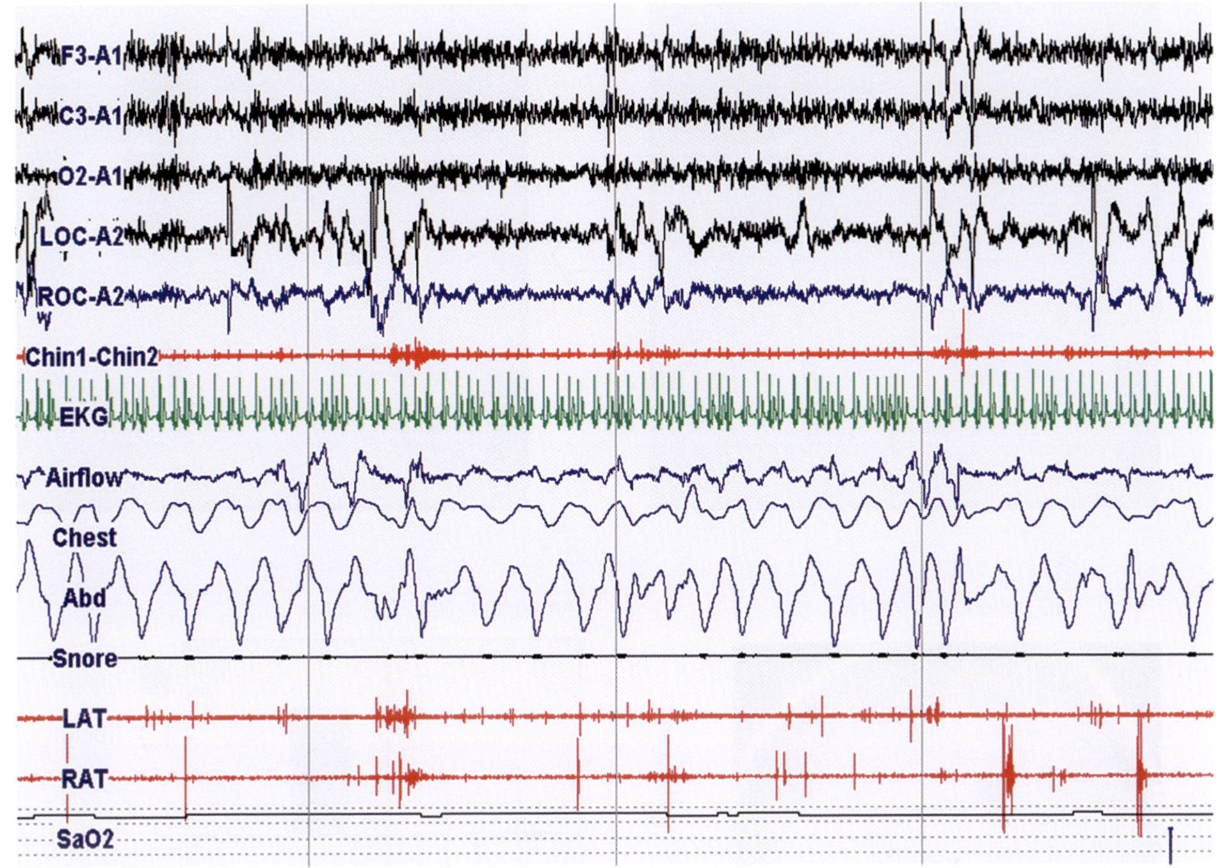

Figure 41.1 Polysomnography of a patient with REM sleep behavior disorder: REM sleep.

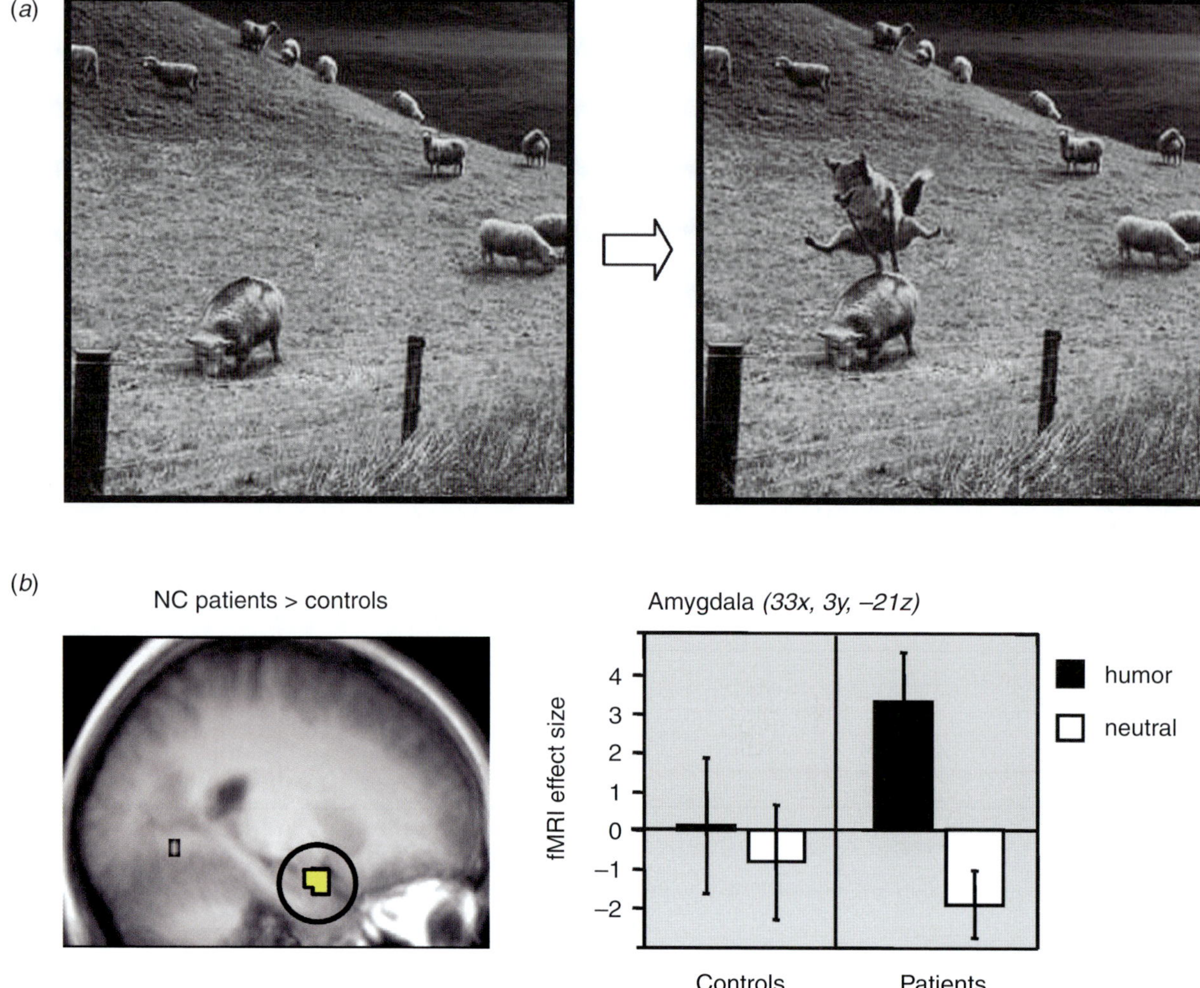

Figure 42.1 Amygdala response to humorous stimuli in narcolepsy–cataplexy (NC) patients. (*a*) Mini-sequence in which a neutral scene was followed by a second picture revealing a new element either neutral or humorous. Here a sequence judged as funny. (*b*) Increased amygdala response to humor in NC patients compared to controls. Parameter estimates show increased fMRI signal to humorous sequences in the patients but not in the controls. (Adapted from Schwartz *et al. Brain* 2008 with permission.)

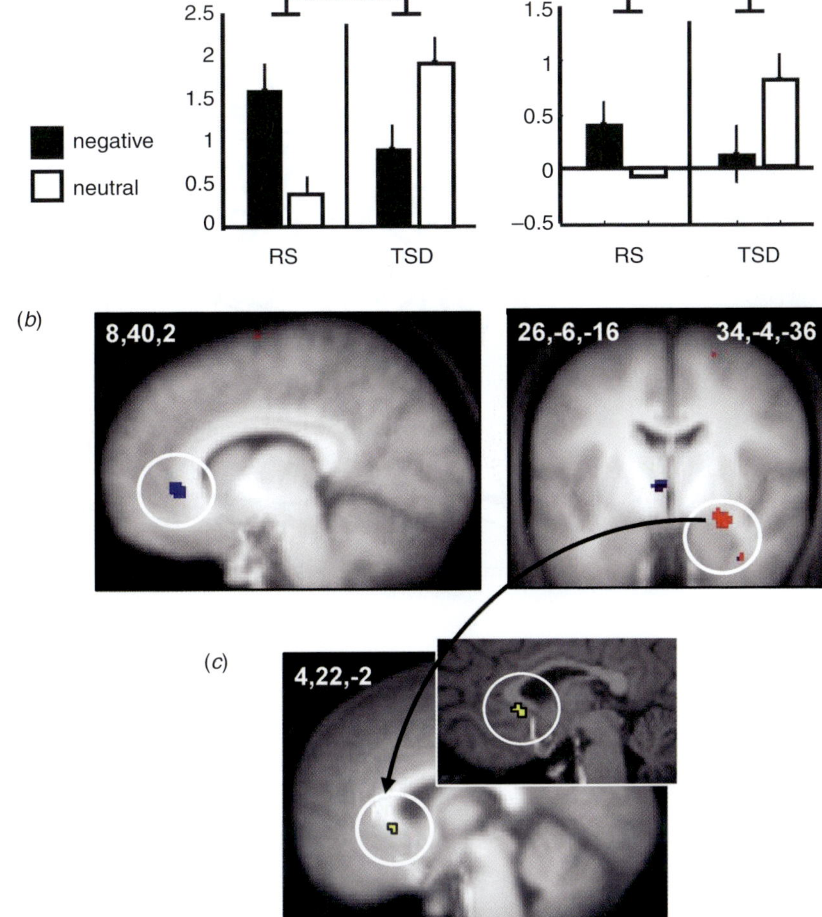

Figure 42.2 Effect of sleep on emotional memory after six months. Sterpenich's fMRI study was performed in three phases: encoding, first retrieval (after three days), and delayed retrieval (after six months). During the incidental encoding session, the subjects rated the valence of 40 negative, 40 positive, and 40 neutral pictures on a seven-point scale (–3, very unpleasant; 0, neutral; +3, very pleasant). During the post-encoding night, one half of the subjects were totally sleep deprived (TSD). The other participants went home and slept as usual (RS). After two additional nights, which allowed sleep-deprived participants to recover, subjects performed a first retrieval session during which 120 previously encoded pictures were presented, randomly mixed with 60 new ones. Six months after the encoding session, the subjects performed a second retest session during which the 120 initially encoded pictures were again mixed with 60 additional new ones. (a) Parameter estimates of activity in the MPFC and amygdala, showing increased activity for negative (black bars) than neutral (white bars) pictures for the RS compared to the TSD group after six months. (b) The amygdala (in red) was more activated by emotional stimuli during encoding, and the ventral medial PFC (in blue) showed a memory by delay interaction. (c) Ventral medial PFC was more connected to the amygdala for negative than neutral correctly recollected pictures and more so in the RS than TSD group (inset, enlarged prefrontal and temporal region in a representative subject). (Adapted from Sterpenich *et al. J Neurosci* 2009 with permission.)

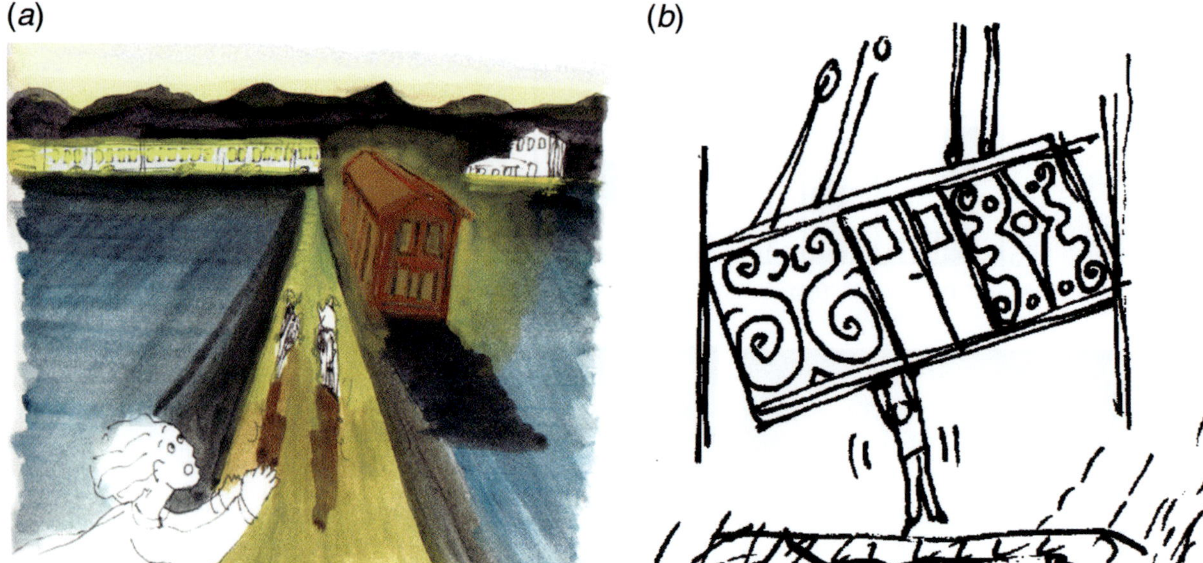

Figure 42.3 Examples of threatening situations associated with strong emotions in dreams. (*a*) Terrified, the dreamer tries to escape a danger by catching a train. (*b*) The dreamer is trapped in a space beneath an elevator, threatened to get crushed by the weight of the elevator. Drawings selected from a dream diary extensively analyzed elsewhere (S. Schwartz, Doctoral thesis).

The role of tuberomammillary nucleus histaminergic neurons, and of their receptors, in the regulation of sleep and waking

Jaime M. Monti

Summary

Neuroanatomical, neurochemical, genetic, and neuropharmacological evidence presently indicates a role for histamine (HA) in the control of behavioral states. The known neuroanatomical connections of the HA-ergic pathways resemble those of the ascending noradrenergic and serotonergic components of the reticular activating system. Also, the arousing effect of intracerebroventricular (icv) HA administration indicates an important role for HA in this system as a major determinant of the waking state. This is further supported by findings in which 2-(3-trifluoromethylphenyl)histamine, the selective H_1 receptor agonist, and thioperamide, the H_3 receptor antagonist, increase waking while the HA synthesis inhibitor α-FMH, the H_1 receptor antagonists mepyramine, diphenhydramine, chlorpheniramine, and promethazine, and the H_3 receptor agonist AMH produce the opposite effects.

It has been proposed that HA may act to modulate REM sleep, such that inhibition of HA functional activity would be followed by increased amounts of REM sleep (permissive role). Accordingly, during REM sleep HA-containing neurons become silent. Moreover, rats treated with α-FMH and HD-KO mice show a significant increase of REM sleep. However, stimulation or blockade of the H_1 or H_3 receptor suppresses REM sleep. These seemingly conflicting sets of data could be partly related to the lack of specificity of drugs that modify HA transmission. However, experimental manipulations involving direct interactions with receptors may not necessarily have the same consequences for REM sleep as would manipulations that result in reduced HA availability. In this respect, the suppression of REM sleep after stimulation of H_1 receptors could be related to the activation of GABAergic interneurons located within and around the LDT/PPT that express these receptors. On the other hand, the reduction of REM sleep after activation of H_3 heteroreceptors located in cholinergic and glutamatergic neurons of the LDT/PPT and the mPRF involved in the induction and maintenance of REM sleep could be related to the inhibition of the release of ACh and GLU.

Introduction

Histamine was first synthesized by Winders and Vogt in 1907, but its pharmacological activity was recognized only a few years later when it was shown to stimulate smooth muscle.

Although much of the attention since has been given to HA in peripheral tissues, allergic reactions, and injury, knowledge of its presence in the central nervous system (CNS) goes back as far as that of norepinephrine.

Kwiatkowski (1943) was the first to detect the amine in the brain, mainly in gray matter, while Harris *et al.* (1952) found relatively higher amounts of HA in the hypothalamus than in other brain areas. The successful synthesis of HA in the brain from labeled histidine and the development of compounds with HA-blocking properties and marked sedative effects, later to be called H_1 receptor antagonists, strongly suggested that the amine might be in histaminergic neurons.

Further advances in our understanding of HA as a neurotransmitter in the CNS were made possible by (1) the development of antibodies against both HA and the HA-synthesizing enzyme L-histidine decarboxylase (HD); (2) the finding that the amine occurs in

REM Sleep: Regulation and Function, eds. Birendra N. Mallick, S. R. Pandi-Perumal, Robert W. McCarley, and Adrian R. Morrison. Published by Cambridge University Press. © Cambridge University Press 2011.

neurons located in the tuberomammillary nucleus of the posterior hypothalamus and is released by depolarization; (3) the characterization in brain of three distinct subclasses of HA receptors, H_1, H_2, and H_3; and (4) the availability of new pharmacological tools capable of interfering with HA synthesis or of activating or selectively blocking HA receptors.

Neural structures and neurotransmitters involved in the regulation of sleep and waking

The neural structures involved in the promotion of the waking (W) state are located in (1) the brain stem (dorsal raphe nucleus, DRN; median raphe nucleus, MRN; locus coeruleus, LC; laterodorsal and pedunculopontine tegmental nuclei, LDT/PPT; and medial-pontine reticular formation, mPRF); (2) hypothalamus (tuberomammillary nucleus, TMN; and lateral hypothalamus, LH); (3) basal forebrain, BFB (medial septal area, nucleus basalis of Meynert); and (4) midbrain ventral tegmental area (VTA) and substantia nigra pars compacta (SNc) (Jones, 2003). The following neurotransmitters function to promote W: (1) acetylcholine (ACh: LDT/PPT, BFB); (2) noradrenaline (NA: LC); (3) serotonin (5-HT: DRN, MRN); (4) histamine (HA: TMN); (5) glutamate (GLU: mPRF, BFB, thalamus); (6) orexin (OX: LH); and (7) dopamine (DA: VTA, SNc).

The neural structures involved in the regulation of W give rise to mainly ascending projections that follow a dorsal and a ventral route. The dorsal route terminates in non-specific thalamic nuclei, which in turn project to the cerebral cortex; glutamate is involved in this step. The ventral route passes through the hypothalamus and continues into the BFB, where cells in turn project to the cerebral cortex and hippocampus; acetylcholine participates in this step. In addition, a number of neural structures send descending projections to the spinal cord that modulate muscle tone.

Neurons in the BFB, preoptic area, and anterior hypothalamus constitute the sleep-inducing system. A majority of these neurons contain γ-aminobutyric acid (GABA) and galanin, two inhibitory neurotransmitters, and project to the BFB and to brain-stem and hypothalamic areas involved in the promotion of W (Szymusiak *et al.*, 2001). A similar role has been proposed for the melanin-concentrating hormone (MCH). Accordingly, MCH-containing neurons located in the zona incerta, perifornical nucleus, and lateral hypothalamus tend

to facilitate sleep occurrence by inhibiting 5-HT, NA, ACh, and OX neurons involved in the promotion of W (Lagos *et al.*, 2009).

Adenosine has been proposed to induce sleep by inhibiting cholinergic neurons of the BFB and the brain stem via A_1 receptors, and infusion of antisense oligonucleotides into the BFB prevents the sleep rebound that occurs following sleep deprivation.

Cholinergic neurons of the LDT/PPT act to promote rapid-eye movement (REM) sleep. The predominantly glutamatergic neurons of the REMS-induction region of the mPRF are in turn activated by cholinergic cells; this activation results in the occurrence of tonic and phasic components of REM sleep. It should be mentioned that in addition to the mPRF the most ventral and rostral part of the pontine reticular nucleus, the perilocus coeruleus alpha nucleus of the mediodorsal pontine tegmentum, and the dorsal part of the rostral pontine tegmentum have been proposed to be critical for REM sleep generation. All these neurons are inhibited by serotonergic (DRN), noradrenergic (LC), histaminergic (TMN), orexinergic (LH), and dopaminergic (VTA, SNc) cells.

Histamine synthesis and metabolism

Labeled HA does not cross the blood–brain barrier, indicating that the CNS depends upon local neuronal biosynthesis. Histamine in the brain is formed from L-histidine, this being actively transported into the brain. Histidine is decarboxylated by HD, a pyridoxal 5′-phosphate-dependent enzyme. Histidine decarboxylase is not saturated, and consequently administration of L-histidine increases brain HA levels. Histamine content is highest in the hypothalamus, intermediate in the basal ganglia and thalamus, and lowest in the brain stem and cerebellum. Because no high-affinity uptake system seems to exist for HA, its inactivation occurs solely by catabolic pathways. In the mammalian brain HA is methylated to tele-methylhistamine by the enzyme HA-N-methyltranferase. Tele-methylhistamine is further deaminated by monoamine oxidase (MAO)-B into tele-methylimidazolacetic acid. Studies using the rate of decline of HA levels after irreversible inhibition of HD by the compound α-fluoromethylhistidine (α-FMH), tend to indicate that brain HA turnover is rapid, with a half-life of about 30 minutes. Of note, HA synthesis and release are under the control of inhibitory H_3 autoreceptors located on the soma and axon terminals of HA cells.

In the brain, HA is contained in both a neuronal and a non-neuronal pool. The latter corresponds to the mast cells that make only a minor contribution to HA at central sites.

Histamine release in the hypothalamus follows a circadian rhythm both in nocturnal and diurnal animals. In this respect, the release of HA from the anterior and the posterior hypothalamus is higher during the dark period compared to the light period in the freely moving rat (Prast *et al.*, 1992). On the other hand, in the rhesus monkey, a diurnal animal, HA release is higher during the daytime than at night. Strecker *et al.* (2002) measured extracellular HA levels in the cat preoptic/anterior hypothalamic area during the different sleep–waking states. Histamine levels fluctuated across the sleep–wake cycle with the lowest levels observed during REM sleep followed by non-rapid-eye movement (NREM) sleep and the highest level during W. HA-ergic neuron activity was assessed also using c-Fos protein in predominantly sleeping or awake rats. c-Fos expression in histaminergic neurons of three TMN subnuclei was higher during periods of W.

Efferent and afferent connections of the tuberomammillary nucleus

The location of histaminergic neurons and of their projection axons was achieved after the development of specific and sensitive antibodies to HD and HA (Panula *et al.*, 1984). With these methods histaminergic neurons were identified in the tuberal region of the posterior hypothalamus of the rat. The histaminergic neuronal system consists of a single group of diffusely distributed neurons in the TMN, where Ericson *et al.* (1987) proposed the existence of three main subgroups of cells: (1) the medial tuberomammillary subgroup located on either side of the mammillary recess; (2) the ventral tuberomammillary subgroup located at the ventral surface of the brain, rostral and caudal to the mammillary bodies; and (3) the diffuse part of the TMN, which consists of a relatively small number of cells scattered within various hypothalamic nuclei.

Histamine immunoreactive neurons were found also in the tuberomammillary complex of the guinea pig, cat, tree shrew, and human. In the guinea pig HA neurons are more numerous than in the rat, being also found between the medial and lateral mammillary nuclei. In the tree shrew the majority of cell bodies are located laterally in the ventral part of the tuberomammillary nucleus. In the human distinct clusters of HA neurons are seen between the ventromedial nucleus and the third ventricle, and in the basal hypothalamus in areas corresponding to the tuberomammillary nucleus.

Some TMN neurons exhibit also immunoreactivity for adenosine deaminase (the enzyme that catalyzes the conversion of adenosine to inosine), glutamic acid decarboxylase (GAD), galanin, proenkephalin-derived peptides, thyrotropin releasing hormone (TRH), and substance P (SP).

The HA-containing neurons in the TMN project practically to the entire brain. Panula *et al.* (1988) recognized one descending and two ascending pathways. The ventral ascending pathway runs close to the major hypothalamic nuclei towards the nucleus of the diagonal band, the medial septal nucleus, and the olfactory tubercle and bulb. The dorsal ascending pathway runs along the lateral side of the third ventricle and sends branches to the thalamic nuclei and rostral forebrain structures including the limbic system and the cerebral cortex. These tracts remain largely ipsilateral, although there is a crossing over at the level of the retrochiasmatic area, the optic chiasma, and the supramammillary region. The descending pathway provides innervation to the brain stem (VTA, SNc, LDT/PPT, DRN, LC) and spinal cord.

Several laboratories have shown afferents to HA-immunoreactive neurons from the prefrontal cortex, septal nuclei, olfactory tubercle, hippocampus, medial septal area, hypothalamus, particularly preoptic/anterior areas, and brain stem. Thus, there is a reciprocal interaction between the TMN HA-containing neurons and cells in the brain stem (LDT/PPT, LC, DRN), the hypothalamus (LH, ventrolateral/preoptic area, VLPA) and the BFB (diagonal band of Broca) that participate in the regulation of sleep and W.

Inhibitory and facilitatory influences of other neurotransmitter systems on HA-containing TMN neurons

GABAergic neurons that project to the TMN are located in the BFB and the hypothalamus (LH, VLPA). GABA reduces the activity of HAergic cells by acting on both $GABA_A$ and $GABA_B$ receptors. Galanin is coexpressed by a number of GABAergic cells located in the preoptic area that project to the TMN. Galanin exerts also an inhibitory effect on the HA-containing neurons.

The adenosine A_1 receptor is expressed in HAergic neurons of the rat TMN. Histamine release at postsynaptic sites is reduced following the micro-injection into the TMN of adenosine, an adenosine A_1 receptor agonist or an inhibitor of adenosine deaminase. All these findings tend to indicate that adenosine inhibits the HA-ergic system via A_1 receptors.

Glutamatergic inputs to the TMN have been described that originate in several hypothalamic nuclei and the cerebral cortex. The presence of GLU receptors – NMDA and AMPA receptors – in TMN neurons has been determined in the rat and electrical stimulation of lateral preoptic area and lateral hypothalamus induces the appearance of glutamatergic excitatory potentials in presumed HA-ergic cells.

Rodent studies have shown that cholinergic cell bodies project from the mesopontine tegmentum to the TMN. In addition, HA-ergic neurons endowed with nicotinic receptors, predominantly of the α_7 subtype, have been detected in the TMN and their activation has been proposed to affect the HA-induced arousal.

Efferent projections from the DRN have been found to reach the TMN, and 5-HT has been shown to depolarize HAergic neurons via the 5-HT_{2C} receptor.

There is an anatomical relationship between the LC and the TMN. However, NA does not directly affect the firing rate of HA cells in vitro. In fact, NA inhibits GABAergic inhibitory postsynaptic potentials in HAergic neurons through the activation of α_2 adrenoceptors.

Dopamine D_2 receptors have been characterized on cell bodies in the TMN, and their selective activation increases the firing rate of HA-containing neurons.

Chemelli *et al.* (1999) characterized a direct projection from orexin-immunoreactive neurons localized within the lateral and posterior hypothalamus to the TMN. It has been determined, in addition, that orexins (A and B) cause an increase in firing frequency of HAergic neurons through the orexin type II receptor.

Prostaglandin (PG)E_2 and PGD_2 are positional stereoisomers that exhibit opposite biological actions (Hayaishi and Huang, 2004). Prostaglandin E_2 perfusion in the TMN has been shown to increase HA synthesis and release in the preoptic area and the frontal cortex of the rat. Administration of an EP_4 receptor agonist, one of the four functionally distinct subtypes of PGE_2 receptors, has been shown to reproduce the effect of PGE_2 on HA synthesis and release in the brain.

Thus, presently available evidence tends to indicate that GABA, galanin, and adenosine inhibit the activity of HA neurons whereas GLU, ACh, NA, 5-HT, OX, and PGE_2 induce the opposite effect.

Histamine receptors

The HAergic H_1, H_2, and H_3 receptors are prominently expressed in the brain. Recently, a fourth HA receptor (H_4) has been identified in peripheral tissues. The presence of the H_4 receptor on leukocytes and mast cells led to the proposal that it is mainly involved in the modulation of the immune system. However, experimental evidence provided by Strakhova *et al.* (2009) tends to indicate that the H_4 receptor is localized also in CNS anatomical structures involved in the regulation of the behavioral state. Accordingly, in rat H_4 mRNA has been detected in the cerebral cortex, dorsal striatum, amygdala, thalamus, brain stem, and cerebellum. Very low levels of H_4 mRNA were found in the hypothalamus, and no H_4 signal was detected in the rat hippocampus. Transcripts of H_4 receptor were present also in the human CNS including the cerebral cortex, limbic system (hippocampus, amygdala), thalamus, and spinal cord.

Histamine-related functions in the CNS are regulated at postsynaptic sites by the H_1 and the H_2 receptors. On the other hand, the H_3 receptor shows the features of a presynaptic autoreceptor, mediating the synthesis and release of HA, and of a presynaptic heteroreceptor, controlling the release of several neurotransmitters, including 5-HT, NE, DA, ACh, GLU, GABA, and a number of neuropeptides (Haas *et al.*, 2008). The three types of receptors differ in their molecular properties, distribution in the CNS, electrophysiological responses, and affinity for HA and synthetic agonists and antagonists.

The H_1 receptor is related to the enzyme phospholipase C via a $G_{q/11}$ protein and acts primarily by increasing the Ca^{2+} concentration in the target cell. The process is linked to the hydrolysis of inositol phospholipids by the enzyme phospholipase C with the production of inositol-1,4,5-triphosphate, that mobilizes Ca^{2+}, and 1,2-diacylglycerol that activates protein kinase C.

The H_1 receptor is widely distributed in the CNS. However, its density and regional distribution vary between species. In the guinea pig, the H_1 receptor is present in: (1) all areas and layers of the cerebral cortex with a higher density in the deep layers; (2) the limbic system, including the hippocampus, amygdala, and medial and lateral septal nuclei; (3) the caudate-putamen and the nucleus accumbens, which are moderately and highly labeled, respectively; (4) the thalamus, with a higher distribution of receptors in the anterior, median, and lateral nuclei; (5) the hypothalamus, including the medial preoptic area, dorsolateral and ventromedial nuclei, and the tuberomammillary complex; (6) the midbrain and brain stem where H_1 receptors predominate on the DA-, ACh-, NA-, and 5-HT-containing neurons, cerebellum and area postrema; (7) the spinal cord, predominantly the dorsal horn.

Histamine acting through the H_2 receptor, activates a stimulatory G_s protein, which in turn stimulates adenylate cyclase. Increased cAMP levels lead to activation of protein kinase A and to a physiological response.

The H_2 receptor is distributed extensively and in a heterogeneous fashion. In the rodent brain the H_2 receptor is present in: (1) the superficial layers of the cerebral cortex; (2) the limbic system including the hippocampus and the amygdala; (3) the basal ganglia, where very high densities have been detected in the nucleus accumbens, the caudate-putamen, and the olfactory tubercle; (4) the thalamus (medial group of nuclei); (5) the hypothalamus where the density is very low; (6) the mesencephalon where relatively high densities have been found at the level of the superior and inferior colliculi, central gray matter, and substantia nigra; and (7) the lower brain stem, with the highest density observed in the raphe nuclei (Schwartz *et al.*, 1991). In the human and rhesus monkey brain H_2 receptor sites are predominantly localized in the basal ganglia, although they are also present in the cerebral cortex.

The H_3 receptor signals through $G_{i/o}$ proteins. It is negatively coupled to adenylate cyclase and its stimulation induces a decrease of cAMP. The $G_{i/o}$ protein may activate also the mitogen-activated protein kinase and phosphatidylinositol 3-kinase.

The distribution of H_3 receptor in the rodent brain is highly heterogeneous and not exactly the same as that of histaminergic terminals, which is in accordance with its presence on non-HAergic nerve endings. Thus, it has been localized on HAergic axons, but also on 5HTergic and NAergic nerve endings. In rodents the H_3 receptor is found in: (1) all layers of the cerebral cortex, especially in the deep layers; (2) structures corresponding to the limbic system, including the hippocampus and the amygdala; (3) the striatum, nucleus accumbens, anterior olfactory nuclei, and olfactory tubercles; (4) the thalamus, mainly its medial part; (5) the hypothalamus at the level of the TMN; (6) the mesencephalon, where a relatively high density is found in the SN pars reticulata, the VTA, and the superior and inferior colliculi; (7) the lower brain stem where low to moderate densities are found in the LC, the raphe nuclei, and the vestibular nuclei (Schwartz *et al.*, 1991). In the human and rhesus monkey brain H_3 receptors predominate in the basal ganglia, mainly the globus pallidus.

Effects of histamine at the cellular level

The evidence obtained from an extensive series of studies tends to indicate that HA H_1 receptors mediate excitatory actions in the CNS. The H_2 receptors predominantly activate neural systems at central sites although inhibitory effects have been described also. The H_3 receptors have an inhibitory effect on the synthesis and release of HA and, in addition, on the release of several inhibitory and facilitary neurotransmitters.

The effects of HA and of H_1, H_2, or H_3 receptor agonists and antagonists on CNS neurons have been studied in tissue slices and anesthetized as well as unanesthetized animals. The excitatory responses related to H_1 or H_2 receptor activation manifest as depolarization, increase in firing rate, and facilitation of signal transmission. Excitatory actions mediated via H_1 receptors have been found in the brain stem (mPRF, LC, DRN), hypothalamus (supraoptic, suprachiasmatic, ventromedial, dorsomedial and arcuate nuclei, preoptic area, lateral hypothalamic area), BFB (medial septal nucleus, nucleus basalis of Meynart), basal ganglia (nucleus accumbens) and cerebral cortex (pyramidal neurons, visual relay neurons) (Brown *et al.*, 2001). Excitatory effects mediated via H_2 receptors have been characterized in the brain stem (LC), hippocampus (CA1, CA2, and CA3 areas), basal ganglia (nucleus accumbens), and cerebral cortex (visual relay neurons). Inhibitory effects of HA mediated by H_2 receptors are due to the hyperpolarization and decrease in the firing rate of the corresponding neuron (direct effect), or to the activation of GABAergic interneurons that induce the inhibition of the postsynaptic cell (indirect effect). Inhibitory actions mediated via H_2 receptors have been found in the spinal cord, hypothalamus (supraoptic and suprachiasmatic nuclei), and cerebral cortex (pyramidal neurons) (Haas *et al.*, 2008).

The H_3 receptor mediates the inhibitory response of HA on the TMN neurons.

Rates of firing of histaminergic neurons involved in the regulation of sleep and waking

Single-unit extracellular recordings in the ventrolateral posterior hypothalamus of the freely moving cat or

TMN of urethane-anesthetized and freely behaving rats have defined a population of histaminergic cortically projecting neurons that show a relatively long-lasting action potential and a slow conduction velocity (Vanni-Mercier *et al.*, 1985). Histaminergic neurons display a slow and regular discharge during quiet W (1.4 spikes/s) in the cat. When the animal is moving (active W) the mean discharge rate increases to 2.3 spikes/s. As the cat enters SWS the mean discharge rate shows a progressive decrease (0.43 spikes/s). During deep SWS and REM sleep all the neurons become silent (Vanni-Mercier *et al.*, 1985). A similar pattern has been described for NAergic LC and 5-HTergic DRN neurons. There is also evidence that orexinergic LH neurons discharge at their maximal rate during W, decrease firing during SWS, and cease firing during REM sleep. Unlike 5-HT, NA, and OX cells, DA neurons in the VTA and the SNc show a change in the temporal pattern rather than the firing rate during W. It manifests as burst firing and is accompanied by a more efficient release of DA.

Role of histamine in the regulation of sleep and waking

The data pertinent to the role of HA in the regulation of sleep and waking has been obtained mainly from: (1) lesion studies of the posterior hypothalamus; (2) animals with irreversible inhibition of HD activity; (3) HD knock-out mice and HAergic H_1 and H_3 receptor knock-out mice; (4) pharmacological studies in which selective HA receptor agonists and antagonists were administered to laboratory animals (Table 23.1).

Lesion studies

Long before it was known that HA-immunoreactive neurons are located in the TMN, it was established that damage, lesioning, or cooling of the posterior hypothalamus of several species, including human, gives rise to a state of somnolence or hypersomnia.

In the study of the Vienna epidemic of encephalitis lethargica, Von Economo (1926) established that somnolence was present in only those patients with lesions of the caudal part of the hypothalamus. The experiments by Ranson (1939) on monkeys showed that bilateral lesions in the area of the mammillary bodies caused the same marked somnolence observed in patients with epidemic encephalitis. Naquet *et al.* (1965) and Swett and Hobson (1968) found that electrolytic lesions of the posterior hypothalamus in cats were followed by a behavioral state of somnolence; the animals had at least twice as much SWS as those with medial lesions. Temporary inhibition of the posterior hypothalamus by means of a thermode permitting a light progressive cooling gave way to slowing of cortical rhythms and to the appearance of bilateral spindles accompanied by behavioral sleep (Naquet *et al.*, 1966). Relevant to our topic is the report by Sallanon *et al.* (1987) that insomnia induced in cats after neurotoxic lesions of the paramedial preoptic area with ibotenic acid could be reversed by pharmacological inactivation of the posterior hypothalamus with the GABAergic agonist muscimol. Moreover, microinjection of muscimol into the posterior hypothalamus causes somnolence in normal cats.

In the rat complete bilateral transection of the posterior hypothalamus interfered with the maintenance of the waking state (Nauta, 1946). Accordingly, the animals slept uninterrupted for several days in the absence of external stimuli. Bilateral electrolytic lesions of the posterior hypothalamus and adjacent subthalamic area in rats produced a continuous sleep-like state that lasted from one to four days. Electroencephalogram (EEG) patterns were of large amplitude and low frequency. REM sleep was completely suppressed during the continuous phase of somnolence. Recovery from somnolence was gradual but complete, thus suggesting the rapid development of compensatory mechanisms (McGinty, 1969).

In conclusion, electrolytic lesions, complete bilateral transection, light, progressive cooling, or pharmacological inactivation of the posterior hypothalamus in cats and rats induced behavioral sleep, and in those studies where the EEG was recorded an increase in the number of spindles and slow-wave activity were observed.

Histamine synthesis inhibition

α-Fluoromethylhistidine is a highly specific, irreversible inhibitor of HD. α-FMH does not inhibit other decarboxylases, such as dopa and glutamate decarboxylase, or the HA-metabolizing enzyme, HA-N-methyltransferase. Single injection of α-FMH (10–50 mg/kg) produced an 80 to 95% inhibition of HD activity at central sites within three days in the hypothalamus, but was incomplete in the cerebral cortex after four days. In the studies by Monti *et al.* (1985, 1988), where rats were given α-FMH 50 mg/kg, ip, and recorded for three days, ten hours per day in the light period, W and

Table 23.1 The role of histamine in the regulation of sleep and wakefulness: neuroanatomical, neurochemical, genetic, and pharmacological data

Experimental approach	W	SWS	REMS	Comments	References
Lesion and pharmacological inactivation of the posterior hypothalamus (TMN)	?	+	?	Behavioral state of somnolence	1,2,3,4,5,6, 7,8
Histamine synthesis inhibition (irreversible inhibition of HD with α-FMH)	–	+	+	Systemic administration	9
HD knock-out mice	n.s.	n.s.	+	Reduction in cortical EEG power in θ-rhythm	10
H_1 receptor knock-out mice	n.s.	n.s.	n.s.	Decrease in ambulation	11
H_3 receptor knock-out mice	Data not provided			Reduction of spontaneous locomotor activity	12
Pharmacological studies – intracerebral administration of HA	Data not provided			Increase of spontaneous locomotor activity	13
– HA H_1 receptor agonist [(2-(3 -trifluoromethylphenyl)histamine)]	+	–	n.s.	Prevented by H_1 receptor antagonist	14
– HA H_3 receptor agonists (AMH, BP 2.04)	–	+	–	Prevented by H_3 receptor antagonists	15

Abbreviations: α-FMH, α-fluoromethylhistine; AMH, R- α-methylhistamine; HA, histamine; HD, histidine decarboxylase; REMS, REM sleep; SWS, slow-wave sleep; TMN, tuberomammillary nucleus; W, waking; n.s., non-significant; +, increased; –, reduced.

References: 1. Ranson, 1939; 2. Naquet *et al.*, 1965; 3. Swett and Hobson, 1968; 4. Naquet *et al.*, 1966; 5. Sallanon *et al.*, 1987; 6. Lin *et al.*, 1990; 7. Nauta, 1946; 8. McGinty, 1969; 9. Monti *et al.*, 1985; 10. Parmentier *et al.*, 2002; 11. Huang *et al.*, 2006; 12. Toyota *et al.*, 2002; 13. Monnier *et al.*, 1970; 14. Monti *et al.*, 1986; 15. Monti *et al.*, 1991.

light sleep were significantly decreased, while SWS and REM sleep showed the opposite changes. In rats housed under 16 h light/8 h dark compared with 12 h light/12 h dark conditions, W increased significantly during the dark period. Under these conditions α-FMH decreased W and increased SWS during the dark period (Monti *et al.*, 1988).

Bilateral injection of α-FMH (50 μg) into the ventrolateral posterior hypothalamus of the cat resulted in a significant increase in deep SWS and decrease of W, without a change in REM sleep; these effects appeared as early as the second hour after injection. Similar results were obtained when α-FMH (20 mg/kg) was given ip, the effect being apparent early after drug administration.

Histidine decarboxylase knock-out mice and HAergic H_1 and H_3 receptor knock-out mice

The sleep–wake cycle, cortical EEG, and a variety of behaviors have been examined in HD knock-out (HD-KO) mice. Compared to wild-type (WT) mice, HD-KO mice showed an increase of REM sleep that occurred predominantly during the light phase and was related to a greater number of REM sleep periods. In addition, SWS and REM sleep latencies were decreased. Values corresponding to W and SWS were not significantly modified over 24 h (Parmentier *et al.*, 2002). Notwithstanding this, the increase of W that normally precedes and follows lights-off was significantly reduced in the HD-KO animals. Moreover, HD-KO mice showed a reduction in the cortical EEG power in θ-rhythm during W, and a decreased SWS/W power ratio. Administration of α-FMH or the H_3 receptor antagonist ciproxifan induced no significant changes of sleep variables in the HD-KO animals (Parmentier *et al.*, 2002).

HD-KO mice also showed hypoactivity and increased measures of anxiety in the open field, elevated plus-maze, height-fear task, and the graded anxiety test. Interestingly, they had also higher ACh levels and a significantly higher 5-HT turnover in the frontal cortex.

The sleep–wake characteristics and behavior have been examined, in addition, in HAergic H_1 receptor knock-out (H_1-KO) mice. Compared to WT mice,

H_1-KO mice had fewer brief awakening episodes and a shorter SWS latency. However, no significant differences could be detected in the total amount of SWS and REM sleep between both genotypes of mice (Huang *et al.*, 2006). Systemic administration of mepyramine or ciproxifan did not result in quantitative changes of sleep variables in the H_1-KO animals.

H_1-KO mice showed a significant decrease in ambulation in an open field and on an activity field. The transfer latency in the elevated plus-maze test was significantly longer in the H_1-KO mice than in the WT animals, thus indicating that the H_1 receptor is involved in the control of anxiety. There was no increase of aggressiveness (isolation-induced aggression test), or an antidepressant effect (forced swimming test) in the mutant mice.

Toyota *et al.* (2002) have characterized the behavior of mice lacking HAergic H_3 receptors (H_3-KO). H_3-KO mice showed a reduction of spontaneous locomotor activity, wheel running behavior, and body temperature during the dark phase but maintained a normal circadian rhythm. As expected, the wake-promoting effect of the selective H_3 receptor antagonist thioperamide was absent in the H_3-KO animals. 5-HT, NA and DA levels in the cerebral cortex were not significantly different from those obtained in WT mice. On the other hand, HA levels showed a significant reduction. No attempts were made by the study authors to quantify values corresponding to sleep and W in the H_3-KO mice.

Toyota *et al.* (2002) contend that an increase of spontaneous motor activity should have occurred in the H_3-KO mice; the opposite effect could have been related to a compensatory reduction of histaminergic neurotransmission. However, further studies are needed to resolve this issue.

Pharmacological studies

Intracerebral administration of HA

Histamine infusion (150–300 µg) into the third ventricle of the conscious rabbit has been shown to elicit a marked electrographic arousal reaction and a decrease in spectral power in the delta band. Pretreatment with the H_1 receptor antagonist mepyramine (1.5 mg/kg) abolished the cortical EEG activation. This observation led Monnier *et al.* (1970) to postulate that HA may have a role in the modulation of EEG arousal. Histamine was administered also into the lateral cerebral ventricle of the conscious and pentobarbital-anesthetized

rat. In the freely moving rat HA (0.25–25 µg) induced a significant increase in spontaneous motor activity; in the anesthetized rat, it induced a dose-related decrease in narcosis duration. Histamine-induced behavioral arousal was blocked by ip administration of the H_1 receptor antagonists chlorpheniramine (5 mg/kg) or diphenhydramine (5 mg/kg). On the other hand, intracerebral injection of the H_2 receptor antagonist cimetidine did not alter HA-induced behavioral response.

As mentioned earlier, the cholinergic neurons of the magnocellular regions of the BFB receive histaminergic projections from the TMN. In order to test the hypothesis that histaminergic neurons excite the cholinergic cells of the BFB to induce W and cortical arousal, Thakkar *et al.* (2000) perfused HA for six hours in the horizontal diagonal band (HDB) of the rat. Histamine perfused in the cholinergic HDB significantly increased W and reduced SWS during the perfusion period. REM sleep showed no change.

All these findings support the postulate that HA may have a physiological function in modulating arousal.

H_1 receptor agonists and antagonists

It was initially shown that the relatively selective H_1 receptor agonist 2-thiazolylethylamine (64.5–258 µg) dose-dependently increases W and reduces SWS and REM sleep when delivered by an icv route in rats prepared for chronic sleep recordings. The H_1 receptor antagonist mepyramine (1–2 mg/kg) prevented both the increase of W and reduction of SWS (Monti *et al.*, 1986). More recently, the effect of the selective HAergic H_1 agonist 2-(3-trifluoromethylphenyl)histamine (80–120 µg) injected by the icv route on sleep variables was assessed in freely moving rats. The compound increased W and reduced SWS whereas REM sleep remained unchanged. The effects on W and SWS were prevented by mepyramine (2 mg/kg) (Monti *et al.*, 1994).

The H_1 receptor antagonists mepyramine (1–5 mg/kg), diphenhydramine (1.6–10 mg/kg), chlorpheniramine (2–10 mg/kg), and promethazine (5–20 mg/kg) decreased W and REM sleep and augmented SWS in rats and dogs (Monti *et al.*, 1985, 1986, Wauquier, 1983). A decrease in W and increase in SWS in cats followed bilateral injection of mepyramine (120 µg) into the ventrolateral posterior hypothalamus. Although mepyramine has anticholinergic and membrane-stabilizing effects, the results obtained after its direct administration into the TMN do not seem to be related to non-specific mechanisms, since neither atropine nor tetracaine reproduced the actions of the H_1 receptor antagonist on sleep variables.

The second generation HAergic H_1 antagonists astemizole, terfenadine, and loratadine (3 mg/kg, per oral) given to cats and dogs at doses similar to those effective as antihistamines in humans were devoid of any significant effect on the sleep–wakefulness pattern. Even slightly greater amounts of astemizole (10 mg/kg, per oral) did not alter sleep variables in dogs (Wauquier, 1983). On the other hand, doses of astemizole or terfenadine in the order of 30 mg/kg po reduced SWS and/or REM sleep in cats. The lack of an effect of astemizole, terfenadine, or loratadine on sleep–waking patterns of laboratory animals after doses similar to those effective in man could be related to their poor penetration through the blood–brain barrier and weaker affinity for central H_1 receptors.

H_2 receptor agonists and antagonists

Following icv administration of either the H_2 receptor agonist, dimaprit, or the H_2 receptor antagonists metiamide, cimetidine, or ranitidine, hypersynchronous electrocortical activity was induced in the frontal and occipital areas of the rat cortex. The cortical discharges showed sustained high-voltage spikes, which lasted ten seconds to five minutes. These electrographic changes were not accompanied by motor manifestations (Monti et al., 1986). When cimetidine was given by the intraperitoneal (ip) route, sleep and W showed slight but inconsistent changes that did not attain significance. It is possible that factors other than those related to H_2 receptors contribute to effects of these drugs on rat cortical EEG activity.

The benzthiazole derivative zolantidine, which is a potent antagonist of H_2 receptors, penetrates the brain. Zolantidine (0.25–8.0 mg/kg) had no significant effect on sleep parameters in rats (Monti et al., 1990). Although these results tend to suggest that H_2 receptors are not involved in sleep regulation, the absence of selective, brain-penetrating H_2 receptor agonists leaves the matter of their effects on sleep and W unresolved.

H_3 receptor agonists and antagonists

The effect of the H_3 receptor agonist R-α-methylhistamine (AMH) has been compared with that of the H_3 receptor antagonist thioperamide in freely moving rats. AMH (1–4 μg) injected bilaterally into the premammillary area of the rat, where HA immunoreactive neurons are located, increased SWS whereas W and REM sleep were reduced. On the other hand, thioperamide (1–20 mg/kg) increased W and reduced SWS and REM sleep. Pretreatment with thioperamide (4 mg/kg) prevented the effect of AMH (2 μg) on sleep and W (Monti et al., 1991). Moreover, the arousal effect of thioperamide (2 mg/kg) was prevented by pretreatment with mepyramine (1 mg/kg) in cats (Lin et al., 1990).

More recent studies with newly developed H_3 receptor agonists and antagonists confirmed the results obtained with AMH and thioperamide. In this respect, the H_3 receptor agonist BP 2.04 given by oral route produced a significant increase of SWS in the rat that was related to slight decrease in W, light sleep, and REM sleep. In contrast, the H_3 receptor antagonist carboperamide significantly increased W and reduced SWS and REM sleep. Pretreatment with carboperamide prevented the effect of BP 2.04 on SWS (Monti et al., 1996). The H_3 receptor antagonist ciproxifan has been shown to increase W and cortical EEG fast rhythms in mice, whereas the H_3 receptor agonist imetit enhanced SWS and attenuated the ciproxifan-induced increase of W. Similar effects have been observed following the administration of the novel non-imidazole H_3 receptor antagonist JNJ-5207852 in mice and rats; however, the compound failed to modify sleep variables in H_3-KO mice.

Of note, a correlation has been found between ex vivo receptor occupancy and wake-promoting activity of the selective H_3 receptor antagonists thioperamide, ciproxifan, GSK 189254, and ABT-239.

The effects of the H_3 receptor agonists and antagonists on sleep and W could depend on changes in the availability of HA at the postsynaptic H_1 receptor. Alternatively, activation or blockade of H_3 heteroreceptors found in central catecholamine, indolamine, acetylcholine, glutamate, and orexin nerve endings could inhibit or increase the release of NA, DA, 5-HT, ACh, GLU, and OX, which would secondarily result in changes of sleep variables (Monti et al., 1996).

References

Brown, R. E., Stevens, D. R. & Haas, H. L. (2001) The physiology of brain histamine. *Prog Neurobiol* **63**: 637–72.

Chemelli, R. M., Willie, J. T., Sinton, C. M. et al. (1999) Narcolepsy in orexin knockout mice: molecular genetics of sleep regulation. *Cell* **98**:437–451

Ericson, H., Watanabe, T. & Kohler, C. (1987) Morphological analysis of the tuberomammillary nucleus in the rat brain: delineation of subgroups with antibody against L-histidine decarboxylase as a marker. *J Comp Neurol* **263**: 1–24.

Haas, H. L., Sergeeva, O. A. & Selbach, O. (2008) Histamine in the nervous system. *Physiol Rev* **88**: 1183–241.

Harris, G. W., Jacobson, D. & Kahlson, G. (1952) The occurrence of histamine in the cerebral regions related to the hypophysis. In *CIBA Foundation Colloquia on Endocrinology*, ed. G. E. W. Wolstenholme. New York: Blakiston, pp. 186–93.

Hayaishi, O. & Huang, Z. L. (2004) Role of orexin and prostaglandin E(2) in activating histaminergic neurotransmission. *Drug News Perspect* **17**: 105–9.

Huang, Z.-L., Mochizuki, T., Qu, W.-M. *et al.* (2006) Altered sleep–wake characteristics and lack of arousal response to H3 receptor antagonist in histamine H_1 receptor knockout mice. *PNAS* **103**: 4687–92.

Jones, B. E. (2003) Arousal systems. *Front Biosci* **8**: 438–51.

Kwiatkowski, H. (1943) Histamine in nervous tissues. *J Physiol* **102**: 32–41.

Lagos, P., Torterolo, P., Jantos, H. *et al.* (2009) Effects on sleep of melanin-concentrating hormone (MCH) microinjections into the dorsal raphe nucleus. *Brain Res* **1265**: 103–10.

Lin, J. S., Sakai, K., Vanni-Mercier, G. *et al.* (1990) Involvement of histaminergic neurons in arousal mechanisms demonstrated with H3-receptor ligands in the cat. *Brain Res* **523**: 325–30.

McGinty, D. J. (1969) Somnolence, recovery and hyposomnia following ventromedial diencephalic lesions in the rat. *Electroencephalogr Clin Neurophysiol* **26**: 70–9.

Monnier, M., Sauer, R. & Hatt, A. M. (1970) The activating effect of histamine on the central nervous system. *Int Rev Neurobiol* **12**: 265–305.

Monti, J. M., Pellejero, T., Jantos, H. *et al.* (1985) Role of histamine in the control of sleep and waking. In *Sleep: Neurotransmitters and Neuromodulators*, eds. A. Wauquier, J. M. Gaillard, J. M. Monti & M. Radulovacki. New York: Raven, pp. 197–209.

Monti, J. M., Pellejero, T. & Jantos, H. (1986) Effects of H_1- and H2-histamine receptor agonists and antagonists on sleep and wakefulness in the rat. *J Neural Transm* **66**: 1–11.

Monti, J. M., D'Angelo, L., Jantos, H. *et al.* (1988) Effects of α-fluoromethylhistidine on sleep and wakefulness in the rat. *J Neural Transm* **72**: 141–5.

Monti, J. M., Orellana, C., Boussard, M. *et al.* (1990) Sleep variables are unaltered by zolantidine in rats: are histamine H_2-receptors not involved in sleep regulation? *Brain Res Bull* **25**: 229–31.

Monti, J. M., Jantos, H., Boussard, M. *et al.* (1991) Effects of selective activation or blockade of the histamine H_3

receptor on sleep and wakefulness. *Eur J Pharmacol* **205**: 283–7.

Monti, J. M., Jantos, H., Leschke, C. *et al.* (1994) The selective histamine H1-receptor agonist 2-(3-trifluoromethylphenyl) histamine increases waking in the rat. *Eur Neuropharmacol* **4**: 459–62.

Monti, J. M., Jantos, H., Ponzoni, A. *et al.* (1996) Sleep and waking during acute histamine H_3 agonist BP 2.94 or H3 antagonist carboperamide (MR 16155) administration in rats. *Neuropsychopharmacology* **15**: 31–5.

Naquet, R., Denavit, M., Lanoir, J. *et al.* (1965) Alterations transitoires ou définitives de zones diencéphaliques chez le chat. Leurs effets sur l´activité électrique corticale et le sommeil. In *Aspects anatomofonctionnels de la physiologie du sommeil*. ed. M. Jouvet. Paris: CNRS, pp. 107–31.

Naquet, R., Denavit, M. & Albe-Fessard, D. (1966) Comparison entre le róle du subthalamus et celui des différentes structures bulbomésencéphaliques dans le maintien de la vigilance. *Electroencephalogr Clin Neurophysiol* **20**: 149–64.

Nauta, W. J. H. (1946) Hypothalamic regulation of sleep in rats. An experimental study. *J Neurophysiol* **9**: 285–316.

Panula, P., Yang, H. Y. & Costa, E. (1984) Histamine-containing neurons in the rat hypothalamus. *Proc Natl Acad Sci* **81**: 2572–6.

Panula, P., Häppölä, O., Airaksinen, M. S. *et al.* (1988) Carbodiimide as a tissue fixative in histamine immunocytochemistry and its application in developmental neurobiology. *J Histochem Cytochem* **36**: 259–69.

Parmentier, R., Ohtsu, J., Djebbara-Hannas, Z. *et al.* (2002) Anatomical, physiological and pharmacological characterististics of histidine decarboxylase knock-out mice: evidence for the role of brain histamine in behavioral and sleep-wake control. *J Neurosci* **22**: 7695–711.

Prast, H., Dietl, H. & Philippu, A. (1992) Pulsatile release of histamine in the hypothalamus of conscious rats. *Auton Nerv Syst* **39**: 105–10.

Ranson, S. W. (1939) Somnolence caused by hypothalamic lesion in the monkey. *Arch Neurol Psychiatry* **41**: 1–2.

Sallanon, M., Aubert, C., Denoyer, M. *et al.* (1987) L'insomnie consécutive á la lésion de la région préoptique paramédiane est réversible par inactivation de l'hypothalamus postérieur chez le chat. *C R Acad Sci* **305**: 561–7.

Schwartz, J. C., Arrang, J. M., Garbarg, M. *et al.* (1991) Histaminergic transmission in the mammalian brain. *Physiol Rev* **71**: 1–51.

Strakhova, M. I., Nikkel, A. L., Manelli, A. M. *et al.* (2009) Localization of histamine H4 receptors in the central nervous system of human and rats. *Brain Res* **1250**: 41–8.

Strecker, R. E., Nalwalk, J., Dauphin, L. J. *et al.* (2002) Extracellular histamine levels in the feline preoptic/anterior hypothalamic area during natural sleep–wakefulness and prolonged wakefulness: an in vivo microdialysis study. *Neuroscience* **113**: 663–70.

Swett, C. P. & Hobson, J. A. (1968) The effects of posterior hypothalamic lesions on behavioral and electrographic manifestations of sleep and waking in cats. *Arch Ital Biol* **106**: 279–83.

Szymusiak, R., Steininger, T., Alam, N. *et al.* (2001) Preoptic area sleep-regulating mechanisms. *Arch Ital Biol* **139**: 77–92.

Thakkar, R. V., Cape, M. M., Strecker, W. S. *et al.* (2000) Microdialysis perfusion of histamine in rat basal forebrain increases wakefulness. *Sleep* **23**(Suppl 2): 1715.

Toyota, H., Dugovic, C., Koehl, M. *et al.* (2002) Behavioral characterization of mice lacking histamine H3 receptors. *Mol Pharmacol* **62**: 389–97.

Vanni-Mercier, G., Sakai, K., Salvert, D. *et al.* (1985) Waking-state specific neurons in the posterior hypothalamus of the cat. In *Sleep 84*. eds. W. P. Koella, S. Rüther & H. Schulz. Stuttgart: Fischer, pp. 238–40.

Von Economo, C. (1926) Die Pathologie des Chlafes. In *Handbuch der normalen und pathologischen psychologie*. vol 17, eds. A. Berthe, G. von Bergmann, G. Embden & A. Ellinger. Berlin: Springer, pp. 591–610.

Wauquier, A. (1983) Drug effects on sleep–wakefulness patterns in dogs. *Neuropsychobiology* **10**: 60–4.

Winders, A. & Vogt, W. (1907) Synthese des imidazolylethylamins. *Ber Dtsch Chem Ges* **40**: 3691–5.

Chapter 24

Hypocretinergic system: role in REM-sleep regulation

Md. Noor Alam, Ronald Szymusiak, and Dennis McGinty

Summary

The hypocretins (HCRTs) are two hypothalamic peptides that have been implicated in a variety of functions including the regulation of behavioral arousal. In the brain, HCRT-expressing neurons are localized within the perifornical-lateral hypothalamic area, where they are intermingled with various other neuronal groups, including GABAergic, glutamatergic, and melanin-concentrating hormone containing neurons. Hypocretin neurons are active during behavioral arousal and are quiet during non-REM and REM sleep. Deficiency of HCRTergic signaling is linked to the symptoms of narcolepsy in humans, dogs, and rodents. Narcolepsy is a debilitating sleep disorder characterized by excessive daytime sleepiness, disrupted night-time sleep, sleep-onset REM sleep, and sudden loss of muscle tone during waking (cataplexy). Hypocretin neurons project extensively to brain structures, especially to those that are involved in arousal and motor control as well as receive extensive inputs from areas regulating emotions, autonomic tone, appetite, circadian rhythms, and sleep–wake behavior. Therefore, HCRT neurons are well positioned to integrate a variety of interoceptive and homeostatic signals to increase behavioral arousal and suppress REM sleep and its atonia. This chapter provides a brief review of the HCRTergic system, its interactions with other neuronal systems involved in sleep–wake regulation, and the neuronal circuitry and the potential mechanism(s) by which the HCRTergic system promotes behavioral arousal and suppresses REM sleep and its muscle atonia.

Introduction

The hypocretins, also called orexins, are hypothalamic peptides that were discovered barely a decade ago and have been implicated in multiple physiological functions including sleep–wake regulation. Soon after their discovery, a role of HCRTergic system in the regulation/maintenance of behavioral arousal and suppression of REM sleep and muscle atonia became evident from studies linking a loss of HCRT signaling with symptoms of narcolepsy in human and experimental animals. Narcolepsy is a sleep disorder characterized by excessive daytime sleepiness, sleep-onset REM sleep, and cataplexy, i.e., sudden loss of muscle tone without impairment of consciousness.

In the brain, HCRT-expressing neurons are localized within the perifornical-lateral hypothalamic area (PF-LHA). Hypocretin neurons are most active during behavioral arousal and are quiet during non-REM and REM sleep. Hypocretin neurons project widely to brain structures implicated in sleep–wake regulation, especially to those regions that are involved in arousal and motor control, where HCRTs exert excitatory effects via two receptors, namely, HCRT-R1 and HCRT-R2. In turn, HCRT neurons receive extensive inputs from areas regulating emotions, autonomic tone, appetite, circadian rhythms, and sleep–wake behavior. Anatomical and electrophysiological studies suggest that HCRT neurons integrate a variety of interoceptive and homeostatic signals to increase behavioral arousal and suppress REM sleep and its atonia.

During the last decade our understanding about the role of the HCRTergic system in physiological sleep–wake regulation and the mechanisms involved has improved significantly. There are many excellent reviews on the HCRTergic system and their role in various neurological functions including sleep–wake regulation (Eriksson *et al.*, 2010; Kukkonen *et al.*, 2002; Ohno and Sakurai, 2008; Siegel, 2004). This chapter is aimed at providing an overview of the HCRTergic system, its physiological role in sleep–wake regulation,

REM Sleep: Regulation and Function, eds. Birendra N. Mallick, S. R. Pandi-Perumal, Robert W. McCarley, and Adrian R. Morrison. Published by Cambridge University Press. © Cambridge University Press 2011.

and the neuronal circuitry and the mechanism by which the HCRTergic system enhances behavioral arousal and suppresses REM sleep and its muscle atonia.

Discovery of the hypocretinergic system

The HCRTergic or orexinergic system of the hypothalamus was discovered almost simultaneously barely a decade ago by two independent group of researchers (de Lecea *et al.*, 1998; Sakurai *et al.*, 1998) utilizing completely different research strategies. de Lecea and colleagues using a substrative RNA hybridization technique, identified a hypothalamic mRNA encoding a precursor peptide, preprohypocretin. They predicted two neuropeptides to originate from this precursor and named them as HCRT-1 and HCRT-2, for their hypothalamic location and their proposed sequence similarity to the secretin family of peptides. Sakurai and colleagues, using the reverse pharmacology technique, identified the same two peptides as endogenous ligands for two orphan G-protein coupled receptors. They named these peptides as orexin-A and orexin-B, based on the hypothalamic location of their synthesizing neurons and the finding that intracerebroventricular (icv) administration of these peptides increased food intake. Since their discovery, there has been spectacular progress in our understanding of the HCRTergic/orexinergic system and its roles in the regulation of various neurological functions including energy homeostasis, reward and addiction, and the most prominent and extensively documented function, sleep–wake regulation. Given that the HCRTergic/orexinergic system has been implicated in multiple neurological functions (Nishino *et al.*, 2010; Ohno and Sakurai, 2008; Siegel, 2004), the term orexins for these peptides seems restrictive. Therefore, a name, which is functionally less restrictive, i.e., HCRT, is used throughout this chapter.

Overview of the hypocretinergic system

Chemistry (structure) of HCRTs

Hypocretins are unique hypothalamic peptides with no significant homology with any previously known peptides. Both HCRT-1 and HCRT-2 are derived from a common 130- (rodent) to 131- (human) amino-acid precursor, preprohypocretin (Kukkonen *et al.*, 2002;

Ohno and Sakurai, 2008). Hypocretin-1 is a 33-amino acid peptide with two intramolecular disulfide bonds in the N-terminal region. This structure, so far, is known to be fully conserved across several mammalian species. Hypocretin-2 is a linear 28-amino acid peptide with 46% of its amino acid sequence identical to HCRT-1. The C-terminal half of HCRT-2 is very similar to that of HCRT-1, while the N-terminal half is more variable. Hypocretin peptides co-localize within secretory vesicles, implying that both HCRT-1 and HCRT-2 are co-released at terminals. Hypocretin-1 seems to be much more stable than HCRT-2 in the physiological milieu.

Anatomy of HCRT neurons

In the brain, HCRT-expressing neurons are localized within the hypothalamus, including the perifornical nucleus, lateral hypothalamic area (LH), dorsomedial hypothalamic nucleus (DMH), and posterior hypothalamic (PH) areas (Figure 24.1) (de Lecea *et al.*, 1998; Peyron *et al.*, 1998; Sakurai *et al.*, 1998). The number of HCRT neurons has been estimated to be around 5,800 to 6,800 in the rat brain and 50,000 to 70,000 in the human brain (Henny and Jones, 2006; Thannickal *et al.*, 2000). The size of the HCRT cell body ranges from 15 to 40 μm and their shape could be spherical, fusiform, or multipolar (Kukkonen *et al.*, 2002; Ohno and Sakurai, 2008).

In the PF-LHA, HCRT neurons are intermingled with other neuronal phenotypes, including neurons expressing melanin-concentrating hormone (MCH), gamma-aminobutyric acid (GABA) and glutamate. Hypocretin neurons do not co-localize MCH and these neurons constitute two distinct populations. Hypocretin neurons do not express GAD-67 mRNA as well. Both MCH and GABAergic neurons in the PF-LHA have also been implicated in the regulation of sleep (Fort *et al.*, 2009; Kumar *et al.*, 2005). HCRT co-localizes with glutamate, dynorphin, galanin, and neuronal activity-regulated pentraxin. Evidence indicates that HCRT neuronal activation is driven by glutamate (Li *et al.*, 2002).

Hypocretin receptors and signal transduction

The actions of HCRTs are mediated by two known G protein-coupled receptors, namely, HCRT-R1 and HCRT-R2. HCRT-R1 has ten times higher affinity for HCRT-1 than HCRT-2, whereas HCRT-R2 is a

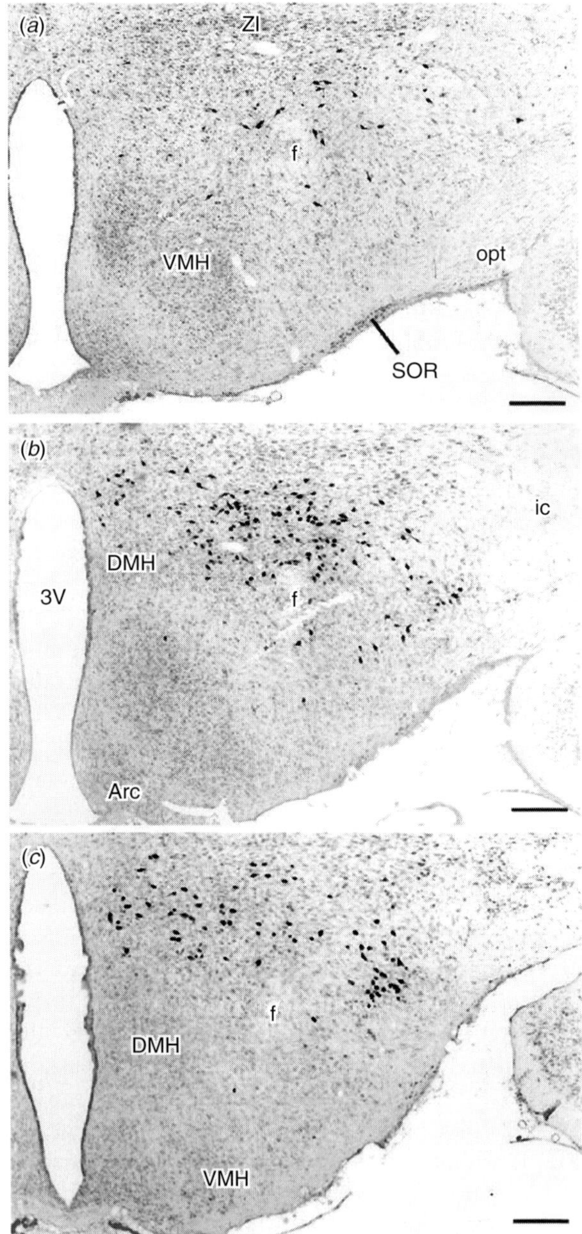

Figure 24.1 Distribution of HCRT neurons at three rostrocaudal levels of the tuberal region of the hypothalamus. 3V, 3rd ventricle; Arc, arcuate nucleus; DMH, dorsomedial hypothalamic nucleus; f, fornix; ic, internal capsule; opt, optic tract; SOR, retrochiasmatic part of the supraoptic nucleus; VMH, ventromedial hypothalamic nucleus; ZI, zona incerta. Scale bars, 275 μm. (Adapted from Peyron *et al.*, 1998, *J. Neuroscience*, with permission.) (See plate section for color version.)

non-selective receptor with similar affinities for both peptides. HCRT-R1 is coupled exclusively to the G_q subclass of heterotrimeric G proteins, whereas HCRT-R2 is coupled to $G_{i/o}$ and/or G_q, suggesting that while

HCRT-R1 mediated signaling is excitatory, HCRT-R2 mediated signaling could be excitatory or inhibitory (Kukkonen *et al.*, 2002; Ohno and Sakurai, 2008).

The anatomical distribution of HCRT-R1 and HCRT-R2 are somewhat distinct, although partially overlapping and consistent with HCRT projections (Marcus *et al.*, 2001; Trivedi *et al.*, 1998). Hypocretin-R1 is highly expressed in the prefrontal and infralimbic cortex, bed nucleus of stria terminalis (BNST), paraventricular thalamus, ventromedial hypothalamus (VMH), arcuate nucleus (ARC), dorsal raphe nucleus (DRN), and locus coeruleus (LC). The HCRT-R2 is a predominant type in septal nuclei, hippocampus, medial thalamic groups, dorsal and medial raphe nuclei, and many hypothalamic nuclei including dorsomedial hypothalamus (DMH) and tuberomammillary nucleus (TMN). Hypocretins exert excitatory effects on several state-controlling neuronal populations including LC neurons exclusively expressing HCRT-R1 and TMN neurons exclusively expressing HCRT-R2, suggesting that both receptor signaling are excitatory on wake-promoting systems.

Hypocretin neurons: efferents and afferents

Projections of HCRT neurons that mediate its actions on the sleep–wake function

Hypocretin neurons project extensively to brain nuclei implicated in the control of behavioral state, appetite, and autonomic functions (Figure 24.2) (Peyron *et al.*, 1998). Major effector sites, as demonstrated by HCRT projections as well as the presence of its receptors, that mediate its actions in the regulation of behavioral state include: (a) brain-stem and hypothalamic nuclei with monoaminergic neurons, i.e., LC (noradrenergic neurons), ventral tegmental area (VTA, dopaminergic neurons), DRN (serotonergic neurons), and TMN (histaminergic neurons); (b) brain-stem pontine reticular formation; (c) major cholinergic neurons in the brain stem, i.e., laterodorsal tegmental/pedunculopontine tegmental nucleus (LDT/PPT) and the basal forebrain (BF); and (d) moderate projections to the preoptic region (POA) of the hypothalamus.

Anatomical inputs that modulate HCRT neurons

Hypocretin neurons receive projections from a large number of brain regions implicated in the regulation of homeostatic drives, behavioral states, and

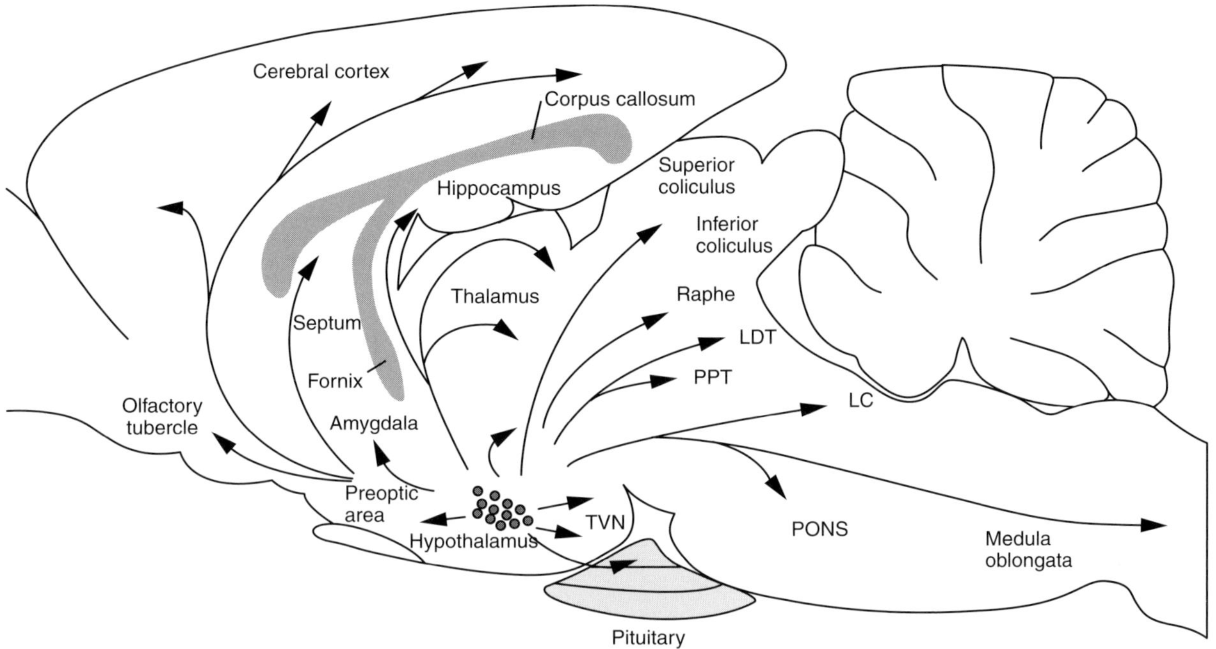

Figure 24.2 Schematic drawing of HCRT neuronal projections. (Adapted from Ohno and Sakurai, 2008, *Frontiers in Neuroendocrinology*, with permission.)

autonomic tone (Figure 24.3) (Sakurai *et al.*, 2005; Yoshida *et al.*, 2006). Some of the notable inputs with known and expected involvement in the regulation of HCRT neuronal activity in relation to behavioral states include extensive input coming from other parts of the hypothalamus including the POA, BF, PH, LH, DMH; infralimbic cortex; the lateral septum, BNST; and modest innervation from periaqueductal gray matter (PAG), DRN, and lateral parabrachial nucleus of the brain-stem region. Furthermore, hypothalamic regions preferentially innervate HCRT neurons in the medial and perifornical parts of the field, but most projections from the brain stem target the lateral part of the field (Yoshida *et al.*, 2006). Direct input from the suprachiasmatic nucleus (SCN) is sparse, although HCRT neurons receive abundant innervations from the BST, supraventricular zone, and the DMH, thereby receiving indirect inputs from the SCN.

Physiology of hypocretin neurons

Hypocretin neurons are wake-active/REM-off neurons

Although HCRT neurons were initially shown to exhibit wake-associated Fos protein-immunoreactivity

(IR), a marker of neuronal activation, the behavior of HCRT neurons during REM sleep was not conclusively known until unit activity of identified HCRT neurons was reported (Lee *et al.*, 2005; Mileykovskiy, 2005). Mileykovskiy and colleagues used electrophysiological properties of HCRT neurons in anesthetized animals to characterize their sleep–wake discharge properties in freely behaving animals. At the same time, Lee and colleagues used juxtacellular labeling with neurobiotin of neurons recorded in head-restrained animals and post-hoc HCRT immunohistochemistry to characterize the sleep–wake profile of HCRT neurons (Figure 24.4). As suggested by an earlier study (Alam *et al.*, 2002) both of these studies confirmed that HCRT neurons are active during waking, particularly during active waking, when postural muscle tone is high in association with movement, decrease discharge during quiet waking, and virtually cease firing during non-REM and REM sleep. Hypocretin neurons exhibit elevated discharge during REM sleep by several seconds prior to the return of waking . The discharge profile of HCRT neurons is consistent with a role in maintaining arousal in particular active arousal, while antagonizing sleep including REM sleep and REM muscle atonia. Consistent with its discharge activity, higher levels of HCRT in the cerebrospinal fluid (CSF)

Inputs to the medial part of the orexin field

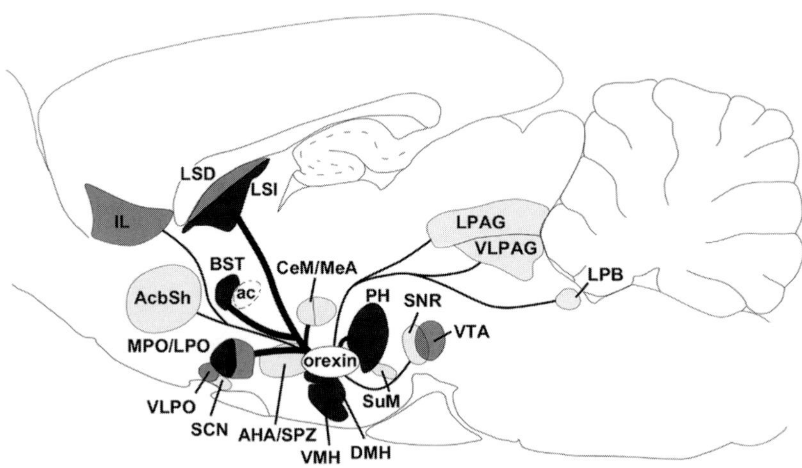

Inputs to the lateral part of the orexin field

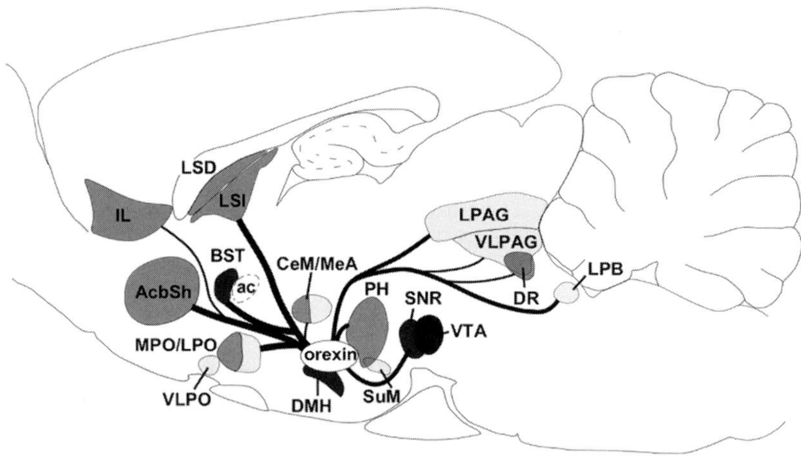

Figure 24.3 Schematic drawing of afferents to the HCRT neurons. Regions labeled in dark, medium, and light gray innervate >45%, 25 to 44%, or 5 to 24% of the HCRT neurons. Inputs that innervate <5% of the HCRT neurons are not included. Line thickness indicates the relative number of retrogradely labeled neurons. (Adapted from Yoshida *et al.*, 2006, *J. Comp. Neurology*, with permission.)

have been reported during active waking in various species (Nishino *et al.*, 2010). Optogenetic photostimulation of HCRT neurons increased the probability of transition to wakefulness from either non-REM or REM sleep (Adamantidis *et al.*, 2007).

Excitatory and inhibitory influences on HCRT neurons

Electrophysiological, mostly *in vitro*, studies have identified several neurotransmitters, neuromodulators, and peripheral metabolic cues that influence the activity of HCRT neurons (Kukkonen *et al.*, 2002; Ohno and Sakurai, 2008). Those with

excitatory effects include, glutamate, acetylcholine (ACh), ghrelin, CCK, neurotensin, vasopressin, oxytocin, glucagon-like peptide-1, corticotrophin-releasing factor, and ATP. On the other hand, GABA, dopamine (DA), noradrenaline (NA), serotonin (5-HT), adenosine, glucose, neuropeptide Y, and leptin inhibit HCRT neurons. The relative effects of the majority of these factors on HCRT neurons in intact animals and in influencing behavioral states, especially REM sleep, remain poorly understood. Notable neurotransmitters and neuromodulators that influence the activity of HCRT neurons with significant implications in sleep–wake regulation are as follows.

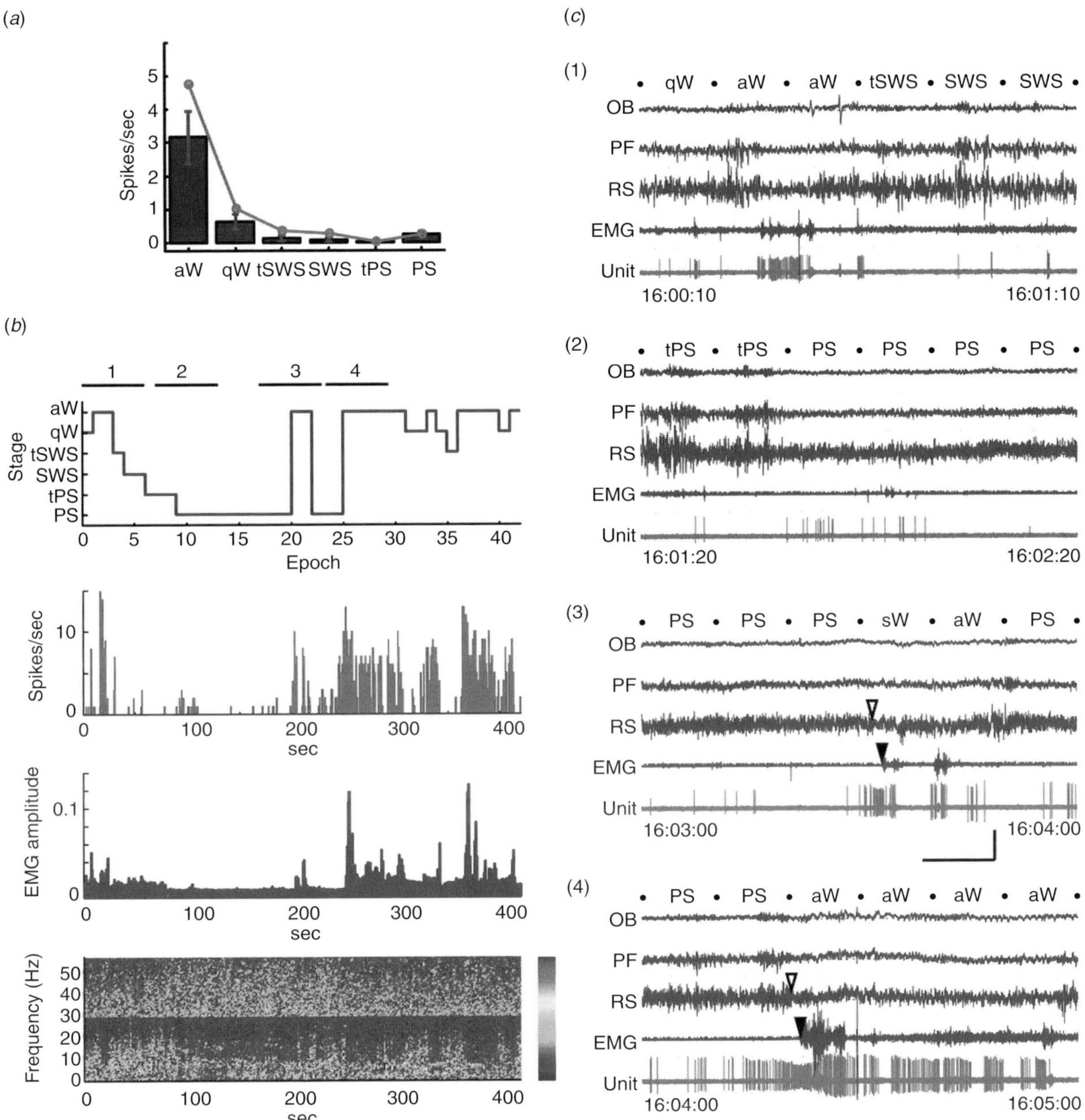

Figure 24.4 Sleep–wake discharge profile of identified HCRT neuron. (*a*) Bar diagram showing mean spike rate. The line drawing shows the discharge rate of an individual HCRT neuron shown in (*b*) and (*c*). (*b*) Hypnogram, spike-rate histogram, and EMG amplitude and EEG frequency spectra over the recording session. (*c*) One-minute segments of unit, EEG, and EMG activity during state transitions. The increase in firing before arousal from REM sleep (in 3 and 4) anticipates the transition from REM to waking judged by EEG (open arrowhead) and also EMG (filled arrowhead). OB, Olfactory bulb; PF, prefrontal cortex; RS, retrosplenial cortex. (Adapted from Lee *et al.*, 2005, *J. Neuroscience*, with permission.) (See plate section for color version.)

Glutamatergic influences

Glutamate is the principal excitatory neurotransmitter in the brain. The PF-LHA contains local glutamatergic neurons and HCRT neurons also express glutamate and its vesicular transporters and thus may release glutamate by itself. Electrophysiological *in vitro* studies of identified HCRT neurons suggest that glutamate, acting via ionotropic glutamate receptors (AMPA and NMDA), activates HCRT neurons (Li *et al.*, 2002; Torrealba *et al.*, 2003).

Applications of HCRTs depolarize and increase the discharge of HCRT neurons, although these peptides have no direct postsynaptic effects on these neurons (Li *et al.*, 2002; Torrealba *et al.*, 2003). The mechanism for this activation appears to be HCRT-mediated activation of local glutamatergic neurons that regulate HCRT neuronal activity, in part, by presynaptic facilitation of glutamate release (Li *et al.*, 2002). Hypocretin neurons also receive a substantial glutamatergic input from the BF. It is proposed that these BF glutamatergic neurons are wake-on/REM-off neurons and exert significant excitatory influences on HCRT neurons (Henny and Jones, 2006). Hypocretin neurons project extensively to the BF as well. These glutamatergic positive-feedback loops may be important for maintaining higher arousal and muscle tone.

Monoaminergic and cholinergic influnces

Presumed monoaminergic neurons, i.e., NA neurons in the LC, 5-HT neurons in the DRN, histaminergic neurons in the TMN are wake-on/REM-off neurons. Evidence suggests that the monoaminergic arousal system sends inhibitory feedback projections to the HCRT neurons, and might contribute to increasing sleepiness accompanying prolonged arousal (Ohno and Sakurai, 2008). Noradrenaline and 5-HT inhibit HCRT neurons via α_2 and $5HT_{1A}$ receptors, respectively. Interestingly, histamine has little/no effect on HCRT neurons. Acetylcholine seems to exert excitatory effects on HCRT neurons.

GABAergic influences

Hypocretin neurons are subject to strong GABAergic inhibition. Both $GABA_A$ and $GABA_B$ receptors have been implicated (Alam *et al.*, 2005; Li *et al.*, 2002; Matsuki *et al.*, 2009). Microdialysis perfusion of a $GABA_A$ receptor antagonist into the PF-LHA dose-dependently increased cFos-IR in HCRT neurons and produced arousal with concomitant suppression of non-REM and REM sleep (Alam *et al.*, 2005). A recent study of mice lacking the $GABA_B$ receptor specifically on HCRT neurons (oxGKO) suggests that $GABA_B$ receptors on HCRT neurons are essential for stabilizing and consolidating sleep–wake states. oxGKO mice exhibit severe fragmentation of sleep–wake states and HCRT neurons from these mice exhibit decreased sensitivity to both excitatory and inhibitory inputs in *in vitro* preparation (Matsuki *et al.*, 2009).

A major source of GABAergic input to HCRT neurons are projections from sleep-active GABAergic neurons in the POA region including the median preoptic nucleus (MnPN), ventrolateral preoptic area (VLPO), and BF (Gong *et al.*, 2004; Henny and Jones, 2006; Suntsova *et al.*, 2002; Uschakov *et al.*, 2006). Hypocretin neurons may receive inputs from local GABAergic neurons as well. Recent evidence suggests that MnPN sleep-active neurons inhibit HCRT neurons (Kumar *et al.*, 2008; Suntsova *et al.*, 2007). Median preoptic nucleus electrical and chemical stimulation suppressed the discharge activity of most PF-LHA neurons including putative wake-active HCRT neurons. Local inactivation of MnPN increased Fos-IR in HCRT neurons in anesthetized rats. It is likely that POA/BF-induced GABAergic inhibition of HCRT neurons is crucial for sleep initiation.

Melanin-concentrating hormone influences

Much evidence suggests that MCH-containing neurons of the PF-LHA play a role in the regulation of REM sleep. Extracellular unit recording and Fos-IR studies suggest that MCH neurons are active during REM sleep (Hassani *et al.*, 2009; Modirrousta *et al.*, 2005; Verret *et al.*, 2003). Intracerebroventricular administration of MCH induces sleep, specifically REM sleep. Melanin-concentrating hormone is an inhibitory peptide and MCH neurons also contain GABA. Since MCH neurons project to arousal systems as well as make contacts with HCRT neurons, it is hypothesized that MCH neurons promote non-REM and REM sleep via MCH/GABA inhibitory actions on HCRT and other arousal systems including the monoaminergic system (Fort *et al.*, 2009).

Adenosinergic influences

Recent studies suggest that adenosine acting via the A_1 receptor on HCRT neurons may play a role in the homeostatic regulation of sleep. An *in vitro* study suggests that adenosine inhibits HCRT neurons, most potently via presynaptic inhibition of the glutamatergic input or excitatory postsynaptic potentials, and that this effects is mediated via A_1 receptors (Liu and Gao, 2007). Adenosine A_1 receptor antagonist, when microinjected into the PF-LHA produces arousal and suppresses non-REM and REM sleep in spontaneously sleeping animals as well as during recovery sleep after sleep deprivation (Thakkar *et al.*, 2008).

Hypocretinergic system and REM sleep

Much evidence supports a hypothesis that activation of HCRT neurons is critical for the maintenance of active arousal with muscle tone, whereas inactivation/switching off of these neurons is necessary for maintaining consolidated non-REM and REM sleep and REM muscle atonia. These lines of studies include (1) genetic alterations linking a loss of HCRTergic signaling to narcolepsy with cataplexy; (2) the wake-active/REM-off discharge profile of HCRT neurons as discussed above; and (3) the pharmacological studies supporting the wake-promoting and REM sleep/atonia suppressing effects of the peptide.

Hypocretin and narcolepsy

The initial evidence for a role of HCRT in the regulation of arousal/motor activity and suppression of REM sleep and its atonia came from two landmark studies, one on the genetic form of canine narcolepsy (Lin *et al.*, 1999) and another on prepro-orexin knock-out mice (Chemelli *et al.*, 1999). Lin and colleagues found that inherited canine narcolepsy was caused by a mutation in the HCRT-2 gene. Chemelli and colleagues found that prepro-orexin knock-out mice exhibited periods of behavioral arrests that strongly resembled cataplexy in both narcoleptic dogs and humans.

Narcolepsy is a chronic sleep disorder with an estimated prevalence of about 1 in 2,000 individuals. The core symptoms of the disease are excessive daytime sleepiness, or inability to sustain alertness, and cataplexy. Hypnagogic hallucinations, sleep paralysis, and fragmented nocturnal sleep are often present. Excessive daytime sleepiness manifests in irresistible sleep attacks that are often relieved by napping. As a result the subject falls asleep at inappropriate times. The latency to REM sleep is markedly reduced and sleep-onset REM period can occur during the middle of a daytime nap. In narcolepsy–cataplexy syndrome, waking is often interrupted by episodes of cataplexy. Cataplexy is a sudden loss of muscle tone without loss of consciousness and is usually triggered by situations that require sudden action or strong emotions, e.g., laughing, embarrassment, and anger.

The hypothesis that a lack of HCRTergic signaling contributed to narcolepsy was further confirmed in studies of post-mortem brains of human narcolepsy–cataplexy patients, which showed dramatic loss of HCRT mRNA and HCRT immunoreactivity (Peyron *et al.*, 2000; Thannickal *et al.*, 2000). Hypocretin-1 level is undetectable in the cerebrospinal fluid of most human narcoleptic patients (Nishino *et al.*, 2010). Many narcolepsy symptoms, e.g., rapid state-transitions or inability to remain awake for long, and sudden episodes of cataplexy during waking behavior, are also exhibited by HCRT-receptor knock-out mice and HCRT/ataxin-3 transgenic mice and rats with ablated HCRT neurons (Ohno and Sakurai, 2008; Siegel, 2004). It is pertinent to note that prepro-orexin knock-out mice and double-receptor knock-out mice exhibit similar and more severe behavioral abnormalities than HCRT-R2 or HCRT-R1 knock-out (severity is least) mice suggesting that a loss of signaling through both receptor pathways is necessary for the emergence of a complete narcoleptic phenotype (Ohno and Sakurai, 2008). These findings further suggest that HCRT normally facilitates alertness and muscle tone and inhibits REM sleep and atonia.

Hypocretin promotes arousal and suppresses REM sleep and atonia by acting on several brain regions and multiple cell types

Administration of HCRTs into the lateral ventricle promotes behavioral arousal and suppresses non-REM and REM sleep. The anatomical projections, receptor distribution, and pharmacological studies suggest that this HCRT-induced arousal and suppression of REM sleep is predominantly mediated via its excitatory effects on multiple systems, including the cerebral cortex, non-specific thalamocortical projection system, BF, hypothalamic, and brain-stem arousal systems, as well as sympathetic and motor circuits in the spinal cord (Eriksson *et al.*, 2010; Jones, 2008; McCarley, 2007; Ohno and Sakurai, 2008; Siegel, 2004).

Monoaminergic system

Hypocretin neurons project heavily to the DRN, LC, and TMN, and monoaminergic neurons in these regions express HCRT receptors suggesting that the activities of these neuronal groups are, at least, partly regulated by HCRT (Jones, 2008; McCarley, 2007; Ohno and Sakurai, 2008; Siegel, 2004). Applications of HCRT into the LC, TMN, and DRN increase the time spent in waking, and decrease the time spent in non-REM and REM sleep. Consistent with the behavioral response, HCRTs have been shown to excite NA cells of the LC, dopaminergic cells of the VTA, 5-HT cells of the DRN, and histaminergic cells of the TMN. In a recent study, locomotor activity in a novel environment, dopamine turnover, and psychostimulant-induced hyperlocomotion were found to be significantly lower in HCRT-deficient mice than in wild-type mice (Mori *et al.*, 2009). Therefore, it is generally believed that HCRT-induced behavioral arousal is mediated, in part, via the activation of monoaminergic neurons. Of these neuronal groups, the activation of histaminergic neurons via the H_1 receptor seems to be predominantly involved in HCRT-mediated behavioral arousal. The H_1 receptor antagonist attenuates HCRT-induced arousal considerably. The HCRT-induced arousal is practically absent in histamine H_1-receptor deficient mice; and histamine concentrations are low in narcoleptic dogs (Huang *et al.*, 2001; Ohno and Sakurai, 2008).

Cholinergic system

Hypocretin neurons provide robust projections to cholinergic systems in the BF and LDT/PPT. Most BF and LDT/PPT neurons are wake-REM active, i.e., they discharge in association with cortical activation. A subset of cholinergic neurons in the LDT/PPT (30–40%) are REM-on neurons, i.e., increase their firing just prior to and during REM sleep (Eriksson *et al.*, 2010; Fort *et al.*, 2009; Jones, 2008; McCarley, 2007). Application of HCRT into the BF and the LDT produces arousal and suppress REM sleep. Consistent with these findings, HCRT excites cholinergic neurons in these structures *in vitro*. Hypocretin also increases local glutamate release within the BF, suggesting an additional indirect effect of HCRT on BF cholinergic activity (Jones, 2008). Hypocretin may also inhibit cholinergic neurons in the PPT via activation of GABAergic local interneurons. It is likely that HCRT promotes and modulates components of arousal via complementary and synergistic effects on both BF and brain-stem cholinergic systems. Acetylcholine also excites HCRT neurons *in vitro*, suggesting a feed-forward mechanism implicated in cortical activation, behavioral arousal, and gating of REM sleep.

GABAergic system

Hypocretin neurons project moderately to sleep-promoting POA regions. The POA regions also contain few HCRT receptors. Thus HCRT neurons do not seem to have mutually inhibitory interactions with POA neurons. However, monoaminergic afferents to the POA (VLPO) express HCRT receptors, and thus HCRT may inhibit POA neurons presynaptically by enhancing those effects (Saper *et al.*, 2005). Hypocretin neurons project to and excite identified or presumed GABAergic neurons in the substantia nigra pars reticulata, DRN, VTA, arcuate nucleus, medial septum, ventrolateral periaqueductal gray matter (vlPAG), and lateral pontine tegmentum (LPT). Evidence suggests that activation of the vlPAG/LPT by HCRT neurons may also contribute significantly to HCRT-induced behavioral arousal and increased muscle activity.

REM sleep generation: role of the HCRTergic system

The mechanism(s) of REM-sleep generation have been described in detail in other chapters in this book. In brief, according to the widely accepted hypothesis, a reciprocal inhibitory interaction between cholinergic REM-on and monoaminergic REM-off neurons plays a critical role in REM onset and maintenance (McCarley, 2007). In this model, generation of REM sleep depends on the activation of cholinergic REM-on neurons in the LDT/PPT, which partly is due to the disinhibition from wake-on LC/DRN neurons. The ascending projections of these neurons produce active thalamocortical signaling of REM sleep. These neurons also trigger muscle atonia of REM sleep via its projections to neurons in the caudal pons and medulla.

The sublaterodorsal nucleus (SLD; equivalent to the subcoeruleus area or peri-LC alpha in cats) just ventral to the LC, has been linked to the muscle atonia component of REM sleep. Its stimulation triggers, whereas its lesions block, REM atonia. The SLD may produce REM atonia by direct inhibition of motor neurons or via descending excitatory projections to glycine/GABA neurons in the ventral medulla, which in turn inhibit spinal motoneurons during REM sleep.

Recently a parallel mutually inhibitory GABAergic model of REM sleep has been proposed (Fort *et al.*, 2009; Lu *et al.*, 2006; McCarley, 2007). In this model, GABAergic REM-on neurons localized in the SLD inhibit GABAergic wake-on/REM-off neurons, localized in the vlPAG/LPT and vice versa, suggesting a flip-flop arrangement. It was also reported that one set of glutamatergic neurons projects to the BF and regulates EEG phenomena of REM sleep, while another group of glutamatergic neurons in the ventral SLD projects to the ventromedial medulla and spinal cord and regulates atonia of REM sleep. Cell-specific lesions or inhibition of the vlPAG/LPT are reported to increase the amount of REM sleep and produce cataplexy-like periods of atonia during wakefulness (Lu *et al.*, 2006).

Role of hypocretin

Local injections of carbachol in the SLD induce REM sleep and its atonia. The SLD also receives HCRTergic and monoaminergic inputs that can antagonize the cholinergic action of eliciting REM sleep and its atonia (Jones, 2008; McCarley, 2007). Application of antisense oligonucleotides against HCRT-R2 mRNA in the SLD/ adjoining area increased REM sleep and induced cataplexy-like attacks (Thakkar *et al.*, 1999). Many neurons in this region bear the HCRT-R2, which is mutated in narcoleptic dogs (Lin *et al.*, 1999). In this area some HCRT-R2 bearing neurons also bear M2 receptors, associated with hyperpolarizing responses to ACh. Therefore, through the inputs to SLD neurons, HCRT would facilitate and ACh would inhibit muscle tone. It is likely that by such opponent processes, HCRT could override any inhibitory effects of ACh on muscle atonia (Jones, 2008). Thus, concurrent release of ACh in the BF and brain stem would be associated with cortical activation in the presence of muscle tone and activity during waking when HCRT is also released, but it would be associated with cortical activation in the absence of muscle tone during REM sleep when HCRT signaling is naturally absent (Jones, 2008).

GABAergic neurons in the vlPAG and LPT are strongly innervated by HCRT neurons as well as POA GABAergic neurons. VlPAG/LPT neurons project extensively to the SLD. Activation of HCRT neurons may inhibit atonia and REM sleep by activating vlPAG/ LPT GABAergic wake-active/REM-off neurons and associated pathways.

The potential neuronal circuits and the mechanisms by which the HCRTergic system enhances behavioral arousal and suppresses REM sleep and its muscle atonia are summarized below.

Waking

Hypocretin neurons are activated in response to stress, hunger, circadian signals, and autonomic challenges to increase behavioral arousal. The activated HCRT neurons in turn enhance arousal and motor activity predominantly by exciting and sustaining the activities of monoaminergic neurons in the LC, DRN, and TMN; cholinergic neurons in the LDT/PPT and BF; GABAergic wake-active neurons in the vlPAG/LPT as well as thalamic neurons. The activated NA and 5-HT neurons may increase motor tone by inhibiting

atonia- and REM sleep-producing neurons of the SLD, reticular formation, and LDT/PPT. In addition, NA and 5-HT may increase muscle tone by directly exciting motor neurons. The activated vlPAG/LPT GABAergic neurons would inhibit REM and atonia-producing SLD neurons. These activated systems thus act synergistically to promote overall arousal and higher muscle tone. Hypocretin neurons also activate glutamatergic neurons present locally and in the BF, which in turn activate HCRT neurons.

The HCRTergic system does not seem to have a mutually inhibitory relationship with VLPO/MnPN/ BF sleep-active neurons, but may exert its influences via activation of monoaminergic and cholinergic wake-promoting systems that inhibit GABAergic putative sleep-promoting neurons in the POA region (Gallopin *et al.*, 2000). Basal forebrain sleep-active GABAergic neurons bear an α-2 receptor indicating that these neurons would be hyperpolarized by NA, in contrast to cholinergic neurons that would be excited by NA via α-1 receptors (Jones, 2008). This relationship allows HCRT neurons to actively reinforce monoaminergic/ cholinergic arousal tone during waking. Rapid state-transitions, including transitions into REM-like states of muscle atonia directly from wakefulness, in animals with loss of HCRTergic signaling, suggest that HCRT neurons normally reinforce the activity of the waking side of the flip-flop switch, thus stabilizing it and preventing sudden and inappropriate transitions between wakefulness and sleep (Saper *et al.*, 2005).

Non-REM sleep

In vitro studies suggest that HCRT neurons fire spontaneously through an intrinsic depolarization (Eggermann *et al.*, 2003). Therefore, HCRT neurons need to be inhibited during non-REM and REM sleep. Major sources of this inhibition include inputs from the MNPN/VLPO and BF sleep-active GABAergic neurons as well as local accumulation of adenosine as a consequence of HCRT neuronal activation during arousal.

The MNPN/VLPO and BF neurons are activated at sleep onset in response to circadian and homeostatic cues including several sleep-promoting agents. The activated MNPN/VLPO sleep-promoting system strongly inhibits HCRTergic and other arousal systems including putative monoaminergic neurons with inhibitory influences on POA/BF neurons. Therefore the POA sleep-promoting system is in a position to unbalance the flip-flop for switching from waking to non-REM sleep. The activated POA sleep-promoting system can control EEG spindles and slow waves of non-REM sleep by directly hyperpolarizing thalamic neurons as well as by inhibiting HCRT and monoaminergic neurons that facilitate thalamic depolarization (Szymusiak and McGinty, 2008). Sleep-related GABAergic inhibition of the HCRT neurons provides a basis for sleep-related deactivation of autonomic and motor functions as well.

Reversible inactivation or lesions of the PF-LHA/ PH counteract the insomnia that follows POA lesions, suggesting that inhibition of HCRT neurons is a critical component of the sleep-promoting mechanism. The inhibition of HCRT neurons disfacilitates multiple arousal systems, further supplementing POA actions and thus consolidating non-REM sleep.

REM sleep

The majority of sleep-active neurons in the POA exhibit REM > non-REM > waking discharge profiles. The POA also contains REM-active GABAergic neurons. Therefore, it is possible that the sustained activation of POA/BF GABAergic neurons and consequent inhibition of HCRTergic and monoaminergic activities triggers the activation of brain-stem REM sleep-generating neuronal circuitries, i.e., activation of the LDT/PPT and SLD REM-on neurons. Increased HCRTergic and monoaminergic tones would normally inhibit those REM-on neurons. Consistent with this idea, microdialysis studies have shown progressively increasing levels of GABA (REM > non-REM > waking) in the PF-LHA/LH, DRN, and LC (Siegel, 2004; Szymusiak and McGinty, 2008). In addition, MCH neurons in the PF-LHA become active and may exert inhibitory influences on HCRT neurons as well as on GABAergic wake-on/REM-off neurons in the vlPAG thereby facilitating the activation of SLD atonia/ REM-on neurons. A POA-mediated cessation of HCRT neurons in this cascade of events seems central to the onset and maintenance of REM sleep and its atonia.

Acknowledgments

Supported by the US Department of Veterans Affairs Medical Research Service and US National Institutes of Health grant, NS-050939.

References

Adamantidis, A. R., Zhang, F., Aravanis, A. M., Deisseroth, K. & de Lecea, L. (2007) Neural substrates of awakening probed with optogenetic control of hypocretin neurons. *Nature* **450**: 420–4.

Alam, M. N., Gong, H., Alam, T., Jaganath, R., McGinty, D. & Szymusiak, R. (2002) Sleep–waking discharge patterns of neurons recorded in the rat perifornical lateral hypothalamic area. *J Physiol* **538**: 619–31.

Alam, M. N., Kumar, S., Bashir, T. *et al.* (2005) GABA-mediated control of hypocretin- but not melanin-concentrating hormone immunoreactive neurones during sleep in rats. *J Physiol* **563**: 569–82.

Chemelli, R. M., Willie, J. T., Sinton, C. M. *et al.* (1999) Narcolepsy in orexin knockout mice: molecular genetics of sleep regulation. *Cell* **98**: 437–51.

de Lecea, L., Kilduff, T. S., Peyron, C. *et al.* (1998) The hypocretins: hypothalamus-specific peptides with neuroexcitatory activity. *Proc Natl Acad Sci U S A* **95**: 322–7.

Eggermann, E., Bayer, L., Serafin, M. *et al.* (2003) The wake-promoting hypocretin-orexin neurons are in an intrinsic state of membrane depolarization. *J Neurosci* **23**: 1557–62.

Eriksson, K. S., Sergeeva, O. A., Haas, H. L. & Selbach, O. (2010) Orexins/hypocretins and aminergic systems. *Acta Physiol (Oxf)* **198**: 263–75.

Fort, P., Bassetti, C. L. & Luppi, P. H. (2009) Alternating vigilance states: new insights regarding neuronal networks and mechanisms. *Eur J Neurosci* **29**: 1741–53.

Gallopin, T., Fort, P., Eggermann, E., *et al.* (2000) Identification of sleep-promoting neurons in vitro. *Nature* **404**: 992–5.

Gong, H., McGinty, D., Guzman-Marin, R., *et al.* (2004) Activation of c-fos in GABAergic neurones in the preoptic area during sleep and in response to sleep deprivation. *J Physiol* **556**: 935–46.

Hassani, O. K., Lee, M. G. & Jones, B. E. (2009) Melanin-concentrating hormone neurons discharge in a reciprocal manner to orexin neurons across the sleep–wake cycle. *Proc Natl Acad Sci U S A* **106**: 2418–22.

Henny, P. & Jones, B. E. (2006) Innervation of orexin/ hypocretin neurons by GABAergic, glutamatergic or cholinergic basal forebrain terminals evidenced by immunostaining for presynaptic vesicular transporter and postsynaptic scaffolding proteins. *J Comp Neurol* **499**: 645–61.

Huang, Z. L., Qu, W. M., Li, W. D. *et al.* (2001) Arousal effect of orexin A depends on activation of the histaminergic system. *Proc Natl Acad Sci U S A* **98**: 9965–70.

Jones, B. E. (2008) Modulation of cortical activation and behavioral arousal by cholinergic and orexinergic systems. *Ann N Y Acad Sci* **1129**: 26–34.

Kukkonen, J. P., Holmqvist, T., Ammoun, S. & Akerman, K. E. (2002) Functions of the orexinergic/hypocretinergic system. *Am J Physiol Cell Physiol* **283**: C1567–91.

Kumar, S., Szymusiak, R., Bashir, T. *et al.* (2008) Inactivation of median preoptic nucleus causes c-Fos expression in hypocretin- and serotonin-containing neurons in anesthetized rat. *Brain Res* **1234**: 66–77.

Kumar, S., Szymusiak, R., Methippara, M. M. *et al.* (2005) GABAergic and glutamatergic neurons in the perifornical lateral hypothalamic area exhibit differential Fos expression after sleep deprivation vs. recovery sleep. *Sleep* **29**: A146.

Lee, M. G., Hassani, O. K. & Jones, B. E. (2005) Discharge of identified orexin/hypocretin neurons across the sleep–waking cycle. *J Neurosci* **25**: 6716–20.

Li, Y., Gao, X. B., Sakurai, T. & van den Pol, A. N. (2002) Hypocretin/Orexin excites hypocretin neurons via a local glutamate neuron: a potential mechanism for orchestrating the hypothalamic arousal system. *Neuron* **36**: 1169–81.

Lin, L., Faraco, J., Li, R. *et al.* (1999) The sleep disorder canine narcolepsy is caused by a mutation in the hypocretin (orexin) receptor 2 gene. *Cell* **98**: 365–76.

Liu, Z. W. & Gao, X. B. (2007) Adenosine inhibits activity of hypocretin/orexin neurons by the A1 receptor in the lateral hypothalamus: a possible sleep-promoting effect. *J Neurophysiol* **97**: 837–48.

Lu, J., Sherman, D., Devor, M. & Saper, C. B. (2006) A putative flip-flop switch for control of REM sleep. *Nature* **441**: 589–94.

Marcus, J. N., Aschkenasi, C. J., Lee, C. E. *et al.* (2001) Differential expression of orexin receptors 1 and 2 in the rat brain. *J Comp Neurol* **435**: 6–25.

Matsuki, T., Nomiyama, M., Takahira, H. *et al.* (2009) Selective loss of GABA(B) receptors in orexin-producing neurons results in disrupted sleep/wakefulness architecture. *Proc Natl Acad Sci U S A* **106**: 4459–64.

McCarley, R.W. (2007) Neurobiology of REM and NREM sleep. *Sleep Med* **8**: 302–30.

Mileykovskiy, B. Y., Kiyashchenko, L. I. & Siegel, J. M. (2005) Behavioral correlates of activity in identified hypocretin/orexin neurons. *Neuron* **46**: 787–98.

Modirrousta, M., Mainville, L. & Jones, B. E. (2005) Orexin and MCH neurons express c-Fos differently after sleep deprivation vs. recovery and bear different adrenergic receptors. *Eur J Neurosci* **21**: 2807–16.

Mori, T., Ito, S., Kuwaki, T., Yanagisawa, M. & Sawaguchi, T. (2009)Monoaminergic neuronal changes in orexin deficient mice. *Neuropharmacology*.

Nishino, S., Okuro, M., Kotorii, N. *et al.* (2010)Hypocretin/orexin and narcolepsy: new basic and clinical insights, *Acta Physiol (Oxf)* **198**: 209–22.

Ohno, K. & Sakurai, T. (2008) Orexin neuronal circuitry: role in the regulation of sleep and wakefulness. *Front Neuroendocrinol* **29**: 70–87.

Peyron, C., Faraco, J., Rogers, *et al.* (2000) A mutation in a case of early onset narcolepsy and a generalized absence of hypocretin peptides in human narcoleptic brains. *Nat Med* **6**: 991–7.

Peyron, C., Tighe, D. K., van den Pol, A. N., *et al.* (1998) Neurons containing hypocretin (orexin) project to multiple neuronal systems. *J Neurosci* **18**: 9996–10,015.

Sakurai, T., Amemiya, A., Ishii, M. *et al.* (1998) Orexins and orexin receptors: a family of hypothalamic neuropeptides and G protein-coupled receptors that regulate feeding behavior. *Cell* **92**: 573–85.

Sakurai, T., Nagata, R., Yamanaka, A. *et al.* (2005) Input of orexin/hypocretin neurons revealed by a genetically encoded tracer in mice. *Neuron* **46**: 297–308.

Saper, C. B., Cano, G. & Scammell, T. E. (2005) Homeostatic, circadian, and emotional regulation of sleep. *J Comp Neurol* **493**: 92–8.

Siegel, J. M. (2004a) Hypocretin (orexin): role in normal behavior and neuropathology. *Ann Rev Psychol* **55**: 125–48.

Siegel, J.M. (2004b) The neurotransmitters of sleep, *J Clin Psychiatry*, **65** Suppl 16: 4–7.

Suntsova, N., Guzman-Marin, R., Kumar, S. *et al.* (2007) The median preoptic nucleus reciprocally modulates activity of arousal-related and sleep-related neurons in the perifornical lateral hypothalamus. *J Neurosci* **27**: 1616–30.

Suntsova, N., Szymusiak, R., Alam, M. N., Guzman-Marin, R. & McGinty, D. (2002) Sleep–waking discharge patterns of median preoptic nucleus neurons in rats. *J Physiol* **543**: 665–77.

Szymusiak, R. & McGinty, D. (2008) Hypothalamic regulation of sleep and arousal. *Ann N Y Acad Sci* **1129**: 275–86.

Thakkar, M. M., Engemann, S. C., Walsh, K. M. & Sahota, P. K. (2008) Adenosine and the homeostatic control of sleep: effects of A1 receptor blockade in the perifornical lateral hypothalamus on sleep–wakefulness. *Neuroscience* **153**: 875–80.

Thakkar, M. M., Ramesh, V., Cape, E. G. *et al.* (1999) REM sleep enhancement and behavioral cataplexy following orexin (hypocretin)-II receptor antisense perfusion in the pontine reticular formation. *Sleep Res Online* **2**: 112–20.

Thannickal, T. C., Moore, R. Y., Nienhuis, R. *et al.* (2000) Reduced number of hypocretin neurons in human narcolepsy. *Neuron* **27**: 469–74.

Torrealba, F., Yanagisawa, M. & Saper, C. B. (2003) Colocalization of orexin a and glutamate immunorcactivity in axon terminals in the tuberomammillary nucleus in rats. *Neuroscience* **119**: 1033–44.

Trivedi, P., Yu, H., MacNeil, D. J., Van der Ploeg, L. H. &
Guan, X. M. (1998) Distribution of orexin receptor
mRNA in the rat brain. *FEBS Lett* **438:** 71–5.

Uschakov, A., Gong, H., McGinty, D. & Szymusiak, R. (2006)
Sleep-active neurons in the preoptic area project to the
hypothalamic paraventricular nucleus and perifornical
lateral hypothalamus. *Eur J Neurosci* **23:** 3284–96.

Verret, L., Goutagny, R., Fort, P. *et al.* (2003) A role of
melanin-concentrating hormone producing neurons in
the central regulation of paradoxical sleep. *BMC Neurosci*
4: 19.

Yoshida, K., McCormack, S., Espana, R. A., Crocker, A. &
Scammell, T. E. (2006) Afferents to the orexin neurons of
the rat brain. *J Comp Neurol* **494:** 845–61.

Chapter

25

Neuropeptides and REM sleep

Oscar Prospéro-García, Mónica Méndez-Díaz, Alejandra E. Ruiz-Contreras, and Marcel Pérez-Morales

Summary

Sleep is a process occurring in all living animals. Although it is still controversial whether insects and other animals sleep alike; there is no doubt that they rest, as many studies in *Drosophila melanogaster* have shown. In this context, several seminal studies have documented species-dependent variations in sleep patterns. These findings along with obvious non-learned characteristics of sleep in general, such as the total time of sleep, the alternating NREM–REM sleep pattern, among many others, suggest strong regulation by genes. Clearly, the way genes may influence sleep physiology is via proteins. Hence, the importance of proteins in the regulation of sleep is observed in every minute event occurring to trigger or to maintain sleep. In this chapter we discuss families of proteins that are grouped by their effect on food ingestion, immuno-logical response, trophic activity, and intracellular signaling, all of them affecting the sleep–waking cycle. Although we do not fully discuss the mechanisms of action, we put our effort in highlighting their effects on sleep. Along with the proteins and their effects we have listed those genes encoding them. We also show examples of proteins and the way they affect sleep. Hence, we hope that the overall message that readers will gather from this chapter is the importance of several proteins in the regulation of sleep. Also, by observing the effects of each family of proteins we can infer at least some functions of sleep and, finally, that sleep is a multigenic trait.

Introduction

An extensive literature currently demonstrates that the sleep–waking cycle is regulated by several mole-cules classified as neurotransmitters, neuropeptides, amino acids, and lipids, among others. The group integrated by a large amount of molecules is the one of neuropeptides; its members can be classified con-sidering their action mechanisms, their effects on the physiology and behavior (Table 25.1). In this context, some peptides, besides their involvement in the regu-lation of the sleep–waking cycle, regulate food intake, such as the vasoactive intestinal polypeptide (VIP), cholecystokinin-8 (CCK-8), and corticotropin-like intermediate lobe peptide (CLIP). Hormones are also involved in these actions, such as somatostatin, insulin, ghrelin and leptin, and orexins. Cortistatin is also a sleep- and food intake-regulating peptide. There are neuropeptides classified as mediators in the immunological systems. For example, interleukins 1β (IL-1 β) and IL-4; however, these are more involved in the facilitation of slow-wave sleep (SWS) and are considered as rapid-eye-movement (REM) sleep suppressors. Finally, there are those named trophic factors, like the growth hormone (GH) and the brain-derived neurotrophic factor (BDNF) that participate in neuronal survival and restoration. All these neu-ropeptides regulate the sleep–waking cycle. Since neuropeptides are encoded by genes, frequently they acquire their active form after post-transcriptional or post-translational modifications, we would like to emphasize that sleep, in general, and REM sleep, in particular, is a polygenic trait. Moreover, we believe that, by highlighting the effects exerted by each fam-ily of peptides on the body, we can suggest a potential function of such an enigmatic behavioral state as is REM sleep.

Neuropeptides regulating sleep and food intake

There are several neuropeptides that besides regulat-ing food intake, during waking, they modulate the

REM Sleep: Regulation and Function, eds. Birendra N. Mallick, S. R. Pandi-Perumal, Robert W. McCarley, and Adrian R. Morrison. Published by Cambridge University Press. © Cambridge University Press 2011.

Table 25.1 Neuropeptides affecting REM sleep and their chromosomal loci

Neuropeptide	W	SWS	REM	Gene	Human chromosome position
Neuropeptides and hormones involved in food ingestion					
Vasoactive intestinal polypeptide (VIP)	↓	=	↑	VIP	6q25
Cholecystokinin octapeptide (CCK-8)	↓	=	↑	CCK	3p22–p21.3
Corticotropin-like intermediate lobe peptide (CLIP)	↓	=	↑	POMC	2p23.3
Somatostatin (SRIF)	↓	=	↑	SST	3q28
Insulin	↓	↑	=	INS	11p15.5
Leptin	=	↑	↓	LEP	7q31.3
Ghrelin	↓	↑	=	GHRL	3p26–p25
Neuropeptide Y (NPY)	↓	↑	=	NPY	7p15.1
Cortistatin	=	↑	↑↓	CORT	1p36.22
Proteins of the immunological system					
Tumor necrosis factor (TNF-α)	↓	↑	↓	TNF	6p21.3
Interleukin 1β (IL-1β)	=	↑	↑	IL1B	2q14
Trophic factors					
Growth hormone releasing hormone (GHRH)		↑	↑		
Growth hormone (GH)	↓		↑	GH1	17q24.2
Prolactin (PRL)			↑	PRL	6p22.2–p21.3
Brain-derived neurotrophic factor (BDNF)	↓	↑		BDNF	11p13
Nerve growth factor (NGF-β and γ)	↓	↑	↑	NGFB NGFG	1p13.1 19q13.3
Neurotrophin-3 and 4 (NT-3 and NT-4)	↓	↑	↑	NTF3 NTF4	12p13 19q13.3

↑↓ means increase or decrease of REM sleep on dependence on the circadian cycle.

sleep–waking cycle, suggesting that one of the functions of sleep is to regulate the body's energy.

Vasoactive intestinal peptide and prolactin hormone

Vasoactive intestinal peptide (VIP) is a 28 amino acid (aa) long peptide released during food ingestion. It exerts its actions by binding to VPAC1 and VPAC2 receptors. Both of them are G-coupled receptors, extensively distributed in the central nervous system (CNS).

In 1981, Jouvet's group reported (Riou *et al.*, 1982) that VIP induces REM sleep in rats. A few years later, several other groups supported this finding by reproducing this effect in cats and rabbits (Drucker-Colín *et al.*, 1984; Obál *et al.*, 1986). Further studies demonstrated that VIP was capable of restoring REM sleep in cats rendered insomniac by either serotonin synthesis inhibitor, parachlorophenylalanine (PCPA) (Prospéro-García *et al.*, 1986), or a lesion in the basal forebrain (Pacheco-Cano *et al.*, 1990). Additionally, it was shown that cats subjected to REM-sleep deprivation exhibited an increase in both the concentration of VIP in the cerebrospinal fluid (CSF) and the VIP receptors' expression in the mesopontine structures involved in the generation and maintenance of REM sleep (Jiménez-Anguiano *et al.*, 1993).

In 1988, Mirmiran *et al.* (1988) reported that VIP antagonists reduced REM sleep in rats; a fact earlier suggested by Jouvet's group when they reported that anti-VIP antibodies induced a similar effect (Riou *et al.*, 1982).

Later, in a series of interesting studies, Krueger and his colleagues showed that VIP increases prolactin hormone (PrH) and, by inactivating PrH with antibodies, VIP's REM sleep-inducing effect could be abolished (Obál Jr. *et al.*, 1994). The same group indicated that VIP increases PrH mRNA, suggesting that somehow VIP triggers a cascade of transcription-promoting factors that activate Prl (gene encoding PrH) transcription. Krueger's group went further by characterizing the sleep–waking cycle of Prl-knock-out mice, clearly showing that these animals had reduced, albeit not abolished, expression of REM sleep. Additionally, they showed that the exogenous administration of PrH for 11 to 12 days restored REM sleep to a normal amount (Obál Jr. *et al.*, 2005). Interestingly, it has been suggested that orexin A (Orex A) seems to reduce PrH synthesis and release in sheep (Molik *et al.*, 2008), indicating that Orex A exerts an inhibitory effect on REM-sleep mechanisms. Orexin A also prevents the synthesis and release of growth hormone, a hormone that also increases REM sleep; further supporting that Orex A plays an inhibitory regulation on REM sleep. Additionally, it is known that VIP and acetylcholine (ACh) are co-localized in pontine structures. Vasoactive intestinal peptide administration in the reticularis pontis oralis nucleus (PON) induces an increase in REM sleep (Bourgin *et al.*, 1997), very likely through the activation of cholinergic neurons (Kohlmeier and Reiner, 1999). Later, Simón-Arceo *et al.* (2003) demonstrated that VIP administration into the central and basal amygdaloid nuclei induces a long-lasting enhancement in SWS and REM sleep. These findings strongly suggest that this neuropeptide is involved in REM-sleep generation, very likely through the interaction with many other peptides, such as PrH, and neurotransmitters, such as ACh.

Cholecystokinin-8

The 33-aa cholecystokinin (CCK) is released by the intestine, causing gall bladder contraction, pancreatic enzyme secretion, and it participates in inducing a satiety syndrome. The brain contains larger amounts of its octapeptide form, CCK-8. In particular, the cerebral cortex, hippocampus, hypothalamus, and pons have high concentrations of CCK-8 as compared to the cerebellum (Beresford *et al.*, 1986). This octapeptide exerts its action by binding to its protein G-coupled receptors, CCKA and CCKB, which are also widely distributed in the CNS.

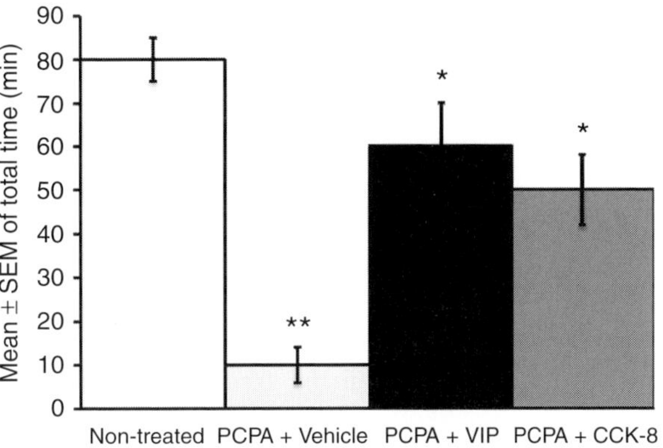

Figure 25.1 Illustration of the effects induced by VIP or CCK-8 on the insomnia induced by PCPA in cats. Observe the almost total restoration of REM sleep in the otherwise insomniac cats. VIP and CCK-8 still remained with less REM sleep (these groups are still statistically different from the control non-treated cats, but definitively they are different from the cats under PCPA and additionally treated with vehicle).

Very early work indicated that CCK-8 diminishes the latency to slow-wave sleep (SWS), during the light phase of the photoperiod (Mansbach and Lorenz, 1983; Rojas-Ramirez *et al.*, 1982). Back in those days, we also reported that CCK-8 restores REM sleep in PCPA-treated cats (Prospéro-García *et al.*, 1987) (see Figure 25.1). Later, in 2001, Shemyakin and Kapás showed that the administration of a CCKA receptor antagonist, L-364,718, prevented SWS and REM sleep that appear after eating, suggesting that CCKA is implicated in the expression of postprandial sleep (Shemyakin and Kapás, 2001). However, a few studies have indicated that the blockade of CCK-8 receptors, i.e., CCKB receptor, improves slow-wave and REM sleep in aged rats. Hence, the role of CCK-8 in the regulation of sleep remains controversial. No definitive results have been generated to accept or rule out its participation in sleep modulation.

Melanin-concentrating hormone

Melanin-concentrating hormone (MCH) is a 19-aa neuropeptide. Although MCH has been reported to exert its effects through two metabotropic receptors, known as MCH1R and MCH2R (Tan *et al.*, 2002), it seems that in rodents only MCH1R is active; however, in many other mammals, including humans, both are active. MCH-ergic neurons are located principally in the hypothalamus, just as orexinergic neurons and like them, they project abundantly to several areas in the CNS; this suggests that MCH, as other peptides, is involved in food ingestion and sleep. In fact, in 2003, Verret *et al.* (2003) demonstrated that the icv administration of MCH causes a 200% increase in REM-sleep expression in rats; whereas the subcutaneous administration of MCH1R antagonists increase waking and decrease REM sleep in rats (Ahnaou *et al.*, 2008). In addition, MCH-ergic neurons are hyperactive after REM-sleep deprivation (Hanriot *et al.*, 2007). Recently, Jones and her colleagues (Hassani *et al.*, 2009), in one of her typically elegant studies, showed that MCH-ergic neurons increase their firing frequency in relation to REM sleep, whereas orexinergic neurons increase their firing rate during waking, indicating that Orex is more related to waking whereas MCH is more related to REM sleep (Hassani *et al.*, 2009). Since Bayer *et al.* (2005) found that MCH neurons may be hyperpolarized by noradrenaline or acetylcholine agonists, it is very likely MCH is regulating REM sleep through the interaction with noradrenergic and cholinergic systems.

Orexin A and orexin B (or hypocretin-1 and hypocretin-2)

These neuropeptides play an important role in the promotion of wakefulness and feeding. They were described simultaneously by de Lecea *et al.* (1998) and Yanagisawa's group (1998). These neuropeptides are the subject of other chapters in this book; hence, we will not go into detail here. We would just like to say that the activity of orexinergic neurons is rather related to the induction of waking than of REM sleep or any other sleep stage. It is fascinating to acknowledge that the orexinergic neurons' activity not only promotes waking but also, by doing so, they repress REM sleep occurrence. Hence, when their action is banned by some, until now, unknown pathological mechanisms, REM sleep intrudes into the waking period. This is narcolepsy, a disease that shows that the mechanisms that regulate waking oppose those regulating REM sleep and vice versa.

Cortistatin

Cortistatin (CST) is a neuropeptide whose mRNA is expressed in the cerebral cortex and the hippocampus of mice, rats, and humans, in neurons that contain GAD_{67}, hence GABAergic (de Lecea *et al.*, 1996). Cortistatin is structurally similar to somatostatin (SST). Both share the same aa sequence, which SST

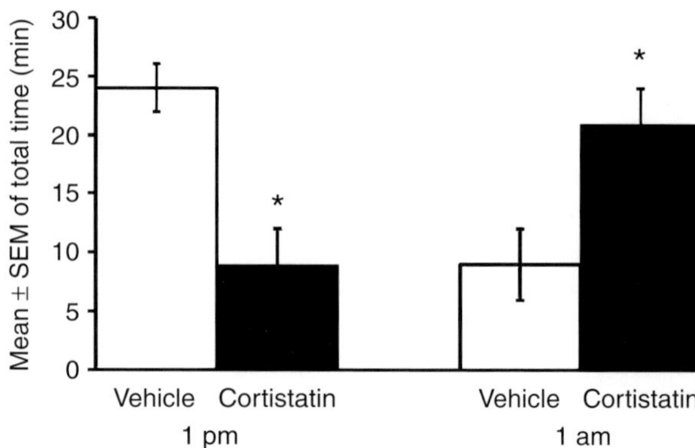

Figure 25.2 This illustration depicts the biphasic effect induced by cortistatin. Observe that the very same dose of cortistatin induces an increase or a decrease of REM sleep in rats depending on the hour of the day.

uses to bind to its own receptors. In fact, CST binds to all SST receptors. However, the existence of a specific receptor for CST, the MrgX2a, in the hippocampus, hypothalamus, and substantia nigra has been suggested (Robas *et al.*, 2003). Cortistatin antagonizes acetylcholine excitatory actions in the cerebral cortex and hippocampus (de Lecea *et al.*, 1996). Therefore, involvement of cortistatin in the modulation of memory processes (Méndez-Díaz *et al.*, 2005; Sánchez-Alavez *et al.*, 2000) and sleep (de Lecea *et al.*, 1996; Méndez-Díaz *et al.*, 2005) has been suggested. Our first report describes that CST induces only SWS (de Lecea *et al.*, 1996). However, later we observed that CST increases REM sleep during the dark phase of the cycle (Méndez-Díaz *et al.*, 2005). This finding suggested a dependence of the CST REM sleep-inducing effect on the dark–light cycle. In addition, we have observed that CST increases food intake (Méndez-Díaz *et al.*, 2008) (Figure 25.2).

Cocaine-and-amphetamine-regulated transcript

This is a neuropeptide principally expressed in the CNS and intestine. Its mRNA is upregulated, principally in the hypothalamus, after the administration of cocaine and amphetamine in rats (Douglass *et al.*, 1995). Cocaine-and-amphetamine-regulated transcript (CART) has been implicated in a variety of physiological processes; but its major effect is the induction of hyporexia (Kristensen *et al.*, 1998). In humans, obesity has been related to a low serum concentration of CART. This condition seems to be a consequence of a mutation in the gene CARTPT (del Giudice *et al.*, 2001). We have recently shown that CART is involved in the regulation of the sleep–waking cycle. The icv administration of 0.3 nmol of CART during the light induces an increase of REM sleep in rats, as a consequence of augmenting the frequency of REM bouts. This increase in REM sleep was associated to an increase in c-Fos expression in several hypothalamic nuclei (arcuate, ventromedial, and dorsomedial) involved in the regulation of food intake (Méndez-Díaz *et al.*, 2009).

Neuropeptides regulating sleep and stress

Most of the neuropeptides that regulate stress and the sleep–waking cycle are pro-opiomelanocortin (POMC) derivatives. Among them are the adrenocorticotropin hormone (ACTH), α-melanocyte-stimulating hormone (α-MSH), also known as $ACTH_{1-13}$ fragment, and corticotropin-like intermediate lobe peptide (CLIP), also considered an $ACTH_{18-39}$ fragment.

Adrenocorticotropin hormone and corticotropin-releasing factor

Both hormones seem to increase waking. The original studies by Chastrette and Cespuglio (1985) indicated that ACTH at a 1 ng dose does not modify the sleep–waking cycle. However, later, they published that 1 µg increases waking (Chastrette *et al.*, 1990a). Similar doses of CRH also increase waking.

α-melanocyte-stimulating hormone

In 1976, Kastin and his group indicated that α-MSH increases SWS in rats (Panskepp *et al.*, 1976). This finding was reproduced by Chastrette and Cespuglio almost ten years later (Chastrette and Cespuglio, 1985). By that time Krueger and his colleagues reported that α-MSH reduces REM sleep (Opp *et al.*, 1988), as well as SWS, although its main effect is on REM sleep. The main difference between the experimental paradigms of these research groups lies in the amount of α-MSH injected. While Kastin and his group and Chastrette and Cespuglio injected an amount in the order of nanograms; Krueger's group injected 100 ng and up to 50 µg. We believe that the former group utilized a dose closer to the physiological concentration than the latter group.

It is interesting to note that these neuropeptides seem to suppress actively the expression of REM sleep. Supporting this notion are those studies performed by Jouvet's group, in which they showed that the induction of stress by immobilization of rats was followed by an increase in REM sleep, once the stressor had disappeared (release of the rat from the immobilization) (Rampin *et al.*, 1991). It is highly possible that as ACTH is released as a response to the stressor, at the end it is broken down into α-MSH and CLIP; the former would increase SWS, while the latter, REM sleep.

Corticotropin-like intermediate lobe peptide

This neuropeptide is found primarily in the pituitary intermediate lobe but also in the arcuate nucleus of the basal hypothalamus. The REM-sleep inducing effect of CLIP was first demonstrated by Chastrette and Cespuglio (1985) and later Chastrette *et al.* (1990b) reported that CLIP was able to induce REM sleep in otherwise insomniac rats. Rats were maintained insomniac by the administration of apormorphine (D1/D2 agonist) or 8-OH-DPAT (serotonin agonist). Also the icv administration of CLIP during the dark period of the light–dark cycle increased REM sleep in rats. Immunohistological studies found CLIP-positive cells in the preoptic area, amygdala and pons; all nuclei involved in sleep regulation. In addition, Jouvet *et al.* suggested that the effect of CLIP on REM-sleep generation may be on the dorsal raphe nucleus through a serotonergic action, since local administration of CLIP releases serotonin and increases REM sleep (Chastrette and Cespuglio, 1985; Chastrette *et al.*, 1990a).

Neuropeptides that act as trophic factors and regulate sleep

This group of peptides involved in REM sleep includes growth hormone (GH), nerve growth factor (NGF), and neurotrophin 3 and 4 (NT-3 and NT-4). It has been shown that GH promotes REM sleep in several species including humans. The ip administration of GH increases REM sleep in cats and rats (Drucker-Colín *et al.*, 1975; Stern *et al.*, 1975) while transgenic mice that overproduce GH exhibit an enhancement in REM-sleep expression (Hajdu *et al.*, 2002). In humans, the nocturnal secretion of GH occurs during SWS, during the first part of the night, and it seems that both GH secretion and SWS expression are dependent on the reciprocal interaction with the GH-releasing hormone (GHRH). Actually, there is some experimental evidence indicating that GHRH increases SWS and

REM sleep, suggesting that GHRH facilitates SWS and the consequent release of GH increases REM sleep. Earlier, we discussed PrH, as a REM-sleep facilitating hormone. However, it is also known that PrH facilitates the neurogenesis associated to maternal behavior (Shingo *et al.*, 2003) and prevents the decrease in hippocampal neurogenesis induced by stress (Torner *et al.*, 2009). Hence, it seems to have neurotrophic properties. It is possible that one of the actions of PrH in facilitating REM sleep is exerted through its neurotrophic properties.

In this context, microinjection of NGF and NT-3 into the rostral pontine tegmentum of adult cats promptly induces long-lasting episodes of REM sleep (Yamuy *et al.*, 1995). Neurons that contain neurotrophin receptors (p75, trkA, trkB, and trkC) are present in the regions involved in the generation and control of REM sleep, the pons and mesencephalon in cats, suggesting that neurotrophin receptors may modulate the electrical activity of neurons in the rostral pontine tegmentum, which are responsible for the generation of REM sleep (Yamuy *et al.*, 2000).

Intracellular proteins and sleep

Intracellular signaling is very important in understanding the functions of sleep. What kind of cytoplasmic proteins are activated by secreted neuropeptides and neurotransmitters when they bind to their receptor in the plasma membrane is a crucial question. For example, we have observed that pharmacological blockade of ERK (extracellular signal-regulated kinase) activation by blocking the protein kinase MEK (MAP-ERK kinase) or blocking the alternative pathway mediated by p38 MAPK (mitogen-activated protein kinase) prevents the occurrence of REM sleep (Díaz-Ruiz *et al.*, 2001) (Figure 25.3). In addition, endocannabinoids, such as anandamide, which activate the MAPK intracellular pathway (Derkinderen *et al.*, 2001), increase REM sleep (Murillo-Rodríguez *et al.*, 1998). Since this pathway has been involved in brain plasticity, it seems likely that along with the trophic factors, they are able to exert a restorative effect while the subject is asleep and in this particular case during REM sleep.

Based on this information and much more mounting evidence generated by several research groups worldwide, we can safely conclude that neuropeptides are involved in the regulation and generation of such a fascinating state as is REM sleep. Secondly, since neuropeptides as proteins are the result of a command

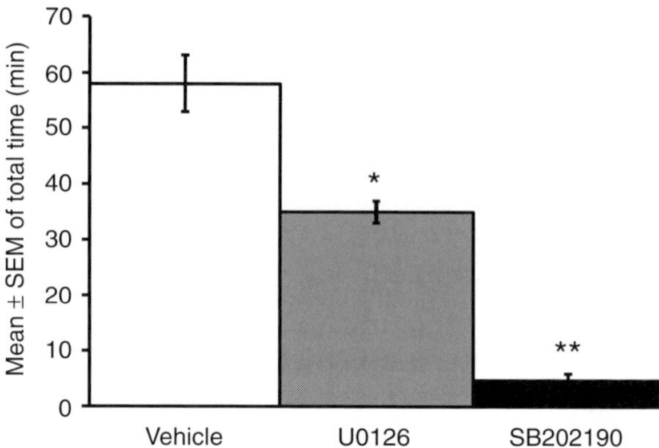

Figure 25.3 Illustration of the effects of two drugs that interfere with the MAPK pathway. U0126 inhibits MEK, the activating enzyme of ERK; while SB202190 inhibits MAPK-p38. Both inhibit REM-sleep expression, although at the dose used SB202190 seems to be more potent in inhibiting REM sleep than U0126.

encoded in the genes, we can also conclude that REM sleep, as well as the other sleep stages, and their interaction resulting in a regular cycling across the hours of sleep, arise from the action of multiple genes. REM sleep, then, is a polygenetic trait. Hence, many more neuropeptides and proteins regulating this sleep stage are expected to be described. In this context, it is highly possible that many sleep disorders may have a genetic origin. Epigenetic modulation of genes encoding for these REM-sleep-promoting neuropeptides may occur across a subject's lifetime. For instance, methylation of specific genes as a result of a subject's interaction with an unfriendly or frankly hostile environment in crucial stages of ontogeny, could remain this way for the rest of the subject's life. As an example, we can say that improper maternal care of rat puppies (unfriendly environment) facilitates the methylation of the gene encoding for the glucocorticoid receptor, with quite impressive consequences on the performance of rats in several behavioral tests. Likewise, both the synthesis and release of several neurotransmitters and the availability of their receptors are modified in these rats. Unpublished observations made in our laboratory have indicated that these type of rats exhibit significantly reduced REM-sleep expression.

REM-sleep expression is the result of a genetic load and environmental pressure. In this context, it is very likely that nobody sleeps in the same way every night. Particularly, if we take into account that one of the main sources of stimulation to the brain is learning, and we learn something about our environment every single day. Neuropeptides, then, are the heralds of genes regulating sleep including REM sleep (and many other physiological states and behaviors), whose bioavailability is regulated by epigenetic mechanisms.

Acknowledgments

This work was supported by Grant 49797 to OPG and Grant 80148 to MMD from CONACYT, and Grant IN209808 to AERC from PAPIIT-DGAPA.

References

Ahnaou, A., Drinkenburg, W. H., Bouwknecht, J. A. *et al.* (2008) Blocking melanin-concentrating hormone MCH1 receptor affects rat sleep–wake architecture. *Eur J Pharmacol* **579**(1/3): 177–88.

Bayer, L., Eggermann, E., Serafin, M. *et al.* (2005) Opposite effects of noradrenaline and acetylcholine upon hypocretin/orexin versus melanin concentrating hormone neurons in rat hypothalamic slices. *Neuroscience* **130**: 807–11.

Beresford, I. J. M., Clarck, C. R. & Hughes, J. (1986) Measurement and characterization of neuronal cholecystokinin using a novel radioreceptor assay. *Brain Res* **398**(2): 313–23.

Bourgin, P., Lebrand, C., Escourrou, P. *et al.* (1997) Vasoactive intestinal polypeptide microinjections into the oral pontine tegmentum enhance rapid eye movement sleep in the rat. *Neuroscience* **77**(2): 351–60.

Chastrette, N. & Cespuglio, R. (1985) Influence of proopiomelanocortin-derived peptides on the sleep-waking cycle of the rat. *Neurosci Lett* **62**(3): 365–70.

Chastrette, N., Cespuglio, R. & Jouvet, M. (1990a) Proopiomelanocortin (POMC)-derived peptides and sleep in the rat. Part 1 – Hypnogenic properties of ACTH derivatives. *Neuropeptides* **15**(2): 61–74.

Chastrette, N., Cepuglio, R., Lin, Y. L. & Jouvet, M. (1990b) Proopiomelanocortin (POMC)-derived peptides and sleep in the rat. Part 2 – aminergic regulatory processes. *Neuropeptides* **15**(2): 75–88.

de Lecea, L., Criado, J. R., Prospéro-García, O. *et al.* (1996) A cortical neuropeptide with neuronal depressant and sleep-modulating properties. *Nature* **381**(6579): 242–5.

de Lecea, L., Kilduff, T. S., Peyron, C. *et al.* (1998) The hypocretins: hypothalamus-specific peptides with neuroexcitatory activity. *Proc Natnl Acad Sci (USA)* **95**(1): 322–7.

del Giudice, E. M., Santoro, N., Cirillo, *et al.* (2001) Mutational screening of the CART gene in obese children. Identifying a mutation (Leu34Phe) associated with reduced resting energy expenditure and cosegregating with obesity phenotype in a large family. *Diabetes* **50**(9): 2157–60.

Derkinderen, P., Ledent, C., Parmentier, M., Girault, J. A. (2001) Cannabinoids activate p38 mitogen-activated protein kinases through CB1 receptor in hippocampus. *J Neurochem* **77**(3): 957–60.

Díaz-Ruiz, O., Navarro L., Méndez-Díaz, M. *et al.* (2001) Inhibition of the ERK pathway prevents HIVgp120-induced REM sleep increase. *Brain Res* **913**(1): 78–81.

Douglass, J., McKinzie, A. M. & Couceyro, P. (1995) PCR differential display identifies a rat brain mRNA that is transcriptionally regulated by cocaine and amphetamine. *J Neurosci* **15**(3/2): 2471–81.

Drucker-Colín, R., Spanis, C. W., Hunyadi, J. & McGaugh, J. L. (1975) Growth hormone effects on sleep and wakefulness in the rat. *Neuroendocrinology* **18**(1): 1–8.

Drucker-Colín, R., Bernal-Pedraza, J., Fernández-Cancino, F. & Oksenberg, A. (1984) Is vasoactive intestinal polypeptide (VIP) a sleep factor? *Peptides* **5**(4): 837–40.

Estabrooke, I. V., McCarthy, M. T., Ko, E. *et al.* (2001) Fos expression in orexin neurons varies with behavioral state. *J Neurosci* **21**(5): 1656–62.

Hajdu, I., Obal, F. Jr., Fang, J., Krueger, J. M. & Rollo, C. D. (2002) Sleep of transgenic mice producing excess rat growth hormone. *Am J Physiol-Reg I* **282**(1): R70–6.

Hanriot, L., Camargo, N., Courau, A. C. *et al.* (2007) Characterization of the melanin-concentrating hormone neurons activated during paradoxical sleep hypersomnia in rats. *J Compar Neurol* **505**(2): 147–57.

Hassani, O. K., Lee, M. G. & Jones, B. E. (2009) Melanin-concentrating hormone neurons discharge in a reciprocal manner to orexin neurons across the sleep–wake cycle. *Proc Natnl Acad Sci (USA)* **106**(7): 2418–22.

Jiménez-Anguiano, A., Báez-Saldaña, A. & Drucker-Colín R. (1993) Cerebrospinal fluid (CSF) extracted immediately after REM sleep deprivation prevents REM rebound and contains vasoactive intestinal peptide (VIP). *Brain Res* **631**(2): 345–8.

Kohlmeier, K. A. & Reiner, P. B. (1999) Vasoactive intestinal polypeptide excites medial pontine reticular formation neurons in the brainstem rapid eye movement sleep-induction zone. *J Neurosci* **19**(10): 4073–81.

Kristensen, P., Judge, M. E., Thim, L. *et al.* (1998) Hypothalamic CART is a new anorectic peptide regulated by leptin. *Nature* **393**(6680): 72–6.

Mansbach, R. S. & Lorenz, D. N. (1983) Cholecystokinin (CCK-8) elicits prandial sleep in rats. *Physiol Behavi* **30**(2): 179–83.

Méndez-Díaz, M., Irwin, L., Gómez-Chavarín, M. *et al.* (2005) Cortistatin modulates memory evocation in rats. *Eur J Pharmacol* **507**(1/3): 21–8.

Méndez-Díaz, M., Domínguez Martín, E., Sanchez Galvez, X., Pérez Pérez, L. & Prospéro-García, O. (2008) Cortistatin and CART modulates sleep and food intake. In *38 Annual Meeting. Society for Neuroscience.* Washington, D.C.

Méndez-Díaz, M., Domínguez Martín, E., Pérez Morales, M. *et al.* (2009) The anorexigenic peptide cocaine-and-amphetamine-regulated transcript modulates REM-sleep in rats. *Neuropeptides* **43**(6): 499–505.

Mirmiran, M., Kruisbrink, J., Bos, N. P., Van der Werf, D. & Boer, G. J. (1988) Decrease of rapid-eye-movement sleep in the light by intraventricular application of a VIP-antagonist in the rat. *Brain Res* **458**(1): 192–4.

Molik, E., Zieba, D. A., Misztal, T. *et al.* (2008) The role of orexin A in the control of prolactin and growth hormone secretions in sheep: in vitro study. *J Physiol Pharmacol* **59**(Suppl 9): 91–100.

Murillo-Rodríguez, E., Sánchez-Alavez, M., Navarro, L. *et al.* (1998) Anandamide modulates sleep and memory in rats. *Brain Res* **812**(1/2): 270–4.

Obál, F. Jr., Sáry, G., Alföldi, P., Rubicsek, G. & Obál, F. (1986) Vasoactive intestinal polypeptide promotes sleep without effects on brain temperature in rats at night. *Neurosci Lett* **64**(2): 236–40.

Obál, F. Jr., Payne, L., Kacsoh, B. *et al.* (1994) Involvement of prolactin in the REM sleep-promoting activity of systemic vasoactive intestinal peptide (VIP). *Brain Res* **645**(1/2): 143–9.

Obál J. F, García-García F., Kacsóh, B. *et al.* (2005) Rapid eye movement sleep is reduced in prolactin-deficient mice. *J Neurosci* **25**(44): 10,282–9.

Opp, M.R., Obal, F. Jr., Krueger, J.M. (1988) Effects of α-MSH on sleep, behavior, and brain temperature: interactions with IL-1. *Am J Physiol* **255** (6Pt 2): R914–22.

Pacheco-Cano, M. T., García-Hernández, F., Prospéro-García, O. & Drucker-Colín, R. (1990) Vasoactive intestinal polypeptide induces REM recovery in insomniac forebrain lesioned cats. *Sleep* **13**(4): 297–303.

Panskepp, J., Reilly, P., Bishop, P. *et al.* (1976) Effects of alpha-MSH on motivation, vigilance and brain respiration. *Pharmacol Biochem Behav* **5**(Suppl 1): 59–64.

Prospéro-Garcia, O., Morales, M., Arankowsky-Sandoval, G. & Drucker-Colin, R. (1986) Vasoactive intestinal polypeptide (VIP) and cerebrospinal fluid (CSF) of sleep-deprived cats restores REM sleep in insomniac recipients. *Brain Res* **385**(1): 169–73.

Prospéro-García, O., Ott, T. & Drucker-Colín, R. (1987) Cerebroventricular infusion of cholecystokinin (CCK-8) restores REM sleep in parachlorophenylalanine (PCPA)-pretreated cats. *Neurosci Lett* **78**(2): 205–10.

Rampin, C., Cespuglio, R., Chastrette, N. & Jouvet, M. (1991) Immobilization stress induces a paradoxical sleep rebound in rat. *Neurosci Lett* **126**(2): 113–18.

Riou F., Cespuglio, R. & Jouvet, M. (1982) Endogenous peptides and sleep in the rat. III. The hypnogenic properties of vasoactive intestinal polypeptide (VIP). *Neuropeptides* **2**(5): 265–77.

Robas, N., Mead, E. & Fidock, M. (2003) MrgX2 is a high potency cortistatin receptor expressed in dorsal root ganglion. *J Biol Chem* **278**(45): 44,400–4.

Rojas-Ramirez, J. A., Crawley, J. N. & Mendelson, W. B. (1982) Electroencephalographic analysis of the sleep-inducing actions of cholecystokinin. *Neuropeptides* **3**(2): 129–38.

Sakurai, T., Amemiya, A., Ishii, M. *et al.* (1998) Orexins and orexin receptors: a family of hypothalamic neuropeptides and G protein-coupled receptors that regulate feeding behavior. *Cell* **92**(4): 573–85.

Sánchez-Alavez, M., Gómez-Chavarín, M., Navarro, L. *et al.* (2000) Cortistatin modulates memory processes in rats. *Brain Res* **858**(1): 78–83.

Shemyakin, A. & Kapás, L. (2001) L-364,718, a cholecystokinin-A receptor antagonist, suppresses feeding-induced sleep in rats. *Am J Physiol- Reg I* **280**(5): R1420–6.

Shingo, T., Gregg, C., Enwere, E. *et al.* (2003) Pregnancy-stimulated neurogenesis in the adult female forebrain mediated by prolactin. *Science* **299**(5603): 117–20.

Simón-Arceo, K., Ramírez-Salado, I. & Calvo, J. M. (2003) Long-lasting enhancement of rapid eye movement sleep and pontogeniculooccipital waves by vasoactive intestinal peptide microinjection into the amygdala temporal lobe. *Sleep* **26**(3): 259–64.

Stern, W. C., Jalowiec, J. E., Shabshelowitz, H. & Morgane, P. J. (1975) Effects of growth hormone on sleep–waking patterns in cats. *Horm Behav* **6**(2): 189–96.

Tan, C. P., Sano, H., Iwaasa, H. *et al.* (2002) Melanin-concentrating hormone receptor subtypes 1 and 2: species-specific gene expression. *Genomics* **79**(6): 785–92.

Torner, l., Karg, S., Blume, A., *et al.* (2009) Prolactin prevents chronic stress-induced decrease of adult hippocampal neurogenesis and promotes neuronal fate. *J Neurosci* **29**(6): 1826–33.

Verret, L., Goutagny, R., Fort, P. *et al.* (2003) A role of melanin-concentrating hormone producing neurons in the central regulation of paradoxical sleep. *Bio Med Central Neuroscience* [online] **4**(19). Available at www.biomedcentral.com/1471-2202/4/19 [Accessed May 19, 2006].

Yamuy, J., Morales, F. R. & Chase, M. H. (1995) Induction of rapid eye movement sleep by the microinjection of nerve growth factor into the pontine reticular formation of the cat. *Neuroscience* **66**(1): 9–13.

Yamuy, J., Sampogna, S. & Chase, M. H. (2000) Neurotrophin-receptor immunoreactive neurons in mesopontine regions involved in the control of behavioral states. *Brain Res* **866**(1/2): 1–14.

Chapter

26 Adenosine and glycine in REM-sleep regulation

Mahesh M. Thakkar, Rishi Sharma, Samuel C. Engemann, and Pradeep Sahota

Summary

The discovery of rapid eye movement (REM) sleep revolutionized the field of sleep research. REM sleep is that state in which most of our dreams occur. During REM sleep, the brain is active, while the body is asleep. These characteristics make REM sleep a unique and a paradoxical state. While we are struggling to understand the function of REM sleep, major advances have been made in understanding the cellular mechanisms responsible for REM-sleep control. In this chapter, we have described two neurochemical substrates involved in REM-sleep regulation. One of them is adenosine and the other is glycine.

Adenosine is implicated to be the homeostatic regulator of sleep. It has been suggested that adenosine acts via A_1 receptors to inhibit wake-promoting neurons and promote the transition from wakefulness to sleep. Adenosine acts on multiple wake-promoting systems including the basal forebrain cholinergic and the noncholinergic systems, namely the orexinergic, and the histaminergic systems. There are reports suggesting that adenosine may act via A_{2A} receptors and activate sleep-promoting neurons of the preoptic region. In addition, studies suggest a direct role of adenosine in the modulation of REM sleep.

During REM sleep, there is a tonic muscle atonia coupled with phasic muscle twitches. This phenomenon is regulated by the dorsolateral pons and ventromedial medulla along with local neurons within the spinal cord. Glycinergic mechanisms are responsible for the control of muscle tone during REM sleep. However, the exact role is under debate.

Introduction

In the middle of the twentieth century, the notion that sleep is a passive homogeneous state of the brain was disregarded when rhythms in eye movements were observed during sleep and linked to dreaming in humans (Aserinsky and Kleitman, 1953). Subsequently, Dement and Kleitman characterized the electroencephalographic (EEG) activity during dreaming in humans and recorded rapid eye movements (REMs) during sleep in animals (Dement, 2000). These discoveries established the presence of a non-REM (NREM)–REM sleep cycle. However, it was only after Jouvet demonstrated the presence of muscle atonia (total suppression of muscle tone) and the importance of the pontine reticular formation in REM sleep, which he termed as "sommeil paradoxal" or paradoxical sleep, that finally established REM sleep as a distinct state of behavior along with wakefulness and NREM sleep. This was the beginning of a new era in the history of modern sleep (Dement, 2000).

REM sleep is characterized by an ensemble of events including desynchronized, low-amplitude EEG, complete loss of activity in the antigravity muscles, frequent bursts of eye movements, tonic hippocampal theta activity, increased metabolic rate, muscle twitches, and ponto-geniculo-occipital (PGO) waves. Other striking features of REM sleep are cardiovascular and respiratory irregularities, irregular sympathetic activity, increased parasympathetic tone, and an inhibited thermoregulatory responsiveness.

REM sleep latency is another striking feature of REM sleep. In normal conditions, REM sleep is always preceded by NREM sleep. The duration of NREM sleep from sleep onset to the onset of the first REM sleep period is defined as the latency to REM sleep. Changes in REM sleep latency are considered to be a significant pathological feature in various sleep disorders and psychiatric illnesses.

The neuronal mechanisms involved in the generation and the maintenance of REM sleep are beginning

REM Sleep: Regulation and Function, eds. Birendra N. Mallick, S. R. Pandi-Perumal, Robert W. McCarley, and Adrian R. Morrison. Published by Cambridge University Press. © Cambridge University Press 2011.

to be understood at both the cellular and molecular level (Datta and Maclean, 2007; McCarley, 2007). Current theory suggests that REM sleep is produced by two cholinergic cell groups at the junction of the mid-brain and pons, the laterodorsal tegmental nucleus (LDT), and the pendunculopontine tegmental (PPT) nucleus, which provide cholinergic innervation to the pontine (PRF) and bulbar reticular formation. These reticular neurons, in turn, likely act as effectors for many REM-sleep phenomena, including the muscle atonia, rapid eye movements, muscle twitches, and initiation of PGO waves. This brain-stem REM-generating machinery is tightly regulated by inputs from the forebrain including the orexinergic, cholinergic, histaminergic, and GABAergic systems. Multiple neurotransmitters and neuromodulators are responsible for orchestrating the REM-sleep phenomenon.

In this chapter, we will focus on the role of adenosine and glycine in the regulation of REM sleep. Adenosine, an endogenous purine nucleoside, modulates many physiological processes in the brain. Although there is little evidence to suggest that adenosine has a direct role in controlling REM sleep, there is convincing evidence implicating adenosine as a homeostatic modulator of sleep with a critical role in the transition from wakefulness to NREM sleep. Glycine, on the other hand, is the simplest of the amino acids and a major inhibitory neurotransmitter in the brain stem and spinal cord. Glycine has been implicated in the control of muscle atonia during REM sleep.

Adenosine and the regulation of sleep

The effect of adenosine on the circulation was first discovered in 1929 by Drury and Szent-Györgyi. Since then the role of adenosine has been extensively investigated in different tissues and we now know that adenosine is a ubiquitous nucleoside and has a pivotal role in the regulation of many bodily functions. Adenosine serves as a building block of nucleic acids and energy storage molecules. Adenosine is a substrate for multiple enzymes and, most importantly, serves as an extracellular modulator of cellular activity (Basheer *et al.*, 2004). The endogenous release of adenosine exerts powerful effects on a wide range of organ systems including the circulatory and the nervous system. Since adenosine is a central substance in energy metabolism, it can effectively regulate neuronal activity. While the excitatory actions are mediated by ATP

via P2-receptors, adenosine has been implicated to mediate inhibitory activity correlated with low energy reserve. The most profound effect of adenosine in the central nervous system is the inhibitory modulation of neuronal activity and neurotransmitter release. One intriguing possibility for physiological action is adenosine's function as a regulator of sleep.

The sedative action of adenosine was first described in the early 1950s (reviewed in Basheer *et al.*, 2004). Subsequently, extensive research conducted by Radulovacki and his coworkers demonstrated the sleep-inducing effects of systemic and central administrations of adenosine and its agonists, and wake-inducing effects of caffeine and theophylline, powerful blockers of adenosine receptors (Radulovacki, 1985). Furthermore, REM-sleep deprivation was reported to affect adenosine metabolism and adenosine receptor (Thakkar and Mallick, 1996).

Multiple lines of evidence exist to suggest that an extracellular adenosine concentration is linked to metabolic and neuronal activity. For example, extracellular glucose levels are higher during NREM sleep suggesting glucose utilization/breakdown decreases during NREM sleep as compared to wakefulness (reviewed by Basheer *et al.*, 2004). Extracellular adenosine levels in the neo-striatum and hippocampus were higher during the circadian active period when the animal is awake, and lower during the circadian inactive period when the animal is sleeping (Huston *et al.*, 1996). Thus, high neuronal activity results in increased adenosine release.

Adenosine modifies neuronal activity by acting at membrane-bound, G-protein coupled receptors. Four distinct adenosine receptors, A_1, A_{2A}, A_{2B}, and A_3, have been identified and their relative distributions examined. Of these, the A_1 and the A_{2A} are highly expressed within the rat brain, whereas, intermediate expression of A_3 has been found in the hippocampus and cerebellum. The A_1 receptor is negatively coupled to adenylyl cyclase activity, while the A_{2A} receptor is positively coupled to this enzyme.

The brain contains multiple neuronal systems that are responsible for evoking wakefulness from sleep and also generating and maintaining wakefulness. These arousal systems include the cholinergic neurons of the basal forebrain and mesopontine tegmentum, histaminergic and orexinergic neurons of the posterior and lateral hypothalamus, glutamatergic neurons of the pontine reticular formation, serotonergic raphe neurons, and the noradrenergic locus coeruleus neurons. All these wakefulness-promoting systems display increased neuronal activity during wakefulness. Does adenosine promote sleep by acting globally on wakefulness-promoting centers or does adenosine act on selective wakefulness or sleep centers to promote sleep? Subsequent sections provide a detailed description of adenosine on multiple sleep–wakefulness regulatory regions of the brain.

Adenosine and the cholinergic basal forebrain

The basal forebrain (BF) is the rostral-most extension of a distributed network of neurons implicated in regulating cortical activation. The BF contains a mixed phenotype of neurons, some of which are cholinergic. The BF cholinergic neurons send their projections to the cortex and provide a major source of acetylcholine to the cortex. There is a strong correlation between the discharge activity of the BF cholinergic neurons and cortical arousal.

In vivo studies conducted in freely behaving cats and rats revealed that reverse microdialysis administration of adenosine in the cholinergic BF produced a significant reduction in wakefulness (Basheer *et al.*, 2004). Porkka-Heiskanen and her coworkers were the first to show spontaneous fluctuations in extracellular levels of adenosine in the BF across behavioral states (Porkka-Heiskanen *et al.*, 1997).

Extracellular levels of adenosine were higher during wakefulness in the BF when compared with NREM sleep. Furthermore, extending wakefulness resulted in a progressive increase in extracellular adenosine that slowly declined during subsequent recovery sleep (Porkka-Heiskanen *et al.*, 1997). The monotonic rise in adenosine concentrations with each hour of prolonged wakefulness and the slow decline with recovery sleep led to the hypothesis that adenosine was a key mediator of the sleep propensity following extended wakefulness. Finally, using local perfusion of an adenosine transporter inhibitor, Porkka-Heiskanen *et al.* (1997) demonstrated that an increase in endogenous adenosine levels in the BF is associated with a significant increase in time spent in sleep with a concomitant decrease in the amount of time spent in wakefulness.

Increased extracellular adenosine in the cholinergic BF, whether by prolonged wakefulness or by local increase in adenosine (exogenous or endogenous) strongly correlated with increased power in the delta (1–4 Hz) frequency of the EEG. Increased power in the delta band is a marker of sleep pressure behaviorally manifested as sleepiness (reviewed in Basheer *et al.*, 2004). This behavioral effect was not observed following perfusion of the same transporter inhibitor into the thalamus despite a similar elevation of local extracellular adenosine levels. The thalamus also sends projections to the cortex. However, unlike those in the BF, thalamocortical projections are non-cholinergic.

There is evidence in support of both A_1 and A_{2A} receptor subtypes in mediating the somnogenic effects of adenosine. However, *in-situ* hybridization and real-time polymerase chain reaction (RT-PCR) studies suggested the presence of only A_1 receptors and not A_{2A} receptors in the cholinergic BF (Basheer *et al.*, 2004). Furthermore, extracellular single-unit recording of BF neurons in conjunction with local in vivo microdialysis administration of A_1 selective agonist decreased and A_1 selective antagonist increased the discharge activity of the wake-active neurons in the BF (Alam *et al.*, 1999; Thakkar *et al.*, 2003). In vitro studies also demonstrated that adenosine acts via activation of postsynaptic A_1 receptors and reduces the discharge activity of cholinergic as well as a subset of non-cholinergic neurons in the BF. The importance of the BF A_1 receptor in mediating the homeostatic regulation of sleep was also demonstrated by antisense studies. Bilateral microdialysis perfusion of antisense against adenosine A_1 receptor in the BF produced a transient "knockdown" or downregulation of A_1 receptor resulting in a significant reduction of the amount of time spent in recovery sleep and delta activity following six hours of sleep deprivation. However, that constitutive A_1 receptor knock-out mice did not display any alterations in the spontaneous sleep–wake cycle or recovery sleep following six hours of sleep deprivation may be due to developmental compensation (Basheer *et al.*, 2004).

In summary, prolonged wakefulness results in a selective increase of extracellular adenosine in the BF. The primary effect of the increased extracellular adenosine in cholinergic BF, whether by prolonged wakefulness or by local increase in adenosine (exogenous or endogenous), was to track sleep debt. In simple terms, the more awake you are, the more extracellular adenosine is present in the BF, the more power in the EEG, and the sleepier you feel.

Adenosine and the histaminergic posterior hypothalamus

The histamine-containing neurons are exclusively localized within the tuberomammillary nucleus (TMN) and innervate all the major regions of the central nervous system including the spinal cord. There is strong evidence to suggest that the histaminergic system may play a pivotal role in the modulation and maintenance of wakefulness (Takahashi *et al.*, 2006; Thakkar and McCarley, 2008).

The histamine-containing TMN neurons are known to express high levels of adenosine deaminase, a major enzyme involved in adenosine catabolism and A_1 receptors. Activation of A_1 receptors or inhibition of adenosine degradation (by selective adenosine deaminase inhibitor) in the TMN induced a dose-dependent decrease in the histamine release in the frontal cortex and increased the amount of time spent in NREM sleep and the EEG delta power density. However, REM sleep remained unaffected. Furthermore, activation of A_1 receptors in the TMN did not induce NREM sleep in A_1 receptor and histamine H_1 receptor knock-out mice (Oishi *et al.*, 2008).

These results indicate that endogenous adenosine, via the A_1 receptor, suppresses the TMN histaminergic system to promote sleep.

Adenosine and the orexinergic lateral hypothalamus

Strong evidence exists to suggest that the orexinergic system of the lateral hypothalamus has a foremost role in controlling wakefulness. A reduction or loss of orexinergic tone leads to an increase in REM sleep coupled with cataplexy (Sakurai 2007; Thakkar *et al.*, 1999). In contrast, an increase in orexinergic tone results in increased wakefulness (Thakkar *et al.*, 2001) .

Recently, our laboratory has shown that the orexin-containing neurons express A_1 receptors (Figure 26.1) and blockade of A_1 receptors decreases NREM and REM sleep with a concomitant increase in wakefulness, both during spontaneous bouts of sleep–wakefulness and during recovery sleep after six hours of sleep deprivation. In addition, blockade of A_1 in the orexinergic lateral hypothalamus produced a significant increase in the latency to NREM sleep during recovery sleep, although delta activity during NREM sleep remained unaffected (Thakkar *et al.*, 2002, 2008). Our results were supported by both in vitro and in vivo studies. In vitro studies revealed that adenosine via the A_1 receptor is responsible for the inhibition of excitatory glutamatergic synaptic transmission to orexin neurons resulting in the inhibition of orexin neurons (Liu and Gao, 2007). In vivo studies performed in freely behaving rats showed that activation of the A_1 receptor into the orexinergic zone of the lateral hypothalamus induced sleep (Kumar *et al.*, 2006).

Taken together, these results suggest that endogenous adenosine may be responsible for suppressing orexinergic activity and regulating the expression of NREM and REM sleep.

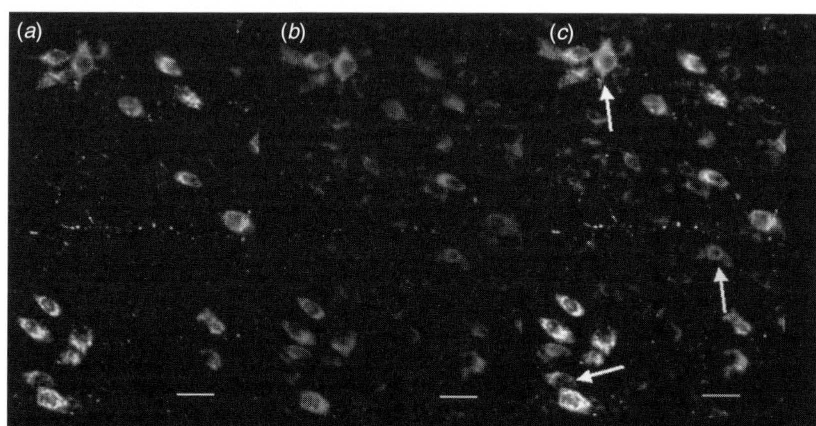

Figure 26.1 (*a*) Orexin-A containing neurons present in the perifornical-lateral hypothalamus region. Orexin-A containing neurons (green) were identified with fluorescence immunohistochemistry using a secondary antibody conjugated to FITC. Numerous cell bodies and fibers containing orexin-A are also visible. Calibration bar = 25 μm. (*b*) Same visual field and section as (*a*), here showing immunoreactivity (red) to the adenosine A_1 receptor in neurons in the perifornical-lateral hypothalamus. The A_1 receptor immunoreactivity is widely distributed and not restricted to orexin-A containing neurons. Calibration bar = 25 μm. (*c*) The same section and visual field, as shown in (*a*) and (*b*) describing double labeling of orexin-A and A_1 receptors. The white arrow indicates a double-labeled neuron, whereas the yellow arrow marks an orexin-A containing neuron without A_1 receptor. The blue arrow indicates a non-orexin containing A_1 receptor-labeled neuron. Calibration bar = 25 μm. (See plate section for color version.)

Adenosine and the cholinergic mesopontine tegmentum

The mesopontine cholinergic neurons are localized in two different nuclei, i.e., LDT/PPT nuclei, located caudolateral to the mid brain and dorsolateral to the oral pons. On the basis of selective discharge during different behavioral states, the presumed cholinergic neurons are categorized in two subgroups, i.e., REM-on and Wake/REM-on neurons. The neuronal subpopulation that preferentially show high discharge rate during REM sleep are termed as REM-on neurons, and those that exhibit high activity during both wakefulness and REM sleep are termed as Wake/REM-on neurons (McCarley, 2007; Thakkar *et al.*, 1998). In vitro studies have shown that the LDT/PPT neurons are under tonic inhibitory control of adenosine, which involves the activation of presynaptic A1 receptors on glutamatergic neurons and postsynaptic A1 receptors on cholinergic neurons in the mesopontine tegmentum. In vivo studies produced conflicting results. Local reverse-microdialysis administration of adenosine in the LDT of cats reduced wakefulness and increased both NREM and REM sleep (Portas *et al.*, 1997). However, local microinjection of adenosine into the PPT of rats did not produce any change in REM sleep (Datta *et al.*, 2003). In addition, sleep deprivation did not produce an increase in extracellular levels of adenosine in the PPT (Porkka-Heiskanen *et al.*, 2000).

In summary, while in vitro studies implicate adenosinergic mechanisms to play an important role in controlling the activity of LDT/PPT neurons, it is yet unclear whether adenosinergic mechanisms in the LDT/PPT have a prominent role in the regulation of sleep, especially REM sleep.

Adenosine and the noradrenergic locus coeruleus

The largest group of norepinephrine (NE)-containing neurons is located within the locus coeruleus (LC). The LC is believed to have an inhibitory role in the modulation of REM sleep. The LC neurons exhibit an REM-off discharge pattern across the sleep–wake cycle with the highest discharge during wakefulness, which reduces during NREM sleep and virtually ceases during REM sleep.

There are reports of adenosinergic involvement in the modulation of NE release in hippocampal slices (Fredholm *et al.*, 1983); however, the role of adenosine in the control of NE neurons across behavioral states is unknown.

Adenosine and the serotonergic dorsal raphe

The dorsal raphe nucleus (DRN) constitutes the rostral-most part of the raphe nuclei and contains the largest number of serotonergic neurons. The DRN neurons, like the NE neurons, exhibit maximal discharge during waking, decreased during NREM and almost no activity during REM sleep. Few studies have evaluated the role of adenosinergic mechanisms on dorsal raphe neurons in the regulation of sleep–wakefulness. There is evidence to suggest that adenosine A_1 receptors are present on dorsal raphe neurons (Clarke *et al.*, 1996). Reverse microdialysis administration of nitrobenzylthioninosine (NBTI) into the DRN induced an increase in REM sleep with a concomitant decrease of waking (W) (McCarley *et al.*, 1997). However, prolonged wakefulness did not induce an increase in extracellular adenosine in the DRN (Porkka-Heiskanen *et al.*, 2000).

While these studies may indicate a role of adenosine, further studies are required to confirm that adenosine acts on dorsal raphe neurons to regulate sleep–wakefulness.

Adenosine and the pontine reticular formation

The role of the reticular formation in the regulation of sleep–wakefulness was first described, almost 60 year ago, by Morruzi and Magoun. Since then tremendous progress has been made and we now have substantial evidence that implicates the PRF as a critical site involved in the control of REM sleep.

Recent pharmacological studies implicate adenosine to act on PRF neurons and regulate REM sleep. While activation of the A_1 or A_{2A} receptor in the PRF resulted in increased REM sleep, activation of the A_{2A} receptor in the PRF induced an increase in acetylcholine (Coleman *et al.*, 2006; Marks *et al.*, 2003). Pretreatment with atropine, a muscarinic receptor antagonist, had no effect on A_1 receptor-induced increase in REM sleep. However, it blocked the A_{2A} receptor agonist-induced increase in REM sleep suggesting that the A_{2A}-induced increased REM sleep requires the activation of the cholinergic receptor.

These studies strongly suggest that adenosine acting on PRF neurons may either directly, or indirectly, play a role in the control of REM sleep.

Adenosine and the sleep-active preoptic region

The preoptic area (POA) of the hypothalamus has been considered to be the main source of sleep-active GABAergic neurons and an important somnogenic center. These sleep-active neurons are distributed in several subregions of the POA, occurring with high density in the ventrolateral preoptic area (VLPO) and the median preoptic nucleus. It was originally considered that the preoptic area may be responsible for NREM sleep only. However, recent studies have identified a population of cells in the regions surrounding the VLPO that display enhanced c-Fos activation during REM sleep. The region, termed as the extended VLPO region, may contain REM-active neurons and may play a role in regulating REM sleep (Szymusiak and McGinty, 2008).

Recent studies implicate adenosine, and its action on POA neurons may have an important role in sleep promotion. Activation of the A_{2A} receptor induced sleep (Methippara *et al.*, 2005). In vitro studies suggest two mechanisms responsible for sleep induction in the POA. The first mechanism suggests direct excitatory effects on POA neurons via activation of its A_{2A} receptor. The second mechanism implicates an indirect excitatory effect via suppression of spontaneous inhibitory postsynaptic potentials (IPSPs) by the activation of A_1 receptors (Gallopin *et al.*, 2005; Morairty *et al.*, 2004). These effects, either individually or in combination, will result in the activation of sleep-active POA neurons leading to the promotion of sleep.

Based on the above-described studies, it appears that adenosine may act to activate sleep-promoting neurons resulting in the promotion of sleep.

Adenosine act on multiple sites to mediate its effects on sleep–wakefulness

In summary, although there are few reports that implicate adenosine to have a direct role in REM-sleep control, strong evidence suggests that adenosine is responsible for regulating the expression of sleep. Based on the studies described above, sufficient evidence exists to suggest that adenosine acts on multiple wakefulness-, NREM-, and REM-promoting systems to regulate sleep.

Glycine and the regulation of REM sleep

Glycine is the simplest, non-essential amino acid commonly found in animal proteins. The role of glycine as a neurotransmitter was first reported in the spinal cord by Aprison and Werman in 1965 (Gundersen *et al.*, 2005). Further investigations have shown that the majority of inhibitory synapses in the spinal cord use glycine as the neurotransmitter. The inhibitory functions of glycine are mediated by a ligand-gated membrane-spanning ion channel with glycine as the prime agonist and strychnine, an alkaloid, as a potent antagonist. Glycine has been implicated to play a major role in the control of muscle activity during REM sleep.

Muscle activity during REM sleep

The majority of our muscles are constantly active and contracting during wakefulness, especially when we maintain a specific posture or perform a specific movement. There is a decrease in muscle activity (tone) during the transition from wakefulness to NREM sleep. However, during REM sleep, there is a complete cessation of somatic muscle activity (Pompeiano, 1975). This phenomenon known as muscle atonia was first reported by Jouvet and coworkers when recording neck-muscle activity across sleep–wake cycle in cats (Chase and Morales, 1990). Subsequently, muscle atonia during REM sleep has been observed in many vertebrate species including humans (reviewed in Thakkar and Datta, 2009). Along with muscle atonia, REM sleep is also characterized by the phasic activation of muscle tone resulting in myoclonic activity, behaviorally manifested as muscle twitches and jerks. Thus, a complex interplay between the excitatory and inhibitory motor commands, originating from the brain stem, is responsible for the control of muscle tone during REM sleep.

In humans, dysfunction of these influences results in REM behavior disorder (RBD). This disorder is characterized by loss of muscle atonia during REM sleep and may result in violent behaviors including yelling, punching, kicking, and jumping out of bed (Schenck and Mahowald, 1996). Long before this syndrome was recognized in humans, it was already established in animals. Jouvet, and subsequently Morrison, had reported that bilateral lesions of the pontine reticular formation resulted in loss of muscle atonia during REM sleep in cats. These cats displayed "oneric behaviors" during REM sleep including locomotion and attack behavior (Hendricks *et al.*, 1982; Jouvet, 1979).

Anatomical substrates regulating muscle activity during REM sleep

Somatic muscle activity is controlled by somatic motor neurons (motoneurons). The motoneuron and its termination onto muscle fibers represent a motor unit, and all muscle fibers connected to a single motoneuron contract synchronously. These muscle units form the "final common pathway" responsible for regulating muscle activity across behavioral states (Chase and Morales, 1990).

Multiple lines of evidence suggest that the dorsolateral pons is the origin and the primary inhibitory site in supra-spinal control of REM-sleep atonia. The medial medullary reticular formation is the second inhibitory site involved in the regulation of muscle control during REM sleep.

The role of excitatory influences emanating from the brain stem in motor control was established with the introduction of decerebrate rigidity. Abolition of decerebrate rigidity by stimulation of the brain-stem reticular formation revealed the importance of disfacilitatory and inhibitory influences in motor control (Lai and Siegel, 1990; Magoun and Rhines, 1946; Pompeiano, 1975). Transection studies demonstrated that the key neuronal centers controlling motoneurons are situated within the confines of the lower brain stem. Lesions and subsequent retrograde tracing studies suggested that the dorsolateral pons, in the immediate vicinity of the nucleus pontis oralis (termed as the subcoeruleus, peri-LCα, or LCα in cats), and its projections to the ventromedial medulla played a pivotal role in controlling muscle atonia during REM sleep (reviewed in Steriade and McCarley, 1990). Electrical stimulation performed in cats and rats also supported the role of the dorsolateral pons and ventromedial medulla (Hajnik *et al.*, 2000; Pompeiano, 1975).

The masseter muscles are postural muscles responsible for the jaw-closure reflex. These muscles are innervated by trigeminal motoneurons and are completely suppressed during REM sleep. Electrophysiological monitoring of trigeminal motoneurons during wakefulness revealed membrane depolarization with sustained spike activity. However, during REM sleep, the membrane potential of trigeminal motoneurons displayed hyperpolarization coupled with phasic spike activity (Chase *et al.*, 1980). Further intracellular investigation of lumbar motoneurons, during REM sleep, revealed that the somatic motoneurons were postsynaptically inhibited by a sustained barrage of IPSPs, and excited by phasic volleys of excitatory postsynaptic potentials, behaviorally manifested as the tonic muscle atonia and phasic muscle twitches observed during REM sleep (Chase and Morales, 1990).

Neurochemical substrates regulating muscle activity during REM sleep

Cholinergic stimulation of the dorsolateral pons elicited muscle atonia and induced REM sleep (Datta and Maclean, 2007; McCarley, 2007). However, within the medullary reticular formation, cholinergic stimulation of the rostra1 medulla produced atonia, whereas glutamatergic stimulation of the caudal medulla produced atonia (Lai and Siegel, 1988).

Microinjection of the glycine receptor antagonist, strychnine, reduced the degree of but did not completely abolish jaw suppression during REM sleep suggesting that glycine may be involved, but is not the exclusive neurochemical substrate responsible for controlling muscle activity during REM sleep (Soja *et al.*, 1987).

Intracellular recording to lumbar motoneurons coupled with microiontophoretic administration of strychnine in the close proximity showed a complete suppression of IPSP activity during REM sleep. This strychnine-suppressing effect was observed in some motoneurons, while in other motoneurons strychnine produced a reduction in the amplitude of the IPSPs but not a complete suppression. In contrast, local microiontophoretic application of the GABAergic antagonists, picrotoxin or bicuculline, had no effect. Since there was no evidence of long monosynaptic inhibitory projections from brain-stem sites, it was suggested that the local glycine-containing interneurons within the spinal cord may be responsible for the inhibition of REM sleep-specific IPSPs resulting in muscle atonia during REM sleep (Chase and Morales, 1990).

As described above, REM sleep is accompanied by tonic muscle atonia and phasic muscle twitches. In order to identify the neurochemical substrates responsible for phasic muscle twitches, Chase and his coworkers performed microiontophoretic application of the excitatory amino acid antagonist, kynurenic acid, in the close proximity to the intracellularly recorded motoneurons, during REM sleep. Kynurenic acid markedly suppressed the excitatory postsynaptic potential without affecting the IPSPs. In contrast, microiontophoresis of the selective N-methyl-D-aspartate (NMDA) antagonist 2-amino-5-phosphonovaleric acid (APV) had no effect (Chase and Morales, 1990).

Based on these results, Chase and his coworkers suggested that glycine is the inhibitory neurotransmitter that mediates REM-sleep atonia, whereas glutamate, acting via a non-NMDA mechanism, may be responsible for muscle twitches that are observed during REM sleep (Chase and Morales, 1990).

Recently, this hypothesis about the role of glycine in the control of muscle activity during REM sleep was challenged (Brooks and Peever, 2008). Reverse-microdialysis administration of strychnine on trigeminal motoneurons had no effect on the jaw-closure reflex during REM sleep suggesting that glycine may not be the mediator of muscle atonia during REM sleep. However, strychnine administration significantly increased the amplitude of muscle twitches during phasic REM sleep suggesting that glycine may be responsible for the presence of aphasic muscle twitches (Brooks and Peever, 2008). While the pros and cons of this study are debated, one thing is certain, the role of glycine in the control of muscle atonia needs to be reevaluated.

Glycinergic regulation of muscle activity during REM sleep

In summary, numerous theories have been proposed to explain the mechanisms responsible for the control of muscle tone during REM sleep (reviewed in Chase and Morales, 1990).

While there are minor differences in individual theories, the common theme suggests that both the tonic and phasic component of muscle control during REM sleep originate from the neurons in the dorsolateral pontine reticular formation and activate the medullary reticular formation (nucleus reticular gigantocellularis). Activation of the medullary reticular formation results in tonic inhibition of somatic motoneurons, which is manifested as muscle atonia. While the role of glycine in mediating muscle activity during REM sleep is under debate, it is clear that GABAergic mechanisms do not control muscle tone during REM sleep.

References

Alam, M. N., Szymusiak, R., Gong, H., King, J. & McGinty, D. (1999) Adenosinergic modulation of rat basal forebrain neurons during sleep and waking: neuronal recording with microdialysis. *J Physiol* **521**(3): 679–90.

Aserinsky, E. & Kleitman, N. (1953) Regularly occurring periods of eye motility and concomitant phenomenon during sleep. *Science* **118**: 273–4.

Basheer, R., Strecker, R. E., Thakkar, M. M. & McCarley, R. W. (2004) Adenosine and sleep-wake regulation. *Progress in Neurobiology* **73**(6): 379–96.

Brooks, P. L. & Peever, J. H. (2008) Glycinergic and GABA(A)-mediated inhibition of somatic motoneurons does not mediate rapid eye movement sleep motor atonia. *J Neurosci* **28**(14): 3535–45.

Chase, M. H., Chandler, S. H. & Nakamura, Y. (1980) Intracellular determination of membrane potential of trigeminal motoneurons during sleep and wakefulness. *J Neurophysiol* **44**(2): 349–58.

Chase, M. H. & Morales, F. R. (1990) The atonia and myoclonia of active (REM) sleep. *Ann Rev Psychol* **41**: 557–84.

Clarke, W. P., Yocca, F. D. & Maayani, S. (1996) Lack of 5-hydroxytryptamine1A-mediated inhibition of adenylyl cyclase in dorsal raphe of male and female rats. *J Pharmacol Exp Ther* **277**(3): 1259–66.

Coleman, C. G., Baghdoyan, H. A. & Lydic, R. (2006) Dialysis delivery of an adenosine A_{2A} agonist into the pontine reticular formation of C57BL/6J mouse increases pontine acetylcholine release and sleep. *J Neurochem* **96**(6): 1750–9.

Datta, S. & Maclean, R. R. (2007). Neurobiological mechanisms for the regulation of mammalian sleep-wake behavior: reinterpretation of historical evidence and inclusion of contemporary cellular and molecular evidence. *Neurosci Biobehav Rev* **31**(5): 775–824.

Datta, S., Mavanji, V., Patterson, E. H. & Ulloor, J. (2003) Regulation of rapid eye movement sleep in the freely moving rat: local microinjection of serotonin, norepinephrine, and adenosine into the brainstem. *Sleep* **26**(5): 513–20.

Dement, W. C. (2000) History of sleep physiology and medicine. In *Principles and Practice of Sleep Medicine*, 3rd edn, ed. M. Kryger, T. Roth & W. Dement. Philadelphia: W. B. Saunders Company, pp. 1–14.

Drury, A. N. & Szent-Györgyi, A. (1929) The physiological activity of adenine compounds with especial reference to their actions upon the mammalian heart. *J Physiol* **68**: 213–37.

Fredholm, B. B., Jonzon, B. & Lindgren, E. (1983) Inhibition of noradrenaline release from hippocampal slices by a stable adenosine analogue. *Acta Physiol Scand Suppl* **515**: 7–10.

Gallopin, T., Luppi, P. H., Cauli, B. *et al.* (2005) The endogenous somnogen adenosine excites a subset of sleep-promoting neurons via A2A receptors in the ventrolateral preoptic nucleus. *Neuroscience* **134**(4): 1377–90.

Gundersen, R. Y., Vaagenes, P., Breivik, T., Fonnum, F. & Opstad, P. K. (2005). Glycine – an important neurotransmitter and cytoprotective agent. *Acta Anaesthesiol Scand* **49**(8): 1108–16.

Hajnik, T., Lai, Y. Y. & Siegel, J. M. (2000) Atonia-related regions in the rodent pons and medulla. *J Neurophysiol* **84**(4): 1942–8.

Hendricks, J. C., Morrison, A. R. & Mann, G. L. (1982) Different behaviors during paradoxical sleep without atonia depend on pontine lesion site. *Brain Res* **239**(1): 81–105.

Huston, J. P., Haas, H. L., Boix, F. *et al.* (1996) Extracellular adenosine levels in neostriatum and hippocampus during rest and activity periods of rats. *Neuroscience* **73**(1): 99–107.

Jouvet, M. (1979) What does a cat dream about? *Trends Neurosci* **2**: 280–2.

Kumar, S., Rai, S., Szymusiak, R., McGinty, D. & Alam, N. (2006) Effects of adenosine A$_1$ receptor agonist into the perifornical lateral hypothalamic area on sleep. Society for Neuroscience Program No. 458.12. 2006.

Lai, Y. Y. & Siegel, J. M. (1988) Medullary regions mediating atonia. *J Neurosci* **8**(12): 4790–6.

Lai, Y. Y. & Siegel, J. M. (1990) Muscle tone suppression and stepping produced by stimulation of midbrain and rostral pontine reticular formation. *J Neurosci* **10**(8): 2727–34.

Liu, Z. W. & Gao, X. B. (2007) Adenosine inhibits activity of hypocretin/orexin neurons by the A1 receptor in the lateral hypothalamus: a possible sleep-promoting effect. *J Neurophysiol* **97**(1): 837–48.

Magoun, H. W. & Rhines, R. (1946) An inhibitory mechanism in the bulbar reticular formation. *J Neurophysiol* **9**:165–71.

Marks, G. A., Shaffery, J. P., Speciale, S. G. & Birabil, C. G. (2003) Enhancement of rapid eye movement sleep in the rat by actions at A1 and A2a adenosine receptor subtypes with a differential sensitivity to atropine. *Neuroscience* **116**(3): 913–20.

McCarley, R., Strecker, R. E., Porkka-Heiskanen, T. *et al.* (1997) Modulation of cholinergic neurons by serotonin and adenosine in the control of REM and non-REM sleep. In *Sleep and Sleep Disorders: From Molecule to Behavior*, eds. O. Hayaishi & S. Inoue. Tokyo: Academic Press, pp. 63–79.

McCarley, R. W. (2007) Neurobiology of REM and NREM sleep. *Sleep Med* **8**(4): 302–30.

Methippara, M. M., Kumar, S., Alam, M. N., Szymusiak, R. & McGinty, D. (2005) Effects on sleep of microdialysis of adenosine A1 and A2a receptor analogs into the lateral preoptic area of rats. *Am J Physiol Regul Integr Comp Physiol* **289**(6): R1715–23.

Morairty, S., Rainnie, D., McCarley, R. & Greene, R. (2004) Disinhibition of ventrolateral preoptic area sleep-active neurons by adenosine: a new mechanism for sleep promotion. *Neuroscience* **123**(2): 451–7.

Oishi, Y., Huang, Z. L., Fredholm, B. B., Urade, Y. & Hayaishi, O. (2008) Adenosine in the tuberomammillary nucleus inhibits the histaminergic system via A1 receptors and promotes non-rapid eye movement sleep. *Proc Natl Acad Sci U S A* **105**(50): 19,992–7.

Pompeiano, O. (1975) The control of posture and movements during REM sleep: neurophysiological and neurochemical mechanisms. *Acta Astronaut* **2**(3/4): 225–39.

Porkka-Heiskanen, T., Strecker, R. E. & McCarley, R. W. (2000) Brain site-specificity of extracellular adenosine concentration changes during sleep deprivation and spontaneous sleep: an in vivo microdialysis study. *Neuroscience* **99**(3): 507–17.

Porkka-Heiskanen, T., Strecker, R. E., Thakkar, M. *et al.* (1997) Adenosine: a mediator of the sleep-inducing effects of prolonged wakefulness. *Science* **276**(5316) 1265–8.

Portas, C. M., Thakkar, M., Rainnie, D. G., Greene, R. W. & McCarley, R. W. (1997) Role of adenosine in behavioral state modulation: a microdialysis study in the freely moving cat. *Neuroscience* **79**(1): 225–35.

Radulovacki, M. (1985) Role of adenosine in sleep in rats. *Rev Clin Basic Pharm* **5**(3/4): 327–39.

Sakurai, T. (2007) The neural circuit of orexin (hypocretin): maintaining sleep and wakefulness. *Nat Rev Neurosci* **8**(3): 171–81.

Schenck, C. H. & Mahowald, M. W. (1996) REM sleep parasomnias. *Neurol Clin* **14**(4): 697–720.

Soja, P. J., Finch, D. M. & Chase, M. H. (1987) Effect of inhibitory amino acid antagonists on masseteric reflex suppression during active sleep. *Exp Neurol* **96**(1): 178–93.

Steriade, M. & McCarley, R. W. (1990) *Brainstem Control of Wakefulness and Sleep*. New York: Plenum Press.

Szymusiak, R. & McGinty, D. (2008) Hypothalamic regulation of sleep and arousal. *Ann N Y Acad Sci* **1129**: 275–86.

Takahashi, K., Lin, J. S. & Sakai, K. (2006) Neuronal activity of histaminergic tuberomammillary neurons during wake-sleep states in the mouse. *J Neurosci* **26**(40): 10,292–8.

Thakkar, M. & Mallick, B. N. (1996) Effect of rapid eye movement sleep deprivation on 5´- nucleotidase activity in the rat brain. *Neurosci Lett* **206**(2/3): 177–80.

Thakkar, M. M. & Datta, S. (2009) The evolution of REM sleep. In *Evolution of Sleep: Phylogenetic and Functional Perspectives*, ed. P. McNamara, R. Barton & C. Nunn. New York: Cambridge University Press 197–217.

Thakkar, M. M., Delgiacco, R. A., Strecker, R. E. & McCarley, R. W. (2003) Adenosinergic inhibition of basal forebrain wakefulness-active neurons: a simultaneous unit recording and microdialysis study in freely behaving cats. *Neuroscience* **122**(4): 1107–13.

Thakkar, M. M., Engemann, S. C., Walsh, K. M. & Sahota, P. K. (2008) Adenosine and the homeostatic control of sleep: effects of A1 receptor blockade in the perifornical lateral hypothalamus on sleep-wakefulness. *Neuroscience* **153**(4): 875–80.

Thakkar, M. M. & McCarley, R. W. (2008) Histamine in the control of sleep-wakefulness. In *Neurochemistry of Sleep and Wakefulness*, ed. J. M. Monti, S. R. Pandi-Perumal &

C. M. Sinton. New York: Cambridge University Press, pp. 144–78.

Thakkar, M. M., Ramesh, V., Cape, E. G. *et al.* (1999) REM sleep enhancement and behavioral cataplexy following orexin (hypocretin)-II receptor antisense perfusion in the pontine reticular formation. *Sleep Res Online* **2**(4): 112–20.

Thakkar, M. M., Ramesh, V., Strecker, R. E. & McCarley, R. W. (2001) Microdialysis perfusion of orexin-A in the basal forebrain increases wakefulness in freely behaving rats. *Arch Ital Biol* **139**(3): 313–28.

Thakkar, M. M., Strecker, R. E. & McCarley, R. W. (1998) Behavioral state control through differential serotonergic inhibition in the mesopontine cholinergic nuclei: a simultaneous unit recording and microdialysis study. *J Neurosci* **18**(14): 5490–7.

Thakkar, M. M., Winston, S. & McCarley, R. W. (2002) Orexin neurons of the hypothalamus express adenosine A1 receptors. *Brain Res* **944**(1/2) 190–4.

Changes in neurotransmitter levels in relation to REM sleep for its regulation

Tohru Kodama

Summary

Research on the REM sleep-generating mechanism has been led by the research of the neuronal discharge (unit) recording and the most remarkable example was the discovery of REM-on neurons. At the current state, because of a technical difficulty, the information obtained from neurotransmitters' changes cannot completely replace the information from unit activity. However, as the changes across sleep–wakefulness are much slower than unit discharges and have more general effects on the entire brain, the contributions of relatively slow-changing factors from neurotransmitters, such as receptor changes, second messenger contribution, or sleep-inducing factors need to be considered when researchers attempt to explain sleep–wake transition mechanisms. The input signal is converted into the neurotransmitter in the synaptic terminal, transmitted, and observed as unit activities. In pharmacological study, the sleep-generating mechanism is verified by investigating the changes of the unit activities (or sleep behavior), induced by external drug administration, instead of an internal neurotransmitter. For instance, it is considered that REM sleep is regulated by an inhibitory mechanism if it is modulated by a GABA agonist. However, the physiological mechanism is not necessarily simple; the neurotransmitters act synergistically as regulating factors, which modulate, buffer, and gate the input signals to regulate REM sleep. Therefore, although changes in the level of individual neurotransmitters are of course crucial, it is even more important to investigate the changes of neurotransmitters simultaneously during sleep–wake cycles. This chapter summarizes some of the recent findings showing sleep-related changes in the levels of neurotransmitters that regulate REM sleep. In addition, the role of neurotransmitters that exist as the background of the REM sleep-generating mechanism are discussed along with two reciprocal models, the flop-flip model and Sakai's mutual-interaction model.

Introduction

The human brain is composed of about 100 billion neuronal cells. In addition, an astonishing fact is that there are about one quadrillion synapses in the brain. Tremendous quantities of information are exchanged constantly using neurotransmitters between these synapses. The field of the synaptic gap is the place where information of the neuronal inputs are summed and interact with each other, contributing to a very complicated transition of information. As described later, the neurotransmitters work synergistically, changing the receptor sensitivity and regulating neurotransmitter release. Firstly, let us recall how the information is transferred from one neuron to another. When electrical signals reach the axonal terminals, the rapid depolarization causes calcium ion channels to open. The calcium increase initiates and directs the vesicles containing the neurotransmitters to move towards the presynaptic membrane. After the vesicle and cell membrane fuse, the packaged neurotransmitters are released into the synaptic gap. The neurotransmitters travel through the synaptic gap to bind to the receptor on the postsynaptic membrane, and then depolarize the postsynaptic membrane to make an output signal, neuronal discharges. This is how, at the synapses, neurons communicate with one another through axons and dendrites, converting electrical impulses into chemical signals. However, the neurotransmitters are known to have additional function(s). They work as a feedback factor through the autoreceptor on the presynaptic membrane, regulate receptor sensitivities to select the signal passage and gain (a kind of gating effect), or they

REM Sleep: Regulation and Function, eds. Birendra N. Mallick, S. R. Pandi-Perumal, Robert W. McCarley, and Adrian R. Morrison. Published by Cambridge University Press. © Cambridge University Press 2011.

(a)

(c)

(b)

(d)

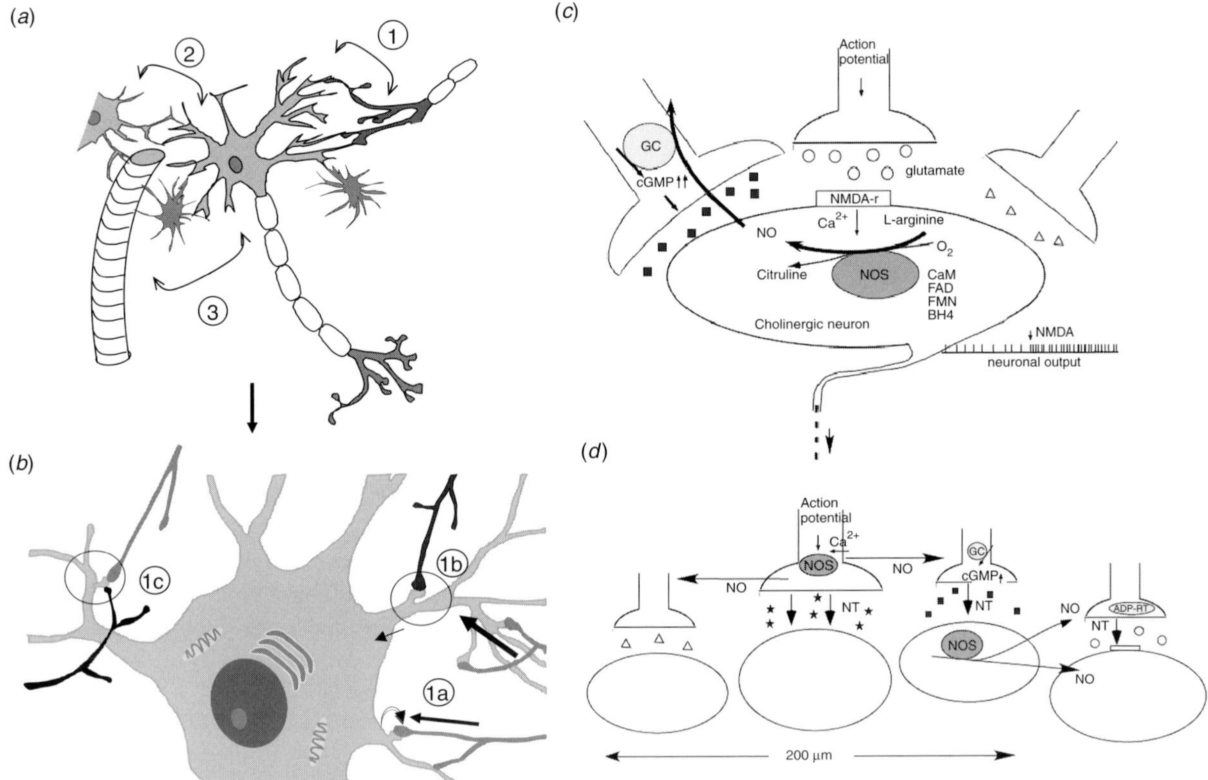

Figure 27.1 The role of the neurotransmitter is not simply passing but processing information from one neuron to the others.

(a) The neurotransmitters transfer the information between axon and dendrite (axo-dendritic) (1), between dendrite and the other dendrites (dendro-dendric) (2), and among neuron, glia, and blood vessel (3).

(b) The neurotransmitters work as a feedback factor through the autoreceptor on the presynaptic membrane (1a), regulate receptor sensitivities to select the signal passage (1b), or affect the input of the other neurons in the spine (triad) (1c).

(c, d) Neurotransmitters' effect on the neurons far from the terminal, for example in the case of nitric oxide (Kodama, 2009).

affect the neurons far from the terminal, for example in the case of nitric oxide (Figure 27.1). It may be said that the neurotransmitters are experienced and important supporting players that regulate and maintain brain activity, including rapid eye movement (REM) sleep, which will be discussed in this chapter.

The importance of neurotransmitters in REM-sleep regulation

Early sleep researchers gathered considerable knowledge using electrophysiological signals, which resulted in the identification of REM sleep (Aserinsky and Kleitman, 1953). Use of microwires for recording single neuronal activities in freely moving, normally behaving animals led the researchers to conclude that the neuronal firing pattern changes across sleep–wake cycles (McGinty *et al.*, 1974). On the other hand, the work of Jouvet's group, followed by that of Hobson

and McCarley's and that of Sakai's, recognized the importance of the roles of neurotransmitters in REM-sleep regulation. Other procedures, such as anatomical, pharmacological, neurochemical, and recent molecular approaches, supplemented their findings. Subsequently, technological advancement made it possible to estimate neurotransmitters in the samples collected from specific region(s) of the brain in relation to states, which allows us to interpret the REM sleep state specific changes in the microenvironment of the neurons.

We now know that the pontine REM-on neurons, which start discharging prior to REM sleep and keep discharging during the REM sleep period, play a significant role in the generation of REM sleep. However, the timing of REM sleep is decided by a few specific conditions, such as circadian rhythm, sleep debt, and so on. Therefore, the success of the investigation into the REM-sleep regulatory mechanism depends to a large extent on how and by what means REM-on neurons are regulated. What kind of input would be responsible for the discharge of the REM-on neurons? Many possibilities have been advocated by many researchers; e.g., the input to the REM-on neurons might simply be a signal from other REM-on neurons, another possibility is, a little more complex though, that the excitatory input from type I neurons and inhibitory input from REM-off neurons may work synergistically to generate an REM-on discharge pattern. These discussions advocated a modified reciprocal-interaction model, for example the flip-flop model (Fuller *et al.*, 2007; Lu, 2006).

As the changes across sleep–wakefulness are much slower than unit discharges and have more general effects on the entire brain, the contributions of relatively slow-changing factors, such as receptor changes, second messenger contribution, or sleep-inducing factors also need to be considered when researchers attempt to explain sleep–wake transition mechanisms. Any kind of these slow-factor changes are mainly caused by neurotransmitter release. Accordingly, further studies of neurotransmitters are necessary to discuss the sleep–wake cycle and consequently the REM-generation mechanisms.

The first step in solving the question of how and by what mechanism REM sleep starts is to measure neurotransmitter release in the targeted regions across the sleep–wake cycle. After the development of the microdialysis technique a method of directly estimating neurotransmitter was established in the 1980s; thereafter, estimation of neurotransmitter in relation to physiological changes has increased significantly. However, compared to the last decade, the number of reports in this decade has not increased significantly even though the sensitivity of the estimation has increased several times. However, as a new promising trend, reports on estimation of chemicals other than the classical transmitter, for example, adenosine or orexin, have increased. The next section summarizes which neurotransmitters show sleep-related changes and what kinds of neurotransmitters are responsible for the REM-sleep-generating mechanism, along with the two reciprocal models advocated.

New models of the REM-generating mechanisms and neurotransimitters

Recent anatomical and neurophysiological studies suggest that, as excitatory inputs, both acetylcholine (ACh) and glutamate in the dorsolateral pontine area are involved in generating REM sleep. Although there are reports that the basal forebrain and the hypothalamus affect REM sleep, transection studies indicate that the inputs from these areas are only the modulator and not required for basic REM phenomena. Therefore, the discussion in this section will be concentrated within the brain-stem mechanism of REM generation.

Cholinoceptive REM-on neurons in the dorsolateral pontine reticular formation are supposed to be important in generating REM sleep. REM sleep starts with the increase of cholinergic or partially glutamatergic excitatory input from other structures in the pons and the medulla. Acetylcholine (ACh) release in peri-locus coeruleus alpha (LCα) is known to increase prior to REM sleep (Kodama, 1990), but the source of this ACh increase is not clear, because cholinergic REM-on neurons are only reported in the pons and medulla. The explanation proposed by sleep researchers is that ACh release from cholinergic neurons in the laterodorsal tegmentum and pedunculopontine tegmentum (LDT/PPT) is somehow regulated by inhibitory input, such as serotonin (5-HT) (Thakkar *et al.*, 1997), norepinephrine (NE) (Semba *et al.*, 1997), or autoreceptors (Baghdoyan *et al.*, 1998; Roth *et al.*, 1996), to make an REM sleep-specific increase in ACh release in the peri-LCα. The 5-HT- and NE-ergic neurons, which are inhibitory and stop firing during REM sleep, are in turn regulated by GABA release (Bjorkum *et al.*, 1997; Nitz and Siegel, 1997a,b) or by adenosine accumulated during wakefulness (Strecker *et al.*, 1997). GABA in the REM-off neuron group may be regulated by other GABA neurons located in other brain regions, for example the basal forebrain. So what regulates these GABA neurons? To avoid this dilemma, it is necessary to use the network-interaction model to explain the generating mechanism of REM-on neurons. There are a couple of proposals to explain REM generation with neuronal interaction. The first famous model is Hobson and McCarley's excitatory–inhibitory model (McCarley and Hobson, 1975), which has been revised recently (McCarley, 2007). Sakai *et al.* (2001) explain it with the mutual-interactive model, and recently, based on available data, Saper's group advocates a modified flip-flop model (Figure 27.2a; Lu *et al.*, 2006). Here I would like to verify the latter two models from the viewpoint of neurotransmitter changes.

Saper's flip-flop model

From the cell-specific lesions at REM executive sites using the excitotoxin ibotenic acid, Saper's group

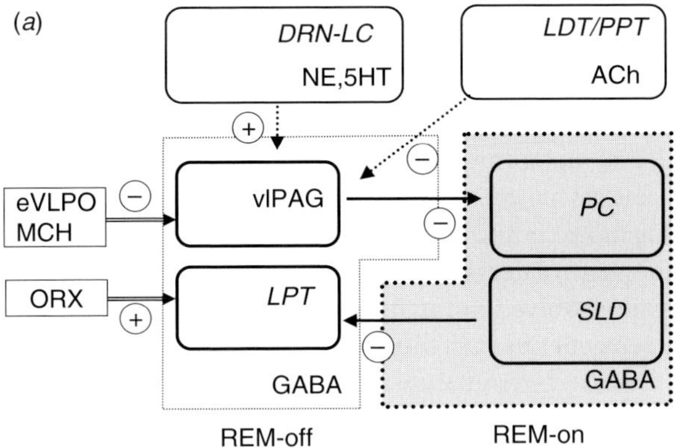

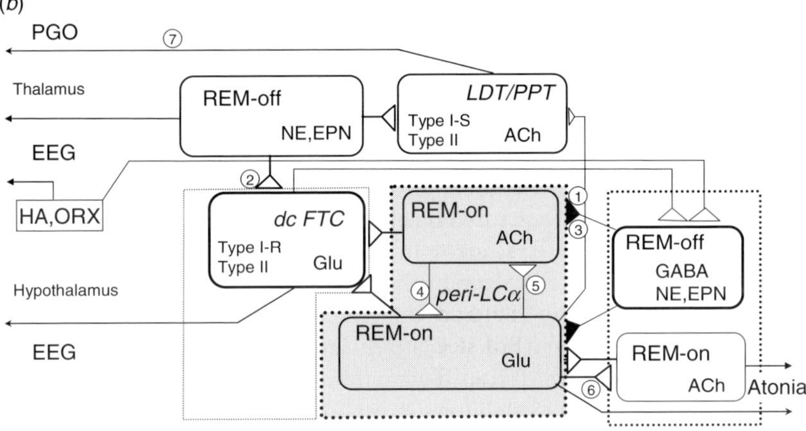

Figure 27.2 Neurotransmitter changes in Saper's flip-flop model (*a*) and Sakai's mutual-interactive model (*b*).

(*a*) The neurons in the vlPAG and LPT have a mutually inhibitory interaction with REM-on GABAergic neurons of the vSLD, but also inhibit REM-generator circuitry in the remainder of the SLD and the PC.
Our microdialysis results indicate that the GABA release in the rostral part of pontine reticular formation, including the dorsal central tegmental field (dcFTC), is high during REM sleep. On the other hand, GABA in the caudal part of pontine reticular formation, including the peri-LCα, is high during the wake state. However, the entire balance is more important than an individual change of neurotransmitters in this model.
vlPAG: the ventrolateral periaqueductal gray; LPT: the lateral pontine tegmentum; SLD: sublaterodorsal nucleus; PC: pre-coeruleus; LDT: laterodorsal tegmentum; PPT: pedunculopontine tegmentum; LC: locus coeruleus; DRN: dorsal raphe nucleus; eVLPO: extended ventrolateral preoptic area. (Revised from Lu *et al.*, 2006.)
(*b*) In Sakai's model, REM sleep is generated by tonic excitation of REM-on neurons (cholinergic and glutamatergic, located in the pons and medulla) and the cessation of REM-off neurons (GABAergic and monoaminergic, in the medulla) inhibiting REM-on neurons during wakefulness and slow-wave sleep.
Our microdialysis results indicate that GABA in the caudal part of the pontine reticular formation, including the peri-LCα, is significantly higher during the wake state than REM sleep (1). Norepinephrine release in the rostral peri-LCα is the lowest during REM sleep and the highest during W (2). Norepinephrine and epinephrine release in the caudal LCα is lowest during REM sleep and highest during W (3). Acetylcholine increase has been reported during REM sleep in the peri-LCα (4). Glutamate shows little change across sleep in all the regions; relatively low during SWS. Glutamate increases toward SWS to REM sleep in the caudal peri-LCα (5), but not in the rostral LCα. In the medullar reticular formation, there is an REM-specific increase of glutamate (6) (Kodama *et al.*, 1998).
LCα: peri-locus coeruleus alpha; dcFTC: dorsal central tegmental field. (Revised from Sakai *et al.*, 2001.)

claims the REM-off regions are the ventrolateral peri-aqueductal gray (vlPAG) or the lateral pontine tegmentum (LPT) and REM-on regions are the sublaterodorsal nucleus (SLD) (equivalent to the subcoeruleus area or peri-locus coeruleus-α in cats) and the periventricular gray matter, including a dorsal extension of the SLD and the pre-coeruleus (PC) region. The mutual inhibition using GABA between these two regions is hypothesized to be responsible for the switch of REM sleep (Figure 27.2a). This is a very simplified model. The main part of the switching is only dependent on the balance of GABA-ergic activities between REM-on regions and REM-off regions. Then, is the circumstantial evidence really obtained from the change in the neurotransmitter? Our microdialysis results indicate that the GABA release in the rostral part of the pontine reticular formation, including the dorsal central tegmental field (dcFTC), is high during REM sleep. On the other hand, GABA in the caudal part of the pontine reticular formation, including the peri-LCα, is high during the wake state. This high GABA release may explain the low activities of the FTC during REM sleep, resulting in relatively high activities in the SLD/peri-LCα. Adversely, high GABA releases in the SLD/peri-LCα inhibit REM-on neurons, keeping relatively high activities in the FTC during wake. This balance may explain Saper's flip-flop switching.

These two regions are, of course, the main factors of the REM-wake switch, but, the difference of the balance between inhibitory and excitatory inputs to each side (REM-on and REM-off) makes the switch turn on to the REM or the wake side. In Saper's model the REM-off region (vlPAG-LPT) receives inputs from the orexin neurons, serotonergic dorsal raphe and noradrenergic LC (DRN–LC) neurons as an activating factor. Cholinergic neurons in the PPT–LDT, melanin-concentrating hormone (MCH) neurons, and extended ventrolateral preoptic area (eVLPO) neurons may inhibit the REM-off region. Therefore the inhibitory and excitatory neurotransmitters are also necessary. We do not discuss further the changes of each neurotransmitter here, because the entire balance is more important than an individual change of neurotransmitters in Saper's model.

Sakai's mutual-interaction model

Sakai proposed the mutual-interaction model (Figure 27.2b) from unit-recording and reverse-microdialysis experiments, in which REM sleep is controlled by two opposite mechanisms, REM-executive and REM-permissive mechanisms (Sakai et al., 2001). REM sleep is generated as a result of a combination of tonic excitation of cholinergic and non-cholinergic (presumably glutamatergic) REM-on neurons and the cessation of activity of monoaminergic and non-monoaminergic (possibly GABA-ergic) REM-off neurons inhibiting REM-on neurons during wakefulness (W) and slow-wave sleep (SWS). In the pons, REM-on neurons in Sakai's schema (Figure 27.2b) are located in the peri-locus coeruleus alpha (peri-LCα; almost the same as the SLD). The rostral part of the peri-LCα contains a dense population of cholinergic neurons that send axons to

the thalamus and/or hypothalamus, whereas the caudal peri-LCα contains mainly non-cholinergic and non-monoaminergic descending neurons (Sakai, 1991). REM-off neurons in both the serotonergic (5-HT-ergic) dorsal raphe and the NE-ergic LC nuclei are not the direct REM-permissive system, but the neurons in the dorsocaudal central tegmental field (dcFTC) just beneath the ventrolateral periaqueductal gray (PAG) are critically involved in the inhibitory mechanisms of REM-sleep generation in their model (Crochet et al., 2006).

Our microdialysis results of neurotransmitter release support some part of their model. GABA in the caudal part of the pontine reticular formation, including the peri-LCα, is significantly higher during the wake state than in REM sleep (Figure 27.2b-1). Norepinephrine release in the rostral peri-LCα is lowest during REM sleep and highest during W (Figure 27.2b-2). Norepinephrine and epinephrine (EPN) release in the caudal LC-α is lowest during REM sleep and highest during W, showing the involvement of monoaminergic REM-off regulation (Figure 27.2b-3). Acetylcholine increase has also been reported during REM sleep in the peri-LCα (Fig 27.2b-4). Glutamate shows little change across sleep in all the regions, however, and is relatively low during SWS. Toward SWS to REM sleep, glutamate increases in the caudal peri-LCα (Figure 27.2b-5), but, does not increase in the rostral LC-α. In the medullar reticular formation, there is an REM-specific increase of glutamate (Figure 27.2b-6). From the observation of neurotransmitter changes, it is plausible to say their model is quite reasonable.

Sakai et al. also concluded that the dorso-caudal FTC, but not the vlPAG, is critically implicated in the inhibitory mechanisms of REM-sleep generation, and that these neurons are under the control of GABA-ergic, glutamatergic, epinephrinergic, and histaminergic systems. The activation of presumably glutamatergic dcFTC neurons during W may excite brain-stem REM-off neurons, inhibiting REM-sleep generation. During SWS, the reduction of their activity would decrease the excitatory drive on REM-off neurons (disfacilitation), leading to their cessation of discharge, which in turn would promote REM-sleep generation. This mutual-interaction model is also supported by other reports (Mallick et al., 2004; Thankachan et al., 2001). During REM sleep, the gradual increase of dcFTC neurons would progressively drive REM-off neurons resulting in the end of the REM episode.

We also pay attention to the dorsocaudal FTC and hypothesized in a previous review that when 5-HT

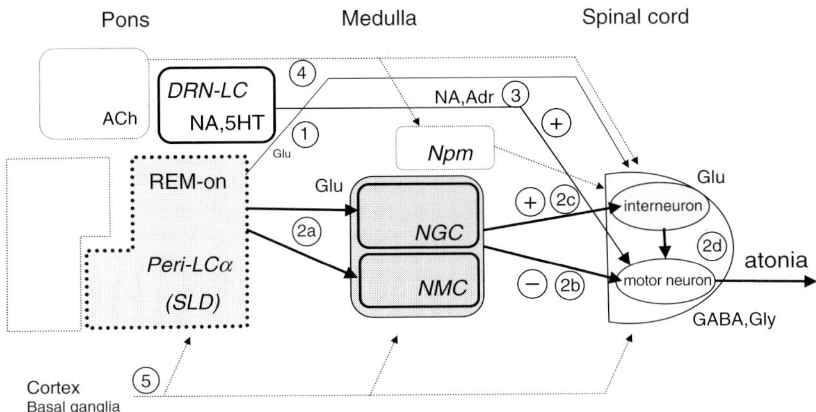

Figure 27.3 Neurotransmitter changes in the pathway of muscle atonia
Direct glutamatergic projections from the pontine reticular formation (SLD/peri-LCα) to the interneurons in the spinal cord and then glycinergic/GABA-ergic interneurons inhibit motoneurons (1).
Glutamatergic projections from the SLD/peri-LCα to the intermediate ventromedial medulla (NGC/NMC) (2a), which activate the medullary reticulospinal pathways. There are a couple of possibilities of the projection from the medulla to the spinal cord, one is direct glycinergic/GABA-ergic inhibitions from the NMC/NGC to the spinal motor neurons (2b), the other is indirect glutamatergic projection to the motor neurons (2c) via glycinergic/GABA-ergic interneurons (2d). We reported changes in neurotransmitters that indicate glutamate increases in the NMC/NGC and glycine and GABA increases in the ventral horn of the spinal cord during muscle atonia.
There are a couple of subpathways hypothesized; NE-ergic or 5-HT-ergic projections from the brain stem to the motor neurons, facilitate muscle activities (3). From the microdialysis work, it is known that NE and 5-HT increase during the phase of atonia; however, the source of NE and 5-HT is not known yet.
There are minor cholinergic projections from the LDT/PPT to the medullary reticular formation (4). It has also been hypothesized that ACh or dopamine regulate spinal motor neurons.
There are also regulating factors from the cortex, the basal forebrain, and the basal ganglia to not only the pontine atonia executive center, but also the relay neurons in the medulla and spinal motor neurons (5).
NMC: nucleus magnocellularis; NGC: nucleus gigantocellularis; Npm: nucleus paramedianus.

concentration decreases during REM sleep to the critical point of inhibitory/excitatory function, the glia neurons are excited by 5-HT and release glutamate promptly, and that this surge of glutamate depolarizes the arousal neurons to end the REM period (Kodama *et al.*, 1999).

Neurotransmitters change in the pathway of muscle atonia

The REM-on neurons in turn activate an array of brainstem and spinal pathways that produce the phenomena of REM sleep. The main stream of the muscle atonia pathway is constructed in three regions of the brain; the pontine reticular formation, the medullary reticular formation, and the spinal cord (Figure 27.3). This is what almost all sleep researchers agree with. The muscle atonia executive neurons located in the peri-LCα in the pontine reticular formation send the amino acids (presumably glutamatergic) descending fibers which pass though the "tegmento-reticular tract" to the nucleus

magnocellularis (NMC) and gigantocellularis of the medullary reticular formation (NGC). The pathway changes the fiber at the NMC or NGC, passing through the "medullary reticulospinal tract" to the spinal cord. These fibers are considered to be glutamatergic or glycinergic/GABA-ergic. There is a direct projection from the pons to the spinal cord, passing the "pontine reticulospinal tract." The descending pathways can be itemized as follows

(1) Direct, presumably glutamatergic, projections from the pontine reticular formation (SLD/peri-LCα) to the interneurons in the spinal cord and then glycinergic/GABA- ergic interneurons inhibit motoneurons (Vetrivelan *et al.*, 2009). Reports of increased levels of glutamate (Taepavarapruk *et al.*, 2008), glycine and GABA (Kodama *et al.*, 2003) in the ventral horn of the spinal cord during atonia support this pathway.

(2) Presumably glutamatergic projections from the SLD/peri-LCα to the intermediate ventromedial medulla (NGC/NMC), which in turn activate

the medullary reticulospinal pathways. There are a couple of opinions in terms of the projection from the medulla to the spinal cord, one is direct glycinergic/GABA-ergic inhibitions from NMC/NGC to the spinal motor neurons (Siegel, 2005), the other is indirect, presumably glutamatergic, projection to the motoneurons via glycinergic/GABA-ergic interneurons (Brooks and Peever, 2008; Takakusaki *et al.*, 2003). We reported changes in neurotransmitters by using microdialysis; glutamate increases in the NMC/NGC and glycine and GABA increases in the ventral horn of the spinal cord during muscle atonia. However, from the microdialysis observation, it is impossible to say whether GABA/glycine is released from interneurons or not.

To supplement these two main pathways a couple of pathways are hypothesized:

(3) Norepinephrinergic (=NE-ergic) or 5-HT-ergic projections, from the brain stem to the motor neurons, facilitate muscle activities. From the microdialysis work, it is known that NE and 5-HT increase during the phase of atonia (Lai *et al.*, 2001); however, the source of NE and 5-HT is not known yet.

(4) There are minor cholinergic projections from the LDT/PPT to the medullary reticular formation (paramedian nucleus) where the ACh increase was reported during REM sleep (Kodama *et al.*, 1992). It has also been hypothesized that ACh or dopamine (Taepavarapruk *et al*, 2008) regulate spinal motor neurons.

(5) There are also regulating factors from the cortex, the basal forebrain, and the basal ganglia to not only the pontine atonia executive center, but also the relay neurons in the medulla and spinal motor neurons.

The regulation of upper airway muscle is basically the same as the above, but a little more complicated. There are a couple of hypotheses; Neuzeret *et al.* (2009) reported that both 5-HT and histamine (HA), but not NE, have a potent excitatory action on upper airway muscle activity. Kubin proposed that upper airway atonia is caused by withdrawal of excitation mediated by 5-HT and other transmitters rather than by state-dependent inhibition, such as glycine and GABA. Peever's group proposed that the glutamate mechanism is important and NE (and dopamine) triggers muscle tone by amplifying glutamate-driven excitation (Schwarz *et al.*, 2008). In the microdialysis studies, glycine/GABA increase and NE/5-HT decrease, but no change in glutamate level was observed; further studies are needed to clarify which transmitter is mainly responsible for triggering and keeping the upper airway tone.

Supplement: neurotransmitter changes across sleep stages

The number of studies involving neurotransmitters in the brain and their relationships with sleep–waking stages have steadily increased in recent years, even though the physiological changes in their concentrations during the sleep–waking cycles are small compared to those produced by electrical and pharmacological stimulations. A large number of reports on changes in levels of dopamine, NE, 5-HT, amino acids, melatonin, and adenosine in relation to the sleep–wake cycle, as measured by microdialysis, have become available during the past two decades. In this decade changes in the very important sleep factor orexin, and histamine, were reported. But, there are not many reports clarifying the REM-sleep specific change of neurotransmitters. When the contribution of the neurotransmitter to sleep stages is discussed, the point is whether the change comes out as a result or as a cause.

The major neurotransmitters related to sleep stages are summarized briefly in Table 27.1.

Acetylcholine

Changes in ACh release across the sleep–wake cycle in the hippocampus (Kametani and Kawamura, 1990, 1991), the cerebral cortex (Jimenez-Capdeville and Dykes, 1996; Lapierre *et al.*, 2007; Marrosu *et al.*, 1995), thalamus (Williams *et al.*, 1994), and the caudate nucleus (Kodama *et al.*, 1990) are reported, to indicate that ACh release is higher during wakefulness and REM sleep than during SWS. Acetylcholine release in the brain is basically high during both wake and REM sleep as described above. This might correspond to the fact that most of the cholinergic neurons discharge at a higher rate during both wake and REM sleep (type I neurons, classified by Sakai).

In some regions where ACh plays an important role in generating the REM-sleep phenomenon, for example, the pontine reticular formation including the

Table 27.1 Neurotransmitter release across the sleep–wake cycle

Neurotransmitter	Brain area	Sleep–wake cycle	Reference
Acetylcholine	mPRF	**SWS=W<REM**	Kodama *et al.*, 1990
	mPRF	**SWS=W<REM**	Leonard, 1997*
	mPRF	**W<RLS**	Lydic *et al.*, 1991
	hippocampus	SWS<W=REM	Kametani, 1990*
	hippocampus	SWS<REM	Marrosu, 1995*
	thalamus	SWS<W=REM	Williams, 1994*
	LGN	**SWS<W< REM**	Kodama and Honda, 1996
	reticularis thalami	SWS<W=REM	Kodama and Honda, 1996
	caudate	SWS<W=REM	Kodama *et al.*, 1990
	stristum	SWS<W	Gadea-Ciria *et al.*, 1973
	cortex	SWS<REM<W	Marrosu, 1995*
	cortex	SWS<W	Jimenez-Capdeville, 1996*
	cortex	ASWS<QW<AW	Lapierre *et al.*, 2007
	PPT	SWS<W=REM	Kodama, 1999
	NPM	**SWS<W< REM**	Kodama *et al.*, 1992
	NMC	SWS<W=REM	Kodama *et al.*, 1992
	basal forebrain	**SWS<W< REM**	Vazquez and Baghdoyan, 2001; Vazquez *et al.*, 2002
Serotonin	mPRF	REM<SWS<W	Iwakiri, 1993*
	raphe (cat)	REM<SWS<W	Portas, 1994*
	hypothalamus	SWS<W	Auerbach, 1989*
	hypothalamus/preoptic	SWS<W	Wilkinson, 1991*
	hypothalamus	SWS<W	Imeri, 1994*
	medulla	SWS/REM<W	Blanco-Centurion and Salin-Pascual, 2001
	preoptic	REM<SWS<W	Python *et al.*, 2001
	LC/amygdala	REM<SWS<W	Shouse *et al.*, 2000
	hippocampus	AS<QS<QW<AW	Park *et al.*, 1999
	FrCx/DRN (rat)	REM<SWS<W	Portas *et al.*, 1998
	PPT	REM<SWS<W	Strecker *et al.*, 1999
Histamine	frontal cortex	SWS<QW<AW	Chu *et al.*, 2004
	hypothalamus	REM<SWS<W	Strecker *et al.*, 2002
Adenosine	dorsal raphe	SWS<W	Porkka-Heiskanen *et al.*, 1997
	amygdala (human)	SWS=W (diurnal change)	Zeitzer *et al.*, 2006
	basal forebrain/PPT/Cx/ POA/thalamus/DRN	REM=SWS<W	Porkka-Heiskanen *et al.*, 2000
Orexin	hypothalamus	**SWS<W<REM**	Kiyashchenko *et al.*, 2002
	basal forebrain	**SWS<REM**	Kiyashchenko *et al.*, 2002
	LC	W=SWS=REM	Kiyashchenko *et al.*, 2002

Table 27.1 (*cont.*)

Neurotransmitter	Brain area	Sleep–wake cycle	Reference
Nitric oxide	frontal cortex	SWS=REM<W	Burlet, 1997*
	thalamus	W=REM<SWS	Williams, 1997*
NE	LC/amygdala	REM<SWS<W	Shouse *et al.*, 2000
	Fr Cx	SWS<REM<W	Lena *et al.*, 2005
	nucleus accumbens	SWS<REM=W	Lena *et al.*, 2005
	amygdala	AS<QS<QW<AW	Park, 2002
Dopamine	spinal cord ventral horn	REM<SWS<W	Taepavarapruk *et al.*, 2008
	LC/amygdala	W=SWS=REM	Shouse *et al.*, 2000
	Fr Cx/nucleus accumbens	REM<SWS<W	Lena *et al.*, 2005
Glutamate	FCx motor Cx	SWS<W=REM	Dash *et al.*, 2009
	spinal cord ventral horn	W<SWS<REM	Taepavarapruk *et al.*, 2008
	post hypothalamus	NREM<REM	John *et al.*, 2008
	Fr Cx/nucleus accumbens	SWS=REM=W	Lena *et al.*, 2005
	basal forebrain	SWS=W=REM	Azuma, 1997*
	NMC	W<REM	Kodama, 1998*
	PPT	SWS=REM<W	Kodama, 1999
	NPM	SWS=W=REM	Kodama, 1998*
	ventroposterolateral nucleus (VPL)	REM=W<SWS	Kekesi, 1997*
	LDT	SWS<W	Kodama *et al.*, 1997
	mPRF	SWS<W<REM	Hasegawa *et al.*, 1997, 2003
GABA	spinal cord ventral horn	W=SWS<REM	Taepavarapruk *et al.*, 2008
	LC	**SWS=W<REM**	Nitz and Siegel, 1997b
	raphe	**W<SWS<REM**	Nitz and Siegel, 1997a
	hypothalmus	W=REM<SWS	Nitz and Siegel, 1996
	VPL	REM<W<SWS	Kekesi, 1997*
	DRN	**SWS=W<REM**	Porkka-Heiskanen *et al.*, 1997
Glycine	spinal cord ventral horn	W = SWS < REM	Taepavarapruk *et al.*, 2008
	VPL	W=REM<SWS	Kekesi, 1997*
Asparatate	nucleus accumbens	SWS=REM<W	Lena *et al.*, 2005
	Fr Cx	W=REM<SWS	Lena *et al.*, 2005
Gln	VPL	W<REM	Kekesi, 1997*
Thr	VPL	W=REM<SWS	Kekesi, 1997*
Asn	VPL	W=REM<SWS	Kekesi, 1997*
Ser	VPL	W=REM<SWS	Kekesi, 1997*
Tau	VPL	W=REM<SWS	Kekesi, 1997*
cGMP	hippocampus, midbrain, pons, medulla, cerebellum	SWS<REM<W	Ogasawara, 1981*
	striatum	**SWS<W<REM**	Ogasawara, 1981*
	LDT	SWS<REM<W	Kodama, 1997*

Bold letter: REM-sleep specific changes of neurotransmitter are observed.
* Reference not cited in the reference list, please refer Kodama, 1999.

nucleus reticularis pontis oralis (Kodama *et al.*, 1990, Leonard and Lydic, 1997) and the rostral portion of the nucleus reticularis pontis caudalis or the nucleus paramedianus, basal forebrain (Vazquez and Baghdoyan, 2001; Vazquez *et al.*, 2002), enhanced ACh releases during REM sleep were observed.

Glutamate

Glutamate and ACh are the major excitatory inputs to the neurons. Recently in the ventral horn of the spinal cord, glutamate increase during REM sleep has been reported, indicating glutamatergic regulation of muscle atonia (Taepavarapruk *et al.*, 2008). In the hypothalamus, John *et al.* (2008) observed glutamate increase during REM sleep. In the NMC, where our group found the evidence that showed that glutamate might be involved in REM-sleep control, we also detected an REM-sleep related change (11%) of glutamate release. Not the REM specific but the sleep-stage related increases of glutamate in the LDT, cortex, or basal forebrain (Azuma *et al.*, 1997; Dash *et al.*, 2009; Kodama *et al.*, 1997) are reported, but they were also small as in the NMC.

In many cases glutamate release in the brain does not show significant changes across sleep stages. For example, the changes in levels of glutamate in the pontine reticular formation detected by dialysis were smaller than those of ACh and showed no significance across sleep stages, in spite of the fact that glutamate is involved in REM sleep. The most likely explanation for this is that synaptically released glutamate in this area is obscured by the large glial release. Tetrodotoxin (TTX) studies have shown that the neuronal release of glutamate amounts to only 10% (our observation) or less (Westerink *et al.*, 1989) of the ambient level as measured by high performance liquid chromatography (HPLC). The major source of basal glutamate content is presumably the glia cells surrounding the neurons (Villablanca, 1966) and metabolic sources, rather than synaptic releases, which makes it difficult to determine the significant glutamate changes.

GABA

Nitz and Siegel reported GABA increase in the DRN and LC during REM sleep (Nitz and Siegel, 1997a). GABA is supposed to be a strong source to inhibit 5-HT-ergic neurons in the dorsal raphe nucleus during REM sleep (Porkka-Heiskanen *et al.*, 1997). However, Sakai's data suggest that the cessation of dorsal raphe unit activity is caused not by a GABA-ergic mechanism but by the mechanism of disfacilitation resulting from the cessation of discharge of NE- or histamine-containing neurons during REM sleep (Sakai and Crochet, 2000). Therefore there is the possibility that the high GABA release observed is not a function during REM sleep.

In the ventral horn of the spinal cord, there is increase in GABA release, indicating GABA is important for muscle atonia (Kodama *et al.*, 2003; Taepavarapruk *et al.*, 2008). As described above, GABA is the important inhibitory neurotransmitter, working as an essential factor in Saper's flip-flop model. Some REM-on neurons are considered to contain GABA as a transmitter, but GABA-ergic REM-off neurons, which are essential for Saper's model, have not been reported in the pontine reticular formation yet (Crochet *et al.*, 2006). Therefore, further study about GABA-ergic neurons, their releases, and interaction between GABA and other transmitters are desired.

Serotonin

Serotonin release is at its lowest during REM sleep and highest during wakefulness in all the reports with microdialysis, in the mPRF (Iwakiri *et al.*, 1993), raphe (Portas and McCarley, 1994; Portas *et al.*, 1998), medulla (Blanco-Centurion and Salin-Pascual, 2001), preoptic (Python *et al.*, 2001), LC, amygdala (Shouse *et al.*, 2000), hippocampus (Park *et al.*, 1999), cortex (Portas *et al.*, 1998), and the PPT (Strecker *et al.*, 2002). In the atonia pathway, Kubin *et al.* (1994, 1998) reported that 5-HT decreased in the XII nucleus in relation to the atonia during REM sleep. In our reports, 5-HT decreases during muscle atonia in the motor pool, the ventral horn of the spinal cord, and the XII nucleus (Lai *et al.*, 2001). However, Sakai and Crochet (2001) concluded from their findings that DRN 5-HT-ergic activity does not play any crucial role in REM sleep generation, but is involved in the regulation of W and SWS.

Norepinephrine

The discharge rate of NE-ergic neurons is the highest during wake, and NE release is also reported to be highest in wakefulness in the LC/amygdala (Shouse *et al.*, 2000) and cortex/accumbens (Léna *et al.*, 2005). In our reports, NE decreases during muscle atonia in the ventral horn of the spinal cord and XII nucleus (Lai *et al.*, 2001). Sakai's results indicate that NE and epinephrine selectively inhibited REM sleep when applied to the caudal part of the peri-LCα (Crochet and Sakai, 1999).

Dopamine

It was reported that DA release does not change much across the sleep–wake cycle (Shouse *et al.*, 2000) as dopaminergic neurons do not change their discharge rates. Recently, however, it has been reported that DA release in the spinal cord and the frontal cortex are lowest during REM sleep (Léna *et al.*, 2005; Taepavarapruk *et al.*, 2008). This kind of REM sleep-specific decrease may be important for REM-sleep generation because Sakai's results indicate that DA inhibits REM sleep in the peri-LCα via excitation of α_2 adrenoceptors (Crochet and Sakai, 2003).

Histamine

Histamine is considered to relate to wakefulness, and HA release is high during wake in the cortex (Chu *et al.*, 2004) and hypothalamus (Strecker *et al.*, 2002).

Orexin

Orexin is an important transmitter in keeping an animal awake, and its firing rate is highest during wakefulness. However, orexin release in the hypothalamus and thalamus is higher during REM sleep than SWS/W (Kiyashchenko *et al.*, 2002).

Adenosine

Another important finding was reported by Porkka-Heiskanen *et al.* (1997). Adenosine is known as a potent sleep-inducing substance. Adenosine concentration in the basal forebrain increases during wakefulness to inhibit cholinergic neurons in the basal forebrain and decreases in the sleep phase. There was an attempt to collect dialysate from the human brain, which showed no changes in the amygdala across the sleep cycle (a diurnal change is observed) (Zeitzer *et al.*, 2006).

Nitric oxide

Nitric oxide (NO) is a potent enhancer of adenosine in the basal forebrain, regulating sleep. Nitric oxide is now considered to have an important retrograde messenger (Leonard and Lydic, 1999; also Figure 27.1). Our data suggested NO-regulated NE release in the LDT area to coordinate ACh–NE release balance across the sleep–wake cycle (Kodama *et al.*, 1997). Burlet and Cespuglio (1997) reported NO increase during wakefulness in the frontal cortex. Williams *et al.*'s (1997) report indicated an NO increase in the thalamus during SWS . We reported that glutamatergic inputs into cholinergic neurons in the LDT generated NO. Nitric oxide works as a retrograde transmitter to generate cGMP and affect presynapses of NE neurons to regulate NE release (Kodama *et al.*, 1997).

cGMP

cGMP also changes in concentration across the sleep-waking cycle in the LDT (Kodama *et al.*, 1997), hippocampus, pons, medulla, and cerebellum; especially in the striatum, release of cGMP is reported highest (Ogasahara *et al.*, 1981). Although the direct effect on sleep mechanisms is not known now, cGMP plays an important role as a modulator to regulate neuronal release in the presynaptic field (Figure 27.1).

Again, the point that the interaction between neurotransmitters is more important than a single change should be emphasized. In the physiological condition, every neurotransmitter works to affect each other. Just one single neurotransmitter change can never cause the sleep–wake transition, though it tends to be discussed from the pharmacological study, such as the agonist/antagonist of neurotransmitter microinjection study.

References

Aserinsky, E. & Kleitman, N. (1953) Regularly occurring periods of eye motility, and concomitant phenomena during sleep. *Science* **118**: 273–4.

Azuma, A., Kodama, T. Honda, K. & Inoue, S. (1996) State-dependent changes of extracellular glutamate in the medial pre-optic area in freely behaving rats. *Neurosci Lett* **214**: 179–82.

Baghdoyan, H. A., Lydic, R. & Fleegal, M. A. (1998) M2 muscarinic autoreceptors modulate acetylcholine release in the medial pontine reticular formation. *J Pharmacol Exp Therapeutics* **286**: 1446–52.

Bjorkum, A. A., Strecker, R. E., Porkka-Heiskanen, T., Stenberg, D., McCarley, R. W. (1997) GABA modulates the dorsal raphe and alters the pattern of sleep–waking. *Neurosci Abst* **23**: 1065.

Blanco-Centurion, C. A. & Salin-Pascual, R. J. (2001) Extracellular serotonin levels in the medullary reticular formation during normal sleep and after REM sleep deprivation. *Brain Res* **923**: 128–36.

Brooks, P. L. & Peever, J.H. (2008) Unraveling the mechanisms of REM sleep atonia. *Sleep* **31**: 1492–7.

Burlet, S. & Cespuglio, R. (1997) Voltametric detection of nitric oxide(NO) in the rat brain: its variations throughout the sleep–wake cycle. *Neurosci Lett* **226**: 131–5.

Chu, M., Huang, Z. L., Qu, W.-M., *et al.* (2004) Extracellular histamine level in the frontal cortex is positively correlated with the amount of wakefulness in rats. *Neurosci Res* **49**: 417–20.

Crochet, S., Onoe, H. & Sakai, K. (2006) A potent non-monoaminergic paradoxical sleep inhibitory system: a reverse microdialysis and single-unit recording study. *Eur J Neurosci* **24**: 1404–12.

Crochet, S. & Sakai, K. (1999) Effects of microdialysis application of monoamines on the EEG and behavioural states in the cat mesopontine tegmentum. *Eur J Neurosci* **11**: 3738–52.

Crochet, S. & Sakai, K. (2003) Dopaminergic modulation of behavioral states in mesopontine tegmentum: a reverse microdialysis study in freely moving cats. *Sleep* **26**: 801–6.

Dash, M. B., Douglas, C. D., Vyazovskiy, V. V., Cirelli, C. & Tononi, G. (2009) Long-term homeostasis of extracellular glutamate in the rat cerebral cortex across sleep and waking states. *J Neurosci* **29**: 620–9.

Fuller, P. M., Saper, C. B. & Lu, J. (2007) The pontine REM switch: past and present. *J Physiol* **584**: 735–41.

Gadea-Ciria, M., Stadler, H., Lloyd, K. G. & Batholini, G. (1973) Acetylcholine release within the cat striatum during the sleep–wakefulness cycle. *Nature* **43**: 518–19.

Hasegawa, T., Azuma, S., Kimura, M. & Inoue, S. (1997) State dependent changes of amino acids in the rat oral pontine reticular nuclei measured by microdialysis. *Neurosci Abstr* **23**: 2132.

Hasegawa, T., Kohyama, J. & Honda, K. (2003) Amino acid release in the rat oral pontine reticular nucleus across various vigilance states. *Sleep Biol Rhythm* **1**: 195–8.

Iwakiri, H., Matsuyama, K. & Mori, S. (1993) Extracellular levels of serotonin in the medial pontine reticular formation in relation to sleep–wake cycle in cats: a microdialysis study. *Neurosci Res* **18**: 157–70.

Jimenez-Capdeville, M. E. & Dykes, R. W. (1996) Changes in cortical acetylcholine release in the rat during day and night: differences between motor and sensory areas. *Neurosci* **71**: 567–79.

John, J., Ramanathan, L. & Siegel, J. M. (2008) Rapid changes in glutamate levels in the posterior hypothalamus across sleep–wake states in freely behaving rats. *Am J Physiol* **295**: 2041–9.

Kametani, H. & Kawamura, H. (1990) Alterations in acetylcholine release in the rat hippocampus during sleep–wakefulness detected by intracerebral dialysis. *Life Sci* **47**: 421–6.

Kametani, H. & Kawamura, H. (1991) Circadian rhythm of cortical acetylcholine release as measured by in vivo microdialysis in freely moving rats. *Neurosci Lett* **13**: 2263–6.

Kiyashchenko, L. I., Mileykovskiy, B. Y., Maidment, N. *et al.* (2002) Release of hypocretin (orexin) during waking and sleep states. *J Neurosci* **22**: 5282–6.

Kodama, T. (1999) Neurotransmitters changes and REM sleep. In *Rapid Eye Movement Sleep*, eds. B. N. Mallick and S. Inoue. New Delhi: Narosa Publishing House, pp. 194–213.

Kodama, T., Takahashi, Y. & Honda, Y. (1990) Enhancement of acetylcholine release during paradoxical sleep in the dorsal tegmental field of the cat brain stem. *Neurosci Lett* **114**: 277–82.

Kodama, T., Lai, Y. Y. & Siegel, J. M. (1992) Enhancement of acetylcholine release during REM sleep in the caudomedial medulla as measured by in vivo microdialysis. *Brain Res* **580**: 348–50.

Kodama, T. & Honda, Y. (1996) Acetylcholine releases of mesopontine PGO-on cells in the lateral geniculate nucleus in sleep-waking cycle and serotonergic regulation. *Prog Neuro Psychopharmacol & Biol Psychiat* **20**:1213–27.

Kodama, T., Honda, Y. & Koyama, Y. (1997) Glutamate-noradrenergic interaction in the laterodorsal tegmentum neurons mediated by nitric oxide. *Psychiatry Clin Neurosci* **51**: S45.

Kodama, T., Lai, Y. Y. & Siegel, J. M. (1998) Enhanced glutamate release during REM sleep in the rostromedial medulla as measured by in vivo microdialysis. *Brain Res* **780**: 178–81.

Kodama, T. & Honda, Y. (1999) Acetylcholine and glutamate release during sleep-wakefulness in the pedunculopontine tegmental nucleus and norepinephrine changes regulated by nitric oxide. *Psychiatry Clin Neurosci* **53**:109–11.

Kodama, T., Lai, Y.Y. & Siegel, J. M. (2003) Changes in inhibitory amino acid release linked to pontine-induced atonia: an in vivo microdialysis study. *J Neurosci* **23**: 1548–54.

Kubin, L., Reignier, C., Tojima, H. *et al.* (1994) Changes in serotonin level in the hypoglossal nucleus region during carbachol-induced atonia. *Brain Res* **645**: 291–302.

Kubin, L., Davies, R. O. & Pack, A. I. (1998) Control of upper airway motoneurons during REM sleep. *News Physiological Sci* **13**: 91–7.

Lai, Y. Y., Kodama, T. & Siegel, J. M. (2001) Changes in monoamine release in the ventral horn and hypoglossal nucleus linked to pontine inhibition of muscle tone: an in vivo microdialysis study. *J Neurosci* **21**: 7384–91.

Lapierre, J. L., Peter, O., Kosenko, P. O. *et al.* (2007) Cortical acetylcholine release is lateralized during asymmetrical slow-wave sleep in northern fur seals. *J Neurosci* **27**: 11,999–2006.

Léna, I., Parrot, S., Deschaux, O. *et al.* (2005) Variations in extracellular levels of dopamine, noradrenaline, glutamate, and aspartate across the sleep–wake cycle in the medial prefrontal cortex and nucleus accumbens of freely moving rats. *J Neurosci Res* **81**: 891–9.

Leonard, T. O. & Lydic, R. (1997) Pontine nitric oxide modulates acetylcholine release, rapid eye movement sleep generation, amd respiratory rate. *J Neurosci* **17**: 774–85.

Leonard, T. O. & Lydic, R. (1999) Nitric oxide: a diffusible modulator of physiological traits and behavioral states. In *Rapid Eye Movement Sleep*, eds. B. N. Mallick & S. Inoue. New Delhi: Narosa Publishing House, pp. 167–93 .

Lu, J., Sherman, D., Marshall, D. M. & Saper, C. B. (2006) A putative flip–flop switch for control of REM sleep. *Nature* **441**: 589–94.

Lydic, R., Baghdoyan, H. A. & Lorinc, Z. (1991) Microdialysis of cat pons reveals enhanced acetylcholine release during state-dependent respiratory depression. *Am J Physiol* **261**: R766–70.

Mallick, B. N., Thankachan, S. & Islam, F. (2004) Influence of hypnogenic brain areas on wakefulness- and rapid-eye-movement sleep-related neurons in the brainstem of freely moving cats. *J Neurosci Res* **75**: 133–42.

Marrosu, F., Portas, C., Mascia, M. S. *et al.* (1995) Microdialysis measurement of cortical and hippocampal acetylcholine release during sleep–wake cycle in freely moving cats. *Brain Res* **67**: 1329–32.

McCarley, R. W. (2007) Neurobiology of REM and NREM sleep. *Sleep Med* **8**: 302–30.

McCarley, R. W. & Hobson, J. A. (1975) Neuronal excitability modulation over the sleep cycle: a structural and mathematical model. *Science* **189**: 58–60.

McGinty, D. J., Harper, R. M. & Fairbanks, M. K. (1974) Neuronal unit activity and the control of sleep states. *Adv Sleep Res* **1**: 217–50.

Neuzeret, P. C., Sakai, K., Gormand, F. *et al.* (2009) Application of histamine or serotonin to the hypoglossal nucleus increases genioglossus muscle activity across the wake–sleep cycle. *J Sleep Res* **18**: 113–21.

Nitz, D. & Siegel, J. M. (1996) GABA release in posterior hypothalamus across sleep–wake cycle. *Am J Physiol* **271**: R1707–12.

Nitz, D. & Siegel, J. M. (1997a) GABA release in the dorsal raphe nucleus: role in the control of REM sleep. *Am J Physiol* **273**: R451–5.

Nitz, D. & Siegel, J. M. (1997b) GABA release in the locus coeruleus as a function of sleep/wake state. *Neurosci* **78**: 795–801.

Ogasahara, S., Taguchi Y. & Wada, H. (1981) Changes in the levels of cyclic nucleotides in rat brain during the sleep–wakefulness cycle. *Brain Res* **213**: 163–71.

Park, S. P. (2002) In vivo microdialysis measures of extracellular norepinephrine in the rat amygdala during sleep–wakefulness. *J Korean Med Sci* **17**: 395–9.

Park, S. P., Lopez-Rodriguez, F., Wilson, C. L. *et al.* (1999) In vivo microdialysis measures of extracellular serotonin in the rat hippocampus during sleep–wakefulness. *Brain Res* **833**: 291–6.

Porkka-Heiskanen, T., Strecker, R. E., Stenberg, D., Bjorkum, A. A. & McCarley, R. W. (1997) GABA and adenosine inhibit the dorsal raphe nucleus and increase REM sleep as studied by microdialysis. *Sleep Res* **26**: 35.

Porkka-Heiskanen, T., Strecker, R. E. & McCarley, R. W. (2000) Brain site-specificity of extracellular adenosine concentration changes during sleep deprivation and spontaneous sleep: an in vivo microdialysis study. *Neuroscience* **99**: 507–17.

Portas, C. M. & McCarley, R. W. (1994) Behavioral state-related changes of extracelullar serotonin concentration in the dorsal raphe nucleus: a microdialysis study in the freely moving cat. *Brain Res* **648**: 306–12.

Portas, C. M., Bjorvatn, B., Fagerland, S. *et al.* (1998) On-line detection of extracellular levels of serotonin in dorsal raphe nucleus and frontal cortex over the sleep/wake cycle in the freely moving rat. *Neuroscience* **83**: 807–14.

Python, A., Steimer, T., de Saint Hilaire, Z., Mikolajewski, R. & Nicolaidis, S. (2001) Extracellular serotonin variations during vigilance states in the preoptic area of rats: a microdialysis study. *Brain Res* **910**: 49–54.

Roth, M. T., Fleegal, M. A., Lydic, R. & Baghdoyan, H. A. (1996) Pontine acetylcholine release is regulated by muscarinic autoreceptors. *Neuroreport* **7**: 3069–72.

Sakai, K. (1991) Physiological properties and afferent connections of the locus coeruleus and adjacent tegmental neurons involved in the generation of paradoxical sleep in the cat. In Barnes, C. D. & Pompeiano, O. eds., Neurobiology of the locus coeruleus. *Prog Brain Res* **88**: 31–45.

Sakai, K. (1998) Executive mechanisms of paradoxical sleep. *Arch Ital Biol* **126**: 239–57.

Sakai, K. & Crochet, S. (2000) Serotonergic dorsal raphe neurons cease firing by disfacilitation during paradoxical sleep. *Neuroreport* **28**: 3237–41.

Sakai, K. & Crochet, S. (2001) Role of dorsal raphe neurons in paradoxical sleep generation in the cat: no evidence for a serotonergic mechanism. *Eur J Neurosci* **13**: 103–12.

Sakai, K. & Kanamori, N. (1999) Are there non-monoaminergic paradoxical sleep-off neurons in the brainstem? *Sleep Res Online* **2**: 57–63.

Sakai, K., Crochet, S. & Onoe, H. (2001) Pontine structures and mechanisms involved in the generation of paradoxical (REM) sleep. *Arch Ital Biol* **139**: 93–107.

Schwarz, P. B., Yee, N., Mir, S. & Peever, J. H. (2008) Noradrenaline triggers muscle tone by amplifying glutamate-driven excitation of somatic motoneurones in anaesthetized rats. *J Physiol* **586**: 5787–802.

Semba, K., Greene, R. W., Rasmusson, D. D., McCarley, R. W. & Weider, J. (1997) Noradrenergic presynaptic inhibition of acetylcholine release in the rat pontine reticular formation: an in vitro electrophysiological and in vivo microdialysis study. *Neurosci Abstr* **23**: 1065.

Shouse, M. N., Staba, R. J., Saquib, S. F. & Farber, P. R. (2000) Monoamines and sleep: microdialysis findings in pons and amygdala. *Brain Res* **860**:181–9.

Siegel, J. M. (2005) Control of muscle tone across the sleep–wake cycle. In *The Physiologic Nature of Sleep*, eds. P. L. Parmeggiani & R. A. Velluti. Imperial College Press, pp. 281–302.

Strecker, R. E., Porkka-Heiskanen, T., Bjorkum, A. A. & McCarley, R. W. (1997) Adenosine actions of the dorsal raphe nucleus: altered sleep–waking pattern. *Neurosci Abstr* **23**: 1065.

Strecker, R. E., Thakkar, M. M., Porkka-Heiskanen, T. *et al.* (1999) Behavioral state-related changes of extracellular serotonin concentration in the pedunculopontine tegmental nucleus: a microdialysis study in freely moving animals. *Sleep Res Online* **2**: 21–7.

Strecker, R. E., Nalwalk, J., Dauphin, L. J. *et al.* (2002) Extracellular histamine levels in the feline preoptic/anterior hypothalamic area during natural sleep–wakefulness and prolonged wakefulness: an in vivo microdialysis study. *Neuroscience* **113**: 663–70.

Taepavarapruk, N., Taepavarapruk, P., John, J. *et al.* (2008) State-dependent changes in glutamate, glycine, GABA, and dopamine levels in cat lumbar spinal cord. *J Neurophysiol* **100**: 598–608.

Takakusaki, K., Kohyamaa, J. & Matsuyama, K. (2003) Medullary reticulospinal tract mediating a generalized motor inhibition in cats: iii. functional organization of spinal interneurons in the lower lumbar segments. *Neuroscience* **121**:731–46.

Thakkar, M. M., Strecker, R. E. & McCarley, R. W. (1997) A 5HT1A agonist in the laterodorsal tegmental nucleus (LDT) inhibits REM-on neurons but has no effect on wake/REM-on neurons as revealed by combined unit recording and microdialysis. *Neurosci Abstr* **23**: 1065.

Thankachan, S., Islam, F. & Mallick, B. N. (2001) Role of wake inducing brain stem area on rapid eye movement sleep regulation in freely moving cats. *Brain Res Bull* **55**: 43–9.

Vazquez, J. & Baghdoyan, H. A. (2001) Basal forebrain acetylcholine release during REM sleep is significantly greater than during waking. *Am J Physiol Regul Integr Comp Physiol* **280**: R598–601.

Vazquez, J., Lydic, R., Helen, A. & Baghdoyan, H. A. (2002) The nitric oxide synthase inhibitor NG-nitro-L-arginine increases basal forebrain acetylcholine release during sleep and wakefulness. *J Neurosci* **22**: 5597–605.

Vetrivelan, R., Fuller, P. M., Tong, Q. & Lu, J. (2009) Medullary circuitry regulating rapid eye movement sleep and motor atonia. *J Neurosci* **29**: 9361–9.

Villablanca, J. (1966) Behavioral and polygraphic study of "sleep" and "wakefulness" in chronic decerebrate cats. *Electroenceph Clin Neurophysiol* **21**: 562–77.

Westerink, B. H. C., Rollema, H., De Vries, J. B. & Damsma, G. (1989) Levels of neurotransmitters and precursors in microdialysates: criteria for neurogenic origin. *Current Separations* **9**: 76.

Williams, J. A., Comisarow, J., Day, J., Fibiger, H. C. & Reiner, P. B. (1994) State-dependent release of acetylcholine in rat thalamus measured by in vivo microdialysis. *J Neurosci* **14:** 5236–42.

Williams, J. A., Vincent, S. R. & Reiner, P. B. (1997) Nitric oxide production in rat thalmus changes with behavioral states, local depolarization, and brainstem stimulation. *J Neurosci* **17**: 420–7.

Zeitzer, J. M., Morales-Villagran, A., Maidment, N. T. *et al.* (2006) Extracellular adenosine in the human brain during sleep and sleep deprivation: an in vivo microdialysis study. *Sleep* **29**: 455–61.

Chapter

28

Pontine areas inhibiting REM sleep

Priyattam J. Shiromani and Carlos Blanco-Centurion

Summary

In the first half of the twentieth century, research by von Economo and Walle Nauta implicated the hypothalamus in sleep and waking. In the subsequent 50 years the hypothalamus was abandoned and instead the pons was considered to house the neurons regulating states of consciousness. In 1999, the linkage of a hypothalamic peptide, hypocretin, with narcolepsy shifted the emphasis back to the hypothalamus. However, since REM sleep originates from the pons, we sought to identify how the hypothalamus links with the pons, which would elucidate a network map of regions responsible for all three states. In this review we summarize our hypothesis that hypothalamic wake and non-REM sleep active neurons link with a group of i nhibitory pontine neurons to gate the transition to REM sleep. This hypothesis was first publically presented by us at the Society for Neuroscience meeting in 2004. We suggest that the pontine areas inhibiting REM sleep (PAIRS) represent GABA neurons; that these neurons are activated by glucosensing neurons, and neurons involved in emotion and arousal, and that their purpose is to keep the animal upright, mobile, and vigilant as it forages for food.

Introduction

Virtually all living organisms demonstrate periods of rest and activity. It has now been demonstrated that the roundworm (*Caenorhabditis elegans*), fruit fly (*Drosophila melanogaster*), and zebrafish (*Danio rerio*) have distinct bouts of rest and activity and that manipulations that increase the activity periods produce a compensatory increase in the rest periods, just as in mammals (for a review see Zimmerman *et al.*, 2008). In *Drosophila*, stimulants such as caffeine promote periods of arousal, just as in humans (Hendricks

et al., 1999). In birds and mammals these periods have evolved into the electrophysiologically and behaviorally distinct states of wake, non-REM sleep, and REM sleep. How the brain orchestrates the shifts in vigilance states is not known. This is an important question because 70 million Americans suffer from some sort of sleep disorder. A decline in behavioral and psychological well-being results from poor sleep. More importantly, lack of judgment related to sleep loss may contribute to catastrophes (Mitler *et al.*, 1988). There is increasing evidence that lack of sleep may compromise the body's immunocompetence and recuperative abilities (Moldofsky, 1994). By elucidating the neuronal circuit underlying sleep–wakefulness, it will be possible to develop strategies to combat daytime sleepiness and insomnia.

First-order circuit models have emerged as a result of discoveries within the last few years that have identified key neuronal populations in the hypothalamus responsible for non-REM sleep and waking. The non-REM sleep-active neurons in the ventral lateral preoptic nucleus (VLPO) and in the adjacent median preoptic nucleus were initially identified (Sherin *et al.*, 1996) and then the neuropeptide, hypocretin (also known as orexin), whose neurons are located only in the lateral hypothalamus were linked to the sleep disorder narcolepsy (Chemelli *et al.*, 1999; Lin *et al.*, 1999; Peyron *et al.*, 2000; Thannickal *et al.*, 2000). These groups of neurons are now considered to play a prominent role in non-REM sleep and waking since their deletion leads to predictable changes in sleep and wake. The anatomical connections of the non-REM sleep-active and the wake-active neurons are now fairly clear (see Sakurai *et al.*, 2005).

As for REM sleep, Jouvet's transection and lesion studies followed by pharmacological stimulation studies by other investigators demonstrated that it

REM Sleep: Regulation and Function, eds. Birendra N. Mallick, S. R. Pandi-Perumal, Robert W. McCarley, and Adrian R. Morrison. Published by Cambridge University Press. © Cambridge University Press 2011.

originates from the pons (summarized in Jones, 2004). Jouvet and others (Steriade and McCarley, 1990) attempted to place the neurons responsible for wake, non-REM sleep, and REM sleep in the pons. This was not surprising given Moruzzi and Magoun's (1949) finding that electrical stimulation of the reticular formation elicited arousal. Moreover, the pons was found to contain cholinergic, norepinephrine, and serotonin neurons (Dahlstrom and Fuxe, 1964). However, once hypocretin was linked to narcolepsy in 1999 the emphasis shifted away from the pons.

We were part of the discovery of the ventral lateral preoptic area (VLPO) in 1996. A few years earlier (Shiromani *et al.*, 1992) we were the first to advocate for the use of the immediate-early gene, c-FOS, as a neuroanatomical tool to ferret out neurons that were activated during REM sleep. Since then the c-FOS method has been widely used in sleep research and as a result the circuitry underlying sleep–wake is better understood.

Pontine inhibitory neurons as a link between the hypothalamus and the pontine REM sleep generator

With the discovery of the VLPO and hypocretin, the hypothalamus began to assume a prominent role in regulating non-REM sleep and wake. This begged the question: how did the hypothalamus link with the pons where the REM-sleep generator neurons are located? We theorized in 2004 (Blanco-Centurion *et al.*, 2004) that an intermediate group of neurons in the pons gates the generation of REM sleep. To identify these neurons we used the neurotoxin hypocretin-2-saporin to lesion the hypocretin receptor bearing neurons. In that study (Blanco-Centurion *et al.*, 2004) we found an increase (+56.5% during the night) in REM sleep after hypocretin-2-saporin lesions of hypocretin/orexin receptor bearing neurons in the locus subcoeruleus region. This region is also referred to as the sublateral dorsal region by some investigators (Boissard *et al.*, 2003). We theorized that the lesions had killed GABA-ergic neurons inhibitory to REM sleep.

To identify the GABA-ergic neurons we elected to use a transgenic mouse where the GABA-ergic neurons could be easily visualized by the presence of enhanced green fluorescent protein (eGFP). These mice express eGFP under the control of the mouse Gad1 gene promoter, thereby revealing the GABA-ergic neurons

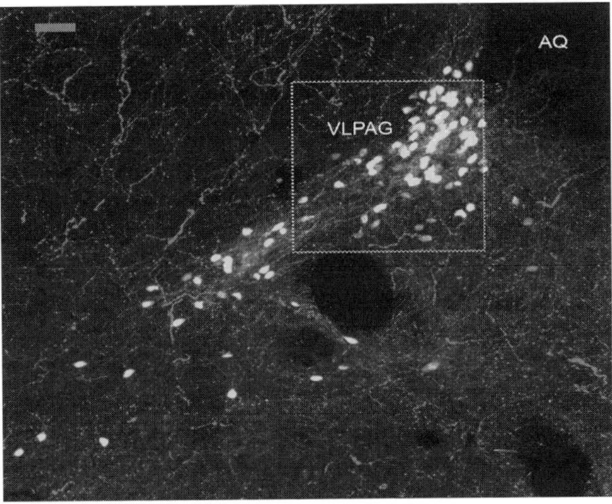

Figure 28.1 GABA neurons (green) in the ventral lateral periaqueductal gray area. These neurons are innervated by hypocretin (red), which activates the GABA neurons thereby inhibiting REM sleep. Lesion of these GABA neurons in the vlPAG releases the inhibition and leads to more REM sleep even in mice that lack hypocretin (Kaur *et al.*, 2009).

Abbreviations: AQ= cerebral aqueduct; VLPAG= ventral lateral periaqueductal gray. (See plate section for color version.)

(Oliva, Jr. *et al.*, 2000). When we examined the pontine brain stem of these mice we noticed a dense cluster of eGFP-labeled neurons in the ventral lateral periaquaductal gray (vlPAG) area. These neurons are innervated by hypocretin terminals (Figure 28.1) and in a recent paper we determined that they possess the hypocretin-2 receptor (Kaur *et al.*, 2009). In that paper we also determined that these neurons were GABA-ergic (Kaur *et al.*, 2009).

Because the vlPAG GABA-ergic neurons possess the hypocretin-2 receptor we utilized hypocretin-2-saporin to lesion them. Mice homozygous for the FVB-TgN (GadGFP) 45704Swn transgene, raised on a FVB background (Jackson Laboratories, Bar Harbor, ME, USA) were used. We found that mice with significant loss (range 55–92%) of the eGFP neurons in the vlPAG had a 79% increase in REM sleep at night compared to mice without lesion (saline group). There was a significant correlation between loss of GFP neurons in the vlPAG and REM sleep at night (r = 0.889; p < 0.001). The increase in REM sleep was a result of more bouts of REM sleep and not lengthening of the bouts. Cataplexy was not triggered by the vlPAG lesions. From these results we concluded that the vlPAG GABA-ergic neurons receive excitatory input from the lateral hypothalamic hypocretin/orexin wake-active neurons, and that because they are GABA-ergic, they would inhibit REM sleep.

We wondered if the vlPAG GABA-ergic inhibitory neurons in mice might also receive other excitatory input, besides hypocretin. To directly test this possibility we lesioned the vlPAG GABA-ergic neurons in mice that lacked hypocretin. We hypothesized that REM sleep should be increased in hypocretin knock-out mice. The hypocretin knock-out mice already have more REM sleep compared to wildtype (Chemelli *et al.*, 1999). In these mice, we injected hypocretin-2-saporin into the vlPAG and two weeks later sleep–wake patterns were recorded for 48 hours. In eight of eleven hypocretin knock-out mice the lesion was localized to the vlPAG. In these mice, REM sleep was increased (+177%) compared to wildtype animals without lesion. Compared to hypocretin knock-out mice without lesion (saline controls), the lesioned mice had a 39% increase in REM sleep. Thus, vlPAG lesions in hypocretin knock-out mice exacerbated the increase in REM sleep. The number of cataplexy bouts in the lesioned hypocretin knock-out mice did not change indicating that such lesions did not trigger cataplexy.

Next, we determined which regions in the brain project to the vlPAG. The retrograde tracer, cholera toxin subunit B, was injected into the vlPAG of the FVB-GFP mice. Moderate to high numbers of retrogradely filled neurons were found in the central nucleus of the amygdala, magnocellular preoptic nucleus, preoptic area, perirhinal cortex, ventromedial hypothalamus (VMH), lateral hypothalamus (LH), tuberomammillary nucleus (TMN), and lateral pontine tegmentum. Some of the CTb-labeled cells in the lateral hypothalamus were immunoreactive for hypocretin and melanin-concentrating hormone (MCH), suggesting that both MCH and hypocretin have inputs to the vlPAG area. From these data we conclude that the hypocretin input is but one input to the vlPAG. We hypothesize that the input from the perirhinal cortex is important for memory (Kaur *et al.*, 2009) while the input from the central nucleus of the amygdala would attach an emotional component to the memory. Both of these inputs may help direct the animal to a familiar food source. The inputs from the VMH and LH would help arouse the animal in response to changing glucose levels. Taken together, we suggest that the projections from areas associated with memory, emotion, glucosensing, and arousal neurons would have an excitatory influence on the vlPAG GABA-ergic neurons. We suggest that the activation of the vlPAG GABA-ergic circuit prevents the animal from entering into REM sleep

thereby enabling it to maintain the proper posture and vigilance required for foraging and feeding.

Are vlPAG neurons active during waking? We have answered this question by directly monitoring the electrophysiology of vlPAG neurons in the hypocretin knock-out mice (Thankachan *et al.*, 2009). We found that 91% of the vlPAG neurons were active during waking (Thankachan *et al.*, 2009). Interestingly, 9% of the recorded neurons were selectively active during REM sleep. This suggests that REM-generator neurons are also located in the vlPAG, and local GABA-ergic neurons do not have to go far to inhibit them.

Pontine areas inhibiting REM sleep

Several groups have proposed models regarding the neurons that regulate REM sleep. Some of these are described in this book. Here we present our model that we refer to as PAIRS (see Figure 28.2). Pontine neurons that inhibit REM sleep are central to our model. We argue that the purpose of these neurons is to keep the animal upright and vigilant during foraging and feeding. When these neurons are active, as during waking, then REM sleep is inhibited. These neurons would also receive input from the sleep-active neurons in the ventral lateral and median preoptic areas. During non-REM sleep activity of the preoptic neurons would release GABA onto the pontine intermediate neurons, so that when sufficient numbers of these neurons are silenced then REM sleep-on neurons become active and REM sleep ensues.

We suggest that the PAIRS neurons are activated primarily during the animal's active period, a time when the bulk of feeding occurs. Thus, loss of these neurons should increase REM sleep during the active period, which it does (Kaur *et al.*, 2009). Indeed, in the FVB mice, lesions of the vlPAG produced a day–night inversion in REM sleep (Kaur *et al.*, 2009). To test our hypothesis these neurons could be lesioned in diurnal rodents to determine whether REM sleep is increased during the day.

Significance

The efforts by us and other researchers around the world have produced a clearer circuit map that underlies the generation of wake, non-REM sleep, and REM sleep. This allows for targeted therapies to treat disorders such as insomnia, excessive sleep, or narcolepsy. For instance, in Parkinson's disease the dopamine neurons die but the therapy is aimed at affecting the target

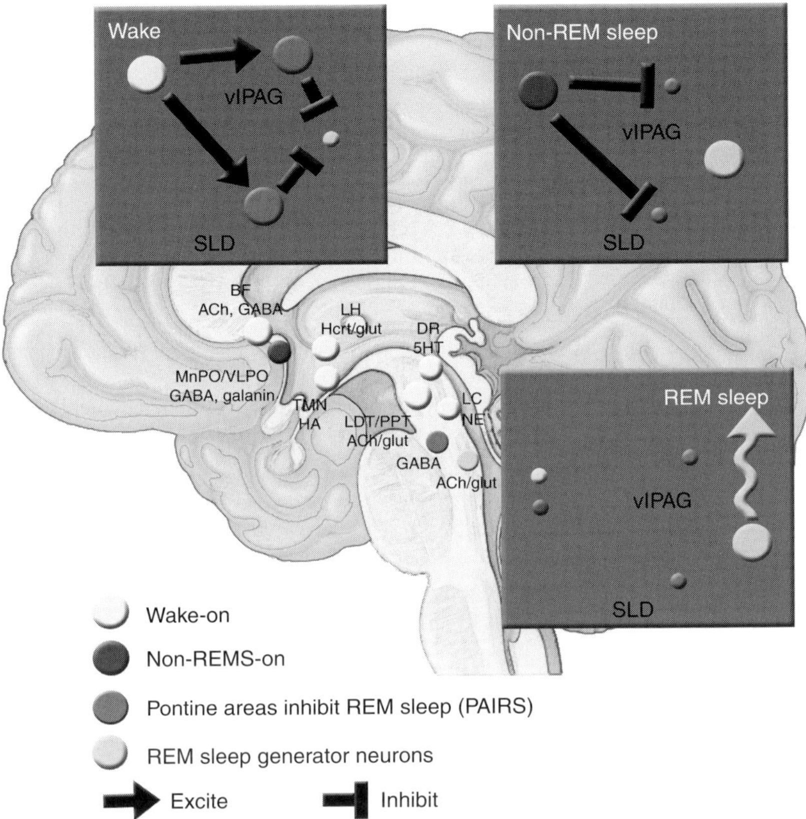

Figure 28.2 Model of neuronal populations that regulate wake, non-REM sleep, and REM sleep (Kaur *et al.*, 2009). This model represents an effort by a number of investigators (for a review see Kaur *et al.*, 2009). There are several neuronal populations that are considered to generate wakefulness and these are identified in yellow. Neurons that are considered to generate non-REM sleep are identified in blue. Both of these neuronal populations act on neurons in the pontine brain stem (red) and influence the generation of rapid-eye movement sleep (REM sleep). Wake-on neurons inhibit REM sleep by activating pontine GABA neurons in the pons. The strength of the excitatory input to the pontine GABA neurons influences REM sleep. A strong input will inhibit REM sleep while a weakened input will facilitate it. This excitatory input to the GABA pontine neurons is from hypocretin and from other sources. The purpose of this excitation is to keep the animal upright and mobile while foraging for food. During non-REM sleep the excitatory input to the pontine GABA neurons is lost and is replaced by a strong inhibitory input. This enables REM-sleep generator neurons (green) to become active and when sufficient numbers of these are activated then REM sleep ensues. The hypothesis that the pontine areas inhibit REM sleep has been tested in two separate studies from our lab (Blanco-Centurion *et al.*, 2004; Kaur *et al.*, 2009). The earlier study tested the hypothesis in rats whereas the second study tested it in mice. In both studies REM sleep increased when the GABA neurons were lesioned with hypocretin-2-saporin thereby supporting the hypothesis of PAIRS. (See plate section for color version.)

Abbreviations: Ach = acetylcholine; BF = basal forebrain; DR = dorsal raphe; GABA = gamma-aminobutyric acid; GLUT = glutamic acid; HA = histamine; HCRT = hypocretin; LC = locus coeruleus; LH = lateral hypothalamus; MnPO = median preoptic nucleus; NE = norepinephrine; LDT = lateral dorsal pontine tegmentum; PPT = pedunculopontine tegmentum; SLD = sublateral dorsal nucleus; TMN = tuberomammillary nucleus; vlPAG = ventral lateral periaqueductal gray; VLPO = ventral lateral preoptic nucleus.

neurons in the striatum as a way of restoring some function. We believe that the same strategy can be employed with sleep disorders, and to do so it is necessary to develop network maps to fully understand the influence of specific neurons on target sites. We have recently shown that hypocretin neurons can be grafted to the pons (Arias-Carrion *et al.*, 2004). However, to be effective we need to know exactly where such transplants, including stem cells or vector-delivered gene therapy, need to be made to reverse specific sleep abnormalities. Toward that end we have embarked on studies to deliver specific genes to treat narcolepsy. In the first of its kind "proof-of-principle" study we found that delivery of the gene for hypocretin into hypocretin knock-out mice significantly decreased narcoleptic behavior (Liu *et al.*, 2008). Such genetic pharmacology approaches are needed now that at least two sleep disorders, narcolepsy (Lin *et al.*, 1999) and restless legs syndrome (Stefansson, *et al.*, 2007; Winkelmann *et al.*, 2007), are linked to specific genes.

Acknowledgments

This work was supported in part by the Department of Veterans Affairs, Veterans Health Administration, Office of Research Development (BLR&D), and NIH grants NS030140, NS052287, MH55772, and HL091363.

References

Arias-Carrion, O., Murillo-Rodriguez, E., Xu, M. *et al.* (2004) Transplantation of hypocretin neurons into the pontine reticular formation: preliminary results. *Sleep* **27**: 1465–70.

Blanco-Centurion, C., Gerashchenko, D., Salin-Pascual, R. J. & Shiromani, P. J. (2004) Effects of hypocretin2-saporin and antidopamine-beta-hydroxylase-saporin neurotoxic lesions of the dorsolateral pons on sleep and muscle tone. *Eur J Neurosci* **19**: 2741–52.

Boissard, R., Fort, P., Gervasoni, D., Barbagli, B. & Luppi, P. H. (2003) Localization of the GABAergic and non-GABAergic neurons projecting to the sublaterodorsal nucleus and potentially gating paradoxical sleep onset. *Eur J Neurosci* **18**: 1627–39.

Chemelli, R. M., Willie, J. T., Sinton, C. M. *et al.* (1999) Narcolepsy in orexin knockout mice: molecular genetics of sleep regulation. *Cell* **98**: 437–51.

Dahlstrom, A. & Fuxe, K. (1964) Evidence for the existence of monoamines in the cell bodies of brain stem neurons. *Acta Physiol* **62**: 1–55.

Hendricks, J. C., Finn, S. M., Panckeri, K. A. *et al.* (1999) Rest in *Drosophila* is a sleep-like state. *Neuron* **25**: 129–38.

Jones, B. E. (2004) Paradoxical REM sleep promoting and permitting neuronal networks. *Arch Ital Biol* **142**: 379–96.

Kaur, S., Thankachan, S., Begum, S. *et al.* (2009) Hypocretin-2 saporin lesions of the ventrolateral periaquaductal gray (vlPAG) increase REM sleep in hypocretin knockout mice. *PLoS ONE* **4**: e6346.

Lin, L., Faraco, J., Li, R. *et al.* (1999) The sleep disorder canine narcolepsy is caused by a mutation in the hypocretin (orexin) receptor 2 gene. *Cell* **98**: 365–76.

Liu, M., Thankachan, S., Kaur, S. *et al.* (2008) Orexin (hypocretin) gene transfer diminishes narcoleptic sleep behavior in mice. *Eur J Neurosci* **28**: 1382–93.

Mitler, M. M., Carskadon, M. A., Czeisler, C.A. *et al.* (1988) Catastrophes, sleep, and public policy: consensus Report. *Sleep* **11**: 100–9.

Moldofsky, H. (1994) Central nervous system and peripheral immune functions and the sleep–wake system. *J Psychiatry Neurosci* **19**: 368–74.

Moruzzi, G. & Magoun, H. W. (1949) Brain stem reticular formation and activation of the EEG. *Electroencephalogr Clin Neurophysiol* **1**: 455–73.

Oliva, A. A. Jr., Jiang, M., Lam, T., Smith, K. L. & Swann, J. W. (2000) Novel hippocampal interneuronal subtypes identified using transgenic mice that express green fluorescent protein in GABAergic interneurons. *J Neurosci* **20**: 3354–68.

Peyron, C., Faraco, J., Rogers, W. *et al.* (2000) A mutation in a case of early onset narcolepsy and a generalized absence of hypocretin peptides in human narcoleptic brains. *Nat Med* **6**: 991–7.

Sakurai, T., Nagata, R., Yamanaka, A. *et al.* (2005) Input of orexin/hypocretin neurons revealed by a genetically encoded tracer in mice. *Neuron* **46**: 297–308.

Sherin, J. E., Shiromani, P. J., McCarley, R. W. & Saper, C. B. (1996) Activation of ventrolateral preoptic neurons during sleep. *Science* **271**: 216–19.

Shiromani, P. J., Kilduff, T. S., Bloom, F. E. & McCarley, R. W. (1992) Cholinergically induced REM sleep triggers Fos-like immunoreactivity in dorsolateral pontine regions associated with REM sleep. *Brain Res* **580**: 351–7.

Stefansson, H., Rye, D. B., Hicks, A. *et al.* (2007) A genetic risk factor for periodic limb movements in sleep. *N Engl J Med* **357**: 639–47.

Steriade, M. & McCarley, R. W. (1990) *Brainstem Control of Wakefulness and Sleep*. New York: Plenum Press.

Thankachan, S., Kaur, S. & Shiromani, P. J. (2009) Activity of pontine neurons during sleep and cataplexy in hypocretin knock-out mice. *J Neurosci* **29**: 1580–5.

Thannickal, T. C., Moore, R. Y., Nienhuis, R. *et al.* (2000) Reduced number of hypocretin neurons in human narcolepsy. *Neuron* **27**: 469–74.

Winkelmann, J., Schormair, B., Lichtner, P. *et al.* (2007) Genome-wide association study of restless legs syndrome identifies common variants in three genomic regions. *Nat Genet* **39**: 1000–6.

Zimmerman, J. E., Naidoo, N., Raizen, D. M. & Pack, A. I. (2008) Conservation of sleep: insights from non-mammalian model systems. *Trends Neurosci* **31**: 371–6.

Chapter 29

Neuronal models of REM-sleep control: evolving concepts

James T. McKenna, Lichao Chen, and Robert W. McCarley

Summary

In this chapter, we will review the recent developments relevant to understanding the neural systems that regulate REM sleep. We will review the initial discovery of REM sleep, followed by a brief description of the polysomnographic characterization of REM sleep. Our discussion will continue with a review of the principal brain-stem executive neurons responsible for REM generation. Pontine reticular formation neurons are involved in the expression of the majority of REM-sleep phenomena, including low-amplitude/high-frequency cortical EEG, the hippocampal theta rhythm, PGO waves/P-waves, and muscle atonia. Cholinergic brain-stem neurons are REM-on, promoting REM sleep; and serotonergic and noradrenergic brain-stem neurons are REM-off, suppressing REM sleep. GABAergic and glutamatergic mechanisms are also integral to REM sleep control. We will also survey the prominent nuclei of the midbrain and forebrain that promote, but do not generate, REM-sleep expression. The conclusion of this chapter will provide a review of three prominent models of REM-sleep regulation: the reciprocal-interaction model; the REM sleep "flip-flop" circuit model; and the revised model of paradoxical (REM) sleep control proposed by Luppi and colleagues.

The discovery of REM sleep

Aserinsky and Kleitman of the University of Chicago were the first to document the sleep state that was accompanied by rapid (R) eye (E) movements (M), and coined the term "REM sleep" (Aserinsky and Kleitman, 1953). This vigilance state was also described in the cat by Jouvet and colleagues (1959a,b,c; for review see Jouvet, 1994), characterized by rapid eye movements, loss of postural muscle tone, and cortical activation similar to that seen during wakefulness (hence termed

"paradoxical sleep", a term still used by groups such as Luppi and colleagues).

Electroencephalographic (EEG) recordings capture field potential activity in the cortex, electromyographic (EMG) recordings reveal general movement and muscle tone, and electrooculographic (EOG) recordings capture eye movement. During REM sleep, the EEG recording is of low-voltage, high-frequency (fast), largely asynchronous activity (LVFA), excluding rhythmicity in higher ranges. This EEG profile is quite similar to that observed during wakefulness. Electromyographic recordings reveal lowest levels of muscle tone, in marked contrast to that seen during wakefulness. Postural muscle movement is suppressed, which is termed muscle atonia. Occasional facial muscle and distant limb twitches occur, as well as regular lateral eye movements, which may be characterized by EOG recording. As well, the physiological phenomena of both hippocampal theta rhythmicity and ponto-geniculo-occipital (PGO) waves are observed.

Brain-stem regulation of REM sleep

Early transection studies

Seminal lesioning experiments by Jouvet and colleagues identified brain-stem nuclei that were responsible for REM-sleep expression (Jouvet *et al.*, 1959c). A transection of the brain at the junction of the midbrain and pons, termed the "pontine cat," abolished the LVFA indicative of REM sleep. Many essential signs of REM sleep were preserved in the brain stem, caudal to this transection, including muscle atonia and rapid eye movements. Also, tegmental neurons increased firing, including the pontine nuclei that generate PGO waves. It was then determined by many investigators that a number of brain-stem nuclei are involved in

REM Sleep: Regulation and Function, eds. Birendra N. Mallick, S. R. Pandi-Perumal, Robert W. McCarley, and Adrian R. Morrison. Published by Cambridge University Press. © Cambridge University Press 2011.

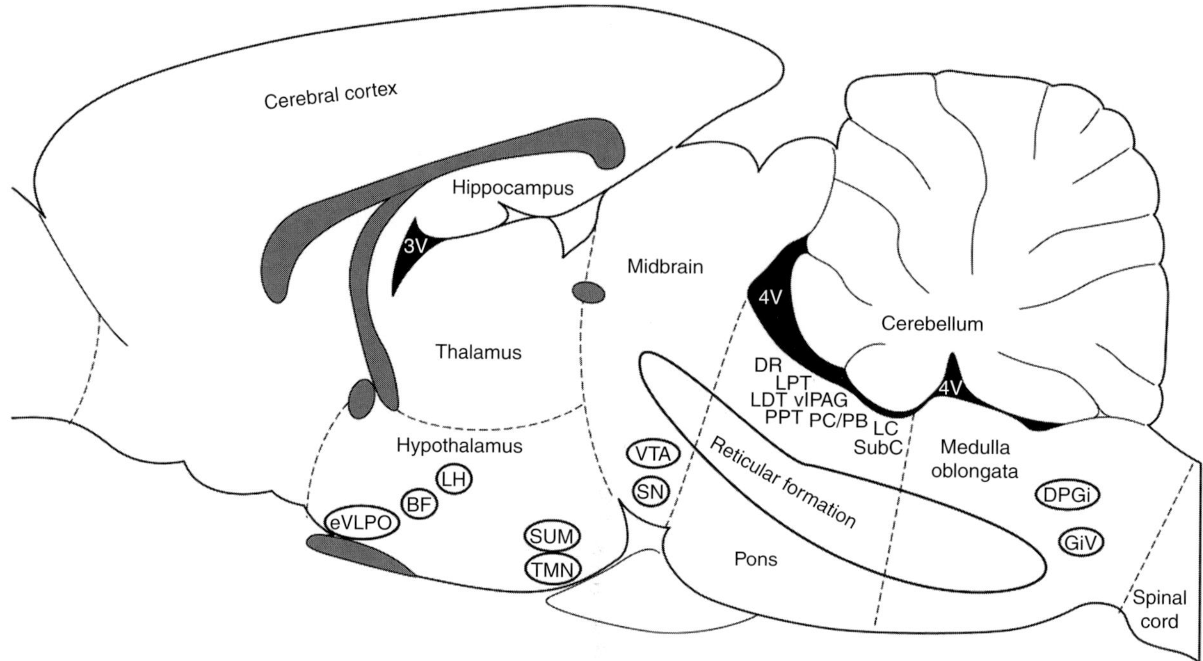

Figure 29.1 A schematic view of nuclei involved in REM-sleep control (adapted from Paxinos and Watson, 1998). Nuclei include: basal forebrain (BF) cholinergic, GABAergic, and putatively glutamatergic; dorsal aspect of the paragigantocellular reticular nucleus (DPGi) GABAergic; dorsal raphe (DR) serotonergic; ventral gigantocellular nucleus (GiV) GABAergic and glycinergic; lateral hypothalamus (LH) orexinergic; extended region of the ventrolateral preoptic nucleus (eVLPO) GABAergic/galaninergic; locus coeruleus (LC) noradrenergic; laterodorsal/pedunculopontine tegmental (PPT/LDT) cholinergic; reticular formation GABAergic and glutamatergic; precoeruleus/parabrachial (PC/PB) glutamatergic; subcoeruleus (SubC, also known as peri-locus coeruleus-alpha or sublaterodorsal nucleus) GABAergic and glutamatergic; substantia nigra (SN) dopaminergic; supramammillary (SUM) glutamatergic; tuberomammillary (TMN) histaminergic; ventrolateral aspect of the periaqueductal gray (vlPAG) GABAergic and glutamatergic; and the ventral tegmental area (VTA) dopaminergic nuclei.

REM sleep generation: the pontine reticular formation (PRF), including the nucleus pontis oralis (PnO) and subcoeruleus (SubC); the REM-on neurons of the cholinergic laterodorsal (LDT) and pedunculopontine tegmental (PPT) nuclei; and the REM-off neurons of the noradrenergic locus coeruleus (LC) and serotonergic raphe nuclei. To help orient the reader to the nuclei important for REM-sleep control, we first present an anatomical schematic of their location (Figure 29.1). Many of the nuclei to be described are anatomically interconnected, acting synergistically in REM-sleep regulation.

The pontine reticular formation, and its role in REM-sleep expression

Early investigations by Moruzzi and Magoun (1949) described the ascending reticular activating system (ARAS). The dorsal ARAS pathway originates in select PRF nuclei, including the PnO, which send glutamatergic projections to midline thalamic nuclei. These thalamic nuclei are reciprocally connected to widespread cortical areas. The ventral ARAS pathway originates in PRF nuclei, which send glutamatergic projections to the basal forebrain and hypothalamic nuclei, which in turn project to the thalamus and cortex. Initial projections of ARAS are largely glutamatergic, although the ventral arousal pathway also includes a number of other neurotransmitter systems, including acetylcholine, norepinephrine, and serotonin. Cholinergic cell populations are active during REM sleep, promoting the LVFA similar to that seen during wakefulness. In addition, it is now known that select midbrain systems are also involved in arousal, including histamine and orexin (also known as hypocretin).

Jouvet and colleagues (1962) were able to produce LVFA by means of electrical stimulation of the PRF and the pontine tegmentum. Many investigations followed, and revealed that PRF activity, particularly PnO, produces many of the physiological events that accompany REM sleep. Lesioning of PRF regions suppressed REM sleep (for a review see McCarley 2004, 2007), and

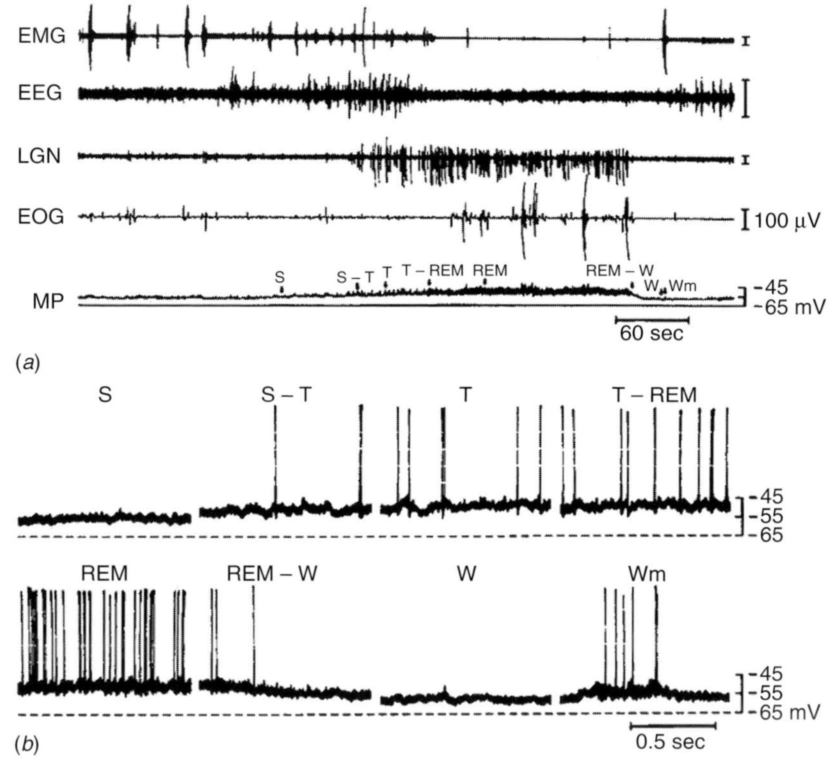

Figure 29.2 Electroencephalograph (EEG) and neuronal recordings of a pontine tegmental neuron over the sleep–wake cycle in the cat. Reticular activity is significantly increased immediately prior to and during REM sleep. (a) The top panel is an electromyogram from the nuchal (neck) muscles, revealing a lack of muscle tone during REM sleep; second trace is an EEG from the frontal cortex, revealing low-amplitude activity during REM sleep; third trace is lateral geniculate nucleus (LGN) activity, showing PGO waves immediately preceding and during REM sleep; fourth trace is an electrooculogram (EOG) from the extra-ocular muscles, revealing eye movement during REM sleep; and the fifth trace is the membrane potential (MP) record of a pontine tegmental neuron. (b) Eight oscilloscope photographs detail the changes in the frequency of action potentials coinciding with MP depolarization. Arrows in the fifth trace of (a) correspond to the eight oscilloscope photographs of (b), which depict tonic neuronal firing during the transition into REM sleep, the REM-sleep episode, and the transition out of REM sleep. Abbreviations: REM, REM sleep; S, sleep; T, transition; W, wake; Wm, wake with movement. (Adapted from Ito et al., 2002.)

extracellular and intracellular recordings in the freely moving cat demonstrated PRF firing during REM sleep (for a review see Steriade and McCarley, 2005). As demonstrated by Ito et al. (2002), little PRF neuronal activity occurs during NREM sleep, for action potentials are not present (Figure 29.2). As REM sleep is entered, the PRF neuronal membrane is depolarized, and action potentials tonically fire as REM sleep progresses. This elevated discharge rate continues throughout REM sleep.

Hippocampal theta rhythm

The theta rhythm is generated by hippocampal field-potential oscillations in the range of 5 to 12 Hz, and is prevalent during REM sleep, as well as during attentional processing, movement, and navigation during wakefulness (for a review see Vertes et al., 2004). The theta rhythm is initially generated in regions of the brain stem, particularly PnO neurons, which tonically fire in relation to the theta rhythm. Some investigators have proposed that the PnO projects to the supramammillary nucleus of the hypothalamus (SUM), where tonic glutamatergic input from the PnO is converted to phasic/rhythmic firing, encoding the theta frequency

that is then transferred to forebrain regions, including the medial septum/vertical limb of the diagonal band in the basal forebrain (MS/DBv) and the hippocampus. GABAergic and cholinergic neurons of the MS/DBv project to the hippocampal formation, as the MS/DBv acts as the "pacemaker" of theta rhythmicity (for a review see Vertes and Kocsis, 1997).

PGO waves/P-waves

Characteristic field potentials in the tegmentum of the pons (P), lateral geniculate nucleus (G), and the occipital cortex (O) coincide with the transitional state that immediately precedes REM sleep (REM-T) (for a review see Steriade and McCarley, 2005). These PGO waves then continue throughout REM sleep, and correlate with the saccadic rapid eye movements of REM sleep, particularly evident during dreaming. Ponto-geniculo-occipital potentials originate in the dorsolateral pons, and these neurons fire in bursts preceding and during PGO waves (Ito et al., 2002; McCarley et al., 1978; Sakai et al., 1976). This pontine activity then propagates via the lateral geniculate nucleus to the occipital cortex. The equivalent of PGO waves during REM sleep in the rat is the "P-wave," for wave propagation from pontine regions to the thalamus has not been shown. Positron emission tomography (PET) scans of the human brain during REM sleep reveal increased activity in both the right geniculate body and occipital cortex of humans during REM sleep (Peigneux *et al.*, 2001), and PGO-like field potentials have been recorded in humans (Lim *et al.*, 2007).

Muscle atonia

Subcoeruleus neurons of the PRF project caudally to medullary glycinergic/GABAergic neurons of the ventral gigantocellular nucleus (GiV) and the spinal cord, and promote muscle atonia during REM sleep. The SubC in the rat brain stem is also defined as the sublaterodorsal nucleus (SLD) and the peri-locus coeruleus-alpha in the cat. Lesions of the SubC suppressed muscle atonia during REM sleep (Sastre and Jouvet, 1979), and lesions that included SubC and neighboring pontine regions elicited "oneiric" (dream-like) behavior, as the cat exhibited attack behavior and postural muscle movement during REM sleep (Hendricks *et al.*, 1982). Subcoeruleus neurons tonically fire immediately prior to and during muscle atonia, and electrical stimulation of the SubC elicited muscle atonia (for a review see Chase and Morales, 1990). Gigantocellular nucleus glycinergic/GABAergic output inhibits the spinal cord motoneurons responsible for postural muscle tone. Muscle atonia results from hyperpolarization of these motoneurons. Therefore, SubC activity during REM sleep promotes GiV glycinergic/GABAergic output. Spinal cord motoneurons are then inhibited, and muscle atonia results.

Cholinergic mechanisms involved in REM-sleep expression

Cholinergic neurons located in the LDT/PPT are integral to REM sleep regulation. Select neurons in the LDT/PPT are "Wake/REM-on," for discharge activity increases during both wakefulness and REM sleep. Other cholinergic LDT/PPT neurons are specifically "REM-on," for these neurons selectively discharge immediately preceding and during REM sleep (El Mansari *et al.*, 1989; Steriade *et al.*, 1990). The LDT/PPT neurons begin to fire immediately preceding REM sleep, and activity continues throughout the REM sleep episode. Injection of muscarinic agonists, acetylcholinesterase inhibitors, or the cholinergic agonist carbachol into the PRF induced an REM-like sleep state (for a review see Steriade and McCarley, 2005). The protein product of the immediate early gene c-Fos may be immunohistochemically labeled, providing a useful tool to document neuronal activity within the preceding hour before sacrifice of the animal (Kovacs, 2008). c-Fos protein expression studies indicated that LDT/PPT neurons are active during REM sleep (Maloney *et al.*, 1999; Merchant-Nancy *et al.*, 1995), although other investigators were not able to replicate these findings (Lu *et al.*, 2006b; Sapin *et al.*, 2009).

Serotonergic and noradrenergic mechanisms involved in REM-sleep suppression

In contrast to cholinergic "REM-on" neurons, other subsets of brain-stem nuclei fire at a high discharge rate during wakefulness, lower rate during NREM sleep, and largely cease activity immediately preceding and during REM sleep. These neurons are REM-off, and include the serotonergic neurons of the raphe nuclei, and the noradrenergic (NA) neurons of the locus coeruleus (LC). The interplay of REM-on and REM-off cell populations allows transition into and out of REM sleep, and provides the basis of the reciprocal-interaction model later described.

The REM-off neuronal activity in the dorsal raphe nucleus (DR) has been documented by many investigators (for a review see McCarley, 2007). Corresponding to this REM-off discharge, levels of serotonin in the DR are highest during wakefulness, decrease during NREM sleep, and reach lowest levels during REM sleep (Portas *et al.*, 1994; Trulson and Jacobs, 1979). Thakkar *et al.* (1998) investigated "Wake/REM-on" and REM-on cell discharge activity of the LDT/PPT in the freely moving cat following infusion of 8-OH-DPAT, a serotonergic auto-receptor agonist. Serotonin levels in the DR were highest during wake, lower during NREM sleep, and lowest during REM sleep, inversely correlated to LDT/PPT neuronal discharge, as well as the corresponding vigilance state expression. Microdialysis infusion of 8-OH-DPAT into the LDT/PPT specifically inhibited REM-on cells, but not "Wake/REM-on" neurons.

Jouvet and colleagues reported that lesions of the locus coeruleus (LC) promoted REM sleep (Jouvet *et al.*, 1965). Locus coeruleus NA neurons were determined to be REM-off in the cat, rat, and monkey (for a review see Mallick *et al.*, 2002; McCarley, 2007). Locus coeruleus neurons, similar to the serotonergic neurons of the raphe, discharge at highest rates during wakefulness, decrease activity during NREM sleep, and largely cease activity during REM sleep. Numerous studies, using reversible inactivation and lesioning techniques, also show that the LC NA neurons are "REM off."

GABAergic mechanisms involved in REM sleep

Recent investigations have suggested that brain-stem GABAergic neurons play a central role in REM-sleep regulation (Fort *et al.*, 2009; Lu *et al.*, 2006b; McCarley, 2007). Brown, McKenna, and colleagues (2008) mapped GABAergic cell populations in the mouse mesopontine junction, including the PnO and SubC, employing a GAD67/green fluorescent protein knock-in mouse model. This distribution of GFP-positive neurons paralleled that described of GABAergic neurons in the rat (Boissard *et al.*, 2003; Ford *et al.*, 1995; Sapin *et al.*, 2009). GABAergic afferent systems to the PRF were distributed throughout the PRF itself, as well as such brain-stem regions as the ventrolateral periaqueductal gray (vlPAG), lateral pontine tegmentum (LPT), and the dorsal aspect of the paragigantocellular reticular nucleus (DPGi) (Boissard *et al.*, 2003).

REM-on GABAergic brain-stem mechanisms

Subpopulations of GABAergic neurons were shown to be involved in REM-sleep regulation. During REM-sleep deprivation (when REM sleep amounts were minimized), GABAergic/c-Fos co-localization increased in regions of the PRF, including the PnO and LPT (Maloney *et al.*, 1999, 2000). During REM sleep-deprivation recovery (when REM sleep amounts were elevated), co-localization in these PRF regions was also particularly high (Lu *et al.*, 2006b; Maloney *et al.*, 1999, 2000; Sapin *et al.*, 2009). These findings suggest that GABAergic subpopulations of the PRF may both promote or suppress REM activity. Consistent with the proposed REM-on role of the PRF GABAergic populations, GABA levels in the PRF are highest during wake, decreased during NREM sleep, and at lowest levels during REM sleep (McCarley, 2004).

A prevalent LDT/PPT cholinergic projection to the PRF is a principal pathway by which REM sleep may be promoted (Mitani *et al.*, 1988). GABAergic SubC neurons were excited by carbachol application in vitro, as well as approximately 65% of PnO GABAergic cells (Brown *et al.*, 2008). During REM sleep, REM-on cholinergic LDT/PPT activity may excite PRF REM-on GABAergic neurons, which may then inhibit such REM-off regions as the DR and LC during REM sleep (McCarley, 2007).

REM-on GABAergic output may inhibit REM-off DR activity during REM sleep. GABAergic input to the DR from preoptic regions, the lateral hypothalamus, vlPAG, PnO, and DPGi has been shown (Gervasoni *et al.*, 2000). In vivo extracellular microdialysis sampling in the cat revealed that GABA levels increased in the DR as REM sleep began (Nitz and Siegel, 1997a). Administration of the GABA agonist muscimol into the DR increased REM sleep, while injection of GABA antagonists (bicuculline) abolished REM sleep, and activated DR neurons that were usually quiet during slow-wave sleep (Gervasoni *et al.*, 1998, 2000; Levine and Jacobs, 1992). Sakai and Crochet (2001) were not able to replicate these effects on DR activity or REM sleep.

GABAergic neurons in the proximity of the LC terminate on LC NA neurons (Aston-Jones *et al.*, 2004), which may provide a direct route by which PRF REM-on GABAergic neurons inhibit LC NA REM-off activity. GABA levels in the LC and the neighboring SubC were significantly increased during REM sleep, when compared to wakefulness or NREM sleep (Nitz and Siegel, 1997b). Microiontophoretic injection of GABA in the LC increased REM sleep (Alam *et al.*, 1993; Mallick *et al.*, 2001), and injection of the GABA antagonist picrotoxin decreased REM sleep amounts (Kaur *et al.*, 2004; Mallick *et al.*, 2001). Bicuculline infusion into the LC during either NREM or REM sleep restored the firing of LC neurons, and during wake increased the discharge firing rate (Gervasoni *et al.*, 1998).

Substantial GABAergic projections to the DR and LC also originate in both the vlPAG/LPT and DPGi (Gervasoni *et al.*, 2000). Retrograde injections into the LC, combined with c-Fos double labeling, revealed a substantial number of double-labeled neurons in these nuclei during REM-sleep rebound (Verret *et al.*, 2006). It was proposed that both GABAergic and non-GABAergic, presumed glutamatergic, populations within the vlPAG/LPT, as well as GABAergic populations of the DPGi, are REM-on, and inhibit REM-off DR and LC (Luppi *et al.*, 2006; Sapin *et al.*, 2009). Bicuculline infusion into the DPGi blocked the discharge of approximately 90% of LC neurons (Ennis and Aston-Jones, 1989a,b), and electrical stimulation of the DPGi promoted REM-sleep expression (Kaur *et al.*, 2001).

REM-off GABAergic brain-stem mechanisms

GABAergic input to the PRF may be regarded as REM-off, inhibiting REM-on PRF neurons and consequently suppressing REM sleep. GABA levels in PRF regions of the cat were lowest during REM sleep (McCarley, 2004). Infusion of GABA or GABA receptor agonists into the SubC or PnO suppressed REM sleep, and promoted wakefulness. Conversely, infusion of GABA-A receptor antagonists induced REM sleep and promoted muscle atonia (Boissard *et al.*, 2002; Xi *et al.*, 1999a,b; 2001a,b). Injection of antisense oligonucleotides for GAD mRNA into the SubC promoted REM-sleep expression (Xi *et al.*, 1999a). Interestingly, Brown *et al.* (2008) also described a GABAergic neuronal subpopulation in the PnO that was inhibited by carbachol in vitro. As suggested, LDT/PPT cholinergic input to the PRF may disinhibit the glutamatergic output of the PRF during REM sleep by means of a GABAergic intermediary (Brown *et al.*, 2006, 2008).

The vlPAG/LPT GABAergic neurons may also play an inhibitory role in REM sleep regulation. Ventrolateral periaqueductal gray lesions and muscimol injections have been shown to produce a large REM-sleep increase (Boissard *et al.*, 2003; Sastre *et al.*, 1996). Accordingly, it was suggested that select vlPAG/LPT neurons may be REM-off. c-Fos protein expression was documented in a subpopulation of GABAergic vlPAG/LPT neurons during REM-sleep deprivation (Sapin *et al.*, 2009), as well as during the REM rebound following deprivation (Maloney *et al.*, 1999; Sapin *et al.*, 2009). REM-off vlPAG/LPT GABAergic neurons may inhibit REM-on SubC activity. The SubC neurons received inhibitory input from local GABAergic neurons within the SubC, as well as from other nuclei (Boissard *et al.*, 2003). Anterograde tracing, combined with c-Fos protein activation studies, found a substantial vlPAG projection to c-Fos-labeled cells in the SubC during REM sleep, and vlPAG projections to the SubC were determined to be GABAergic (Lu *et al.*, 2006a).

As reviewed below, brain-stem GABAergic mechanisms have been integrated into the updated version of the reciprocal-interaction model proposed by McCarley and colleagues. An alternative model has been proposed by Lu *et al.* (2006b), termed the REM sleep "flip-flop" circuit model. These investigators propose that the interplay of REM-off vlPAG/LPT GABAergic and REM-on SubC REM-on GABAergic neurons allows transition into and out of REM sleep.

The revised model of paradoxical sleep control, proposed by Luppi and colleagues, suggests that, during REM sleep, vlPAG and DPGi GABAergic REM-on activity inhibits a number of REM-off nuclei, including the DR, LC, and LPT (Fort *et al.*, 2009).

Non-brain stem nuclei involved in REM-sleep regulation

Following the seminal Jouvet transection study, it was concluded that the nuclei responsible for the generation of REM sleep reside in the brain stem, and nuclei rostral to this transection may promote, but do not generate, REM sleep. Such non-brain stem nuclei are involved in the expression of some of the physiological trademarks of REM sleep, including LVFA, PGO waves, the hippocampal theta rhythm, and muscle atonia.

Orexinergic nuclei of the lateral hypothalamus

The neuropeptide orexin (also called hypocretin), located in the perifornical region of the hypothalamus (LH), may play a unique role in vigilance regulation (for a review see Brown, 2003). Widespread orexinergic input may excite REM sleep-related circuitry, by means of projections to such nuclei as the LC, DR, and SubC (Peyron *et al.*, 1998). Orexinergic neurons fire most during wakefulness, decrease activity during NREM sleep, and largely discontinue firing during REM sleep (Lee *et al.*, 2005; Mileykovskiy *et al.*, 2005). Kiyashchenko *et al.* (2002) described highest levels of orexin in the perifornical region of the hypothalamus, BF, and LC during wakefulness, when compared to NREM sleep. In vitro investigations reported that application of wake-promoting agents excited neurons in the LH (Brown, 2003). In vitro orexin application excites a number of REM-sleep regulatory populations, including serotonergic DR (Brown *et al.*, 2002; Liu *et al.*, 2002) and noradrenergic LC neurons (Hagan *et al.*, 1999; Horvath *et al.*, 1999). Interestingly, GABAergic neurons in both the PnO and SubC were excited by orexin application in vitro (Brown *et al.*, 2008). Orexinergic input to the SubC appears to be important in the regulation of muscle atonia. Luppi and colleagues also propose that orexinergic input to the LPT REM-off GABAergic neurons may play an integral role in REM-sleep transitions (Luppi *et al.*, 2006).

Loss of orexinergic neurons is one of the hallmark features of the sleep disorder narcolepsy. A deficit of the orexin type 2 receptor in narcoleptic dogs was first reported by Lin *et al.* (1999), and in the same year another investigation revealed that orexin knockout mice exhibited decreased wakefulness, as well as behavioral arrest immediately following wakefulness (Chemelli *et al.*, 1999). These abnormal transitions were similar to the narcoleptic symptoms of cataplexy and sleep-onset REM episodes. Lesioning or knockdown of orexinergic neurons produced narcoleptic-like symptoms, including increased transitions between vigilance states, as well as abnormal expression of REM sleep-like characteristics during wakefulness (Chen *et al.*, 2006, 2009; Mochizuki *et al.*, 2004).

Of particular interest, orexin may play a unique role in REM-sleep transition, by means of excitation of REM-off neurons. Infusion of orexin type 2 receptor antisense in the PRF significantly increased REM sleep, and video recordings showed episodes of behavioral cataplexy (Thakkar *et al.*, 1999). Short interfering RNA (siRNA) targeting prepro-orexin mRNA was microinjected into the rat LH, in order to reversibly inactivate orexinergic neurons (Chen *et al.*, 2006). The number of REM-sleep episodes increased during the dark period for four days post-injection. Because these effects were particular to the dark period, it was proposed that orexin may be part of the diurnal gating of REM sleep expression. In support of this suggestion, orexinergic knock-out animals exhibit abnormal circadian modulation of REM sleep (Mochizuki *et al.*, 2004), and orexin neurons are necessary for the circadian suppression of REM sleep (Kantor *et al.*, 2009). An abnormality in diurnal gating due to orexinergic hypofunction, such as seen in narcolepsy, would lead to abnormal expression of REM-sleep related phenomena during inappropriate times, such as when the individual is awake during the day.

Melanin-concentrating hormone nuclei of the lateral hypothalamus

Some investigators have recently proposed that melanin-concentrating hormone (MCH) positive neurons of the lateral hypothalamus may also promote REM sleep (for example, Peyron *et al.*, 2009). Amounts of REM sleep, and to a lesser extent NREM sleep, were increased following icv injection of MCH (Verret *et al.*, 2003). Many neurons within the lateral hypothalamus and the neighboring zona incerta were immunopositive for c-Fos following REM-sleep rebound, and approximately 50% of these neurons were positive

for MCH. Carbachol-induced REM sleep in the cat did not lead to co-localization of the c-Fos protein in MCH neurons though (Torterolo *et al.*, 2006). Hassani *et al.* (2009) recently reported that MCH neurons discharged maximally during REM sleep, and this discharge activity was reciprocal to the firing of a number of REM-off cell populations including that of LH orexinergic neurons.

GABAergic/galaninergic ventrolateral preoptic nuclei

The extended region of the ventrolateral preoptic nucleus (eVLPO) may also play a role in the regulation of LVFA and muscle atonia (Lu *et al.*, 2006b). The VLPO projects to a number of REM sleep-related brain-stem nuclei (for a review see McGinty and Szymusiak, 2001), and these projections were proposed to be GABAergic/galaninergic (Sherin *et al.*, 1998). REM sleep amounts were decreased following lesions in the vicinity of the eVLPO (Lu *et al.*, 2000). Employing dark-exposure enhancement of REM sleep in the rat, Lu and colleagues (2002) reported an elevation of c-Fos activation in the eVLPO. Therefore, it was proposed that the eVLPO promotes REM-sleep expression. Lu and colleagues suggest that eVLPO REM-on galaninergic/GABAergic inhibition of vlPAG REM-off populations may promote REM sleep. In another study, though, retrograde tracer injection into the LC, combined with c-Fos labeling, depicted only sparse co-localization in the eVLPO (Verret *et al.*, 2006). This alternative hypothesis by Lu and colleagues, that the eVLPO may be REM-on, will be described below in our discussion of the REM-sleep "flip-flop" model.

The reciprocal-interaction model

McCarley and Hobson originally proposed the reciprocal-interaction model, in order to explain transitions into and out of REM sleep (Hobson *et al.*, 1975). These transitions were based on the interplay between REM-on and REM-off brain-stem neurons, described by Lotka-Volterra equations, which are derived from population models of prey/predator interaction (McCarley and Hobson, 1975a,b). Updated versions of the model (for example, McCarley, 2007), including the limit cycle model, incorporate the possible role of inhibitory circuitry, such as GABAergic neurons, as well as circadian influences (McCarley and Massaquoi, 1986a,b).

REM-sleep transitions

REM-on neurons of the brain stem include the cholinergic neurons of the LDT/PPT. Certain regions of the PRF, such as the PnO, were first described as REM-on, although more recent versions of the model now describe the LDT/PPT cholinergic neurons as the principal REM-on neurons. The LDT/PPT neurons, by means of projections to the PRF, promote the expression of a number of REM-sleep related characteristics. The transition into an REM-sleep episode begins, as REM-on LDT/PPT neurons become more active. The REM-sleep episode is maintained by the mutually positive feedback between LDT/PPT and PRF neurons. As the REM-sleep episode approaches conclusion, REM-off neurons become active, due to REM-on excitation. REM-off activation reaches a level that REM-on neurons begin to decrease activity, and the REM-sleep episode is eventually terminated.

The updated reciprocal-interaction model

The modified reciprocal-interaction model incorporates GABAergic mechanisms, as now depicted in the updated reciprocal-interaction model (Figure 29.3). It remains to be determined what mechanism may inhibit REM-off neuronal activity, then allowing REM-on neuronal expression at the beginning of the REM-sleep episode. This mechanism may include the recurrent projections within and between LC and DR REM-off neurons. Levels of serotonin and noradrenaline build up during wakefulness and NREM sleep, and REM-off activity consequently decreases as autoreceptors within these systems are activated. As proposed earlier in this chapter, LDT/PPT cholinergic neurons may inhibit GABAergic interneurons of the PRF. In turn, PRF glutamatergic excitatory neurons are disinhibited, and REM sleep is promoted. Some GABAergic PRF PnO and SubC neurons were inhibited by carbachol administration in vitro (Brown *et al.*, 2008). Gerber *et al.* (1991) described in vivo inhibition of some PRF neurons by application of carbachol or another cholinergic agonist, methacholine, although GABAergic phenotyping of these cells was not performed. Also, GABA levels were found to be significantly decreased in the PRF during REM sleep (McCarley, 2004), and application of GABAergic antagonists directly into PRF regions produced REM sleep (Xi *et al.*, 1999a,b, 2001a,b).

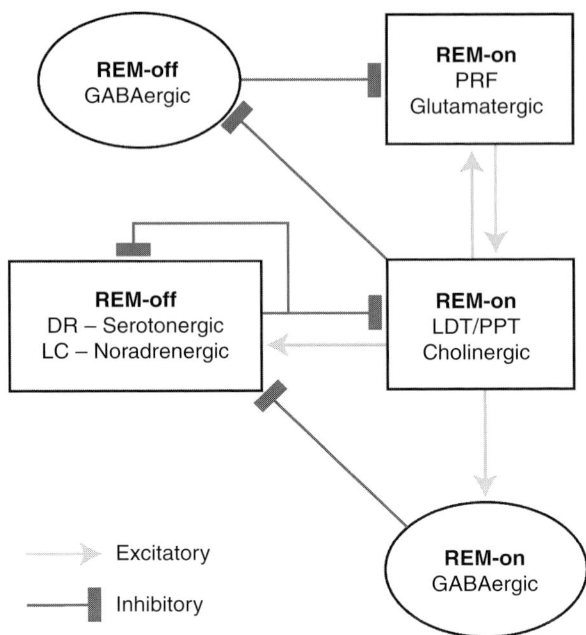

Figure 29.3 Graphic depiction of the modified reciprocal-interaction model of REM-sleep control, originally proposed by McCarley and Hobson (1975a,b), and here modified from McCarley (2007). The dorsal raphe (DR) and locus coeruleus (LC) REM-off neurons inhibit laterodorsal/pedunculopontine tegmental nuclei (LDT/PPT) REM-on neurons during waking and NREM sleep. Self-inhibition of these REM-off neurons leads to disinhibition of REM-on neurons, allowing REM sleep to begin. LDT/PPT REM-on activity excites PRF (pontine reticular formation) glutamatergic REM-on cells that are responsible for muscle atonia, PGO waves, and hippocampal theta rhythmicity during REM sleep. REM-on cells begin to excite the REM-off cells as REM sleep progresses, leading to eventual REM-sleep cessation. REM-on LDT/PPT neurons excite local GABAergic interneurons, in turn inhibiting REM-off neurons. Also, REM-on output inhibits GABAergic REM-off interneurons, which then inhibit REM-on PRF neurons. Red lines denote excitation; blue, inhibition. (See plate section for color version.)

Cholinergic LDT/PPT neurons may also excite GABAergic REM-on cell populations, such as the LC and DR interneurons, which in turn suppress REM-off principal neuronal activity. Cholinergic LDT/PPT neurons project directly to the REM-off neurons described in this chapter, including the LC and DR. Interestingly, carbachol administration into the LC induced wakefulness, as well as increased activity in this region. Such effects were not found in the DR though (Li *et al.*, 1998). Because of this finding, it may be proposed that the LDT/PPT may act directly on NA neurons, but indirectly on DR neurons by means of intermediary PRF excitation. As previously reviewed in this chapter, PRF regions project to both the DR and LC. Interestingly, Mallick and colleagues simultaneously recorded neurons with both "REM-on" and "REM-off" profiles in the same animal preparation (Mallick *et al.*, 1998).

GABA levels increase significantly in the DR and LC during REM sleep (Nitz and Siegel, 1997a,b), and administration of GABAergic agonists into the DR and LC suppressed neuronal activity. Infusion of the GABA antagonist bicuculline led to neuronal discharge in the LC and DR during NREM and REM sleep (Gervasoni *et al.*, 1998, 2000). When REM sleep amounts were elevated, c-Fos protein expression in GAD-positive neurons of the DR and LC was significantly increased (Maloney *et al.*, 1999). Therefore, local GABA interneuronal activity may inhibit DR and LC REM-off activity during REM sleep. It remains to be determined if there is an inverse relation between GABAergic interneuronal vs. principal neuronal (serotonergic DR or noradrenergic LC) firing. Recently, Mallick and colleagues proposed that GABAergic input to the PPT may act to promote REM sleep (Pal and Mallick, 2009).

Circadian variation is evident in the ultradian rhythm of REM-sleep episode cycling. That is, the first REM-sleep episode of the human night is usually of less amplitude and time span, compared to concurrent episodes. According to the reciprocal-interaction model, if no excitatory input is provided to REM-off neurons, the REM-sleep episode is continued. REM-off activity may be high earlier in the night, and decrease as subsequent REM-sleep episodes occur. Orexin may exert a stronger excitatory influence on REM-off populations earlier in the night, and as orexinergic influence wanes, REM-off influences decrease, and REM-sleep episodes consequently increase in amplitude and length as the night progresses. Recent evidence suggests that the dorsomedial suprachiasmatic nucleus, which receives projections from orexin neurons, controls REM-sleep timing (Lee *et al.*, 2009).

Alternative REM-sleep transition models

Lesions of various brain-stem nuclei, reviewed here as the executive neurons involved in REM-sleep generation and maintenance, do not always lead to significant alterations of REM sleep. Therefore, such laboratories as Saper and Luppi have proposed that GABAergic and glutamatergic populations play a central executive role as REM-on and REM-off neurons.

The REM-sleep "flip-flop" circuit model

Lu and colleagues (2006b) proposed an alternative model of REM-sleep regulation (Figure 29.4a). GABAergic vlPAG/LPT REM-off projections inhibit GABAergic SubC (SLD) REM-on neurons. Subcoeruleus neurons then mutually inhibit the vlPAG/LPT neurons, providing a "flip-flop."

GABAergic vlPAG/LPT REM-off projections inhibit GABAergic SubC and glutamatergic PC/PB REM-on neurons during wakefulness and NREM sleep. During REM sleep, REM-on GABAergic/galaninergic eVLPO output inhibits REM-off vlPAG/LPT regions, in turn disinhibiting SubC and PB/PC REM-on neurons. The PB/PC projects rostrally to the basal forebrain, thalamus, and cortex, which, as described, play a crucial role in the generation and maintenance of LVFA and the hippocampal theta rhythm. Alternatively, output of vlPAG/LPT terminating on the SubC may play a role in regulating the muscle atonia of REM sleep. As previously described, SubC glutamatergic output excites the inhibitory GABAergic/glycinergic ventral medulla output to motor neurons in the spinal cord. Lu *et al.* (2006b) propose an alternative route, as SubC (presumed glutamatergic) neurons project to GABAergic interneurons of the spinal cord, bypassing GiV. These interneurons in turn inhibit the spinal cord motor neurons.

The revised model of REM (paradoxical) sleep control (Luppi and colleagues)

Recently, Luppi and colleagues proposed an alternative model of the brain-stem mechanisms responsible for paradoxical (REM) sleep regulation (for a review see Fort *et al.*, 2009). Subcoeruleus (SLD) GABAergic neurons were not determined to be REM-on, which was previously posited (Lu *et al.*, 2006b). Therefore, REM sleep is not generated by the mutually inhibitory "flip-flop" between GABAergic REM-off vlPAG/LPT and GABAergic REM-on SubC neurons. The Luppi revised model is depicted in Figure 29.4b. During REM sleep, vlPAG and DPGi GABAergic REM-on neurons inhibit REM-off activity in the DR, LC, and LPT. During the transition to REM sleep, as well as during REM sleep, this GABAergic "REM-on" input inhibits local interneuronal REM-off GABAergic populations.

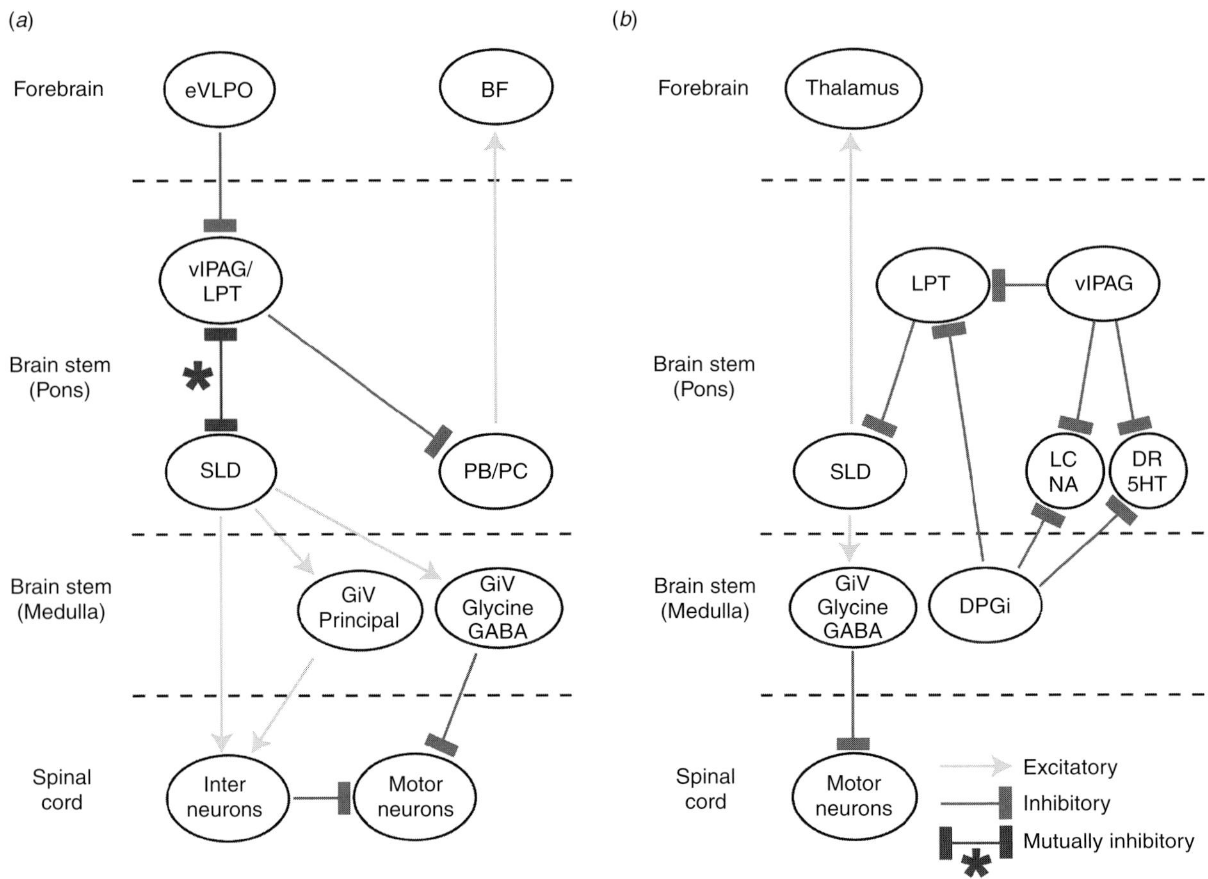

Figure 29.4 Graphic depiction of two suggested models of REM-sleep control. (*a*) The REM-sleep "flip-flop" circuit model of Lu and colleagues (2006b); this REM regulatory model is different from the NREM sleep/wake "flip-flop" switch previously proposed (Saper *et al.*, 2001). During REM sleep, REM-off vlPAG/LPT regions are inhibited by GABAergic/galaninergic eVLPO input, in turn releasing GABAergic and glutamatergic SLD (also known as the subcoeruleus, SubC) and glutamatergic PB/PC neurons. The SLD GABAergic REM-on neurons mutually inhibit vlPAG/LPT GABAergic REM-off neurons, providing a "flip-flop" (asterisk). The PB/PC projects rostrally to the basal forebrain, and plays a crucial role in the expression of LVFA and the hippocampal theta rhythm. The SLD glutamatergic descending output excites GiV principal cells, which in turn excite spinal cord interneurons. These glycinergic/GABAergic interneurons inhibit spinal-cord motoneuronal activity, and muscle atonia results. Also, SLD output excites GiV glycinergic/GABAergic neurons, which directly inhibit the spinal-cord motoneurons. The SLD may also directly excite the inhibitory spinal-cord interneurons, bypassing GiV. (*b*) The revised model of paradoxical sleep control proposed by Luppi and colleagues. During REM sleep, vlPAG and DPGi GABAergic REM-on neurons inhibit DR, LC, and LPT REM-off activity. The SLD glutamatergic output ascends to forebrain regions responsible for LVFA, such as the thalamus, and descends to activate the GiV glycinergic/GABAergic output responsible for muscle atonia. Recent work suggests that GABAergic MCH REM-on hypothalamic neurons may inhibit vlPAG REM-off neurons, thereby promoting REM sleep. We further note that this sketch, adapted from Fort *et al.* (2009, Figure 1), is somewhat less complex than suggested in the Fort *et al.* review's text. Abbreviations: BF, basal forebrain; DPGi, dorsal aspect of the paragigantocellular reticular nucleus; DR, dorsal raphe nucleus; eVLPO, extended region of the ventrolateral preoptic nucleus; GiV, medullary ventral gigantocellular nucleus; LC, locus coeruleus; LPT, lateral pontine tegmentum; PB/PC, parabrachial/precoeruleus nuclei; SLD, sublaterodorsal nucleus, also known as the subcoeruleus SubC; vlPAG, ventrolateral aspect of the periaqueductal gray. Red lines denote excitation; blue, inhibition; and green with asterisk, mutual inhibition. (See plate section for color version.)

The vlPAG REM-on populations inhibit LPT REM-off populations, which usually inhibit SubC REM-on neurons. Therefore, vlPAG REM-on activity disinhibits (releases) SubC REM-on activity during REM. Subcoeruleus glutamatergic output then descends to activate the GiV GABAergic/glycinergic output to the spinal motoneurons responsible for muscle atonia.

Although not shown in Figure 29.4b, Luppi and colleagues also propose that a select group of GABAergic neurons of the lateral hypothalamus and neighboring regions, which are co-localized with MCH, are REM-on, inhibiting TMN histaminergic, LH orexinergic, LC noradrenergic, and raphe serotonergic REM-off neuronal populations (Fort *et al.*, 2009). Also, MCH neurons may inhibit neurons of the VLPO cluster that particularly promote NREM sleep. Lastly, inhibitory MCH connections to the REM-off vlPAG/LPT may also promote REM-sleep expression. In this model, MCH LH, GABAergic vlPAG, and GABAergic DPGi neurons are all REM-on (Fort *et al.*, 2009).

Questions arising

Problems with models of purely inhibitory components

The reader will have noticed that these two models just presented (Lu and colleagues' "flip-flop" model, and Luppi and colleagues' revised model of paradoxical sleep control) have exclusively inhibitory mechanisms at the center of their models for periodic occurrence of REM sleep. These models are mathematically and structurally not capable of cyclic alternation unless some excitatory input is present to drive the model out of a purely quiescent state. This input is not specified. It is thus not clear how transitions may occur between inhibitory populations in the Lu and colleagues' "flip-flop" model (REM-off vlPAG/LPT GABAergic neurons, and REM-on SubC GABAergic neurons) and the Luppi group's model. The system remains "on" or "off" (flipped or flopped) at any point, and a third external agent outside this interaction is needed for state transition. Moreover no explicit timing mechanism is proposed for the generation of rhythmic cycles with regular duration.

Limitations of lesion models

In the "flip-flop" model proposed by Lu and colleagues (Lu *et al.*, 2006b), the neuronal populations described as REM-on and REM-off previously (LDT/PPT cholinergic REM-on, DR serotonergic REM-off, and LC noradrenergic REM-off) are not essential executive neurons involved in REM-sleep generation, but are modulators of REM-sleep activity. Lesioning an area to characterize its role in REM-sleep expression may at times lead to no obvious effect on REM-sleep expression. This does not nullify its role in REM-sleep expression, though, due to the redundancy in REM-sleep generating and sustaining systems, as described here in this chapter.

Limitations of pharmacological experiments

The Luppi group's model relies heavily on pharmacological experiments often without recordings of neuronal activity during natural REM cycles to confirm the role of nuclei in REM-sleep regulation. For example, although abundant recordings of SubC/SLD neurons are available, no recordings of vlPAG neurons during natural REM sleep have been done that would confirm their revised model.

Limitations of c-Fos protein expression as an indicator of neuronal activity

c-Fos expression is an imperfect indicator of neuronal activity. The immunohistochemical localization of the c-Fos protein does not always reflect neuronal activation (Kovacs, 2008). Therefore, investigators should be aware that this technique may lead to "false negative" findings. Both the "flip-flop" model and the revised REM-sleep model of Luppi and colleagues assume that the lack of c-Fos protein expression indicates a lack of neuronal activity. Further evidence such as electrophysiological recordings, including phenotyping of recorded neurons, must be performed in order to conclude that neurons are indeed not active. Lu *et al.* (2006b) acknowledge that electrophysiological recordings of cellular activity are needed to confirm their model.

As reviewed in this chapter, substantial progress has been made in the last fifty years to identify the cell populations, neurotransmitters, and mechanisms responsible for REM-sleep regulation. These investigations utilized a number of newly developed techniques, including pharmacological, lesioning, electrophysiological, and molecular-level technologies. Some questions remain, though, concerning the brain circuitry and mechanisms responsible for REM-sleep regulation. Future investigations will further inform pharmacological and behavioral treatments for sleep disorders such as narcolepsy and REM-sleep behavior disorder.

Acknowledgments

We thank Ritchie E. Brown for editorial review. This research was supported by the US Department of Veterans Affairs Medical Research Awards to RWM; NIH HL060292, MH039683, MH040799.

References

Alam, N. M, Kumari, S. & Mallick, B. N. (1993) Role of GABA in acetylcholine-induced locus coeruleus mediated increases in REM. *Sleep Res* **22**: 541.

Aserinsky, E. & Kleitman, N. (1953) Regularly occurring periods of eye motility, and concomitant phenomena, during sleep. *Science* **118**: 273–4.

Aston-Jones, G., Zhu, Y. & Card, J. P. (2004) Numerous GABAergic afferents to locus ceruleus in the pericerulear dendritic zone: possible interneuronal pool. *J Neurosci* **24**: 2313–21.

Boissard, R., Fort, P., Gervasoni, D., Barbagli, B. & Luppi, P. H. (2003) Localization of the GABAergic and non-GABAergic neurons projecting to the sublaterodorsal nucleus and potentially gating paradoxical sleep onset. *Eur J Neurosci* **18**: 1627–39.

Boissard, R., Gervasoni, D., Schmidt, M. H. *et al.* (2002) The rat ponto-medullary network responsible for paradoxical sleep onset and maintenance: a combined microinjection and functional neuroanatomical study. *Eur J Neurosci* **16**: 1959–73.

Brown, R. E. (2003) Involvement of hypocretins/orexins in sleep disorders and narcolepsy. *Drug News Perspect* **16**: 75–9.

Brown, R. E., McKenna, J. T., Winston, S. *et al.* (2008) Characterization of GABAergic neurons in rapid-eye-movement sleep controlling regions of the brainstem reticular formation in GAD67-green fluorescent protein knock-in mice. *Eur J Neurosci* **27**: 352–63.

Brown, R. E., Sergeeva, O. A., Eriksson, K. S. & Haas, H. L. (2002) Convergent excitation of dorsal raphe serotonin neurons by multiple arousal systems (orexin/hypocretin, histamine and noradrenaline). *J Neurosci* **22**: 8850–9.

Brown, R. E., Winston, S., Basheer, R., Thakkar, M. M. & McCarley, R. W. (2006) Electrophysiological characterization of neurons in the dorsolateral pontine rapid-eye-movement sleep induction zone of the rat: intrinsic membrane properties and responses to carbachol and orexins. *Neuroscience* **143**: 739–55.

Chase, M. H. & Morales, F. R. (1990) The atonia and myoclonia of active (REM) sleep. *Ann Rev Psychol* **41**: 557–84.

Chemelli, R. M., Willie, J. T., Sinton, C. M. *et al.* (1999) Narcolepsy in orexin knockout mice: molecular genetics of sleep regulation. *Cell* **98**: 437–51.

Chen, L., Brown, R. E., McKenna, J. T. & McCarley, R. W. (2009) Animal models of narcolepsy. *CNS Neurol Disord Drug Targets* **8**: 296–308.

Chen, L., Thakkar, M. M., Winston, S. *et al.* (2006) REM sleep changes in rats induced by siRNA-mediated orexin knockdown. *Eur J Neurosci* **24**: 2039–48.

El Mansari, M., Sakai, K. & Jouvet, M. (1989) Unitary characteristics of presumptive cholinergic tegmental neurons during the sleep–waking cycle in freely moving cats. *Exp Brain Res* **76**: 519–29.

Ennis, M. & Aston-Jones, G. (1989a) GABA-mediated inhibition of locus coeruleus from the dorsomedial rostral medulla. *J Neurosci* **9**: 2973–81.

Ennis, M. & Aston-Jones, G. (1989b) Potent inhibitory input to locus coeruleus from the nucleus prepositus hypoglossi. *Brain Res Bull* **22**: 793–803.

Ford, B., Holmes, C. J., Mainville, L. & Jones, B. E. (1995) GABAergic neurons in the rat pontomesencephalic tegmentum: codistribution with cholinergic and other tegmental neurons projecting to the posterior lateral hypothalamus. *J Comp Neurol* **363**: 177–96.

Fort, P., Bassetti, C. L. & Luppi, P. H. (2009) Alternating vigilance states: new insights regarding neuronal networks and mechanisms. *Eur J Neurosci* **29**: 1741–53.

Gerber, U., Stevens, D. R., McCarley, R. W. & Greene, R. W. (1991) Muscarinic agonists activate an inwardly rectifying potassium conductance in medial pontine reticular formation neurons of the rat in vitro. *J Neurosci* **11**: 3861–7.

Gervasoni, D., Darracq, L., Fort, P. *et al.* (1998) Electrophysiological evidence that noradrenergic neurons of the rat locus coeruleus are tonically inhibited by GABA during sleep. *Eur J Neurosci* **10**: 964–70.

Gervasoni, D., Peyron, C., Rampon, C., *et al.* (2000) Role and origin of the GABAergic innervation of dorsal raphe serotonergic neurons. *J Neurosci* **20**: 4217–25.

Hagan, J. J., Leslie, R. A., Patel, S. *et al.* (1999) Orexin A activates locus coeruleus cell firing and increases arousal in the rat. *Proc Natl Acad Sci U S A* **96**: 10,911–16.

Hassani, O. K., Lee, M. G. & Jones, B. E. (2009) Melanin-concentrating hormone neurons discharge in a reciprocal manner to orexin neurons across the sleep–wake cycle. *Proc Natl Acad Sci U S A* **106**: 2418–22.

Hendricks, J. C., Morrison, A. R. & Mann, G. L. (1982) Different behaviors during paradoxical sleep without atonia depend on pontine lesion site. *Brain Res* **239**: 81–105.

Hobson, J. A., McCarley, R. W. & Wyzinski, P. W. (1975) Sleep cycle oscillation: reciprocal discharge by two brainstem neuronal groups. *Science* **189**: 55–8.

Horvath, T. L., Peyron, C., Diano, S. *et al.* (1999) Hypocretin (orexin) activation and synaptic innervation of the locus coeruleus noradrenergic system. *J Comp Neurol* **415**: 145–59.

Ito, K., Yanagihara, M., Imon, H., Dauphin, L. & McCarley, R. W. (2002) Intracellular recordings of pontine medial gigantocellular tegmental field neurons in the naturally sleeping cat: behavioral state-related activity and soma size difference in order of recruitment. *Neuroscience* **114**: 23–37.

Jouvet, M. (1962) [Research on the neural structures and responsible mechanisms in different phases of physiological sleep.] *Arch Ital Biol* **100**: 125–206.

Jouvet, M. (1994) Paradoxical sleep mechanisms. *Sleep* **17**: S77–83.

Jouvet, M., Jeannerod, M. & Delorme, F. (1965) [Organization of the system responsible for phase activity during paradoxal sleep]. *C R Seances Soc Biol Fil* **159**: 1599–604.

Jouvet, M., Michel, F. & Courjon, J. (1959a) [Electric activity of the rhinencephalon during sleep in cats.]. *C R Seances Soc Biol Fil* **153**: 101–5.

Jouvet, M., Michel, F. & Courjon, J. (1959b) [On a stage of rapid cerebral electrical activity in the course of physiological sleep.]. *C R Seances Soc Biol Fil* **153**: 1024–8.

Jouvet, M., Michel, F. & Courjon, J. (1959c) [Recording and stimulation of the subcortical structures in the chronic decorticated animal.] *Rev Neurol (Paris)* **101**: 255–6.

Kantor, S., Mochizuki, T., Janisiewicz, A. M. *et al.* (2009) Orexin neurons are necessary for the circadian control of REM sleep. *Sleep* **32**: 1127–34.

Kaur, S., Panchal, M., Faisal, M. *et al.* (2004) Long term blocking of GABA-A receptor in locus coeruleus by bilateral microinfusion of picrotoxin reduced rapid eye movement sleep and increased brain Na-K ATPase activity in freely moving normally behaving rats. *Behav Brain Res* **151**: 185–90.

Kaur, S., Saxena, R. N. & Mallick, B. N. (2001) GABAergic neurons in prepositus hypoglossi regulate REM sleep by its action on locus coeruleus in freely moving rats. *Synapse* **42**: 141–50.

Kiyashchenko, L. I., Mileykovskiy, B. Y., Maidment, N. *et al.* (2002) Release of hypocretin (orexin) during waking and sleep states. *J Neurosci* **22**: 5282–6.

Kovacs, K. J. (2008) Measurement of immediate-early gene activation- c-fos and beyond. *J Neuroendocrinol* **20**: 665–72.

Lee, M. G., Hassani, O. K. & Jones, B. E. (2005) Discharge of identified orexin/hypocretin neurons across the sleep–waking cycle. *J Neurosci* **25**: 6716–20.

Lee, M. L., Swanson, B. E. & de la Iglesia, H. O. (2009) Circadian timing of REM sleep is coupled to an oscillator within the dorsomedial suprachiasmatic nucleus. *Curr Biol* **19**: 848–52.

Levine, E. S. & Jacobs, B. L. (1992) Neurochemical afferents controlling the activity of serotonergic neurons in the dorsal raphe nucleus: microiontophoretic studies in the awake cat. *J Neurosci* **12**: 4037–44.

Li, X., Rainnie, D. G., McCarley, R. W. & Greene, R. W. (1998) Presynaptic nicotinic receptors facilitate monoaminergic transmission. *J Neurosci* **18**: 1904–12.

Lim, A. S., Lozano, A. M., Moro, E. *et al.* (2007) Characterization of REM-sleep associated ponto-geniculo-occipital waves in the human pons. *Sleep* **30**: 823–7.

Lin, L., Faraco, J., Li, R. *et al.* (1999) The sleep disorder canine narcolepsy is caused by a mutation in the hypocretin (orexin) receptor 2 gene. *Cell* **98**: 365–76.

Liu, R. J., van den Pol, A. N. & Aghajanian, G. K. (2002) Hypocretins (orexins) regulate serotonin neurons in the dorsal raphe nucleus by excitatory direct and inhibitory indirect actions. *J Neurosci* **22**: 9453–64.

Lu, J., Bjorkum, A. A., Xu, M., *et al.* (2002) Selective activation of the extended ventrolateral preoptic nucleus during rapid eye movement sleep. *J Neurosci* **22**: 4568–76.

Lu, J., Greco, M. A., Shiromani, P. & Saper, C. B. (2000) Effect of lesions of the ventrolateral preoptic nucleus on NREM and REM sleep. *J Neurosci* **20**: 3830–42.

Lu, J., Jhou, T. C. & Saper, C. B. (2006a) Identification of wake–active dopaminergic neurons in the ventral periaqueductal gray matter. *J Neurosci* **26**: 193–202.

Lu, J., Sherman, D., Devor, M. & Saper, C. B. (2006b) A putative flip-flop switch for control of REM sleep. *Nature* **441**: 589–94.

Luppi, P. H., Gervasoni, D., Verret, L. *et al.* (2006) Paradoxical (REM) sleep genesis: the switch from an aminergic-cholinergic to a GABAergic-glutamatergic hypothesis. *J Physiol (Paris)* **100**: 271–83.

Mallick, B. N., Kaur, S. & Saxena, R. N. (2001) Interactions between cholinergic and GABAergic neurotransmitters in and around the locus coeruleus for the induction and maintenance of rapid eye movement sleep in rats. *Neuroscience* **104**: 467–85.

Mallick, B. N., Majumdar, S., Faisal, M. *et al.* (2002) Role of norepinephrine in the regulation of rapid eye movement sleep. *J Biosci* **27**: 539–51.

Mallick, B. N., Thankachan, S. & Islam, F. (1998) Differential responses of brain stem neurons during spontaneous and stimulation-induced desynchronization of the cortical EEG in freely moving cats. *Sleep Res Online* **1**: 132–46.

Maloney, K. J., Mainville, L. & Jones, B. E. (1999) Differential c-Fos expression in cholinergic, monoaminergic, and GABAergic cell groups of the pontomesencephalic tegmentum after paradoxical sleep deprivation and recovery. *J Neurosci* **19**: 3057–72.

Maloney, K. J., Mainville, L. & Jones, B. E. (2000) c-Fos expression in GABAergic, serotonergic, and other neurons of the pontomedullary reticular formation and raphe after paradoxical sleep deprivation and recovery. *J Neurosci* **20**: 4669–79.

McCarley, R. W. (2004) Mechanisms and models of REM sleep control. *Arch Ital Biol* **142**: 429–67.

McCarley, R. W. (2007) Neurobiology of REM and NREM sleep. *Sleep Med* **8**: 302–30.

McCarley, R. W. & Hobson, J. A. (1975a) Discharge patterns of cat pontine brain stem neurons during desynchronized sleep. *J Neurophysiol* **38**: 751–66.

McCarley, R. W. & Hobson, J. A. (1975b) Neuronal excitability modulation over the sleep cycle: a structural and mathematical model. *Science* **189**: 58–60.

McCarley, R. W. & Massaquoi, S. G. (1986a) Further discussion of a model of the REM sleep oscillator. *Am J Physiol* **251**: R1033–6.

McCarley, R. W. & Massaquoi, S. G. (1986b) A limit cycle mathematical model of the REM sleep oscillator system. *Am J Physiol* **251**: R1011–29.

McCarley, R. W., Nelson, J. P. & Hobson, J. A. (1978) Ponto-geniculo-occipital (PGO) burst neurons: correlative evidence for neuronal generators of PGO waves. *Science* **201**: 269–72.

McGinty, D. & Szymusiak, R. (2001) Brain structures and mechanisms involved in the generation of NREM sleep: focus on the preoptic hypothalamus. *Sleep Med Rev* **5**: 323–42.

Merchant-Nancy, H., Vazquez, J., Garcia, F. & Drucker-Colin, R. (1995) Brain distribution of c-fos expression as a result of prolonged rapid eye movement (REM) sleep period duration. *Brain Res* **681**: 15–22.

Mileykovskiy, B. Y., Kiyashchenko, L. I. & Siegel, J. M. (2005) Behavioral correlates of activity in identified hypocretin/orexin neurons. *Neuron* **46**: 787–98.

Mitani, A., Ito, K., Hallanger, A. E. *et al.* (1988) Cholinergic projections from the laterodorsal and pedunculopontine tegmental nuclei to the pontine gigantocellular tegmental field in the cat. *Brain Res* **451**: 397–402.

Mochizuki, T., Crocker, A., McCormack, S. *et al.* (2004) Behavioral state instability in orexin knock-out mice. *J Neurosci* **24**: 6291–300.

Moruzzi, G. & Magoun, H. W. (1949) Brain stem reticular formation and activation of the EEG. *Electroencephalogr Clin Neurophysiol* **1**: 455–73.

Nitz, D. & Siegel, J. (1997a) GABA release in the dorsal raphe nucleus: role in the control of REM sleep. *Am J Physiol* **273**: R451–5.

Nitz, D. & Siegel, J. M. (1997b) GABA release in the locus coeruleus as a function of sleep/wake state. *Neuroscience* **78**: 795–801.

Pal, D. & Mallick, B. N. (2009) GABA in pedunculopontine tegmentum increases rapid eye movement sleep in freely moving rats: possible role of GABA-ergic inputs from substantia nigra pars reticulata. *Neuroscience* **164**: 404–14.

Paxinos, G. & Watson, C. (1998) *The Rat Brain in Stereotaxic Coordinates*. San Diego: Academic Press.

Peigneux, P., Laureys, S., Fuchs, S. *et al.* (2001) Generation of rapid eye movements during paradoxical sleep in humans. *Neuroimage* **14**: 701–8.

Peyron, C., Sapin, E., Leger, L., Luppi, P. H. & Fort, P. (2009) Role of the melanin-concentrating hormone neuropeptide in sleep regulation. *Peptides* **30**: 2052–9.

Peyron, C., Tighe, D. K., van den Pol, A. N. *et al.* (1998) Neurons containing hypocretin (orexin) project to multiple neuronal systems. *J Neurosci* **18**: 9996–10,015.

Portas, C. M. & McCarley, R. W. (1994) Behavioral state-related changes of extracellular serotonin concentration in the dorsal raphe nucleus: a microdialysis study in the freely moving cat. *Brain Res* **648**: 306–12.

Sakai, K. & Crochet, S. (2001) Role of dorsal raphe neurons in paradoxical sleep generation in the cat: no evidence for a serotonergic mechanism. *Eur J Neurosci* **13**: 103–12.

Sakai, K., Petitjean, F. & Jouvet, M. (1976) Effects of ponto-mesencephalic lesions and electrical stimulation upon PGO waves and EMPs in unanesthetized cats. *Electroencephalogr Clin Neurophysiol* **41**: 49–63.

Saper, C. B., Chou, T. C. & Scammell, T. E. (2001) The sleep switch: hypothalamic control of sleep and wakefulness. *Trends Neurosci* **24**: 726–31.

Sapin, E., Lapray, D. & Berod, A. *et al.* (2009) Localization of the brainstem GABAergic neurons controlling paradoxical (REM) sleep. *PLoS One* **4**: e4272.

Sastre, J. P., Buda, C., Kitahama, K. & Jouvet, M. (1996) Importance of the ventrolateral region of the periaqueductal gray and adjacent tegmentum in the control of paradoxical sleep as studied by muscimol microinjections in the cat. *Neuroscience* **74**: 415–26.

Sastre, J. P. & Jouvet, M. (1979) [Oneiric behavior in cats]. *Physiol Behav* **22**: 979–89.

Sherin, J. E., Elmquist, J. K., Torrealba, F. & Saper, C. B. (1998) Innervation of histaminergic tuberomammillary neurons by GABAergic and galaninergic neurons in the ventrolateral preoptic nucleus of the rat. *J Neurosci* **18**: 4705–21.

Steriade, M. & McCarley, R. W. (2005) *Brainstem Control of Wakefulness and Sleep*. New York: Plenum Press.

Steriade, M., Pare, D., Datta, S., Oakson, G. & Curro Dossi, R. (1990) Different cellular types in mesopontine cholinergic nuclei related to ponto-geniculo-occipital waves. *J Neurosci* **10**: 2560–79.

Thakkar, M. M., Ramesh, V., Cape, E. G. *et al.* (1999) REM sleep enhancement and behavioral cataplexy following orexin (hypocretin)-II receptor antisense perfusion in the pontine reticular formation. *Sleep Res Online* **2**: 112–20.

Thakkar, M. M., Strecker, R. E. & McCarley, R. W. (1998) Behavioral state control through differential serotonergic inhibition in the mesopontine cholinergic nuclei: a simultaneous unit recording and microdialysis study. *J Neurosci* **18**: 5490–7.

Thakkar, M. M., Strecker, R. E. & McCarley, R. W. (2002) Phasic but not tonic REM-selective discharge of periaqueductal gray neurons in freely behaving animals: relevance to postulates of GABAergic inhibition of monoaminergic neurons. *Brain Res* **945**: 276–80.

Torterolo, P., Sampogna, S., Morales, F. R. & Chase, M. H. (2006) MCH-containing neurons in the hypothalamus of the cat: searching for a role in the control of sleep and wakefulness. *Brain Res* **1119**: 101–14.

Trulson, M. E. & Jacobs, B. L. (1979) Raphe unit activity in freely moving cats: correlation with level of behavioral arousal. *Brain Res* **163**: 135–50.

Verret, L., Fort, P., Gervasoni, D., Leger, L. & Luppi, P. H. (2006) Localization of the neurons active during paradoxical (REM) sleep and projecting to the locus coeruleus noradrenergic neurons in the rat. *J Comp Neurol* **495**: 573–86.

Verret, L., Goutagny, R., Fort, P. *et al.* (2003) A role of melanin-concentrating hormone producing neurons in the central regulation of paradoxical sleep. *BMC Neurosci* **4**: 19.

Vertes, R. P., Hoover, W. B. & Viana di Prisco, G. (2004) Theta rhythm of the hippocampus: subcortical control and functional significance. *Behav Cogn Neurosci Rev* **3**: 173–200.

Vertes, R. P. & Kocsis, B. (1997) Brainstem-diencephalo-septohippocampal systems controlling the theta rhythm of the hippocampus. *Neuroscience* **81**: 893–926.

Xi, M. C., Morales, F. R. & Chase, M. H. (1999a) Evidence that wakefulness and REM sleep are controlled by a GABAergic pontine mechanism. *J Neurophysiol* **82**: 2015–19.

Xi, M. C., Morales, F. R. & Chase, M. H. (1999b) A GABAergic pontine reticular system is involved in the control of wakefulness and sleep. *Sleep Res Online* **2**: 43–8.

Xi, M. C., Morales, F. R. & Chase, M. H. (2001a) Induction of wakefulness and inhibition of active (REM) sleep by GABAergic processes in the nucleus pontis oralis. *Arch Ital Biol* **139**: 125–45.

Xi, M. C., Morales, F. R. & Chase, M. H. (2001b) The motor inhibitory system operating during active sleep is tonically suppressed by GABAergic mechanisms during other states. *J Neurophysiol* **86**: 1908–15.

Significance of deprivation studies

Nishidh Barot and Clete Kushida

Summary

Interest in the effects of total sleep deprivation dates back over one hundred years. After the discovery of rapid eye movement (REM) sleep in the 1950s, selective REM-deprivation studies have been performed in animals and humans. All studies have shown progressively higher pressure for REM sleep as REM deprivation increases. Studies also show that significant REM rebound occurs after selective REM deprivation and total sleep deprivation. Over the past few decades, newer methods have been developed to reduce confounding factors in REM- or paradoxical sleep-deprivation (PSD) studies of animals but, unfortunately, many findings cannot be generalized to humans. Most current PSD studies employ either the gentle handling or forced locomotion technique, and are most often carried out in rats. Forced locomotion techniques like the disk-over-water method have allowed the study of fairly prolonged PSD in rats. Total sleep deprivation (TSD) in rats leads to a host of sleep deprivation effects (SDEs), including eventual death. Development of SDEs seems to correlate with degree of PSD. Paradoxical sleep-deprivation studies in rats show almost identical results, but only occurring over a longer period of time. REM sleep appears to play a vital role in thermoregulation in rats, leading to considerable hypothermia. The heat-loss theory explains the inverse relationship between energy expenditure (EE) and temperature, which eventually is observed in TSD and PSD studies in animals. No human REM sleep-deprivation studies have indicated such profound changes, though no comparable studies have been conducted. From early on, REM sleep-deprivation studies in humans have focused on the cognitive effects of deprivation. Several studies suggest deficits in short-term memory consolidation with REM-sleep deprivation in both humans and animals, though the issue remains controversial. Recent studies suggest that sensitivity to pain increases with selective REM-sleep deprivation in animals, but no convincing evidence is found in human studies.

Introduction

The effects of prolonged total sleep deprivation have been studied as far back as 1894. A study in puppies at this time indicated that extended sleep loss resulted in death (Manaceine, 1894). In 1896, Patrick and Gilbert performed the first sleep-deprivation study in humans, in which they were evaluated for any behavioral and physiologic effects (Patrick and Gilbert, 1896). In the 1920s, Nathaniel Kleitman performed sleep-deprivation studies in humans, which demonstrated an intrinsic human circadian rhythm, which is independent of sleep debt (Dement, 2005). Through the ground-breaking work of Dement, Aserinsky, and Kleitman in the 1950s, the discovery of two different types of sleep, rapid eye movement (REM) and non-REM (NREM) was made (Dement, 2005). Soon afterward, William Dement attempted the first REM sleep selective deprivation study, which he performed in humans (Dement, 1960; Tsien *et al.*, 1996). For five nights, he monitored subjects during sleep and awakened them at the onset of any REMs. There was a significant REM rebound following REM deprivation; this was the first time that there was evidence that suggested a vital role of REM sleep (Dement, 1960; Tsien *et al.*, 1996).

Over the past few decades, extensive research has been conducted on total sleep deprivation (TSD) and sleep state-specific deprivation. Many researchers have embarked upon different sleep-deprivation studies with ambitious hopes of discovering why we have specific stages of sleep or even why we sleep in general (i.e., the function of sleep); unfortunately, the answers to those questions remain elusive, and very few conclusions can be made with certainty. Most sleep-deprivation studies

REM Sleep: Regulation and Function, eds. Birendra N. Mallick, S. R. Pandi-Perumal, Robert W. McCarley, and Adrian R. Morrison. Published by Cambridge University Press. © Cambridge University Press 2011.

have been performed in either humans or rats; however, many of the findings in rats cannot be readily generalized to humans. For one, rats and many other animals have polyphasic sleep patterns as opposed to the monophasic sleep patterns of primates (Hendricks, 2005). Additionally, there have been discrepancies between physiologic findings in rat sleep-deprivation studies and human sleep-deprivation studies that call into question the ability to extrapolate the findings of rat studies to humans (Hendricks, 2005). Additionally, concerns over potential confounding factors have been raised in rat studies, including methodology, the effect of stress as well as circadian rhythms in the paradigms used to deprive these animals of sleep (Hendricks 2005; Rechtschaffen and Bergmann, 2002).

With that being said, the available data do seem to indicate that sleep deprivation in humans as well as other animals leads to higher pressure for slow-wave sleep (SWS) and REM sleep (Bonnet, 2005). A few oft-quoted studies indicate that after one night of total sleep deprivation in young adults, the first recovery night was associated with greater recovery of SWS, whereas the second recovery night was associated with proportionately greater REM rebound (Carskadon and Dement, 1979; Kales *et al.*, 1970). Recovering lost SWS seemed to supersede the need for recovering lost REM sleep; however, in situations in which there was not high delta pressure, such as in older adults, who typically have less SWS, or when partial retention of SWS occurred, REM rebound was more likely to occur earlier while recovering from sleep deprivation (Carskadon and Dement, 1985).

Studies in other animals have also shown a preferential initial rebound in NREM sleep during short-term TSD (Everson *et al.*, 1989); however, in prolonged TSD studies, animals demonstrate a massive, immediate REM sleep (or paradoxical sleep [PS]) rebound. "Studies in rats and other species show that short-term sleep deprivation (< 24 hours) produces a rebound of both NREM sleep and REM sleep, while long-term sleep deprivation (several days) produces mainly a rebound of REM sleep" (Cirelli and Tononi, 2005). This preferential REM rebound during recovery sleep has contributed to the notion that REM sleep serves a very important function, which continues to be explored.

REM deprivation methods in animals

The challenge faced by the designer of any sleep-deprivation study is to perform the intervention without having the methodology affect the results. For example, if I deprive an experimental rat from sleep by applying electric shocks every time it enters sleep, I cannot ascertain if the effect observed is due to the sleep deprivation induced by the electric shock or by the electric shock itself. Modern sleep-deprivation studies have tried to minimize the effect of the methodology. Those aspects of methodology that cannot be avoided are incorporated into one or more control groups.

Of the several different methods for animal PSD, currently, the most widely used fall into two main categories, the gentle handling and forced locomotion methods (Cirelli and Tononi, 2005). These have typically been carried out in rats because of the abilities to monitor sleep and use of such methods for relatively prolonged periods of time, compared with other species (Rechtschaffen and Bergmann, 2002). Gentle handling involves exposing the animal to novel sensory stimuli whenever it enters sleep (Cirelli and Tononi, 2005). It has the advantage of eliminating the potential confound of locomotion (either the motion or the ensuing fatigue/stress). However, it is not successful in sleep deprivation for more than a fairly short period. The forced locomotion technique can involve several different methods, including the rotating wheel, flower-pot/platform method, or disk-over-water (DOW) method. Some studies have used the DOW method, which uses minimal locomotion to enforce sleep deprivation (Cirelli and Tononi, 2005). Compared to other methods, long periods of sleep deprivation, particularly REM-sleep deprivation, can be achieved with this method, though there is also a concomitant partial NREM-sleep deprivation that occurs, particularly as REM-sleep deprivation advances (Landis, 2005). The flower-pot/platform method exclusively deprives the rat of REM sleep. It essentially involves placing an experimental rat on a very small platform (e.g., an upside-down flower pot). This method relies on the loss of muscle tone during PS (paradoxical sleep; the term used by some authors to describe REM sleep), which in turn causes the rat to widen its contact area and come in contact with the water under the platform; this is an excellent way to effectively monitor short periods of REM deprivation without having to perform electrophysiologic monitoring. However, with prolonged REM-sleep deprivation the rat begins to allow immersion/contact with water more and more, and the method becomes less effective after 72 hours (Landis, 2005). It also has the confounds of stress due to sudden water immersion and the physiologic effects of near-constant exposure to water.

Punitive methods have been tried but somewhat surprisingly are not effective as the animals become progressively more sleep deprived. Experimental animals then will still remain asleep during this time, even with very strong painful stimuli (Cirelli and Tononi, 2005). Other less commonly used methods for REM deprivation in animals include direct brain stimulation, a cold ambient environment, and the pendulum or swing technique in which the animal is rocked awake when it enters the "forbidden" state of sleep (Landis, 2005).

Sleep-deprivation considerations in humans

Both homeostatic and circadian factors appear to play a role in determining which stage(s) are restricted during partial sleep deprivation (< 4 hours) in humans. Several human studies have shown that the amount of SWS dominates during partial sleep restriction, with significant reduction in REM occurring. This must be interpreted in light of circadian timing, as REM sleep naturally predominates in the last few hours of one's sleep cycle. If partial sleep deprivation occurs in the last part of the natural sleep cycle, shorter REM sleep latencies and greater amounts of REM are also seen (Landis, 2005). This can have important clinical implications. REM restriction has been shown to improve depression in some cases; if used, the restriction should occur at a time when circadian REM propensity is least (Schilgen and Tolle, 1980).

Studies have shown that after successive nights of REM deprivation, it takes more stimuli to prevent REM sleep, an indication of a homeostatic REM sleep drive/ REM sleep debt (Endo et al., 1998). Additionally, more stimuli are required to inhibit REM if the sleep period occurs in the last third of the night, another sign of the circadian timing of REM (Landis, 2005). Also, during napping after sleep deprivation, the greatest REM pressure occurs early in the day, and declines as the day goes on. It stays at a fairly low level into the first half of the next overnight sleep period until the circadian propensity of the part of the sleep period again. The REM-sleep propensity during partial sleep deprivation and recovery sleep is therefore determined by both homeostatic pressure (REM sleep debt) as well as timing of recovery sleep (circadian propensity) (Brunner et al., 1990; Tilley and Wilkinson, 1984; Webb and Agnew, 1965).

REM deprivation in rats

Early deprivation studies demonstrated that rats would die after both total sleep deprivation (TSD) as well as REM deprivation (paradoxical-sleep deprivation, or PSD). However, the validity of these findings was called into question because of the specific methods used to sleep deprive the animals; there were legitimate concerns that the method by which sleep was inhibited may have been the cause of death or other effects by way of stress, fatigue, etc. (Horne, 1978; Johnson, 1969). These studies used measures such as electrical shocks to keep animals awake. More elaborate methods of sleep deprivation have been developed since that time to address this potential confound. In the 1989 series of rat total-sleep deprivation (TSD) and paradoxical-sleep deprivation (PSD) studies published by Rechtschaffen's group (Bergmann et al., 1989a,b; Everson et al.,1989a,b; Kushida et al., 1989; Rechtschaffen et al., 1989, 2002), the DOW method was employed with the intent of minimizing and controlling for stress and other variables. The experimenters had observed in their own prior TSD studies that those rats who obtained the most amount of PS had fared the best (Rechtschaffen et al., 1983). This finding, and the REM rebound observed in the previously mentioned REM-deprivation study of Dement (Dement, 1960;Tsien et al., 1996) prompted them to perform and pay special attention to PSD (Kushida et al., 1989).

In the DOW method, a yoked control rat was housed in the same glass container as the experimental rat. Each rat was placed upon the same disk, but a divider separated the two rats. Water filled the container to just below the level of the disk. Both rats had continuous physiologic measurements (cortical EEG, muscle EMG), which indicated whether they were in stage wake, REM, low-amplitude NREM sleep (HS1), or high-amplitude NREM sleep (HS2)(Bergmann et al., 1989b). Pontine spike electrodes and additional EMG electrodes were used in the PSD and paradoxical-sleep control (PSC) rats to assist with accurate PS detection. The electrodes all connected to a computer, which analyzed the data in real time and determined stage. The computer sent a signal to a motor adjacent to the disk, which then rotated the disk. Whenever the experimental rat entered the "forbidden state" the motor rotated the disk, at which time both rats would have to move to prevent falling into the water. The control rat would also have to move at this time to avoid immersion in water; however, at other times it was free to sleep (when the experimental rat was eating, exploring, etc.), as long as the experimental rat was not in the "forbidden state" (Bergmann *et al.*, 1989b; Everson *et al.*, 1989a). This method provided a fairly gentle manner of restricting TS or PS and controlled for other variables, such as water immersion, stress, and environment in the control rats. Though the control "yoked" rats did have less sleep than normal (as would be expected), because they were allowed to sleep at other times, they overall had significantly more sleep than the experimental rats.

This series of studies corroborated many findings in previous animal studies (Albert *et al.*, 1970; Karadzic and Dement, 1967). There were even some potential similarities to previous human sleep-deprivation studies, such as the finding of increased appetite during PSD (Dement, 1960; Sampson, 1966; Tsien *et al.*, 1996). Unless given a chance to recover, all sleep-deprived rats eventually died and showed changes in several other physiologic variables (decreased temperature and heart rate, increased energy expenditure). Interestingly, the outcomes were almost identical in both TSD and PSD rats; the major difference being that PSD took a longer time to produce outcomes. For example, PSD rats survived four to six weeks before death compared to two to three weeks in TSD (Kushida *et al.*, 1989). The findings were further corroborated by studies in the years to come. Years later, Rechtschaffen wrote that, "in the rat, sleep and paradoxical sleep are biological necessities and that extended sleep loss reliably produces a syndrome of specific, substantial physiological changes" (Rechtschaffen and Bergmann, 2002). These sleep-deprivation effects (SDEs) included weight loss, increased food intake, increased energy expenditure (EE), lower body temperatures, change in appearance (scrawny, decrepit), ulcerative and hyperkeratotic skin lesions (Rechtschaffen and Bergmann, 2002).

The 1989 studies and studies afterward have indicated that survival time in rats undergoing TSD seems to be associated with the amount of REM sleep achieved during TSD (Rechtschaffen *et al.*, 1983, 1989; Rechtschaffen and Bergmann, 2002). Though the 1989 recovery sleep study had a small sample size (N = 8), the findings were dramatic and deserve attention. The investigators demonstrated a disproportionate PS rebound that occurred when extended TSD was terminated and rats were allowed to obtain recovery sleep. Recovery sleep was initiated when the typical, significant physiological changes had occurred, at which time the rat appeared to be near death. Recovery sleep was allowed by stopping the disk from rotating. Both PSD and

TSD studies demonstrated this massive, immediate PS rebound, which was accompanied by significant reversal of physiologic sleep-deprivation effects (Rechtschaffen *et al.*, 2002). Subsequent TSD studies have shown a preferential, large initial rebound in REM sleep with as little as two to four days of sleep deprivation (Mendelson and Bergmann, 2000; Rechtschaffen *et al.*, 1999). In the 1989 recovery study, rats were monitored during recovery for 15 days, and the five rats that survived during this time almost entirely healed (Everson *et al.*, 1989b). Of note, three out of the eight rats died (2 TSD, 1 PSD), all within a few days of the recovery sleep period. These rats also had the greatest temperature change during the sleep-deprivation period. This suggests that with TSD and PSD there may be a "point of no return," when even if given the opportunity to reverse sleep debt, animals can no longer mobilize the physiological resources to recover from their sleep loss (Everson *et al.*, 1989b).

Very little NREM (HS1 or HS2) was seen during initial recovery from TSD; however, because hypothetically, the SDEs could have been a consequence of sleep restriction in general (and not REM specific), Kushida *et al.* (1989) studied a control group that had a similar amount of total sleep restriction over time. This group survived the entire period and showed no signs of SDEs. These findings collectively suggest PSD as the primary cause of the observed SDEs, and make a strong case for the biologic necessity of PS (at least in rats).

REM sleep and thermoregulation

Several studies have shown that PS appears to be essential for thermoregulation; PSD leads to progressive hypothermia (Landis *et al.*, 1992, Shaw *et al.*, 1998). Findings during the 1989 set of experiments by Rechtschaffen's lab led to the heat loss theory, which explains the inverse relationship between energy expenditure (EE) and temperature observed during the second half of the experimental time period. Essentially, more PSD leads to greater heat loss, which in turn leads to greater EE in an attempt to compensate for heat loss. Initially, EE is somewhat able to compensate for heat loss, but as heat loss progresses, EE cannot keep up (Rechtschaffen *et al.*, 2002). As SD, specifically PSD, progresses, EE inadequately compensates for increasing heat loss, and hypothermia ensues. Though the molecular details of the higher energy expenditure are unclear, studies have indicated that norepinephrine may mediate this increase in metabolic rate and EE (Rechtschaffen *et al.*, 2002). Rats that have comparatively more energy expenditure die more quickly; likewise, rats with a steeper temperature decline die more quickly and are less likely to recover when given the chance. This correlates well with the previous studies of TSD, which have shown that rats that preserve the greatest amount of PS survive the longest (Rechtschaffen *et al.*, 1983).

Apart from the rate of development of SDEs, the only other observable difference between TSD and PSD rats has been the initial temperature profiles (Obermeyer *et al.*, 1991; Prete *et al.*, 1991). Total-sleep deprived rats have shown an initial increase in temperature, followed by a decline. Paradoxical-sleep deprived rats, on the other hand, had continuous decline from the very beginning (Landis *et al.*, 1992; Shaw *et al.*, 1998). Selective NREM deprivation studies have shown temperature to remain at higher levels until the rat approaches death (Gilliland *et al.*, 1989). It has been hypothesized that NREM sleep deprivation raises the hypothalamic temperature set point (Rechtschaffen and Bergmann, 2002), initially leading to higher temperatures. In TSD studies, rats vigorously seek an area of higher ambient temperature because of a higher temperature set point. Paradoxical-sleep deprived rats also show a preference to warmer ambient temperatures; however, mathematical analyses show that this seems to be a response to rapid heat loss rather than a higher temperature set point (Gilliland *et al.*, 1989; Landis *et al.*, 1992; Shaw *et al.*, 1998). As PSD progresses, temperature steadily drops despite significant increases in caloric intake and energy expenditure. This impairment of thermoregulation and heat retention is directly related to the degree of PSD. Higher EE also correlates well with degree of PSD. Rats can develop a higher resting heart rate during sleep (NREM) than even wakefulness (Rechtschaffen and Bergmann, 2002). Furthermore, studies have shown that rats having higher EE in PSD (and TSD) studies have shorter survival times.

Paradoxical-sleep deprivation studies also have shown a reduction in the normal temperature decline that occurs between the wake–sleep transition; as PSD time progresses, the normal difference lessens. In fact, late in PSD, temperatures actually rise in NREM sleep compared to wakefulness; these effects are reversed only after several days of recovery sleep (Feng *et al.*, 1995; Landis *et al.*, 1992; Shaw *et al.*, 1998). Together, these findings support the notion that PSD impairs thermoregulation/heat-retention, which in turn plays a major role in the development of SDEs (Rechtschaffen and Bergmann, 2002).

Significance of deprivation studies: function of REM sleep

Animal studies of REM deprivation and TSD seem to indicate that REM sleep plays a major role in thermoregulation in rats. The story is not so clear in humans. A few studies have shown slight decrement in temperature and/or an increased appetite after sleep deprivation (Dement, 1960; Horne, 1985, 1978; Kant *et al.*, 1984; Sampson, 1966; Tsien *et al.*, 1996). However, the magnitude of these effects, and the host of other physiological SDEs seen with prolonged TSD and PSD in rats, have not been elicited in humans. Certainly, there may be factors that account for this. Firstly, most studies have focused on neuropsychological and behavioral consequences of PSD in humans. Additionally, no study has been performed up to the human equivalent of "rat time." It is highly unlikely that the rate of development of SDEs in humans would be equal to that of rats. Typical total- and REM-sleep requirements, body surface area to BMI ratios, lifespans, basal oxygen requirements (a measure of energy expenditure), and survival time during starvation all differ significantly between rats and humans, and indicate that a much longer period of time would have to elapse in human studies to evaluate for the presence of SDEs (Rechtschaffen *et al.*, 2002). For example, almost all human PSD studies have been less than 16 days in duration. If one were to use survival time during starvation as the measuring stick for comparison between humans and rats, this would correspond to a time where rats showed virtually no SDEs in TSD and PSD studies. The data for prolonged sleep-deprivation effects is therefore not available; for now, it must be said that there are no known significant physiological SDEs from PSD in humans like those observed in rats (Rechtschaffen *et al.*, 2002). It can, however, be said with certainty that in rats PSD is strongly linked with SDEs. It can also be said that in rats REM sleep appears essential for thermoregulation, though much remains to be known about the purpose of REM sleep in humans.

That being said, theories abound regarding the purpose of REM sleep in humans (and other animals). The demonstration of REM-sleep deprivation effects (in other animals), REM rebound after restriction, REM sleep's ultradian rhythm throughout the night, predictable circadian timing, etc., has led to several different theories about its function. We will review a few of these theories.

REM sleep and neurotransmitters

The catecholamine restoration hypothesis is based upon the observation that catecholamine levels are lower during NREM than wake, but are virtually absent during REM sleep. This has led some to believe that REM sleep functions to periodically upregulate mono-amine receptors or regulate local neurotransmitter levels (Bergmann *et al.*, 1994; Stern and Morgane, 1974; Tsai *et al.*, 1993). However, studies have shown no clear differences in numbers of receptors or regional differences of catecholamines after PSD in rats (Bergmann *et al.*, 1994). Because of acetylcholine's essential role in REM sleep, acetylcholine levels have been studied as well. No major changes in regional cholinergic receptors or receptor binding has been found with PSD (Tsai *et al.*, 1994). After death, no major degenerative brain changes, either structurally or chemically, have been found in TSD or PSD rats upon histological examination. This is consistent with the observation that nearly all SDEs are reversed with adequate recovery RS and TS (Rechtschaffen and Bergmann, 2002).

REM-sleep deprivation and memory

One of the more controversial topics regarding REM sleep has been its putative role in learning and memory. Some fairly recent evidence suggests that REM sleep may play a crucial role in learning and memory formation (Graves *et al.*, 2001; Stickgold, 2005; Stickgold and Walker, 2005). It has been well established that total sleep deprivation impairs learning, memory, and other cognitive abilities (Peigneux *et al.*, 2001). Ever since the discovery of REM sleep, and especially because of some apparent similarities it shares with wakefulness, theories have developed about REM sleep's specific role in facilitating memory consolidation. Functional imaging, REM deprivation, and pre- and post-REM studies have all been used to understand the possible cognitive function of REM sleep. Over the past few years there have been REM-deprivation studies, which some feel suggest REM sleep is necessary for consolidation of procedural (implicit) memories (Karni *et al.*, 1994; Smith, 2001). Procedural memories are memories of how to do something, and are typically difficult to verbalize (like skills). For example, one REM-deprivation study showed elimination of the typical overnight improvement in visual discrimination tasks in human subjects (Karni *et al.*, 1994). Procedural memories differ from declarative (explicit) memories, which are facts/things/events, and typically can be verbalized

easily. Many have suggested that declarative memory is dependent on slow-wave sleep (SWS) (Plihal and Born, 1997, 1999). More recent studies indicate that a clear division of labor between SWS and REM sleep may be too simplistic a model (Ambrosini and Giuditta, 2001; Giuditta *et al.*, 1995; Stickgold *et al.*, 2000). In one study human subjects were sleep deprived either in the first half of the night or the second half of the night and then evaluated for episodic (declarative) memory consolidation. In this study design, sleep deprivation in the first half versus the second half of the night was taken to mean SWS versus REM-sleep deprivation, respectively; the study commenced at 10:45 pm. In the REM-deprivation group, the subjects learned, then slept for four hours, then awoke and performed the retrieval tasks, and then slept until 7:15 am. In the SWS-deprivation group, the subjects slept first for four hours, then awoke and learned, then slept again, and then performed the retrieval task until 7:15 am. The authors concluded that episodic (specifically spatial and temporal) memories primarily require REM sleep for consolidation, as the second-half deprived subjects had statistically significant lower scores in retrieval tasks (Rauchs *et al.*, 2004). Methodological issues, however, can be raised, such as the fact that the SWS-deprived group had twice the total amount of sleep (a full night's rest) before the retrieval task.

The hippocampus plays a critical role in memory formation and consolidation. Long-term potential (LTP) in the hippocampus (and elsewhere) is thought to be a cellular mechanism of learning and memory (Tsien *et al.*, 1996). REM-deprivation studies in rats have shown inhibition of LTP in hippocampal cells both in vivo and in vitro (Kim *et al.*, 2005). Kim *et al.* studied induction of rat hippocampal cell LTPs in vivo after a period of REM deprivation. They found a significant impairment in LTP induction that lasted more than 24 hours. To account for stress, they monitored circulating corticosterone levels in the experimental and control group; these levels were similar, which reduced the potential that stress was a confounding variable (Kim *et al.*, 2005). In another study (Ishikawa *et al.*, 2006) LTP was induced in rat hippocampal cells before a period of RSD. The rats were then studied during RSD for 24 to 48 hours after LTP induction, and compared to an unrestricted group and a similar NREM-deprivation group. REM deprivation was enforced by using a brush to stroke the backs of the rats. The LTPs decayed faster, indicating impairment in maintenance of LTPs that had been induced prior to

PSD. Furthermore, after four hours of freedom from RSD (during REM rebound), no appreciable difference was noted in the LTP compared to four hours earlier. This was interpreted to mean that PSD led to impairment in LTP maintenance that could not be overcome with REM rebound (Ishikawa *et al.*, 2006). In another study, Ravassard *et al.* (2009) performed PSD in rats via the platform method to evaluate for any changes in the molecular mechanisms involved in memory formation in hippocampal slices. They showed that during PSD there is reduced synthesis of the proteins that are necessary for adequate synaptic transmission, and for generation and perpetuation of LTPs in hippocampal cells (Ravassard *et al.*, 2009). These findings of LTP changes in hippocampal cells from several different studies collectively lend support to the hypothesis that REM sleep plays a role in short-term memory consolidation (Ishikawa *et al.*, 2006; Kim *et al.*, 2005; Ravassard *et al.*, 2009; Tsien *et al.*, 1996).

For years it remained a dogma in the scientific community that neurogenesis cannot occur in adult mammalian brains; however, recent research has shown otherwise. New neurons actually can and do proliferate in adult mammalian brains (Abrous *et al.*, 2005; Gross, 2000). Two areas of the brain clearly demonstrate adult-onset neuronal proliferation; these are the subependymal zone of the lateral ventricles, and the dentate gyrus of the hippocampus, where progenitor cells can activate and proliferate (Meerlo *et al.*, 2009). Recently, attention has been given to the effects of sleep deprivation on those hippocampal cells that have the ability to proliferate (Meerlo *et al.*, 2009). A few studies have shown that growth factors that stimulate neuronal proliferation in the adult hippocampus are reduced during total sleep deprivation. Additionally, these reductions in neuronal trophic factors were proportionate to the reduction in REM during TSD (Guzman-Marin *et al.*, 2006, 2008). This reduction in growth factors ultimately results in inhibition of cell proliferation. Not surprisingly, the degree of reduction in hippocampal proliferation seems to closely relate to the degree of REM-sleep deprivation during that time. For example, selective REM-sleep deprivation in rats for four days by the platform method has been shown to produce the same reduction in hippocampal proliferation as four days of TSD (Guzman-Marin *et al.*, 2006, 2008).

If sleep truly is necessary for the biologic substrates of memory formation, the available data from PSD studies suggest that REM is more necessary than NREM for initial neuronal proliferation. Some have hypothesized that the initial proliferation of hippocampal cells is dependent exclusively upon REM sleep, whereas further maturation and integration into circuits is both NREM and REM dependent (Meerlo *et al.*, 2009). This correlates with the current theory of sequential or multistep processing of memories. Instead of a clear division of labor for REM (procedural) and NREM (declarative), memory must sequentially go through both REM sleep and SWS to be properly consolidated (Giuditta *et al.*, 1995).

It should be noted that several REM-deprivation studies in humans and animals have also concluded that REM is not essential for memory consolidation (Saxvig *et al.*, 2008; Vertes and Eastman, 2000). Vertes and Eastman provided a compelling case against REM sleep's necessity for memory consolidation with a review in 2000. They highlighted the confounding variables present in several studies, conflicting data on the matter, as well as relative normalcy of pharmacologically (SSRI, MAOI, TCA) and structurally (pontine stroke) REM-restricted people. They posit that REM is a time for periodic stimulation of the brain to maintain an overall level of brain activity throughout the night (Vertes and Eastman, 2000). A more recent study tested 24 graduate students (12 control and 12 experimental) on a wide range of memory tasks after one night of REM deprivation. All subjects were monitored; to increase specificity experimental subjects were awakened whenever an REM occurred; in order to increase REM identification sensitivity ten-second epochs were used. Several aspects of memory were assessed, including verbal, visual, and emotional memory; no significant overall difference was found between the REM-deprived and the control group (Saxvig *et al.*, 2008).

REM-sleep deprivation and pain

Sleep deprivation and its relation to pain sensitivity have been recently attracting more interest. Some studies suggest that REM-sleep deprivation may lower the pain threshold (May *et al.*, 2005). A review of the current literature in 2006 was provided by Lautenbacher *et al.* (2006) who addressed the impact of TSD as well as stage-specific sleep deprivation on pain perception. They concluded that although there are a few discrepancies, in general animal PSD studies seem to indicate heightened pain sensitivity (Asakura *et al.*, 1992; Lautenbacher *et al.*, 2006). For example, some studies on PSD rats showed more tail flicking when given noxious electrical stimuli as compared to control rats

(Hicks *et al.*, 1978, 1979). Ukponmwan *et al.* performed two studies that showed reduced pain modulation in PSD animals. In one study, they used opiate treatment and then compared rat pain responses compared to baseline (Ukponmwan *et al.*, 1984). In another study they potentiated opiate response by applying MAO-B inhibitors to PSD and control groups and then measured response to painful stimuli (Ukponmwan *et al.*, 1986). In both studies, control rats had a higher pain threshold than pre-analgesic baseline, but PSD rats did not demonstrate a change, suggesting elimination of expected analgesic effect. Although these studies and others do suggest enhanced pain sensitivity with REM deprivation in animals, questions have been raised about the methodology that make extrapolation difficult; most studies demonstrated little sleep disruption in controls, making it difficult to determine if the nociceptive effects are due to selective REM deprivation, or to sleep deprivation/fragmentation in general (Lautenbacher *et al.*, 2006).

In human studies, on the other hand, there is little to no evidence of increased pain sensitivity with REM deprivation. One study found that three days of REM deprivation in healthy young men did not lead to increased nociceptive sensitivity, as measured by musculoskeletal pressure pain sensitivity (Moldofsky and Scarisbrick, 1976). Interestingly, the results of this study were used as retrospective control data to a previous study of selective NREM deprivation, the conclusion being that selective SWS deprivation (and not REM-sleep deprivation) lowers the pain threshold (Moldofsky and Scarisbrick, 1976; Moldofsky *et al.*, 1975).

In conclusion, studies on humans and animals have demonstrated that there is a constellation of side effects that occur during total and selective REM-sleep deprivation. Studies have also shown progressively higher pressure for REM sleep during the progression of REM deprivation. Investigators have employed several different methods for depriving humans and animals of REM sleep with variable success. Although there is evidence that REM sleep loss can be associated with neurocognitive deficits and pain sensitivity, further work is necessary to explore these associations and the function of REM sleep, as well as the function of sleep itself.

References

Abrous, D. N., Koehl, M. & Le Moal, M. (2005) Adult neurogenesis: from precursors to network and physiology. *Physiol Rev* **85**(2): 523–69.

Albert, I., Cicala, G. A. & Siegel, J. (1970) The behavioral effects of REM sleep deprivation in rats. *Psychophysiology* **6**(5): 550–60.

Ambrosini, M. V. & Giuditta, A. (2001) Learning and sleep: the sequential hypothesis. *Sleep Med Rev* **5**(6): 477–90.

Asakura, W., Matsumoto, K., Ohta, H. & Watanabe, H. (1992) REM sleep deprivation decreases apomorphine-induced stimulation of locomotor activity but not stereotyped behavior in mice. *Gen Pharmacol* **23**(3): 337–41.

Bergmann, B. M., Everson, C. A., Kushida, C. A. *et al.* (1989a) Sleep deprivation in the rat: V. Energy use and mediation. *Sleep* **12**(1): 31–41.

Bergmann, B. M., Kushida, C. A., Everson, C. A. *et al.* (1989b) Sleep deprivation in the rat: II. Methodology. *Sleep* **12**(1): 5–12.

Bergmann, B. M., Seiden, L. S., Landis, C. A., Gilliland, M. A. & Rechtschaffen, A. (1994) Sleep deprivation in the rat: XVIII. Regional brain levels of monoamines and their metabolites. *Sleep* **17**(7): 583–9.

Bonnet, M. (2005) Acute sleep deprivation. In *Principles and Practice of Sleep Medicine*, eds. M. H. Kryger, T. Roth & W. C. Dement. Philadelphia: Elsevier Saunders, pp. 51–66.

Brunner, D. P., Dijk, D. J., Tobler, I. & Borbély, A. A. (1990) Effect of partial sleep deprivation on sleep stages and EEG power spectra: evidence for non-REM and REM sleep homeostasis. *Electroenceph Clin Neurophysiol* **75**: 492–9.

Carskadon, M. A. & Dement, W. C. (1979) Cumulative effects of total sleep loss on sleep tendency. *Percept Mot Skills* **48**: 495–506.

Carskadon, M. A. & Dement, W. C. (1985) Sleep loss in elderly volunteers. *Sleep* **8**: 207–21.

Cirelli, C. & Tononi, G. (2005) Total sleep deprivation. In *Sleep Deprivation: Clinical Issues, Pharmacology, and Sleep Loss Effects. Vol 193: Lung Biology in Health and Disease*, ed. C. Kushida. New York: Marcel Dekker, pp. 1–27.

Dement, W. C. (1960) The effect of dream deprivation. *Science* **131**: 1705–7.

Dement, W. C. (2005) History of sleep physiology and medicine. In *Principles and Practice of Sleep Medicine*, eds. M. H. Kryger & W. C. Dement. Philadelphia: Elsevier Saunders, pp. 2–12.

Endo, T., Roth, C., Landolt, H. P. *et al.* (1998) Selective REM sleep deprivation in humans: effects on sleep and sleep EEG. *Am Jour Physiol Regulatory Integrative Comp Physiol* **274**: 1186–94.

Everson, C. A., Bergmann, B. M. & Rechtschaffen, A. (1989a) Sleep deprivation in the rat: III. Total sleep deprivation. *Sleep* **12**(1): 13–21.

Everson, C. A., Gilliland, M. A., Kushida, C.A. *et al.* (1989b) Sleep deprivation in the rat: IX. Recovery. *Sleep* **12**(1): 60–7.

Feng, P. F., Shaw, P., Bergmann, B. M. *et al.* (1995) Sleep deprivation in the rat: XX. Differences in wake and sleep temperatures during recovery. *Sleep* **18**(9): 797–804.

Gilliland, M. A., Bergmann, B. M. & Rechtschaffen, A. (1989) Sleep deprivation in the rat: VIII. High EEG amplitude sleep deprivation. *Sleep* **12**(1): 53–9.

Giuditta, A., Ambrosini, M. V., Montagnese, P. *et al.* (1995) The sequential hypothesis of the function of sleep. *Behav Brain Res* **69**(1/2): 157–66.

Graves, L., Pack, A. & Abel, T. (2001) Sleep and memory: a molecular perspective. *Trends Neurosci* **24**(4): 237–43.

Gross, C. G. (2000) Neurogenesis in the adult brain: death of a dogma. *Nat Rev Neurosci* **1**(1): 67–73.

Guzman-Marin, R., Suntsova, N., Bashir, T. *et al.* (2008) Rapid eye movement sleep deprivation contributes to reduction of neurogenesis in the hippocampal dentate gyrus of the adult rat. *Sleep* **31**(2): 167–75.

Guzman-Marin, R., Ying, Z., Suntsova, N. *et al.* (2006) Suppression of hippocampal plasticity-related gene expression by sleep deprivation in rats. *J Physiol* **15**(575/3): 807–19.

Hendricks, J. (2005) Animal models of sleep deprivation. In *Sleep Deprivation: Clinical Issues, Pharmacology, and Sleep Loss Effects, Vol 193: Lung Biology in Health and Disease*, ed. C. Kushida. New York: Marcel Dekker, pp. 1–27.

Hicks, R. A., Coleman, D. D., Ferrante, F., Sahatjian, M. & Hawkins, J. (1979) Pain thresholds in rats during recovery from REM sleep deprivation. *Percept Mot Skills* **48**(3 Pt 1): 687–90.

Hicks, R. A., Moore, J. D., Findley, P., Hirshfield, C. & Humphrey, V. (1978) REM sleep deprivation and pain thresholds in rats *Percept Mot Skills* **47**(3/1): 848–50.

Horne, J. A. (1978) A review of the biological effects of total sleep deprivation. *Biol Psychol* **7**: 55–102.

Horne, J. A. (1985) Sleep function, with particular reference to sleep deprivation. *Ann Clin Res* **17**(5): 199–208.

Ishikawa, A., Kanayama, Y., Matsumura, H. *et al.* (2006) Selective rapid eye movement sleep deprivation impairs the maintenance of long-term potentiation in the rat hippocampus. *Eur J Neurosci* **24**(1): 243–8.

Johnson, L. C. (1969) Physiological and psychological effects following total sleep deprivation. In *Sleep: Pathology and Physiology*, ed. A. Kales. Philadelphia: J. J. Lippincott Company, pp. 206–20.

Kales, A., Tan, T., Kollar, E. J. *et al.* (1970) Sleep patterns following 205 hours of sleep deprivation. *Psychosom Med* **32**: 189–200.

Kant, G. J., Genser, S. G., Thorne, D. R., Pfalser, J. L. & Mougey, E. H. (1984) Effects of 72 hour sleep deprivation on urinary cortisol and indices of metabolism. *Sleep* **7**(2): 142–6.

Karadzic, V. & Dement, W. C. (1967) Heart rate changes following selective deprivation of rapid eye movement (REM) sleep. *Brain Res* **6**(4): 786–8.

Karni, A., Tanne, D., Rubenstein, B. S., Askenasy, J. J. & Sagi, D. (1994) Dependence on REM sleep of overnight improvement of a perceptual skill. *Science* **29**265(5172): 679–82.

Kim, E. Y., Mahmoud, G. S. & Grover, L. M. (2005) REM sleep deprivation inhibits LTP in vivo in area CA1 of rat hippocampus. *Neurosci Lett* **18** 388(3): 163–7.

Kushida, C. A., Bergmann, B. M. & Rechtschaffen, A. (1989) Sleep deprivation in the rat: IV. Paradoxical sleep deprivation. *Sleep* **12**(1): 22–30.

Landis, C. A. (2005) Partial and sleep-state selective deprivation In *Sleep Deprivation: Clinical Issues, Pharmacology, and Sleep Loss Effects, Vol 193: Lung Biology in Health and Disease*, ed. C. Kushida. New York: Marcel Dekker, pp. 20–1.

Landis, C. A., Bergmann, B. M., Ismail, M. M. & Rechtschaffen, A. (1992) Sleep deprivation in the rat: XV. Ambient temperature choice in paradoxical sleep-deprived rats. *Sleep* **15**(1):13–20.

Lautenbacher, S., Kundermann, B. & Krieg, J. C. (2006) Sleep deprivation and pain perception. *Sleep Med Rev* **10**(5): 357–69.

Manaceine, M. (1894) Quelques observations experimentales sur l'influence de l'insomnie absolue. *Arch Ital Biol* **21**: 322–5.

May, M. E., Harvey, M. T., Valdovinos, M. G. *et al.* (2005) Nociceptor and age specific effects of REM sleep deprivation induced hyperalgesia. *Behav Brain Res* **15** 159(1): 89–94.

Meerlo, P., Mistlberger, R. E., Jacobs, B. L., Heller, H. C. & McGinty, D. (2009) New neurons in the adult brain: the role of sleep and consequences of sleep loss. *Sleep Med Rev* **13**(3): 187–94.

Mendelson, W.B. & Bergmann, B. M. (2000) Age-dependent changes in recovery sleep after 48 hours of sleep deprivation in rats. *Neurobiol Aging* **21**(5): 689–93.

Moldofsky, H. & Scarisbrick, P. (1976) Induction of neurasthenic musculoskeletal pain syndrome by selective sleep stage deprivation. *Psychosom Med* **38**(1): 35–44.

Moldofsky, H., Scarisbrick, P., England, R. & Smythe, H. (1975) Musculosketal symptoms and non-REM sleep disturbance in patients with "fibrositis syndrome" and healthy subjects. *Psychosom Med* **37**(4): 341–51.

Obermeyer, W., Bergmann, B. M. & Rechtschaffen, A. (1991) Sleep deprivation in the rat: XIV. Sleep comparison of waking hypothalamic and peritoneal temperatures. **14**(4): 285–93.

Patrick, G. T. W. & Gilbert (1896) On the effect of loss of sleep. *Psychol Rev* **3**: 469–83.

Peigneux, P., Laureys, S., Delbeuck, X. & Maquet, P. (2001) Sleeping brain, learning brain. The role of sleep for memory systems. *Neuroreport* **21** 12(18): A111–24.

Plihal, W. & Born, J. (1997) Effect of early and late nocturnal sleep on procedural and declarative memory. *J Cogn Neurosci* **9**: 544–7.

Plihal, W. & Born, J. (1999) Effects of early and late nocturnal sleep on priming and spatial memory. *Psychophysiology* **36**(5): 571–82.

Prete, F. R., Bergmann, B. M., Holtzman, P., Obermeyer, W. & Rechtschaffen, A. (1991) Sleep deprivation in the rat: XII. Effect on ambient temperature choice. *Sleep* **14**(2): 109–15.

Rauchs, G., Bertran, F., Guillery-Girard, B. *et al.* (2004) Consolidation of strictly episodic memories mainly requires rapid eye movement sleep. *Sleep* **27**(3): 395–401.

Ravassard, P., Pachoud, B., Comte, J. C. *et al.* (2009) Paradoxical (REM) sleep deprivation causes a large and rapidly reversible decrease in long-term potentiation, synaptic transmission, glutamate receptor protein levels, and ERK/MAPK activation in the dorsal hippocampus. *Sleep* **32**(2): 227–40.

Rechtschaffen, A. & Bergmann, B. M. (2002) Sleep deprivation in the rat: an update of the 1989 paper. *Sleep* **25**(1): 18–24.

Rechtschaffen, A., Bergmann, B. M., Everson, C. A., Kushida, C. A. & Gilliland, M. (1989) Sleep deprivation in the rat: I. Conceptual issues. *Sleep* **12**(1): 1–4.

Rechtschaffen, A., Bergmann, B. M., Everson, C. A., Kushida, C. A. & Gilliland, M. A. (2002) Sleep deprivation in the rat: X. Integration and discussion of the findings. *Sleep* **25**(1): 68–87.

Rechtschaffen, A., Bergmann, B. M., Gilliland, M. A. & Bauer, K. (1999) Effects of method, duration, and sleep stage on rebounds from sleep deprivation in the rat. *Sleep* **122**(1): 11–31.

Rechtschaffen, A., Gilliland, M. A., Bergmann, B. M. & Winter, J. B. (1983) Physiological correlates of prolonged sleep deprivation in rats. *Science* **8** 221(4606): 182–4.

Sampson, H. J. (1966) Psychological effects of deprivation of dreaming sleep. *Nerv Ment Dis* **143**(4): 305–17.

Saxvig, I. W., Lundervold, A. J., Grønli, J. *et al.* (2008) The effect of a REM sleep deprivation procedure on different aspects of memory function in humans. *Psychophysiology* **45**(2): 309–17.

Schilgen, B. & Tolle, R. (1980) Partial sleep deprivation as a therapy for depression. *Arch Gen Psychiatry* **37**: 267–71.

Shaw, P. J., Bergmann, B. M. & Rechtschaffen, A. (1998) Effects of paradoxical sleep deprivation on thermoregulation in the rat. *Sleep* **21**(1): 7–17.

Smith, C. (2001) Sleep states and memory processes in humans: procedural versus declarative memory systems. *Sleep Med Rev* **5**(6): 491–506.

Stern, W. C. & Morgane, P. J. (1974) Theoretical view of REM sleep function: maintenance of catecholamine systems in the central nervous system. *Behav Biol* **11**: 1–32.

Stickgold, R. (2005) Sleep-dependent memory consolidation. *Nature* **27** 437(7063):1272–8.

Stickgold, R. & Walker, M. P. (2005) Memory consolidation and reconsolidation: what is the role of sleep? *Trends Neurosci* **28**(8): 408–15.

Stickgold, R., Whidbee, D., Schirmer, B., Patel, V. & Hobson, J. A. (2000) Visual discrimination task improvement: a multi-step process occurring during sleep. *J Cogn Neurosci* **12**(2): 246–54.

Tilley, A. J. & Wilkinson, R. T. (1984) The effects of a restricted sleep regime on the composition of sleep and on performance. *Psychophysiology* **21**: 406–12.

Tsai, L. L., Bergmann, B. M., Perry, B. D. & Rechtschaffen, A. (1993) Effects of chronic total sleep deprivation on central noradrenergic receptors in rat brain. *Brain Res* **5** 602(2): 221–7.

Tsai, L. L., Bergmann, B. M., Perry, B. D. & Rechtschaffen, A. (1994) Effects of chronic sleep deprivation on central cholinergic receptors in rat brain. *Brain Res* **11** 642(1–2): 95–103.

Tsien, J. Z., Huerta, P. T. & Tonegawa, S. (1996) The essential role of hippocampal CA1 NMDA receptor-dependent synaptic plasticity in spatial memory. *Cell* **27** 87(7): 1327–38.

Ukponmwan, O. E., Rupreht, J. & Dzoljic, M. R. (1984) REM sleep deprivation decreases the antinociceptive property of enkephalinase-inhibition, morphine and cold-water-swim. *Gen Pharmacol* **15**(3): 255–8.

Ukponmwan, O. E., Rupreht, J., Dzoljic, M. R. *et al.* (1986) An analgesic effect of enkephalinase inhibition is modulated by monoamine oxidase-B and REM sleep deprivations. *Arch Pharmacol* **332**(4): 376–9.

Vertes, R. P. & Eastman, K. E. (2000) The case against memory consolidation in REM sleep. *Behav Brain Sci* **23**(6):867–76; discussion 904–1121.

Webb, W. B. & Agnew, H. W. (1965) Sleep: effects of a restricted regime. *Science* **150**: 1745–7.

Chapter

31

Modulation of body core temperature in NREM sleep and REM sleep

Pier Luigi Parmeggiani

Summary

The first and most important active defense of homeothermy in non-rapid eye movement (NREM) sleep is both reactive, i.e., depending on actual ambient temperature, and predictive, in that it is set before sleep by behavioral temperature regulation. This behavior provides thermal conditions counteracting the static influence of ambient temperature on the thermal balance of the body. An important passive defense is the thermal inertia of the body, particularly with regard to negative thermal loads. Such inertia is sufficient to buffer temporarily transient thermal imbalances due to sleep processes. In addition, under the influence of thermal loads and in the presence of an important pressure for sleep, autonomic temperature regulation is fully operative during NREM sleep without eliciting immediate awakening from sleep. This defense is energetically expensive, but the advantage is that as a result of the maintenance of brain thermal homeostasis REM sleep onset may also be promoted and then sustained for a while by the thermal inertia of the body. The important tenet is that the more the behavioral temperature regulation and the thermal inertia of the body constrain the activation of autonomic temperature regulation, the more they protect sleep from terminating. Awakening is the extreme defense of body core homeothermy but at the expense of REM sleep initially and, secondarily, of NREM sleep.

More than 40 years have elapsed since it was experimentally shown in cats exposed to cold and warm ambient thermal loads that shivering and panting, respectively, are present in NREM sleep and absent during REM sleep (Parmeggiani and Rabini, 1967). Then, the interaction between sleep and temperature regulation was the object of study in several mammals, and particularly in cats, rabbits, rats, and humans, which will be dealt with in this chapter. Such experiments not

only confirmed the original result but also extended and deepened our knowledge of the changes in temperature regulation that characterize the sleep states. Nevertheless, the physiologic reason why temperature regulation is suspended during REM sleep is still a mystery.

Overview of thermoregulation in sleep

According to the "Glossary of terms for thermal physiology" (IUPS Thermal Commission, 1987) the thermoregulatory responses to external (ambient) and internal (body), positive (warm) and negative (cold) thermal loads are either *behavioral* or *autonomic*. The rationale for this distinction is the following.

(1) *Behavioral temperature regulation* – (the term "behavioral" refers to somato-motor and postural activities) influences passive heat loss by means of changes in posture (e.g., curling or sprawling) and/or location (e.g., to increase or decrease exposure to sun, wind, humidity, etc.) of the body with respect to the thermal environment.

(2) *Autonomic temperature regulation* – (the term "autonomic" is used in its general sense and does not imply that all responses are controlled by the autonomic nervous system) actively influences both physiologic heat production (shivering, non-shivering thermogenesis) and heat loss (vasomotion of heat exchangers, piloerection, thermal tachypnea and panting, and sweating).

In other words, the *behavioral* responses are aimed at establishing appropriate ambient conditions affecting the heat exchange of the body with its environment and the *autonomic* responses, at affecting directly heat production and heat loss to restore and maintain the

---

REM Sleep: Regulation and Function, eds. Birendra N. Mallick, S. R. Pandi-Perumal, Robert W. McCarley, and Adrian R. Morrison. Published by Cambridge University Press. © Cambridge University Press 2011.

balance between the two variables underlying body core homeothermy. The study of long-term changes in thermoregulatory responses, resulting from the acclimatization to low or high ambient temperatures, is beyond the scope of this chapter.

In mammals, body core temperature is controlled by preoptic–hypothalamic integrative mechanisms that drive subordinate brain-stem and spinal somatic and autonomic mechanisms eliciting thermoregulatory responses (see Satinoff, 1978).

The following experimental results show in detail that the thermoregulatory responses to ambient thermal loads are present during NREM sleep and absent during REM sleep.

The cat's posture clearly varies in relation to ambient temperature during NREM sleep, whereas the drop in postural muscle tone during REM sleep is unrelated to ambient temperature (Parmeggiani and Rabini, 1970). Moreover, notwithstanding the same positive thermal load as in NREM sleep, tachypnea and panting in the cat (Parmeggiani and Rabini, 1967, 1970) and heat exchanger vasodilation in the cat (Parmeggiani *et al.*, 1977), rabbit (Franzini *et al.*, 1982), and rat (Alföldi *et al.*, 1990) disappear. Sweating in humans is first suppressed and then depressed during episodes of REM sleep (Dewasmes *et al.*, 1997; Sagot *et al.*, 1987).

A negative thermal load elicits the thermoregulatory responses in NREM sleep. In contrast, shivering in the cat (Parmeggiani and Rabini, 1967, 1970), heat exchanger vasoconstriction in the cat (Parmeggiani *et al.*, 1977), rabbit (Franzini *et al.*, 1982), and rat (Alföldi *et al.*, 1990) and piloerection in the cat (Hendricks *et al.*, 1977) are suppressed during an REM sleep episode. Shivering disappears during REM sleep in a cold ambience also in cats with pontine lesions producing REM sleep without muscle atonia (Hendricks *et al.*, 1977). This crucial result shows that the pontine inhibitory mechanisms eliciting muscle atonia in the normal animal do not underlie the suppression of this thermoregulatory response in REM sleep.

The thermoregulatory responses elicited by positive and negative thermal loads, directly applied to the thermosensitive preoptic–hypothalamic area, are present or absent depending on the state of sleep. In the cat, warming elicits tachypnea and panting (Parmeggiani *et al.*, 1973) and heat exchanger vasodilation (Parmeggiani *et al.*, 1977) during NREM sleep but has no such effects during REM sleep. Likewise, in the kangaroo rat (Glotzbach and Heller, 1976) cooling increases oxygen consumption and metabolic heat production during NREM sleep, whereas it is ineffective during REM sleep.

Experiments of direct thermal stimulation of thermosensitive neurons show the changes in the function of the preoptic–hypothalamic thermostat during sleep in the cat (Alam *et al.*, 1995 b; Parmeggiani *et al.*, 1986, 1987) and kangaroo rat (Glotzbach and Heller, 1984). The thermosensitivity of the majority of such neurons fairly parallels the thermoregulatory responsiveness to central thermal loads during NREM and REM sleep.

In conclusion, the thermoregulatory mechanisms are operative during NREM sleep as during quiet wake in cats, rabbits, rats, kangaroo rats, and humans, albeit there is a difference in the threshold and gain of effector responses to thermal loads. With respect to quiet wake, body and hypothalamic temperatures are downregulated together with energy metabolism in NREM sleep (Brebbia and Altshuler, 1965; Haskell *et al.*, 1981; Parmeggiani *et al.*, 1971, 1975). The lack of thermoregulatory responses observed during REM sleep is not simply the result of state-dependent changes in the threshold and gain of such responses. From the quantitative point of view, REM sleep is characterized by somatic and autonomic activity that is not only functionally inconsistent with the aim of temperature regulation but also lacks any proportional relationship with the intensity of the thermal stimulus. The result is that the temperature of the body changes according to its thermal inertia, as one would expect in a poikilothermic organism (Parmeggiani *et al.*, 1971; Walker *et al.*, 1983).

Table 31.1 shows the most important changes in temperature regulation across the wake–sleep ultradian cycle.

Modulation of body core temperature in sleep

The topic deserves the most attention at this point because the profound changes in temperature regulation across sleep states do not remarkably affect the body core temperature, including that of the brain. For instance, the temperature of the brain decreases in NREM sleep and increases in REM sleep by a few tenths of a degree Celsius in small furry species. Such a slight imbalance between the two sleep states is an effect of different but concurrent factors that constrain body core temperature within narrow limits under moderate positive or negative thermal loads. The question, therefore, is how the physiologic needs of sleep

Table 31.1 Thermoregulatory responses during wake and sleep

Responses		Wake	NREM sleep	REM sleep
	behavioral	locomotion	no locomotion	no locomotion, twitches
		posture	tonic posture	atonic posture
Specific				
	autonomic	vasomotion	vasomotion	inconsistent vasomotion
		piloerection	piloerection	no piloerection
		shivering	shivering	no shivering
		panting	panting	no panting
		sweating	sweating	sweating (suppression, depression)
Non-specific		vigilance	arousal	arousal

and homeothermy are practically reconciled. On the basis of experimental evidence, it appears likely that the operational answer to this question is given in the first instance by the behavioral temperature regulation displayed at the onset of sleep.

In general, mammals display a pre-sleep behavior, that is in part species specific and in part influenced by the actual ambient temperature. This behavior ought to be considered not only *reactive* to actual ambient temperature but also *predictive* (see Moore-Ede, 1986 for this terminology) with respect to the development of the sleep states of the ultradian cycle, since it provides the body core with tolerable and even almost stable thermal conditions. By reducing the preoptic–hypothalamic drive of autonomic temperature regulation, such pre-sleep behavior promotes onset and duration of both NREM sleep and subsequent REM sleep. It has been experimentally shown that even under heavy thermal loads the dramatic suppression of temperature regulation during REM sleep occurs unopposed by arousal if the preoptic–hypothalamic temperature is artificially clamped at the normal physiologic level (Parmeggiani *et al.*, 1974).

In conclusion, the thermoregulatory aspect of the pre-sleep behavior corresponds to the operational definition of *behavioral temperature regulation* of both animals and humans. Such behavior provides thermoneutral conditions particularly to the preoptic–hypothalamic area of the sleeping organism even when the ambient temperature does not correspond exactly to the ambient thermoneutral zone of the species. This zone is defined, on the basis of physiologic criteria, as "The range of ambient temperature at which temperature regulation is achieved only by control of sensible heat loss, i.e. without regulatory changes in metabolic heat production or evaporative heat loss" (IUPS Thermal Commission, 1987, p. 584). This ambient thermal condition promotes the free occurrence of "normal" sleep since the specific decrease in metabolic activity in NREM sleep is not antagonized by a metabolic demand for thermoregulation.

It is beyond the scope of this chapter to enumerate fully the variety of the natural and cultural behavioral measures of animals and humans that provide the sleeping organism with the most favorable thermal condition at a lower energetic cost than that required in wakefulness. Only the basic protective factors, constraining body core temperature within narrow limits, will be considered next in some detail.

Onset of sleep

Both motor and postural patterns characterize the transition from wakefulness to NREM sleep. The motor activity is aimed at finding a safe and thermally comfortable ecological niche to assume the natural sleep posture. The body posture is characterized by the decrease in antigravity muscle activity and by curling up or sprawling, and flexing or extending the limbs in a cold and a warm environment, respectively. As already mentioned, the postural attitude is both reactive to the actual ambient temperature and predictive to protect the controlled decrease in body temperature during NREM sleep.

Heat loss is regulated according to ambient temperature by changing the extension of the body surface that is exposed to the surrounding air or the ground. In particular, curling up and sprawling influence in opposite ways the abdominal thermal stimulation modulating – notably in furry species – the sympathetic vasoconstrictor outflow to the heat exchangers of the body (skin, ear pinna, upper airway mucosa, tail) (Azzaroni and Parmeggiani, 1993). Also, inspired air is thermally conditioned by placing the nose either close to or away from the body surface depending on the posture chosen by the animal at low or high ambient temperatures, respectively. The control of inspired air temperature influences also the temperature of the venous blood flowing from the upper airway vascular bed to the heart. Such blood contributes directly to the regulation of the temperature of the brain before returning to the heart, thanks to countercurrent or conductive mechanisms of heat exchange with the carotid blood supply to the brain (Azzaroni and Parmeggiani, 1993, 1995a,b; Hayward and Baker, 1969; Parmeggiani *et al.*, 2002). The specific body postures thus reduce the energetic cost of temperature regulation in sleep and provide a thermal condition, which is propitious to sleep also when ambient temperature does not correspond precisely to the ambient thermoneutral zone of the species.

NREM sleep

The posture of thermal defense assumed at sleep onset is maintained throughout NREM sleep or modified depending on the persistence or change of the ambient thermal load, respectively. In addition, efficient reactive temperature regulation involving the activity of skeletal muscles (shivering, thermal tachypnea, panting) and the autonomic nervous system (vasomotion, piloerection, sweating), is present during NREM sleep when necessary. Only under the influence of heavy thermal loads is NREM sleep sooner or later interrupted by arousal.

NREM sleep is characterized by decreased body core temperature resulting from both reduced metabolic heat production (Brebbia and Altshuler, 1965; Haskell *et al.*, 1981) and sympathetic activity increasing heat loss (Azzaroni and Parmeggiani, 1993, 1995a,b). In particular, the actual intensity of tonic vasoconstriction of heat exchangers in quiet wakefulness is decreased during NREM sleep as a sleep-dependent event (Azzaroni and Parmeggiani, 1995b). The resulting vasodilatation is shown by an increase in heat exchanger temperature and a related increase in brain cooling that lowers preoptic–hypothalamic temperature during NREM sleep (Azzaroni and Parmeggiani, 1993, 1995b; Hayward and Baker, 1969; Parmeggiani *et al.*, 1975). In conclusion, body and preoptic–hypothalamic temperatures decrease during NREM sleep as a result

of the decrease in metabolic heat production and the regulated increase in heat loss.

Concerning heat loss in particular, in quiet wakefulness the vascular heat exchangers are regulated by the vasoconstrictor sympathetic outflow that varies in intensity depending on ambient and/or preoptic–hypothalamic thermal loads. For instance, in the thermal zone of vasomotor regulation of body temperature (i.e., under moderate negative and positive thermal loads), there is an increase or a decrease in tonic vasoconstriction of the heat exchangers to reduce or enhance heat loss from the body, respectively. In contrast, whatever the actual intensity of such tonic vasoconstrictor sympathetic outflow to heat exchangers may be, there is always a decrease in this intensity during NREM sleep with respect to quiet wakefulness as a sleep-dependent event in the cat (Azzaroni and Parmeggiani, 1995b). The effects of vasodilatation are shown by an increase in heat exchanger temperature and a related increase in brain cooling that lowers brain temperature during NREM sleep (Azzaroni and Parmeggiani, 1993, 1995a,b; Hayward and Baker, 1969; Parmeggiani *et al.*, 1975). Moreover, a sharp decline of preoptic–hypothalamic temperature, e.g., in cats, starts when the head is lowered to assume the sleep posture and is steeper at low ambient temperatures (Parmeggiani *et al.*, 1975). This is a result of the head-down posture (decrease in negative hydrostatic load raising the vascular transmural pressure), which, concomitantly with the decrease of tonic vasoconstrictor sympathetic outflow, contributes to increase heat-exchanger vasodilatation and eventual brain cooling during NREM sleep (Azzaroni and Parmeggiani, 1995a).

In humans, thermal sweating (Sagot *et al.*, 1987) and skin vasodilatation in the lower extremities (Kräuchi *et al.*, 2000) are phenomena consistent with the down-regulation of body core temperature in NREM sleep. Skin vasodilatation in the lower extremities at the onset of NREM sleep indicates a state-dependent change in the central regulation of the sympathetic outflow. The increase in skin temperature, which may also be mimicked by artificial moderate warming, generates a feedback to the central thermostat that positively influences sleep propensity (Kräuchi *et al.*, 2000). This phenomenon, a result of the NREM sleep-related change in preoptic–hypothalamic drive on sympathetic outflow, is analogous to the systemic heat exchanger vasodilatation occurring in furry species that elicits a decrease in preoptic–hypothalamic temperature during NREM sleep (Azzaroni and Parmeggiani, 1993, 1995a,b). The increase and decrease in responsiveness of warm- and cold-responsive neurons, respectively, tested by means of direct thermal stimulation in NREM sleep, underlies the central downregulation of body and brain temperatures (Alam *et al.*, 1995a; Glotzbach and Heller, 1984; Parmeggiani *et al.*, 1986, 1987).

It is a shared tenet that the decrease in metabolic rate and the increase in heat loss are regulated physiologic features of NREM sleep. The NREM sleep-dependent decrease in brain temperature is evidently subliminal as a thermal feedback for thermoregulatory responses across a wide range of ambient temperatures (Parmeggiani *et al.*, 1975). However, in the case of conspicuous thermal loads, autonomic temperature regulation may be normally activated during NREM sleep without eliciting immediate awakening. These facts point to a change in the set point temperature of the thermostat since preoptic–hypothalamic thermosensitive neurons are still responsive to adequate thermal stimulation in NREM sleep (Alam *et al.*, 1995a; Glotzbach and Heller, 1984; Parmeggiani *et al.*, 1986, 1987).

In conclusion, NREM sleep is characterized by somatic quiescence, the functional prevalence of parasympathetic over sympathetic activity, the lowering of metabolic heat production (decrease in muscle tone, and heart and breathing rates) and body temperature (vasodilatation of heat exchangers, sweating). However, all behavioral and autonomic thermoregulatory responses to endogenous and exogenous thermal disturbances may be activated during NREM sleep in order to maintain the selected set point temperature of the body core. The stereotype of phenomena in NREM sleep across mammalian species appears to be the coherent result of a common phylogenetic trend toward development of a pattern of integrated automatic regulation of somatic and autonomic mechanisms that results in minimized energy expenditure.

REM sleep

There is a small increase (up to a few tenths of a degree Celsius) in brain temperature during REM sleep across a wide range of low, neutral, and high ambient temperatures. The increase is not the result of a change in the set point temperature of the thermostat, since the responsiveness of preoptic–hypothalamic thermosensitive neurons is variably altered, up to a clear-cut depression during this state of sleep (Alam *et al.*, 1995b;

Glotzbach and Heller, 1984; Parmeggiani *et al.*, 1986, 1987). Thus, it is neither the expression of a thermoregulatory control, as the decrease in brain temperature observed in NREM sleep, nor a significant sign of the actual cessation of temperature regulation in REM sleep. Surprisingly enough, it depends on (1) brain circulation and (2) body thermal inertia.

Hemodynamic factors

Three main physiologic factors have been considered as possibly underlying the rise in brain temperature related to REM sleep, namely: changes in (1) the metabolic heat production of the nervous tissue; (2) the arterial blood flow; and (3) the arterial blood temperature.

The metabolic heat production of the nervous tissue appears an unlikely candidate as the primary cause of the observed change in brain temperature. Several studies have shown that both brain metabolic rate and arterial blood flow increase in REM sleep with respect to NREM sleep (see Franzini, 1992). Since the increase in brain metabolic heat production is always indirectly related to the rise in brain heat clearance by the increase in arterial blood flow, temperature alone is not a reliable indicator of metabolic heat production (see Hayward and Baker, 1969).

The experimental evidence shows that the proximate cause of the rise of brain temperature in REM sleep is a decrease of the carotid blood supply and an increase of the vertebral blood supply to the circle of Willis (Azzaroni and Parmeggiani, 1993; Parmeggiani *et al.*, 2002). The remote cause of the rise in brain temperature is the instability of autonomic cardiovascular regulation (Calasso and Parmeggiani, 2008) that brings about "stealth" of common carotid artery blood supplying the brain and the systemic heat exchangers of the head. The stealth of common carotid blood flow is counterbalanced in the species studied (cat, rabbit, and rat) by blood flowing to the brain primarily from the vertebral arteries as a result of autoregulation and flow-metabolism coupling. The brain temperature increases because the vertebral blood is warmer than the carotid blood (Azzaroni and Parmeggiani, 1993; Parmeggiani *et al.*, 2002).

Thermal inertia of the body core

The physical factor underlying the passive maintenance of the thermal stability of the brain in NREM sleep and particularly in REM sleep is the thermal inertia of the body core. Such inertia depends primarily on the thermal capacity of body water and the skin thermal conductance in relation to both the surface-to-volume ratio of the body and seasonal factors affecting the heat exchange between body and environment. Among the latter factors are reciprocal changes in the amount of fat and fur with respect to ambient temperature in summer and winter that affect heat loss. The importance of the thermal inertia of the body under moderate thermal loads, in order to protect the state of REM sleep from the arousal response, is shown by a study in cats exposed to low and high ambient temperatures (Parmeggiani *et al.*, 1971). For instance, in a cat exposed to –15°C ambient temperature, about 40°C below the ambient thermal neutrality of the species, a rate of change of body core temperature was measured equal to 0.0017°C/min °C(Tb – Ta) (Tb, body temperature; Ta, ambient temperature) during REM sleep. Such passive cooling, in the absence of thermoregulatory responses like vasoconstriction of heat exchangers, shivering, and piloerection, would correspond to a decrease in body core temperature of 0.68°C in ten minutes of REM sleep duration. The important arousing effect of heavy negative thermal loads, in relation to the progressive cooling of all thermal compartments of the body, is substantially revealed by the decreasing slope of preoptic–hypothalamic temperature during the REM-sleep episode instead of the normal increase (Parmeggiani *et al.*, 1984).

It is worth noting at this point that the length of the sleep cycle positively correlates with the brain weight (Zepelin, 2000), when no exogenous factors (nutritional habits, ecological niche, predator/prey relationship) prevail over temperature regulation as factors affecting the survival of the species. It is theoretically appealing to surmise that this correlation may imply that, besides other factors, a phylogenetic pressure made the maximum duration of REM sleep episodes to fit the thermal inertia of the brain. For instance, in cats (Parmeggiani and Rabini, 1970) and rats (Cerri *et al.*, 2005), the duration of REM-sleep episodes decreases under negative ambient thermal loads. Heavy negative ambient thermal loads readily offset the protective influence of both behavioral temperature regulation and brain thermal inertia on the ultradian sleep cycle, and particularly REM sleep. In such conditions, suppression of REM-sleep episodes is observed (Cerri *et al.*, 2005; Parmeggiani and Rabini, 1970). These conclusions apply also to heavy positive thermal loads that clearly disturb or suppress the occurrence of REM sleep, particularly in small furry species. The fact that

the range of tolerated high temperatures above ambient thermoneutrality is not as wide as that of the negative thermal loads below ambient thermoneutrality confirms the notion that such species are better equipped for the defense against cold than heat.

Ambient temperature and ultradian sleep cycle

In general, the duration of sleep peaks at ambient temperatures close to the upper limit of the ambient thermoneutral zone (Szymusiak and Satinoff, 1981). This pertains to wherever the zone placement may be in the temperature continuum, depending on the species and its acclimatization to the actual ambient temperature. A mild positive preoptic–hypothalamic thermal load promotes both NREM sleep and REM sleep (Parmeggiani *et al.*, 1974; Roberts and Robinson, 1969; Sakaguchi *et al.*, 1979; Von Euler and Söderberg, 1957). The reason is that the effect it induces in somatic (e.g., decrease of muscle tone, posture for heat loss) and autonomic (e.g., vasodilatation due to decrease in sympathetic outflow to heat exchangers, sweating) activities are the same as those occurring in NREM sleep.

In conclusion, sleep duration significantly decreases above and below the ambient thermoneutral zone. Particularly consistent with the physiologic necessity of NREM sleep-regulated decrease in metabolic rate is the fact that without such a zone the decrease in duration of sleep substantially and inversely fits the rate of increase in energy expenditure for temperature regulation (Hensel *et al.*, 1973, p. 533).

The modulation of body core temperature in NREM sleep is a controlled event perfectly consistent with the mammalian repertoire of refined mechanisms of thermal control. In contrast, the teleological significance of the cessation of temperature regulation during REM sleep in mammals is still a mystery more than fifty years after the discovery of REM sleep. However, the inference is appealing that the ultradian fragmentation of REM sleep allows, in practice, physiology to reconcile its dramatic thermoregulatory failure with unknown but surely basic functional needs of the central nervous system: a remarkable example of Cannon's "wisdom of the body."

Acknowledgments

The author is very grateful to Professor Adrian R. Morrison for editing the manuscript.

References

Alam, M. N., McGinty, D. & Szymusiak, R. (1995a) Neuronal discharge of preoptic/anterior hypothalamic thermosensitive neurons: relation to NREM sleep. *Am J Physiol* **269**: R1240–9.

Alam, M. N., McGinty, D. & Szymusiak, R. (1995b) Preoptic/anterior hypothalamic neurons: thermosensitivity in rapid eye movement sleep. *Am J Physiol* **269**: R1250–7.

Alföldi, P., Rubicsek, G., Cserni, G. *et al.* (1990) Brain and core temperatures and peripheral vasomotion during sleep and wakefulness at various ambient temperatures in the rat. *Pflügers Arch* **417**: 336–41.

Azzaroni, A. & Parmeggiani, P. L. (1993) Mechanisms underlying hypothalamic temperature changes during sleep in mammals. *Brain Res* **632**: 136–42.

Azzaroni, A. & Parmeggiani, P. L. (1995a) Postural and sympathetic influences on brain cooling during the ultradian wake–sleep cycle. *Brain Res* **671**: 78–82.

Azzaroni, A. & Parmeggiani, P. L. (1995b) Synchronized sleep duration is related to tonic vasoconstriction of thermoregulatory heat exchangers. *J Sleep Res* **4**: 41–7.

Brebbia, D. R. & Altshuler, K. Z. (1965) Oxygen consumption rate and electroencephalographic stage of sleep. *Science* (Washington DC) **150**: 1621–3.

Calasso, M. & Parmeggiani, P. L. (2008) Carotid blood flow during REM sleep. *Sleep* **31**: 701–7.

Cerri, M., Ocampo-Garcés, A., Amici, R. *et al.* (2005) Cold exposure and sleep in the rat: Effects on sleep architecture and the electroencephalogram. *Sleep* **28**: 694–705.

Dewasmes, G., Bothorel, B., Candas, V. *et al.* (1997) A short-term poikilothermic period occurs just after paradoxical sleep onset in humans: characterization changes in sweating effector activity. *J Sleep Res* **6**: 252–8.

Franzini, C. (1992) Brain metabolism and blood flow during sleep. *J Sleep Res* **1**: 3–16.

Franzini, C., Cianci, T., Lenzi, P. *et al.* (1982) Neural control of vasomotion in rabbit ear is impaired during desynchronized sleep. *Am J Physiol* **243**: R142–6.

Glotzbach, S. F. & Heller, H. C. (1976) Central nervous regulation of body temperature during sleep. *Science* **194**: 537–9.

Glotzbach, S. F. & Heller, H. C. (1984) Changes in the thermal characteristics of hypothalamic neurons during sleep and wakefulness. *Brain Res* **309**: 17–26.

Haskell, E. H., Palca, J. W., Walker, J. M. *et al.* (1981) Metabolism and thermoregulation during stages of sleep in humans exposed to heat and cold. *J Appl Physiol* **51**: 948–54.

Hayward, J. N. & Baker, M. A. (1969) A comparative study of the role of the cerebral arterial blood in the regulation of brain temperature in five mammals. *Brain Res* **16**: 417–40.

Hendricks, J. C., Bowker, R. M. & Morrison, A. R. (1977) Functional characteristics of cats with pontine lesions during sleep and wakefulness and their usefulness for sleep research. In *Sleep 1976*, eds. W. P. Koella & P. Levin. Basel: Karger, pp. 207–10.

Hensel, H., Brück, K. & Raths, P. (1973) Homeothermic organisms. In *Temperature and Life*, eds. H. Precht, J. Christophersen, H. Hensel & W. Larcher. Berlin, Heidelberg, New York: Springer, pp. 503–761.

IUPS Thermal Commission (1987) Glossary of terms for thermal physiology. *Pflugers Arch* **410**: 567–87.

Kräuchi, K., Cajochen, C., Werth, E. *et al.* (2000) Functional link between distal vasodilation and sleep-onset latency. *Am J Physiol* **278**: R741–8.

Moore-Ede, M. C. (1986) Physiology of the circadian timing system: predictive versus reactive homeostasis. *Am J Physiol* **250**: R737–52.

Parmeggiani, P. L. & Rabini, C. (1967) Shivering and panting during sleep. *Brain Res* **6**: 789–91.

Parmeggiani, P. L. & Rabini, C. (1970) Sleep and environmental temperature. *Arch Ital Biol* **108**: 369–87.

Parmeggiani, P. L., Franzini, C., Lenzi, P. *et al.* (1971) Inguinal subcutaneous temperature changes in cats sleeping at different environmental temperatures. *Brain Res* **33**: 397–404.

Parmeggiani, P. L., Franzini, C., Lenzi, P. *et al.* (1973) Threshold of respiratory responses to preoptic heating during sleep in freely moving cats. *Brain Res* **52**: 189–201.

Parmeggiani, P. L., Zamboni, G., Cianci, T. *et al.* (1974) Influence of anterior hypothalamic heating on the duration of fast-wave sleep episodes. *Electroencephalogr Clin Neurophysiol* **36**: 465–70.

Parmeggiani, P. L., Agnati, L. F., Zamboni, G. *et al.* (1975) Hypothalamic temperature during the sleep cycle at different ambient temperatures. *Electroencephalogr Clin Neurophysiol* **38**: 589–96.

Parmeggiani, P. L., Zamboni, G., Cianci, T. *et al.* (1977) Absence of thermoregulatory vasomotor responses during fast wave sleep in cats. *Electroencephalogr Clin Neurophysiol* **42**: 372–80.

Parmeggiani, P. L., Zamboni, G., Perez, E. *et al.* (1984) Hypothalamic temperature during desynchronized sleep. *Exp Brain Res* **54**: 315–20.

Parmeggiani, P. L., Azzaroni, A., Cevolani, D. *et al.* (1986) Polygraphic study of anterior hypothalamic-preoptic neuron thermosensitivity during sleep. *Electroencephalogr Clin Neurophysiol*, **63**: 289–95.

Parmeggiani, P. L., Cevolani, D., Azzaroni, A. *et al.* (1987) Thermosensitivity of anterior hypothalamic-preoptic neurons during the waking–sleeping cycle: a study in brain functional states. *Brain Res* **415**: 79–89.

Parmeggiani, P. L., Azzaroni, A. & Calasso, M. (2002) Systemic hemodynamic changes raising brain temperature in REM sleep. *Brain Res* **940**: 55–60.

Roberts, W. W. & Robinson, T. C. L. (1969) Relaxation and sleep induced by warming of the preoptic region and anterior hypothalalmus in cats. *Exp Neurol* **25**: 282–94.

Sagot, J. C., Amoros, C., Candas, V. *et al.* (1987) Sweating responses and body temperatures during nocturnal sleep in humans. *Am J Physiol*, **252**: R462–70.

Sakaguchi, S., Glotzbach, S. F. & Heller, H. C. (1979) Influence of hypothalamic and ambient temperatures on sleep in kangaroo rats. *Am J Physiol* **237**: R80–8.

Satinoff, E. (1978) Neural organization and evolution of thermal regulation in mammals. *Science* **201**: 16–22.

Szymusiak, R. & Satinoff, E. (1981) Maximal REM sleep time defines a narrower thermoneutral zone than does minimal metabolic rate. *Physiol Behav* **26**: 687–90.

Von Euler, C. & Söderberg, U. (1957) The influence of hypothalamic thermoceptive structures on the electroencephalogram and gamma motor activity. *Electroencephalogr Clin Neurophysiol* **9**: 391–408.

Walker, J. M., Walker, L. E., Harris, D. V. *et al.* (1983) Cessation of thermoregulation during REM sleep in the pocket mouse. *Am J Physiol* **244**: R114–18.

Zepelin, H. (2000) Mammalian sleep. In *Principles and Practice of Sleep Medicine*, eds. M. H. Kryger, T. Roth & W. C. Dement. Philadelphia: Saunders, pp. 82–92.

Chapter 32

Sleep-related hippocampal activation: implications for spatial memory consolidation

Dinesh Pal, Victoria Booth, and Gina R. Poe

Summary

Sleep is implicated in the consolidation of many types of learning and memory tasks. Place cells (hippocampal neurons responding to spatial location of the subject) associated with novel environments on a spatial task reactivate during subsequent sleep (Poe *et al.*, 2000). Such neuronal firing is thought to strengthen memories formed during waking exploration (Huerta and Lisman, 1995). Once the initially novel environment becomes familiar to the animal, place cells *reverse phase* at which they fire with respect to local theta oscillations during REM sleep. Such phase-reversed firing during theta is consistent with patterns that induce the depotentiation of previously potentiated synapses. Depotentiation is important to prevent the saturation of synaptic weights in the hippocampus, keeping the differential weighting structure necessary for memory preservation. These results indicate that sleep in general seems to serve neither an overall synaptic erasing (Tononi and Cirelli, 2001) nor a general synaptic amplification effect. Rather, in a network-by-network manner (Ribeiro and Nicolelis, 2004) and, according to the requirements of the learning phase, REM-sleep reactivation serves to amplify as-yet-unconsolidated memories and erase already transferred networks from the temporary stores of the hippocampus (Best *et al.*, 2007; Booth and Poe, 2006).

Sleep: a brief introduction

Considerable advances in sleep research have brought some semblance of unanimity regarding the mechanisms underlying sleep generation. It is well established now that sleep is an endogenous behavioral state with a circadian periodicity and can be categorized into distinct phases — non-rapid eye movement (NREM) sleep and rapid eye movement (REM) sleep (Pace-Schott and Hobson, 2002). The two states of NREM and REM sleep are not only different in their characteristic electrical signatures but are also governed by different brain regions. Forebrain structures are involved in NREM generation/regulation whereas brain-stem structures are involved in REM-sleep generation/regulation (Pace-Schott and Hobson, 2002; Steriade and McCarley, 2007). Sleep onset is marked by a decrease in the monoaminergic tone through reduced activity of the locus coeruleus (noradrenergic), dorsal raphe (serotonergic), and tubero-mammillary nucleus (histaminergic), which are wake-active nuclei (Pace-Schott and Hobson, 2002; Steriade and McCarley, 2007). With the onset of REM sleep the decreased activity of monoaminergic processes reaches a nadir (Aston-Jones and Bloom, 1981) whereas there is a dominant presence of brain-stem cholinergic mechanisms (Lydic *et al.*, 1991; Lydic and Baghdoyan, 1993).

Given the complexity of sleep as a phenomenon, it is unlikely that it serves only one unique function. Recent emerging evidence overwhelmingly indicates that sleep is required for efficient memory consolidation and that different stages of sleep are involved in the consolidation of different types of memory systems (Frank and Benington, 2006; Stickgold *et al.*, 2001; Walker and Stickgold, 2004). We have preliminary evidence indicating that theta phase-specific firing of hippocampal neurons causes a reformation of the synaptic networks involved in mnemonic processes. Once the memories have been consolidated to the neocortex, phase-specific firing can clear the hippocampal network for future memory formation (Booth and Poe, 2006; Jablonski *et al.*, 2007; Wang *et al.*, 2008).

Memory system classifications

The struggles and the predicaments of the scientific community in coming up with a coherent system

REM Sleep: Regulation and Function, eds. Birendra N. Mallick, S. R. Pandi-Perumal, Robert W. McCarley, and Adrian R. Morrison. Published by Cambridge University Press. © Cambridge University Press 2011.

of memory classification are elegantly described by Squire (2004). Memory systems can be categorized into declarative and non-declarative memory (Squire, 2004). The term "declarative memory" implies the memory used in common parlance and constitutes a recollection of facts and events. These are the things that we can consciously talk about or "declare" as ever existed. Declarative memory is further subcategorized into semantic and episodic memory. Semantic memory encompasses the recollection of factual details e.g., place of birth. In contrast, recollection of an event as it happened – what, where, and when – falls under the domain of episodic memory. "Non-declarative" denotes a large repertoire of life-sustaining activities occurring on a daily basis that are hard to explain and do not register in our conscious recollection. Examples of processes classified under non-declarative memory are procedural skills and habits, such as swimming, emotional responses to a specific stimulus, and reflex actions like salivating at the sound of the dinner bell. Finally, memories can also be divided into short-term memory and long-term memory.

A scheme to classify different types of memory is the human attempt to understand the complex processes underlying learning and memory. In reality, all of these systems interact with each other and do not strictly exist in compartmentalized form. In this chapter, we will elaborate on the hippocampal episodic memory and will develop a thesis for the role of REM sleep in spatial memory consolidation.

Episodic memory formation: an intact hippocampus is a necessity

The well reported case of patient H. M. is a good starting point for discussion on the significance of the hippocampus for intact episodic memory processes. Patient H. M. underwent medial temporal lobe resections at the age of 27 to treat epileptic seizures that were not responding to drug treatment. Although the severity and the frequency of the seizures decreased, an unexpected outcome of the surgery was a global amnesia. The case study by Scoville and Milner (1957) reported that the lobectomy in H. M.'s case also caused extensive damage to the hippocampal structures and that the extent of the hippocampal damage showed a positive correlation with the degree of memory impairment. The patient showed not only complete anterograde amnesia from the time of resection, but also had retrograde amnesia extending back to as many as 11 years prior to the surgery

(Sagar *et al.*, 1985). Further studies over the years confirmed H. M.'s inability to acquire semantic information although H. M. can learn sensorimotor and motor skills (Corkin, 2002). The lesions in the case of H. M. were not limited to the hippocampus, which made it difficult to exclude the role of adjoining extra-hippocampal regions in the memory processes. This study laid the framework for future experimental testing of the role of the hippocampus in memory consolidation. Zola-Morgan and colleagues (1986) reported the case study of a patient named R. B. in which the lesions were limited to the CA1 area of hippocampus. Patient R. B. suffered from moderately severe anterograde amnesia and showed little retrograde amnesia. Neuropsychological and neuropathological testing on a series of such patients confirmed that damage limited to the hippocampus is sufficient to produce significant anterograde and graded retrograde memory impairment, the severity of memory impairment being directly related to the extent and site of damage to the hippocampus (Rempel-Clower *et al.*, 1996).

Experiments in animals confirmed the results obtained from the human data. Lesion of the hippocampus and the adjoining tissue resulted in profound memory impairment in monkeys (Zola-Morgan *et al.*, 1989). Ischemic lesions specific to the hippocampus also resulted in significant memory impairment (Zola-Morgan *et al.*, 1992). Similar results have been obtained from studies in rodents (Martin *et al.*, 2005; Ordy *et al.*, 1988; Volpe *et al.*, 1984).

Memory consolidation and REM sleep

REM sleep has been shown to be important to the performance of many memory tasks (Smith, 1996; Smith and Rose, 1997). Although there are several kinds of learning tasks not dependent on sleep for consolidation, such as word priming, most studies agree that learning tasks requiring synaptic reorganization have a sleep-dependent component (Stickgold *et al.*, 2001; Walker and Stickgold, 2004). The benefit of REM sleep has been shown to be synaptic and specific, e.g., perceptual learning tasks that cause focal synaptic changes to occur need REM sleep for strong, lasting improvements; the gains made by training followed by REM sleep are specific to the circuits trained and do not generally transfer to all other perceptual processing fields (Karni *et al.*, 1994; Mednick *et al.*, 2002). When training intensity is high, the need for REM sleep for memory consolidation is more immediate (Smith, 1996). If REM sleep is prevented in the first few hours after training, memory for the task will be impaired even if the total time spent in REM sleep is not diminished over the sleep period (Smith, 1996; Smith and Rose, 1997). We delayed entrance to REM sleep for four hours in a group of rats after training them on a spatial task every day. Those animals never learned to perform the task in an allocentric, hippocampus-dependent manner. Another group deprived of the same amount of REM sleep in the second four-hour window after training were slowed in their learning relative to controls but were able to perform the task relying on spatial cues (Bjorness *et al.*, 2005).

One explanation for this slowing of learning might be that REM-sleep deprivation inhibits the subsequent ability to induce and/or maintain long-term potentiation (LTP), which, prior to training, could impair the hippocampus in its rapid association role (Campbell *et al.*, 2002; Davis *et al.*, 2003; Marks and Wayner, 2005; McDermott *et al.*, 2003; Romcy-Pereira and Pavlides, 2004). Long-term potentiation is the potentiation (strengthening) of connections from the presynaptic to the postsynaptic cell and is widely considered the building block for learning. Long-term potentiation occurs under conditions of strong depolarization of the postsynaptic cell and simultaneous activity at the presynaptic input. It involves a relatively large influx of calcium ions either through NMDA receptors or voltage-gated calcium channels (or both), which sets up a cascade of intracellular events that ultimately increases the number of postsynaptic glutamate receptors, rendering the postsynaptic cell more sensitive to presynaptic glutamate release (for review, see Blitzer *et al.*, 2005). Long-term potentiation has a counterpart as important as the increase in synaptic efficiency: long-term depression (LTD) or, in the case of prior LTP, depotentiation, which leads to a reduction in postsynaptic glutamate receptors.

Another possibility, and one that is not exclusive of the former, is that reactivation of the cellular assemblies in the hippocampus during REM sleep after learning is important to strengthen synapses newly potentiated during the prior waking period and to consolidate the memory network. Such post-learning function is prevented by disrupting REM sleep. This reactivation during REM sleep needs to occur in concert with NREM sleep events to proceed normally; that is, NREM sleep alone in the first few hours is not sufficient to complete the local strengthening and network consolidation process of hippocampus-dependent memories.

A third possibility is also not exclusive of the prior two mentioned above. REM sleep may also serve to clear the memory assembly place of already consolidated memories, leaving the associative network free again for new learning in subsequent waking periods. Evidence for this idea is presented below.

Hippocampal place-cell activity and sleep

Hippocampal pyramidal cells, which fire in response to specific spatial locations, known as the place fields, are called place cells (O'Keefe and Dostrovsky, 1971). Place fields are formed while an animal is exploring an environment, and these remain stable through LTP mechanisms (Shapiro, 2001). About one-third of an assembly of cells simultaneously recorded in the freely behaving rat will be active (form a place field) in any given environment, and the activity of a cell in one environment does not predict its activity in another. Thus, it is just as likely that a cell with a place field in one environment will fall silent or be active in an unrelated place in the next environment (Figure 32.1).

To date, the best physiological metric of spontaneous LTP that underlies spatial learning is the measure of expansion of place-field size (Mehta *et al.*, 1997, 2000). Specifically, place-cell activity is skewed in the direction opposite to the trajectory of a rat running on a track, indicating that these cells are firing earlier with each pass or lap through the place field. This change in place-field firing distribution is thought to reflect potentiation of inputs to those CA1 place cells (Ekstrom *et al.*, 2001) through the trisynaptic loop originating in the cortex. Place-field expansion is considered a marker of the LTP occurring during exposure to an environment. Backward place-field expansion occurs within the first 15 laps around a track for both familiar and first-exposure places (Mehta *et al.*, 1997, 2000). Since place fields do not expand backward indefinitely upon repeated exposures to an environment, but remain roughly the same size over months (Thompson and Best, 1990), place-field dimensions must reset between track running days. The reversal of this potentiation-induced place field expansion should be through the reversal of LTP, i.e., depotentiation, which, we hypothesize, occurs primarily during REM sleep.

Pavlides and Winson (1989) showed that hippocampal neurons that were active during the waking state increased firing or were "reactivated" in a subsequent sleep session. Reactivation during REM sleep

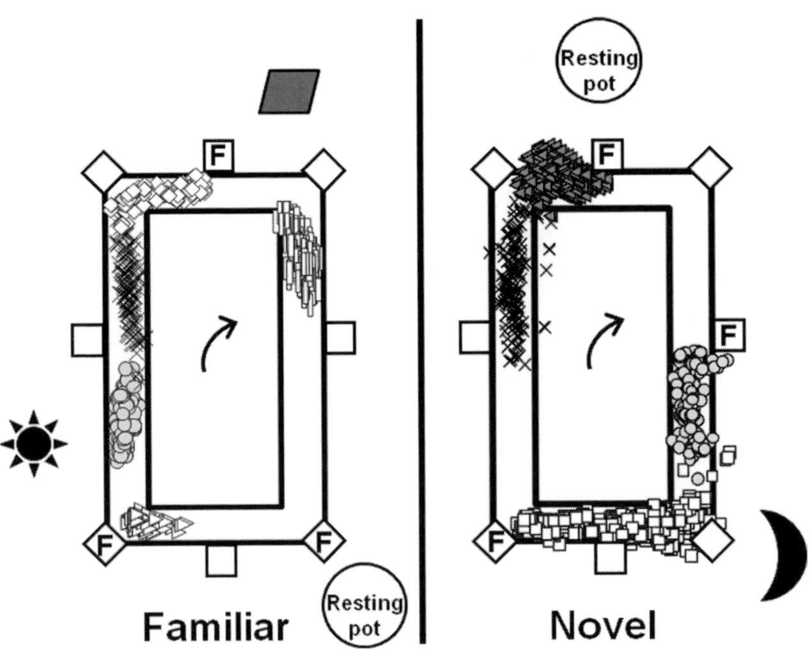

Figure 32.1 The place-mapped firing pattern of seven different place cells recorded over 45 minutes while the rat ran on the familiar (left) and novel (right) sides of a 3-feet-high wooden barrier (black line). Each simultaneously recorded cell is coded by symbol for differentiation and each symbol represents the place where an action potential occurred. Each of the cells shown was active in only one portion of each environment, except two neurons (x's and o's) that showed place-specific activity on both the familiar and novel tracks. The rat ran clockwise on both tracks. The square boxes around the track represent the food boxes, with those that contained the accessible reward (food) labeled with an F on the diagram. The barrier between tracks blocked view of the novel side over days of running the familiar track before the day of the familiar/novel track run recording.

occurs on a timescale and pattern comparable to that of the original behavior, i.e., if it requires 80 seconds to run a lap during wakefulness and cells A, B, and C fire in sequ-ence on that track, the ordered reactivation of those place cells occurs within approximately 80 seconds during REM sleep (Louie and Wilson, 2001). In the zebra finch the higher vocal center (HVC) song-production area also reactivates during sleep in a manner faithful in timescale and pattern to that occurring during the waking state (Dave and Margoliash, 2000). Hippocampal (Wilson and McNaughton, 1994) and neocortical (Siapas *et al.*, 2005) reactivation during NREM sleep occurs at a much accelerated rate on each slow wave (aka sharp wave, or large irregular activity wave, in the hippocampus). Further, during the occurrence of spindles, when noradrenergic neurons are also silent (Aston-Jones and Bloom, 1981) the hippocampus reactivates just prior to bursts of activity in the prefrontal cortex to which hippocampal neurons project (Wierzynski *et al.*, 2009). The functional relevance of this reactivation is unknown, but may serve the prefrontal cortex in much the same manner as reactivation during REM sleep serves the hippocampus. Whether the reactivation during REM and/or NREM sleep has consequences for LTP and depotentiation is the subject of several current investigations.

Hippocampal theta rhythm and memory consolidation

Theta frequency activity (4–9 Hz) is most prominent during active exploration and REM sleep. Disruptions of hippocampal theta impair learning (see Vertes and Kocsis, 1997). Pavlides and colleagues (1988) found that stimulation on the positive phase of the hippocampal theta induced synaptic LTP; stimulation at the opposite phase, the theta trough, induced a decrease in synaptic efficacy in the form of long-term depression, or depotentiation. Both LTP and depotentiation could be induced at the theta peak and trough, respectively, with a burst of four 200-Hz stimuli lasting 20 ms and applied to the Schaeffer collaterals (Huerta and Lisman, 1995). These experiments showed that LTP and depotentiation could be induced with physiologically feasible stimuli when timed to the naturally occurring theta activity.

Place cells fire in a specific relationship to the ongoing theta activity during active waking as well as during REM sleep (known as the "place-cell reactivation" or "replay"). During waking, most spikes occur at the peaks (corresponding to the maximum depolarization of the cell membrane) of theta as the cell discharges through the place field (Buzsáki *et al.*, 1983; Fox *et al.*, 1986). There is a laminar shift of theta phase from the basilar dendrites to the tips of the apical dendrites (Buzsáki *et al.*, 1983) such that at any given time the proximal apical dendrites, where the fast potentiating inputs from CA3 arrive at CA1, are at the opposite phase of theta to the more slowly potentiating distal apical dendritic region, where the direct temperoammonic (TA) inputs from the entorhinal cortex layer III arrive. The CA3 inputs to CA1 are considered novelty encoding, whereas the TA inputs are considered to be an index of consolidation for the memory. These two inputs are highly layer specific. The importance of the theta shift between layers for consolidation during REM will become apparent in the sections below.

Poe *et al.* (2000) showed that during REM sleep there is a progressive experience-dependent shift in the phase of firing of place cells from theta peak to theta trough compared to that observed during the wake state as the animal becomes familiar with the environment and the spatial memory becomes less dependent on the hippocampus. The relationship of place-cell firing with the phase of theta is important because stimulation on the positive phase (peak) induces LTP while stimulation on the negative phase (trough) causes depotentiation (Huerta and Lisman, 1995; Hyman *et al.*, 2003; Pavlides *et al.*, 1988). Thus, the firing phase of place cells can influence whether synapses are strengthened or weakened. The firing of place cells at the theta trough, which occurs only in REM sleep for familiar, consolidated memories, is associated with synaptic depotentiation. If synaptic depotentiation of place cells is associated with theta troughs during REM sleep, then REM sleep should reverse the expansion of place fields from the prior run experience. Conversely, firing of place cells at theta peaks during REM sleep when the environment is novel should maintain the LTP-related expansion of place fields as compared to their size the day prior. Therefore, if the hippocampus is inactivated during subsequent sleep, we propose that there should be no synaptic changes compared to that observed during a day before, and place fields should remain expanded.

Synaptic plasticity: contributions of REM sleep-associated changes in brain monoamine levels

Besides the rhythmic depolarization of neuronal cell membranes underlying theta activity, noradrenaline (NA) is another endogenous modulator of synaptic plasticity. The NA concentration in the hippocampus shows a state-dependent modulation with maximum release during waking and minimum release during REM sleep. Noradrenaline acting at ß receptors blocks depotentiation in the hippocampus and enhances LTP (Katsuki *et al.*, 1997; Thomas *et al.*, 1996; Yang *et al.*, 2002). Enhancing NA concentration in the hippocampus by either stimulation of the locus coeruleus, or icv application of NA to the hippocampus enhances and prolongs LTP (Almaguer-Melian *et al.*, 2005). Thus, the absence of NA during REM sleep may be a key factor and facilitator of depotentiation as evident from the shift of place-cell firing from theta peak to trough during REM sleep.

Serotonin (5-HT) also modulates synaptic plasticity. Kemp and Manahan-Vaughan (2004) found that both depotentiation and habituation to an environment were inhibited by 5-HT_4 agonist application. Another study showed that a 5-HT_4 agonist improved acquisition but impaired memory consolidation (Meneses and Hong, 1997). The latter study showed that the pretraining stimulation of 5-HT_4 receptors enhanced the acquisition of a conditioned response, while post-training activation of postsynaptic 5-HT_4 receptors impaired the consolidation of learning. Thus, it may be that 5-HT_4 receptor activation is beneficial for certain types of information acquisition that depend on LTP and detrimental for other types that depend on depotentiation. Its presence during acquisition, then, should allow early learning processes, and its relative absence during REM sleep should allow network reshaping involving bidirectional plasticity (both LTP and depotentiation) for efficient memory consolidation.

Serotonin also upregulates the hyperpolarization-activated, inward, mixed cation current (I_h) that is present with high density in the distal dendrites of CA1 pyramidal neurons (Gasparini and DiFrancesco, 1999). High levels of I_h in distal dendrites modulate dendritic membrane properties to minimize the effect of distal dendritic input at CA1 cell bodies (Robinson and Siegelbaum, 2003). Thus it is feasible that the specific loss of serotonergic inputs during REM sleep allows the slowly strengthening distal inputs to CA1 (coming in from layer III of the entorhinal cortex) to reach the cell bodies of CA1 neurons and initiate action potentials. The activation of CA1 cells at a time when the proximal CA3 inputs are silent would serve to depotentiate heterosynaptically those presynaptic CA3 inputs. The low levels of serotonin during REM sleep, then, allow the distal entorhinal cortex inputs, marking a level of memory consolidation, to uniquely control CA1

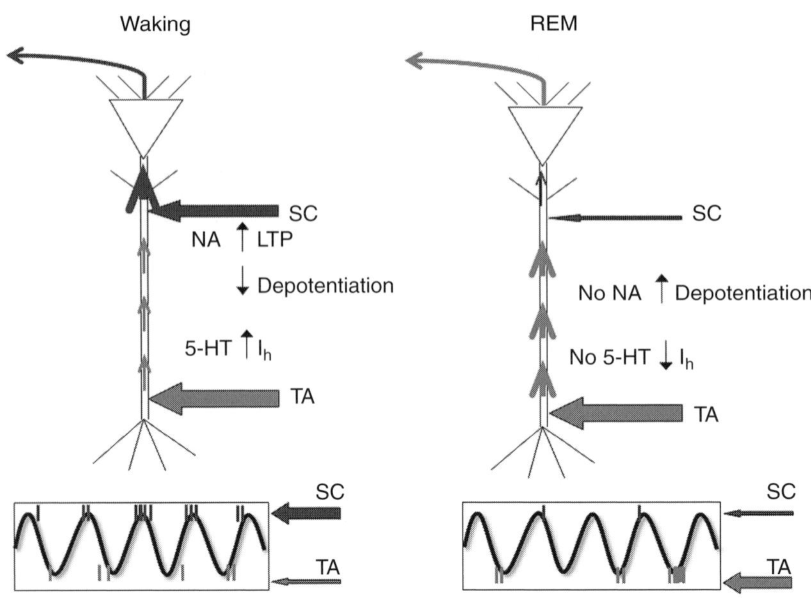

Figure 32.2 Model of proposed contributions of NA and 5-HT to the reformation of synapses in the hippocampal CA1 region. During waking, high levels of 5-HT enhance the I_h current, which attenuates cell response to distal TA–CA1 synaptic inputs and minimizes theta trough firing. SC–CA1 synaptic input dominates cell responses during waking, promoting output firing at the theta peaks. Noradrenaline (NA) (Thomas *et al.*, 1996; Yang *et al.*, 2002), combined with acetylcholine and theta peak activity, act to promote LTP at SC–CA1 synapses and inhibit depotentiation. During REM, the absence of 5-HT decreases the effects of I_h, allowing TA–CA1 synaptic inputs to influence cell activity. In the absence of NA, CA1 activity, when SC inputs are inactive at theta troughs causes heterosynaptic depotentiation of SC–CA1 synapses promoting more theta trough firing in response to TA–CA1 inputs. This model suggests a critical role for REM-associated processes in remodeling inputs during learning.

activity and thus to depotentiate those novelty-encoding CA3-to-CA1 TA synapses.

The importance of synaptic depotentiation for memory consolidation

Hippocampal synapses are more limited in number as compared to the neocortex, where long-term memories are probably stored in a parallel, distributed fashion. Thus, if the hippocampus serves to form associative memories quickly and temporarily store them until they are consolidated in the neocortex, it is expected that the network of weighted synapses involved with those novel memories now transferred to the neocortex should be recycled for future differential weighting of novel associative memories in other hippocampal functional assemblies.

Depotentiation may serve that synaptic recycling function. A growing literature suggests that depotentiation is also critical to cognitive function (Braunewell and Manahan-Vaughan, 2001; Manahan-Vaughan and Braunewell, 1999; Nakao *et al.*, 2002). Depotentiation seems to be associated with the presence of new stimuli in a contextual frame (Kemp and Manahan-Vaughan, 2004). Biphasic changes in synaptic strength could separate the acquisition of different types of information. Novel spatial exploration induces depotentiation of previously induced but irrelevant LTP (Xu *et al.*, 1998), which was prevented by a serotonin 5-HT$_4$ agonist

(Kemp and Manahan-Vaughan, 2004) (see below). However, whether the experience-dependent shift in the theta firing phase of place cells is a cause of synaptic depotentiation, hence, memory consolidation, is not known.

We hypothesize that the absence of NA and 5-HT during REM sleep while the hippocampus reactivates allows for the depotentiation of CA3–CA1 synapses necessary for changing the memory code with the arrival of new information. Specifically, the novelty-encoding CA3–CA1 (Shaffer collateral) synapses would be depotentiated in the absence of NA once the direct entorhinal–CA1 (TA) distal synapses that strengthen with memory consolidation are strong enough to cause, in the absence of 5-HT, the CA1 inputs to fire during REM sleep. The model in Figure 32.2 depicts this combined hypothesis.

Acknowledgments

Research support by the National Institutes of Health Grant MH-60670 and the Department of Anesthesiology, University of Michigan.

References

Almaguer-Melian, W., Rojas-Reyes, Y., Alvare, A. *et al.* (2005) Long-term potentiation in the dentate gyrus in freely moving rats is reinforced by intraventricular application of norepinephrine, but not oxotremorine. *Neurobiol Learn Mem* **83**: 72–8.

Aston-Jones, G. & Bloom, F. E. (1981) Activity of norepinephrine-containing locus coeruleus neurons in behaving rats anticipates fluctuations in the sleep–waking cycle. *J Neurosci* **1**: 876–86.

Best, J., Diniz Behn, C., Poe, G.R. & Booth, V. (2007) Neuronal models for sleep–wake regulation and synaptic reorganization in the sleeping hippocampus. *J Biol Rhythms* **22**: 220–32.

Bjorness, T. E., Riley, B. T., Tysor, M. K. & Poe, G. R. (2005) REM restriction persistently alters strategy used to solve a spatial task. *Learn Mem* **12**(3) 352–9.

Blitzer, RD., Iyengar, R. & Landau, E.M. (2005) Postsynaptic signaling networks: cellular cogwheels underlying long-term plasticity. *Biol Psych* **57**:113–39.

Booth, V. & Poe, G. R. (2006). Input source and strength influences overall firing phase of model hippocampal CA1 pyramidal cells during theta: relevance to REM sleep reactivation and memory consolidation. *Hippocampus* **16**: 161–73.

Braunewell, K. H. & Manahan-Vaughan, D. (2001) Long-term depression: a cellular basis for learning? *Rev Neurosci* **12**: 121–40.

Buzsáki, G., Leung, L.W. & Vanderwolf, C.H. (1983) Cellular bases of hippocampal EEG in the behaving rat. *Brain Res* **287**: 139–71.

Campbell, I. G., Guinan, M. J. & Horowitz, J. M. (2002). Sleep deprivation impairs long-term potentiation in rat hippocampal slices. *J Neurophysiol* **88**: 1073–6.

Corkin, S. (2002) What's new with the amnesic patient H. M.? *Nat Rev Neurosci* **3**: 153–60.

Dave, A. S. & Margoliash, D. (2000) Song replay during sleep and computational rules for sensorimotor vocal learning. *Science* **290**: 812–16.

Davis, C. J., Harding, J. W. & Wright, J. W. (2003) REM sleep deprivation-induced deficits in the latency-to-peak induction and maintenance of long-term potentiation within the CA1 region of the hippocampus. *Brain Res* **973**: 293–7.

Ekstrom, A. D., Meltzer, J., McNaughton, B. L. & Barnes, C. A. (2001) NMDA receptor antagonism blocks experience dependent expansion of hippocampal "place fields". *Neuron* **31**: 631–8.

Fox, S. E., Wolfson, S. & Ranck, J. B. Jr. (1986). Hippocampal theta rhythm and the firing of neurons in walking and urethane anesthetized rats. *Exp Brain Res* **62**: 495–508.

Frank, M. G. & Benington, J. H. (2006) The role of sleep in memory consolidation and brain plasticity: dream or reality? *Neuroscientist* **12**: 477–88.

Gasparini, S. & DiFrancesco, D. (1999) Action of serotonin on the hyperpolarization-activated cation current (Ih) in rat CA1 hippocampal neurons. *Eur J Neurosci* **11**: 3093–100.

Huerta, P. T. & Lisman, J. E. (1995). Bidirectional synaptic plasticity induced by a single burst during cholinergic theta oscillation in CA1 in vitro. *Neuron* **15**: 1053–63.

Hyman, J. M., Wyble, B. P., Goyal, V., Rossi, C. A. & Hasselmo, M. E. (2003) Stimulation in hippocampal region CA1 in behaving rats yields long-term potentiation when delivered to the peak of theta and long-term depression when delivered to the trough. *J Neurosci* **23**: 11,725–31.

Jablonski, P., Poe, G. R. & Zochowski, M. (2007) Structural network heterogeneities and network dynamics: a possible dynamical mechanism for hippocampal memory reactivation. *Phys Rev E Stat Nonlin Soft Matter Phys* **75**: 011912.

Karni, A., Tanne, D., Rubenstein, B. S., Askenasy, J. J. M. & Sagi, D. (1994) Dependence on REM sleep of overnight improvement of a perceptual skill. *Science* **265**: 679–82.

Katsuki, H., Izumi, Y. & Zorumski, C. F. (1997) Noradrenergic regulation of synaptic plasticity in the hippocampal CA1 region. *J Neurophysiol* **77**: 3013–20.

Kemp, A. & Manahan-Vaughan, D. (2004) Hippocampal long-term depression and long-term potentiation encode different aspects of novelty acquisition. *Proc Natl Acad Sci U S A* **101**: 8192–7.

Louie, K. & Wilson, M.A. (2001) Temporally structured replay of awake hippocampal ensemble activity during rapid eye movement sleep. *Neuron* **29**: 145–56.

Lydic, R. & Baghdoyan, H. A. (1993) Pedunculopontine stimulation alters respiration and increases ACh release in the pontine reticular formation. *Am J Physiol* **264**: R544–54.

Lydic, R., Baghdoyan, H. A. & Lorinc, Z. (1991) Microdialysis of cat pons reveals enhanced acetylcholine release during state-dependent respiratory depression. *Am J Physiol* **261**: R766–70.

Manahan-Vaughan, D. & Braunewell, K. H. (1999). Novelty acquisition is associated with induction of hippocampal long-term depression. *Proc Natl Acad Sci U S A* **96**: 8739–44.

Marks, C. A. & Wayner, M. J. (2005) Effects of sleep disruption on rat dentate granule cell LTP in vivo. *Brain Res Bull* **66**: 114–19.

Martin, S. J., de Hoz, L. & Morris, R. G. (2005) Retrograde amnesia: neither partial nor complete hippocampal lesions in rats result in preferential sparing of remote spatial memory, even after reminding. *Neuropsychologia* **43**: 609–24.

McDermott, C. M., LaHoste, G. J., Chen, C., *et al.* (2003) Sleep deprivation causes behavioral, synaptic, and membrane excitability alterations in hippocampal neurons. *J Neurosci* **23**: 9687–95.

Mednick, S. C., Nakayama, K., Cantero, J. L., *et al.* (2002) The restorative effect of naps on perceptual deterioration. *Nat Neurosci* **5**: 677–81.

Mehta, M. R., Barnes, C. A. & McNaughton, B. L. (1997) Experience-dependent, asymmetric expansion of hippocampal place fields. *Proc Natl Acad Sci U S A* **94**: 8918–21.

Mehta, M. R., Quirk, M. C. & Wilson, M. A. (2000) Experience-dependent asymmetric shape of hippocampal receptive fields. *Neuron* **25**: 707–15.

Meneses, A. & Hong, E. (1997) Effects of 5-HT4 receptor agonists and antagonists in learning. *Pharmacol Biochem Behav* **56**: 347–51.

Nakao, K., Ikegaya, Y., Yamada, M. K., Nishiyama, N. & Matsuki, N. (2002) Hippocampal long-term depression as an index of spatial working memory. *Eur J Neurosci* **16**: 970–4.

O'Keefe, J. & Dostrovsky, J. (1971) The hippocampus as a spatial map. Preliminary evidence from unit activity in the freely-moving rat. *Brain Res* **34**: 171–5.

Ordy, J. M., Thomas, G. J., Volpe, B. T., Dunlap, W. P. & Colombo, P. M. (1988) An animal model of human-type memory loss based on aging, lesion, forebrain ischemia, and drug studies with the rat. *Neurobiol Aging* **9**: 667–83.

Pace-Schott, E. F. & Hobson, J. A. (2002) The neurobiology of sleep: genetics, cellular physiology and subcortical networks. *Nat Rev Neurosci* **3**: 591–605.

Park, S. P., Lopez-Rodriguez, F., Wilson, C. L. *et al.* (1999) In vivo microdialysis measures of extracellular serotonin in the rat hippocampus during sleep–wakefulness. *Brain Res* **833**: 291–6.

Pavlides, C., Greenstein, Y. J., Grudman, M. & Winson, J. (1988) Long-term potentiation in the dentate gyrus is induced preferentially on the positive phase of theta-rhythm. *Brain Res* **439**: 383–7.

Pavlides, C. & Winson, J. (1989) Influences of hippocampal place cell firing in the awake state on the activity of these cells during subsequent sleep episodes. *J Neurosci* **9**: 2907–18.

Pedemonte, M., Barrenechea, C., Nuñez, A., Gambini, J. P. & García-Austt, E. (1998) Membrane and circuit properties of lateral septum neurons: relationships with hippocampal rhythms. *Brain Res* **800**: 145–53.

Poe, G. R., Nitz, D. A, McNaughton, B. L. & Barnes, C. A. (2000) Experience-dependent phase-reversal of hippocampal neuron firing during REM sleep. *Brain Res* **855**: 176–80.

Rempel-Clower, N. L., Zola, S. M., Squire, L. R. & Amaral, D. G. (1996) Three cases of enduring memory impairment after bilateral damage limited to the hippocampal formation. *J Neurosci* **16**: 5233–55.

Ribeiro, S., Mello, Nicolelis, M. A. L. (2004) Reverberation, storage, and postsynaptic propagation of memories during sleep. *Learn Mem* **11**: 686–96.

Robinson, R. B. & Siegelbaum, S. A. (2003) Hyperpolarization-activated cation currents: from molecules to physiological function. *Ann Rev Physiol* **65**: 453–80.

Romcy-Pereira, R. & Pavlides, C. (2004) Distinct modulatory effects of sleep on the maintenance of hippocampal and medial prefrontal cortex LTP. *Eur J Neurosci* **20**: 3453–62.

Sagar, H. J., Cohen, N. J., Corkin, S. & Growdon, J. H. (1985) Dissociations among processes in remote memory. *Ann N Y Acad Sci* **444**: 533–5.

Scoville, W. B. & Milner, B. (1957) Loss of recent memory after bilateral hippocampal lesions. *J Neurol Neurosurg Psych* **20**: 11–21.

Shapiro, M. (2001) Plasticity, hippocampal place cells, and cognitive maps. *Arch Neurol* **58**: 874–81.

Siapas, A. G., Lubenov, E. V. & Wilson, M. A. (2005) Prefrontal phase locking to hippocampal theta oscillations. *Neuron* **46**: 141–51.

Smith, C. (1996) Sleep states, memory processes and synaptic plasticity. *Behav Brain Res* **78**: 49–56.

Smith, C. & Rose, G. M. (1997) Posttraining paradoxical sleep in rats is increased after spatial learning in the Morris water maze. *Behav Neurosci* **111**: 1197–204.

Squire, L. R. (2004) Memory systems of the brain: a brief history and current perspective. *Neurobiol Learn Mem* **82**: 171–7.

Steriade, M. & McCarley, R. W. (2007) *Brain Stem Control of Wakefulness and Sleep*. New York: Plenum.

Stickgold, R., Hobson, J. A., Fosse, R. & Fosse, M. (2001) Sleep, learning, and dreams: off-line memory reprocessing. *Science* **294**: 1052–7.

Thomas, M. J., Moody, T. D., Makhinson, M. & O'Dell, T. J. (1996) Activity dependent beta-adrenergic modulation of low frequency stimulation induced LTP in the hippocampal CA1 region. *Neuron* **17**: 475–82.

Thompson, L. T. & Best, P. J. (1990) Long-term stability of the place-field activity of single units recorded from the dorsal hippocampus of freely behaving rats. *Brain Res* **509**: 299–308.

Tononi, G. & Cirelli, C. (2001) Modulation of brain gene expression during sleep and wakefulness: a review of recent findings. *Neuropsychopharmacology* **25**: S28–35.

Vertes, R. P. & Kocsis, B. (1997) Brainstem-diencephalo-septohippocampal systems controlling the theta rhythm of the hippocampus. *Neuroscience* **81**: 893–926.

Volpe, B. T., Pulsinelli, W. A., Tribuna, J. & Davis, H. P. (1984) Behavioral performance of rats following transient forebrain ischemia. *Stroke* **15**: 558–62.

Walker, M. P. & Stickgold, R. (2004) Sleep-dependent learning and memory consolidation. *Neuron* **44**: 121–33.

Wang, J. X., Poe, G. & Zochowski, M. (2008) From network heterogeneities to familiarity detection and hippocampal memory management. *Phys Rev E Stat Nonlin Soft Matter Phys* **78**: 41905.

Wierzynski, C. M., Lubenov, E. V., Gu, M. & Siapas, A. G. (2009) State-dependent spike-timing relationships between hippocampal and prefrontal circuits during sleep. *Neuron* **61**: 587–96.

Wilson, M. A. & McNaughton, B. L. (1994) Reactivation of hippocampal ensemble memories during sleep. *Science* **265**: 676–9.

Xu, L., Anwyl, R. & Rowan, M. J. (1998) Spatial exploration induces a persistent reversal of long-term potentiation in rat hippocampus. *Nature* **394**: 891–4.

Yang, H. W., Lin, Y. W., Yen, C. D. & Min, M. Y. (2002) Change in bi-directional plasticity at CA1 synapses in hippocampal slices taken from 6-hydroxydopamine-treated rats: the role of endogenous norepinephrine. *Eur J Neurosci* **16**: 1117–28.

Zola-Morgan, S., Squire, L. R. & Amaral, D. G. (1986) Human amnesia and the medial temporal region: enduring memory impairment following a bilateral lesion limited to field CA1 of the hippocampus. *J Neurosci* **6**: 2950–67.

Zola-Morgan, S., Squire, L. R. & Amaral, D. G. (1989) Lesions of the hippocampal formation but not lesions of the fornix or the mammillary nuclei produce long-lasting memory impairment in monkeys. *J Neurosci* **9**: 898–913.

Zola-Morgan, S., Squire, L. R., Rempel, N. L., Clower, R. P. & Amaral, D. G. (1992) Enduring memory impairment in monkeys after ischemic damage to the hippocampus. *J Neurosci* **12**: 2582–96.

Chapter 33

The role of REM sleep in memory consolidation, enhancement, and integration

Robert Stickgold

Summary

The last decade has seen a dramatic increase in our understanding of the role of sleep in off-line memory reprocessing, with published articles on sleep and memory increasing more than five-fold from the 1990s to 2008. While there is now clear evidence that sleep can enhance performance on previously learned tasks, several key questions remain unanswered. Chief among these are (1) the types of learning and memory that are enhanced; (2) the nature of the enhancement; (3) the differential roles of the various sleep stages; and (4) the cellular, molecular, and neurophysiological processes that mediate this enhancement. In this chapter, we review our current state of knowledge in regard to each of these questions, and then focus on the specific role of REM sleep.

Types of learning and memory enhanced by sleep

Memory systems

Asking what types of memory are enhanced by sleep obviously requires a clear understanding of the types of memory that exist and how they can be measured. Unfortunately, this is not a settled matter. Yet without some agreement on the categorization of memory systems, no meaningful progress can be made in answering this question.

Memories are most commonly classified according to the system of Schacter and Tulving (1994), which divides memories into two major systems, declarative and non-declarative, and then into subcategories. Declarative memories are defined as those that can be brought into consciousness and reported to an observer. These include episodic memories, consisting of autobiographical memories of specific events in one's life, and semantic memories, consisting of general knowledge and facts. Thus, a memory of what one had for dinner last night constitutes an episodic memory, while that of the capital of France is a semantic memory. Tests of declarative memory require explicit reporting of the contents of the memory, and as such can only be carried out with humans.

In contrast, non-declarative memories, by definition, cannot be brought into consciousness or reported explicitly, and tests of non-declarative memory are, of necessity, implicit. Several subcategories of non-declarative memory have been defined, including procedural skills. Procedural skills include memories of how to perform various tasks. These commonly include motor skills, such as how to tie one's shoes or play the piano, and perceptual skills, such as how to judge distances and speeds of approaching objects or to read Braille. But procedural skills include more sophisticated skills as well, such as surgical skills and medical diagnostic skills.

Other subcategories of non-declarative memory include classical conditioning, non-associative learning, and priming. Classical conditioning refers to the linking of new stimuli to expected outcomes, for example, learning that a light or tone predicts a subsequent shock or presentation of food. Non-associative learning encompasses even more basic forms of learning, including habituation and sensitization. Priming is yet more basic, reflecting the ability of earlier stimuli to affect responses to a subsequent stimulus. In one classic example, stem completion, subjects are asked to report the first word they can think of that starts with some string of characters, such as "t-h-r". The earlier presentation of a matching word (e.g., "thoroughbred") will greatly increase the likelihood of that word

REM Sleep: Regulation and Function, eds. Birendra N. Mallick, S. R. Pandi-Perumal, Robert W. McCarley, and Adrian R. Morrison. Published by Cambridge University Press. © Cambridge University Press 2011.

being reported, regardless of whether or not the subject explicitly recalls the earlier presentation of the word.

In thinking about these systems, two caveats must be kept in mind. Firstly, while these categories of memories are considered to be separate and distinct, in reality it is uncommon for a given event to be encoded in only one of these systems. Thus, semantic memories always are based on episodic memories, and almost all procedural skill learning includes a phase of declarative learning. Hence the aphorism that chess is a game that takes an hour to learn (i.e., declarative encoding of the rules) and a life to master (i.e., the procedural, non-declarative development of strategic skills). It can thus be unclear which system a particular subject is actually utilizing. In the example of stem completion given above, reporting the word "thoroughbred" in response to the stem "t-h-r" may have been mediated by the explicit, declarative recall to consciousness of having heard the word earlier, in the study phase, but may also have occurred without any conscious awareness of this fact and without activation of any declarative memory.

This leads us to the second caveat, which is related to the concept of "implicit" and "explicit" memories. Different researchers use these words in very different ways. In their seminal work on memory systems, Schacter and Tulving (1994) carefully define "implicit" and "explicit" not in terms of memory systems, but of memory tests. Using the example of stem completion again, asking subjects to report "the first word that comes to mind" matching the stem is an implicit test of memory, because one can only imply from the subject's response the existence of a memory of hearing the word earlier. In contrast, asking subjects to report "a word from the list you just heard" matching the stem is an explicit test of memory, since the subject is reporting the conscious accessing of a memory. The confound here is that implicit tests, according to these definitions, do not tell us what memory system has been accessed. Retrieval could have come through either a declarative or non-declarative system.

This becomes further confused when other researchers use these same words to refer not to recall tests but the memory systems themselves. For these researchers "explicit" and "implicit" are simply synonyms for "declarative" and "non-declarative", and they refer, for example, to explicit memories as opposed to explicit tests of memory. Still other researchers use these terms to refer to the encoding process, that is, to whether subjects are consciously aware of the fact

that they are encoding the information during training. Thus, on a serial reaction time test, subjects may be explicitly informed of the presence of a repeating sequence in the stimuli, or they may become explicitly aware of such a sequence without having been forewarned, or they may never be aware of its presence. In all three cases, however, training results in faster performance when the sequence is present than when it is absent, implicitly confirming that the subject has some form of memory for the sequence.

All of these factors make our original question of what types of memory benefit from sleep less clear than one would like. But despite these impediments, considerable progress has been made.

Sleep enhances declarative memory

The seminal study of sleep and memory was performed by Jenkins and Dallenbach (1924), who reported better recall of nonsense syllables after a period of sleep than after an equivalent time spent awake. However, their conclusion rejected the possibility that the memories were actually enhanced during sleep. Instead, they interpreted their findings in light of Ebbinghaus' theory of memory decay (Ebbinghaus, 1885), concluding that the deterioration of memory over time resulted from daytime interference (for example, from other words heard between training and retest) rather than some simple decay, and that the better recall after sleep merely reflected a blockade of interference during sleep. Thus, they concluded that the benefit seen after sleep resulted from a passive protection against the ravages of interference, rather than the active consolidation of the memories. Some 85 years later, it now appears that sleep offers both passive protection and active consolidation of declarative memory.

Verbal memory

Early evidence of active consolidation of declarative memory came from a study by Plihal and Born (1997), demonstrating that cued recall of word pairs was enhanced by sleep early in the night (when slow-wave sleep [SWS] predominates), but not by sleep late in the night (when SWS is often absent). Thus, it appears that specific aspects of sleep other than some uniform passive protection against interference are responsible for its benefits. Furthermore, word pair memory appears to be more resistant to experimentally introduced interference after a night of sleep than after an equivalent period of daytime wake (Ellenbogen *et al.*, 2006).

Emotional memory

Emotional declarative memory also benefits from sleep, and appears to benefit preferentially from REM rather than SWS. Such benefits from REM have been seen both with emotional texts (Wagner *et al.*, 2001) and emotional pictures (Nishida *et al.*, 2009). The selective retention of emotional material could arguably reflect a specific evolutionary adaptation based on the consistent salience of such information. Thus REM sleep, during which midline limbic structures involved with emotional processing are preferentially activated (Maquet *et al.*, 1996), may have evolved, at least in part, to specifically consolidate emotional declarative memory.

Spatial memory

Spatial memory, which, like declarative memories in general, is hippocampally mediated and, in human studies presumed to be declarative, also benefits from sleep, and, again, from SWS. Thus, when subjects learned to navigate through a virtual maze, overnight improvement correlated with increases in hippocampal activation (seen with positron emission tomography) during SWS the night after training (Peigneux *et al.*, 2004). In a very different spatial learning task, Rudoy *et al.* (2009) had subjects memorize the positions of 50 objects on a two-dimensional grid. During training, each object was associated with an ecologically appropriate sound, such as mewing with a cat. During a post-training nap, the sounds associated with half of the objects were replayed during SWS (without EEG evidence of awakenings). Subsequent testing showed significantly more accurate spatial memories for those objects whose associated sounds had been played during SWS in the intervening nap. In light of earlier considerations, it should be noted that both of these spatial tasks rely on implicit tests of memory, and the enhancement of specifically declarative aspects of the memories was not confirmed.

Selective enhancement

Sleep-dependent enhancement of memories need not be an all-or-none phenomenon. Thus, in the two studies of emotional memory noted above, only the emotional text elements (Wagner *et al.*, 2001) and emotional pictures (Nishida *et al.*, 2009) benefited from post-encoding sleep, while emotionally neutral content did not. A more dramatic example of this was reported by Payne *et al.* (2008), who found that post-encoding sleep led to retention of emotional objects seen against neutral background scenes, but not of their backgrounds, and not of either neutral objects or their backgrounds. Thus sleep appears capable of unbinding episodic memories and selectively retaining what are arguably the most salient aspects of the memory. No evidence of similar unbinding or selective retention was seen across periods of wake.

Such selective retention of salient material during sleep is not limited to emotional memories. It has also been seen in the retention of gist information, extracted during a declarative memory task. Using the Deese–Roediger–McDermott (DRM) false memory paradigm (Roediger and McDermott, 1995), Payne *et al.* observed selective recall following sleep of "false" memories of words representing the gist of studied word lists (Payne *et al.*, 2009). In a pattern reminiscent of the emotional object study just described (Payne *et al.*, 2008), sleep led to the recall of these gist words at rates equal to or higher than immediately after training, while memory for the actual studied words deteriorated. In contrast, time spent awake led to diminished reporting of both gist words and studied words. Curiously, Fenn and colleagues (2009) carried out a similar study using word recognition (identifying presented words as "old" or "new") instead of recall (writing down all remembered words) and obtained the opposite result, with false recognition being lower after sleep than after an equal time spent awake. Since both papers included multiple studies with similar outcomes, the difference likely reflects differences in the processes involved in recall and recognition. Interestingly, none of these sleep effects seen for gist memory were seen for the studied words, again indicating that sleep treats gist and detail memory differently, and can selectively retain one over the other.

Presumably, the effects of sleep on gist memory have evolved to specifically maintain forms of information that are of most value for the organism. While the mechanisms underlying this selectivity are unknown, a piece of the process can be gleaned from the spatial memory study described above (Rudoy *et al.*, 2009). In that study, the replay of sounds associated with individual item memories led to the selective retention or enhancement of those memories. Since such replay presumably triggers the reactivation of those specific item memories, such reactivation during SWS appears sufficient to initiate the consolidation and enhancement process.

Sleep enhances perceptual and motor procedural memory

Perhaps the clearest evidence of active memory consolidation during sleep comes from studies of perceptual and motor procedural memory. Declarative memory almost invariably shows deterioration over time, and the benefits of sleep are most often seen as decreased deterioration over sleep, which leaves open the question of the relative contribution of active consolidation and passive protection against interference. In tests of procedural memory, however, absolute improvement is often seen across a nap or a night of sleep. Such findings provide unequivocal evidence of active memory enhancement during sleep. Examples of sleep-dependent enhancement of perceptual and motor skill learning abound. On a visual texture discrimination task, subjects show robust improvements after either a night of sleep (e.g., Karni and Sagi, 1991) or a nap (Mednick *et al.*, 2003). Similar absolute sleep-dependent improvements have been seen with an auditory pitch memory task (Gaab *et al.*, 2004), and with both motor sequence (Walker *et al.*, 2002a) and motor adaptation (Huber *et al.*, 2004) tasks.

Selective enhancement

As with declarative memories, sleep-dependent benefits gained by procedural memories can also be selective. In one case, subjects were trained on an auditory tone sequence discrimination task, in which the pitch of one of five notes in the sequence was altered on 13% of trials by approximately one whole step. When tested 48 and 72 hours later, subjects who were sleep deprived the night after training showed improvements in performance speed and accuracy equivalent to those who had slept normally (Atienza *et al.*, 2004). But when event-related brain potentials (ERPs) were recorded during unattended presentation of the tone sequences, those cortical responses directly associated with the automatic shift of attention to unexpected stimuli (MMN and P3a) failed to develop in sleep-deprived subjects (Atienza *et al.* 2004). In this particular case, sleep appears to enhance the sensitivity of the deviation-detector system not while attention is focused on the task, but when attention is focused elsewhere. In so doing, sleep facilitates the alerting of the brain's attentional mechanisms, as well as the conscious mind, to the presence of meaningful stimuli within the environment.

Even the much simpler motor sequence task mentioned earlier (Walker *et al.*, 2002a) shows selective enhancement. In this task, subjects repeatedly typed a numeric sequence (e.g., 4–1–3–2–4) on a computer keyboard as quickly and accurately as possible. Both speed (Walker *et al.*, 2002a) and accuracy (Walker

et al., 2003b) show sleep-dependent improvement. But when examined more closely, selective sleep-dependent enhancement was observed for the reaction times of specific keystrokes (Kuriyama *et al.*, 2004). When learning the task, subjects typically break the sequence into two "chunks", typing, for example 413–24 or 41–324. Behaviorally, chunking is identified by longer keystroke intervals at the start of a chunk. When performance was re-measured after a night of sleep, a selective shortening of the inter-chunk keystroke interval was observed, apparently reflecting the uniting of the chunks into a single unit (Kuriyama *et al.*, 2004). Such selective improvement was not seen across an equal time spent awake, or during the initial training session, when overall speed increased over 50%.

Whether this selective enhancement of only certain elements of recently encoded memories is part of a larger brain strategy that uses sleep-dependent processes to identify meaning in the events that make up an organism's life remains to be seen. It is noteworthy that such selective processing of memories during sleep has now been seen in multiple instances for both procedural and declarative memories.

Sleep enhances complex cognitive procedural memory

Nowhere is sleep's predilection for identifying the meaning of events more apparent than in the realm of what Carlyle Smith has referred to as "complex cognitive procedural" memory. Such procedural learning shares with the more classic perceptual and motor skill learning the properties of being non-declarative and built up over numerous similar trials (unlike episodic memories, which typically form after a single event). If sleep acts to bind together motor-sequence chunks to optimize performance (Kuriyama *et al.*, 2004), while it acts on declarative memories of emotional scenes to "unbind" unified scenes and selectively retain the most salient elements (Payne *et al.*, 2009), then the findings described below for these more complex tasks may not seem so surprising.

Tower of Hanoi

In one of the seminal studies of such tasks, Smith and Smith (2003) demonstrated that REM suppression the night after training on the Tower of Hanoi task (induced by pre-sleep ethanol ingestion) suppressed subsequent improvement in performance. The classic task, which involves moving a series of disks of diminishing size from one peg to another without placing a larger disk on top of a smaller one, required 40% fewer steps to complete at retest than at initial training, eight days earlier. But when REM sleep was suppressed the night after training, only a non-significant 10% improvement was seen. While learning was again measured implicitly, it was clear that subjects in both groups failed to attain an explicit (declarative) understanding of the optimal algorithm for performing the task, since, at retest, members of the two groups on average made 72% (control) and 97% (REM suppressed) more moves than required for optimal performance.

Number reduction task

More recently, a series of studies have impressively extended the range of cognitive procedural learning that benefits from sleep. Wagner *et al.* (2004) taught subjects a rote algorithm for solving a class of mathematical problems, but withheld information about the existence of a simpler and faster algorithm. While only 10% of subjects discovered the shortcut during 90 training trials, and only 25% of the remaining subjects did so if retested either immediately or after eight hours of wakefulness, more than twice as many (59%) did so after a night of sleep. Thus, sleep appeared to continue processing the information gained during training and facilitated the subsequent discovery of this shortcut, despite the lack of explicit instructions that such a shortcut existed.

Remote associates task

Wagner *et al.* (2004) described this outcome as the sleep-dependent enhancement of insight, where insight can be defined as the sudden appearance in conscious awareness of a new understanding of previously known information. Another example of sleep-dependent enhancement of insight involves the remote associates task (RAT) of Mednick (1962), in which subjects are presented with various three-word sets and instructed to find a remote associate that links all three words. For example, the words HEART, SIXTEEN, and COOKIES are all associates of the word SWEET (i.e., *sweetheart, sweet sixteen, sweet cookies*). Cai *et al.* (2009) reported that a 90-minute nap led to enhanced discovery of remote associates that subjects had failed to find prior to the nap period, and more specifically, only naps containing REM sleep produced this benefit. While subjects with naps containing REM sleep improved significantly, and by nearly 40%, at retest, those with naps consisting only of NREM sleep and

those in a wake control group showed no significant improvement. (To be more accurate, priming of solution words before the nap was necessary; see Cai *et al.*, 2009 for details.)

That REM sleep may specifically enhance such insightful problem solving is also suggested by a study of Walker *et al.* (2002b), which demonstrated that subjects were significantly more successful at solving anagrams when awakened from REM than following awakening from stage 2 NREM, and another study finding that semantic priming by weak associates was significantly greater than by normally strong associates following awakenings from REM sleep (Stickgold *et al.*, 1999).

Transitive inference

The development of transitive inference is also facilitated by sleep (Ellenbogen *et al.*, 2007). Transitive inference refers to the construction of assumptions about relationships between recently studied objects. Classically, subjects are taught to select, for example, stimulus A over stimulus B (A $\supset$ B), and to select stimulus B over stimulus C (B $\supset$ C), but are given no information about how to respond when stimuli A and C are presented (A **?** C). Transitive inference is the inferring that if A $\supset$ B and B $\supset$ C, then A $\supset$ C. Both humans and rats make such inferences.

When human subjects are trained on a series of five "premise pairs" (A $\supset$ B, B $\supset$ C, C $\supset$ D, D $\supset$ E, and E $\supset$ F), at immediate retest they show no evidence of transitively inferring B $\supset$ D, C $\supset$ E, or, more complexly, B $\supset$ E. In contrast, when tested 12 hours later, either across the day or over a night of sleep, they showed significant transitive inference for both the simpler, first-degree inferences (B $\supset$ D and C $\supset$ E, each of which bridges two premise pairs) and the more complex second-degree inference (B $\supset$ E, which bridges three). But while similar amounts of improvement were seen across wake and sleep for the first-degree inferences, the extent of inference was nearly doubled across sleep for the second-degree inference. Thus, there was a selective, sleep-dependent enhancement of these more complex inferences, both compared to the simpler inferences across sleep and compared to both the simpler and more complex inferences across wake.

Probabilistic learning

As a final example, sleep enhances learning of a probabilistic weather prediction task, in which subjects attempt to learn to predict the outcomes of various stimuli (Djonlagic *et al.*, 2009). In one form of the task, the "feedback" mode, subjects first see one, two, or three of four possible "cards," and then must predict whether it will be sunny or rainy, before finally being shown the actual outcome. In observation mode, the cards and outcome are presented together, and subjects are instructed to respond by indicating the outcome. Both forms of the task involve 200 training trials, over which they are simply instructed to try to learn how to predict the weather outcome.

The probabilistic nature of the task, of which they are not informed, lies in the fact that each card has a certain probability, ranging from 20% to 80% of being associated with the sunny or rainy outcome. Thus no combination of cards reliably predicts a given outcome. Following training, subjects are given 100 test trials with no outcome feedback, and 12 hours later, either across the day or over a night of sleep, they are retested with the identical 100 trials.

While no significant change in performance is seen between test and retest across the day, subjects show significant absolute improvement across a night of sleep, amounting to 11% greater predictive power for the feedback form of the task and 7% greater power for the observation mode (Djonlagic *et al.*, 2009).

Sleep enhances multiple forms of memory

Taken together, the findings described above, reported from ten laboratories over the last decade, provide overwhelming evidence of sleep-dependent memory processing both for episodic and semantic declarative memories, and for perceptual, motor, and cognitive procedural memories. Other forms of procedural memory also show sleep-dependent processing, including classical conditioning (Pace-Schott *et al.*, 2009) and priming (Stickgold *et al.*, 1999), leaving only non-associative learning (habituation and sensitization) undocumented. It thus seems fair to predict that all forms of learning and memory are capable of sleep-dependent processing.

The nature of sleep-dependent enhancement of learning and memory

The previous section has made passing reference to many of the stages of post-encoding memory processing that occur in humans. In the past, the term memory "consolidation" has been used to refer to some or all of these processes, although its original meaning was restricted to the stabilization of initially labile

memories. Because of this ambiguity, and because the term carries an implication of the implacable preservation of memories in their original forms, we have begun referring to the processes of "memory evolution," which mediate changes in memories that continue over decades, and which perform, at different times, the contradictory functions of stabilizing and modifying memories. While the exact list of processes included probably varies depending on the anatomic substrate of the memories, many of these processes are most likely utilized by all memory systems.

Two forms of post-encoding processing can occur at the level of the original encoded memory. Stabilization, or classic consolidation, can be produced by simply stabilizing the changes in synaptic weights produced during the original memory encoding, regardless of the anatomical location or physiological structure of the memory. This could occur by identifying at the cellular level recently altered synapses and further modifying them to increase their stability. The process of protein-synthesis dependent long-term potentiation (LTP) could neatly fill this role. If this process not only stabilized these changes but also amplified them, magnifying changes in synaptic weights that occurred during encoding, memory stabilization would result in the functional enhancement of the memory as well.

Most other forms of post-encoding memory processing, many of which also produce functional enhancement and which account for the bulk of the overall process of memory evolution, appear to be more complex, involving either the translocation of a memory from one brain region to another or the development of associative links between a recently encoded memory and other memories. Each of these, in turn, can have various forms, serving distinct functions. For example, procedural learning requires the formation of associative links between large numbers of recently formed memories, not just for perceptual and motor skill learning, but for complex cognitive procedural tasks, such as the Tower of Hanoi (Smith and Smith, 2003) and probabilistic weather prediction (Djonlagic *et al.*, 2009) tasks, as well. In other cases, links may form between new item memories and a dense network of older memories, as seen in the gist extraction of the DRM false memory task (Payne *et al.*, 2009). Similarly, for declarative tasks, memories are known to be initially dependent on the hippocampus for recall and recognition, but, over time, are thought to develop independence from the hippocampus, a process that has been hypothesized to be sleep dependent (McClelland *et al.*, 1995). In contrast, procedural memories of motor (Walker *et al.*, 2005a) and perceptual (Walker *et al.*, 2005b) skills appear to shift between regions within the cortex and cerebellum. All of these processes have been reported to benefit from sleep and, in some paradigms, appear to occur only during sleep. A final form of memory evolution is mediated by a process known as memory "reconsolidation," wherein stable memories are relabilized by their reactivation and must then go through a process of reconsolidation to become stable again. Sleep modulates this process as well (Walker *et al.*, 2003a).

Thus, as with the many types of memory, the multiple known stages of memory evolution all appear to benefit from sleep. Whether this will continue to be true, as more details of the overall process of memory evolution are brought to light, remains to be seen. But, to date, no aspect of post-encoding memory processing that has been investigated from sleep dependency has failed to show a role for sleep.

The role of the various sleep stages in memory processing

Given the fact that this chapter is nominally about the role of REM sleep in memory processing, it may initially have seemed strange that this question has been reserved for the final portion of the chapter. But, hopefully, by now the reader appreciates the necessity of these preceding sections. Not only must a discussion of the roles of individual sleep stages occur within the context of the multiple forms of memory and stages of memory evolution, but the functions of individual sleep stages in memory evolution are less clear than the types of memory and stages of memory evolution affected by sleep. Nevertheless, we now turn our attention to this question.

Wake

It is important to begin by discussing how the wake state contributes to various forms of memory and memory evolution. Surprisingly, our understanding of wake's role is probably less clear than for sleep stages. Many forms of memory processing do occur during wake. For example, on the motor sequence task described earlier, training on a new sequence ten minutes after initial sequence training blocks overnight improvement on the first sequence. But allowing six hours of wake between training on the two sequences appears to

consolidate learning of the initial sequence so that normal overnight improvement is seen for both sequences (Walker *et al.*, 2003a). Brasher-Krug *et al.* (1996) have likewise reported daytime stabilization of a motor adaptation task similar to that of Huber *et al.* (2004), noted above, which showed sleep-dependent enhancement. As noted by others (Krakauer and Shadmehr, 2006), these two forms of motor memory processing, stabilization and enhancement, may represent very different processes, one of which is sleep dependent and the other of which is not.

A more complex picture emerges from studies of a third motor task, the serial reaction time task (SRTT). In this task, subjects press four keys in response to the lighting of four squares located above the keys, so that the order of lighting of the squares must be repeated on the keyboard. But while responding to what may appear to be a random sequence of lights, subjects are actually responding to a complex sequence that is repeated over and over. Learning of the sequence is reflected in a slowing of response times when a truly random sequence is suddenly introduced. Robertson *et al.* (2004) have found that when subjects are informed prior to training that a sequence is present, they show only delayed, sleep-dependent improvement. But when they remain unaware of the sequence's presence, delayed improvement is seen across periods of both wake and sleep. Thus, depending on the subject's understanding of the task and, presumably, the strategy they adopt, sequence learning may or may not be facilitated by the passing of time spent awake. A somewhat similar pattern was seen on the transitive inference task described above, on which subjects show equal improvement in making first-order inferences across periods of wake and sleep, but show significantly more improvement in second-order inferences over sleep than over wake (Ellenbogen *et al.*, 2007). In contrast, no improvement was seen across wake for either the remote associates task (Cai *et al.*, 2009) or the probabilistic learning task (Djonlagic *et al.*, 2009). It thus remains unclear what determines when a given form of memory processing will occur during extended periods of wake.

Slow-wave sleep and REM

While there is general consensus that SWS and REM play different roles in memory processing, there is little agreement about what these roles are. Three distinct models have been proposed (Table 33.1). The "memory type" model proposes that SWS and REM contribute

Table 33.1 Putative roles of SWS and REM in memory processing

Memory type model: SWS and REM support the processing of different types of memory – SWS supports processing of most declarative (hippocampal) memory, while REM supports procedural memory and emotional declarative memory processing (Diekelmann *et al.*, 2009; Plihal and Born, 1997; Wagner *et al.*, 2001).

Memory process specificity model: SWS and REM support different forms of memory processing – SWS supports the stabilization of memories while REM supports their enhancement and integration (Mednick *et al.*, 2003; Stickgold, 2009).

Sequential (two-step) model: Memory processing requires SWS followed by REM – individual memories are processed through two stages, with SWS acting to weaken or eliminate spurious information, and REM then acts to integrate the prevailing new memories into pre-existing memory networks (Giuditta *et al.*, 1995).

to the processing of different types of memories, while the "memory process" model argues that they contribute to different aspects of memory evolution. Finally, the "sequential model" argues that SWS and REM must work together for the effective processing of memories. In reality, all three models may simply represent variants of the "memory process" model. For example, the apparently distinct patterns of sleep-stage dependence reported for declarative and procedural memories may result from the tendency for these memory systems to be tested with different experimental paradigms. Tests of declarative memory tend to require subjects to report back the exact stimulus they initially encoded. In such circumstances, the stabilization of the initially encoded memory during SWS would enhance subsequent performance (since all declarative memory tends to deteriorate over time), while integrating this information during REM, either with other recently encoded information or with older information, could lead to increased errors. In contrast, procedural memory is commonly built up over tens or hundreds of trials, and the integration of these trials, with identification or extraction of their commonalities during REM, would be beneficial, while strengthening of individual, possibly non-optimal individual trials could actually impair performance. From this perspective, the apparent correlation of SWS with declarative memory processing and of REM with procedural memory processing would merely reflect the different stages of processing normally tested in declarative and procedural tasks.

Such an explanation is supported by notable exceptions to the simple memory-type model: (1) sleep-dependent improvement on a procedural visual discrimination task requires both SWS and REM (Stickgold *et al.*, 2000b), which appear to make specific contributions to its stabilization and enhancement respectively (Mednick *et al.*, 2003); (2) emotional declarative memory appears to benefit selectively from REM (Wagner *et al.*, 2001); and (3) recall on the DRM false memory task, which depends on gist rather than detailed item memory, shows a negative correlation with the amount of post-training SWS obtained, whether over a full night of sleep or in a shorter nap (Payne *et al.*, 2009).

NREM Stages 1 and 2

Much less is known about the role of the lighter stages of NREM sleep. Spindle activity in Stage 2 and, perhaps, in all NREM, correlates with motor sequence learning (Nishida and Walker, 2007), but also with performance IQ (Fogel *et al.*, 2007). Studying Stage 2 is problematic because it cannot be easily manipulated, and is distributed relatively evenly throughout the night. Nap studies, where total sleep time can be limited to preclude both SWS and REM, are probably the best approach at least for the time being. In any case, more work is needed to clarify whether Stage 2 NREM has a unique role to play here, although the large amount of time spent in this stage argues that it must serve some valuable function.

Whether Stage 1 NREM has any role in memory processing is completely unknown. One might argue that Stage 1 is merely transitional between wake and Stage 2 NREM, but the presence of hypnagogic dream reports from this stage, whose frequency exceeds even that of REM, suggests that something more interesting than a simple slide into sleep is occurring. Add to this the high frequency with which recent learning experiences can be replayed in these dreams (Stickgold *et al.*, 2000a), and the tendency of the sleep-onset period to fill with cognitive review of both incomplete actions from the preceding day and planned activities for the next, and we are led to suggest that this phase of sleep might serve to identify and mark specific memories for further processing during sleep. Indeed, Wamsley *et al.* (2010) have recently reported significant correlations between reports of hypnagogic dreams about a pre-nap learning task and subsequent sleep-dependent improvement in task performance. Nonetheless, a concrete role for Stage 1 NREM in memory processing does not yet exist.

Cellular, molecular, and neurophysiological processes in REM

There are strong physiological grounds on which to support the claim that SWS plays an important role in hippocampally mediated memory consolidation (Walker, 2009), with a combination of slow waves and sharp wave-ripple activity repeatedly replaying hippocampal representations of declarative memories back to neocortical regions in which the detailed features of a memory are stored. But while synchronous hippocampal and neocortical activity during SWS provides a mechanism for the specific processing of declarative memories, REM sleep may process hippocampal memories as well. Hippocampal theta waves, seen during REM sleep, can facilitate hippocampal LTP (Huerta and Lisman, 1995), and information flow, which predominantly flows from the hippocampus to the cortex during SWS, reverses direction and brings cortically stored information back into the hippocampus during REM, producing what Buzsáki has referred to as the hippocampo–neocortical dialogue (Buzsáki, 1996). In addition, the critical role of acetylcholine in memory processing (Hasselmo, 2006), taken together with the dramatically elevated levels of hippocampal acetylcholine during REM (Kametani and Kawamura, 1990) argues for an important role of REM in processing of hippocampally dependent memories.

While much more could be said about the cellular, molecular, and neurophysiological processes that underlie sleep-dependent memory evolution, we lack a clear and coherent picture. Indeed, cognitive neuroscience still lacks any clear picture of how memory encoding, short-term consolidation, or recall is instantiated in the brain during wake. It is an exciting possibility that sleep research may end up leading the larger cognitive neuroscience research community in answering these questions.

Conclusion

Over the last decade, the role of sleep in memory evolution has been slowly elucidated. Perhaps the strongest conclusions that can be made are the following: (1) all classes of memory that have been studied have shown significant benefits from post-encoding sleep; (2) similarly, all stages of memory evolution appear to show significant benefits from post-encoding sleep; and finally (3) a combination of correlational and experimental studies has demonstrated that all stages of sleep, with the exception of Stage 1 NREM, contribute to sleep-dependent memory processing, with each stage (REM, Stage 2 NREM, and SWS) having its own unique profile of contributions. But still unclear are (1) the characteristics of any given memory task that determine which sleep stages will contribute to its evolution; and (2) the cellular, neurochemical, and neurophysiological characteristics of the individual sleep stages that underlie their unique contributions to the overall process of sleep-dependent memory evolution. Understanding the role of REM sleep in this process will depend not only on studies specifically of REM sleep and memory, but on studies that help to clarify the overall evolutionary strategy and physiological mechanisms of sleep-dependent memory processing.

Acknowledgments

Preparation of this chapter was supported by NIH grant MH48832.

References

Atienza, M., Cantero, J. L. & Stickgold, R. (2004) Posttraining sleep enhances automaticity in perceptual discrimination. *J Cogn Neurosci* **16**: 53–64.

Brashers-Krug, T., Shadmehr, R. & Bizzi, E. (1996) Consolidation in human motor memory. *Nature* **382**: 252–5.

Buzsáki, G. (1996) The hippocampo-neocortical dialogue. *Cerebr Cortex* **6**: 81–92.

Cai, D. J., Mednick, S. A., Harrison, E. M. *et al.* (2009) REM, not incubation, improves creativity by priming associative networks. *Proc Natl Acad Sci U S A* **106**:10,130–4.

Diekelmann, S., Wilhelm, I. & Born, J. (2009) The whats and whens of sleep-dependent memory consolidation. *Sleep Med Rev* **13**: 309–21.

Djonlagic, I., Rosenfeld, A., Shohamy, D. *et al.* (2009) Sleep enhances category learning. *Learn Mem* **16**: 751–5.

Ebbinghaus, H. (1885) *Über das Gedachtnis*. New York: Teachers' College Press.

Ellenbogen, J. M., Hu, P. T., Payne, J. D. *et al.* (2007) Human relational memory requires time and sleep. *Proc Natl Acad Sci U S A* **104**:7723–8.

Ellenbogen, J. M., Hulbert, J. C., Stickgold, R. *et al.* (2006) Interfering with theories of sleep and memory: sleep, declarative memory, and associative interference. *Curr Biol* **16**: 1290–4.

Fenn, K. M., Gallo, D. A., Margoliash, D. *et al.* (2009) Reduced false memory after sleep. *Learn Mem* **16**: 509–13.

Fogel, S. M., Nader, R., Cote, K. A. *et al.* (2007) Sleep spindles and learning potential. *Behav Neurosci* **121**:1–10.

Gaab, N., Paetzold, M., Becker, M. *et al.* (2004) The influence of sleep on auditory learning: a behavioral study. *Neuroreport* **15**: 731–4.

Giuditta, A., Ambrosini, M. V., Montagnese, P. *et al.* (1995) The sequential hypothesis of the function of sleep. *Behav Brain Res* **69**: 157–66.

Hasselmo, M. E. (2006) The role of acetylcholine in learning and memory. *Curr Opin Neurobiol* **16**: 710–5.

Huber, R., Ghilardi, M. F., Massimini, M. *et al.* (2004) Local sleep and learning. *Nature* **430**: 78–81.

Huerta, P. T. & Lisman, J. E. (1995) Bidirectional synaptic plasticity induced by a single burst during cholinergic theta oscillation in CA1 in vitro. *Neuron* **15**:1053–63.

Jenkins, J. G. & Dallenbach, K. M. (1924) LXXII. Obliviscence during sleep and waking. *Am J Psychol* **35**: 605–12.

Kametani, H. & Kawamura, H. (1990) Alterations in acetylcholine release in the rat hippocampus during sleep–wakefulness detected by intracerebral dialysis. *Life Sciences* **47**: 421–6.

Karni, A. & Sagi, D. (1991) Where practice makes perfect in texture discrimination: evidence for primary visual cortex plasticity. *Proc Natl Acad Sci U S A* **88**: 4966–70.

Krakauer, J. W. & Shadmehr, R. (2006) Consolidation of motor memory. *Trends Neurosci* **29**: 58–64.

Kuriyama, K., Stickgold, R. & Walker, M. P. (2004) Sleep-dependent learning and motor-skill complexity. *Learn Mem* **11**: 705–13.

Maquet, P., Peters, J., Aerts, J. *et al.* (1996) Functional neuroanatomy of human rapid-eye-movement sleep and dreaming. *Nature* **383**: 163–6.

McClelland, J. L., Mcnaughton, B. L. & O'Reilly, R. C. (1995) Why there are complementary learning systems in the hippocampus and neocortex: insights from the successes and failures of connectionist models of learning and memory. *Psychol Rev* **102**: 419–57.

Mednick, S., Nakayama, K. & Stickgold, R. (2003) Sleep-dependent learning: a nap is as good as a night. *Nat. Neurosci* **6**: 697–8.

Mednick, S. A. (1962) The associative basis of the creative process. *Psychol Rev* **69**: 220–32.

Nishida, M., Pearsall, J., Buckner, R. L. *et al.* (2009) REM sleep, prefrontal theta, and the consolidation of human emotional memory. *Cereb Cortex* **19**: 1158–66.

Nishida, M. & Walker, M. P. (2007) Daytime naps, motor memory consolidation and regionally specific sleep spindles. *PLoS ONE* **2**: e341.

Pace-Schott, E. F., Milad, M. R., Orr, S. P. *et al.* (2009) Sleep promotes generalization of extinction of conditioned fear. *Sleep* **32**: 19–26.

Payne, J. D., Schacter, D. L., Propper, R. E. *et al.* (2009) The role of sleep in false memory formation. *Neurobiol Learn Mem* **92**: 327–34.

Payne, J. D., Stickgold, R., Swanberg, K. *et al.* (2008) Sleep preferentially enhances memory for emotional components of scenes. *Psychol Sci* **19**: 781–8.

Peigneux, P., Laureys, S., Fuchs, S. *et al.* (2004) Are spatial memories strengthened in the human hippocampus during slow wave sleep? *Neuron* **44**: 535–45.

Plihal, W. & Born, J. (1997) Effects of early and late nocturnal sleep on declarative and procedural memory. *J Cogn Neurosci* **9**: 534–47.

Robertson, E. M., Pascual-Leone, A. & Press, D. Z. (2004) Awareness modifies the skill-learning benefits of sleep. *Curr Biol* **14**: 208–12.

Roediger, H. L. & McDermott, K. B. (1995) Creating false memories: remembering words not presented in lists. *J Exp Psychol Learn Mem Cogn* **21**: 803–14.

Rudoy, J. D., Voss, J. L., Westerberg, C. E. *et al.* (2009) Strengthening individual memories by reactivating them during sleep. *Science* **326**:1079.

Schacter, D. L. & Tulving, E. (1994) *Memory Systems 1994*. Cambridge, MA: MIT Press.

Smith, C. & Smith, D. (2003) Ingestion of ethanol just prior to sleep onset impairs memory for procedural but not declarative tasks. *Sleep* **26**:185–91.

Stickgold, R. (2009) How do I remember? Let me count the ways. *Sleep Med Rev* **13**: 305–8.

Stickgold, R., Scott, L., Rittenhouse, C. *et al.* (1999) Sleep-induced changes in associative memory. *J Cogn Neurosci* **11**: 182–93.

Stickgold, R., Malia, A., Maguire, D. *et al.* (2000a) Replaying the game: hypnagogic images in normals and amnesics. *Science* **290**: 350–3.

Stickgold, R., Whidbee, D., Schirmer, B. *et al.* (2000b) Visual discrimination task improvement: A multi-step process occurring during sleep. *J Cogn Neurosci* **12**: 246–54.

Wagner, U., Gais, S. & Born, J. (2001) Emotional memory formation is enhanced across sleep intervals with high amounts of rapid eye movement sleep. *Learn Mem* **8**: 112–19.

Wagner, U., Gais, S., Haider, H. *et al.* (2004) Sleep inspires insight. *Nature* **427**: 352–5.

Walker, M. P. (2009) The role of slow wave sleep in memory processing. *J Clin Sleep Med* **5**: S20–6.

Walker, M. P., Brakefield, T., Morgan, A. *et al.* (2002a) Practice with sleep makes perfect: sleep-dependent motor skill learning. *Neuron* **35**: 205–11.

Walker, M. P., Liston, C., Hobson, J. A. *et al.* (2002b) Cognitive flexibility across the sleep-wake cycle: REM-sleep enhancement of anagram problem solving. *Cogn Brain Res* **14**: 317–24.

Walker, M. P., Brakefield, T., Hobson, J. A. *et al.* (2003a) Dissociable stages of human memory consolidation and reconsolidation. *Nature* **425**: 616–20.

Walker, M. P., Brakefield, T., Seidman, J. *et al.* (2003b) Sleep and the time course of motor skill learning. *Learn Mem* **10**: 275–84.

Walker, M. P., Stickgold, R., Alsop, D. *et al.* (2005a) Sleep-dependent motor memory plasticity in the human brain. *Neuroscience* **133**: 911–17.

Walker, M. P., Stickgold, R., Jolesz, F. A. *et al.* (2005b) The functional anatomy of sleep-dependent visual skill learning. *Cerebr Cortex* **15**: 1666–75.

Wamsley, E. J., Tucker, M., Payne, J. D. *et al.* (2010) Dreaming of a learning task is associated with enhanced sleep-dependent memory consolidation. *Curr Biol* **20**: 850–55.

Chapter 34

The role of REM sleep in emotional brain processing

Matthew P. Walker

Summary

Cognitive neuroscience continues to build meaningful connections between affective behavior and human brain function. Within the biological sciences, a similar renaissance has taken place, focusing on the role of sleep in various neurocognitive processes and, most recently, the interaction between sleep and emotional regulation. In this chapter, I survey an array of diverse findings across basic and clinical research domains, resulting in a convergent view of sleep-dependent emotional brain processing. Based on the unique neurobiology of sleep, I outline a model describing the overnight modulation of affective neural systems and the (re)processing of recent emotional experiences, both of which appear to redress the appropriate next-day reactivity of limbic and associated autonomic networks. Furthermore, an REM sleep hypothesis of emotional-memory processing is proposed, the implications of which may provide brain-based insights into the association between sleep abnormalities and the initiation and maintenance of mood disturbances.

Introduction

The ability of the human brain to generate, regulate, and be guided by emotions represents a fundamental process governing not only our personal lives, but our mental health as well as our societal structure. The recent emergence of cognitive neuroscience has ushered in a new era of research connecting affective behavior with human brain function. Additionally it has provided a systems-level view of emotional information processing, translationally bridging animal models of affective regulation and relevant clinical disorders (Labar and Cabeza, 2006).

Independent of this research area, a recent resurgence of interest in the functional impact of sleep on neurocognitive processes has also taken place within the basic sciences (Walker and Stickgold, 2006). However, surprisingly less research attention has been given to the interaction between sleep and affective brain function. I say surprising considering the remarkable overlap between the known physiology of sleep, especially REM sleep, and the associated neurochemistry and network anatomy that modulate emotions, as well as the prominent co-occurrence of abnormal sleep (including REM sleep) in almost all affective psychiatric and mood disorders.

Despite the relative historical paucity of research, recent work has begun to describe a consistent and clarifying role for sleep in the selective modulation of emotional information and the affective regulation. In the following chapter, I provide a synthesis of these findings, describing an intimate relationship between sleep, emotional brain function, and clinical mood disorders, and offer a tentative first theoretical framework that may account for these observed interactions.

Sleep and emotional-memory processing

The impact of sleep has principally been characterized at two different stages of memory (1) before learning, in the initial formation (encoding) of new information; and (2) after learning, in the long-term solidification (consolidation) of new memories. I now consider each of these stages, and focus on reports involving affective learning.

Sleep and affective memory encoding

Sleep and emotional-memory formation

At a behavioral level, pre-training sleep deprivation in rodents has been shown to impair encoding of

REM Sleep: Regulation and Function, eds. Birendra N. Mallick, S. R. Pandi-Perumal, Robert W. McCarley, and Adrian R. Morrison. Published by Cambridge University Press. © Cambridge University Press 2011.

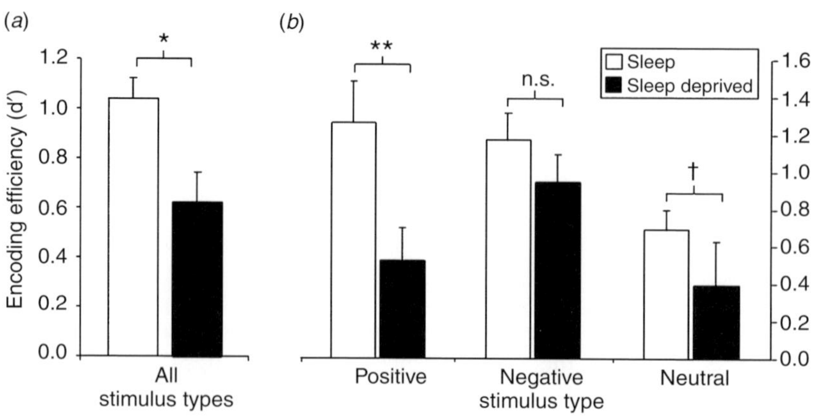

Figure 34.1 Sleep deprivation and encoding of emotional and non-emotional declarative memory. Effects of 38 hours of total-sleep deprivation on encoding of human declarative memory: (*a*) when combined across all emotional and non-emotional categories; (*b*) when separated by emotional (positive and negative valence) and non-emotional (neutral valence) categories, demonstrating a significant group (sleep, sleep-deprivation) x emotion category (positive, negative, neutral) interaction. (F(1,18) 3.58, $p < 0.05$). Post-hoc t-test comparisons:

$\dagger p < 0.08$, $^*p < 0.05$, $^{**}p < 0.01$, n.s. not significant, error bars represent s.e.m.

numerous memory tasks – the evidence for which is not covered here for brevity, due to a focus on humans (for reviews, see Walker and van der Helm, 2009). Critically, however, many if not all of these animal studies involve either appetitive or aversive learning paradigms; meaning these tasks are of an emotional nature.

While early studies investigating the role of sleep-dependent memory in humans focused primarily on *post*-learning consolidation (see later sections), more recent data similarly support the need for adequate *pre*-learning sleep in the formation of new human episodic memories. Some of the first studies of sleep deprivation and human-memory encoding focused on neutral forms of learning, indicating that "temporal memory" (memory for when events occur) was significantly disrupted by a night of pre-training sleep deprivation (Harrison and Horne, 2000; Morris *et al.*, 1960); even when caffeine was administered to overcome non-specific effects of lower arousal.

More recent investigations have examined the importance of pre-training sleep for the formation of emotional and neutral memories (Walker *et al.*, unpublished findings). Subjects were either sleep deprived for 36 hours or allowed to sleep normally prior to a learning session composed of emotionally negative, positive, and neutral words. Participants were then tested following two recovery nights of sleep so that in both groups, recollection was tested in a sleep-rested state. Therefore, any differences observed in performance observed could not be accounted for by the effects of sleep deprivation on retrieval, since neither group was sleep deprived at later testing. Averaged across all memory categories, subjects who were sleep deprived demonstrated a 40% deficit in memory encoding, relative

to subjects who had slept normally prior to learning (Figure 34.1*a*). However, when these data were separated into the three emotional categories (negative, positive, or neutral), selective dissociations became apparent (Figure 34.1*b*). In subjects that had slept (control group), both positive and negative stimuli were associated with superior retention levels relative to the neutral condition, consistent with the notion that emotion facilitates memory encoding. In the sleep-deprived group, a severe encoding impairment was evident for neutral and especially positive emotional memories, exhibiting a significant 59% retention deficit, relative to the control condition. Most interesting was the relative resistance of negative emotional memory to sleep deprivation, showing a markedly smaller and non-significant impairment.

These data indicate that sleep loss impairs the ability to commit new experiences to memory, and has recently been associated with dysfunction throughout the hippocampal complex (Yoo *et al.*, 2007b). They also suggest that, while the effects of sleep deprivation are directionally consistent across emotional subcategories, the most profound impact is on the encoding of positive emotional stimuli, and to a lesser degree, emotionally neutral stimuli. In contrast, the encoding of negative memory appears to be more resistant to the effects of prior sleep loss. Moreover, such results may offer novel learning and memory insights into affective mood disorders that express co-occurring sleep abnormalities. Indeed, if one compares the two profiles of memory encoding in Figure 34.1*b*, it is clear that the sleep control group completes the encoding session with a balanced mix of both positive and negative memories. However, those in the deprivation group have a skewed distribution, finishing the encoding session with an overriding dominance of negative memories, and far fewer positive or neutral memories; an issue with clinical relevance discussed below.

In summary, studies indicate that prior sleep loss significantly impairs the ability for effective next-day learning of new experiences across numerous species. Furthermore, sleep loss appears to disrupt the learning of different affective categories to different extents, potentially creating an imbalance in negative emotional memory dominance. Most intriguing, animal models indicate that affective learning demonstrates a particular sensitivity to REM-sleep deprivation, suggesting a dependency on a specific physiological stage of prior sleep for next-day emotional learning.

Sleep and affective memory consolidation

Mechanisms of emotional-memory consolidation

In addition to substantial evidence suggesting that emotion facilitates initial memory encoding, emotion is also known to modulate the subsequent stage of latent memory consolidation. A number of behavioral studies in humans have demonstrated diminished forgetting of emotional compared to neutral stimuli. This benefit of emotion on later memory retention increases as the time delay between learning and testing increases. This effect of offline retention has been shown over varying post-learning intervals, including comparisons between recollection at: 20 minutes to 1 week, immediate to 1 hour, immediate to 24 hours and 15 minutes to 2 weeks (Walker and van der Helm, 2009).

With the knowledge that emotion triggers improvements in memory performance over time, elegant work in animal models has substantively characterized the underlying anatomical and neurochemical mechanisms contributing to these effects; findings with implications relevant to the role of sleep neurobiology in emotional-memory processing. It is now proposed that stress hormones constitute a plausible protracted means of modifying latent consolidation by way of emotional arousal, promoting the adaptive reorganization of long-term memory representations. Recent human studies have confirmed these predictions. Using post-training pharmacological and pain manipulations to elicit responses involving the amygdala

(Cahill and Alkire, 2003; Cahill et al., 2003), Cahill and coworkers have demonstrated that induction of stress hormones can selectively enhance long-term memory of emotional stimuli when retested several days later (and see later sections). Thus, the hormones adrenaline and corticosterone appear to offer two important adaptive functions in response to arousing experiences: (1) they aid immediate responses to a potentially stressful experience; and (2) they aid future responses by enhancing consolidation of declarative memory for those arousing events.

In addition to neurohormonal effects, there is also substantial evidence that several neurotransmitters coregulate the effects of emotion on consolidation; including adrenergic transmitters and acetylcholine (ACh). The cholinergic effects are of particular note in relationship to sleep and specifically REM sleep discussed later. Acetylcholine appears to enhance amygdala-dependent memory consolidation. For example, in rats, post-training infusions of muscarinic cholinergic agonists and antagonists into the amygdala enhance and impair, respectively, memory across numerous tasks, including inhibitory avoidance, fear conditioning, and change in reward magnitude (Walker and van der Helm, 2009). Furthermore, post-training cholinergic stimulation of the amygdala using either muscarinic cholinergic agonists or the acetylcholinesterase inhibitor physostigmine has been shown to attenuate this emotional-memory impairment (Power and McGaugh, 2002).

Sleep and emotional-memory consolidation

The role of sleep after learning in subsequent memory consolidation has now been demonstrated across a range of phylogeny (Walker and Stickgold, 2004, 2006). Here I focus on affective learning paradigms, especially in humans.

Animal models support a role for sleep in the consolidation of both contextual fear and shock-avoidance tasks (for more detailed reviews beyond the scope of the current chapter, see Walker and Stickgold, 2004; Walker and van der Helm, 2009), all known to depend on intact hippocampal function. Daytime training on these tasks triggers alterations in sleep-stage characteristics, especially REM sleep (Ambrosini et al., 1988, 1993; Hennevin and Hars, 1987; Mandai et al., 1989; Sanford et al., 2001, 2003; Smith et al., 1980), possibly reflecting homeostatic

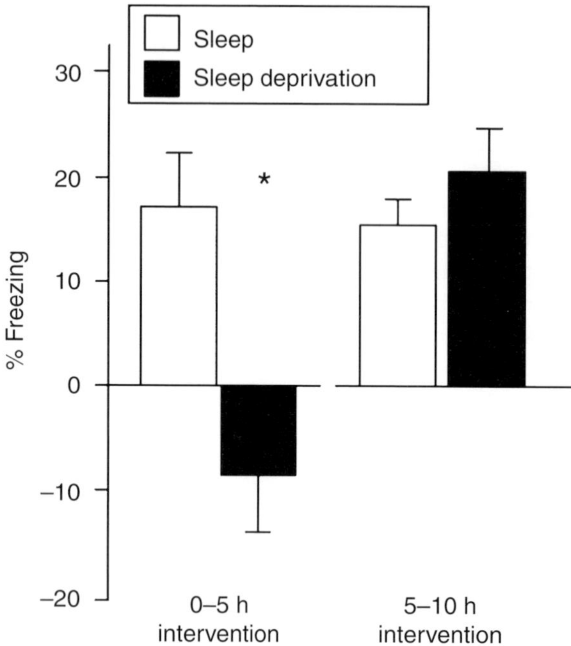

Figure 34.2 Difference in percent freezing during contextual-fear conditioning with or without sleep deprivation, across either zero to five hours post-training, or five to ten hours post-training (Graves *et al.*, 2003).

*$p < 0.05$, error bars represent s.e.m.

demands on REM sleep-dependent mechanisms of consolidation. Conversely, sleep deprivation after learning of such tasks has also been shown to disrupt consolidation and impair next-day memory retention (Smith, 1985; Walker and Stickgold, 2004). Moreover, these effects are apparent following selective REM-sleep deprivation, rather than total-sleep deprivation (Beaulieu and Godbout, 2000; Fishbein *et al.*, 1974; Hennevin and Hars, 1987; Marti-Nicolovius *et al.*, 1988; Oniani *et al.*, 1987; Pearlman, 1969; Shiromani *et al.*, 1979; Smith and Kelly, 1988).

Interestingly, the timing of when sleep deprivation occurs appears to be important. For example, Graves *et al.* (2003) have demonstrated that sleep deprivation zero to five hours post-training selectively impairs consolidation of contextual fear conditioning (as measured at a later 24-hour retest; Figure 34.2). However, sleep deprivation five to ten hours post-training did not block consolidation, resulting in similar memory performance at retest (Figure 34.2). These findings suggest that the consolidation of fear-associated memory occurs soon after learning with implications at a clinical treatment perspective; a situation perhaps most pertinent to conditions such as PTSD (discussed below).

In humans, the role of sleep in declarative-memory consolidation, rather than being absolute, may depend on more intricate aspects of the information being learned, such as novelty, meaning to extract, and also the affective salience of the material. The wealth of evidence demonstrating that human emotional experiences tend to be remembered better than neutral ones may help clarify the potential contribution of sleep to episodic-memory processing (Walker and van der Helm, 2009).

Based on the coincident neurophysiology that REM sleep provides and the neurobiological requirements of emotional-memory processing, work has now begun to test a selective REM sleep-dependent hypothesis of affective human-memory consolidation. For example, Hu *et al.* have compared the consolidation of emotionally arousing and non-arousing picture stimuli following a 12-hour period across a day or following a night of sleep (Hu *et al.*, 2006). A specific emotional-memory benefit was observed only following sleep and not across an equivalent time awake.

Wagner and colleagues (2001) have also shown that sleep selectively favors the retention of previously learned emotional texts relative to neutral texts, and that this affective-memory benefit is only present following late-night sleep (a time period rich in REM sleep). This emotional-memory benefit was found to persist in a follow-up study performed four years later (Wagner *et al.*, 2006). It has also been demonstrated that the speed of recognizing emotional face expressions presented prior to sleep is significantly improved the next day, a benefit that is positively correlated with the amount of intervening REM sleep (Wagner *et al.*, 2007).

Sleep has been shown to target the consolidation of specific aspects of emotional experiences, as well as mediate the extinction of human-fear memories. By experimentally varying the foreground and background elements of emotional picture stimuli, Payne *et al.* have demonstrated that sleep can target the strengthening of negative emotional objects in a scene, but not the peripheral background (Payne *et al.*, 2008). In contrast, equivalent time awake did not afford any benefit to emotional-object memory (or the background scene). This may suggest that sleep-dependent processing can selectively separate episodic experience into component parts, preferentially consolidating those of greatest affective salience.

Using a nap paradigm, Nishida *et al.* recently demonstrated that sleep, and specifically REM sleep neurophysiology, may underlie such consolidation benefits (Nishida *et al.*, 2009). Subjects performed two study sessions in which they learned emotionally arousing negative and neutral picture stimuli; one four hours prior, and one 15 minutes prior to a recognition memory test. In one group, participants slept (90-minute nap) after the first study session, while in the other group, participants remained awake. Thus, items from the first (four-hour) study sessions transitioned through different brain states in each group prior to testing, containing sleep in the nap group and no sleep in the no-nap group, yet experienced identical brain-state conditions following the second (15-minute) study session prior to testing. No change in memory for emotional (or neutral) stimuli occurred across the offline delay in the no-nap group. However, a significant and selective offline enhancement of emotional memory was observed in the nap group (Figure 34.3*a*), the extent of which was correlated with the amount of REM sleep (Figure 34.3*b*), and the speed of entry into REM sleep (latency; not shown in figure). Most striking, spectral analysis of the EEG demonstrated that the

magnitude of right-dominant prefrontal theta power during REM sleep (activity in the frequency range of 4.0 to 7.0 Hz) exhibited a significant and positive relationship with the amount of emotional-memory improvement (Figure 34.3*c,d*).

These findings move beyond demonstrating that affective memories are preferentially enhanced across periods of sleep, and indicate that the extent of emotional-memory improvement is associated with specific REM-sleep characteristics – both quantity and quality (and independent of nocturnal hormonal changes). Corroborating these correlations, it has previously been hypothesized that REM sleep represents a brain state particularly amenable to emotional memory consolidation, based on its unique biology (Hu *et al.*, 2006). Neurochemically, levels of limbic and forebrain ACh are markedly elevated during REM sleep (Vazquez and Baghdoyan, 2001), reportedly quadruple those seen during NREM and double those measured in quiet waking (Marrosu *et al.*, 1995). Considering the known importance of ACh in the long-term consolidation of emotional learning (Walker and van der Helm,

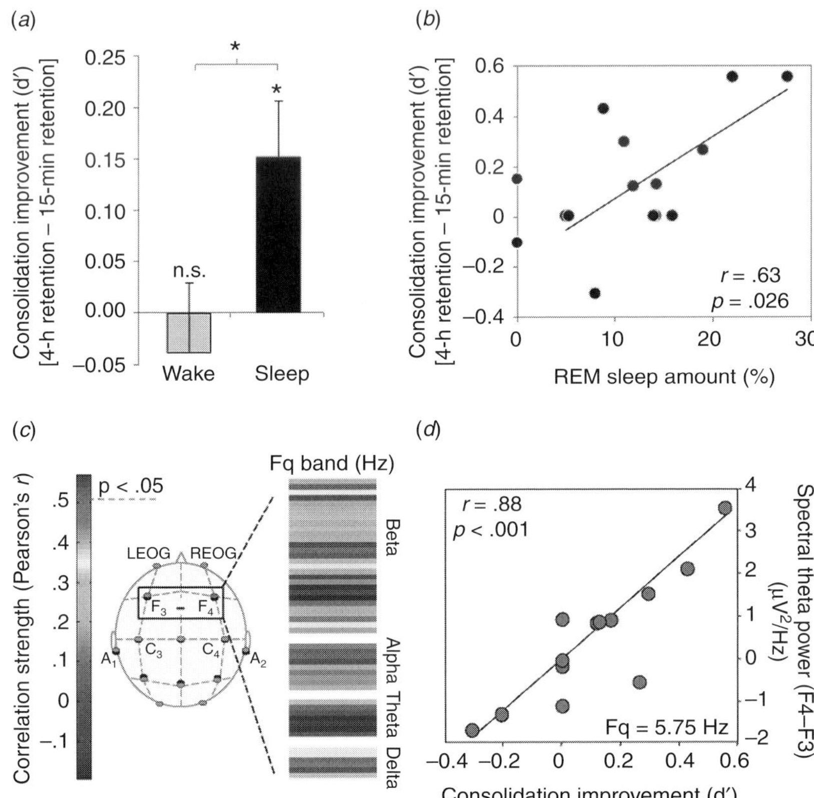

Figure 34.3 REM-sleep enhancement of negative emotional memories. (*a*) Offline benefit (change in memory recall for 4 hours versus 15 minutes old memories) across the day (wake, grey bar) or following a 90-minute nap (sleep, filled bar). (*b*) Correlation between the amount of offline emotional memory improvement in the nap group (i.e., the offline benefit expressed in filled bar of figure (*a*), and the amount of REM sleep obtained within the nap. (*c*) Correlation strength (Pearson's *r*-value) between offline benefit for emotional memory in the sleep group (the benefit expressed in filled bar of figure (*a*)) and the relative right versus left prefrontal spectral-band power (F4–F3) within the delta, alpha, theta, and beta spectral bands, expressed in average 0.5 Hz bin increments. Correlation strength is represented by the color range, demonstrating significant correlations within the theta frequency band (hot colors), and (*d*) exhibiting a maximum significance at the 5.75 Hz bin. $*p < 0.05$; error bars indicate s.e.m. (Modified from Nishida *et al.*, 2009). (See plate section for color version.)

343

2009), this pro-cholinergic REM-sleep state may promote the selective memory facilitation of affective memories, similar to that reported using experimental manipulations of ACh (Walker and van der Helm, 2009). Neurophysiologically, theta oscillations have been proposed as a carrier frequency, allowing disparate brain regions that initially encode information to selectively interact offline, in a coupled relationship. By doing so, REM-sleep theta may afford the ability to strengthen distributed aspects of specific memory representations across related but different anatomical networks.

Sleep and emotional regulation

Despite substantial research focusing on the interaction between sleep and affective memory, the impact of sleep loss on basic emotional regulation and perception has received limited research attention. This absence of research is also striking considering that nearly all psychiatric and neurological mood disorders express co-occurring abnormalities of sleep, suggesting an intimate relationship between sleep and emotion. Nevertheless, a number of studies evaluating subjective as well as objective measures of mood and affect, combined with insights from clinical domains, offer an emerging understanding for the critical role sleep plays in regulating emotional brain function.

Sleep loss, mood stability, and emotional brain (re)activity

Together with impairments of attention and alertness, sleep deprivation is commonly associated with increased subjective reports of irritability and affective volatility (Horne, 1985). Using a sleep-restriction paradigm (five hours per night), Dinges *et al.* have reported a progressive increase in emotional disturbance across a one-week period on the basis of questionnaire mood scales and daily journals (Dinges *et al.*, 1997). Zohar *et al.* have investigated the effects of sleep disruption on emotional reactivity to daytime work events in medical residents (Zohar *et al.*, 2005), demonstrating amplified negative emotional consequences of disruptive daytime experiences while blunting the positive benefit associated with rewarding or goal-enhancing activities.

While these findings help to characterize the behavioral irregularities imposed by sleep loss, evidence for the role of sleep in regulating psychophysiological reactivity and emotional brain networks is

only now starting to emerge. To date, only two studies have addressed this interaction. Using functional MRI (fMRI), Yoo and colleagues examined the impact of one night of sleep deprivation on emotional brain reactivity in healthy young adults (Yoo *et al.*, 2007a). During scanning, participants performed an affective stimulus-viewing task involving the presentation of picture slides ranging in a gradient from emotionally neutral to increasingly negative and aversive. While both groups expressed significant amygdala activation in response to increasingly negative picture stimuli, those in the sleep-deprivation condition exhibited a remarkable +60% greater magnitude of amygdala reactivity, relative to the control group (Figure 34.4a,b). In addition to this increased intensity of activation, there was also a three-fold increase in the extent of amygdala volume recruited in response to the aversive stimuli in the sleep-deprivation group (Figure 34.4b). Perhaps most interestingly, relative to the sleep-control group, there was a significant loss of functional connectivity identified between the amygdala and the medial prefrontal cortex (mPFC) in those who were sleep deprived – a region known to have strong inhibitory top-down projections to the amygdala (Figure 34.4c,d). In contrast, significantly greater connectivity was observed between the amygdala and the autonomic-activating centers of the locus coeruleus in the deprivation group. Thus, without sleep, an amplified hyperlimbic reaction by the human amygdala was observed in response to negative emotional stimuli. Furthermore, this altered magnitude of amygdala activity was associated with a loss of functional connectivity with the mPFC in the sleep-deprivation condition; implying a failure of top-down inhibition by the prefrontal lobe. Interestingly, a similar pattern of anatomical dysfunction has been implicated in a number of psychiatric mood disorders, which express co-occurring sleep abnormalities (Davidson *et al.*, 2002), and directly raises the issue of whether such factors (sleep loss and clinical mood disorders) are causally related.

More recently, Franzen *et al.* measured the impact of total-sleep deprivation on pupil-diameter responses (a measure of autonomic reactivity) during a passive affective picture-viewing task containing positive, negative, and neutral stimuli (Franzen *et al.*, 2009). Relative to a sleep control group, there was a significantly larger pupillary response to negative pictures compared to positive or neutral stimuli in the deprivation group. Furthermore, those in the sleep-deprived condition expressed earlier reactivity to negative images prior to

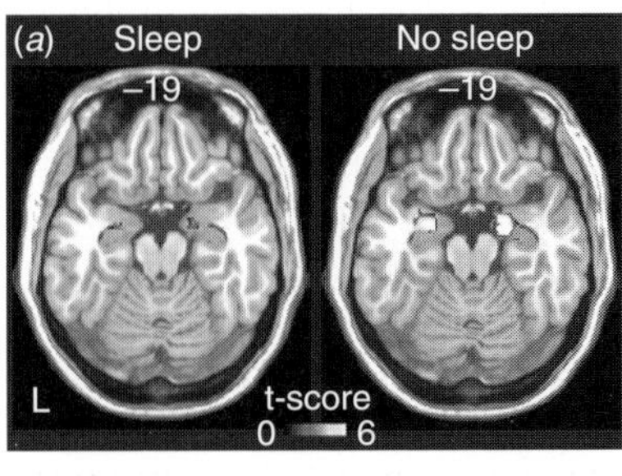
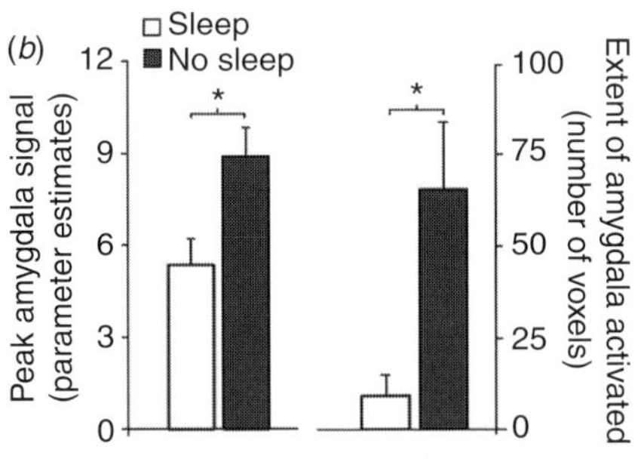
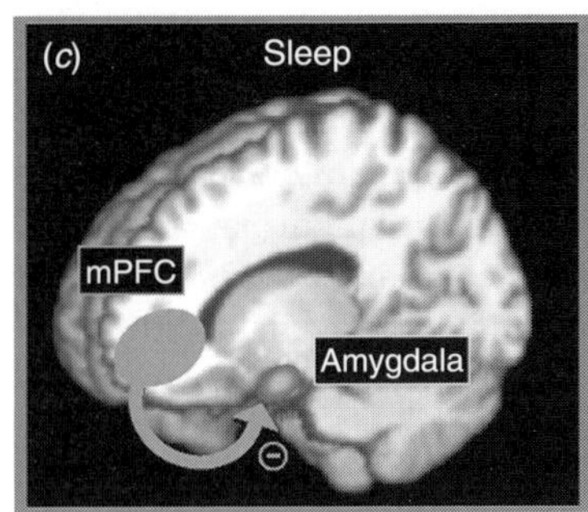
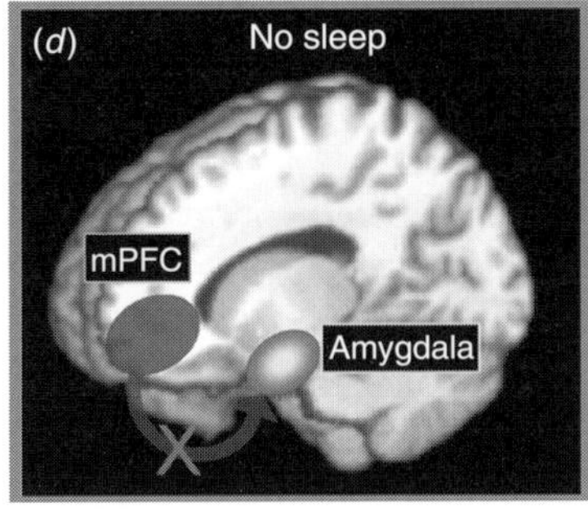

Figure 34.4 The impact of sleep deprivation on emotional-brain reactivity and functional connectivity. (*a*) Amygdala response to increasingly negative emotional stimuli in the sleep-deprivation and sleep-control groups, and (*b*) corresponding differences in intensity and volumetric extent of amygdala activation between the two groups (average ± s.e.m. of left and right amygdala). (*c*) Depiction of associated changes in functional connectivity between the medial prefrontal cortex (mPFC) and the amygdala. With sleep, the prefrontal lobe was strongly connected to the amygdala, regulating and exerting an inhibitory top-down control. (*d*) Without sleep, however, amygdala-mPFC connectivity was decreased, potentially negating top-down control and resulting in an overactive amygdala.

*$p < 0.01$; error bars indicate s.e.m. (See plate section for color version.)

the stimulus onset cue. These data suggest that sleep deprivation not only alters emotional reactivity, but may also change the anticipation of these events.

A heuristic model of sleep-dependent emotional processing: explanatory clinical insights and predictive associations

Based on the emerging interaction between sleep and emotion at the basic experimental as well as clinical level, I next provide a synthesis of these findings, which converge on a functional role for sleep in affective brain modulation. I describe a model of sleep-dependent emotional information processing, offering provisional brain-based explanatory insights regarding the impact of sleep abnormalities in the initiation and maintenance of certain mood disorders, and leading to testable predictions for future experimental investigations.

Emotional-memory processing: a sleep to *forget* and sleep to *remember* (SFSR) hypothesis

Founded on the emerging interaction between sleep and emotion, below I outline a model of affective information processing that may offer brain-based

explanatory insights regarding the impact of sleep abnormalities, particularly REM sleep, for the initiation or maintenance of mood disturbance.

Although there is abundant evidence to suggest that emotional experiences persist in our autobiographies over time, an equally remarkable but far less noted change is a reduction in the affective tone associated with their recall. The reason that affective experiences appear to be encoded and consolidated more robustly than neutral memories is due to autonomic neurochemical reactions elicited at the time of the experience, creating what I commonly term an "emotional memory." However, the later recall of these memories tends not to be associated with anywhere near the same magnitude of autonomic (re)activation as that elicited at the moment of experience – suggesting that, over time, the affective "blanket" previously enveloped around the memory during learning has been removed, whereas the information contained within that experience (the memory) remains.

For example, neuroimaging studies have shown that initial exposure and learning of emotional stimuli is associated with substantially greater activation in the amygdala and hippocampus, relative to neutral stimuli (Dolcos *et al.*, 2004, 2005). In one of these studies (Dolcos *et al.*, 2004), however, when participants were re-exposed to these same stimuli during recognition testing many months later, a change in the profile of

345

activation occurred (Dolcos *et al.*, 2005). Although the same magnitude of differential activity between emotional and neutral items was observed in the hippocampus, this was not true in the amygdala. Instead, the difference in amygdala (re)activity to emotional items compared with neutral items had dissipated over time. This would support the idea that the strength of the memory (hippocampal-associated activity) remains at later recollection, yet the associated emotional reactivity to these items (amygdala activity) is reduced over time.

The hypothesis predicts that this decoupling preferentially takes place overnight, such that we *sleep to forget* the emotional tone, yet *sleep to remember* the tagged memory of that episode (SFSR model; Figure 34.5). The model further argues that if this process is not achieved, the magnitude of affective "charge" remaining within autobiographical memory networks would persist, resulting in the potential condition of chronic anxiety.

Based on the unique neurobiology of REM, here I propose an REM-sleep hypothesis of emotional brain processing (Figure 34.5a). It is suggested that the state of REM provides an optimal biological theater, within which can be achieved a form of affective "therapy." Specifically, increased activity within limbic and paralimbic structures (including the hippocampus and amygdala) during REM sleep may first offer the ability for reactivation of previously acquired affective experiences. Secondly, the neurophysiological signature of REM sleep involving dominant theta oscillations within subcortical as well as cortical nodes may offer large-scale network cooperation at night, allowing the integration and, as a consequence, greater understanding of recently experienced emotional events in the context of pre-existing neocortically stored semantic memory. Thirdly, these interactions during REM sleep (and perhaps through the conscious process of dreaming) critically and perhaps most importantly take place within a brain that is devoid of aminergic neurochemical concentration, particularly noradrenergic input from the locus coeruleus; the influence of which has been linked to states of high stress and anxiety disorders.

In summary, the described neuroanatomical, neurophysiological, and neurochemical conditions of REM sleep offer a unique biological milieu in which to achieve, on one hand, a balanced neural facilitation of the informational core of emotional experiences (the memory), yet may also depotentiate and ultimately ameliorate the autonomic arousing charge originally acquired at the time of learning (the emotion), negating a long-term state of anxiety (Figure 34.5).

Predictions of the model

If this process of divorcing emotion from memory were not achieved across the first night following such an experience, the model would predict that a repeat attempt of affective demodulation would occur on the second night, since the strength of the emotional "tag" associated with the memory would remain high. If this process failed a second time, the same events would continue to repeat across ensuing nights. It is just such a cycle of REM-sleep dreaming (nightmares) that represents a diagnostic key feature of post-traumatic stress disorder (PTSD). It may not be coincidental, therefore, that these patients continue to display hyperarousal reactions to associated trauma cues (Harvey *et al.*, 2003), indicating that the process of separating the affective tone from the emotional experience has not been accomplished. The reason why such an REM mechanism may fail in PTSD remains unknown, although the exceptional magnitude of trauma-induced emotion at the time of learning may be so great that the system is incapable of initiating/completing one or both of these processes, leaving some patients unable to integrate and depotentiate the stored experience. Alternatively, it may be the hyperarousal status of the brain during REM sleep in these patients, potentially lacking sufficient aminergic demodulation, that prevents the processing and separation of emotion from memory.

This model also makes specific experimental predictions as to the fate of these two components – the memory and the emotion. As partially demonstrated, the first prediction would be that, over time, the veracity of the memory itself would be maintained or improved, and the extent to which these (negative) emotional experiences are strengthened would be proportional to the amount of post-experience REM sleep obtained, as well as how quickly it is achieved (REM latency).

Secondly, using physiology measures, these same predictions would hold in the inverse direction for the magnitude of emotional reactivity induced at the time of recall. Together with the neuroimaging studies of emotional memory recall over time, and psychological studies investigating the role of REM-sleep dreaming in mood regulation, a recent fMRI study offers perhaps the strongest preliminary support of

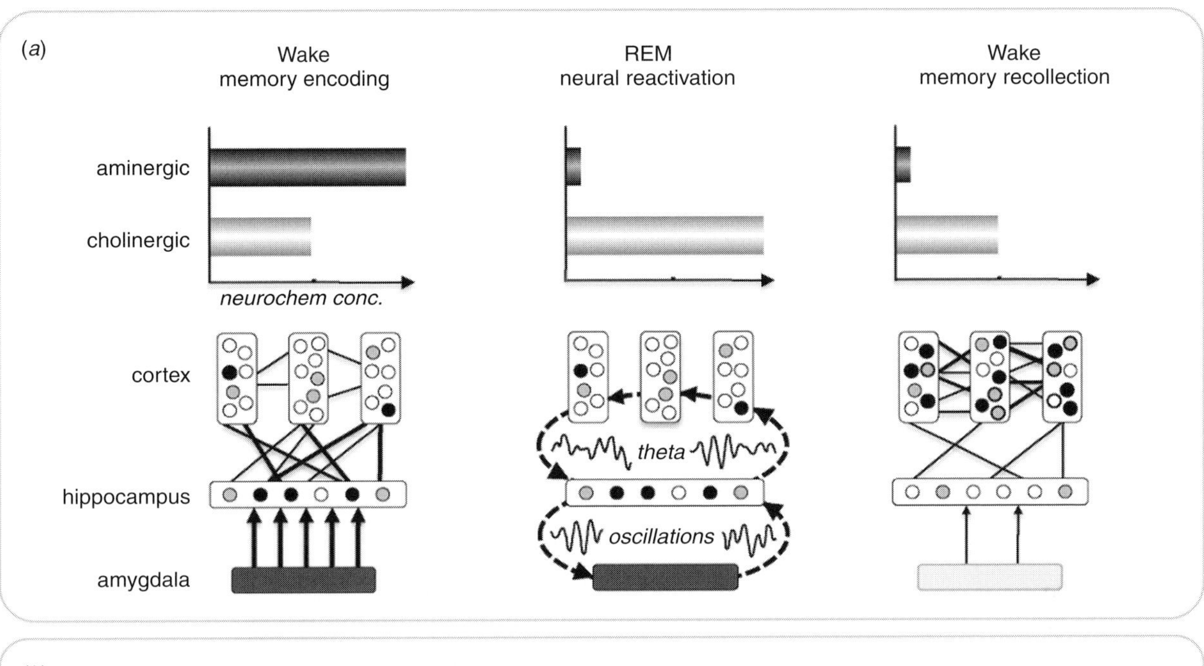

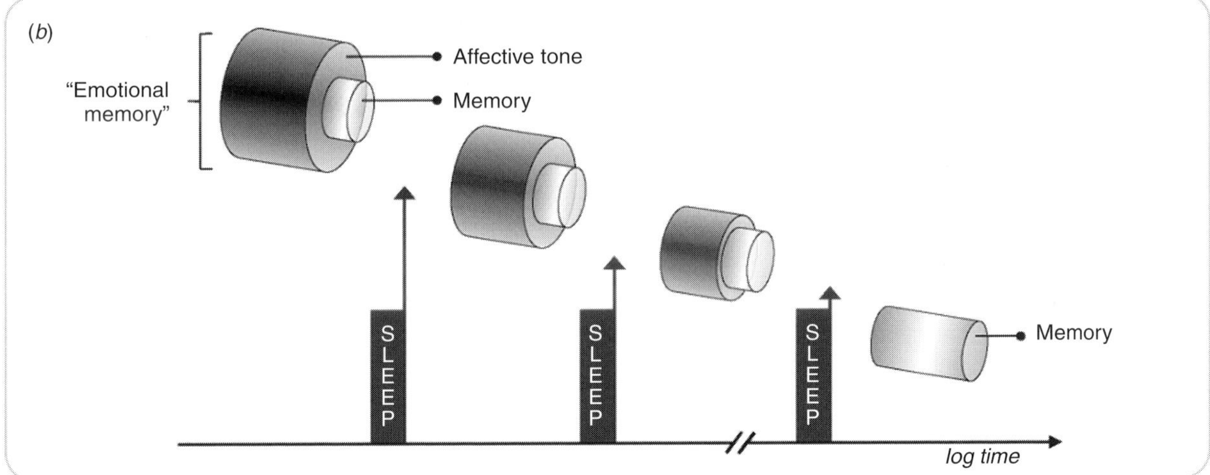

Figure 34.5 The sleep to *forget* and sleep to *remember* (SFSR) model of emotional-memory processing. (*a*) Neural dynamics. Waking formation of an episodic emotional memory involves the coordinated encoding of hippocampal-bound information within cortical modules, facilitated by the amygdala, and modulated by high concentrations of aminergic neurochemistry. During subsequent REM sleep, these same neural structures are reactivated, the coordination of which is made possible by synchronous theta oscillations throughout these networks, supporting the ability to reprocess previously learned emotional experiences. However, this reactivation occurs in a neurochemical milieu devoid of aminergic modulation, and dominated by cholinergic neurochemistry. As a consequence, emotional-memory reprocessing can achieve, on the one hand, a depotentiation of the affective tone initially associated with the event(s) at encoding, while on the other, a simultaneous and progressive neocortical consolidation of the information. The latter process of developing stronger cortico-cortical connections additionally supports integration into previous acquired autobiographical experiences, further aiding the assimilation of the affective event(s) in the context of past knowledge, the conscious expression of which may contribute to the experience of dreaming. Cross-connectivity between structures is represented by the number and thickness of lines. Circles within cortical and hippocampal structures represent information nodes; shade reflects extent of connectivity: strong (filled), moderate (gray), and weak (clear). Color fill of amygdala and arrow thickness represents magnitude of co-activation with and influence on the hippocampus. (*b*) Conceptual outcome. Through multiple iterations of this REM mechanism across the night, and/or across multiple nights, the long-term consequence of such sleep-dependent reprocessing would allow for the strengthening and retention of salient information previously tagged as emotional at the time of learning. However, recall no longer maintains an affective, aminergic charge, allowing for post-sleep recollection with minimal autonomic reactivity (unlike encoding), thereby preventing a state of chronic anxiety.

this sleep-dependent model of emotional-memory processing (Sterpenich *et al.*, 2007). Relative to a control group that slept, participants who were deprived of sleep the first night after learning arousing emotional picture slides not only showed reduced recall of the information 72 hours later (the sleep to remember component of the hypothesis), but also showed a lack of reduction in amygdala reactivity when re-exposed to these same negative emotional picture slides at recognition testing (the sleep to forget component of the hypothesis). Thus, sleep after learning facilitated improved recollection of these prior emotional experiences, yet this later recollection was conversely associated with a reduction in amygdala reactivity. In contrast, those who did not sleep the first night after the emotional learning session, despite obtaining two full recovery nights of sleep, exhibited no such depotentiation of subsequent amygdala reactivity.

The third tenet of the model predicts that a pathological increase in REM, as commonly occurs in depression (Armitage, 2007), may disproportionately amplify the strength of negative memories, so much so that, despite concomitant attempts at ameliorating the associated affective tone, would still create a perceived autobiographical history dominated by negative memory excess (which may also facilitate disadvantageous waking rumination). In contrast, the selective decrease of REM, as occurs with many antidepressants, would predict a reduction of such negative memory consolidation and bias, although it may curtail the degree of affective decoupling that can occur. Long term, the balanced extent of accumulated REM should therefore correlate not only with the persistence, in memory, of the emotional experience, it should also be associated with a decreased magnitude of autonomic response associated with recall – all of which are testable experimental questions.

When viewed as a whole, findings at the cellular, systems, cognitive, and clinical level all point to a crucial role for sleep in the affective modulation of human brain function. Based on the remarkable neurobiology of sleep, and REM sleep in particular, a unique capacity for the overnight modulation of affective networks and previously encountered emotional experiences may be possible, redressing and maintaining the appropriate connectivity and hence next-day reactivity throughout limbic and associated autonomic systems. Ultimately, the timeless wisdom of mothers alike may never have been more relevant: that is, when troubled "get to bed, you'll feel better in the morning."

References

Ambrosini, M. V., Mariucci, G., Colarieti, L. *et al.* (1993) The structure of sleep is related to the learning ability of rats. *Eur J Neurosci* **5**: 269–75.

Ambrosini, M. V., Sadile, A. G., Gironi Carnevale, U. A., Mattiaccio, M. & Giuditta, A. (1988) The sequential hypothesis on sleep function. I. Evidence that the structure of sleep depends on the nature of the previous waking experience. *Braz J Med Biol Res* **21**: 141–5.

Armitage, R. (2007) Sleep and circadian rhythms in mood disorders. *Acta Psychiatr Scand Suppl* 104–15.

Beaulieu, I. & Godbout, R. (2000) Spatial learning on the Morris Water Maze Test after a short-term paradoxical sleep deprivation in the rat. *Brain Cogn* **43**: 27–31.

Cahill, L. & Alkire, M. T. (2003) Epinephrine enhancement of human memory consolidation: interaction with arousal at encoding. *Neurobiol Learn Mem* **79**: 194–8.

Cahill, L., Gorski, L. & Le, K. (2003) Enhanced human memory consolidation with post-learning stress: interaction with the degree of arousal at encoding. *Learn Mem* **10**: 270–4.

Davidson, R. J., Pizzagalli, D., Nitschke, J. B. & Putnam, K. (2002) Depression: perspectives from affective neuroscience. *Annu Rev Psychol* **53**: 545–74.

Dinges, D. F., Pack, F., Williams, K., *et al.* (1997) Cumulative sleepiness, mood disturbance, and psychomotor vigilance performance decrements during a week of sleep restricted to 4–5 hours per night. *Sleep* **20**: 267–77.

Dolcos, F., Labar, K. S. & Cabeza, R. (2004) Interaction between the amygdala and the medial temporal lobe memory system predicts better memory for emotional events. *Neuron* **42**: 855–63.

Dolcos, F., Labar, K. S. & Cabeza, R. (2005) Remembering one year later: role of the amygdala and the medial temporal lobe memory system in retrieving emotional memories. *Proc Natl Acad Sci U S A* **102**: 2626–31.

Fishbein, W., Kastaniotis, C. & Chattman, D. (1974) Paradoxical sleep: prolonged augmentation following learning. *Brain Res* **79**: 61–75.

Franzen, P. L., Buysse, D. J., Dahl, R. E., Thompson, W. & Siegle, G. J. (2009) Sleep deprivation alters pupillary reactivity to emotional stimuli in healthy young adults. *Biol Psychol* **80**: 300–5.

Graves, L. A., Heller, E. A., Pack, A. I. & Abel, T. (2003) Sleep deprivation selectively impairs memory consolidation for contextual fear conditioning. *Learn Mem* **10**: 168–76.

Harrison, Y. & Horne, J. A. (2000) Sleep loss and temporal memory. *Q J Exp Psychol* **53**: 271–9.

Harvey, A. G., Jones, C. & Schmidt, D. A. (2003) Sleep and posttraumatic stress disorder: a review. *Clin Psychol Rev* **23**: 377–407.

Hennevin, E. & Hars, B. (1987) Is increase in post-learning paradoxical sleep modified by cueing? *Behav Brain Res* **24**: 243–9.

Horne, J. A. (1985) Sleep function, with particular reference to sleep deprivation. *Ann Clin Res* **17**: 199–208.

Hu, P., Stylos-Allen, M. & Walker, M. P. (2006) Sleep facilitates consolidation of emotionally arousing declarative memory. *Psychol Sci* **17**: 891–8.

Labar, K. S. & Cabeza, R. (2006) Cognitive neuroscience of emotional memory. *Nat Rev Neurosci* **7**: 54–64.

Mandai, O., Guerrien, A., Sockeel, P., Dujardin, K. & Leconte, P. (1989) REM sleep modifications following a Morse code learning session in humans. *Physiol Behav* **46**: 759–62.

Marrosu, F., Portas, C., Mascia, M. S. *et al.* (1995) Microdialysis measurement of cortical and hippocampal acetylcholine release during sleep–wake cycle in freely moving cats. *Brain Res* **671**: 329–32.

Marti-Nicolovius, M., Portell-Cortes, I. & Morgado-Bernal, I. (1988) Improvement of shuttle-box avoidance following post-training treatment in paradoxical sleep deprivation platforms in rats. *Physiol Behav* **43**: 93–8.

Morris, G. O., Williams, H. L. & Lubin, A. (1960) Misperception and disorientation during sleep. *Arch Gen Psychiatry* **2**: 247–54.

Nishida, M., Pearsall, J., Buckner, R. L. & Walker, M. P. (2009) Prefrontal theta during REM sleep enhances emotional memory. *Cereb Cortex* **19**: 1158–66.

Oniani, T. N., Lortkipanidze, N. D. & Maisuradze, L. M. (1987) Interaction between learning and paradoxical sleep in cats. *Neurosci Behav Physiol* **17**: 304–10.

Payne, J. D., Stickgold, R., Swanberg, K. & Kensinger, E. A. (2008) Sleep preferentially enhances memory for emotional components of scenes. *Psychol Sci* **19**: 781–8.

Pearlman, C. A. (1969) Effect of rapid eye movement (dreaming) sleep deprivation on retention of avoidance learning in rats. Rep No 563. *Rep US Nav Submar Med Cent*, 1–4.

Power, A. E. & McGaugh, J. L. (2002) Cholinergic activation of the basolateral amygdala regulates unlearned freezing behavior in rats. *Behav Brain Res* **134**: 307–15.

Sanford, L. D., Silvestri, A. J., Ross, R. J. & Morrison, A. R. (2001) Influence of fear conditioning on elicited ponto-geniculo-occipital waves and rapid eye movement sleep. *Arch Ital Biol* **139**: 169–83.

Sanford, L. D., Tang, X., Ross, R. J. & Morrison, A. R. (2003) Influence of shock training and explicit fear-conditioned cues on sleep architecture in mice: strain comparison. *Behav Genet* **33**: 43–58.

Shiromani, P., Gutwein, B. M. & Fishbein, W. (1979) Development of learning and memory in mice after brief paradoxical sleep deprivation. *Physiol Behav* **22**: 971–8.

Smith, C. (1985) Sleep states and learning: a review of the animal literature. *Neurosci Biobehav Rev* **9**: 157–68.

Smith, C. & Kelly, G. (1988) Paradoxical sleep deprivation applied two days after end of training retards learning. *Physiol Behav* **43**: 213–16.

Smith, C., Young, J. & Young, W. (1980) Prolonged increases in paradoxical sleep during and after avoidance-task acquisition. *Sleep* **3**: 67–81.

Sterpenich, V., Albouy, G., Boly, M. *et al.* (2007) Sleep-related hippocampo-cortical interplay during emotional memory recollection. *PLoS Biol* **5**: e282.

Vazquez, J. & Baghdoyan, H. A. (2001) Basal forebrain acetylcholine release during REM sleep is significantly greater than during waking. *Am J Physiol Regul Integr Comp Physiol* **280**: R598–601.

Wagner, U., Gais, S. & Born, J. (2001) Emotional memory formation is enhanced across sleep intervals with high amounts of rapid eye movement sleep. *Learn Mem* **8**: 112–19.

Wagner, U., Hallschmid, M., Rasch, B. & Born, J. (2006) Brief sleep after learning keeps emotional memories alive for years. *Biol Psychiatry* **60**: 788–90.

Wagner, U., Kashyap, N., Diekelmann, S. & Born, J. (2007) The impact of post-learning sleep vs. wakefulness on recognition memory for faces with different facial expressions. *Neurobiol Learn Mem* **87**: 679–87.

Walker, M. P. & Stickgold, R. (2004) Sleep-dependent learning and memory consolidation. *Neuro* **44**: 121–33.

Walker, M. P. & Stickgold, R. (2006) Sleep, memory and plasticity. *Annu Rev Psychol* **10**: 139–66.

Walker, M. P. & van der Helm, E. (2009) Overnight therapy? The role of sleep in emotional brain processing. *Psychol Bull* **135**: 731–48.

Yoo, S. S., Gujar, N., Hu, P., Jolesz, F. A. & Walker, M. P. (2007a) The human emotional brain without sleep – a prefrontal amygdala disconnect. *Curr Biol* **17**: R877–8.

Yoo, S. S., Hu, P. T., Gujar, N., Jolesz, F. A. & Walker, M. P. (2007b) A deficit in the ability to form new human memories without sleep. *Nat Neurosci* **10**: 385–92.

Zohar, D., Tzischinsky, O., Epstein, R. & Lavie, P. (2005) The effects of sleep loss on medical residents' emotional reactions to work events: a cognitive-energy model. *Sleep* **28**: 47–54.

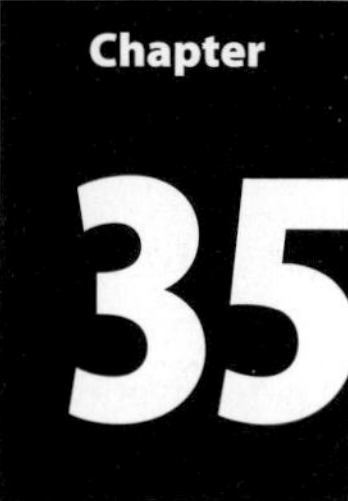

Chapter

35

REM-sleep loss, oxidative damage, and apoptosis

Sudipta Biswas and Anupama Gopalakrishnan

Summary

Rapid eye movement (REM) sleep is present across species and is considered essential for an animal's survival. However, loss of sleep, including REM sleep, occurs in many conditions and has been thought to have detrimental effects on the well-being of the individual. Many neurological and neuropathological disorders are associated with sleep loss and changes in the cellular oxidative status independently. In this chapter, we have made an effort to discuss the possible role of REM sleep deprivation-induced oxidative stress and cellular apoptosis in the etiology of the neurological diseases. A brief discussion of the effects of sleep and REM-sleep deprivation (REMSD) is followed by an account of various neurodegenerative disorders that are characterized by apoptotic cell loss caused by oxidative stress and also by sleep disturbances. Several animal studies, which have observed the indices of oxidative stress following sleep deprivation, have varied conclusions. Upon analysis, we observed that a high number of experimental variables such as species, method of sleep deprivation, duration of sleep deprivation, brain areas, and choice of apoptosis markers studied, has led to a lack of concordance between experimental reports. Therefore a detailed systematic study exploring the relationships between REM-sleep deprivation, oxidative stress, and apoptosis is required to help us gain a better understanding of many neuropathological disorders.

REM sleep is a stage of sleep that is present across species of most mammals (Frank, 1999). It serves important functions such as maintaining brain excitability (Mallick *et al.*, 2002), memory consolidation (Graves *et al.*, 2003) and is considered to be essential for survival of the organism (Kushida *et al.*, 1989). Most researchers now believe that one of the functions of REM sleep is to consolidate recent memories and to facilitate the learning process (Graves *et al.*, 2003). Loss of REM sleep or sleep deprivation in general is a phenomenon that occurs in neurological and neuropathological disorders and in jobs that involve loss of sleep such as nursing, airline pilots and cabin crews, call center employees, etc. Many of these neurological diseases are also associated with changes in oxidative status of cells. Therefore, the physiological, behavioral, and molecular changes associated with REM-sleep deprivation are of great interest to researchers worldwide. Hence, this article reviews the literature to determine the specific effects of REM-sleep deprivation and total-sleep deprivation on the oxidative status of cells and apoptosis mechanisms. We start with a brief description of REM-sleep deprivation in animal models and the loss of REM sleep that is observed in neuropathological disorders. This is followed by a discussion of the various studies that have investigated oxidative stress and cell damage following sleep deprivation, specifically deprivation of REM sleep. We end with our views on the physiological significance of REM-sleep deprivation induced cellular changes.

REM-sleep deprivation

REM sleep is characterized by low-voltage EEG, muscle atonia, and rapid eye movements and occupies about 15 to 20% of total sleep in adults. In spite of its low occurrence, it is very important and distinct as evidenced by the biochemical, physiological, and molecular changes observed following REM-sleep deprivation. The classical method of REM-sleep deprivation as described by Jouvet *et al.*, (1964) and Mendelson *et al.*, (1974), involved the platform method, with the large platform, recovery group, and caged animals serving as controls. Although this method has been under criticism as a stress inducer, it remains the most popular and effective method of REM-sleep deprivation. Other popular methods include grid-over-water and disk-over-water techniques (reviewed in Gulyani *et al.*, 2000).

REM Sleep: Regulation and Function, eds. Birendra N. Mallick, S. R. Pandi-Perumal, Robert W. McCarley, and Adrian R. Morrison. Published by Cambridge University Press. © Cambridge University Press 2011.

REM-sleep deprivation leads to physiological, biochemical, and molecular changes. When total-sleep deprivation (TSD) or REMSD is enforced in rats for one to several weeks, pathologies develop that lead to significant morbidity. Collectively referred to as "sleep deprivation effects" (reviewed in Rechtschaffen and Bergmann, 2002), the cluster of syndromes was first described by Rechtschaffen *et al.* (1983) using the sophisticated disk-over-water (DOW) paradigm. The pathologies are reliably produced and include hyperphagia, weight loss, elevated energy expenditure, increased plasma catecholamines, hypothyroidism, reduction in core temperature, deterioration in physical appearance, reduced levels of anabolic hormones, and declines in the integrity of the immune system (Everson and Toth, 2000). The importance of sleep is underlined by the fact that it is not possible to adapt to sleep deprivation, though one can recover from short-term sleep loss. Prolonged sleep deprivation is always fatal, whether the sleep deprivation is total (Everson *et al.*, 1989) or selective for REM sleep (Kushida *et al.*, 1989).

Loss of REM sleep in neurodegenerative disorders

There have been numerous studies that have reported changes in REM-sleep pattern and REM-sleep loss in various diseases such as Alzheimer's disease, Huntington's chorea, and Parkinson's disease. Onen and Onen (2003) have reported that the sleep architecture in Alzheimer's disease is marked by decreases in slow-wave sleep and further decreases in REM sleep. The EEG recorded during REM sleep in these patients has been observed by spectral analysis to slow down significantly as compared to controls. Christos (1993) had hypothesized that one of the side effects of REM-sleep deprivation observed in Alzheimer's disease is short-term memory loss. Further, REM-sleep related cholinergic neurons in the hippocampus and nucleus basalis of Meynert are damaged in this disease thereby affecting the cognitive processes. Sleep apneas and REM-sleep behavior disorders are present in 15 to 59% of people with Parkinson's disease (De Cock *et al.*, 2008). REM-sleep behavior disorders (RBD) are vigorous, complex movements corresponding to enacted dreams. They may disturb sleep, and injure patients or their bed partners (Comella, 2007). REM-sleep behavior disorders are frequently associated with neurodegenerative diseases, especially synucleopathies. They can precede Parkinsonism or dementia by five to ten years.

Oxidative stress and cellular damage in neurodegenerative disorders

The brain is particularly sensitive to oxidative damage. The brain is preferentially susceptible to oxidative damage since it is under very high oxygen tension and highly enriched in reactive oxygen species (ROS), susceptible proteins, lipids, and poor DNA repair. Oxidative stress, resulting in glutathione loss and oxidative DNA and protein damage, has been implicated in many neurodegenerative disorders, including Alzheimer's disease, Parkinson's disease, and Huntington's disease. Long-term hypoxia/reoxygenation events in adult mice, simulating oxygenation patterns of moderate to severe sleep apnea, result in lasting hypersomnolence, oxidative injury, and proinflammatory responses in wake-active brain regions (Zhan *et al.*, 2005; Zhu *et al.*, 2007).

Oxidative stress is believed to be one of the principal players in the etiology of neurodegenerative diseases. Coppede and Migliore (2009) reported that markers of DNA damage, particularly oxidative DNA damage, have been found in brain areas of Alzheimer's patients. Oxidative DNA damage and an impaired DNA repair mechanism is one of the earliest detectible events during the progression of dementia in both Alzheimer's and Parkinson's diseases (Rao, 2009). Oxidative stress induces macroautophagy of Aβ proteins in Alzheimer's disease and induces cell death by destabilizing lysosomal enzymes (Zheng *et al.*, 2009). REM-sleep behavior disorder associated with Alzheimer's disease may also lead to development of Lewy bodies and monoaminergic cell loss (Schenck *et al.*, 1996). Postmortem examinations have revealed that Lewy bodies, Lewy neurites, and α-synuclein are found in brain-stem nuclei in both Parkinsonism and REM-sleep behavior disorder patients (Lai and Siegel, 2003). Also recent studies have reported that there is loss of hypocretin (orexin) cells in Parkinson's disease. Hypocretin cells are also lost in narcolepsy, an REM-sleep behavior disorder (Thannickal *et al.*, 2007). While it is difficult to speculate whether REM-sleep disturbance is a cause or effect of the disease process, it is still important to determine if REM-sleep deprivation would lead to changes in the indices of oxidative stress and apoptotic machinery of the neurons.

Cellular and physiological implications of oxidative stress

It is indeed a strange paradox that the biomolecules, which consist primarily of carbon, hydrogen, oxygen,

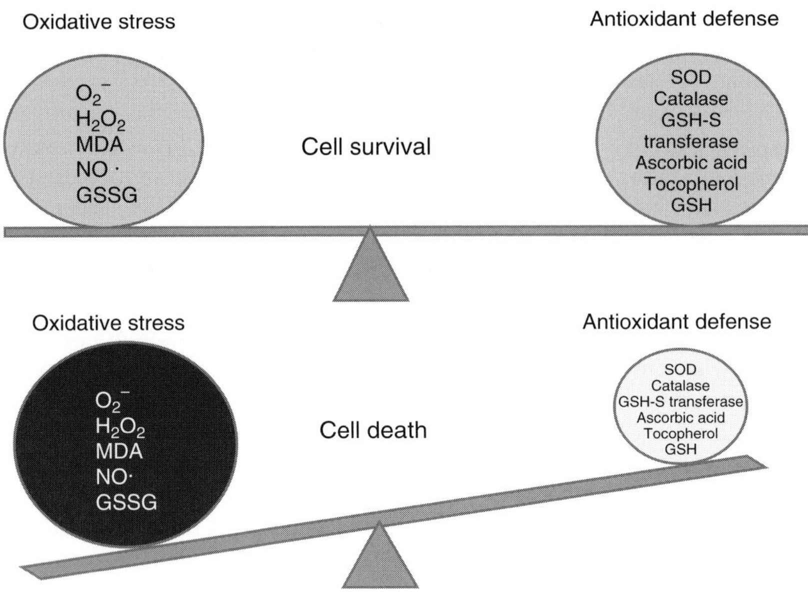

Figure 35.1 Cartoon representation of the oxidative balance in the cell. In a healthy cell, a balance between the oxidant production and antioxidant response is maintained. However, an increase in oxidant production, if uncompensated by an increase in antioxidant response, leads to oxidative damage and cell death. (See plate section for color version.)

nitrogen and sulfur, are disrupted by the presence of oxygen (O$_2$) (Schulz *et al.*, 2001). A wide variety of reactive oxygen species (ROS) can be found in biological systems. Mitochondria, nitric oxide synthase, arachidonic acid metabolism, xanthine oxidase, monoamine oxidase, and P450 enzymes are sources of ROS in the brain. The high metabolic rate of neurons implies a high baseline ROS production. Correspondingly, healthy brain cells possess high concentrations of both enzymatic and small-molecule antioxidant defenses (Figure 35.1). The enzymes include Cu-Zn-superoxide dismutase and Mn-superoxide dismutase, GSH peroxidase and catalase, as well as the small molecules glutathione, ascorbic acid, vitamin E, and a number of dietary flavonoids. Under normal physiological conditions, cells thereby cope with the flux of ROS. Cellular oxidative stress arises due to an imbalance in the production of ROS and antioxidative defense, and describes a condition in which cellular antioxidant defenses are insufficient to keep the levels of ROS below a toxic threshold. This may be either due to excessive production of ROS, loss of antioxidant defenses, or both (Schulz *et al.*, 2001).

Oxygen free radicals are highly reactive and have the capacity to damage cellular components such as proteins, lipids, and nucleic acids. Hydrogen peroxide is an important ROS and is generated predominantly by the mitochondria. In combination with reduced trace metals such as iron or copper, hydrogen peroxide

is transformed into the highly reactive hydroxyl radical, which causes damage to virtually all macromolecules. Oxidation of nucleic acids results in mutations, while protein denaturation leads to enzyme defects and impairment of the cytoskeleton. Lipid peroxidation in cell membranes is strongly involved in the perturbation of ion homeostasis. Because this cell damage ultimately causes cell death, oxidative stress is thought to play an important role in the initiation of several diseases. Mitochondria play a major role in this context because they are the main source of endogenous oxidative stress and additionally function as an inducer of programmed cell death (apoptosis). Several strategies of antioxidative defense exist; while transition metals can be inactivated by chelating proteins (e.g., ferritin), ROS can be reduced enzymatically (e.g., by the glutathione peroxidase) or non-enzymatically by antioxidants (e.g., by vitamin E, vitamin C, and glutathione). Oxidative stress may lead to cell injury and, if not repaired, to cell death by apoptosis or by necrosis. Many biochemical effects, following sleep deprivation, are believed to be induced by neurochemical and hormonal abnormalities that are often associated with oxidative stress.

Cells die through either of two distinct processes: necrosis or apoptosis. Necrosis is death due to unexpected and accidental cell damage. A number of toxic chemical or physical events can cause necrosis such as toxins, radiation, heat, trauma, lack of oxygen due the blockage of blood flow, etc. These physical or chemical *insults* can lead to the lethal disruption of cell structure and activity. As necrotic cells begin to die, they swell – holes appear in the plasma membrane and intracellular materials spill out into the surrounding environment. Apoptosis, also called programmed cell death, is a way to remove unwanted cells from the body. During apoptosis, there is no inflammation and cellular components are not released. Apoptotically dying cells activate a set of degrading enzymes called caspases that mediate the controlled disassembly and degradation of the cell. The cell forms apoptotic bodies, which are subsequently engulfed by phagocytes (Kerr *et al.*, 1995).

Sleep-deprivation induced changes in indices of oxidative stress

Results from total-sleep deprivation studies

In an attempt to explain the mechanism of sleep-deprivation induced metabolic disturbances, Chang *et al.* (2008) estimated phosphatidylcholine levels in the rat liver by MALDI-TOF-MS (matrix-assisted laser desorption/ionisation-time of flight mass spectrometry) and found a significant decrease in the levels following total-sleep deprivation. This was also accompanied by increases in the levels of hepatic malondialdehyde and 25 heat shock proteins. Similarly, Singh and Kumar (2008) also reported significant changes in the indices of oxidative stress following total-sleep deprivation in mice using the grid-over-water technique. They reported a decrease in reduced glutathione and catalase activity, apart from an increase in lipid peroxidation and nitrite levels in the homogenate and post-nuclear fraction prepared from whole brain. This was corroborated by results of another study, where prolonged sleep deprivation using the disk-over-water technique led to a significant decrease in Cu/Zn superoxide dismutase activity in the hippocampus and brain stem (Ramanathan *et al.*, 2002).

Everson *et al.* (2005) performed long-term sleep deprivation and studied indices of oxidative stress and cellular damage in the liver, heart, and lungs. Results showed decreases in both liver glutathione and catalase activity in sleep-deprived animals, without detectable increases in recycling activities, suggesting uncompensated oxidative stress. Also, marked increases in serum aminotransferase concentrations were observed, indicative of cell damage. When the animals were allowed to recover from sleep deprivation, the result was restoration or accentuation of antioxidant activities, and antioxidant capacity was observed in both the liver and the heart.

However, Gopalakrishnan *et al.* (2004) conducted a comprehensive study of oxidative stress indices following total-sleep deprivation using the disk-over-water technique and found no significant changes in oxidant production, superoxide dismutase activity, lipid peroxidation, and protein oxidation in the cerebral cortex and peripheral tissues, thus concluding that sleep deprivation does not lead to increase in free radicals or oxidative damage and there is no change in antioxidant response.

Results from REM-sleep deprivation studies

Different groups studying changes in oxidative stress parameters following selective REM-sleep deprivation have also reported varying results. D'Almeida's study (1997, 1998) revealed decreases in glutathione levels in the hippocampus only, while the other brain areas were not affected. In a study by Hipólide *et al.* (2002) when total brain levels of SOD, catalase, glutathione peroxidase, total glutathione, and malondialdehyde (MDA) were compared between controls, small-platform, and large-platform groups, no differences were observed.

Singh *et al.* (2008) used the classic flower-pot method for REM-sleep deprivation for 72 hours and found differences in response of various brain regions to sleep deprivation. While the cerebral cortex and brain stem showed a decrease in oxidative stress (evidenced by a decrease in lipid peroxidation and an increase in SOD), the hippocampus, thalamus, and hypothalamus showed an increase in lipid peroxidation and decrease in SOD. This fits nicely with another study by Silva *et al.* (2004) where mice, REM-sleep deprived for 72 hours with the multiple-platform method, showed increases in hippocampal oxidation, glutathione levels, and lipid peroxidation. Interestingly, Das *et al.* (2008) found a decrease in lipid peroxidation level following four days of REM-sleep deprivation using the flower-pot method. The authors concluded that REM-sleep deprivation induced an increase in norepinephrine, which decreased lipid peroxidation in an alpha-1-adrenoceptor-mediated and calcium-mediated mechanism. In a related study, plasma homocysteine was reduced in sleep-deprived rats as compared with the control group and did not revert to normal levels after 24 or 48 hours of sleep recovery. A trend was observed toward decreased glutathione and increased thiobarbituric acid reactive substance levels in sleep-deprived rats. The authors concluded that the observed decreases in homocysteine levels may represent a self-correcting response to depleted glutathione in sleep-deprived animals, which would contribute to the attenuation of the deleterious effects of sleep deprivation (de Oliveira *et al.*, 2002).

Therefore, it may be possible that REM-sleep deprivation affects different brain regions inversely and these variations are not apparent while studying whole brain preparations.

REM sleep deprivation- and total sleep deprivation-induced cell damage and apoptosis

There are conflicting reports regarding the role of sleep deprivation (both selective REM-sleep deprivation and total-sleep deprivation) on indices of cell damage and apoptosis. Cirelli *et al.* (1999) found no evidence of brain-cell degeneration following total-sleep deprivation ranging from 8 hours to 14 days in rats. Their study found no difference in brain sections of total-sleep deprived rats when stained with apoptotic markers, such as TUNEL (terminal deoxynucleotidyl transferase dUTP nick end labeling) and Fluoro-Jade staining, as compared to controls. Hippólide *et al.* (2002) did not find indices of either apoptosis or necrosis in rat brains following 96 hours of REM-sleep deprivation. Their study used necrosis markers, such as benzodiazepine ligand binding to reactive astrocytes, and apoptosis markers, such as TUNEL staining and changes in mRNA levels of apoptosis-related genes bcl-2 and bax in the hypothalamus, amygdala, and cortex, and found no significant differences in REM sleep-deprived animals compared to controls. Similarly Landis *et al.* (1993) had also failed to find an overall increase in immediate early gene Egr-1 expression in prolonged sleep-deprived rat brains and concluded that there was no evidence for the hypothesis that sleep protected the brain from massive global damage, fatigue, or dysfunction.

Eiland *et al.* (2002) were the first to report that a significant increase in amino cupric silver staining (a marker for degenerated neurons) was observed in the supraoptic nucleus (SON) of the hypothalamus of rats with high sleep loss (> 45 hours) vs. their yoked controls. Follow-up experiments by the same group showed that staining was not significantly different in rats sleep deprived for less than 45 hours, suggesting that injurious sleep-deprivation-related processes occur above a threshold quantity of sleep loss. Following this, many groups have subsequently found indices of cell loss and apoptosis after REM-sleep deprivation. Morrissey *et al.* (2004) observed that following prolonged REM-sleep deprivation in rats by using clonidine, an α-2 adrenergic agonist, amino-cupric silver positive (degenerated) neurons were present in the cortex, thalamus, dorsal hippocampus, amygdala, and other limbic areas of the brain. In Biswas *et al.* (2006), one of the present authors systematically studied various parameters of neuronal degeneration and apoptosis following 6 days (144 hours) of REM-sleep deprivation in rats. Using various techniques such as amino-cupric silver staining (for neuronal degeneration) and TUNEL (Figure 35.2), bcl-2/bax (for apoptosis), and visualizing apoptosis under electron and confocal microscopes after staining with tubulin and Hoechst dyes, increased apoptotic neurons were observed in the locus coeruleus, LDT/PPT, and medial preoptic areas of REM sleep-deprived rats. Increased apoptosis was not found in the lateral septum, which is an area not related to REM sleep, and after 96 hours of REM-sleep deprivation. The authors therefore concluded that prolonged sleep deprivation was necessary in order to observe the changes that were more evident in areas of the brain that were functionally important for the generation of REM sleep.

A few recent studies have also found evidence of cellular degeneration after REM-sleep deprivation. Jiang *et al.* (2006) found increased CB1 receptor mRNA expression and observed neural apoptosis under the electron microscope in the REM-sleep deprived rat hippocampus as compared to controls. Andersen *et al.* (2009) have recently observed that in rats REM-sleep deprived for 24 and 96 hours, DNA damage was evident following single-cell gel comet assay in blood cells and excessive genotoxic damage was observed in brain tissue. The damage was more pronounced in the 96-hour group. Hence, various studies have reported indices of apoptosis after REM-sleep deprivation. However, the extent of damage and the brain areas affected differ with the duration of REM sleep and the variety of techniques used to study neuronal degeneration.

Physiological significance of REM sleep deprivation-induced changes in oxidative stress and apoptosis

As discussed earlier in this chapter, the results of various studies do not seem to corroborate each other, and

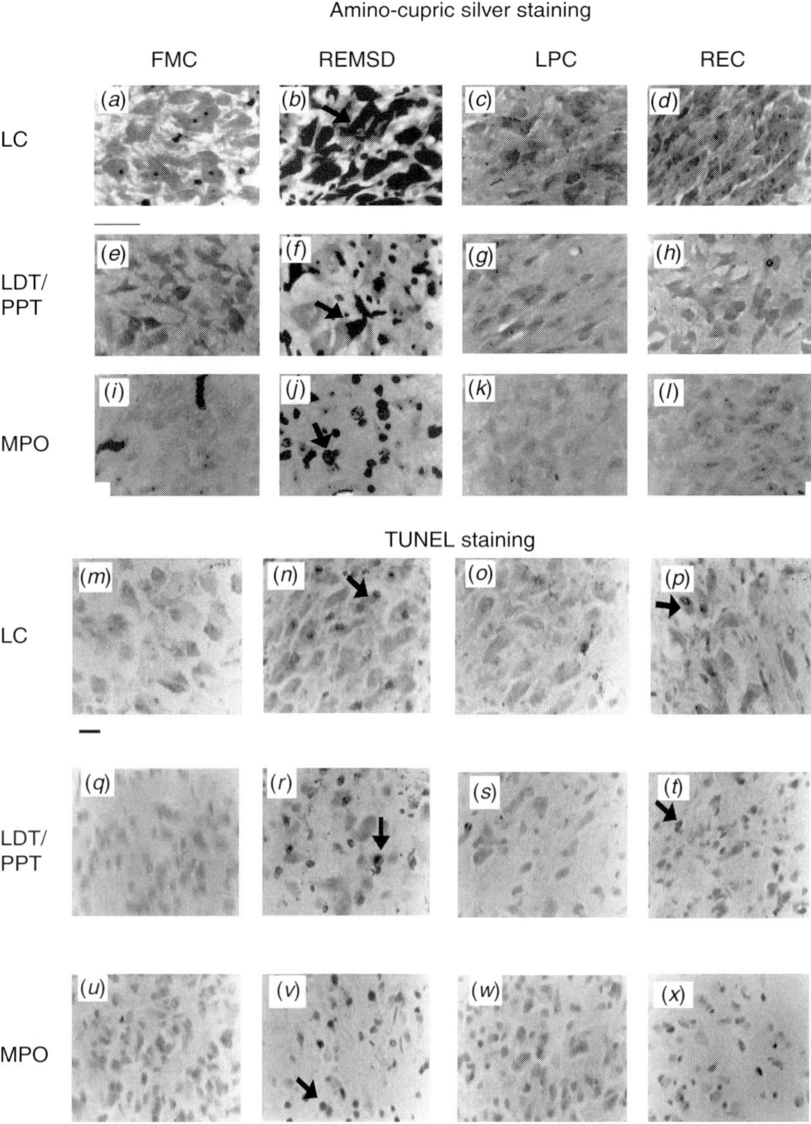

Figure 35.2 Representative photomicrographs of amino-cupric silver stained (*a–l*) and TUNEL stained (*m–x*) sections in the LC, LDT/PPT, and MPO under different conditions. (See plate section for color version.)

Top panel (*a–l*): Following amino-cupric silver staining, degenerated neurons seen as black–silver deposited stains (black arrows) were observed after REMSD in the LC (*b*), LDT/PPT (*f*), and MPO (*j*). Scale bar = 40 μm.

Bottom panel (*m–x*): Significant increased number of TUNEL-positive neurons can be observed following REMSD in the LC (*n*), LDT/PPT (*r*), and MPO (*v*) suggesting increased apoptosis in the REM sleep-related areas. Black arrows point to TUNEL-stained apoptotic neurons. Scale bar = 20 μm. (Modified from Biswas *et al.*, 2006.)

therefore it is difficult to conclude if sleep deprivation (total or REM sleep) affects indices of oxidative stress and apoptosis. However, the experimental conditions in the various studies were different with regards to the animal model studied, strain of the animal, length and method of sleep deprivation, and, finally, the brain areas/tissues studied. Results from the various studies discussed above indicate that various regions of the brain respond to loss of sleep (total/REM sleep) in a differential manner. We have attempted to combine the various views in this chapter and to arrive at a working model (Figure 35.3). In terms of sleep deprivation-induced changes in oxidative stress, the brain areas seem to also differ in their response to the nature of the experimental paradigm. The response of the cerebral cortex (Gopalakrishnan *et al.*, 2004; Singh *et al.*, 2008) differs from the response of the hippocampus (Ramanathan *et al.*, 2002; Singh *et al.*, 2008) and since these responses to sleep deprivation were opposite, it is not surprising that total brain homogenate did not show any differences between the control and sleep-deprived animals. In the apoptotic studies, there were also variations in the reported incidences of apoptosis by different groups. Generally, those groups

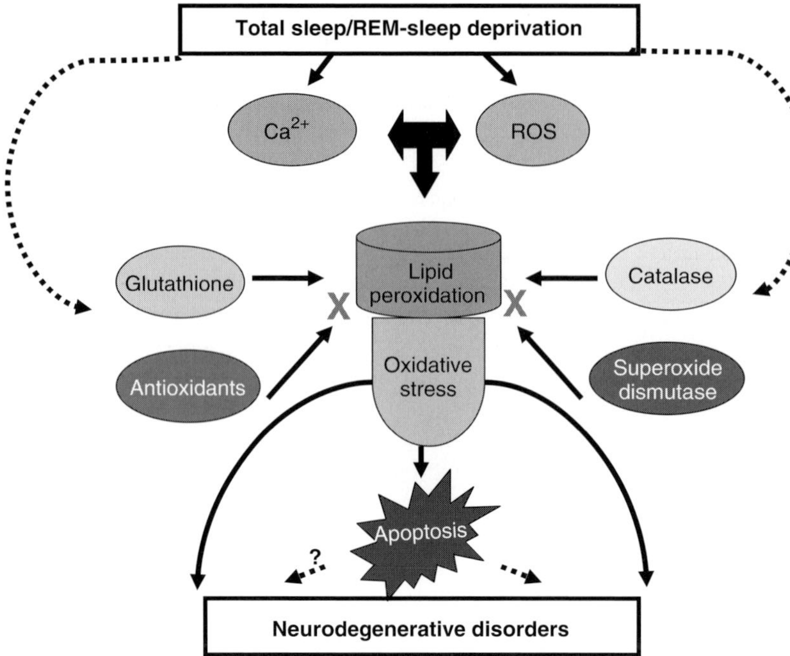

Figure 35.3 Effect of sleep deprivation (TSD and REMSD) on oxidative stress and apoptosis: a working model. Sleep deprivation, including REM-sleep deprivation, may induce lipid peroxidation and oxidative stress leading to apoptosis in some brain regions and may be the underlying cause of several neurodegenerative disorders. In contrast, it may also elevate the levels of protective enzymes such as glutathione, SOD, and antioxidants and prevent lipid peroxidation. (See plate section for color version.)
The model was compiled based on the following studies: Singh and Kumar (2008); Ramanathan *et al.* (2002); Singh *et al.* (2008); Das *et al.* (2008); Biswas *et al.* (2006); Andersen *et al.* (2009); Lai and Siegel (2003); Coppede and Migliore (2009).

that did study sleep deprivation for longer durations (96 hours or more) reported observing apoptotic neurons while others did not. Also, there was no generalized neuronal damage to all brain areas. Brain areas that play a major role in the generation and maintenance of sleep, specifically REM sleep, seem to sustain more cell damage. Hence, indices of apoptosis, such as oxidative damage, seem to have region specificity and differences in the responses to different experimental paradigms.

As of now, it is difficult to make a definite statement that REM-sleep or total-sleep deprivation affects oxidative stress levels and induces apoptosis, due to the reasons discussed above. However, the cellular implications of oxidative stress and cell damage cannot be ignored. Sleep deprivation leads to changes in receptors, enzyme activities such as monamine oxidase (MAO), Na-K-ATPase, acetylcholinesterase, mRNA of various transcripts, hormonal levels, immune response, stress proteins, etc. (Gulyani *et al.*, 2000). All these parameters listed above are susceptible to changes in oxidative status of the cells. For example, oxidative challenge affects calcium levels, which in turn affects Na-K-ATPase activity, thereby affecting membrane excitability. This change can further affect a whole myriad of events, such as neurotransmitter release, receptor internalization, cellular structure and volume (Majumdar and Mallick, 2005), and further lead to change in structural proteins leading to cell death (Biswas *et al.*, 2006).

In conclusion, the interrelationships between oxidative stress, sleep deprivation, and neurodegenerative disorders are complex and further studies need to be undertaken to determine the significance of sleep or REM sleep deprivation-induced changes in oxidative status of the cell and changes in vulnerability of the affected cells to undergo apoptosis, thereby increasing the propensity of the animal to develop neuropathalogies.

Acknowledgments

The photographs in Figure 35.2 were originally published in a different format in the journal *Neuroscience* (2006). The authors thank Elsevier Ltd for their kind permission.

References

Andersen, M. L., Ribeiro, D.A., Bergamaschi, C.T. *et al.* (2009) Distinct effects of acute and chronic sleep loss on DNA damage in rats. *Prog Neuro-psychopharmacol Biol Psychiat* 33: 562–7.

Biswas, S., Mishra, P. & Mallick, B. N. (2006) Increased apoptosis in rat brain after rapid eye movement sleep loss. *Neuroscience* 142: 315–31.

Chang, H. M., Mai, F. D., Chen, B. J. *et al.* (2008) Sleep deprivation predisposes liver to oxidative stress and phospholipid damage: a quantitative molecular imaging study. *J Anat* **212**(3): 295–305.

Christos, G. A. (1993) Is Alzheimer's disease related to a deficit or malfunction of rapid eye movement (REM) sleep? *Med Hypoth* **41**: 435–9.

Cirelli, C., Shaw, P. J., Rechtschaffen, A. & Tononi, G. (1999) No evidence of brain cell degeneration after long-term sleep deprivation in rats. *Brain Res* **840**: 184–93.

Comella, C. (2007) Sleep disorders in Parkinson's disease: an overview. *Movement Disord* **22**: S367–73.

Coppede, F. & Migliore, L. (2009) DNA damage and repair in Alzheimer's disease. *Curr Alzheimer Res* **6**(1): 36–47.

D'Almeida, V., Hipólide, D. C., Azzalis, L. A. *et al.* (1997) Absence of oxidative stress following paradoxical sleep deprivation in rats. *Neurosci Lett* **235**(1/2): 25–8.

D'Almeida, V., Lobo, L. L., Hipólide, D.C. *et al.* (1998) Sleep deprivation induces brain region-specific decreases in glutathione levels. *Neuroreport* **9**(12): 2853–6.

Das, G., Gopalakrishnan, A., Faisal, M. & Mallick, B. N. (2008) Stimulatory role of calcium in rapid eye movement sleep deprivation-induced noradrenaline-mediated increase in Na-K-ATPase activity in rat brain. *Neuroscience* **155**(1): 76–89.

De Cock, V. C., Vidailhet, M. & Arnulf, I. (2008) Sleep disturbances in patients with parkinsonism. *Nat Clin Pract Neurol* **4**(5): 254–66.

de Oliveira, A. C., D'Almeida, V., Hipólide, D. C., Nobrega, J. N. & Tufik, S. (2002) Sleep deprivation reduces total plasma homocysteine levels in rats. *Can J Physiol Pharmacol* **80**(3): 193–7.

Eiland, M. M., Ramanathan, L., Gulyani, S. *et al.* (2002) Increases in amino-cupric-silver staining of the supraoptic nucleus after sleep deprivation. *Brain Res* **945**: 1–8.

Everson, C. A. & Toth, L. A. (2000) Systemic bacterial invasion induced by sleep deprivation. *Am J Physiol Regul Integr Comp Physiol* **278**: R905–16.

Everson, C. A., Bergmann, B. M. & Rechtschaffen, A. (1989) Sleep deprivation in the rat. III. Total sleep deprivation. *Sleep* **12**: 13–21.

Everson, C. A., Laatsch, C. D. & Hogg, N. (2005) Antioxidant defense responses to sleep loss and sleep recovery. *Am J Physiol Regul Integr Comp Physiol* **288**(2): R374–83.

Frank, M. G. (1999) Phylogeny and evolution of rapid eye movement (REM) sleep. In *Rapid Eye Movement*, eds. B. N. Mallick & S. Inoue. New York: Marcel Dekker Inc., pp. 17–38.

Gopalakrishnan, A., Ji, L. L. & Cirelli, C. (2004) Sleep deprivation and cellular responses to oxidative stress. *Sleep* **27**(1): 27–35.

Graves, L. A., Heller, E. A., Pack, A. I. & Abel, T. (2003) Sleep deprivation selectively impairs memory consolidation for contextual fear conditioning. *Learn Mem* **10**: 168–76.

Gulyani, S., Majumdar, S. & Mallick, B. N. (2000) Rapid eye movement sleep and significance of its deprivation studies: a review. *Sleep Hypn* **2**: 49–68.

Hipólide, D. C., D'Almeida, V., Raymond, R., Tufik, S. & Nobrega, J. N. (2002) Sleep deprivation does not affect indices of necrosis or apoptosis in rat brain. *Intern J Neurosci* **112**: 155–66.

Jiang, P. F., Zu, T. & Xia, J. J. (2006) Cannabinoid receptor 1 expression and pathological changes in rat hippocampus after deprivation of rapid eye movement sleep. *Zhejiang Da Xue Xue Bao Yi Xue Ban* **35**(5): 535–40.

Jouvet, D., Vimont, P., Delorme, F. & Jouvet, M. (1964) Etude de la privation selective de la phase paradoxale de sommeil chez le chat. *CR Soc Biol* **158**: 756–9.

Kerr, J. F. R., Gobe, G. C., Winterford, C. M. & Harman, B. V. (1995) Anatomical methods in cell death. In Schwartz, L. M., Osborne, B. A. (ed) *Methods in Cell Biology*, Academic Press, New York, pp. 1–27.

Kushida, C. A., Bergmann, B. M. & Rechtschaffen, A. (1989) Sleep deprivation in the rat. IV. Paradoxical sleep deprivation. *Sleep* **12**: 22–30.

Lai, Y. Y. & Siegel, J. M. (2003) Physiological and anatomical link between Parkinson-like disease and REM sleep behavior disorder. *Mol Neurobiol* **27**(2): 137–51.

Landis, C. A., Collins, B. J., Leanne, L. L. *et al.* (1993) Expression of Egr-1 in the brain of sleep deprived rats. *Mol Brain Res* **17**: 300–6.

Mendelson, W. B., Guthrie, R. D., Frederick, G. & Wyatt, R. J. (1974) The flowerpot technique of Rapid Eye Movement (REM) sleep deprivation. *Pharmacol Biochem Behav* **2**: 553–6.

Majumdar, S. & Mallick, B. N. (2005) Cytomorphometric changes in rat brain neurons after rapid eye movement sleep deprivation. *Neuroscience* **135**: 679–90.

Mallick, B. N., Majumdar, S., Faisal, M. *et al.* (2002) Role of norepinephrine in the regulation of rapid eye movement sleep. *J Biosci* **27**: 539–51.

Morrisey, M. J., Duntley, S. P., Anch, A. M. & Nonneman, R. (2004) Active sleep and its role in the prevention of apoptosis in the developing brain. *Med Hypoth* **62**: 876–9.

Onen, F. & Onen, S. H. (2003) Sleep rhythm disturbances in Alzheimer's disease. *Rev Med Interne* **24**: 165–71.

Ramanathan, L., Gulyani, S., Nienhuis, R. & Siegel, J. M. (2002) Sleep deprivation decreases superoxide dismutase activity in rat hippocampus and brainstem. *Neuroreport* **13**(11):1387–90.

Rao, K. S. (2009) Free radical induced oxidative damage to DNA: relation to brain aging and neurological disorders. *Indian J Biochem Biophys* **46**(1): 9–15.

Rechtschaffen, A., Gilliland, M. A., Bergmann, B. M. & Winter, J. B. (1983) Physiological correlates of prolonged sleep deprivation in rats. *Science* **221**: 182–4.

Rechtschaffen, A. & Bergmann, B. M. (2002) Sleep deprivation in the rat: an update of the 1989 paper. *Sleep* **25**: 18–24.

Schenck, C. H., Garcia-Rill, E., Skinner, R. D., Anderson, M. L. & Mahowald, M. W. (1996) A case of REM sleep behavior disorder with autopsy-confirmed Alzheimer's disease: postmortem brainstem histochemical analyses. *Biol Psychiat* **40**: 422–5.

Schulz, J. B., Lindenau, J., Seyfried, J. & Dichgans, J. (2001) Glutathione, oxidative stress and neurodegeneration. *Euro J Biochem* **267**(16): 4904–11.

Silva, R. H., Abílio, V. C., Takatsu, A. L. *et al.* (2004) Role of hippocampal oxidative stress in memory deficits induced by sleep deprivation in mice. *Neuropharmacology* **46**(6): 895–903.

Singh, A. & Kumar, A. (2008) Protective effect of alprazolam against sleep deprivation-induced behavior alterations and oxidative damage in mice. *Neurosci Res* **60**(4): 372–9.

Singh, R., Kiloung, J., Singh, S. & Sharma, D. (2008) Effect of paradoxical sleep deprivation on oxidative stress parameters in brain regions of adult and old rats. *Biogerontology* **9**(3): 153–62.

Thannickal, T. C., Lai, Y. Y. & Siegel, J. M. (2007) Hypocretin (orexin) cell loss in Parkinson's disease. *Brain* **130**: 1586–95.

Zhan, G., Serrano, F., Fenik, P. *et al.* (2005) NADPH oxidase mediates hypersomnolence and brain oxidative injury in a murine model of sleep apnea. *Am J Respir Crit Care Med* **172**: 921–9.

Zheng, L., Kagedal, K., Dehvari, N. *et al.* (2009) Oxidative stress induces macroautophagy of amyloid B-protein and ensuring apoptosis. *Free Rad Biol Med* **46**: 422–9.

Zhu, Y., Fenik, P., Zhan, G. *et al.* (2007) Selective loss of catecholaminergic wake–active neurons in a murine sleep apnea model. *J Neurosci* **27**: 10, 060–71.

36 The role of REM sleep in maintaining neuronal excitability and its possible mechanism of action

Vibha Madan and Birendra N. Mallick

Summary

Sleep has been generally divided into rapid eye movement (REM) sleep and non-REM (NREM) sleep in higher order mammals, including humans. Several theories have proposed various functions of different stages of sleep. We hypothesized that *REM sleep maintains brain excitability*. In this chapter, we discuss the significance of REM sleep in the maintenance of neuronal electrochemical homeostasis, which governs brain excitability. Selective REM-sleep loss increases the activity of Na-K ATPase, a membrane-bound enzyme that maintains neuronal Na^+ and K^+ homeostasis and, thus, the neuronal resting membrane potential. Further, the REM sleep deprivation-induced increase in Na-K ATPase activity has been attributed to an increased level of norepinephrine in the brain.

Introduction

Sleep is regarded as a natural state of rest during which voluntary body movements and awareness of surroundings are greatly reduced. The concept of the essential nature of sleep has evolved over the past century from an intuitively appealing but erroneous belief that sleep is simply a passive phenomenon required to provide rest to the fatigued body, to a view of sleep as a complex state that is actively induced as well as maintained by specific brain neuronal circuitry and also regulated by the biological clock (Zeplin *et al.*, 2005). Further, sleep is not a unitary state, but based on characteristic electrophysiological signs it has been classified into two stages: REM sleep and non-REM sleep. Sleep is likely to perform an essential function for the body, given the fact that all organisms including humans spend a significant portion of their daily life

in sleep. However, what distinct purpose would REM sleep serve, in which we spend such a small time, is an intriguing question. REM sleep has been identified phylogenetically at least in avian and mammalian species; its quantity varies ontogenetically; it has a precise cyclic regulation and its duration increases in subsequent cycles at least in humans. Further, REM sleep is affected in various diseases and its loss is associated with several disorders. Its importance in brain maturation, memory processing, memory consolidation, etc. has also been reported (please see related chapters in this volume for references). Hence, we argue that REM sleep cannot be a remnant of vestigial significance and it must serve a defined function, which may be analogous to the functions of the housekeeping genes in a cell.

During the past 50 years or so, substantial research has been carried out to understand the specific function(s) of sleep as a whole, or of REM sleep. Most of the experimental studies that have contributed to elucidate the possible function(s) of REM sleep are interpretations and conclusions based on experiments involving REM-sleep deprivation (REMSD) approach (Gulyani *et al.*, 2000). It has been observed that REMSD affects the levels of various neurotransmitters and hormones in the body and it also alters several biochemical and psycho-physiological processes (Mallick *et al.*, 2005). For example, REMSD increases aggressiveness, fighting, confusion; however, it decreases body temperature and impairs mental concentration and memory consolidation. Based on these observations we proposed earlier that REM sleep possibly maintains the excitability of the neurons in the brain (Mallick *et al.*, 1994, 1999), which we will discuss in detail along with its mechanism of action.

REM sleep and its importance

One fundamental housekeeping role of REM sleep could be the maintenance of fundamental neuronal properties. For example, REMSD during early life reduced the stability of neuronal circuitry in the hippocampus suggesting that REM sleep provides cues for the expression of the specific synaptic components necessary for stabilization of neuronal circuitry during development. However, a question that still awaits an answer is what happens in the brain in the absence of REM sleep that leads to the destabilization of the neuronal circuitries. Although several factors may be associated, one potential factor that may be involved with REM sleep-dependent changes in the neuronal circuitries and behavioral modifications could be the alteration in neuronal excitability, which is known to affect synaptic plasticity (Gall and Lynch, 2004; Wheal *et al.*, 1998).

REM sleep may play an important role for maintaining several behaviors. Dement and Fisher (1963) deprived human subjects of REM sleep for two to seven nights and all showed signs of anxiety, irritability, and inability to concentrate. Deprivation of REM sleep has been reported to increase shock-induced fighting behavior in rats (Morden *et al.*, 1968). REM sleep-deprived rats showed heightened aggressiveness and increased sensitivity to tactile stimuli as shown by flinching, jumping, and squealing when touched (Rechtschaffen *et al.*, 1989). In cats, REMSD by the treadmill arousal technique showed an increase in sexual behavior, and a decrease in motivation to obtain food and in grooming behavior. These REM sleep-deprived cats showed episodes of violent facial and limb muscle twitches as if the animals were in a state of seizure; however, during the REM sleep-rebound phase, the intensity of the phasic motor activity subsided (Dement, 1965). Dewson *et al.* reported that there was an accelerated auditory recovery in cats deprived of REM sleep for five or more days (Dewson *et al.*, 1965). Further, the threshold for electroconvulsive shock decreased significantly after REMSD (Cohen and Dement, 1965). Single neuronal activity recorded from the brain stem after REMSD showed a decreased and increased waking discharge rates of REM-off and REM-on neurons, respectively (Mallick *et al.*, 1990). Additionally, REMSD altered neuronal sensitivity towards auditory stimulation. In many dorsolateral pontine neurons, auditory stimulation produced an initial excitation followed by inhibition; however, after REMSD, when the cats were exposed to the auditory tone, the same neurons showed a significantly reduced auditory evoked inhibitory period, suggesting overt responses to the same stimulation (Mallick *et al.*, 1991).

REM-sleep deprivation and neuronal excitability

A precise regulation of neural excitability is essential for proper functioning of the brain. Neurons are able to compensate for various perturbations and maintain appropriate levels of excitability by modulating their transmembrane ionic composition and distribution. In a complex multisynaptic neuronal circuitry, the mechanisms of compensation are diverse, including regulated changes in synaptic size, synaptic strength, and ion-channel properties in the plasma membrane. The neurons must face and adapt to changing patterns of synaptic drive and such adaptations seem to be essential to prevent neurons from either falling silent or being sensitized or desensitized or, conversely, becoming saturated during periods of intense neuronal activity. Some of the important ways that neurons show such adaptability is by modulating synaptic long-term potentiation/depression (LTP/LTD) neurotransmitters' receptor upregulation or downregulation (Cirelli, 2006). However, these phenomena ultimately alter the neuronal threshold or transmembrane potential leading to alterations in neuronal excitability.

Long-lasting stresses or presentation of persistent stimuli to the neurons alter the neuronal milieu unrelentingly resulting in modulation of neuronal excitability or responsiveness, which, however, depends on the situational (direct and/or consequential) demands. The membrane-bound enzyme Na-K ATPase is the primary factor to exchange intracellular Na^+ with extracellular K^+, which attempts to restore transmembrane ionic homeostasis and neuronal excitability to its original level. Thus, it is reasonable that alterations in Na^+/K^+ exchange and/or any variation in the Na-K ATPase activity would modulate neuronal excitability. The activity of Na-K ATPase significantly decreases during the initial stage of LTP induction (Wyse *et al.*, 2004), after ischemic brain injury and emotional painful stress accompanied with preservation of defensive conditioned reflexes (Sazontova *et al.*, 1984). Although it is not clear how sleep helps in maintaining neuronal homeostasis, we first showed that REMSD increases the activity of the Na-K ATPase enzyme suggesting that REMSD would compromise the excitability of the neurons.

As mentioned above, the Na-K ATPase exchanges Na^+ and K^+ across membranes and thus maintains neuronal ionic homeostasis. Thus the level of Na-K ATPase activity is a reasonable estimate of the neuronal excitability status. In order to support the hypothesis that *REM sleep maintains brain excitability*, ideally it was desirable that transmembrane potential of the same neuron in the brain be recorded in vivo in freely behaving animals before, during, and after an REM-sleep episode or after varying periods of REMSD. However, there are technical limitations of estimating the transmembrane potential from the same neuron in vivo, in freely moving animals, for days before, during, and after REMSD. In the absence of such recording, we estimated the Na-K ATPase activity in the membranes prepared from control and REM sleep-deprived rat brains.

REM-sleep deprivation and changes in Na-K ATPase activity

Rats were subjected to REMSD by the flower-pot method and several control studies were conducted. The Na-K ATPase activity in the brain was elevated after REMSD. The enzyme activity increased in all the brain regions, i.e., the cerebrum, the cerebellum, and the brain stem, with a maximum rise in the brain stem (Gulyani and Mallick, 1993) (Figure 36.1*a*,*b*). Interestingly, REMSD affected the neuronal and glial Na-K ATPase activities in an opposite direction; while the activity increased in the neurons, the enzyme activity decreased in the glia. These observations are significant since the glia is known to take up excess K^+ extruded by the neurons during repolarization and help in maintaining neuronal excitability and functioning (Baskey *et al.*, 2009).

Enzyme kinetic study showed that REMSD increased both the K_m and V_{max} of Na-K ATPase; hence, it was proposed that in addition to allosteric modulation, REMSD would also at least partly increase the turnover of Na-K ATPase molecules (Adya and Mallick, 2000). The Na-K ATPase is a tetramer and contains two each of alpha and beta chains having molecular weights of 110 and 55 kDa, respectively. The specific activity of the enzyme as well as the quantity of Na-K ATPase molecules were estimated using monoclonal antibody against the alpha-1 subunit of rat Na-K ATPase and it was observed that there was an increased number of Na-K ATPase molecules in the rat brain after REMSD (Majumdar *et al.*, 2003). Thus, REMSD-mediated increase in Na-K ATPase activity could be attributed to both an allosteric modulation as well as an increased turnover of the enzyme molecules in the brain.

Some of the intrinsic factors that regulate the Na-K ATPase activity are intracellular ATP, Na^+, and Mg^{++}, and extracellular K^+ and Ca^{++} concentrations (Kaplan, 2002). Additionally, it is also regulated by other factors, for example, changes in membrane fluidity (Lebel and Schatz, 1990), membrane lipid peroxidation (Morel *et al.*, 1998), and hormones including insulin and thyroxine as well as neurotransmitters such as norepinephrine (NE) and serotonin, the levels of some of which are reported to alter after REMSD as well (Kushida, 2005).

Norepinephrine: relationship with REM sleep and its deprivation

Neuronal excitability must be compromised due to enhanced Na-K ATPase activity after REMSD. Recent direct evidence showed that intracellular (synaptosomal) potential indeed increased after REMSD suggesting increased depolarization of the neurons after deprivation (Das and Mallick, 2008). The intriguing question is "which one or more of the signaling pathway(s) is/are responsible for the enhanced Na-K ATPase activity and how do they get activated upon REMSD?" Since REM sleep is regulated by the brain stem and after REMSD a more pronounced increase in Na-K ATPase enzyme activity was observed in the brain stem, we argued that altered functioning of the REM-sleep regulating neurons and associated factors must be responsible for inducing certain changes, which in turn would increase the Na-K ATPase activity.

Although the precise neural mechanism for REM-sleep generation is not yet understood, it is known that NE-ergic neurons located in the locus coeruleus, the REM-off neurons, are continuously active in all stages except during REM sleep. Cessation of these REM-off neurons is a prerequisite for the initiation and maintenance of REM sleep (reviewed in Pal *et al.*, 2005). Since these REM-off neurons remain active during REMSD, the NE level is likely to increase in the brain after REMSD. The metabolism of NE has been reported to remain elevated after REMSD and increased turnover of NE after REMSD has been reported (Pujol *et al.*, 1968; Sinha *et al.*, 1973; Stern *et al.*, 1971). We have shown that activity of monoamine oxidase-A (MAO-A), which degrades synaptic NE, decreased after REMSD. Further, after REMSD, the level of tyrosine hydroxylase (TH), the first rate-limiting enzyme in the NE biosynthesis pathway, and the amount of TH-mRNA also increased

(a) Na-K ATPase activity after REM-sleep deprivation

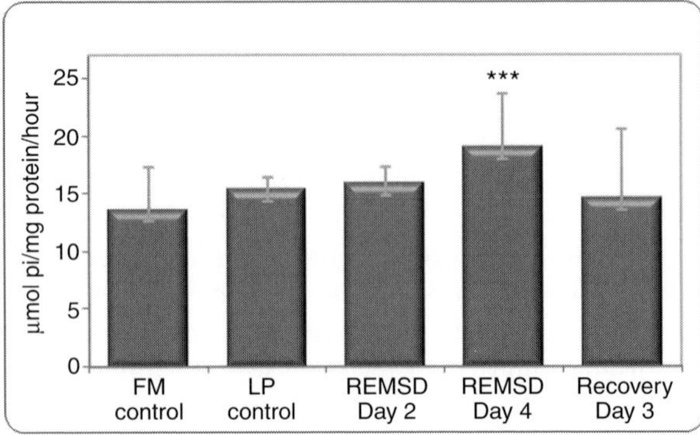

(b) Na-K ATPase activity in different brain areas after REM-sleep deprivation and its modulation through NE-ergic receptors

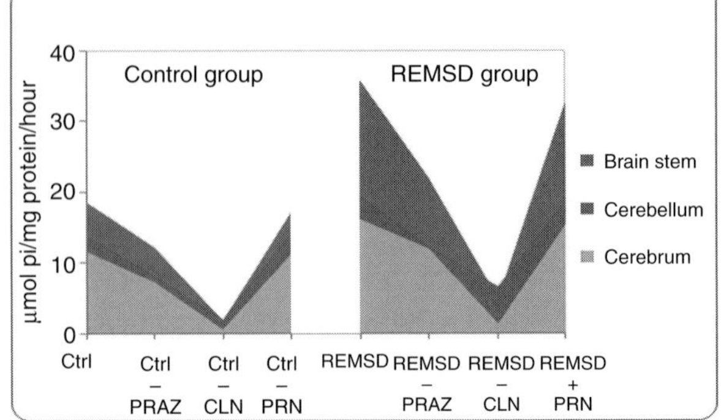

(c) Na-K ATPase activity in the presence of NE and inhibitors of second messenger signaling system

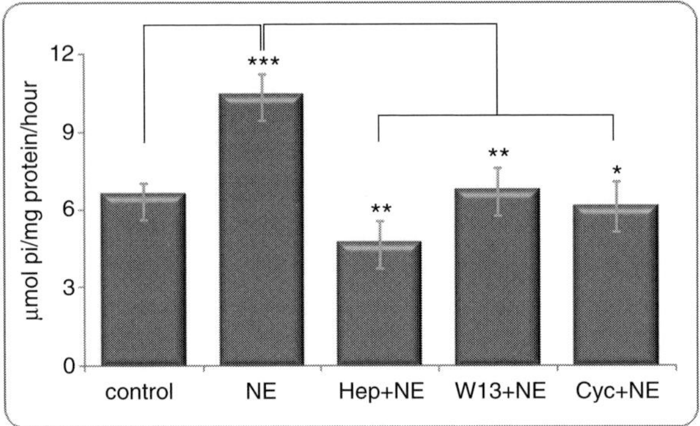

(d) Changes in Na-K ATPase activity and intra-synaptosomal DiSC$_2$ fluorescence after REM-sleep deprivation

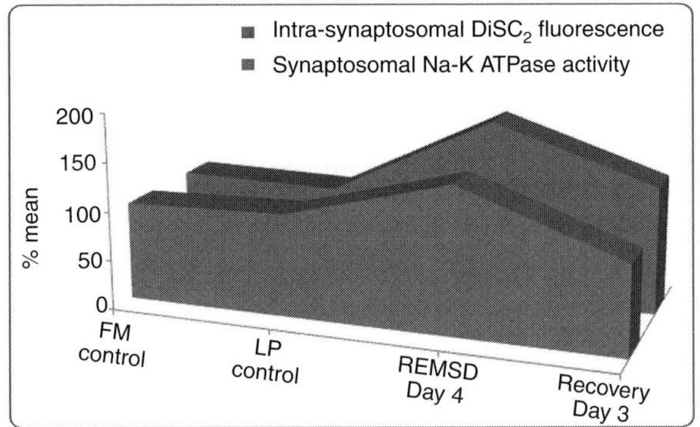

Figure 36.1 REM sleep deprivation-induced increase in the Na-K ATPase activity and intrasynaptosomal potential as a reflection of intracellular potential. (a) Four days of REMSD significantly increased the Na-K ATPase activity as compared to the free moving (FM) control. The enzyme activity did not alter significantly after two days of REMSD and in large-platform (LP) control animals. The increased activity returned to its normal level after three days of recovery of REM-sleep loss. (b) Significant increase in Na-K ATPase activity after REMSD were observed in all three regions studied, i.e., the cerebrum, cerebellum, and brain stem. However, maximum changes were observed in the brain-stem region. The increase in Na-K ATPase activity was modulated by NE specifically through its action via the alpha-1 NE-ergic receptors in both the control and REM sleep-deprived groups. (Abbreviations: PRAZ, prazosin; CLN, clonidine; PRN, propranolol). (c) Na-K ATPase activity was significantly inhibited by heparin (an IP3 antagonist), W13 (a calmodulin antagonist), and Cyc (a calcineurin inhibitor) suggesting that the NE-mediated increase in the enzyme activity involves intracellular calcium for signaling. (Abbreviations: NE, norepinephrine; Hep, heparin; Cyc, cyclosporin A). (d) Na-K ATPase activity and intra-synaptosomal positive potential increased significantly after four days of REMSD. Intra-synaptosomal positive potential (as a reflection of intracellular potential) was estimated using the membrane permeable mono-cationic fluorescent dye, 3,3′-diethylthiacarbocyanine iodide (DiSC$_2$). Significance level: * $p<0.05$; ** $p< 0.01$; *** $p<0.001$. Figures reconstructed based on previous reports from this lab; Gulyani and Mallick, 1993 (a); Gulyani and Mallick, 1995 (b); Mallick *et al.*, 2000 (c); Das and Mallick, 2008 (d). (See plate section for color version.)

(Porkka-Heiskanen *et al.*, 1995) suggesting an increased turnover of NE. Also, several other reports support the view that the NE level increases in the brain after REMSD (Pal *et al.*, 2005). Thus, the findings mentioned above suggest that normally during REM sleep the NE level reduces in the brain; however, it increases after REMSD, therefore we reasoned that REMSD-induced increase in Na-K ATPase activity could be mediated by NE (Mallick *et al.*, 2002).

Mechanism of action of norepinephrine in stimulating Na-K ATPase activity

In a series of in vivo and in vitro experiments, it was shown that prazosin (an alpha-1 NE-ergic receptor antagonist) and clonidine (an alpha-2 NE-ergic receptor agonist) prevented the REMSD-induced elevated activity of Na-K ATPase, while propranolol (a beta

NE-ergic receptor antagonist) was ineffective (Figure 36.1*b*) (Gulyani and Mallick, 1995). These results suggested that the increase in Na-K ATPase activity after REMSD is mediated by NE by its action on alpha-1 adrenergic receptors. Subsequently, it was observed in an in vitro synaptosome preparation study that the NE-induced increase in Na-K ATPase activity was prevented by pretreating the sample with either WB4101 (an alpha-1A NE-ergic receptor specific antagonist), heparin (an IP3 antagonist), W13 (a calmodulin inhibitor), or cyclosporin A (a calcineurin inhibitor) (Figure 36.1*c*). These findings led us to trace the intracellular pathway of NE action in stimulating the Na-K ATPase activity as follows. The NE acting on alpha-1A adrenoceptors activates phospholipase C leading to stimulation of Ca-calmodulin causing activation of calcineurin and finally resulting in stimulation of the Na-K ATPase activity (Mallick *et al.*, 2000). Our subsequent in vivo and in vitro studies confirmed that increased NE after REMSD indeed dephosphorylated the Na-K ATPase and increased its activity (Das *et al.*, 2008). Recently we reported that REMSD elevated intracellular positivity (Figure 36.1*d*) reflecting depolarization and an increased excitability of the neurons (Das and Mallick, 2008). Hence, we propose that REMSD increases neuronal depolarization (excitation), although the exact cause needs to be established. However, simultaneous elevation of NE increases Na-K ATPase activity possibly as a compensation to restore the ionic balance across the neuronal membranes.

Relationship with calcium in norepinephrine-mediated stimulation of Na-K ATPase activity

Increased calcium concentration is known to decrease Na-K ATPase activity (Davis and Vincenzi, 1971); in support we reported that REMSD decreased synaptosomal Ca^{++} levels (Mallick and Gulyani, 1996). Further, isolated studies showed that NE-stimulated increase in Na-K ATPase activity was mediated on one hand by chelation of extracellular Ca^{++} (Adya and Mallick, 1998) and on the other hand by releasing membrane bound Ca^{++} (Mallick and Adya, 1999). A closer look trying to integrate all the findings mentioned above revealed that there was an inherent contradiction as follows. Reduction of intracellular Ca^{++} is a necessity for the activation of Na-K ATPase; however, we found that after REMSD although there was reduced intracellular Ca^{++} level, at the same time some Ca^{++}, which may be released from the Na-K ATPase or the membrane in which the enzyme molecule remains embedded, was necessary to activate the calmodulin for dephosphorylation and activation of the enzyme.

Comprehensive studies in vivo as well as in vitro using nifedipine (an L-type Ca-channel blocker), cyclopiazonic acid (a Ca-channel activator), and NE-ergic agonists and antagonists were conducted. Also, membrane lipid peroxidation, Ca^{++} concentration, Na-K ATPase activity as well as phosphorylated state of Na-K ATPase were estimated in the presence and absence of NE in vitro as well as in control and REM sleep-deprived rat brain synaptosomes. It was observed that NE as well as REMSD reduced synaptosomal lipid peroxidation and simultaneously decreased Ca^{++} influx by blocking the L-type calcium channels (Das *et al.*, 2008). On the other hand, it was already reported that NE by acting on alpha-1A adrenoceptors induced the release of membrane-bound Ca^{++} (Mallick and Adya, 1999), which dephosphorylated the Na-K ATPase causing its stimulation; the latter is possibly a coupled reaction by activation of Ca^{++}-dependent calmodulin (Das *et al.*, 2008). Hence, it is reasonable to suggest that REMSD increases NE in the brain, which on one hand reduces Ca^{++} influx into the neurons by decreasing neuronal membrane lipid peroxidation (Lu *et al.*, 2002), while at the same time, the NE-ergic activation of alpha-1A adrenoceptor leads to the activation of phospholipase C, which possibly releases Ca^{++} from the Na-K ATPase structure spanning the membrane. The increased Ca^{++} in the presence of calmodulin activates calcineurin (a calmodulin dependent phosphatase), which then dephosphorylates Na-K ATPase, the active form of the enzyme. The entire mechanism has been compiled and presented as a model shown in Figure 36.2.

Significance of REM sleep in maintaining neuronal excitability

The Na-K ATPase enzyme activity is one of the determinants that modulate neuronal excitability; hence its modulation is likely to affect neural signaling and communication in the brain. Activity-dependent acquisition of learning tasks and consolidation of memory, which usually take place during alertness, induce synaptic potentiation and are dependent on

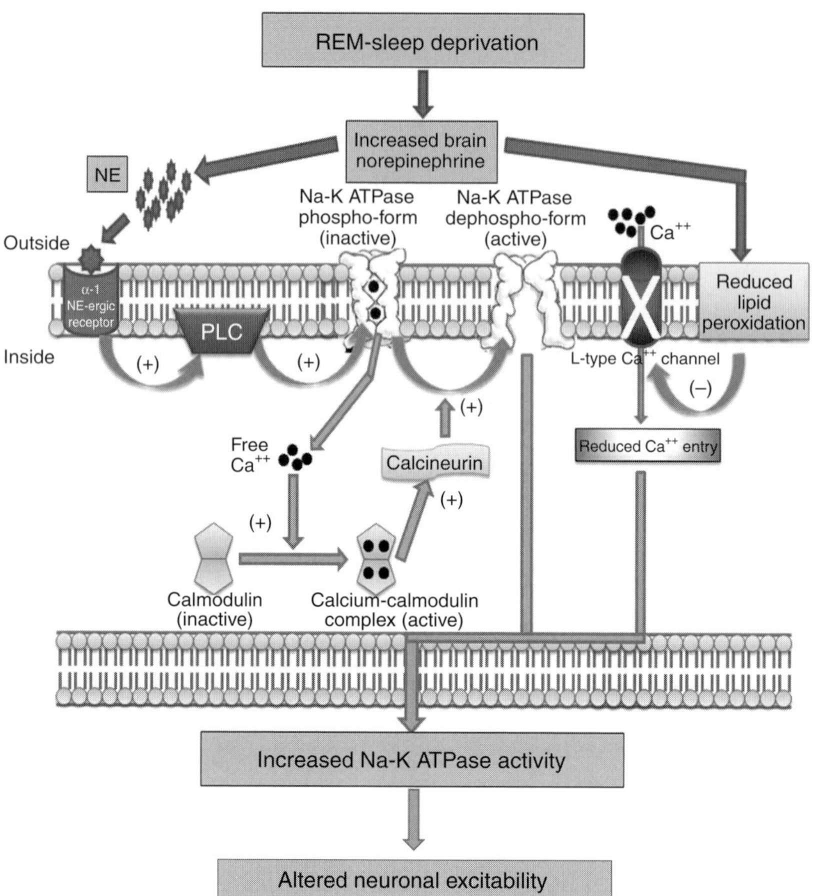

Figure 36.2 Schematic representation of the underlying mechanism of REMSD-induced changes in Na-K ATPase activity. Norepinephrine (NE) concentration increases in the brain after REMSD. The increased NE binds to the alpha-1A adrenoceptor on the neuronal membrane and activates PLC, which then releases membrane-bound calcium that activates calcineurin causing dephosphorylation of the Na-K ATPase, the active form of the enzyme. Additionally, the increased NE in the brain decreases the neuronal membrane lipid peroxidation causing a reduction in Ca++ influx into the neurons possibly by closing the L-type calcium channels, which also activates the Na-K ATPase activity. Figure reconstructed based on several reports cited in the text. (See plate section for color version.)

synaptic strength (Benington and Frank, 2003). The latter is known to be modulated by changes in Na-K ATPase activity, which decreases during memory consolidation (Wyse *et al.*, 2004). On the other hand it has been reported that inhibition of Na-K ATPase by ouabain impairs learning and memory (Zhan *et al.*, 2004) and inhibition of ouabain-like substances around the locus coeruleus by local microinfusion of antibodies against digitalis-like substances decreases REM sleep (Jaiswal *et al.*, 2009). Also, REM sleep plays a crucial role in memory consolidation and its deprivation impairs performance (Benington and Frank, 2003). Although the underlying mechanism of such behavioral and memory deficiency after REMSD are not yet clearly known, subject to verification, it appears that REMSD-induced increased Na-K ATPase activity may be involved in deprivation-associated impairment of memory and performance. Further, the REMSD-associated increased excitability of the neurons in the brain may be the cause of deprivation-associated psycho-behavioral changes, e.g., hyperactivity, aggressiveness, confusion, mood disorder, and so on (Kushida, 2005).

The above model may be supported by indirect isolated evidence that repeated presentation of similar but strong stimuli to the neurons may cause synaptic silencing. Although the neurons regain their activities with the passage of time, it has been observed that sleep can turn them on faster. At the cellular level it has been reported that chick neurons, which were responsive to imprinting stimuli, became non-responsive to the stimuli just one hour after training; the change was attributed to the silencing of the synapse. However, a few hours later, when the chicks underwent undisturbed sleep, responsiveness of the synapses to the imprinting stimuli recouped (Jackson *et al.*, 2008). In an earlier study it was observed that the inhibitory response of the brain-stem neurons that was lost after REMSD, was regained after REM-sleep recovery (Mallick *et al.*, 1991). Pending verification, we propose that persistent depolarization of neurons after REMSD may fatigue the neurons and eventually turn them silent; increased NE may be the culprit. However, during REM sleep since the NE-ergic REM-off neurons cease firing, the excess NE level is washed off and the neurons are protected from long-term alterations. Further, depolarization has been suggested to play a crucial role in apoptosis in dopaminergic neurons in rats by releasing factors such as cytochrome c, which activate the caspase cascade (Moon *et al.*, 2005). Since we have observed neuronal depolarization (Das and Mallick, 2008) and morphological changes as well as apoptosis in neurons after REMSD (Biswas *et al.*, 2006), we propose that the former may be the cause for inducing the latter. The studies reviewed here suggest that in the absence of REM sleep neuronal excitability is enhanced and upon recovery from REM-sleep loss the altered functions are reclaimed. Thus, the findings support our hypothesis that *one of the vital and basic functions of REM sleep is to maintain neuronal excitability and thus help homeostatic regulation by the brain.*

In conclusion, REMSD induces neuronal excitability by increasing neuronal depolarization. Further, on one hand, the NE level increases in the brain following REMSD, and on the other hand, we have shown by a series of in vivo and in vitro studies that REMSD-induced increase in NE significantly activates the Na-K ATPase enzyme. These findings put together support our hypothesis that *one of the functions of REM sleep is to maintain brain excitability.*

Acknowledgments

VM was financially supported by NIH grant (RO1-MH072897) to Dr. Adrian Morrison, UPENN, Philadelphia. BNM's research was funded by DST, ICMR, and UGC-Networking, India.

References

Adya, H. V. & Mallick, B. N. (1998) Comparison of Na-K ATPase activity in rat brain synaptosome under various conditions. *Neurochem Int* **33**: 283–6.

Adya, H. V. & Mallick, B. N. (2000) Uncompetitive stimulation of rat brain Na-K ATPase activity by rapid eye movement sleep deprivation. *Neurochem Int* **36**: 249–53.

Baskey, G., Singh, A., Sharma, R. & Mallick, B. N. (2009) REM sleep deprivation-induced noradrenaline stimulates neuronal and inhibits glial Na-K ATPase in rat brain: in vivo and in vitro studies. *Neurochem Int* **54**: 65–71.

Benington, J. H. & Frank, M. G. (2003) Cellular and molecular connections between sleep and synaptic plasticity. *Prog Neurobiol* **69**: 71–101.

Biswas, S., Mishra, P. & Mallick, B. N. (2006) Increased apoptosis in rat brain after rapid eye movement sleep loss. *Neuroscience* **142**: 315–31.

Cirelli, C. (2006) Cellular consequences of sleep deprivation in the brain. *Sleep Med Rev* **10**: 307–21.

Cohen, H. B. & Dement, W. C. (1965) Sleep: changes in threshold to electroconvulsive shock in rats after deprivation of "paradoxical" phase. *Science* **150**: 1318–19.

Das, G., Gopalakrishnan, A., Faisal, M. & Mallick, B. N. (2008) Stimulatory role of calcium in rapid eye movement sleep deprivation-induced noradrenaline-mediated increase in Na-K-ATPase activity in rat brain. *Neuroscience* **155**: 76–89.

Das, G. & Mallick, B. N. (2008) Noradrenaline acting on alpha1-adrenoceptor mediates REM sleep deprivation-induced increased membrane potential in rat brain synaptosomes. *Neurochem Int* **52**: 734–40.

Davis, P. W. & Vincenzi, F. F. (1971) Ca-ATPase activation and NaK-ATPase inhibition as a function of calcium concentration in human red cell membranes. *Life Sci II* **10**: 401–6.

Dement, W. & Fisher, C. (1963) Experimental interference with the sleep cycle. *Can Psychiatr Assoc J* **257**: 400–5.

Dement, W. C. (1965) Recent studies on the biological role of rapid eye movement sleep. *Am J Psychiatry* **122**: 404–8.

Dewson, J. H., 3rd, Dement, W. C. & Simmons, F. B. (1965) Middle ear muscle activity in cats during sleep. *Exp Neurol* **12**: 1–8.

Gall, C. M. & Lynch, G. (2004) Integrins, synaptic plasticity and epileptogenesis. *Adv Exp Med Biol* **548**: 12–33.

Gulyani, S., Majumdar, S. & Mallick, B. N. (2000) Rapid eye movement sleep and significance of its deprivation studies – a review. *Sleep Hypn* **2**: 49–68.

Gulyani, S. & Mallick, B. N. (1993) Effect of rapid eye movement sleep deprivation on rat brain Na-K ATPase activity. *J Sleep Res* **2**: 45–50.

Gulyani, S. & Mallick, B. N. (1995) Possible mechanism of rapid eye movement sleep deprivation induced increase in Na-K ATPase activity. *Neuroscience* **64**: 255–60.

Jackson, C., McCabe, B. J., Nicol, A. U. *et al.* (2008) Dynamics of a memory trace: effects of sleep on consolidation. *Curr Biol* **18**: 393–400.

Jaiswal, M. K., Dvela, M., Lichtstein, D. & Mallick, B. N. (2009) Endogenous ouabain-like compounds in locus coeruleus modulate rapid eye movement sleep in rats. *J Sleep Res.* DOI: 10.1111/j.1365–2869.2009.00781.

Kaplan, J. H. (2002) Biochemistry of Na,K-ATPase. *Annu Rev Biochem* **71**: 511–35.

Kushida, C. A. (2005) *Sleep Deprivation: Basic Science, Physiology and Behavior*. Marcel-Dekker.

Lebel, C. P. & Schatz, R. A. (1990) Altered synaptosomal phospholipid metabolism after toluene: possible relationship with membrane fluidity, Na$^+$,K$(^+)$-adenosine triphosphatase and phospholipid methylation. *J Pharmacol Exp Ther* **253**: 1189–97.

Lu, C., Chan, S. L., Fu, W. & Mattson, M. P. (2002). The lipid peroxidation product 4-hydroxynonenal facilitates opening of voltage-dependent Ca^{2+} channels in neurons by increasing protein tyrosine phosphorylation. *J Biol Chem* **277**: 24, 368–75.

Majumdar, S., Faisal, M., Madan, V. & Mallick, B. N. (2003) Increased turnover of Na-K ATPase molecules in rat brain after rapid eye movement sleep deprivation. *J Neurosci Res* **73**: 870–5.

Mallick, B. N. & Adya, H. V. (1999) Norepinephrine induced alpha-adrenoceptor mediated increase in rat brain Na-K ATPase activity is dependent on calcium ion. *Neurochem Int* **34**: 499–507.

Mallick, B. N. & Gulyani, S. (1996) Alterations in synaptosomal calcium concentrations after rapid eye movement sleep deprivation in rats. *Neuroscience* **75**: 729–36.

Mallick, B. N., Siegel, J. M. & Fahringer, H. (1990) Changes in pontine unit activity with REM sleep deprivation. *Brain Res* **515**: 94–8.

Mallick, B. N., Fahringer, H. M., Wu, M. F. & Siegel, J. M. (1991) REM sleep deprivation reduces auditory evoked inhibition of dorsolateral pontine neurons. *Brain Res* **552**: 333–7.

Mallick, B. N., Thakkar, M. & Gulyani, S. (1994) Rapid eye movement sleep deprivation induced alteration in neuronal excitability : possible role of norepinephrine. In *Environment and Physiology*, eds. B. N. Mallick & R. Singh. Narosa Publishing House, pp. 196–203.

Mallick, B. N., Adya, H. V. & Thankachan, S. (1999) REM sleep deprivation alters factors affecting neuronal excitability: role of norepinephrine and its possible mechanism of action. In *Rapid Eye Movement Sleep*, eds. B. N. Mallick & S. Inoué. Marcel Dekker, pp. 338–54.

Mallick, B. N., Adya, H. V. & Faisal, M. (2000) Norepinephrine-stimulated increase in Na$^+$, K$^+$-ATPase activity in the rat brain is mediated through alpha1A-adrenoceptor possibly by dephosphorylation of the enzyme. *J Neurochem* **74**: 1574–8.

Mallick, B. N., Majumdar, S., Faisal, M., *et al.* (2002). Role of norepinephrine in the regulation of rapid eye movement sleep. *J Biosci* **27**: 539–51.

Mallick, B. N., Madan, V. & Faisal, M. (2005) Biochemical changes. In *Sleep Deprivation: Basic Science, Physiology and Behavior*, ed. C. A. Kushida. Marcel-Dekker, pp. 339–57.

Moon, Y., Lee, K. H., Park, J. H., Geum, D. & Kim, K. (2005) Mitochondrial membrane depolarization and the selective death of dopaminergic neurons by rotenone: protective effect of coenzyme Q10. *J Neurochem* **93**: 1199–208.

Morden, B., Conner, R., Mitchell, G., Dement, W. & Levine, S. (1968) Effects of rapid eye movement (REM) sleep deprivation on shock-induced fighting. *Physiol Behav* **3**: 425–32.

Morel, P., Tallineau, C., Pontcharraud, R., Piriou, A. & Huguet, F. (1998) Effects of 4-hydroxynonenal, a lipid peroxidation product, on dopamine transport and Na$^+$/K$^+$ ATPase in rat striatal synaptosomes. *Neurochem Int* **33**: 531–40.

Pal, D., Madan, V. & Mallick, B. N. (2005) Neural mechanism of rapid eye movement sleep generation: cessation of locus coeruleus neurons is a necessity. *Sheng Li Xue Bao* **57**: 401–13.

Porkka-Heiskanen, T., Smith, S. E., Taira, T. *et al.* (1995) Noradrenergic activity in rat brain during rapid eye movement sleep deprivation and rebound sleep. *Am J Physiol* **268**: R1456–63.

Pujol, J. F., Mouret, J., Jouvet, M. & Glowinski, J. (1968) Increased turnover of cerebral norepinephrine during rebound of paradoxical sleep in the rat. *Science* **159**: 112–14.

Rechtschaffen, A., Bergmann, B. M., Everson, C. A., Kushida, C. A. & Gilliland, M. A. (1989) Sleep deprivation in the rat: X. Integration and discussion of the findings. *Sleep* **12**: 68–87.

Sazontova, T. G., Arkhipenko Iu, V. & Meerson, F. Z. (1984) [Increased brain Na, K-ATPase activity of rats under stress]. *Biull Eksp Biol Med* **97**: 556–8.

Sinha, A. K., Ciaranello, R. D., Dement, W. C. & Barchas, J. D. (1973) Tyrosine hydroxylase activity in rat brain following "REM" sleep deprivation. *J Neurochem* **20**: 1289–90.

Stern, W. C., Miller, F. P., Cox, R. H. & Maickel, R. P. (1971) Brain norepinephrine and serotonin levels following REM sleep deprivation in the rat. *Psychopharmacologia* **22**: 50–5.

Wheal, H. V., Chen, Y., Mitchell, J. *et al.* (1998) Molecular mechanisms that underlie structural and functional changes at the postsynaptic membrane during synaptic plasticity. *Prog Neurobiol* **55**: 611–40.

Wyse, A. T., Bavaresco, C. S., Reis, E. A. *et al.* (2004) Training in inhibitory avoidance causes a reduction of Na$^+$, K$^+$-ATPase activity in rat hippocampus. *Physiol Behav* **80**: 475–9.

Zeplin, H., Siegel, J. M. & Tobler, I. (2005) Mammalian sleep. In *Principles and Practice of Sleep Medicine*, eds M. Kryger, T. Roth & W. Dement. Elsevier Saunders, pp. 91–100.

Zhan, H., Tada, T., Nakazato, F., Tanaka, Y. & Hongo, K. (2004) Spatial learning transiently disturbed by intraventricular administration of ouabain. *Neurol Res* **26**: 35–40.

Chapter 37

Comparison of REM sleep-deprivation methods: role of stress and validity of use

Deborah Suchecki and Sergio Tufik

Summary

Sleep-deprivation protocols are useful to examine the consequences of inadequate or insufficient sleep on health. By employing different paradigms of sleep deprivation or sleep restriction in humans and animals, numerous laboratories have come to the conclusion that insufficient sleep is stressful. Particularly, activation of stress response systems – the locus coeruleus/ adrenal medulla and the hypothalamic–pituitary– adrenal (HPA) axis – appears to be a caveat of instrumental methods to induce REM-sleep deprivation. However, not all effects of REM-sleep deprivation are mediated by increased secretion of glucocorticoids (the final outcome of HPA axis activation) nor are these effects common to other protracted stressors. Therefore, the present chapter presents an overview of the very peculiar form of stress represented by inadequate or insufficient sleep, by means of REM-sleep deprivation.

Introduction

Deprivation of total sleep or of REM sleep (REMSd) represents one of the most widely used strategies to investigate the functions of sleep in general or that of specific phases of sleep. By preventing a human being or an experimental animal from sleeping, it is possible to observe the consequences on numerous systems and infer the function of sleep on these systems.

The first study involving REMSd was carried out in human beings and consisted of waking up the volunteers every time they entered into REM sleep (REMS). This classical study demonstrated the occurrence of a well known phenomenon after the end of the deprivation period, i.e. an increase in the time spent in REMS (Dement, 1960). The same phenomenon was described in rats (Morden *et al.*, 1967) as well. After REMSd, the latency to initiate REMS was sensibly reduced, indicating the need to compensate for the lost time in sleep; this compensatory event is denominated as sleep rebound.

The body of work on the effects of REMSd on functions that vary from sleep homeostasis to learning and memory, from neurotransmission to neuroendocrinology and neurogenesis is quite impressive. However, the question of how useful these methods are in terms of modeling the sleep pathologies in human beings is still unanswered. For instance, in sleep apnea patients the sleep stages that are most impaired are delta and REMS; insomnia patients, in turn, exhibit long sleep latency, early awakening or they wake in the midst of their sleep, so their sleep is fragmented. In this sense, these methods could be valuable because they mimic, at least partially, the human condition. It is important, nonetheless, to bear in mind that these methods do not model entirely any of these pathologies, simply because, among many factors, these are long-lasting conditions that afflict the patients for many years before they seek treatment.

Despite these considerations, it is interesting that some of the alterations observed in sleep apnea and insomniac patients, such as changes in biological systems of stress response, have also been described in rats submitted to prolonged REMSd. Both sleep apnea and insomniac patients exhibit increased levels of circulating cortisol and adrenaline indicating that sleep loss may be stressful (Carneiro *et al.*, 2008; Vgontzas *et al.*, 1998, 2001). Under laboratory conditions, healthy volunteers that are subjected to sleep curtailment (four hours of sleep per night, during seven nights) also present increased cortisol levels, and increased sympathovagal balance (Spiegel *et al.*, 1999). Thus, it seems that hindering normal sleep represents stress to the organism.

REM Sleep: Regulation and Function, eds. Birendra N. Mallick, S. R. Pandi-Perumal, Robert W. McCarley, and Adrian R. Morrison. Published by Cambridge University Press. © Cambridge University Press 2011.

The conundrum of REM-sleep deprivation and stress

A common source of criticism in sleep-deprivation studies involving instrumental methods is the possible induction of stress and whether or not activation of stress mediators, such as the HPA axis and the sympathetic nervous system, could participate or even be responsible for the biochemical, neurochemical, and behavioral alterations.

Stress can be defined in several different, but somewhat related, ways. The classical definition is that stress represents a threat to homeostasis, and recruitment of biological systems that respond to a stressor is of primordial importance to restore internal balance. The main response systems are the locus coeruleus (LC)/adrenal medulla and the HPA axis, which are described below. These systems which must be correctly activated for either hypo- or hyper-responsiveness represent inadequate reactions that may, ultimately, impose a demand on the organism; this increased demand is also considered stress. These systems may respond inadequately by being incapable of adapting to the stressful situation, such that repeated or prolonged exposure to the stressor will result in surges of hormone release of equal or increased magnitude. Failure to shut off the HPA axis, by means of the glucocorticoid negative feedback (the main regulator of the axis activity), also represents a threat to health, given the detrimental effects of sustained glucocorticoid release – immune suppression, changes in glucose and lipid metabolism, proteolysis, and inhibition of hippocampal neurogenesis, to mention but a few (McEwen, 2006).

Thus, according to the classical definition of stress, REM- and total-sleep deprivation should be viewed as a stressor, because preventing an organism from engaging in such essential function is incompatible with life. Moreover, prolonged, unremitting sleep deprivation stimulates the activity of both biological systems' responses to stress, the LC/medulla adrenal and the HPA axis, as is shown in Table 37.2. In fact, rats cannot survive beyond 20 to 30 days of unremitting sleep deprivation. In the very first study on this matter, Madame Marie de Manacéine reported that four to six days of sleep deprivation was sufficient to lead dog pups to death, in contrast to the much longer period required for food deprivation to produce the same effect.

The first study that raised the issue of REMSd methods, and not suppression of REMS per se, as being stressful was carried out by Kovalzon and Tsibulsky (1984), who compared two forms of REMSd – direct stimulation of the midbrain reticular formation and the flower-pot method (explanation about this method is given below). The reticular formation is also called the reticular activating system. It mediates various levels of alertness and projects to the thalamus, which also plays a role in wakefulness. The authors reported that rats exposed to either the flower-pot or to cold stress exhibited changes in classical stress indices, i.e., an increased number of ulcers, heavier adrenals, and decreased thymus weight, whereas stimulation of the reticular formation did not produce these changes. These results led the authors to postulate that the method, and not the lack of REMS, would induce stress. However, they can also be interpreted as evidence that the need to sleep as well as the REMS are essential and not being able to do so constitutes the stressful stimulus.

In this chapter we will review numerous methods of REMSd and discuss whether it is possible to surpass the stressful nature of this condition. We will also show that REMSd may be yet another form of stress, and that some of the outcomes of REMSd are not entirely dependent on glucocorticoid (GC) circulating levels.

Stress response: biological systems involved

In the face of either a physical or psychological threatening stimulus, the organism responds by activating two main systems, whose major function is to promote behavioral and metabolic adaptations to the situation so as to guarantee survival. These systems are briefly described below (for review, see Gunnar and Quevedo, 2007; Morilak et al., 2005; Sapolsky et al., 2000).

Locus coeruleus/adrenal medulla

The LC/adrenal medulla is also known as the sympathetic-adrenomedullary system and is part of the sympathetic nervous system. The preganglionic neurons constitute the cell bodies and are located in the interomediolateral (IML) cell column, which exits the spinal cord via the ventral root to form cholinergic synapses on the chromaffin cells of the adrenal medulla. When the chromaffin cells are stimulated, epinephrine (Epi – 80%) and norepinephrine (NE – 20%) secretion ensues and these catecholamines affect organs and tissues by binding to specific alpha and beta adrenergic receptors. The net result of activation of these receptors involves

Table 37.1 Features of glucocorticoid and mineralocorticoid receptors (GR and MR, respectively) in regards to their affinity to natural and synthetic glucocorticoids (GC), distribution and the main functions

Mineralocorticoid receptors (MR)	Glucocorticoid receptors (GR)
High affinity for natural GC (cortisol or corticosterone) and for aldosterone	Low affinity for natural GC and high affinity for synthetic GC (dexamethasone)
Full occupation throughout the day (90 to 100%)	Low occupation during the nadir of the circadian rhythm (10%) and high occupation during the peak of the rhythm or during stressful situations (~ 70%)
High receptor density in the hypothalamus, hippocampus, lateral septum, medial and central amygdala, olfactory nucleus (for corticosterone), and in the circumventricular organ (aldosterone)	Widely distributed in the central nervous system (CNS), pituitary, and periphery. In the CNS, GR are located in the prefrontal cortex, hippocampus (but CA3 area), septum, amygdala, paraventricular and supra-optic nuclei
Associated with permissive and basal functions (↑ digestive enzymatic activity, fibrinogen production, enzyme involved in the conversion of norepinephrine to epinephrine)	Associated with the effects of stressful situations (suppressive effects) and responsible for the GC negative feedback

vasodilatation of muscle and vasoconstriction of skin blood vessels, increased blood pressure and heart rate, increased oxygen and glucose supply to skeletal muscles and the brain, so as to assure the best conditions for the fight or flight reaction.

The LC is the main noradrenergic nucleus in the central nervous system and is strategically located in the brain stem where it controls brain and peripheral functions mediated by the sympathetic nervous system. Although neither Epi nor NE cross the blood–brain barrier, activation of the LC parallels the peripheral actions of these catecholamines so that vigilance, arousal, and increased attention to the source of the stressful stimulus is ensured. In addition, this system also stimulates, and is stimulated by, the neuroendocrine limb of the stress response, represented by the HPA axis.

Hypothalamic–pituitary–adrenal axis

The paraventricular nucleus (PVN) of the hypothalamus conveys information from ascending pathways originating in the brain stem and midbrain, more specifically from the nucleus of the solitary tract, the LC, and raphe nucleus, and from descending pathways originating in the limbic system (hippocampus and amygdala) and prefrontal cortex, which signal, respectively, physical and psychological threats to homeostasis. Stimulation of the PVN triggers a cascade of neuroendocrine events, which involves the release of corticotrophin-releasing factor (CRF) and vasopressin (AVP), which stimulates the synthesis and release of adrenocorticotropin (ACTH) from the

anterior pituitary. Adrenocorticotropin reaches the adrenal cortex and induces the synthesis and secretion of GC – cortisol in human beings and primates, and corticosterone (CORT) in rodents. Glucocorticoids regulate the activity of the HPA axis by means of a feedback signal at the prefrontal cortex, hippocampus, hypothalamus, and pituitary that results from the steroid binding to the low affinity glucocorticoid receptor (GR or type II), ubiquitously distributed throughout the body. These receptors are involved with the suppressive effects of GC, including immune suppression, increased waking (suppression of sleep), and the negative feedback regulatory function (suppression of HPA axis activity). In addition to these receptors, high-affinity mineralocorticoid receptors (MR or type I) are also involved in the basal, permissive effects of GC. These effects include the induction of digestive enzymes, stimulation of fibrinogen production (in case of tissue injury), regulation of memory consolidation, and regulation of REM sleep. Binding of GC to their cytoplasmic receptors leads to changes in gene transcription, which explains the long time lag for initiation of their effects. A description of the features for these receptors appears in Table 37.1.

The effects of stress hormones on several functions, including REMS regulation, depend on the balance of MR and GR occupancy. Because MR presents high affinity for the natural ligand, it is saturated throughout the day, but GR shows low affinity for endogenous GC, so it is occupied by 50 to 70% during the peak of the circadian rhythm or after a stressor. At this point (100% MR, and 50 to 70% GR occupation) the best performance is seen. Either hypo- (lower than 50% GR occupation) or hyper-responsiveness (higher then 70% GR occupation) for extended periods of time will result in poor performance of a given system (De Kloet *et al.*, 1998).

Methods of REM-sleep deprivation and the stressors involved

The first method developed to produce selective REMSd was the flower-pot or single platform method, which is based on the muscle atonia typically observed during REMS. In this method, the animal is individually placed on top of a platform (for rats, 6.5 to 7 cm in diameter; for mice, 3 cm), surrounded by water. Once the animal enters REMS, it loses balance and touches the water, being awakened (Figure 37.1).

This method was first tested in cats in 1964 and adapted to rats in the following year. Some modifications to the method have been introduced since, but the basic rationale remains: once the animal initiates REMS, muscle atonia ensues and the rat falls into the water waking up. However, the presence of stressful stimuli, such as social isolation, movement restriction, and excessive humidity that are inherent to the original flower-pot method, led some authors to suspect that the outcomes were not due to loss of REMS per se, but to these confounding environmental adverse stimuli. Thus, a proposed change to the original method included the placement of one animal in a larger water tank, containing five or more platforms on which the rat can ambulate (multiple platform method). Still, the

animal remains alone, which may yet represent a source of stress. To overcome this adversity, the modified multiple platform was introduced, and in this case, socially stable groups of animals (four to ten animals) are placed onto several platforms, the number of which exceeds that of the animals, and that allows the animals to interact and to move between the platforms (Figure 37.2).

All these methods were validated by polysomnographic recordings as to their ability to suppress REMS. A comparison between the flower-pot and the modified multiple platform method showed a complete elimination of REMS and a reduction of approximately 40% of slow-wave sleep, throughout a 96-hour sleep-deprivation period, indicating that these methods also impact other sleep phases, especially when muscle relaxation occurs, as is the case of deep slow-wave sleep (Machado *et al.*, 2004).

The disk-over-water method also relies on muscle atonia as the rationale but, in this case, rats are implanted with recording electrodes and when the experimental rat enters into REMS, a motor initiates the rotation of the disk and the rat must wake and walk in the opposite direction so as not to fall into the water. The yoked animal, which for many years was used as a control, must also walk when the experimental rat enters into REMS, thus, it may also be sleep deprived in an unspecific sleep phase (Figure 37.3).

The use of a slowly rotating treadmill has gained some popularity in the last years. This method can be used to selectively deprive rats or mice of REMS, by placing the animal in the apparatus set up to turn on when REMS is detected by polysomnographic recordings,

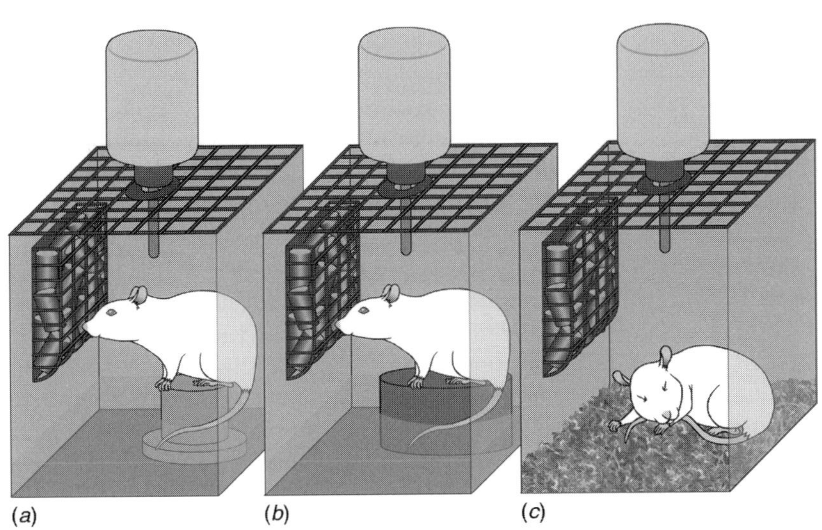

(a)   (b)   (c)

Figure 37.1 The single platform method (SPM), including the narrow platform (*a*), large platform, which has been used as a form of stress control (*b*), and the cage control, in which rats are placed in the same container as REMsd rats, but are allowed to sleep freely, lying down on a bedding made of sawdust (*c*). Water and food are available throughout the entire sleep-deprivation period, and the water inside the chambers is changed once or twice a day, depending on the study. (See plate section for color version.)

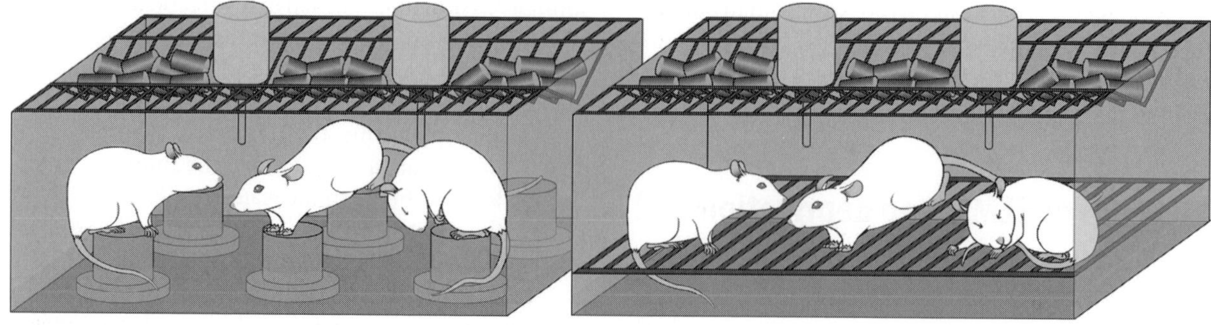

Figure 37.2 The modified multiple platform method (MMPM) was elaborated based on the SPM, but with sufficient platforms so the rats would be allowed to move around the water tank. Rats are placed in the large water tanks as a socially stable group, to prevent additional, non-sleep related stressors. One possible stress-control group consists of placing large platforms, but alternatively, a grid can be placed inside the water tank, so the rats can lie down and sleep freely. Previous results show some loss of sleep in the grid, but far less than that seen in large platforms (Machado *et al.*, 2004). (See plate section for color version.)

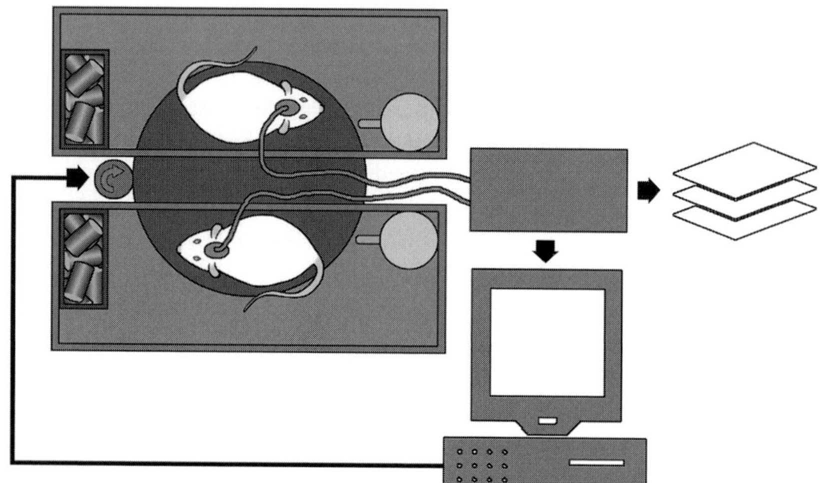

Figure 37.3 The disk-over-water (DOW) method involves the implant of electrodes for sleep monitoring. Because a computer detects the sleep phase, it is possible to deprive rats of specific sleep phases. Therefore, upon sleep (or REM sleep) onset, the disk turns on and the rat walks counterwise to avoid falling in the water. The yoked rat is also obliged to walk regardless of whether it is awake or not. (See plate section for color version.)

whereas yoked rats are wakened up regardless of the stage of the sleep–wake cycle. Total-sleep deprivation is accomplished by turning the treadmill on for 3 seconds and off for 12 seconds, whereas the control animal is placed on the apparatus set up to turn on for 15 minutes and off for 60 minutes. Thus, the distance "walked" is the same, but the control animals can rest. Usually the deprived animals remain awake for 92% of the time, and the controls, 60%, whereas home-cage animals remain awake 50% of the time. One bias of this method, however, is that control animals will engage in longer periods of physical activity (15 minutes), which may represent some kind of stress, although the nature of this stressor is quite different from REMSd. The former is a physical stressor and, as such, will most certainly elicit some activation of the HPA axis; the latter

is a mixed physical/psychological stressor, and may therefore elicit a higher stress response.

Finally, gentle handling is a procedure that is widely used in many laboratories, although the length of deprivation accomplished by this method is usually short. In this method, the animals are prevented from sleeping by placing new objects in the cage, or by gently tapping the cage or by waking the animal with a soft brush. If sleep is being monitored, it is possible to specifically deprive the animal of REMS, but total-sleep deprivation is more frequently used with this method.

Other forms of REMSd that do not involve instrumental techniques, and therefore avoid some of the stressors present in these methods, such as movement restriction and frequent contact with water, have also been used successfully to study the regulation of this sleep phase. For instance, mild electrical stimulation of the pontine tegmentum around the LC produces a significant reduction of REMS, comparable to that produced by the single platform method (Singh and Mallick, 1996). Release of the LC from GABAergic tonic inhibition is another method that results in reduction of REMS and that can be used to assess the consequences of REMSd on the neurotransmitters involved in the regulation of this sleep phase (Kaur *et al.*, 2004).

The data presented in Table 37.2 resulted from the selection of studies that employed any method of unremitting total or REMSd and their effects on physiological, neurochemical, and behavioral stress responses. The general conclusion that can be drawn from these studies is that in order to produce a reliable stress response, the length of deprivation must be at least 12 hours. What this probably means is that the unfulfilled homeostatic need to sleep represents a stress to the organism, regardless of the method used to induce sleep deprivation.

Appropriate control groups: are there any?

The choice of appropriate control groups in sleep-deprivation studies has proved a much more difficult matter than initially thought, especially when the final outcome is some measurement of stress response. In general, control groups are composed of animals exposed to the adverse situation without being sleep deprived so any difference between the stress control and the sleep-deprived group can be inferred to be due to sleep deprivation and not to some unspecific stressor contained in the method.

Usually, for the flower-pot method, placement of animals onto a large platform (from 14 to 28 cm) immersed in water has been used for the control group, the idea being that on the large platform, the animal would be able to sleep, because despite the muscle atonia, the platform would be large enough to allow the animal to lie down, so it would be exposed to the same stressful environment, without being sleep deprived. However, although reasonable in theory, it proved not to be so in practice, because rats tend to sleep on the edge of the platform and if there is enough room between the platform and the walls of the container, the rat will fall into the water. In fact, a comparative study showed that rats placed onto large platforms, either individually or in a group, exhibit approximately 50% suppression of REMS (Machado *et al.*, 2004) and the magnitude of

sleep rebound after 90 hours in large or narrow platforms in the modified multiple platform method is 99% and 184%, respectively, indicating that stress control rats are also sleep deprived (Suchecki *et al.*, 2000).

Another important control aspect when using the flower-pot method (single or multiple platforms) is to habituate the animals to the environment. The fact that this method requires that the animals balance on small platforms requires that they be trained to do so, to prevent excessive falls in the water, which would constitute an additional stressor. Therefore, it is recommended that the rats be placed onto the platform for 30 to 60 minutes per day, for two to three days before the onset of the actual REMSd procedure, because they learn to balance very quickly. Moreover, comparison between the effects of REMSd and those of other stressors has been employed as a strategy to discriminate the impact of REMSd on numerous functions from those of possible stressors associated with the method. For instance, it has been reported that REMSd increases NA-K-ATPase activity in the brain stem, cerebellum, and cerebrum, but movement restriction and swimming stressors do not, indicating that this effect is not associated to stress, but rather, to the loss of sleep (Gulyani and Mallick, 1993).

With regard to the disk-over-water method, yoked rats, which are awakened at unspecific moments during their sleep, are also subjected to sleep fragmentation. Maybe they are not sleep deprived as much as the experimental rats, but they are, nonetheless, subjected to sleep loss, and recent findings have shown that sleep fragmentation can be as detrimental to health as sleep deprivation. This may explain why yoked and sleep-deprived rats exhibit similar CORT levels, leading, sometimes, to the erroneous conclusion that this method is not stressful. However, it is important to emphasize that both yoked and sleep-deprived groups exhibit hormone levels that are above acceptable basal, non-stress, concentrations.

The involvement of stress on the effects of REM-sleep deprivation: two approaches

Comparison with acute and chronic stressors

One strategy that has been used to distinguish the effects of REMSd and stress is to compare their effects on distinct systems. Despite being an indirect way of

Table 37.2 Studies that employ methods to induce total- or selective REM-sleep deprivation and their outcomes related to the neurobiology of stress

Reference	Method / type of deprivation	Length	Variable	Outcome (compared to control or otherwise specified)	Control group / species
1982 – Murison *et al., Physiol Behav* 29(4): 693	SPM – REMSd Handling / almost TSD	24 h	Gastric ulcers CORT plasma levels	↑ (vs. handling and HC) ↑	HC control rats
1983 – Tobler *et al., Neurosci Lett* 35(3): 297	Forced locomotion in slowly rotating drums / TSD	21.5 h and 2.5 h of sleep recovery	CORT plasma levels	↑ after 21.5 h of TSD and = after 2.5 h of recovery	HC control rats
1983 – Abel *et al., Brain Res Bull* 11(6): 729	SPM / REMSd	72 h and 24 h of sleep recovery	Binding to cortical β adrenoceptors	= controls	HC control and stress control (22 h/day in the water for 3 days) rats
1985 – Coenen *et al., Physiol Behav* 35(4): 501	Pendulum method / REMSd SPM / REMSd Multiple platforms / REMSd	72 h	Relative adrenal / thymus weight Body weight Gastric ulcers	↑ in all methods and respective controls (vs. HC) ↓ in all methods and control for SPM (vs. HC) = controls	HC control, large platform (LP – SPM and multiple platforms) and tilted cage (pendulum technique) rats
1989 – Kushida *et al., Sleep* 12(1): 22	DOW / REMSd	Until death	Relative adrenal weight Heart rate	↑ ↑	Yoked control rats
1991 – Patchev *et al., Homeost Health Dis* 3(3): 97	SPM / REMSd	7–9 days	Food intake / Body weight Rectal temperature CORT plasma levels	↑ / ↓ ↓ ↑	Note: based on information given in the abstract. The paper is inaccessible
1994 – Moulin *et al., Mol Brain Res* 22(1/4): 113	SPM / REMSd	24 h and 4 h of sleep recovery	Glutamine synthase CORT plasma levels	↑ cortex and LC/ ↓ rebound ↑ / ↓ rebound	Individual HC control rats
1994 – Brock *et al., Physiol Behav* 55(6): 997	SPM / REMSd	96 h	NA levels Body weight / Food intake Time of immobility	↑ Parietal cortex (vs. HC) and lateral hypothalamus ↓ ↑	HC and LP control rats
1995 – Porkka-Heiskanen *et al., Am J Physiol* 268 (6 Pt 2): R1456	SPM / REMSd	8 h, 24 h, 72 h	NA levels Tyrosine hydroxylase mRNA	24 h – ↓ neocortex, hippocampus, posterior hypothalamus, 72 h – ↑ levels 72 h – ↑ levels in LC	HC controls
1997 – Fadda & Fratta, *Pharmacol Res* 35: 443	SPM / REMSd	72 h	CRH hypothalamic content CRH receptors	↑ striatum, limbic areas and pituitary, ↓ hypothalamus ↓ striatum and pituitary	HC control rats

Table 37.2 (*cont.*)

Reference	Method / type of deprivation	Length	Variable	Outcome (compared to control or otherwise specified)	Control group / species
1998 – Hipólide *et al.*, *Neuroscience* 86(3): 977	MMPM / REMSd	96 h	Autoradiography of α and β adrenoceptors in the brain	α_1 and α_2 receptors = HC $\downarrow \beta_1$ and $\uparrow \beta_2$ anterior olfactory nucleus, lateral septum, dentate gyrus, entorhinal cortex, amygdala–hippocampal nucleus and infralimbic cortex	Group HC control rats
1998 – Suchecki *et al.*, *J Sleep Res* 7(4): 276	SPM and mixed groups in the MPM / REMSd	24 h and 96 h	ACTH plasma levels CORT plasma levels	24 h = HC and LP / $\uparrow$ 96 h $\uparrow$ 24 h and 96 h	Individual and group LP rats
2000 – Suchecki & Tufik, *Physiol Behav* 68: 309	MMPM / REMSd	96 h	ACTH and CORT plasma levels Relative adrenal weight	= / $\uparrow$ SPM and grid $\uparrow$ (vs. HC and grid)	Grouped HC and grid control rats
2001 – Hairston *et al.*, *Neurosci Lett* 315(1/2): 29	Gentle handling / TSD	70, 90, 140, or 180 min	CORT plasma levels	$\uparrow$ in 12-, 16-, 20- and 24-day old pups	HC, separated rat pups
2002 – Campbell *et al.*, *J Neurophysiol* 88(2): 1073	Forced locomotion in slowly rotating drums / TSD	12 h	CORT plasma levels Hippocampal LTP	$\uparrow$ $\downarrow$	Rats placed inside non-rotating drums
2002 – Meerlo *et al.*, *J Neuroendocrinol* 14(5): 397	Forced locomotion in slowly rotating wheels / TSD	48 h	ACTH plasma levels CORT plasma levels Hormone response to restraint	$\uparrow$ by 24 h, = by 48h $\uparrow$ by 6h and remained $\uparrow$ $\downarrow$ ACTH / = CORT	Rats placed in non-rotating wheels
2002 – Pokk & Väli, *Prog Neuropsycho-pharmacol Biol Psychiatry* 26(2): 241	SPM / REMSd	24 h	Anxiety-type behavior in the elevated plus maze (EPM)	$\downarrow$	HC control mice
2002 – Suchecki *et al.*, *J Neuroendocrinol* 14(7): 549	SPM and MMPM / REMSd	96 h	Time course of ACTH response to EPM Time course of CORT response to EPM Anxiety-type behavior	$\uparrow$ post-REMSd / = stress response $\uparrow$ post-REMSd / $\downarrow$ MMPM $\downarrow$ MMPM / = flower-pot, $\uparrow$ individual controls	HC, individual control and grid control rats
2002 – Suchecki *et al.*, *Neurosci Lett* 320(1/2): 45	SPM and MMPM / REMSd	96 h	Time course of ACTH response to saline injection Time course of CORT response	$\uparrow$ post-REMSd / = stress response $\uparrow$ post-REMSd, $\uparrow$ 5 min, $\downarrow$ 20 and 60 min	HC and grid control rats

Table 37.2 (*cont.*)

Reference	Method / type of deprivation	Length	Variable	Outcome (compared to control or otherwise specified)	Control group / species
2003 – Irie *et al.*, *Int Arch Allergy Immunol* 130(4): 300	SPM / REMSd	72 h	Immediate asthmatic response Late asthmatic response Histamine plasma levels Adrenaline plasma levels	↑ ↑ ↓ ↑	HC and LP control rats
2003 – McDermott *et al.*, *J Neurosci* 23(29): 9687	SPM and MMPM / REMSd	72 h	CORT plasma levels Contextual fear conditioning Cue fear conditioning	↑ (vs. HC) Impaired =	HC and LP control rats. Note: LP group exhibited elevated CORT plasma levels compared to HC controls
2003 – Suchecki *et al.*, *J Neuroendocrinol* 15(9): 815	SPM / REMSd	96 h	ACTH / CORT plasma levels Relative adrenal weight Body weight Food intake Sucrose intake	↑ / ↑ ↑ ↓ ↑ ↑	HC control rats
2003 – Papakonstantinou *et al.*, *Physiol Behav* 78(4–5): 759	SPM / REMSd	48 or 96 h	CORT plasma levels Body temperature TNF-α	↑ 2 and 4 days ↑ 2 days ↓ 4 days	HC control rats
2004 – Martinez-Gonzalez *et al.*, *Sleep* 27(4): 609	Multiple platforms / REMSd	5 days	Fear-related behaviors: EPM (time in open arms) OF (time in center) Shock-induced freezing Defensive burying	↑ ↑ ↓ ↓	LP control rats
2005 – Andersen *et al.*, *J Sleep Res* 14(1): 83	SPM / REMSd	96 h of REMSd and 96 h of sleep recovery	Prolactin plasma levels ACTH and CORT plasma levels Noradrenaline plasma levels	↑ day 4 and ↓R1 ↑ day 1–day 4 and ↓R1 ↑ day 4 and ↓R1	Grouped HC control rats
2005 – Kim *et al.*, *Neurosci Lett* 388(3): 163	SPM / REMSd	5 days	CORT plasma levels LTP in hippocampal CA1	= ↓	LP control rats
2006 – Cirelli *et al.*, *J Neurochem* 98(5): 1632	DOW / TSD	7 days	Gene transcripts in cerebral cortex, stress response proteins: macrophage inhibitor factor-related protein 14, heat-shock protein 27, alpha-B-crystallin	↑	HC and yoked rats

Table 37.2 (*cont.*)

Reference	Method / type of deprivation	Length	Variable	Outcome (compared to control or otherwise specified)	Control group / species
2006 – Hipólide *et al.*, *J Neuroendocrinol* 18(4): 231	SPM / REMSd	96 h of REMSd and 96 h of sleep recovery	Body weight Food intake Insulin plasma levels ACTH plasma levels CORT plasma levels	↓ in REMSd / = recovery ↑ in REMSd / = recovery ↓ in REMSd / ↓ recovery ↑ in REMSd / = recovery ↑ in REMSd / ↑ recovery	Individual HC control rats
2006 – Koban *et al.*, *Endocrinology* 147(1): 421	SPM / REMSd	5, 10, 20 days	CRH immunoreactivity and mRNA expression	↑ at days 5 and 10 (peak at day 5)	Grouped HC control rats
2006 – Kopp *et al.*, *J Neurosci* 26(48): 12456	Gentle handling by knocking on the cage and nesting change / TSD	4 h	CORT plasma levels	=	Grouped HC control mice
2006 – Palshykova *et al.*, *Neurobiol Learn Mem* 85(3): 263	Gentle handling and nesting change / TSD	6 h	ACTH and CORT plasma levels	↑ / ↑	Grouped HC control mice
2006 – Palshykova *et al.*, *Physiol Behav* 87(1): 144	Gentle handling / TSD	30 min or 4 h	ACTH and cortisol plasma levels	= / =	Novelty (30 min) and HC hamsters
2006 – Sgoifo *et al.*, *Psychoneuro-endocrinology* 31(2): 197	Forced locomotion in slowly rotating drums / TSD	48 h	ACTH and CORT plasma levels ACTH and CORT responses to restraint Heart rate	↑ / ↑ ↓ / = ↑	HC rats
2006 – Wada *et al.*, *Brain Res Bull* 69(4): 388	Gentle handling with a soft brush / TSD	6 h	Heat shock protein 70 mRNA in the hippocampus	↑	HC control rats
2007 – Fenzl *et al.*, *J Neurosci Methods* 166(2): 229	Gentle handling and automated rotating drum / TSD	6 h	CORT plasma levels	=	HC mice Note: levels of sleep-deprived mice were twice as that of controls, but probably due to the high variability, no statistical difference was detected

Table 37.2 (cont.)

Reference	Method / type of deprivation	Length	Variable	Outcome (compared to control or otherwise specified)	Control group / species
2007 – Sánchez-Alavez et al., Brain Res 1158(1): 71	Gentle handling, introduction of novel objects / TSD	24 h	ACTH and CORT plasma levels	↑ / ↑	Baseline levels Prion protein knock-out mice
2008 – Everson et al., Am J Physiol 295(6): E2067	DOW / TSD	5 or 10 days	CORT plasma levels	=	Yoked rat Note: baseline levels were extremely high (four-fold the acceptable non-stress value). Yoked and sleep-deprived rats exhibited similarly high values
2008 – Machado et al., Psychoneuro-endocrinology 33(9): 1211	SPM / REMSd	96 h	ACTH and CORT plasma levels Prolactin plasma levels Heart rate	↑ / ↑ ↑ ↑	HC control rat
2008 – Mueller et al., Am J Physiol 294(5): R1693	SPM and MMPM / REMSd	96 h	CORT plasma levels Hippocampal neurogenesis	↑ ↓	HC control and stress control rat
2008 – Tiba et al., Sleep 31(4): 505	MMPM / REMSd	96 h	CORT plasma levels Contextual fear conditioning	↑ Impairment	HC control rat placed in the water tank for 1 h/day
2009 – Galvão et al., Psychoneuro-endocrinology 34(8): 1176	SPM / REMSd	96 h	ACTH and CORT plasma levels CRH immunoreactivity Orexin immunoreactivity	↑ / ↑ ↑ ↑	HC control rat
2009 – Tartar et al., Behav Brain Res 197(2): 450	Forced locomotion on the treadmill / TSD	24 h	CORT plasma levels Behavior in the OF	↑ ↓ anxiety	Exercise control and HC control rat

Abbreviations used: ACTH: adrenocorticotropic hormone; CORT: corticosterone; CRH: corticotropin-releasing factor; DOW: disk-over-water; EPM: elevated plus maze test; HC: home-cage; LC: locus coeruleus; LP: large platform; LTP: long-term potentiation; MMPM: modified multiple platform method; NA: noradrenaline; OF: open-field test; R1: Day 1 of sleep recovery; REMSd: REM sleep-deprivation; SPM: single platform method; TNF: tumour necrosis factor; TSD: total-sleep deprivation.

telling these events apart, there are a few studies that employ this approach. These studies are presented in Table 37.3; however, contrary to Table 37.2, we narrowed down the studies to fit two criteria: the studies must employ methods of REMSd and the duration must be at least 12 hours.

Involvement of glucocorticoids

Glucocorticoids represent the link between the periphery and the CNS under stressful conditions. Therefore, it is only natural to think that the effects of REMSd on numerous functions and systems could be mediated by

Table 37.3 Comparative effects of different types of stressors and REMSd on several sleep and physiological parameters

Reference	Method of REMSd	Length of REMSd	Comparative stressors	Measurement	Result
1994 – Corsi-Cabrera *et al.*, *Physiol Behav* 55(6): 1021–7	SPM	72 h and 24 h of sleep recovery	Swimming (SWIM) in cold water – 30 min/day	Waking EEG	REMSd: ↑ alpha band ↓ theta band (at 24 h) SWIM: ↓ theta band (at 24 h)
1995 – Nathan *et al.*, *Physiol Behav* 58(1): 181–4	Not used	–	Footshock (FS) – 1 h, twice/day/4 days SWIM – 1h, twice/day/4 days Immobilization (IMMO) – 22 h/4 days	Drug-induced yawning	Suppression by REMSd and IMMO
1996 – Pokk *et al.*, *Naunyn Schmiedebergs Arch Pharmacol* 354(6):703–8	SPM	24 h	Isolation SWIM	Cortical BDZ binding sites GABA-stimulated Cl⁻ uptake	REMSd: ↓ BDZ binding and ↓ Cl⁻ uptake Stressors had no effect
2000 – Palma *et al.*, *Brain Res* 861(1): 97–104	SPM	18 h	IMMO – 1 h FS – 1 h Cold (4°C) – 1 h	Stress-induced sleep rebound (for 6 h)	REMSd: ↑ NREM and REM sleep FS: ↑ sleep latency, ↓ NREM and REM sleep IMMO: ↑ NREM and REM sleep Cold: ↑ NREM sleep
2004 – Velazquez-Moctezuma *et al.*, *Neuroimmunomodulation* 11(4): 261–7	SPM	24 h (short-term) and 240 h (long-term)	IMMO – same periods	Lymphocyte distribution in peripheral blood	REMSd: Short- and long-term ↓ T lymphocytes and ↑ NK cells. Short-term IMMO: ↑ B lymphocytes and ↓ T lymphocytes. Long-term IMMO: no effect
2004 – Andersen *et al.*, *Braz J Med Biol Res* 37: 791–7	MMPM	96 h	IMMO – 1 h, twice for 1 day FS – 1 h, twice for 1 day Cold (4°C) – 1 h, twice for 1 day SWIM – 1 h, twice for 1 day	Testosterone, progesterone, estradiol plasma levels	
2005 – Papale *et al.*, *Brain Res* 1060(1/2): 47–54	Not used	–	IMMO – 22 h/day, for 4 days FS – 1 h, twice/day, for 4 days Cold (4° C) – 1 h, twice/day for 4 days SWIM – 1 h, twice/day for 4 days	Sleep pattern	IMMO: ↓ NREM and REM sleep on all days FS: ↓ NREM and REM sleep on days 3 and 4 Cold: No changes SWIM: ↓ NREM and ↑ REM on day 1, = baseline thereafter

List of abbreviations: BDZ: benzodiazepines; FS: footshock; GABA: gamma-aminobutyric acid; IMMO: immobilization stress; MMPM: modified multiple platform method; NREM: non-REM sleep; REM: rapid eye movement; REMSd: REM sleep deprivation; SPM: single platform method; SWIM: swimming stress.

increased levels of circulating GC. However, we have recently performed a series of studies that may indicate otherwise. Some of these functions and systems do indeed seem to be modulated by GC levels, whereas some appear to be partially modulated and others are not modulated at all.

One of the most replicable effects of REMSd is loss of body weight despite an increase in food intake (Elomaa, 1985; Everson and Wehr, 1993; Hipolide *et al.*, 2006; Koban *et al.*, 2008). Because the hypothalamus is the brain's homeostatic site that regulates, among other functions, sleep and feeding, we hypothesized that REMSd would result in changes in nuclei simultaneously involved in waking (since REMSd represents forced waking) and feeding. Body-weight variation, ACTH, and plasma CORT levels were also assessed throughout a four-day period of REMSd in the same animals, so correlations between these parameters could be done. The results of this study showed that REMSd produced activation of the HPA axis in its entirety, i.e., at the hypothalamic, pituitary, and adrenal levels, since we observed increased immunoreactivity to CRH at the end of the deprivation period, and peak secretion of ACTH and CORT by 24 hours of REMsd, with a gradual reduction of these levels toward the end of the experiment, but no return to control levels. The correlation test showed that rats that secreted more CORT during the REMSd period were the ones that also lost more weight (Galvao *et al.*, 2009). Moreover, by inhibiting the activity of CORT enzyme synthesis 11-βHSD, loss of body weight is prevented (Tiba *et al.*, 2008), indicating that body-weight variation during REMSd is modulated by GC.

The second study is related to the fact that some types of acute stress (immobilization, restraint, cold) produce a sleep rebound some hours after the end of the event (Cespuglio *et al.*, 1995; Palma *et al.*, 2000; Tiba *et al.*, 2004), whereas chronic stress impairs sleep (Cano *et al.*, 2008; Sanford *et al.*, 2003). Since prolonged REMSd produces sleep rebound, we tested whether the association with a chronic stressor could alter the stress response so as to impact on sleep pattern; our prediction being that chronic footshock would prevent the sleep rebound. Contrary to this prediction, chronic intermittent footshock given throughout REMSd resulted in a much greater REMS rebound, due to very long REMS episodes. Assessment of stress hormone levels, including ACTH, CORT, and prolactin demonstrated that REMS-deprived rats subjected to chronic footshock exhibited optimum CORT levels

(i.e., intermediate levels between basal and excessive stress response) associated with the highest prolactin levels (Machado *et al.*, 2008). These results suggest that moderate levels of CORT are important for REMS manifestation, which may be further increased by the association with high prolactin levels.

REM-sleep deprivation accomplished by either the single or modified multiple platform methods impairs the performance of rats in several memory tasks (Bueno *et al.*, 1994; Dametto *et al.*, 2002; Moreira *et al.*, 2003; Smith *et al.*, 1998; Youngblood *et al.*, 1997). Because some of the tasks used are related to the hippocampus, and the hippocampus is an important site of GC action, we asked whether REMSd-induced memory impairment in the contextual fear conditioning could be mediated by elevated GC levels. To answer this question, we administered metyrapone, twice per day, during the sleep-deprivation period. The results showed that although metyrapone was effective in maintaining GC levels close to basal, memory impairment was not prevented, being similar between saline- and drug-treated sleep-deprived groups, thus indicating that GC are not involved in this effect of REMSd and that impaired performance in this memory test is most likely due to loss of sleep (Tiba *et al.*, 2008). Similar results were reported after adrenalectomy, but because this intervention eliminates both GC and adrenaline, it was not possible to attribute the effect to one or other hormone with certainty (Ruskin *et al.*, 2006).

This brief review chapter has emphasized the inseparable nature of prolonged and unremitting REMSd from stress. From the studies presented in Table 37.2, it is possible to conclude that sleep-deprivation paradigms that last 12 hours or more do result in increased secretion of stress hormones. There are very few studies that fail to show this increase, most likely because levels of control rats are as high as those of sleep-deprived ones. Ideal resting basal levels of CORT in rats should not be above 5 µg/dl, but in these studies, yoked rats' values are usually two-fold higher (see Table 37.2).

It is important to emphasize that systems other than the HPA axis also play an important part in the stress response, including the sympathetic nervous system and prolactin. Most studies indicate that sleep deprivation results in augmented activity of the LC/medulla adrenal system, but there seems to be no consensus as to whether sleep deprivation induces prolactin secretion. Possibly, REMSd does induce prolactin secretion, whereas total-sleep deprivation reduces the release of this hormone. These differential effects could underlie the resulting sleep rebound that follows each type of deprivation.

Despite the subtleties that characterize the different methods of REMSd and total-sleep deprivation, all seem to be comparable with regard to the activation of classical hormonal stress response. Considering that sleep is essential to survival, sleep deprivation represents a threat to the organism, and therefore prompts the stress response to take place in order to restore homeostasis.

Acknowledgments

The authors are indebted to Lia Assae Esumi for drawing the figures and to Paula Ayako Tiba for her critical reading of this manuscript. The authors are recipients of fellowships from Conselho Nacional de Desenvolvimento Científico e Tecnológico (CNPq). This work is supported by grants from Fundação de Amparo à Pesquisa do Estado de São Paulo (FAPESP, Grant # 98–14303/3) and Associação Fundo de Incentivo à Psicofarmacologia (AFIP).

References

Bueno, O. F., Lobo, L. L., Oliveira, M. G., *et al.* (1994) Dissociated paradoxical sleep deprivation effects on inhibitory avoidance and conditioned fear. *Physiol Behav* **56**: 775–9.

Cano, G., Mochizuki, T. & Saper, C. B. (2008) Neural circuitry of stress-induced insomnia in rats. *J Neurosci* **28**: 10,167–84.

Carneiro, G., Togeiro, S. M., Hayashi, L. F. *et al.* (2008) Effect of continuous positive airway pressure therapy on hypothalamic-pituitary-adrenal axis function and 24-h blood pressure profile in obese men with obstructive sleep apnea syndrome. *Am J Physiol Endocrinol Metab* **295**: E380–4.

Cespuglio, R., Marinesco, S., Baubet, V., Bonnet, C. & El Kafi, B. (1995) Evidence for a sleep-promoting influence of stress. *Adv Neuroimmunol* **5**: 145–54.

Dametto, M., Suchecki, D., Bueno, O. F. *et al.* (2002) Social stress does not interact with paradoxical sleep deprivation-induced memory impairment. *Behav Brain Res* **129**: 171–8.

De Kloet, E. R., Vreugdenhil, E., Oitzl, M. S. & Joels, M. (1998) Brain corticosteroid receptor balance in health and disease. *Endocr Rev* **19**: 269–301.

Dement, W. (1960) The effect of dream deprivation. *Science* **131**: 1705–7.

Elomaa, E. (1985) Effects of rapid eye movement sleep deprivation on the feeding behavior in the laboratory rat with a description of the cuff pedestal technique. *Acta Physiol Scand Suppl* **545**: 1–35.

Everson, C. A. & Wehr, T. A. (1993) Nutritional and metabolic adaptations to prolonged sleep deprivation in the rat. *Am J Physiol* **264**: R376–87.

Galvao, M. D., Sinigaglia-Coimbra, R., Kawakami, S. E., Tufik, S. & Suchecki, D. (2009) Paradoxical sleep deprivation activates hypothalamic nuclei that regulate food intake and stress response. *Psychoneuroendocrinology* **34**: 1176–83.

Gulyani, S. & Mallick, B. N. (1993) Effect of rapid eye movement sleep deprivation on rat brain Na-K ATPase activity. *J Sleep Res* **2**: 45–50.

Gunnar, M. & Quevedo, K. (2007) The neurobiology of stress and development. *Annu Rev Psychol* **58**: 145–73.

Hipolide, D. C., Suchecki, D., Pimentel de Carvalho Pinto, A., *et al.* (2006) Paradoxical sleep deprivation and sleep recovery: effects on the hypothalamic-pituitary-adrenal axis activity, energy balance and body composition of rats. *J Neuroendocrinol* **18**: 231–8.

Kaur, S., Panchal, M., Faisal, M., *et al.* (2004) Long term blocking of GABA-A receptor in locus coeruleus by bilateral microinfusion of picrotoxin reduced rapid eye movement sleep and increased brain Na-K ATPase activity in freely moving normally behaving rats. *Behav Brain Res* **151**: 185–90.

Koban, M., Sita, L. V., Le, W. W. & Hoffman, G. E. (2008) Sleep deprivation of rats: the hyperphagic response is real. *Sleep* **31**: 927–33.

Kovalzon, V. M. & Tsibulsky, V. L. (1984) REM-sleep deprivation, stress and emotional behavior in rats. *Behav Brain Res* **14**: 235–45.

Machado, R. B., Hipolide, D. C., Benedito-Silva, A. A. & Tufik, S. (2004) Sleep deprivation induced by the modified multiple platform technique: quantification of sleep loss and recovery. *Brain Res* **1004**: 45–51.

Machado, R. B., Tufik, S. & Suchecki, D. (2008) Chronic stress during paradoxical sleep deprivation increases paradoxical sleep rebound: association with prolactin plasma levels and brain serotonin content. *Psychoneuroendocrinology* **33**: 1211–24.

McEwen, B. S. (2006) Protective and damaging effects of stress mediators: central role of the brain. *Dialogues Clin Neurosci* **8**: 367–81.

Morden, B., Mitchell, G. & Dement, W. (1967) Selective REM sleep deprivation and compensation phenomena in the rat. *Brain Res* **5**: 339–49.

Moreira, K. M., Hipolide, D. C., Nobrega, J. N. *et al.* (2003) Deficits in avoidance responding after paradoxical sleep deprivation are not associated with altered [3H] pirenzepine binding to M1 muscarinic receptors in rat brain. *Brain Res* **977**: 31–7.

Morilak, D. A., Barrera, G., Echevarria, D. J. *et al.* (2005) Role of brain norepinephrine in the behavioral response to stress. *Prog Neuropsychopharmacol Biol Psychiatry* **29**: 1214–24.

Palma, B. D., Suchecki, D. & Tufik, S. (2000) Differential effects of acute cold and footshock on the sleep of rats. *Brain Res* **861**: 97–104.

Ruskin, D. N., Dunn, K. E., Billiot, I., Bazan, N. G. & Lahoste, G. J. (2006) Eliminating the adrenal stress response does not affect sleep deprivation-induced acquisition deficits in the water maze. *Life Sci* **78**: 2833–8.

Sanford, L. D., Tang, X., Ross, R. J. & Morrison, A. R. (2003) Influence of shock training and explicit fear-conditioned cues on sleep architecture in mice: strain comparison. *Behav Genet* **33**: 43–58.

Sapolsky, R. M., Romero, L. M. & Munck, A. U. (2000) How do glucocorticoids influence stress responses? Integrating permissive, suppressive, stimulatory, and preparative actions. *Endocr Rev* **21**: 55–89.

Singh, S. & Mallick, B. N. (1996) Mild electrical stimulation of pontine tegmentum around locus coeruleus reduces rapid eye movement sleep in rats. *Neurosci Res* **24**: 227–35.

Smith, C. T., Conway, J. M. & Rose, G. M. (1998) Brief paradoxical sleep deprivation impairs reference, but not working, memory in the radial arm maze task. *Neurobiol Learn Mem* **69**: 211–17.

Spiegel, K., Leproult, R. & Van Cauter, E. (1999) Impact of sleep debt on metabolic and endocrine function. *Lancet* **354**: 1435–9.

Suchecki, D., Duarte Palma, B. & Tufik, S. (2000) Sleep rebound in animals deprived of paradoxical sleep by the modified multiple platform method. *Brain Res* **875**: 14–22.

Tiba, P. A., Tufik, S. & Suchecki, D. (2004) Effects of maternal separation on baseline sleep and cold stress-induced sleep rebound in adult Wistar rats. *Sleep* **27**: 1146–53.

Tiba, P. A., Oliveira, M. G., Rossi, V. C., Tufik, S. & Suchecki, D. (2008) Glucocorticoids are not responsible for paradoxical sleep deprivation-induced memory impairments. *Sleep* **31**: 505–15.

Vgontzas, A. N., Tsigos, C., Bixler, E. O. *et al.* (1998) Chronic insomnia and activity of the stress system: a preliminary study. *J Psychosom Res* **45**: 21–31.

Vgontzas, A. N., Bixler, E. O., Lin, H. M. *et al.* (2001) Chronic insomnia is associated with nyctohemeral activation of the hypothalamic-pituitary-adrenal axis: clinical implications. *J Clin Endocrinol Metab* **86**: 3787–94.

Youngblood, B. D., Zhou, J., Smagin, G. N., Ryan, D. H. & Harris, R. B. (1997) Sleep deprivation by the "flower pot" technique and spatial reference memory. *Physiol Behav* **61**: 249–56.

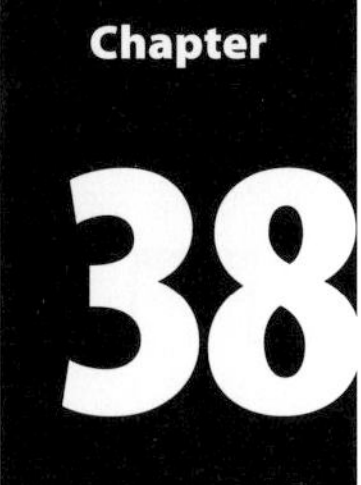

Chapter

38

REM sleep in patients with depression

Axel Steiger and Harald Murck

Summary

Disinhibition of REM sleep is a characteristic finding in patients with major depression. REM disinhibition includes shortened REM latency, prolonged first REM periods, and increased REM density (measure of the frequency of rapid eye movements). REM latency, but not REM density, is influenced by age. REM-sleep changes appear to be closely related to the development and the course of depression. A relationship between REM-sleep changes before treatment and treatment outcome is suggested by several studies. REM density is elevated in healthy subjects who have a high genetic load for affective disorders. Most antidepressants suppress REM sleep in patients, normal controls, and laboratory animals. REM-sleep suppression appears to be a distinct hint for the antidepressive properties of a substance, whereas it is not absolutely required. REM-sleep variables during treatment with antidepressants appear to predict the course of the illness. The noradrenergic locus coeruleus and the serotonergic dorsal raphe nuclei, the cholinergic nuclei, and the nucleus of the solitary tract (NTS) are involved in sleep and mood regulation. Hyperaldosteronism has been demonstrated in major depression. Subchronic aldosterone administration can induce anxiety-like behavior. Because of the unusual presence within the brain of both mineralocorticoid receptors and 11-β hydroxysteroid dehydrogenase (11-β HSD), the NTS can act as the gate of the influence of peripheral aldosterone into the brain. Importantly, aldosterone secretion is closely related to the REM/non-REM cycle and is sensitive to sleep manipulations. Hypersecretion of corticotropin-releasing hormone (CRH), the key hormone of the hypothalamo–pituitary–adrenocortical system appears to participate in the pathophysiology of REM-sleep disinhibition. This is supported by increased time spent in REM sleep in mice overexpressing corticotropin-releasing hormone (CRH) in the brain. Furthermore CRH-receptor-type 1 antagonism seems to induce normalization of the REM-sleep changes related to the depression.

Introduction

Two observations in the 1970s stimulated the interest of psychiatrists in sleep research and particularly in REM sleep. Firstly, David Kupfer suggested that a shortened REM latency, the interval between sleep onset and the first REM episode, is an indicator of depression (Kupfer and Foster, 1972). On the other hand, it was observed that most antidepressant drugs suppress REM sleep (Chen, 1979). These findings stimulated the ongoing research in various laboratories revealing complex results. This chapter aims to present the state of the art in this field.

Phenomenology of REM sleep in depression

In nearly all patients with major depression, sleep is impaired (Armitage, 2007). Characteristically REM sleep is disinhibited. The REM latency is shortened or sleep-onset REM periods (SOREMs) occur (REM latency 0 to 20 minutes). The first REM period is prolonged. The REM density (measure of the frequency of rapid eye movements) is increased, particularly during the first REM period. Other sleep-EEG changes in depression are impaired sleep continuity (prolonged sleep latency, increased intermittent awakenings, early morning awakening), and changes of non-REM sleep (decreases in slow-wave sleep [SWS], slow-wave activity [SWA], and stage 2 sleep; in younger patients a shift of SWS and SWA from the first to the second non-REM period) (Armitage, 2007) is frequently observed.

In patients with depression, and in normal control subjects as well, sleep is influenced by age. In two studies

REM Sleep: Regulation and Function, eds. Birendra N. Mallick, S. R. Pandi-Perumal, Robert W. McCarley, and Adrian R. Morrison. Published by Cambridge University Press. © Cambridge University Press 2011.

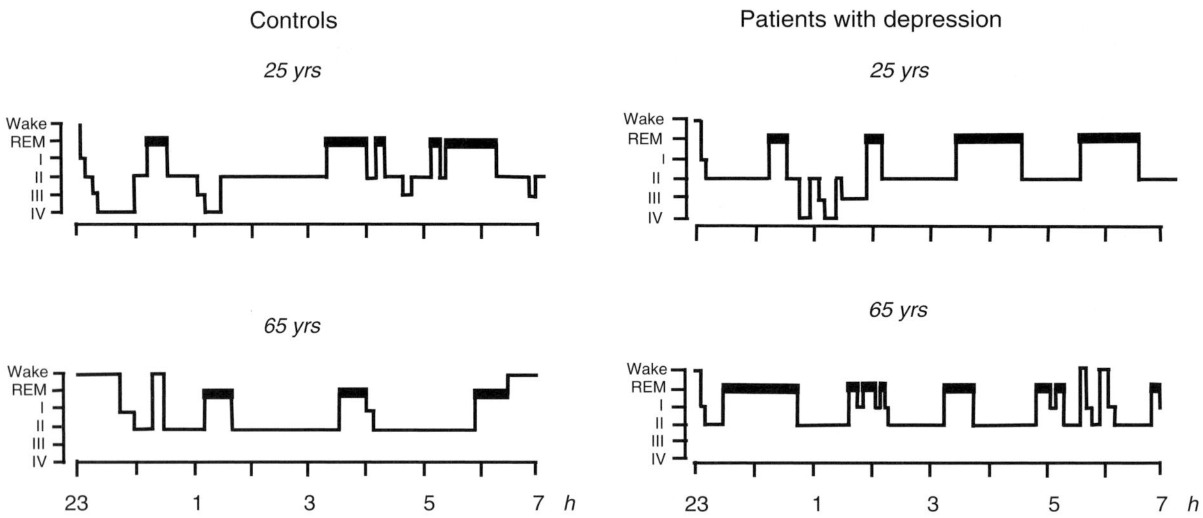

Figure 38.1 Hypnograms of young and older normal controls and patients with depression (Steiger, 2002, Fig. XXIV-3.1. Copyright John Wiley & Sons, Ltd, London. Reproduced with permission).

(Lauer *et al.*, 1991; Riemann *et al.*, 1991) age-related sleep-EEG changes were obvious in both patients with depression and in aged normal control subjects. REM latency was clearly affected by age, but until the middle of the fourth decade of the lifespan there were no differences between patients and controls. REM density, however, was not influenced by age and was higher in the patients than in the controls. Figure 38.1 depicts characteristic hypnograms in young and older normal controls and depressed patients.

A bimodal distribution of REM latency was found in patients with depression. Sleep-onset REM periods were observed in 20 to 30% of the patients, whereas REM latency between 20 and 40 minutes is rare. Between 40 and 60 minutes a second peak occurs, just below the normal range. In older patients and in patients with psychotic depression SOREMs are found frequently. No bimodal distribution of REM latency exists in these samples. REM sleep is disinhibited in depressed patients with insomnia and hypersomnia as well. Two studies compared sleep EEG between acute depression and stable remission for several weeks. At the initial examination the patients were drug free, than treated with antidepressants and were drug free again for several weeks at the second examination. Sleep-EEG variables, including REM-sleep measures did not differ between acute depression and recovery. Existing sleep-EEG changes in remitted patients may represent a biological scar. REM latency was permanently shortened, whereas depression improved in a sample of 12 drug-free patients who were investigated during three weeks every night (Steiger and Kimura, 2010).

An inverse correlation was found between REM latency and the severity of depression according to the Hamilton Depression (HAMD) score (Spiker *et al.*, 1978). In contrast in another report no relationship between sleep EEG and the severity of depression was found (Feinberg *et al.*, 1982). Most studies report no differences in the REM-sleep variables of depressed children and adolescents when compared to normal controls (Puig-Antich *et al.*, 1982), whereas other studies report increased REM-density and reduced REM-latency, similar to adults, but highlight the effect of age on REM-latency. (Lahmeyer *et al.*, 1983).

Several reports challenge the hypothesis that a shortened REM latency is a specific marker of depression. These have cited evidence of reduced REM latencies in schizophrenia, schizoaffective disorders, mania, panic disorders, obsessive–compulsive disorders, eating disorders, and sexual impotence (for a review see Steiger and Kimura, 2010). The observation of persisting REM-sleep changes in remitted patients suggests that a history of depression or a comorbidity with depression may explain a shortened REM latency in these disorders. This view is supported by two studies by Lauer and colleagues. These authors compared normal controls with three groups of patients with major depression, anorexia, and bulimia. The patients with eating disorders were never depressed. REM density was elevated in the patients with depression, whereas other variables did not differ between groups (Lauer *et al.*, 1990). In their other study, patients with depression, patients with panic disorder who were never depressed, and normal control subjects were compared. REM latency was shortened in both groups of patients compared to controls (Lauer *et al.*, 1992).

REM-sleep changes appear to be closely related to the development and the course of depression. An increasing abnormality of REM-sleep variables during subsequent episodes of depression was described in a long-term investigation. REM latency did not distinguish between first and recurrent episodes. However, increased phasic REM sleep was found in patients with recurrent unipolar depression. A relationship between REM-sleep changes before treatment and treatment outcome is suggested by several studies. Several reports found an association between shortened REM latency before treatment and the response to antidepressant drug therapy. A cluster of several disturbed sleep-EEG variables (REM latency, REM density, and sleep efficiency) improved the predicted power for treatment response to psychotherapy. The most robust predictor for remission after psychotherapy was low REM density, whereas REM density before psychotherapy was higher in patients who did not remit (Steiger and Kimura, 2010).

REM sleep in high-risk probands for affective disorders

A prospective high-risk design was applied in the Munich vulnerability study on affective disorders. In this study, healthy subjects who had a high genetic load for affective disorders because of a positive family history of the disease were investigated. The study's aim was to identify premorbid vulnerability factors. In these high-risk probands REM density was elevated and the amount of SWS during the first non-REM period was decreased at the index investigation when compared to normal controls from families without an elevated risk for affective disorders (Lauer *et al.*, 1995). These findings were stable in a follow-up investigation, which was performed about four years later (Modell *et al.*, 2002).

During the follow-up period of the Munich vulnerability study, 20 subjects of an initial sample of 82 high-risk probands exhibited signs of an affective disorder. At baseline the sleep EEGs of the high-risk probands showed an increased REM density during the total night and during the first REM period when compared with normal control subjects (Modell *et al.*,

2005). These results suggest that increased REM density meets all major requirements for a biological vulnerability marker for affective disorder: (i) it is found in patients with depression during the acute episode as well as in remission; (ii) it occurs already in healthy first-degree relatives of patients with affective disorders; (iii) it remains stable over time; and (iv) it is of predictive value for the onset of the disorder. REM density is recommended by the authors as a possible endophenotype in family studies (Modell *et al.*, 2005).

Effects of antidepressants on REM sleep

A common effect of most antidepressants is the suppression of REM sleep in patients, normal controls, and laboratory animals. In humans this effect is shared by tricyclics (with the exception of trimipramine and iprindol), by irreversible and short-acting reversible monoaminoxidase inhibitors, tetracyclics, selective serotonin reuptake inhibitors (SSRIs), selective noradrenaline reuptake inhibitors (NARIs), and selective serotonin and noradrenaline reuptake inhibitors (SNRIs) (for reviews see Chen, 1979; Steiger and Kimura, 2010).

Some studies show that early changes of REM-sleep parameters, especially REM latency and the percentage of REM time during the sleep period, might predict treatment outcome with substances that have an acute effect on REM sleep such as amitriptyline (Kupfer *et al.*, 1981), clomipramine, and imipramine (Sonntag *et al.*, 1996); but there are studies that could not confirm this, for example in the case of clomipramine. In a study comparing the effect of tianeptine vs. paroxetine, an inverse correlation between changes in REM density and changes in the HAMD score in patients who received paroxetine were reported, but no such correlation was found for tianeptine (see Figure 38.4) (Murck *et al.*, 2003b).

A few antidepressants lack a suppressive effect on REM sleep. These include bupropione, the serotonin reuptake enhancer tianeptine, and the noradrenergic and specific serotonergic antidepressant mirtazapine. REM suppression is characterized by increased REM latency and decreases of the amount of REM sleep and of REM density. After cessation of REM-suppressing antidepressants an REM rebound occurs (see Figure 38.2). During REM rebound REM latency decreases, and the amount of REM sleep and REM density increase exceeding baseline values. In healthy volunteers who received various antidepressants for two weeks the REM rebound after withdrawal of the substances still

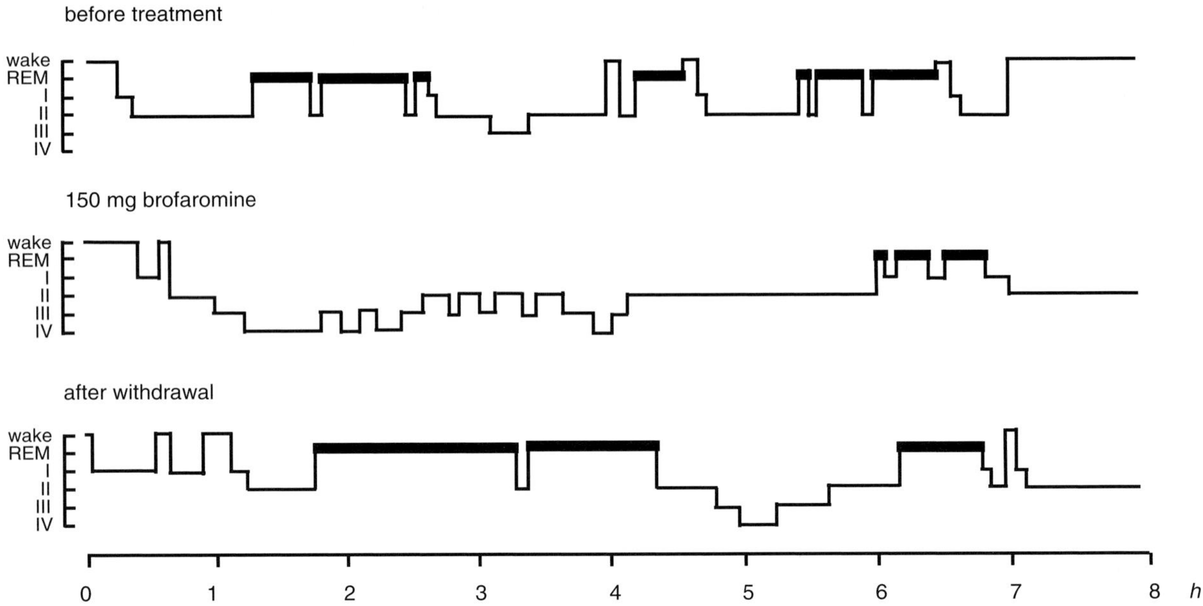

Figure 38.2 Sleep EEG before, during, and after treatment of a depressed patient with the reversible monoamine oxidase inhibitor brofaromine. (Steiger *et al.*, 1987, Fig. 2. © Georg Thieme Verlag Stuttgart, New York. Reproduced with permission).

persisted after one week. The potency of various antidepressants to suppress REM sleep differs. Clomipramine and the irreversible monoaminoxidase inhibitors phenelzine and tranylcypromine exert distinct suppressing effects on REM sleep. These substances are capable of abolishing REM sleep totally. This effect can last up to one week after the cessation of these monoaminoxidase inhibitors, at which time a REM rebound occurs. Similarly, REM sleep has been found to be suppressed nearly totally in normal control subjects following a single dose of the combined SSRI and serotonin 5-HT_{1A} receptor agonist vilazodone (formerly EMD 68843). In addition to differences between substances, the dosage and plasma concentration have been shown to influence the amount of REM-sleep suppression (for a review see Steiger and Kimura, 2010) (Figure 38.3).

REM suppression is shared by alcohol, amphetamines, and barbiturates. After subchronic administration of these substances an adaptation of REM sleep is found, whereas after antidepressants REM sleep remains suppressed for longer periods (Vogel, 1983). A weak adaptation was found after tricyclics. In two studies irreversible monoaminoxidase inhibitors totally suppressed REM sleep for several months. In contrast, small amounts of REM sleep were found to reoccur after three to six months of treatment with phenelzine in a group of three patients (for a review see Steiger and Kimura, 2010).

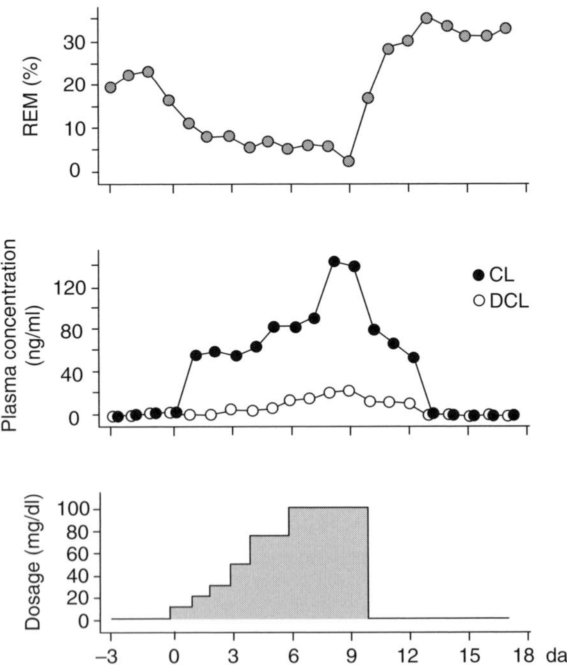

Figure 38.3 Courses of the percentage of REM sleep and the plasma concentration of clomipramine and desmethylclomipramine in a normal subject before, during, and after administration of clomipramine. (Steiger, 1999, Fig. 1. Copyright Wissenschaftliche Verlagsgesellschaft mbH, Stuttgart, 1999. Reproduced with permission).

Selective REM-sleep deprivation by awakenings, but not selective non-REM sleep deprivation for three weeks, promoted antidepressive effects (Vogel *et al.*, 1975). This finding, plus the observation that most antidepressants suppress REM sleep, support the view that REM suppression is a mechanism of the action of these drugs. However, the findings by Vogel *et al.* (1975) were not reproduced by another study (Grözinger *et al.*, 2002). Furthermore, this hypothesis is challenged by the fact that some antidepressants do not suppress REM sleep. Trimipramine and mirtazapine even increase REM sleep in patients with depression.

REM suppression appears to facilitate the antide-pressive properties of a compound, but it is not abso-lutely required. However, the importance of REM suppression is illustrated by studies comparing the effects of stereoisomers of oxaprotiline, R(–) oxapro-tiline and S(+) oxaprotiline. S(+) oxaprotiline was superior to R(–) oxaprotiline in its antidepressive effects. S(+) oxaprotiline, but not R(–) oxaprotiline, suppressed REM sleep in patients with depression (Steiger *et al.*, 1993a).

REM-sleep variables as predictors of the course of depression

Sleep-EEG profiles of patients with depression were investigated in order to determine whether (i) the retrospective clinical course as reflected by the num-ber of depressive episodes, and (ii) the prospective long-term outcome during the follow-up as reflected by the occurrence of further episodes, are associated with certain sleep-EEG variables (Hatzinger *et al.*, 2004). In this exploratory follow-up study 15 depressed patients were enrolled who participated in an earl-ier trial with trimipramine over six weeks. The study showed an association between sleep-EEG variables during acute depressive episodes as well as the long-term course of depression. At the end of drug treat-ment an association between elevated REM density (by trend), less SWS particularly during the first third of the sleep period, and the number of previous episodes is found. A clear association was shown between sleep EEG and the prospective long-term course of depres-sion: increased REM density and decreased SWS and the end of treatment were related to an increased recur-rence rate between the treatment study and the follow up. In addition the sleep-EEG variables were related to hypothalamo–pituitary–adrenocortical (HPA) system disturbance as mirrored by abnormal dexamethasone/corticotropin-releasing hormone (DEX/CRH) test results. Taken together, the evidence of this study dem-onstrates that patients with an unfavorable long-term course of depression show increasing aberrations in sleep regulation. These alterations could be of predict-ive value not only for treatment response during an acute episode of depression but also for the long-term outcome of depression. Furthermore the predictive sleep-EEG markers of the long-term course of depres-sion are closely related to HPA-system activity. The more the sleep EEG is disturbed, the more the HPA system shows deterioration. This finding is in line with the hypothesis that HPA overactivity contributes to sleep-EEG changes in depressed patients.

Neurophysiology of REM-sleep regulation

The implications of the sleep-EEG studies in patients with depression as well as in vulnerable subjects point to a dysfunction of REM-sleep regulation in a group of patients with major depression. In order to under-stand the potential implications for the physiological changes in major depression it is useful to understand the basic principles of REM-sleep regulation and how the involved systems may be dysregulated in depres-sion. The most relevant data are summarized in the reciprocal-interaction model, which was originally presented by Hobson *et al.* (1975).

This model describes the interplay between noradrenergic, serotonergic, and cholinergic pontine nuclei in the regulation of the ultradian non-REM–REM cycles. It is important in the current context, inas-much as most of the currently available conventional antidepressant substances affect the regulation of the pons-based transmitter systems. The model has been extended over time, but its original predictions are still valid. In short, the first element is a group of the cholin-ergic nuclei (pedunculopontine tegmental [PPT] and laterodorsal tegmental [LDT] nuclei), which project to the monoaminergic nuclei and excite them. The second element is established by the monoaminergic nuclei, i.e., the noradrenergic locus coeruleus (LC) and the seroton-ergic dorsal raphe nuclei (DRN), which reciprocally pro-ject to the cholinergic nuclei and inhibit them. The third element is a system of autoactivating cholinergic pro-jections to cholinergic nuclei, and the fourth is autoin-hibitory monoaminergic projections to monoaminergic nuclei. When these nuclei act in coordination, a repeti-tive cycle of REM and non-REM sleep occurs.

387

Important implications of this interplay include the close relation of sleep stages with the activity level of the noradrenergic LC (Aston-Jones and Bloom, 1981) and of the serotonergic DRN (Trulson and Jacobs, 1979). Both nuclei cease their electrical activity during REM sleep, have low activity during deep SWS, increase firing in light SWS, and have the highest rate during waking. Of note is that from this perspective REM sleep and SWS, which are often regarded as opposite ends of the spectrum of sleep, are in fact rather closely related. Furthermore, cholinergic activity is high in both REM sleep and wakefulness; however, there is also evidence that some wakefulness- and REM-inducing neurons are differentially regulated from purely REM-inducing neurons (Thakkar *et al.*, 1998).

Given these features it appears that there is a functional cholinergic overactivity during sleep in patients with depression. There could be different reasons for this: (i) increased activity of the cholinergic nuclei during the night; and (ii) increased sensitivity of cholinergic receptors on the basis of a low cholinergic activity during the day (counter-regulatory). In the depressive subtype with the most pronounced sleep disturbances, which include changes in REM sleep, i.e., melancholic depression, there is an apparent overactivity of the noradrenergic system as determined by the concentration of cerebrospinal norepinephrine (NE), the main neurotransmitter of the LC (Wong *et al.*, 2000). According to the reciprocal-interaction model this should indeed be related to a reduced activity of the cholinergic nuclei. This is, however, not in line with the increase in REM sleep. An overactive LC during the day, which is related to

high stress levels and high sympathetic nervous system activity, would induce a cholinergic sensitization due to the reduced cholinergic activity. A test of this hypothesis is the cholinergic REM-sleep induction test. In this test a cholinergic substance is administered before sleep and its effect on REM sleep is observed. In previous studies cholinergic stimulation has been found to produce REM-sleep induction in patients with depression, which was more pronounced than that of healthy controls (Berger *et al.*, 1985; Gillin *et al.*, 1979; Jones *et al.*, 1985) or euthymic patients with a history of major depression (Sitaram *et al.*, 1980). Interestingly, this increased sensitivity was also observed in high-risk probands of the Munich vulnerability study for depression: at baseline REM latency did not differ between high-risk probands and normal control subjects. However, after cholinergic stimulation REM latency was distinctly shortened in the high-risk probands (Schreiber *et al.*, 1992). This finding suggests a threshold cholinergic dysfunction in high-risk probands for affective disorders. Their response pattern in the cholinergic REM-sleep induction test was predictive for the onset of the first depressive episode (Lauer *et al.*, 2004). This suggests that a cholinergic deficit during the day, as a consequence of a high noradrenergic activity, could induce a cholinergic supersensitivity during the night with the consequence of disinhibited REM-sleep generation. This is in line with observations that the administration of the cholinergic antagonist scopolamine, given in the morning for three consecutive days, leads to REM-sleep changes similar to those seen in depression. The reason for this cholinergic dysfunction during the day

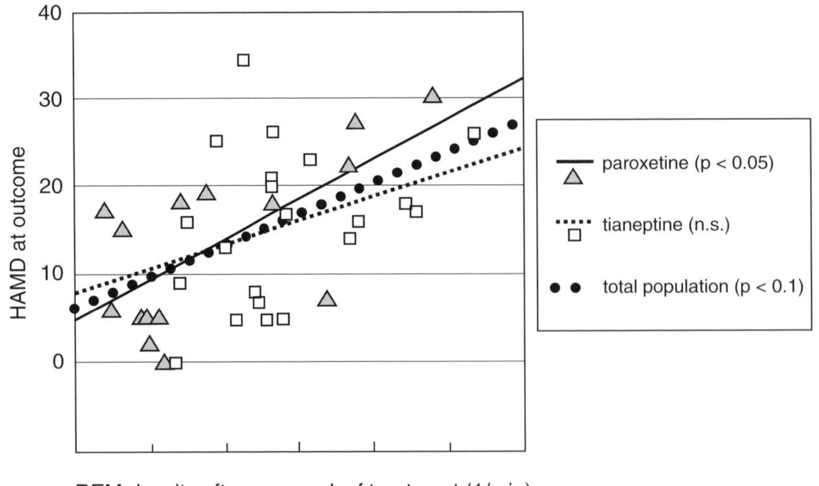

Figure 38.4 Hamilton Depression (HAMD) score at day 42 in relation to the REM density at day 7. With paroxetine REM density at day 7 is correlated to treatment outcome, whereas with tianeptine no significant correlation is found. (Murck *et al.*, 2003b, Fig. 3).

may be related to increased LC activity, as discussed above. In this context it has recently been proposed that all antidepressant interventions are associated with decreased LC activity (West *et al.*, 2009), which is also a consequence of sleep deprivation, in particular REM-sleep deprivation (Mallick *et al.*, 1990; Porkka-Heiskanen *et al.*, 1995) .

The role of neuroendocrine systems in REM-sleep changes in depression

Enhanced sleep-associated levels of cortisol (Linkowski *et al.*, 1987; Steiger *et al.*, 1989) and ACTH (Linkowski *et al.*, 1987) are state markers of acute depressive episodes. Increased HPA axis activity appears to be related to sleep disturbances, in particular reduced sleep duration and reduced SWS (Hubain *et al.*, 1998). The central neuropeptide corticotropin-releasing hormone (CRH) is a key hormone regulating humoral and behavioral adaptation to stress (De Kloet *et al.*, 2005). Prolonged CRH hypersecretion is thought to play a key role in the development and course of depression. In order to investigate the specific effects of CRH overexpression in the CNS on sleep Kimura *et al.* (2009) used conditional mouse mutants that overexpress CRH in the entire central nervous system (CRH-COE-Nes) or only in the forebrain, including limbic structures (CRH-COE-Cam). Compared with the wildtype or control mice, homozygous CRH-COE-Nes (see Figure 38.5) and -Cam mice showed increased REM sleep throughout 24 hours at baseline. Non-REM sleep was suppressed only in the CRH-COE-Nes mice during the light period. After sleep deprivation increased REM sleep

was found also in heterocygous CRH-COE-Nes and -Cam mice, in comparison to control mice, during recovery sleep. This effect was reversed by treatment with a CRH receptor type 1 antagonist (DNP696) in heterozygous and homozygous CRH-COE-Nes mice. The peripheral stress hormone levels were neither elevated at baseline nor after sleep deprivation across genotypes. Therefore the sleep-EEG changes, in particular the elevated REM sleep in these models, are most likely induced by the forebrain CRH via activation of CRH receptor type 1. Corticotropin-releasing hormone hypersecretion in the forebrain appears to drive REM sleep and to contribute to REM-sleep disinhibition in depression.

This view is supported by a clinical trial in which the CRH-1-receptor type 1 antagonist R121919 was administered in two different dosages to inpatients with major depression over a four-week period. Three sleep-EEG recordings were performed in a random subgroup of ten patients (baseline before treatment, at the end of the first week, and at the end of the fourth week of active treatment). Compared with baseline after one week and after four weeks REM density and the number of awakenings showed a decreasing trend. During the same period the time spent in SWS increased. Separate evaluation of these changes for two dosages of R121919 showed no significant effects of the lower dose, whereas at the higher dose REM density decreased and SWS increased significantly between baseline and the fourth week (Held *et al.*, 2004). These data suggest that CRH-1-receptor type 1 antagonism exerts a normalizing influence on the sleep EEG in patients with depression. A significant association was found between REM density during the first half

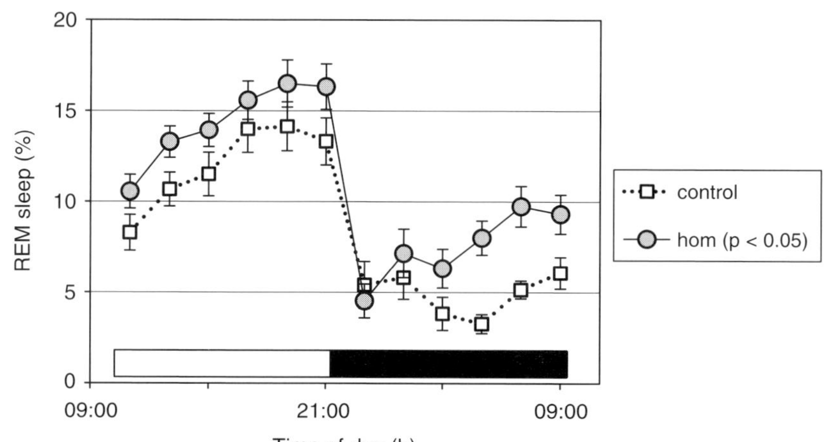

Figure 38.5 Enhanced REM sleep in CNS-specific corticotropin-releasing hormone conditionally overexpressing (CRH-COE-Nes) mice. Data points ± SEM indicates 2-hour average in time spent in REM sleep during a baseline recording day: squares, CRH-COE-Nes control mice (n = 20); circles, CRH-COE-Nes homozygous (hom) mice (n = 21). Compared with control mice, CRH-COE-Nes hom mice showed significant increases in REM sleep throughout a day. Open and closed bars indicate the light and dark period, respectively.

of the night at baseline and the relative improvement of HAMD scores after four weeks of treatment with R121919 (Holsboer and Ising, 2010).

It is important to keep in mind that CRH-stimulated ACTH release triggers in turn not only the release of cortisol, but also of aldosterone, as demonstrated by the reduction of aldosterone by the synthetic glucucorticoid dexamethasone (Takeda *et al.*, 1984). Angiotensin II (ATII) has an additional stimulatory effect on aldosterone, which itself is relased by renin. In fact, in addition to increases in HPA axis activity, an increase in aldosterone secretion in patients with depression has been reported (Murck *et al.*, 2003a) and independently confirmed (Emanuele *et al.*, 2005).

With regard to REM-sleep regulation it is important to note that the highest correlation between the REM–non-REM sleep changes with any neuroendocrine system is that of renin and aldosterone release. Both hormones show peaks related to SWS and are low during REM-sleep (Brandenberger *et al.*, 1994; Charloux *et al.*, 1999).

In order to elucidate the interaction of steroid hormones in REM-sleep regulation the following observations are important. Steroid hormones have clear effects on REM sleep. (1) The administration of the glucocorticoid (GR) and mineralocorticoid (MR) agonist cortisol leads to a reduction in REM sleep, accompanied by an increase in SWS (Born *et al.*, 1987; Friess *et al.*, 1994). (2) Administration of the selective GR-agonist dexamethasone after four to six days leads to a reduction of both REM and SWS duration (Born *et al.*, 1991). (3) Short-term administration of dexamethasone and the combination of dexamethasone and the MR antagonist spironolactone lead to a similar reduction in REM sleep (Wiedemann *et al.*, 1994). This shows that one of the effects of dexamethasone is to reduce GR- and MR-activation by depleting cortisol and aldosterone from the system. (4) Administration of aldosterone (Born *et al.*, 1987) or of the mineralocorticoid deoxycorticosterone (Steiger *et al.*, 1993b) at the beginning of the sleep period, i.e., a period of already high RAAS activity, does not have a major effect on the sleep EEG. (5) Administration of the synthetic glucocorticoid and weak mineralocorticoid receptor agonist methylprednisolone to female patients with multiple sclerosis results in REM-sleep changes similar to those found during acute depression (increased REM density, shortened REM latency). Furthermore,

SWS and SWA shift from the first to the second sleep cycle (Antonijevic and Steiger, 2003).

These data are confusing and difficult to interpret, when the assumption is made that the observed effects are direct consequences of GR or MR engagement. It is important to take the close interaction between GR- and MR-regulating systems into account. (1) Mineralocorticoid antagonism leads to an increase in cortisol by reducing the MR-mediated hippocampal feedback inhibition of the HPA system. (2) Aldosterone itself has a direct influence on MR receptors only in areas that contain 11-beta hydroxysteroid dehydrogenase (type 2) (11-beta HSD-2), as otherwise the higher concentrations of cortisol occupy MR receptors. This is the case for most situations in the hippocampus. There is primarily one anatomical region that contains both MR and 11-beta-HSD, i.e., the nucleus tractus solitarius (NTS) (Geerling *et al.*, 2006). This is a potentially extremely important insight, because the NTS is centrally involved in both REM- and slow wave-sleep regulation (Gottesmann, 1999) as well as in mood regulation (Nemeroff *et al.*, 2006), as it acts as the first-line target of vagus nerve stimulation, which has antidepressant efficacy. In this context it is important to note that stimulation of the vagus nerve leads to pronounced changes in sleep EEG, in particular an increase in REM activity in the cat (Valdes-Cruz *et al.*, 2002). (3) Peripherally administered GR-agonists lead to suppression of both cortisol and aldosterone and therefore can lead to a reduced activation of MR both in the hippocampus and the NTS. Mineralocorticoid receptors in the NTS are probably more sensitive to this change than hippocampal ones, inasmuch as the latter can still be activated by low cortisol concentrations.

How can the influences of the activation of MR vs. GR be dissected, taking the anatomical locations into account? Following the above-reviewed findings one emerging pattern is that all interventions that reduce MR activation at the level of the NTS (or other aldosterone sensitive areas), but not reduction at the level of the hippocampus (or other areas where the MR is mainly occupied by cortisol) lead to reduced REM activity. On this basis we propose the following working hypothesis: MR activation, in particular at the level of the NTS, is a requirement for REM-sleep generation. High MR activation at the hippocampal level seems to be required for SWS, this may be counteracted by high GR activation.

This hypothesis is in line with most of the reviewed observations, in detail:

- Combined acute administration of dexamethasone and/or spironolactone (depletion of cortisol and aldosterone from the brain) leads to:

  at the NTS: low MR activation ⇒ reduced REM sleep;

  at the hippocampus: low MR activation, intermediate GR activation ⇒ no significant SWS change.

- Cortisol administration depletes aldosterone and leads to:

  at the NTS: low MR activation ⇒ reduced REM sleep;

  at the hippocampus: high MR activation, high GR activation ⇒ high SWS.

- Long-term dexamethasone leads to a direct GR activation and reduction of aldosterone from the brain:

  at the NTS: low MR activation ⇒ reduced REM sleep;

  at the hippocampus: low MR activation, high GR activation ⇒ reduced SWS.

- Administration of canrenoate (at doses increasing cortisol and aldosterone) leads to:

  at the NTS: potentially low MR activation (but increased aldosterone has to be considered) ⇒ no change in REM (unexpectedly);

  at the hippocampus: low MR activation, high GR activation ⇒ reduced SWS.

- Subchronic administration of methylprednisolone leads to:

  at the NTS: high MR activation ⇒increased REM activity;

  at the hippocampus: high MR activation, very high GR activation ⇒ reorganized SWS.

The contrast of the effect of long-term (10 days) methylprednisolone administration (primarily GR, but a weak MR agonist) with that of dexamethasone (pure GR agonist) are particularly interesting, as the changes in REM sleep are opposite: methylprednisolone leads to increased REM activity, and dexamethasone to REM-sleep suppression.

The evidence for this regulation is nevertheless only circumstantial at present. Direct local blockade of the systems would be required for a final proof. Nevertheless it makes biological sense that sleep is influenced by MR located at the NTS, given the close synchronicity between aldosterone secretion and REM–non-REM rhythmicity. It is also in line with the general fact that SWS-related aldosterone release may be required before REM sleep can occur, as is the case during sleep in healthy subjects. With the finding of increased aldosterone secretion in depression (see above), this hypothesis would also account for disinhibited REM sleep in major depression. It is finally also in line with the observation that sleep deprivation, which is associated with an absence of the sleep-related aldosterone surge (Charloux *et al.*, 2001), leads to a reduced REM activity during recovery sleep in depression, and is further accompanied by a rebound in renin release (Murck *et al.*, 2006).

Conclusions

REM-sleep changes occur in many, but not all, patients with a depressive syndrome. Many, but not all, antidepressant compounds lead to a suppression of REM sleep. The neuronal areas that are involved in sleep regulation overlap broadly with those involved in mood regulation. Neuroendocrine signals influence these systems, but the interactions are complex. Besides the classic role of the monoaminergic nuclei LC, DRN, and the cholinergic REM-generating neurons a recently rediscovered neuronal influence is established by the nucleus of the solitary tract (NTS). This nucleus is linked to broad autonomic regulation, including neuroendocrine signaling. It may also be the gate of influence of peripheral aldosterone, which is closely related to sleep regulation as well as to some forms of depression. Corticotropin-releasing hormone hypersecretion in the basal forebrain appears to promote REM sleep. CRH-receptor-type 1 antagonists seem to help to normalize REM-sleep disinhibition related to depression.

In general, REM-sleep changes have an important role in determining the neurobiology of depression, as well as the action of antidepressant compounds. This is based on the overlap between REM-sleep regulation and mood-regulating anatomical areas as well as its close interaction with neuroendocrine systems.

Acknowledgments

We thank Dr Mayumi Kimura for preparing Figure 38.5.

References

Antonijevic, I. A. & Steiger, A. (2003) Depression-like changes of the sleep-EEG during high dose corticosteroid treatment in patients with multiple sclerosis. *Psychoneuroendocrinol* **28**: 780–95.

Armitage, R. (2007) Sleep and circadian rhythms in mood disorders. *Acta Psychiatr Scand* **115**(Suppl. 433): 104–15.

Aston-Jones, G. & Bloom, F. E. (1981) Activity of norepinephrine-containing locus coeruleus neurons in behaving rats anticipates fluctuations in the sleep–waking cycle. *J Neurosci* **1**:876–86.

Berger, M., Höchli, D., Zulley, J., Lauer, C. & von Zerssen, D. (1985) Cholinomimetic drug RS 86, REM sleep, and depression. *Lancet* **1**: 1385–6.

Born, J., De Kloet, E. R., Wenz, H., Kern, W. & Fehm, H. L. (1991) Gluco- and antimineralocorticoid effects on human sleep: a role of central corticosteroid receptors. *Am J Physiol: Endocr Metab* **260**: E183–8.

Born, J., Zwick, A., Roth, G., Fehm-Wolfsdorf, G. & Fehm, H. L. (1987) Differential effects of hydrocortisone, fluocortolone, and aldosterone on nocturnal sleep in humans. *Acta Endocrinol (Copenhagen)* **116**: 129–37.

Brandenberger, G., Follenius, M., Goichot, B. *et al.* (1994) Twenty-four-hour profiles of plasma renin activity in relation to the sleep-wake cycle. *J Hypertension* **12**: 277–83.

Charloux, A., Gronfier, C., Lonsdorfer-Wolf, E., Piquard, F. & Brandenberger, G. (1999) Aldosterone release during the sleep-wake cycle in humans. *Am J Physiol* **276**: E43–9.

Charloux, A., Gronfier, C., Chapotot, F., *et al.* (2001) Sleep deprivation blunts the night time increase in aldosterone release in humans. *J Sleep Res* **10**: 27–33.

Chen, C. N. (1979) Sleep, depression and antidepressants. *Br J Psychiatry* **135**: 385–402.

De Kloet, E. R., Joels, M. & Holsboer, F. (2005) Stress and the brain: from adaptation to disease. *Nat Rev Neurosci* **6**: 463–75.

Emanuele, E., Geroldi, D., Minoretti, P., Coen, E. & Politi, P. (2005) Increased plasma aldosterone in patients with clinical depression. *Arch Med Res* **36**: 544–8.

Feinberg, M., Gillin, J. C., Carroll, B. J., Greden, J. F. & Zis, A. P. (1982) EEG studies of sleep in the diagnosis of depression. *Biol Psychiatry* **17**: 305–16.

Friess, E., von Bardeleben, U., Wiedemann, K., Lauer, C. & Holsboer, F. (1994) Effects of pulsatile cortisol infusion on sleep-EEG and nocturnal growth hormone release in healthy men. *J Sleep Res* **3**: 73–9.

Geerling, J. C., Kawata, M. & Loewy, A. D. (2006) Aldosterone-sensitive neurons in the rat central nervous system. *J Comp Neurol* **494**: 515–27.

Gillin, J. C., Sitaram, N. & Duncan, W. C. (1979) Muscarinic supersensitivity: a possible model for the sleep disturbance of primary depression? *Psychiatry Res* **1**: 17–22.

Gottesmann, C. (1999) The neurophysiology of sleep and waking: intracerebral connections, functioning and ascending influences of the medulla oblongata. *Prog Neurobiol* **59**: 1–54.

Grözinger, M., Kogel, P. & Röschke, J. (2002) Effects of REM sleep awakenings and related wakening paradigms on the ultradian sleep cycle and the symptoms in depression. *J Psychiatric Res* **36**: 299–308.

Hatzinger, M., Hemmeter, U. M., Brand, S., Ising, M. & Holsboer-Trachsler, E. (2004) Electroencephalographic sleep profiles in treatment course and long-term outcome of major depression: association with DEX/CRH-test response. *J Psychiatric Res* **38**: 453–65.

Held, K., Künzel, H., Ising, M. *et al.* (2004) Treatment with the CRH1-receptor antagonist R121919 improves sleep EEG in patients with depression. *J Psychiatric Res* **38**: 129–36.

Hobson, J. A., McCarley, R. W. & Wyzinski, P. W. (1975) Sleep cycle oscillation: reciprocal discharge by two brainstem neuronal groups. *Science* **189**: 55–8.

Holsboer, F. & Ising, M. (2010) Stress hormones and stress hormone regulation: Biological role and behavioral effects. *Ann Rev Psychol* **61**: 81–109.

Hubain, P. P., Staner, L., Dramaix, M. *et al.* (1998) The dexamethasone suppression test and sleep electroencephalogram in nonbipolar major depressed inpatients: a multivariate analysis. *Biol Psychiatry* **43**: 220–9.

Jones, D., Kelwala, S., Bell, J. *et al.* (1985) Cholinergic REM sleep induction response correlation with endogenous major depressive subtype. *Psychiatry Res* **14**: 99–110.

Kimura, M., Müller-Preuss, P., Lu, A. *et al.* (2009) Conditional corticotropin-releasing hormone overexpression in the mouse forebrain enhances rapid eye movement sleep. *Mol Psychiatry* doi:10.1038/mp.2009.54.

Kupfer, D. J. & Foster, F. G. (1972) Interval between onset of sleep and rapid-eye-movement sleep as an indicator of depression. *Lancet* **2**: 684–6.

Kupfer, D. J., Spiker, D. G., Coble, P. A. *et al.* (1981) Sleep and treatment prediction in endogenous depression. *Am J Psychiatry* **138**: 429–34.

Lahmeyer, H. W., Poznanski, E. O. & Bellur, S. N. (1983) EEG sleep in depressed adolescents. *Am J Psychiatry* **140**: 1150–3.

Lauer, C. J., Krieg, J. C., Riemann, D., Zulley, J. & Berger, M. (1990) A polysomnographic study in young psychiatric inpatients: major depression, anorexia nervosa, bulimia nervosa. *J Affect Disord* **18**: 235–45.

Lauer, C., Riemann, D., Wiegand, M. & Berger, M. (1991) From early to late adulthood. Changes in EEG sleep of depressed patients and healthy volunteers. *Biol Psychiatry* **29**: 979–93.

Lauer, C. J., Krieg, J. C., Garcia-Borreguero, D., Özdaglar, A. & Holsboer, F. (1992) Panic disorder and major depression: A comparative electroencephalogramic sleep study. *Psychiatry Res* **44**: 41–54.

Lauer, C. J., Schreiber, W., Holsboer, F. & Krieg, J. C. (1995) In quest of identifying vulnerability markers for psychiatric disorders by all-night polysomnography. *Arch Gen Psychiatry* **52**: 145–53.

Lauer, C. J., Modell, S., Schreiber, W., Krieg, J. C. & Holsboer, F. (2004) Prediction of the development of a first major depressive episode with a rapid eye movement sleep induction test using the cholinergic agonist RS 86. *J Clin Psychopharmacol* **24**: 356–7.

Linkowski, P., Mendlewicz, J., Kerkhofs, M. *et al.* (1987) 24-hour profiles of adrenocorticotropin, cortisol, and growth hormone in major depressive illness: effect of antidepressant treatment. *J Clin Endocrinol Metab* **65**: 141–52.

Mallick, B. N., Siegel, J. M. & Fahringer, H. (1990) Changes in pontine unit activity with REM sleep deprivation. *Brain Res* **515**: 94–8.

Modell, S., Ising, M., Holsboer, F. & Lauer, C. J. (2002) The Munich Vulnerability Study on Affective Disorders: stability of polysomnographic findings over time. *Biol Psychiatry* **52**: 430–7.

Modell, S., Ising, M., Holsboer, F. & Lauer, C. J. (2005) The Munich vulnerability study on affective disorders: premorbid polysomnographic profile of affected high-risk probands. *Biol Psychiatry* **58**: 694–9.

Murck, H., Held, K., Ziegenbein, M., Koch, K. & Steiger, A. (2003a) The renin-angiotensin-aldosterone system in patients with depression compared to controls – a sleep endocrine study. *BMC Psychiatry* **29**: 3–15.

Murck, H., Nickel, T., Künzel, H. *et al.* (2003b) State markers of depression in sleep EEG: Dependency on drug and gender in patients treated with tianeptine or paroxetine. *Neuropsychopharmacol* **28**: 348–58.

Murck, H., Uhr, M., Ziegenbein, M. *et al.* (2006) Renin–Angiotensin–Aldosterone system, HPA-axis, and sleep-EEG changes in unmedicated patients with depression after total sleep deprivation. *Pharmacopsychiatry* **39**: 1–7.

Nemeroff, C. B., Mayberg, H. S., Krahl, S. E. *et al.* (2006) VNS therapy in treatment-resistant depression: clinical evidence and putative neurobiological mechanisms. *Neuropsychopharmacol* **31**: 1345–55.

Porkka-Heiskanen, T., Smith, S. E., Taira, T. *et al.* (1995) Noradrenergic activity in rat brain during rapid eye movement sleep deprivation and rebound sleep. *Am J Physiol Reg, Integr Comp Physiol* **268**: R1456–R63.

Puig-Antich, J., Goetz, R., Hanlon, C. *et al.* (1982) Sleep architecture and REM sleep measures in prepubertal children with major depression: a controlled study. *Arch Gen Psychiatry* **39**: 932–39.

Riemann, D., Hohagen, F., Lauer, C. & Berger, M. (1991) Long-term evolution of sleep in depression. In *Sleep and Aging*, eds. S. Smirne, M. Franceschi & L. Ferini-Strambi. Paris: Masson, pp. 195–204.

Schreiber, W., Lauer, C. J., Krumrey, K., Holsboer, F. & Krieg, J. C. (1992) Cholinergic REM sleep induction test in subjects at high risk for psychiatric disorders. *Biol Psychiatry* **32**: 79–90.

Sitaram, N., Nurnberger, J. I., Jr., Gershon, E. S. & Gillin, J. C. (1980) Faster cholinergic REM sleep induction in euthymic patients with primary affective illness. *Science* **208**: 200–2.

Sonntag, A., Rothe, B., Guldner, J. *et al.* (1996) Trimipramine and imipramine exert different effects on the sleep EEG and on nocturnal hormone secretion during treatment of major depression. *Depression* **4**: 1–13.

Spiker, D. G., Coble, P., Cofsky, J., Foster, F.G. & Kupfer, D. J. (1978) EEG sleep and severity of depression. *Biol Psychiatry* **13**: 485–8.

Steiger, A. (1999) Unterschiede in den Wirkungen von Antidepressiva auf den Schlaf. *Psychopharmakotherapie* **3**: 91–5.

Steiger, A. (2002) Neuroendocrinology of sleep disorders. In *Textbook of Biological Psychiatry*. eds. H. d'Haenen, J. A. den Boer, H. Westenberg & P. Willner. London: John Wiley & Sons, pp. 1229–46.

Steiger, A. & Kimura, M. (2010) Wake and sleep-EEG provide biomarkers in depression. *J Psychiatric Res* **44**(4): 242–52.

Steiger, A., Holsboer, F., Gerken, A., Demisch, L., Benkert, O. (1987) Results of an open clinical trial of brofaromine (CGP 11 305 A), a competitive, selective, and short-acting inhibitor of MAO-A in major endogenous depression. *Pharmacopsychiatry* **20**: 262–9.

Steiger, A., von Bardeleben, U., Herth, T. & Holsboer, F. (1989) Sleep EEG and nocturnal secretion of cortisol and growth hormone in male patients with endogenous depression before treatment and after recovery. *J Affect Disord* **16**: 189–95.

Steiger, A., Gerken, A., Benkert, O. & Holsboer, F. (1993a) Differential effects of the enantiomers R(–) and S(+) oxaprotiline on major endogenous depression, the sleep EEG and neuroendocrine secretion: studies on depressed patients and normal controls. *Eur Neuropsychopharmacol* **3**: 117–26.

Steiger, A., Rupprecht, R., Spengler, D. *et al.* (1993b) Functional properties of deoxycorticosterone and spironolactone: molecular characterization and effects on sleep-endocrine activity. *Journal of Psychiatric Research* **27**: 275–84.

Takeda, R., Miyamori, I., Ikeda, M. *et al.* (1984) Circadian rhythm of plasma aldosterone and time dependent alterations of aldosterone regulators. *J Steroid Biochem* **20**: 321–3.

Thakkar, M. M., Strecker, R. E. & McCarley, R. W. (1998) Behavioral state control through differential serotonergic inhibition in the mesopontine cholinergic nuclei: a simultaneous unit recording and microdialysis study. *J Neurosci* **18**: 5490–7.

Trulson, M. E. & Jacobs, B. L. (1979) Raphe unit activity in freely moving cats: correlation with level of behavioral arousal. *Brain Res* **163**: 135–50.

Valdes-Cruz, A., Magdaleno-Madrigal, V. M., Martinez-Vargas, D. *et al.* (2002) Chronic stimulation of the cat vagus nerve: effect on sleep and behavior. *Prog Neuro-Psychopharmacol Biol Psychiatry* **26**: 113–18.

Vogel, G. W. (1983) Evidence for REM sleep deprivation as the mechanism of action of antidepressant drugs. *Prog Neuro-Psychopharmacol Biol Psychiatry* **7**: 343–9.

Vogel, G. W., Thurmond, A., Gibbons, P., Sloan, K. & Walker, M. (1975) REM sleep reduction effects on depression syndromes. *Arch Gen Psychiatry* **32**: 765–77.

West, C. H. K., Ritchie, J. C., Boss-Williams, K. A. & Weiss, J. M. (2009) Antidepressant drugs with differing pharmacological actions decrease activity of locus coeruleus neurons. *Int J Neuropsychopharmacol* **12**: 627–41.

Wiedemann, K., Lauer, C., Pollmächer, T. & Holsboer, F. (1994) Sleep-endocrine effects of antigluco- and antimineralocorticoids in healthy males. *Am J Physiol Endocrin Metab* **267**:E109–E14.

Wong, M. L., Kling, M. A., Munson, P. J. *et al.* (2000) Pronounced and sustained central hypernoradrenergic function in major depression with melancholic features: relation to hypercortisolism and corticotropin-releasing hormone. *Proc Natnl Acad Sci USA* **97**: 325–30.

Chapter 39

Proteins and neuropeptides in REM-sleep regulation and function

Radhika Basheer

Summary

Rapid eye movement sleep (REMS), first described by Aserinsky and Kleitman (1953), is a distinct state during sleep when the electroencephalographic (EEG) recordings appear similar to those observed during wake with low-voltage, high-frequency asynchronous activity, whereas the electromyographic (EMG) recordings, unlike wake, show lowest levels of muscle tone (muscle atonia), accompanied by rapid eye movements detectable by electro-oculographic (EOG) recordings. This paradoxical vigilant state combining wake-like cortical activation and inactive state-like muscle atonia with rapid eye movements has been extensively studied using animal model systems since the 1950s. Today much is known about the brain regions, neuronal networks, and neurotransmitters involved in REMS regulation (Fort *et al.*, 2009; Jones, 2004; Luppi *et al.*, 2006; McCarley, 2007). However, promising discoveries about the mechanisms depend on the identification of molecular processes that are involved in the transition and maintenance of different vigilant states, especially REMS, which is recognized for its brevity. The recent advances in molecular biology, instrumentation, and bioinformatics further extend novel opportunities to understand the mechanisms involved in REMS regulation and its function. Currently, no study has identified a single specific protein needed for REM generation or maintenance, but several proteins have been identified as changing either during REMS or following REMS deprivation, indicating their involvement in REMS. This chapter will begin with a brief review of the genomic and proteomic studies on sleep followed by a review of reports on REMS describing these different proteins, which include transcription factors, receptors, enzymes, and small peptides, and how they have contributed significantly towards the anatomical localization of REMS-associated brain regions and neurotransmitter phenotype of neurons, and toward a better understanding of REMS regulation and function.

Introduction

As early as 1909 and 1910 the idea of sleep induction by accumulating endogenous chemical substances was tested by injecting either substances extracted from the brain or the cerebrospinal fluid from sleep-deprived dogs into naïve recipients (Ishimori, 1909; Legendre and Pieron, 1910). Since then, the twentieth century has witnessed remarkable progress in the investigations of such an idea in different animal models suggesting the "endogenous sleep substances" are likely to be polypeptide hormones or proteins (Inoue, 1989). With the advent of microarray technology, the last decade has witnessed several reports on genomic expression analysis in rodents, birds, and flies associated with the sleep–wake state and alterations induced by sleep deprivation (Cirelli, 2009; Mackiewicz *et al.*, 2007). The changes in gene expression are suggestive of potential cellular alterations associated with different vigilant states; however, the complexity of the regulation of downstream processes such as translation of mRNA into protein, post-translational modifications of translated proteins, protein–protein interactions etc., prevents a direct assessment of the effect of gene expression on physiological processes. Since proteins are the ultimate players capable of influencing vigilance states it is important to understand the significance of proteomics. Proteomics is an experimental approach to explain the information contained in the genomic sequences in terms of the structure, function, and control of biological processes and pathways. The proteome indicates the quantitative expression profile of a cell, an organism, or a tissue under defined conditions. In contrast to the temporally constant genome,

---

REM Sleep: Regulation and Function, eds. Birendra N. Mallick, S. R. Pandi-Perumal, Robert W. McCarley, and Adrian R. Morrison. Published by Cambridge University Press. © Cambridge University Press 2011.

the proteome is dependent on intracellular and extracellular parameters, dynamics, and variables. Thus, the analysis of a proteome represents an important supplementation to genome analysis.

The use of various proteomic approaches for investigating the regulation of vigilant states is relatively new. As the efficiency of proteomic methodology is being refined for increased sensitivity and inclusion of a wider range of proteins, a few attempts have already been made to explore overall protein changes during sleep–wake state and prolonged waking (Basheer *et al.*, 2005; Cirelli *et al.*, 2009; Pawlyk *et al.*, 2007; Poirrier *et al.*, 2008; Vazquez *et al.*, 2008). Most of these studies in the cortex, basal forebrain, or hippocampus of the rat brain have compared protein profiles of sleep with prolonged sleep deprivation. So far only two studies have examined protein changes after ten minutes of spontaneous sleep or wake (Vazquez *et al.*, 2008, 2009) and no studies have examined proteomic changes selective to REMS. Major challenges for such studies originate from the short durations of REMS episodes in rodents, a model system that has proven ideal for such profiling. Nevertheless, the short duration of this vigilant state dictates that rapid activation/inactivation of the proteins involved in membrane receptors and intracellular signaling as well as protein–protein interactions are key to transitions into and maintenance of REMS.

An association of protein synthesis during the REMS state was described as early as the 1970s. Sleep-associated increased levels of mRNA of proteins involved in protein synthesis (observed in genome-wide gene expression studies) strongly suggest that protein synthesis is enhanced during sleep (Cirelli, 2009; Mackiewicz *et al.*, 2007). Further supportive evidence is made available from the positive correlation between protein synthesis and sleep reported in several studies (Drucker-Colin *et al.*, 1975; Nakanishi *et al.*, 1997; Ramm and Smith, 1990; Reich *et al.*, 1967, 1973; Voronka *et al.*, 1971). In particular, administration of protein synthesis inhibitors such as chloramphenicol reduced REM sleep in rats (Kitahama and Valatx, 1975; Rojas-Ramirez *et al.*, 1977). Moreover, REM-sleep rebound during withdrawal from chronic amphetamine administration was blocked by suggesting protein synthesis is essential for REMS (Drucker-Coli and Benitez, 1977). These reports strongly indicated the need for protein synthesis in REMS and the occurrence of quantitative and qualitative changes in proteins during REMS. Although no studies have

succeeded in assessing changes in the entire proteome during REMS in any part of the brain region, there are several proteins that have been selectively examined and shown to be involved in REMS and are associated with the functions of REMS as described in the following sections.

Transcription factors and neurotransmitter synthesizing proteins

Since the landmark reports in 1975 on the reciprocal-interaction model of REMS by Robert McCarley and Allan Hobson (Hobson *et al.*, 1975; McCarley and Hobson, 1975a,b) describing the balance between the REM-on (neurons active during REMS) and REM-off (neurons that cease firing during REMS) components in the regulation of REMS, many reports have used specific proteins for the anatomical localization of neuronal activation during REMS and for identifying the neurotransmitter phenotype of such neurons. While discussing the proteins associated with REM, these neuroanatomical studies utilizing protein immunohistochemical approaches lead REMS investigation.

Several intracellular proteins have been used in immunohistochemical techniques in attempts to establish REMS circuitry. These studies parallel and complement the electrophysiological characterization of neurons during REMS. One such protein widely used for REMS studies is c-Fos. The transcription factor c-Fos is an archetype of the set of cellular immediate–early proteins that are responsible for coupling short-term signals elicited by extracellular environments to alterations in the cellular phenotype by orchestrating changes in expression of several target genes (Morgan and Curran, 1991). Induction of c-Fos and its detection in neuronal nuclei is considered suggestive of neuronal activation. Thus, with some exceptions (Kovacs, 2008), many have successfully utilized induction of c-Fos expression and nuclear detection of phosphorylated (activated) c-Fos protein as a tool for functional anatomical mapping within the brain (Dragunow and Faull, 1989; Sagar *et al.*, 1988). Immunohistochemical techniques to identify c-Fos expressing cells often used double labeling for the neurotransmitters (GABA or serotonin, etc.) or the biosynthetic proteins (enzymes) for a specific neurotransmitter, such as tyrosine hydroxylase (TH for noradrenergic neurons), choline acetyl transferase (ChAT for cholinergic neurons), and glutamic acid decarboxylase (GAD for GABAergic neurons).

The initial studies that used c-Fos protein induction for localization of REMS-associated areas, used carbachol microinjection into the pontine reticular formation (PRF) in cats. This induced REMS-like state was accompanied by the presence of c-Fos immunoreactivity in brain-stem areas such as the locus coeruleus (LC), dorsal raphe nucleus (DRN), pedenculopontine tegmentum (PPT), laterodorsal tegmentum (LDT), medial PRF, and medulla (Shiromani *et al.*, 1992; Yamuy *et al.*, 1993). Later, several studies in rats utilized c-Fos immunohistochemistry for identification of REM-on neurons by performing three days of REM deprivation using the widely used flower-pot technique (Mendelson *et al.*, 1974) followed by a recovery REMS rebound period. Most studies used double-labeling immunohistochemistry of c-Fos with either specific neurotransmitter or their biosynthetic proteins (enzymes) to identify the neurotransmitter nature of the neurons that are activated during REMS recovery. These approaches identified the pontomes-encephalic cholinergic neurons using ChAT, pon-tomedullary reticular neurons to be GABAergic using GAD, and raphe neurons using serotonin (Ser) double labeling as components of REMS circuitry (Maloney *et al.*, 1999, 2000; Verret *et al.*, 2005). Using the same paradigm of REMS rebound, other studies used double labeling of c-Fos with retrograde tracer cholera toxin injected into the LC. The results showed that the dorsal and lateral paragigantocellular reticular nucleus and the ventrolateral periaqueductal gray send inhibitory GABAergic projections to the LC resulting in inhibition of noradrenergic neurons during REMS (Luppi *et al.*, 2006; Verret *et al.*, 2006).

A recent study demonstrated the use of a transcriptional activator, cyclic AMP response element binding protein (CREB), in the identification of REMS-associated activated neurons (Datta *et al.*, 2009). The phosphorylated form of CREB (pCREB) is an important transcriptional activator in neurons that transduces the effects of receptor activations associated with cyclic AMP production in the cell (Brindle and Montminy, 1992) and is much recognized for its role in synaptic plasticity, long-term potentiation, and memory (Silva *et al.*, 1998). Datta *et al.* (2009) showed that there exists a positive correlation between the increased REMS and the number of pCREB-positive cells in REM-active areas of the medial pontine reticular formation (mPRF), pontine reticular nucleus oral (PnO), and dorsal subcoeruleus nucleus (SubCD); whereas very little pCREB staining is observed in the LC and DRN where neuronal activity almost ceases during REMS. Thus protein immunohistochemistry for transcription factors in combination with neurotransmitter markers have been extensively used in the anatomical localization of brain regions and neurons involved in REMS.

Signal transduction and membrane-associated proteins

Intracellular enzymes that catalyze reactions in order to transduce extracellular signals following specific cell-surface receptor activation constitute an important class of proteins that impact downstream processes, such as protein phosphorylation, protein synthesis, or transcription of genes. A few such proteins have been identified and shown to be involved in REMS-associated processes.

The inhibitory $G_{(i/o)}$-coupled enzyme adenylate cyclase has been shown to play a role in mediating GABA-receptor effects in the REM-associated brain-stem region of the PPT. Inhibition of adenylate cyclase due to the action of GABA on GABAb receptors on REM-on neurons in the PPT leads to REMS suppression (Datta and Prutzman, 2005). This mechanism is suggested to involve another intracellular enzyme, protein kinase A (PKA), whose activation is dependent on cyclic-adenosine monophosphate (cAMP) – a product of the reaction catalyzed by activated adenylate cyclase. Pharmacologically enhanced activation of PKA in the PPT also enhances REMS induction, whereas suppression of cAMP production resulting in decreased activation of PKA leads to REMS suppression (Bandyopadhya *et al.*, 2006; Datta, 2007). Contrary to the effect of PKA on REMS, activation of calcium/calmodulin- dependent enzyme, CaM-Kinase II has been shown to decrease REMS and increase waking. This effect is suggested to be in response to the activation of the NMDA receptor in PPT neurons and subsequent increase in intracellular calcium availability (Stack *et al.*, 2010). CaM-Kinase II, quite abundant in the brain, is a serine/threonine kinase, recognized for its crucial role in aspects of plasticity at glutamatergic synapses. Sustained activation of CaM-Kinase II localized at the postsynaptic density results in phosphorylation of numerous synaptic substrates including ion channels, other signaling molecules, and scaffolding proteins, to modulate synaptic transmission within minutes (Soderling *et al.*, 2001). Increased expression of CaM-Kinase II protein and its activity in the PPT has been shown to correlate positively with waking and negatively with REMS (Stack *et al.*, 2010).

The LC noradrenergic system is an integral component of REMS. The expression of proteins responsible for the biosynthesis of norepinephrine, TH, and the membrane norepinephrine transporter (NET) are regulated in the LC in response to REMS induction or deprivation. These neurons almost cease firing during REM sleep (McCarley and Hobson, 1975a,b). On the contrary, during REMS deprivation they continue to fire, releasing an excessive amount of norepinephrine. The activity of TH in the brain was first shown to increase following REMS deprivation (Sinha *et al.*, 1973). Later experiments showed that the mRNA expression of TH and NET are upregulated during such prolonged REMS deprivation (Basheer *et al.*, 1998). A differential effect on the activities of monoamine oxidase (MOA) with a direct bearing on the noradrenergic system was observed in rat brain regions following REMS deprivation (Thakkar and Mallick, 1993b). Overactivation of the LC also results in an upregulation of the protein, $Na^+K^+ATPase$, responsible for the maintenance of the membrane ionic gradient in neurons (Mallick *et al.*, 2010). Both the activity and the expression of this protein increase following REMS deprivation (Adya and Mallick, 2000). These authors have recently shown that REMS-specific increase in $Na^+K^+ATPase$ activity is specific to the neuronal fraction, whereas the glial enzyme shows a decrease in activity (Baskey *et al.*, 2009). Thus this membrane protein is likely involved in regulation of REM sleep that is dependent on the norepinephrine release from the LC neurons.

The activity of acetylcholinesterase, an enzyme responsible for the breakdown of acetylcholine, has been shown to increase in brain-stem pontine regions but not in the cerebellum (Thakkar and Mallick, 1991). The activity of energy-regulating metabolic enzymes, such as glucose 6-phosphate and hexokinase, have also been shown to be altered by REMS deprivation. The former showed decreased activity with short term (one day), whereas the latter showed an increased activity following four days of REMS deprivation (Thakkar and Mallick, 1993a). Although the changes in the activities of these enzyme proteins in brain-stem areas provide supporting evidence for the involvement of the pontine region in REM regulation, the mechanistic role is not clear and needs further investigation.

Neuropeptides

Neuropeptides are short-length polypeptide (protein-like) molecules that are expressed and released by neurons and modulate neuronal communication by acting on cell-surface receptors. Several such neuropeptides have been recognized for their role in modulating REMS (de Lecea and Bourgin, 2008). The most important neurotransmitter associated with REMS is orexin (or hypocretin), first described by two independent groups (de Lecea *et al.*, 1998; Sakurai *et al.*, 1998) and later shown to be associated with the sleep disorder, narcolepsy (Chemelli *et al.*, 1999; Lin *et al.*, 1999). A decade of intense research has confirmed its role in waking. Orexin deficiency leads to sleep fragmentation with direct entry in REMS during waking and is suggestive of its action at REM-on neurons during wake. The role of orexin in regulating the REM gate is a complex one and is discussed in detail by other authors in this book.

Two additional peptides, pituitary adenylate cyclase activating polypeptide (PACAP) or vasoactive intestinal peptide (VIP) when administered into the ventricles, enhance REMS that lasts for several days (Ahnaou *et al.*, 1999; Bourgin *et al.*, 1999). The actions of these peptides are suggested to be mediated through the PAC1 receptors located at the pontine reticular formation (Ahnaou *et al.*, 1999). Immunohistochemistry demonstrated a dense network of PACAP-staining cell bodies and fibers in the pontine reticular formation, whereas VIP cell bodies and fibers are located in the dorsal raphe (Ahnaou *et al.*, 2006). Thus the activity of neurons at two pontine REM-associated areas is modulated by PACAP and VIP. Another neuropeptide hormone, prolactin, has been suggested to be involved in enhancing the REM-promoting activity of VIP (Roky *et al.*, 1995).

Urotensin II (UII), a cyclic peptide with a core structure (a hydrophobic tetrad FWKY) that shares similarities with somatostatin and cortistatin, and another closely related peptide, urotensin related peptide (URP) have been shown to modulate REMS through their actions on brain-stem cholinergic neurons (Huitron-Resendiz *et al.*, 2005). Urotensin II receptor mRNA colocalizes with ChAT in the PPT and LDT but is not detected in basal forebrain cholinergic neurons (Clark *et al.*, 2001). Localized injection of UII into the PPT but not in the LC induced significant increase in REMS and an increase in theta and gamma activities during REM and wakefulness, respectively (Huitron-Resendiz *et al.*, 2005). Whole-cell recordings from the brain slices showed that, like orexin, UII also selectively excites cholinergic neurons in the PPT and increases cholinergic tone (Clark *et al.*, 2005).

REMS and memory: proteins involved in synaptic plasticity and long-term potentiation

One of the presumed functions of REMS is to enhance memory consolidation both in humans and animals (Siegel, 2001; Stickgold and Walker, 2007) and REMS has been associated with protein synthesis. Both short-term memory and long-term memory involve protein modifications. The former depends on modification of pre-existing proteins, whereas the latter requires transcription and synthesis of new proteins (Costa-Mattioli *et al.*, 2009). In rodents the mechanisms involved in memory formation are studied at the cellular level using a model that measures changes in synaptic strength, termed long-term potentiation (LTP) and long-term depression (LTD) (Kandel, 2001). Long-term potentiation and memory share similar molecular and cellular mechanisms (Neves *et al.*, 2008). Early LTP (E-LTP) is similar to short-term memory lasting one to two hours, and is typically induced by a single train of high-frequency (titanic) stimulation of an efferent pathway. The late-LTP (L-LTP) persists for many hours and is induced by repeated titanic trains (Costa-Mattioli *et al.*, 2009). Several proteins have been identified as participants in the process of synaptic potentiation, and REMS deprivation has been shown to reduce the levels of these proteins and thus LTP. For example, REMS deprivation performed during early development results in decreased levels of N-methyl-D-aspartate receptor subunits 2A and 2B (NR2A and NR2B), AMPA receptor subunit 1 (GluR1), postsynaptic density protein 95 (PSD-95), and CaMkinase II in the hippocampus leading to reduced stability of LTP (Lopez *et al.*, 2008). In adult rats 72 hours of REMS deprivation results in similar reduction in GluR1 and NMDA receptor subunit NR1, but not in NR2B and the phosphorylated extracellular signal-regulated kinases (pERK) leading to specific impairments in L-LTP in the dorsal hippocampus (Ravassard *et al.*, 2009). Contrary to synaptic proteins, in the hippocampus, the activity of cytosolic protein calcineurin increases with REMS deprivation (Wang *et al.*, 2009). Calcineurin is a phosphatase dependent on calcium/calmodulin, which is abundant in brain. This phosphatase dephosphorylates pCREB and inhibits the expression of proteins needed for long-term memory (Mansuy, 2003). Thus, REMS deprivation-induced increased activity of calcineurin is suggested to inhibit processes involved in memory, specifically spatial memory. Together, these reports clearly demonstrate the regulation of important proteins with a bearing on the function of REMS in memory formation and consolidation. This exciting area will be explored widely for other molecular players in the future.

REM sleep, apoptosis, and neurogenesis

Disturbances in the mitochondrial proteins in hippocampus CA1 pyramidal neurons have been reported following REMS deprivation. One of the major components of the oxidative phosphorylation, cytochrome c, is released into the cytoplasm following REMS deprivation along with an increased transport of a membrane-pore forming protein, Bax (Yang *et al.*, 2008). Bax is known to respond to proapoptotic stimuli by increasing the permeabilization of the outer mitochondrial membrane, allowing intermembrane proteins such as cytochrome c to escape into the cytosol and induce capsase activation (Antignani and Youle, 2006). Increased transport of Bax to mitochondria accompanied by increased cytosolic release of cytochrome c and changes in the structural proteins such as tubulin and actin during REMS deprivation may underlie the increase in apoptotic markers observed in the rat brain (Biswas *et al.*, 2006). REMS deprivation also contributes to the reduction in neurogenesis in rat dentate gyrus (Guzman-Marin *et al.*, 2008). These reports indicate that REMS is important not only for preventing deterioration of cellular health and causing cell death, but is also essential for proliferation and differentiation of progenitor cells into neurons in the adult brain.

In summary, research in the last 25 years has succeeded in identifying several proteins that either modulate REMS or are associated with one or more functions of REMS. Proteomic technology is fast evolving and this method of investigation not only promises information on a larger number of proteins that will help toward a better understanding of the mechanisms involved in the regulation of physiological processes such as REM sleep, but will also be essential to design treatment strategies for REMS disorders.

References

Adya, H. V. & Mallick, B. N. (2000) Uncompetitive stimulation of rat brain Na-K ATPase activity by rapid eye movement sleep deprivation. *Neurochem Int* **36**: 249–53.

Ahnaou, A., Basille, M., Gonzalez, B. *et al.* (1999) Long-term enhancement of REM sleep by the pituitary adenylyl cyclase-activating polypeptide (PACAP) in the pontine reticular formation of the rat. *Eur J Neurosci* **11**: 4051–8.

Ahnaou, A., Yon, L., Arluison, M. *et al.* (2006) Immunocytochemical distribution of VIP and PACAP in the rat brain stem: implications for REM sleep physiology. *Ann N Y Acad Sci* **1070**: 135–42.

Antignani, A. & Youle, R. J. (2006) How do Bax and Bak lead to permeabilization of the outer mitochondrial membrane? *Curr Opin Cell Biol* **18**: 685–9.

Aserinsky, E. & Kleitman, N. (1953) Regularly occurring periods of eye motility, and concomitant phenomena, during sleep. *Science* **118**: 273–4.

Bandyopadhya, R. S., Datta, S. & Saha, S. (2006) Activation of pedunculopontine tegmental protein kinase A: a mechanism for rapid eye movement sleep generation in the freely moving rat. *J Neurosci* **26**: 8931–42.

Basheer, R., Magner, M., McCarley, R. W. & Shiromani, P. J. (1998) REM sleep deprivation increases the levels of tyrosine hydroxylase and norepinephrine transporter mRNA in the locus coeruleus. *Brain Res Mol Brain Res* **57**: 235–40.

Basheer, R., Brown, R., Ramesh, V., Begum, S. & McCarley, R. W. (2005) Sleep deprivation-induced protein changes in basal forebrain: implications for synaptic plasticity. *J Neurosci Res* **82**: 650–8.

Baskey, G., Singh, A., Sharma, R. & Mallick, B. N. (2009) REM sleep deprivation-induced noradrenaline stimulates neuronal and inhibits glial Na-K ATPase in rat brain: in vivo and in vitro studies. *Neurochem Int* **54**: 65–71.

Biswas, S., Mishra, P., Mallick, B. N. (2006) Increased apoptosis in rat brain after rapid eye movement sleep loss. *Neuroscience* **142**: 315–31.

Bourgin, P., Ahnaou, A., Laporte, A. M., Hamon, M. & Adrien, J. (1999) Rapid eye movement sleep induction by vasoactive intestinal peptide infused into the oral pontine tegmentum of the rat may involve muscarinic receptors. *Neuroscience* **89**: 291–302.

Brindle, P. K. & Montminy, M. R. (1992) The CREB family of transcription activators. *Curr Opin Genet Dev* **2**: 199–204.

Chemelli, R. M., Willie, J. T., Sinton, C. M. *et al.* (1999) Narcolepsy in orexin knockout mice: molecular genetics of sleep regulation. *Cell* **98**: 437–51.

Cirelli, C. (2009) The genetic and molecular regulation of sleep: from fruit flies to humans. *Nat Rev Neurosci* **10**: 549–60.

Cirelli, C., Pfister-Genskow, M., McCarthy, D., Woodbury, R. & Tononi, G. (2009) Proteomic profiling of the rat cerebral cortex in sleep and waking. *Arch Ital Biol* **147**: 59–68.

Clark, S. D., Nothacker, H. P., Wang, Z. *et al.* (2001) The urotensin II receptor is expressed in the cholinergic mesopontine tegmentum of the rat. *Brain Res* **923**: 120–7.

Clark, S. D., Nothacker, H. P., Blaha, C. D. *et al.* (2005) Urotensin II acts as a modulator of mesopontine cholinergic neurons. *Brain Res* **1059**: 139–48.

Costa-Mattioli, M., Sossin, W. S., Klann, E. & Sonenberg, N. (2009) Translational control of long-lasting synaptic plasticity and memory. *Neuron* **61**: 10–26.

Datta, S. (2007) Activation of pedunculopontine tegmental PKA prevents GABAB receptor activation-mediated rapid eye movement sleep suppression in the freely moving rat. *J Neurophysiol* **97**: 3841–50.

Datta, S. & Prutzman, S. L. (2005) Novel role of brain stem pedunculopontine tegmental adenylyl cyclase in the regulation of spontaneous REM sleep in the freely moving rat. *J Neurophysiol* **94**: 1928–37.

Datta, S., Siwek, D. F. & Stack, E. C. (2009) Identification of cholinergic and non-cholinergic neurons in the pons expressing phosphorylated cyclic adenosine monophosphate response element-binding protein as a function of rapid eye movement sleep. *Neuroscience* **163**: 397–414.

de Lecea, L. & Bourgin, P. (2008) Neuropeptide interactions and REM sleep: a role for Urotensin II? *Peptides* **29**: 845–51.

de Lecea, L., Kilduff, T. S., Peyron, C. *et al.* (1998) The hypocretins: hypothalamus-specific peptides with neuroexcitatory activity. *Proc Natl Acad Sci U S A* **95**: 322–7.

Dragunow, M. & Faull, R. (1989) The use of c-fos as a metabolic marker in neuronal pathway tracing. *J Neurosci Methods* **29**: 261–5.

Drucker-Coli, R. & Benitez, J. (1977) REM sleep rebound during withdrawal from chronic amphetamine administration is blocked by chloramphenicol. *Neurosci Lett* **6**: 267–71.

Drucker-Colin, R. R., Spanis, C. W., Cotman, C. W. & McGaugh, J. L. (1975) Changes in protein levels in perfusates of freely moving cats: relation to behavioral state. *Science* **187**: 963–5.

Fort, P., Bassetti, C. L. & Luppi, P. H. (2009) Alternating vigilance states: new insights regarding neuronal networks and mechanisms. *Eur J Neurosci* **29**: 1741–53.

Guzman-Marin, R., Suntsova, N., Bashir, T. *et al.* (2008) Rapid eye movement sleep deprivation contributes to reduction of neurogenesis in the hippocampal dentate gyrus of the adult rat. *Sleep* **31**: 167–75.

Hobson, J. A., McCarley, R. W. & Wyzinski, P. W. (1975) Sleep cycle oscillation: reciprocal discharge by two brainstem neuronal groups. *Science* **189**: 55–8.

Huitron-Resendiz, S., Kristensen, M. P., Sanchez-Alavez, M. *et al.* (2005) Urotensin II modulates rapid eye movement sleep through activation of brainstem cholinergic neurons. *J Neurosci* **25**: 5465–74.

Inoue, S. (1989) Mechanism of sleep and insomnia. *Kangogaku Zasshi* **53**: 754–60. (Japanese. No abstract available).

Ishimori, K. (1909) The demonstration of intracerebral substances in sleep-deprived animals: sleep-inducing substances as the true cause of sleep. *Chuo Igakkai Zasshi* **84**: 1–47.

Jones, B. E. (2004) Paradoxical REM sleep promoting and permitting neuronal networks. *Arch Ital Biol* **142**: 379–96.

Kandel, E. R. (2001) The molecular biology of memory storage: a dialogue between genes and synapses. *Science* **294**:1030–8.

Kitahama, K. & Valatx, J. L. (1975) [Effects of chloramphenicol and thiamphenicol on sleep of the mouse]. *C R Seances Soc Biol Fil* **169**: 1522–5.

Kovacs, K. J. (2008) Measurement of immediate-early gene activation- c-fos and beyond. *J Neuroendocrinol* **20**: 665–72.

Legendre, R. & Pieron, H. (1910) Le probleme des facteurs du sommeil: resultats d'injections vasculaires et intra-cerbrales de liquides insomniques. *C R Soc Biol* **68**: 1077–9.

Lin, L., Faraco, J., Li, R. *et al.* (1999) The sleep disorder canine narcolepsy is caused by a mutation in the hypocretin (orexin) receptor 2 gene. *Cell* **98**: 365–76.

Lopez, J., Roffwarg, H. P., Dreher, A. *et al.* (2008) Rapid eye movement sleep deprivation decreases long-term potentiation stability and affects some glutamatergic signaling proteins during hippocampal development. *Neuroscience* **153**: 44–53.

Luppi, P. H., Gervasoni, D., Verret, L. *et al.* (2006) Paradoxical (REM) sleep genesis: the switch from an aminergic-cholinergic to a GABAergic-glutamatergic hypothesis. *J Physiol Paris* **100**: 271–83.

Mackiewicz, M., Shockley, K. R., Romer, M. A. *et al.* (2007) Macromolecule biosynthesis: a key function of sleep. *Physiol Genomics* **31**: 441–57.

Mallick, B. N., Singh, S. & Singh, A. (2010) Mechanism of noradrenaline-induced stimulation of Na-K ATPase activity in the rat brain: implications on REM sleep deprivation-induced increase in brain excitability. *Mol Cell Biochem.* **336**: 1–16.

Maloney, K. J., Mainville, L. & Jones, B. E. (1999) Differential c-Fos expression in cholinergic, monoaminergic, and GABAergic cell groups of the pontomesencephalic tegmentum after paradoxical sleep deprivation and recovery. *J Neurosci* **19**: 3057–72.

Maloney, K. J., Mainville, L. & Jones, B. E. (2000) c-Fos expression in GABAergic, serotonergic, and other neurons of the pontomedullary reticular formation and raphe after paradoxical sleep deprivation and recovery. *J Neurosci* **20**: 4669–79.

Mansuy, I. M. (2003) Calcineurin in memory and bidirectional plasticity. *Biochem Biophys Res Commun* **311**: 1195–208.

McCarley, R. W. (2007) Neurobiology of REM and NREM sleep. *Sleep Med* **8**: 302–30.

McCarley, R. W. & Hobson, J. A. (1975a) Neuronal excitability modulation over the sleep cycle: a structural and mathematical model. *Science* **189**: 58–60.

McCarley, R. W. & Hobson, J. A. (1975b) Discharge patterns of cat pontine brain stem neurons during desynchronized sleep. *J Neurophysiol* **38**: 751–66.

Mendelson, W. B., Guthrie, R. D., Frederick, G. & Wyatt, R. J. (1974) The flower pot technique of rapid eye movement (REM) sleep deprivation. *Pharmacol Biochem Behav* **2**: 553–6.

Morgan, J. I. & Curran, T. (1991) Stimulus-transcription coupling in the nervous system: involvement of the inducible proto-oncogenes fos and jun. *Annu Rev Neurosci* **14**: 421–51.

Nakanishi, H., Sun, Y., Nakamura, R. K. *et al.* (1997) Positive correlations between cerebral protein synthesis rates and deep sleep in Macaca mulatta. *Eur J Neurosci* **9**: 271–9.

Neves, G., Cooke, S. F. & Bliss, T. V. (2008) Synaptic plasticity, memory and the hippocampus: a neural network approach to causality. *Nat Rev Neurosci* **9**: 65–75.

Pawlyk, A. C., Ferber, M., Shah, A., Pack, A. I. & Naidoo, N. (2007) Proteomic analysis of the effects and interactions of sleep deprivation and aging in mouse cerebral cortex. *J Neurochem* **103**: 2301–13.

Poirrier, J. E., Guillonneau, F., Renaut, J. *et al.* (2008) Proteomic changes in rat hippocampus and adrenals following short-term sleep deprivation. *Proteome Sci* **6**:14.

Ramm, P. & Smith, C. T. (1990) Rates of cerebral protein synthesis are linked to slow wave sleep in the rat. *Physiol Behav* **48**: 749–53.

Ravassard, P., Pachoud, B., Comte, J. C. *et al.* (2009) Paradoxical (REM) sleep deprivation causes a large and rapidly reversible decrease in long-term potentiation, synaptic transmission, glutamate receptor protein levels, and ERK/MAPK activation in the dorsal hippocampus. *Sleep* **32**: 227–40.

Reich, P., Driver, J. K. & Karnovsky, M. L. (1967) Sleep: effects on incorporation of inorganic phosphate into brain fractions. *Science* **157**: 336–8.

Reich, P., Geyer, S. J., Steinbaum, L., Anchors, M. & Karnovsky, M. L. (1973) Incorporation of phosphate into rat brain during sleep and wakefulness. *J Neurochem* **20**: 1195–205.

Rojas-Ramirez, J. A., Aguilar-Jimenez, E., Posadas-Andrews, A., Bernal-Pedraza, J. G., Drucker-Colin, R. R. (1977) The effects of various protein synthesis inhibitors on the sleep-wake cycle of rats. *Psychopharmacology (Berl)* **53**: 147–50.

Roky, R., Obal, F., Jr., Valatx, J. L. *et al.* (1995) Prolactin and rapid eye movement sleep regulation. *Sleep* **18**: 536–42.

Sagar, S. M., Sharp, F. R. & Curran, T. (1988) Expression of c-fos protein in brain: metabolic mapping at the cellular level. *Science* **240**: 1328–31.

Sakurai,T., Ameniya, A., Ishii, M. *et al.* (1998) Orexins and orexin receptors: a family of hypothalamic neuropeptides and G protein-coupled receptors that regulate feeding behavior. *Cell* **92**: 573–85.

Shiromani, P. J., Kilduff, T. S., Bloom, F. E. & McCarley, R. W. (1992) Cholinergically induced REM sleep triggers Fos-like immunoreactivity in dorsolateral pontine regions associated with REM sleep. *Brain Res* **580**: 351–7.

Siegel, J. M. (2001) The REM sleep-memory consolidation hypothesis. *Science* **294**: 1058–63.

Silva, A. J., Kogan, J. H., Frankland, P. W. & Kida, S. (1998) CREB and memory. *Annu Rev Neurosci* **21**: 127–48.

Sinha, A. K., Ciaranello, R. D., Dement, W. C. & Barchas, J. D. (1973) Tyrosine hydroxylase activity in rat brain following "REM" sleep deprivation. *J Neurochem* **20**: 1289–90.

Soderling, T. R., Chang, B. & Brickey, D. (2001) Cellular signaling through multifunctional Ca^{2+}/calmodulin-dependent protein kinase II. *J Biol Chem* **276**: 3719–22.

Stack, E. C., Desarnaud, F., Siwek, D. F. & Datta, S. (2010) A novel role for calcium/calmodulin kinase II within the brainstem pedunculopontine tegmentum for the regulation of wakefulness and rapid eye movement sleep. *J Neurochem* **112**: 271–81.

Stickgold, R. & Walker, M. P. (2007) Sleep-dependent memory consolidation and reconsolidation. *Sleep Med* **8**: 331–43.

Thakkar, M. & Mallick, B. N. (1991) Effect of REM sleep deprivation on rat brain acetylcholinesterase. *Pharmacol Biochem Behav* **39**: 211–14.

Thakkar, M. & Mallick, B. N. (1993a) Rapid eye movement sleep-deprivation-induced changes in glucose metabolic enzymes in rat brain. *Sleep* **16**: 691–4.

Thakkar, M. & Mallick, B. N. (1993b) Effect of rapid eye movement sleep deprivation on rat brain monoamine oxidases. *Neuroscience* **55**: 677–83.

Vazquez, J., Hall, S. C. & Greco, M. A. (2009) Protein expression is altered during spontaneous sleep in aged Sprague Dawley rats. *Brain Res* **1298**: 37–45.

Vazquez, J., Hall, S. C., Witkowska, H. E. & Greco, M. A. (2008) Rapid alterations in cortical protein profiles underlie spontaneous sleep and wake bouts. *J Cell Biochem* **105**: 1472–84.

Verret, L., Leger, L., Fort, P. & Luppi, P. H. (2005) Cholinergic and noncholinergic brainstem neurons expressing Fos after paradoxical (REM) sleep deprivation and recovery. *Eur J Neurosci* **21**: 2488–504.

Verret, L., Fort, P., Gervasoni, D., Leger, L. & Luppi, P. H. (2006) Localization of the neurons active during paradoxical (REM) sleep and projecting to the locus coeruleus noradrenergic neurons in the rat. *J Comp Neurol* **495**: 573–86.

Voronka, G., Demin, N. N. & Pevzner, L. Z. (1971) [Total protein content and quantity of basic proteins in neurons and neuroglia of rat brain supraoptic and red nuclei during natural sleep and deprivation of paradoxical sleep]. *Dokl Akad Nauk SSSR* **198**: 974–7.

Wang, G. P., Huang, L. Q., Wu, H. J. *et al.* (2009) Calcineurin contributes to spatial memory impairment induced by rapid eye movement sleep deprivation. *Neuroreport* **20**: 1172–6.

Yamuy, J., Mancillas, J. R., Morales, F. R. & Chase, M. H. (1993) C-fos expression in the pons and medulla of the cat during carbachol-induced active sleep. *J Neurosci* **13**: 2703–18.

Yang, R. H., Hu, S. J., Wang, Y. *et al.* (2008) Paradoxical sleep deprivation impairs spatial learning and affects membrane excitability and mitochondrial protein in the hippocampus. *Brain Res* **1230**: 224–32.

Chapter 40

Narcolepsy and REM sleep

Seiji Nishino

Summary

Narcolepsy is characterized by excessive daytime sleepiness (EDS), cataplexy, and/or other dissociated manifestations of rapid eye movement (REM) sleep (hypnagogic hallucinations and sleep paralysis).

The major pathophysiology of human narcolepsy has been recently elucidated based on the discovery of narcolepsy genes in animals. Using forward (i.e., positional cloning in canine narcolepsy) and reverse (i.e., mouse gene knock-out) genetics, the genes involved in the pathogenesis of narcolepsy (hypocretin/orexin ligand and its receptor) in animals have been identified. Hypocretins/orexins are novel hypothalamic neuropeptides also involved in various hypothalamic functions such as energy homeostasis and neuroendocrine functions. Mutations in hypocretin-related genes are rare in humans, but hypocretin-ligand deficiency is found in many narcolepsy–cataplexy cases.

After the discovery of sleep-onset REM periods (SOREMs) in narcolepsy, narcolepsy has often been referred as an "REM-sleep disorder." REM sleep can intrude in active wake or at sleep onset, resulting in cataplexy, sleep paralysis, and hypnagogic hallucinations; these three symptoms are often categorized as "dissociated manifestations of REM sleep." Although cataplexy and REM-sleep abnormalities are the hallmarks of narcolepsy and these symptoms differentiated narcolepsy from other types of hypersomnia, it is now conceived that impairments of hypocretin neurotransmission cause both the EDS (possibly due to the sleep–wake fragmentation) and REM-sleep abnormalities in narcolepsy; it is impossible to discuss these mechanisms independently.

While sleep paralysis and hypnagogic hallucinations exist in other sleep disorders (such as obstructive sleep apnea) and even in normal subjects, since cataplexy is tightly associated with hypocretin impairments, cataplexy is likely to be pathophysiologically distinct from other dissociated manifestations of REM sleep.

In this review, the clinical and pathophysiological aspects of sleep abnormalities in narcolepsy, with a special focus on those of REM sleep-related symptoms, are discussed.

Introduction

Gélineáu, first coined the term "narcolepsy," in 1880 with the complete description of a patient with excessive daytime sleepiness (EDS), sleep attacks, and episodes of muscle weakness triggered by emotions (Gélineau, 1880). In the current international classification, narcolepsy is characterized by "excessive daytime sleepiness that is typically associated with cataplexy (i.e., narcolepsy with cataplexy) and/or with abnormal rapid eye movement (REM) sleep phenomena such as sleep paralysis and hypnagogic hallucinations" (ICSD-2, 2005).

After the discovery of sleep-onset REM periods (SOREMs) in the 1960s (Dement *et al.*, 1966; Takahashi and Jimbo, 1963; Vogel, 1960), narcolepsy has often been referred to as an "REM-sleep disorder." It was interpreted that REM sleep can intrude in active wake or at sleep onset, resulting in cataplexy, sleep paralysis, and hypnagogic hallucinations, and these three symptoms are often categorized as "dissociated manifestations of REM sleep" (see Nishino and Mignot, 1997).

The major pathophysiology of human narcolepsy has been recently elucidated based on the discovery of narcolepsy genes in animals. Mutations in hypocretin-related genes are rare in humans, but hypocretin-ligand deficiency is found in many cases (Nishino *et al.*, 2000b; Peyron *et al.*, 2000). It is therefore conceivable that impairment of the hypocretin system results in EDS, cataplexy, and other REM-sleep abnormalities. In this chapter, REM-sleep abnormalities of

REM Sleep: Regulation and Function, eds. Birendra N. Mallick, S. R. Pandi-Perumal, Robert W. McCarley, and Adrian R. Morrison. Published by Cambridge University Press. © Cambridge University Press 2011.

narcolepsy are described followed by discussions on the possible mechanisms involved. Since the REM-sleep abnormalities seen in narcolepsy cannot be explained independently from the occurrence of EDS and sleep fragmentations, pathophysiological aspects of these symptoms are also discussed.

Clinical characteristics of narcolepsy

Excessive daytime sleepiness and cataplexy are considered to be the two primary symptoms of narcolepsy, with EDS often being the most disabling symptom (Nishino and Mignot, 1997). EDS in narcolepsy is most often relieved by short naps (15 to 30 minutes), but in most cases, the refreshed sensation only lasts a short time after waking. Sleepiness also occurs in irresistible waves in these patients, a phenomenon best described as "sleep attacks." EDS is usually the first symptom to appear, followed by cataplexy, sleep paralysis, and hypnagogic hallucinations (Billiard *et al.*, 1983; Honda, 1988). EDS, cataplexy, sleep paralysis, and hypnagogic hallucinations are often referred as the narcolepsy tetrad.

Although some people confuse cataplexy with sleep attack, cataplexy is distinct from EDS and sleep attacks and is pathognomonic of the disease (Guilleminault *et al.*, 1974). Cataplexy is defined as a sudden episode of muscle weakness triggered by emotional factors, most often in the context of positive emotions (such as laughter), and less frequently by negative emotions (most typically anger or frustration). All antigravity muscles can be affected, leading to a progressive collapse of the subject, but respiratory and eye muscles are not affected. The patient is typically awake at the onset of the attack but may experience blurred vision or ptosis. The attack is almost always bilateral and usually lasts a few seconds. Neurological examination performed at the time of attack shows suppression of the patellar reflex and sometimes of Babinski's sign.

Sleep paralysis is present in 20 to 50% of all narcoleptic subjects (Hishikawa, 1976), and is often associated with hypnagogic hallucinations. Sleep paralysis is best described as a brief inability to perform voluntary movements at the onset of sleep, upon awakening during the night, or in the morning. Contrary to simple fatigue or locomotion inhibition, the patient is unable to perform even a small movement, such as lifting a finger. Sleep paralysis may last a few minutes and is often finally interrupted by noise or other external stimuli. The symptom is occasionally bothersome in narcoleptic subjects, especially when associated with frightening hallucinations (Rosenthal, 1939).

Abnormal visual (most often) or auditory perceptions that occur while falling asleep (hypnagogic) or upon waking up (hypnopompic) are frequently observed in narcoleptic subjects (Ribstein, 1976). These hallucinations are often unpleasant and are typically associated with a feeling of fear or threat (Hishikawa, 1976; Rosenthal, 1939). Polygraphic studies indicate that these hallucinations occur most often during REM sleep (Hishikawa, 1976). These episodes are often difficult to distinguish from nightmares or unpleasant dreams, which also occur frequently in narcolepsy. These hallucinations are usually easy to distinguish from the hallucinations observed in schizophrenia or related psychotic conditions.

One of the most frequently associated symptoms is insomnia, best characterized as a difficulty to maintain nighttime sleep (Nishino and Mignot, 1997). Typically, narcoleptic patients fall asleep easily, only to wake up after a short nap and unable to fall asleep again for an hour or so. Other frequently associated problems are REM-behavior disorder, other parasomnias (Mayer *et al.*, 1993), periodic leg movements (Mosko *et al.*, 1984), and obstructive sleep apnea (Mosko *et al.*, 1984).

Objective measures of sleep abnormalities in narcolepsy

The primary sleep abnormality observed in narcoleptic subjects is extremely short sleep latency during night and day. In addition, patients have the abnormal tendency to fall asleep into REM sleep very quickly, a phenomenon called SOREMs (Dement *et al.*, 1966; Takahashi and Jimbo, 1963; Vogel, 1960). SOREMs are initially found during nighttime polysomnography (PSG), but also seen during daytime naps (Figure 40.1). REM sleep usually appears 90 to110 minutes after sleep onset and reappears every 90 to 110 minutes in humans, but if the first REM-sleep episode occurs within 15 minutes after sleep onset, these episodes are defined as SOREMs (Figure 40.1).

These sleep abnormalities in narcoleptic subjects are objectively evaluated with a multiple sleep latency test (MSLT). The PSG nap test consists of four or five 20-minute nap opportunities that are scheduled two hours apart (Carskadon and Dement, 1987). A mean sleep latency of less than eight minutes on the MSLT is usually considered diagnostic for excessive sleepiness (Moscovitch *et al.*,

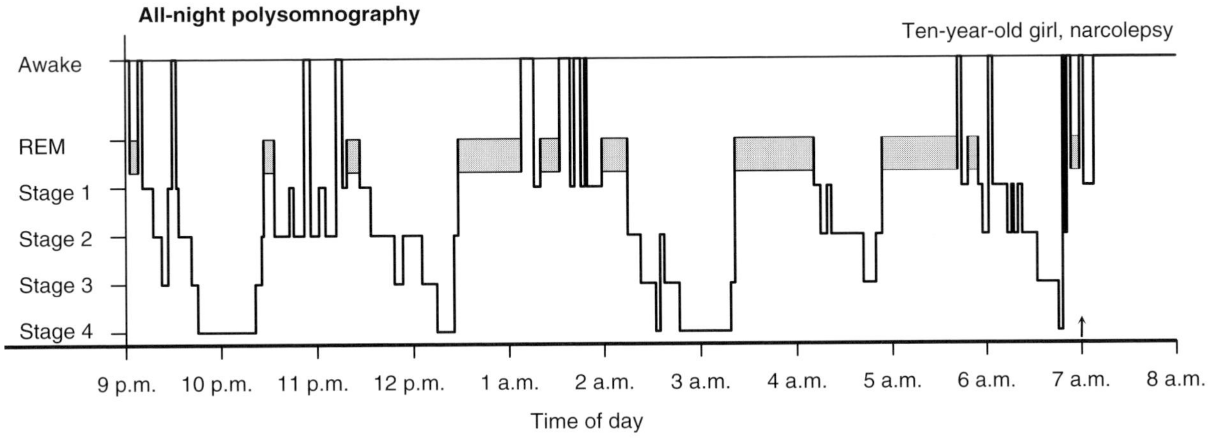

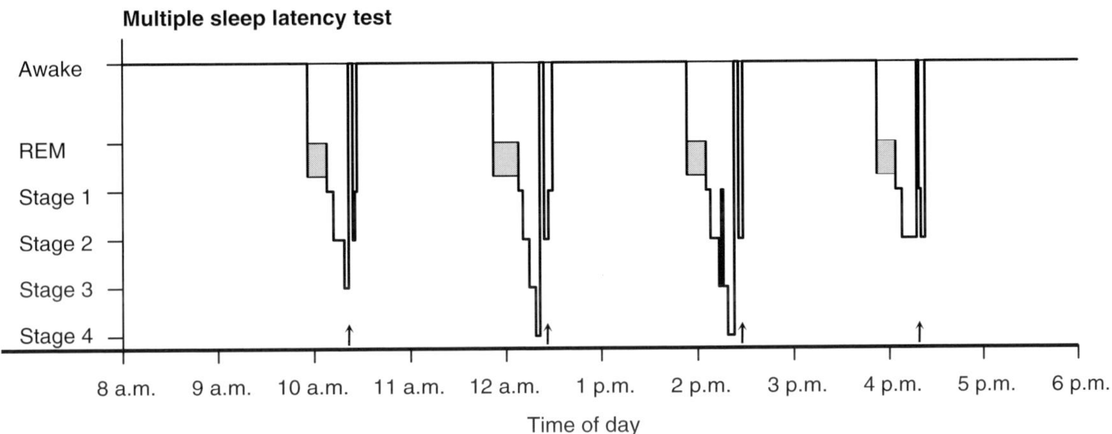

Figure 40.1 All-night polysomnography and MSLT of a narcoleptic patient (adapted from Honda, 1988). (See plate section for color version.)

1993). A total of more than two transitions to REM sleep out of the four to five naps (SOREMs) is usually considered diagnostic for narcolepsy (Figure 40.1).

Despite the sleep tendency during the daytime (frequent sleep episodes) in narcolepsy, narcoleptic patients do not usually sleep more than normal individuals over the 24-hour cycle (Broughton *et al.*, 1988; Hishikawa *et al.*, 1976; Montplaisir *et al.*, 1978) and frequently have a very disrupted nighttime sleep (Broughton *et al.*, 1988; Hishikawa *et al.*, 1976; Montplaisir *et al.*, 1978). Sleep efficiency during nocturnal PSG may also be normal or low due to the frequent wake episodes at night.

Just as animal models of narcolepsy significantly contributed to the discovery of narcolepsy genes and the major pathophysiology of human narcolepsy (i.e., hypocretin-ligand deficiency), animal models also contribute to our understanding of the physiological and pathophysiological mechanisms involved in sleep abnormalities in human narcolepsy (Chemelli *et al.*, 1999; Hara *et al.*, 2001; Nishino and Mignot, 1997). This research was initiated from the detailed characterizations of sleep phenotypes in narcoleptic dogs, followed by those in rodent models.

Narcoleptic Dobermans showed shortened sleep latency and reduced latency to REM sleep during multiple daytime naps by a canine version of the MSLT (Nishino *et al.*, 2000a), suggesting that these dogs have a very similar phenotype to those in human narcolepsy. A series of polygraphic studies clearly demonstrated a difference in sleep patterns between narcoleptic dogs and control dogs. Compared to age- and breed-matched dogs, narcoleptic dogs exhibit an increased frequency in sleep state changes, their sleep–wake pattern is more fragmented and shorter, and their wake–sleep bouts much shorter than in the control dogs (Figure 40.2) (Nishino *et al.*, 2000a; Kaitin *et al.*, 1986).

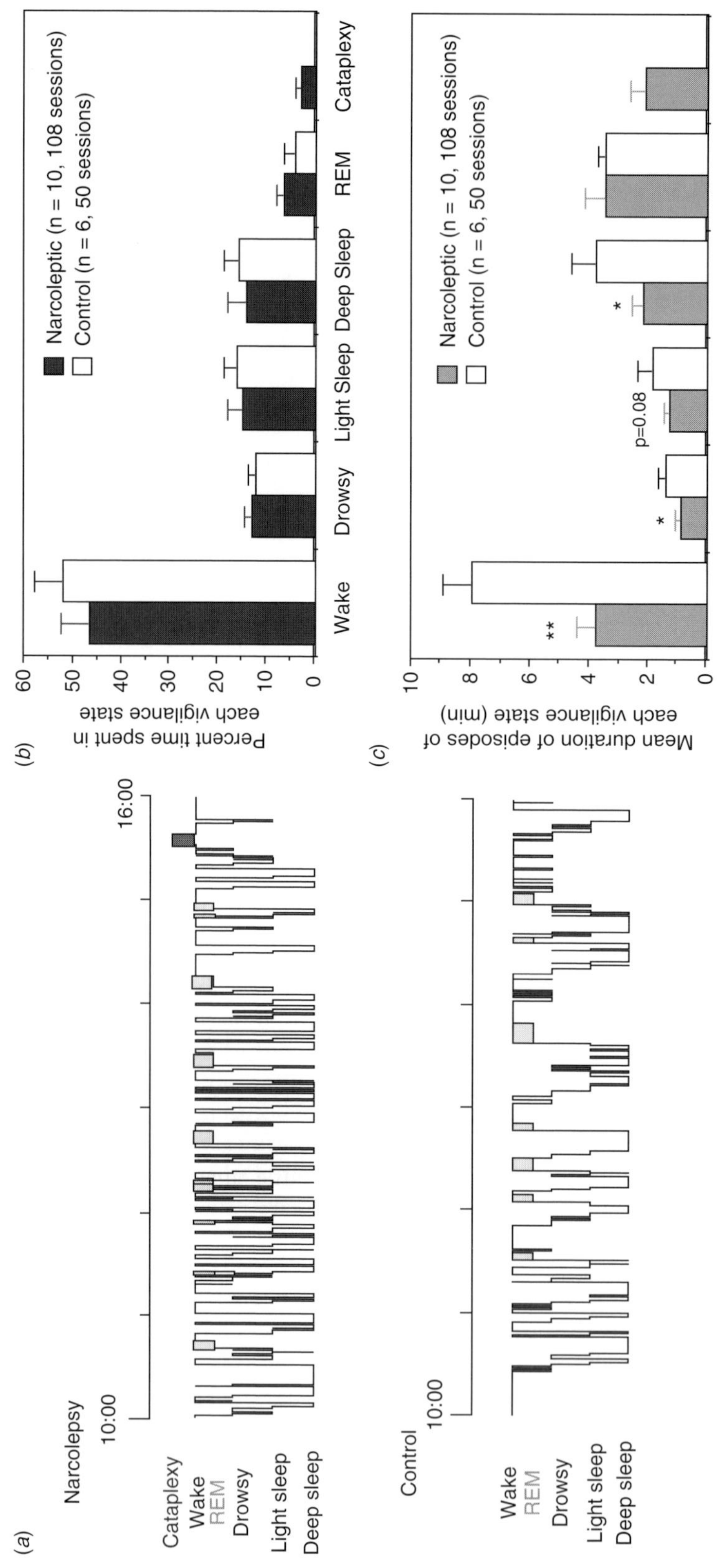

Figure 40.2 (a) Typical hypnograms from a narcoleptic and a control Doberman. (b, c) Percentage of time spent in, mean frequency of, and mean duration for each vigilance state of narcoleptic and control Dobermans during daytime six-hour recordings (10:00 to 16:00). No significant difference was found in the percentage of time spent in each vigilance state between narcoleptic and control dogs. However, the mean duration of wake, drowsy state, and deep-sleep episodes were significantly shorter in the narcoleptics, suggesting a fragmentation of the vigilance states (wake and sleep) in these animals. To compensate for the influence of cataplectic episodes on wake and drowsiness, those episodes interrupted by the occurrence of cataplexy were excluded. (See plate section for color version.)

Abnormal sleep patterns of prepro-orexin (prepro-hypocretin) gene knock-out (KO) mice and hypocretin neuron-ablated (*orexin/ataxin-3 transgenic*) mice were also characterized, and these mice exhibit highly fragmented vigilance states, occasional direct transition to REM sleep from wakefulness, and behavioral arrest similar to cataplexy (Chemelli *et al.*, 1999; Hara *et al.*, 2001). It appears that sleep–wake fragmentation is therefore the primary symptom of narcolepsy across different species. In other words, narcoleptic subjects could not maintain long bouts of both wakefulness and sleep, which also explains why most narcoleptic humans are insomniac at night while they have EDS during the daytime (see Nishino and Mignot, 1997). Interestingly, however, animal studies have demonstrated that REM sleep in narcoleptic subjects is not fragmented and the mean bout length of REM sleep is the same or slightly longer that that of controls (Figure 40.2) (see also Chemelli *et al.*, 1999; Hara *et al.*, 2001), suggesting that REM-sleep maintenance is not affected in a similar way to wake and slow-wave sleep (SWS) maintenance.

Pathophysiological considerations of sleep abnormalities in narcolepsy

Several authors have proposed the pathophysiological aspects of sleep abnormalities and sleep-related symptoms in hypocretin-deficient narcoleptics. These include (1) unstable sleep–wake circuit; (2) abnormal timing of circadian distribution of sleep and wake; (3) insufficient non-rapid eye movement sleep (non-REMS) intensity; and (4) enhanced strength of the REM oscillator. The former two theories come from the results of animal studies, while the latter two theories are from human studies, and these concepts are introduced and discussed.

Unstable sleep–wake switch

Human and animal studies suggested that problems with the maintenance of the vigilance stage (i.e., fragmented sleep–wake pattern) together with cataplexy are the primary symptoms in narcolepsy. However, no apparent abnormalities have been found in sleep homeostasis and SCN function in human narcoleptics (i.e., they show compensatory responses to sleep loss and show normal entrainment to light–dark cycles) (Tafti *et al.*, 1992; Dantz *et al.*, 1994; Broughton *et al.*, 1988). Thus, loss of hypocretin signaling itself may directly contribute to instability of vigilance states independent from the circadian and homeostasis regulatory mechanisms of sleep. In this regard, hypocretin may stabilize the sleep–wake switch, and loss of hypocretin signaling may induce abnormally unstable sleep–wake transitions (Saper *et al.*, 2001).

The hypocretin neurons are mainly active during wakefulness and especially during motor activity when animals actively explore their environment (Estabrooke *et al.*, 2001; Lee *et al.*, 2005; Mileykovskiy *et al.*, 2005). They have ascending projections to the cerebral cortex, as well as descending projections to all the monoaminergic and cholinergic cell groups of the arousal systems (Peyron *et al.*, 1998). There are mutual projections between the ventrolateral preoptic (VLPO) sleep-active neurons and the hypocretin neurons, directly or indirectly (Gallopin *et al.*, 2000; Yoshida *et al.*, 2006). The sleep-producing neurons of the VLPO receive substantial aminergic inputs (Chou *et al.*, 2002), and are inhibited by norepinephrine, acetylcholine, and serotonin (Gallopin *et al.*, 2000). During wakefulness, high monoaminergic activity likely inhibits the VLPO, thus reducing inhibition of the arousal regions, which further enhances their activity. Conversely, during sleep, VLPO neurons are active and inhibit the arousal regions, thus disinhibiting and reinforcing their own firing. This mutual inhibitory relationship may create a bistable feedback loop that avoids intermediate states and inappropriate transitions between states when input signals to the VLPO or the arousal regions transiently fluctuate. This asymmetric relationship could help stabilize the flip-flop switch (circuits familiar to electrical engineers) like a "finger" on the switch that might prevent unwanted transitions into sleep. The increase in homeostatic sleep drive due to consolidated wakefulness might, in turn, help produce consolidated sleep. When animals switch between behavioral states, they spend little time in intermediate states. This is adaptive for survival since an animal performing daily tasks in a state of muddled drowsiness, neither fully awake nor asleep, would be in danger from predators and would be unable to carry out essential tasks. Narcoleptic people and animals lacking the hypocretin inputs may behave as if their sleep flip-flop switch has been destabilized. They do not sleep more than normal individuals, but easily doze off during the day and wake more often from sleep at night, as the flip-flop model would also predict.

Although this hypothesis by Saper *et al.* (2001) explains well the mechanisms of the sleep fragmentation in narcoleptic animals whose sleep–wake are not consolidated, it is uncertain if this mechanism can also explain the sleep abnormalities in human narcolepsy, since normal subjects can stay awake over 16 hours without naps. Similarly this hypothesis does not predict the abnormal occurrence of REM sleep (and its related symptoms) in narcolepsy, and REM sleep in narcoleptic subjects is not fragmented.

Hypocretin injection promotes wakefulness (Hagan *et al.*, 1999), and hypocretin levels stay high during forced wakefulness in experimental animals (Fujiki *et al.*, 2001). Hypocretin levels in the cerebrospinal fluid are also correlated with locomotor activity in normal and suprachiasmatic nucleus (SCN)-lesioned animals (Zhang *et al.*, 2004). The hypocretin system may thus generate a positive feedback loop for maintaining active wakefulness, and thus a lack of this system may also contribute to difficulties of maintaining wakefulness during the active period in narcoleptic subjects. Experiments using squeal monkeys, which are wake-consolidating animals like humans, however, pointed out that locomotion is rather unnecessary for CSF hypocretin-1 to increase throughout the daytime in wake-consolidating animals, but high levels of locomotion are likely to provide a small positive feedback into the hypocretin system (Zeitzer *et al.*, 2004).

Loss of circadian wake signal

The circadian process sets the time for sleep and wakefulness to occur and helps to consolidate wakefulness during the active period, and sleep during the rest period (Dijk and Czeisler, 1994; Edgar *et al.*, 1993). It achieves this by opposing or compensating the homeostatic process; towards the end of the active period, despite a strong drive to initiate sleep (i.e., high levels of "S"), wakefulness can remain consolidated through an "alerting" circadian signal that reaches peak levels at this time of the day (Dijk and Czeisler, 1994). This circadian signal originates from the suprachiasmatic nucleus (SCN), since consolidated episodes of sleep and wakefulness were absent in SCN-lesioned animals (Edgar *et al.*, 1993). Thus, both circadian and homeostatic processes likely contribute to the ability to maintain wakefulness throughout the active period (and sleep throughout the rest period).

As stated above, the hypocretin system is at least activated by a circadian-independent reactive homeostatic mechanism. It is likely that the hypocretin system is also regulated by the circadian pacemaker. Hypocretin levels in the brain extracellular fluids and in the CSF increase during the active period, with highest levels at the end of the active period, declining with the onset of sleep (Yoshida *et al.*, 2001). Fluctuation of hypocretin levels in the CSF disappeared in SCN-lesioned rats, while a weak (but significant) fluctuation in activity and temperature was still observed in these rats, suggesting that a daily oscillation of hypocretin tonus is also controlled by a circadian clock (Zhang *et al.*, 2004).

Unstable sleep–wake behavior is the hallmark of narcolepsy, but narcoleptic subjects also have disturbed circadian timing of sleep and wakefulness (Broughton *et al.*, 1998; Dantz *et al.*, 1994). In normal individuals, wakefulness is strongly promoted through much of the day, and REM sleep occurs mainly between 2 a.m. and 8 a.m. (Dijk and Czeisler, 1995). Narcoleptic subjects have difficulty maintaining wakefulness, and their naps often include bouts of REM sleep, regardless of the time of day (Dantz *et al.*, 1994; Lavie, 1991). As stated before, this marked attenuation of the normal sleep–wake rhythm in narcolepsy is not caused by an underlying defect in the generation of circadian rhythms, because the rhythms of body temperature, cortisol, and melatonin under the constant-dark condition are essentially normal (Bourgine *et al.*, 1986; Mayer *et al.*, 1997). Altered circadian distribution of sleep and wakefulness is also not caused by a simple disinhibition of sleep because narcoleptic subjects have normal amounts of sleep over 24 hours (Broughton *et al.*, 1988, 1998; Dantz *et al.*, 1994). The hypocretin neurons may thus play a critical role in diurnal distributions of sleep and wakefulness.

Animal studies demonstrated that diurnal non-REM sleep distribution in hypocretin-deficient narcolepsy seems to be intact (Beuckmann *et al.*, 2004; Hara *et al.*, 2001), while distribution of REM sleep is impaired significantly (the animals have a large amount of REM sleep during the active phase) (Figure 40.3). It thus appears that distribution patterns of REM sleep are highly dependent on the availability of the hypocretin system and on the changes in neuronal activities. Hypocretin deficiency may therefore result in disinhibition of REM sleep, especially during the active phase, therefore narcoleptic subjects may have various REM sleep-related abnormalities during the daytime (such as frequent REM-sleep episodes during daytime naps) as well as sleep onset and offset (if the SCN function is intact) (Figure 40.3).

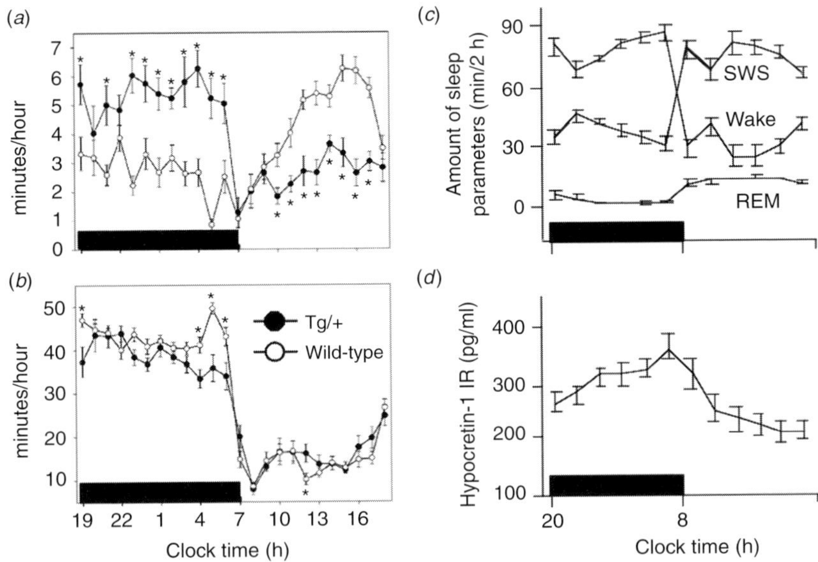

Figure 40.3 Time spent each hour (in minutes; mean ± SEM) in wakefulness (*a*) and REM sleep (*b*) for wild-type rats and their *orexin/ataxin-3* hemizygous transgenic littermates (*c*) in relation to fluctuation of hypocretin-1 levels in the extracellular space in normal rats. Significant differences between the genotypes (*t* test; $p < 0.05$) are marked by asterisks. The dark phase is denoted by the horizontal bar. Although *orexin/ataxin-3* hemizygous transgenic animals exhibit clear diurnal distribution patterns of non-REM sleep, total wakefulness time is reduced during the dark phase in these narcoleptic rats. The results of the microdialysis experiment in rats by Yoshida *et al.*, demonstrate that hypocretin-1 levels build up toward the end of active phase, and thus lack of the build up of hypocretin may contribute to this difference. The diurnal distribution of REM sleep in hypocretin neuron-ablated rats was significantly impaired, and it appears that distribution patterns of REM sleep are highly dependent on the availability of the hypocretin system. (Adapted from Yoshida *et al.*, 2001 and Beuckmann *et al.*, 2004.)

Insufficient non-rapid eye movement sleep (NREMS) intensity

From the results of human PSG studies, Khatami *et al.* (2007) proposed that insufficient non-REM sleep intensity contributes to disturbed nocturnal sleep in patients with narcolepsy. The authors addressed the changes in homeostatic sleep regulation as a possible mechanism underlying nocturnal sleep fragmentation in narcolepsy. These authors reported that REM-sleep cycles were longer in patients with narcolepsy than in controls. Mean slow-wave activity (SWA) declined in both groups across the first three NREM-sleep episodes. The rate of decline, however, appeared to be steeper in patients with narcolepsy–cataplexy than in controls. The steeper decline of SWA in narcolepsy–cataplexy compared to controls was related to an impaired build up of slow-wave activity in the second cycle. Build up of SWA after sleep deprivation in narcolepsy was normal, suggesting that sleep homeostasis is intact. Since the increased non-REM sleep intensity in recovery sleep postpones sleep fragmentation, these authors speculate that sleep fragmentation in narcolepsy is directly related to insufficient non-REM sleep.

Sleep deprivation in narcoleptic subjects also increased the duration of SOREMs, and the authors also suggest an abnormal interaction between non-REM sleep and REM sleep regulatory processes in narcolepsy (Khatami *et al.*, 2008).

Altered REM-on/REM-off interaction

Another human study by Ferrillo *et al.* (2007) presented a mathematical model of sleep-EEG structure applied to the analysis of sleep patterns in narcoleptics by combining the two-process model of sleep regulation and the reciprocal-interaction model of REM. The REM oscillator, characterized by two coupled differential equations (Lotka-Volterra type), has been added on the basis of the reciprocal-interaction model suggested by McCarley and Hobson (Hobson *et al.*, 1975). It consists of two coupled, non-linear differential equations describing the dynamics of REM-on and REM-off variables, where the strength of interactions is denoted by the coupling parameters. The mathematical model was fitted to quantitative EEG data by an optimization procedure. The sleep model was fitted to the SWA profile for each recording and to the averaged SWA profile for each group. Bartlett and Kolmogorov-Smirnov tests were used to evaluate the goodness of the fit and the accuracy of model predictions. In both controls and narcoleptics, the optimization procedure produced a good fit of SWA raw data, but significant differences in the REM-on/REM-off coupling parameters between the groups were observed, suggesting an enhanced strength of the REM oscillator in narcoleptics. The authors suggested that this difference can explain the occurrence of SOREMs and variations of the REM–NREM sleep cycle duration in narcoleptic subjects, also reported by other authors.

Pathophysiological considerations of cataplexy

After the discoveries of SOREMs in narcolepsy (Dement *et al.*, 1966; Takahashi and Jimbo, 1963; Vogel, 1960), it was thought that in narcolepsy REM sleep can intrude in active wake or at sleep onset, resulting in cataplexy, sleep paralysis, and hypnagogic hallucinations, and these three symptoms are often categorized as "dissociated manifestations of REM sleep" (see Nishino and Mignot, 1997).

The similarity between cataplexy and REM-sleep atonia (the presence of frequent episodes of hypnagogic hallucinations and of sleep paralysis, and the propensity for narcoleptics to go directly from wakefulness into REM sleep), suggests that narcolepsy is primarily a "disease of REM sleep" (Dement *et al.*, 1966). This hypothesis may, however, be too simplistic and does not explain the presence of sleepiness during the day and the short latency to both NREM and REM sleep during nocturnal and nap recordings. Another complementary hypothesis is that narcolepsy results from the disruption of the control mechanisms of both sleep and wakefulness or, in other words, of vigilance-state boundary problems (Broughton *et al.*, 1986). According to this hypothesis, a cataplectic attack represents an intrusion of REM-sleep atonia during wakefulness, while the hypnagogic hallucinations appear as dream-like imagery taking place in the waking state, especially at sleep onset in patients who frequently have SOREMs.

Another important pathophysiological consideration of cataplexy is that chronic hypocretin deficiency is likely required for the occurrence of narcolepsy. In other word, acute hypocretin deficiency is not sufficient to cause cataplexy. Excessive daytime sleepiness

is the first symptom to occur in most cases of narcolepsy, and hypocretin deficiency is already evident at the onset of EDS even before the onset of cataplexy (Arii *et al.*, 2004). Cataplexy most typically occurs several months after the onset of EDS (Billiard *et al.*, 1983; Honda, 1988). This suggests that chronic loss of hypocretin neurotransmission may be required for the occurrence of cataplexy. In addition, we have experienced several symptomatic cases of EDS associated with multiple sclerosis (MS) and neuromyelitica optica (NMO) (Kanbayashi *et al.* 2009; Nishino and Kanbayashi, 2005). In some of these cases, CSF hypocretin levels became undetectably low during the course of the disease, but they never developed cataplexy (but displayed SOREMs). This contrasts with symptomatic narcolepsy–cataplexy cases associated with a dozen MS cases appearing in the old literature. Of note, most recent MS/NMO cases are treated with steroids at the early stage of the disease, and EDS and hypocretin levels are completely recovered in most cases. The reason for the delays in the cataplexy onset (after that of EDS) is not known, and an additional pathologic process secondary to hypocretin deficiency may possibly be involved. Similarly, the mechanisms of emotional induction of cataplexy are completely unknown, and this should be elucidated.

REM sleep, but not cataplexy, is governed by an ultradian REM sleep cyclicity in narcolepsy

In order to understand mechanisms of cataplexy and REM-sleep abnormalities in narcolepsy, it is essential to examine whether REM-sleep generation in narcolepsy is impaired. We have first analyzed the REM sleep and cataplexy cyclicity in narcoleptic and control canines to observe whether the cyclicity at which REM sleep occurs is disturbed in narcoleptic canines (Figure 40.4) (Nishino *et al.*, 2000a). Interval histograms for REM-sleep episodes revealed that a clear 30-minute cyclicity exists in both narcoleptic and control animals, suggesting that the system controlling REM-sleep generation is intact in narcoleptic dogs (Figure 40.4). In contrast to REM sleep, cataplexy can be elicited at any time upon emotional stimulation (i.e., no 30-minute cyclicity is observed) (Nishino *et al.*, 2000a). These results, together with the results of extensive human studies, show that cataplexy is tightly associated with hypocretin-deficiency status (cataplexy appears now

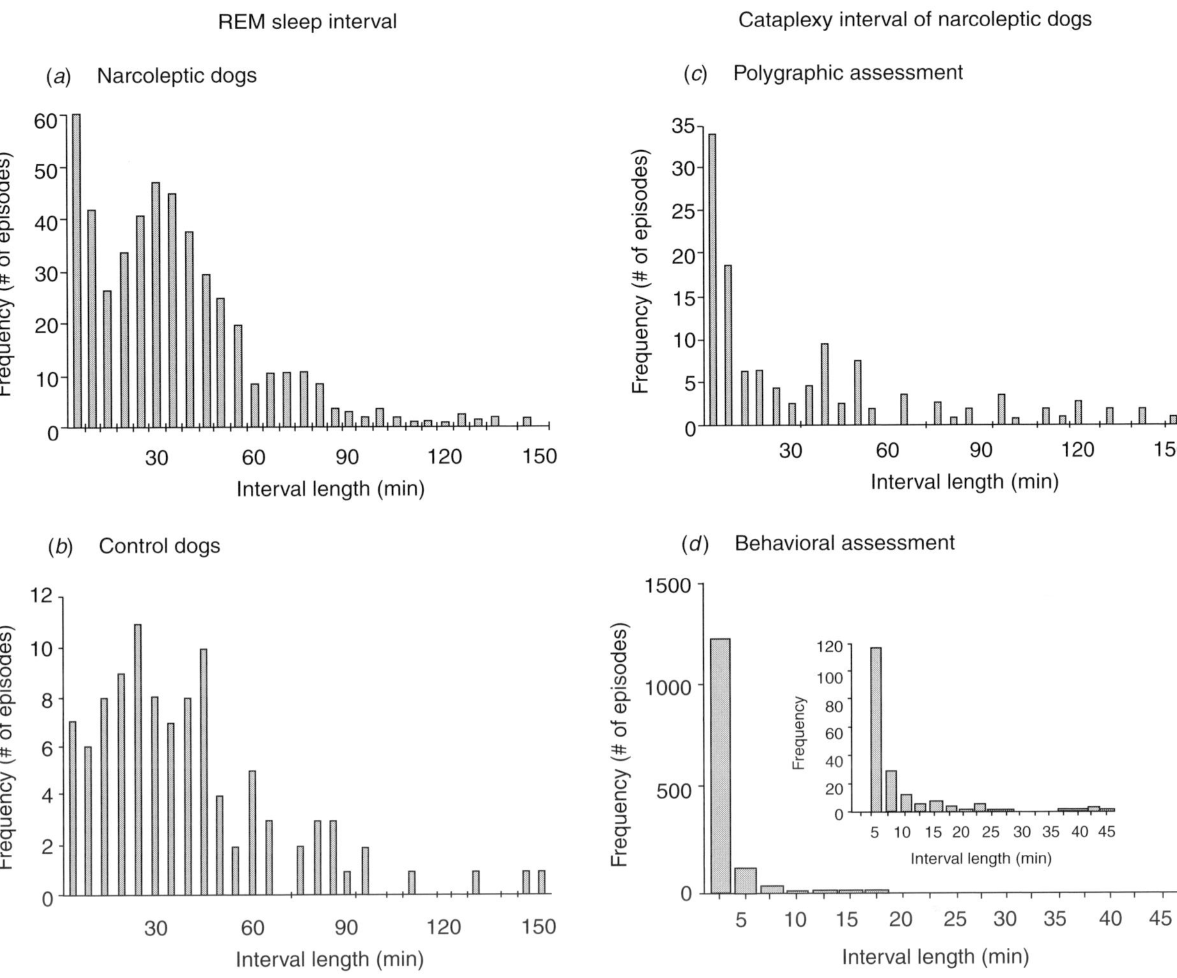

Figure 40.4 Frequency of interval lengths between consecutive REM-sleep episodes in narcoleptic and control dogs and cataplexy interval lengths in narcoleptic canines. (*a*) REM-sleep intervals are shown in 5-minute bins, while cataplexy intervals are shown in 2.5-minute bins. (*b*) A clear 30-minute interval between consecutive REM-sleep episodes is present in both narcoleptic and control animals. (*c*) No such cyclicity is present for spontaneous cataplectic attacks that occurred during daytime six-hour sleep recordings. (*d*) Cyclicity of emotionally stimulated cataplectic attacks was also evaluated during a separate behavioral assay session, the Play Elicited Cataplexy Test. Two dogs were brought into a procedure room (3 m × 6 m), and dogs were allowed to play freely with each other and with toys provided. These interactions resulted in multiple cataplectic attacks. The occurrence of cataplexy was continuously monitored for two hours. More than 90% of cataplectic attacks occurred within short intervals of each other (five minutes), suggesting that cataplexy can be elicited at any time with emotional excitation. The frequencies that occurred at intervals of more than five minutes are magnified and replotted inside the frame; no 30-minute cyclicity was observed. (Adapted from Nishino *et al.*, 2000a.)

to be a unique pathological condition caused by a loss of hypocretin neurotransmission) (Mignot *et al.*, 2002) suggesting that the mechanisms for the triggering of cataplexy and REM sleep are distinct.

The fact that patients with other sleep disorders such as sleep apnea, and even healthy controls, can manifest SOREMs, hypnagogic hallucinations, and sleep paralysis when their sleep–wake patterns are sufficiently disturbed, yet these subjects never develop cataplexy, provides further support to the proposal that

cataplexy may be unrelated to other REM-associated symptoms (Aldrich *et al.*, 1997; Bishop *et al.*, 1996; Fukuda *et al.*, 1987).

However, previous electrophysiological data have also demonstrated various similarities between REM-sleep atonia and cataplexy (Guilleminault, 1976). Since H-reflex activity (one of the monosynaptic spinal electrically induced reflexes) profoundly diminishes or disappears during both REM sleep and cataplexy, it is likely that the motor inhibitory components of REM sleep are also responsible for the atonia during cataplexy (Guilleminault, 1976). Thus, the executive systems for the induction of muscle atonia during cataplexy and REM sleep are likely to be the same. This interpretation is also supported by the pharmacological findings that most compounds that significantly reduce or enhance REM sleep reduce and enhance cataplexy respectively. However, some exceptions, such as the discrepant effects of dopamine D2/D3 antagonists on REM sleep and cataplexy, also exist (Okura *et al.*, 2000).

Preceding REM-sleep episodes influence on occurrence of cataplexy

Although cataplexy is likely to be a unique pathological condition and is distinct from physiological REM-sleep atonia, our results in narcoleptic dogs also suggest that short-term feedback mechanisms resulting from the occurrence of physiological REM sleep on cataplexy also exists.

We have examined whether the amount and timing of preceding REM sleep or slow-wave sleep (SWS) may affect the occurrence of cataplexy in narcoleptic Dobermans (Nishino *et al.*, 2004). Four narcoleptic Dobermans implanted with polygraph-recording electrodes were used. The dogs were left alone in the recording room in the afternoon (1 to 5 p.m.), and their sleep was monitored polygraphically for ten minutes. Immediately after every sleep-recording session, an experimenter came into the recording room and tried to initiate cataplexy for ten minutes (using the presentation of appetitive food). The occurrence of cataplexy (starting time, number of attacks, and duration) was recorded during five minutes of testing. The occurrence of cataplexy (TSC; total time spent in cataplexy) was negatively correlated with amounts of REM sleep (but not SWS and wake) observed during ten-minute (p = 0.008) sleep-recording sessions prior to cataplexy testing (Figure 40.5). REM sleep amount in the ten-minute preceding periods was also statistically correlated with the latency to the first cataplexy attacks (positively) and the duration of the first cataplectic attacks (negatively) (Figure 40.5). It thus appears that low REM-sleep propensity (after spontaneous REM sleep) prevents the occurrence of cataplexy.

Although the timing of occurrence of cataplexy is not governed by a 30-minute ultradian REM-sleep cyclicity (see Figure 40.4), REM-sleep propensity may also influence the occurrence of cataplexy.

Muscle activity during REM sleep in narcolepsy and RBD

REM sleep behavior disorder (RBD) is a neurological condition well known to be associated with the synucleinopathies in middle-aged patients. It is reported that more than one in three adult patients suffering from narcolepsy–cataplexy experience RBD, while RBD in childhood is extremely rare. Bonakis *et al.* (2008) report two patients aged less than 33 years who presented with clinical and polysomnographical features of RBD, both of whom proved to have previously undiagnosed narcolepsy. Nevsimalova *et al.* (2007) also present the cases of two girls (aged 9 and 7 years old) with narcolepsy–cataplexy, in whom RBD was one of the first symptoms of the disease. These authors claim that narcolepsy should be included in the differential diagnosis of young patients presenting with abnormal behavior during sleep compatible with RBD.

Dauvilliers *et al.* (2007) recently quantified REM-sleep parameters in patients with narcolepsy in relation to RBD and found higher percentages of REM sleep without atonia, phasic electromyographic (EMG) activity, and REM density in patients with narcolepsy than normal controls (Figure 40.6). In contrast, idiopathic RBD patients had a higher percentage of REM sleep without atonia but a lower REM density than patients with narcolepsy and normal controls (Figure 40.6). Based on a threshold of 80% for percentage of REM sleep with atonia, 50% of narcoleptics and 87.5% of RBD patients had abnormal REM-sleep muscle activity. However, no significant behavioral manifestation in REM sleep was noted in narcoleptics. Therefore, abnormalities in REM-sleep motor regulation with an increased frequency of REM sleep without atonia, phasic EMG events, and PLMS are more frequently observed in narcoleptic patients when compared to controls. These abnormalities were seen more prominently in patients with RBD than in narcoleptics, with the exception of the PLMS index. Since dopaminergic mechanisms are believed to be involved in sleep-related motor dyscontrol, the authors proposed that dysfunctions in the hypocretin–dopaminergic system may lead to motor dyscontrol in REM sleep that results in dissociated sleep–wake states. This hypothesis is consistent with the findings in narcoleptic dogs: (1) narcoleptic dogs are very sensitive to D2/3 receptor agonist to exhibit cataplexy and drowsiness (Nishino *et al.*, 1991); (2) they also exhibit PLMS-like involuntary movement (Okura *et al.*, 2001). The study demonstrated some

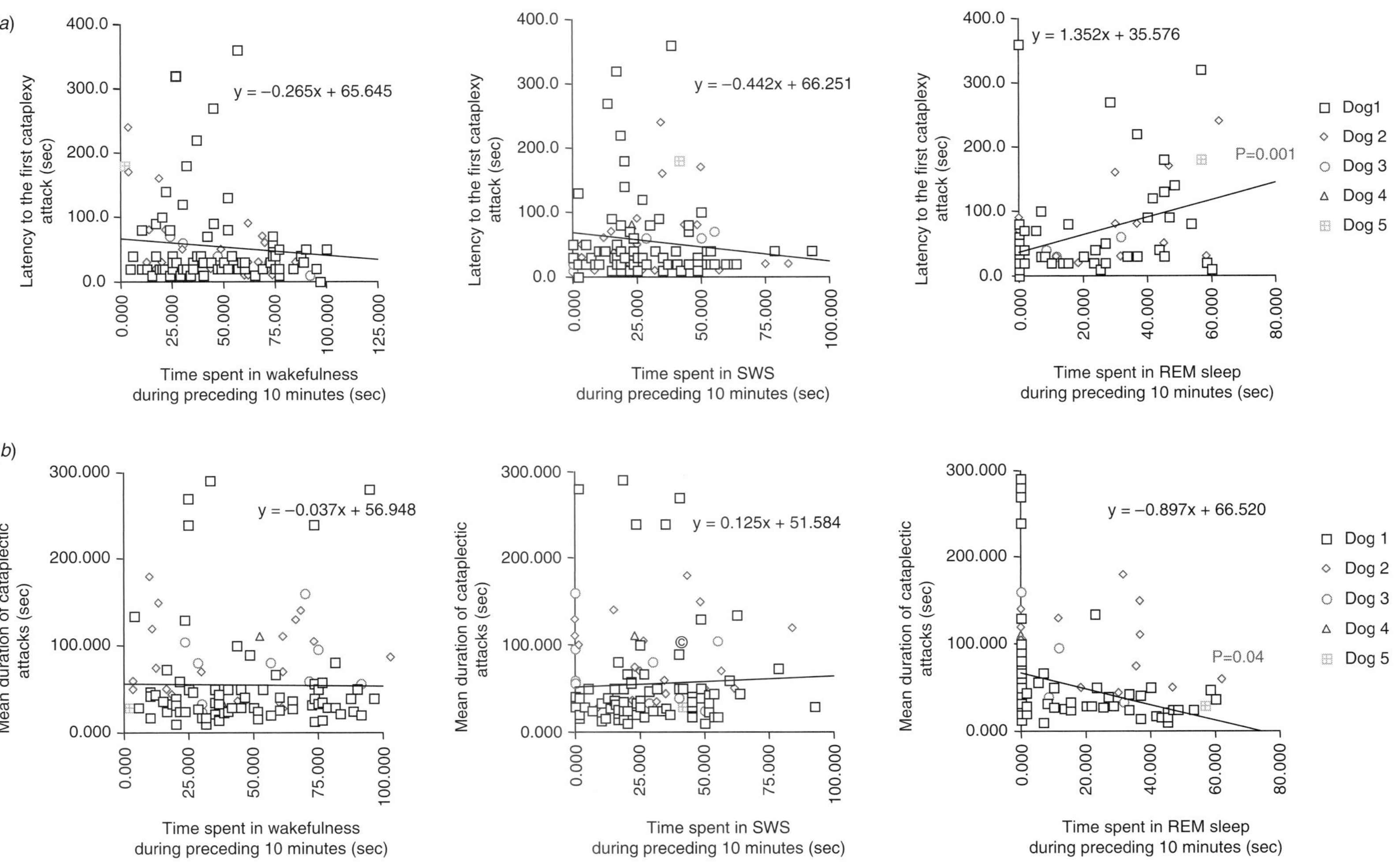

Figure 40.5 (*a*) Correlation between ten minutes preceding amount of wakefulness, SWS and REM sleep, and latencies to the first cataplectic attacks and (*b*) mean duration of cataplectic attacks. Preceding REM-sleep amount is positively correlated to the latency to the first cataplectic attack (p = 0.001), and is negatively correlated with the mean duration of cataplectic attacks (p = 0.04). Preceding REM-sleep amount is also negatively correlated with the duration of the first cataplectic attacks and total time spent in cataplexy (TSC) (data not shown). In contrast, preceding wake and SWS amount do not influence these parameters. (See plate section for color version.)

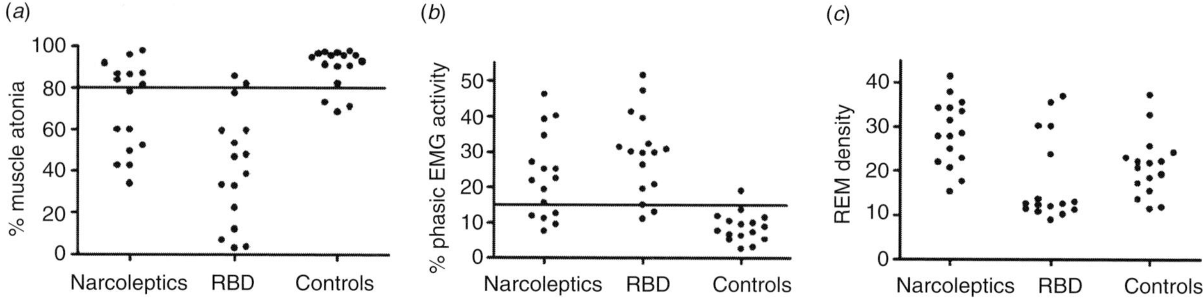

Figure 40.6 Distribution of (*a*) REM-sleep muscle atonia; (*b*) REM-sleep phasic EMG activity and (*c*) REM density in 16 patients with narcolepsy, 16 patients with "idiopathic" RBD, and 16 normal controls. Cut-offs at 80% and 15% were noted for the normal percentage of REM-sleep muscle atonia and chin phasic EMG in REM sleep, respectively. (Adapted from Dauvilliers *et al.*, 2007)

similarities in motor dyscontrol in REM sleep between narcolepsy and RBD, but clear distinctions were also noted.

Conclusion

Although REM-sleep abnormalities were initially emphasized as the major characteristics of narcolepsy, these abnormalities cannot be discussed separately from other sleep abnormalities, namely EDS and sleep–wake fragmentation. Several authors are studying proposed models for sleep abnormalities in narcolepsy. These include (1) unstable sleep–wake circuit; (2) abnormal timing of circadian distribution of sleep and wake; (3) insufficient non-REM sleep intensity; and (4) enhanced strength of the REM oscillator. These theories explain some aspects of symptoms well, but there are still incompatibilities to explain other aspects of the symptoms. There are also limitations in human studies, and the models mostly describe the phenomenon and do not address the mechanisms underlying the abnormal sleep regulation in narcolepsy much.

Since the hypocretin system is likely involved in both sleep homeostasis and circadian control of occurrence of sleep and wake, complex mechanisms are likely involved for the pathological manipulations of sleep and its related phenomena.

Even more complexly, cataplexy is likely to be distinct from other dissociated manifestations of REM sleep (i.e., sleep paralysis and hypnagogic hallucinations). The observation that prepubertal narcolepsy-cataplexy cases are almost always hypocretin deficient suggests that hypocretin deficiency occurs at cataplexy onset. In addition, acute ablation of hypocretin ligands by focal hypothalamic lesions associated with immune-related inflammatory encephalopathies, such as those in MS and NMO, rarely induce cataplexy. Chronic and selective loss of hypocretin ligand may be required to exhibit cataplexy. The consequence of the chronic and selective loss of hypocretin ligand (vs. the acute loss of hypocretin neurotransmission) involved in the induction of cataplexy is not known. The mechanisms of emotional induction of cataplexy remain to be studied.

References

Aldrich, M. S., Chervin, R. D. & Malow, B. A. (1997) Value of the multiple sleep latency test (MSLT) for the diagnosis of narcolepsy. *Sleep* **20**: 620–9.

Arii, J., Kanbayashi, T., Tanabe, Y. *et al.* (2004) CSF hypocretin-1 (orexin-A) levels in childhood narcolepsy and neurologic disorders. *Neurology* **63**: 2440–2.

Beuckmann, C. T., Sinton, C. M., Williams, S. C. *et al.* (2004) Expression of a poly-glutamine-ataxin-3 transgene in orexin neurons induces narcolepsy-cataplexy in the rat. *J Neurosci* **24**: 4469–77.

Billiard, M., Besset, A. & Cadilhac, J. (1983) The clinical and polygraphic development of narcolepsy. In *Sleep/Wake Disorders: Natural History, Epidemiology and Long-term Evolution*, eds. C.Guilleminault & E. Lugaresi. New York: Raven Press.

Bishop, C., Rosenthal, L., Helmus, T., Roehrs, T. & Roth, T. (1996) The frequency of multiple sleep onset REM periods among subjects with no excessive daytime sleepiness. *Sleep* **19**: 727–30.

Bonakis, A., Howard, R. S. & Williams, A. (2008) Narcolepsy presenting as REM sleep behaviour disorder. *Clin Neurol Neurosurg* **110**: 518–20.

Bourgine, N., Claustrat, B., Besset, A. & Billiard, M. (1986) Melatonin plasma concentrations during day-time and night-time in narcoleptic subjects and controls. *Sleep Res* **15**: 46.

Broughton, R., Dunham, W., Newman, J. *et al.* (1988) Ambulatory 24 hour sleep-wake monitoring in narcolepsy-cataplexy compared to matched control. *Electroenceph Clin Neurophysiol* **70**: 473–81.

Broughton, R., Krupa, S., Boucher, B., Rivers, M. & Mulligan, J. (1998) Impaired circadian waking arousal in narcolepsy-cataplexy. *Sleep Res Online* **1**: 159–65.

Broughton, R., Valley, V., Aguirre, M. *et al.* (1986) Excessive daytime sleepiness and pathophysiology of narcolepsy-cataplexy: a laboratory perspective. *Sleep* **9**: 205–15.

Carskadon, M. A. & Dement, W. C. (1987) Daytime sleepiness: quantification of a Behavioral State. *Neurosci Biobehav Rev* **11**: 307–17.

Chemelli, R. M., Willie, J. T., Sinton, C. M. *et al.* (1999) Narcolepsy in orexin knockout mice: molecular genetics of sleep regulation. *Cell* **98**: 437–51.

Chou, T. C., Bjorkum, A. A., Gaus, S. E. *et al.* (2002) Afferents to the ventrolateral preoptic nucleus. *J Neurosci* **22**: 977–90.

Dantz, B., Edgar, D. M. & Dement, W. C. (1994) Circadian rhythms in narcolepsy: studies on a 90 minute day. *Electroceph Clin Neurophy* **90**: 24–35.

Dauvilliers, Y., Rompre, S., Gagnon, J. F. *et al.* (2007) REM sleep characteristics in narcolepsy and REM sleep behavior disorder. *Sleep* **30**: 844–9.

Dement, W., Rechtschaffen, A. & Gulevich, G. (1966) The nature of the narcoleptic sleep attack. *Neurology* **16**: 18–33.

Dijk, D. J. & Czeisler, C. A. (1994) Paradoxical timing of the circadian rhythm of sleep propensity serves to consolidate sleep and wakefulness in humans. *Neurosci Lett* **166**: 63–8.

Dijk, D. J. & Czeisler, C. A. (1995) Contribution of the circadian pacemaker and the sleep homeostat to sleep propensity, sleep structure, electroencephalographic slow waves, and sleep spindle activity in humans. *J Neurosci* **15**: 3526–38.

Edgar, D. M., Dement, W. C. & Fuller, C. A. (1993) Effect of SCN-lesions on sleep in squirrel monkeys: evidence for opponent processes in sleep-wake regulation. *J Neurosci* **13**: 1065–79.

Estabrooke, I. V., McCarthy, M. T., Ko, E. *et al.* (2001) Fos expression in orexin neurons varies with behavioral state. *J Neurosci* **21**: 1656–62.

Ferrillo, F., Donadio, S., De Carli, F., Garbarino, S. & Nobili, L. (2007) A model-based approach to homeostatic and ultradian aspects of nocturnal sleep structure in narcolepsy. *Sleep* **30**: 157–65.

Fujiki, N., Yoshida, Y., Ripley, B. *et al.* (2001) Changes in CSF hypocretin-1 (orexin A) levels in rats across 24 hours and in response to food deprivation. *NeuroReport* **12**: 993–7.

Fukuda, K., Miyasita, A., Inugami, M. & Ishihara, K. (1987) High prevalence of isolated sleep paralysis: Kanashibari phenomenon in Japan. *Sleep* **10**: 279–86.

Gallopin, T., Fort, P., Eggermann, E., *et al.* (2000) Identification of sleep-promoting neurons in vitro. *Nature* **404**: 992–5.

Gélineau, J. B. E. (1880) De la narcolepsie. *Gazette des hôpitaux* **53**: 626–8.

Guilleminault, C. (1976) Cataplexy. In *Narcolepsy (Advances in Sleep Research Vol. 3)*. pp. 125–43.

Guilleminault, C., Wilson, R. A. & Dement, W. C. (1974) A study on cataplexy. *Arch Neurol* **31**: 255–61.

Hagan, J. J., Leslie, R. A., Patel, S. *et al.* (1999) Orexin A activates locus coeruleus cell firing and increases arousal in the rat. *Proc Natl Acad Sci U S A* **96**: 10,911–16.

Hara, J., Beuckmann, C. T., Nambu, T. *et al.* (2001) Genetic ablation of orexin neurons in mice results in narcolepsy, hypophagia, and obesity. *Neuron* **30**: 345–54.

Hishikawa, Y. (1976) Sleep paralysis. In *Narcolepsy*, eds. C. Guilleminault & P. Passpouant. New York: Spectrum.

Hishikawa, Y., Wakamatsu, H., Furuya, E. *et al.* (1976) Sleep satiation in narcoleptic patients. *Electroencephalogr Clin Neurophysiol* **41**: 1–18.

Hobson, J. A., McCarley, R. W. & Wyzinski, P. W. (1975) Sleep cycle oscillation: reciprocal discharge by two brainstem neuronal groups. *Science* **189**: 55–8.

Honda, Y. (1988) Clinical features of narcolepsy. In *HLA in Narcolepsy*, eds. Y. Honda & T. Juji. Berlin: Springer-Verlag.

ICSD-2 (ed.) (2005) *ICSD-2-International Classification of Sleep Disorders*, 2nd edn. *Diagnostic and Coding Manual*. Westchester, Illinois: American Academy of Sleep Medicine.

Kaitin, K. I., Kilduff, T. S. & Dement, W. C. (1986) Evidence for excessive sleepiness in canine narcoleptics. *Electroencephalogr Clin Neurophysiol* **64**: 447–54.

Kanbayashi, T., Shimohata, T., Nakashima, I. *et al.* (2009) Symptomatic narcolepsy in MS and NMO patients; new neurochemical and immunological implications. *Arch Neurol* **66**: 1563–6

Khatami, R., Landolt, H. P., Achermann, P. *et al.* (2008) Challenging sleep homeostasis in narcolepsy-cataplexy: implications for non-REM and REM sleep regulation. *Sleep* **31**: 859–67.

Khatami, R., Landolt, H. P., Achermann, P. *et al.* (2007) Insufficient non-REM sleep intensity in narcolepsy-cataplexy. *Sleep* **30**: 980–9.

Lavie, P. (1991) REM periodicity under ultrashort sleep/wake cycle in narcoleptic patients. *Can J Psychol* **45**: 185–93.

Lee, M. G., Hassani, O. K. & Jones, B. E. (2005) Discharge of identified orexin/hypocretin neurons across the sleep-waking cycle. *J Neurosci* **25**: 6716–20.

Mayer, G., Hellmann, F., Leonhard, E. & Meier-Ewert, K. (1997) Circadian temperature and activity rhythms in unmedicated narcoleptic patients. *Pharmacol Biochem Behav* **58**: 395–402.

Mayer, G., Pollmächer, T., Meier-Ewert, K. & Schulz, H. (1993) Zur Einschätzung des Behinderungsgrades bei Narkolepsie. *Gesundh-Wes* **55**: 337–42.

Mignot, E., Lammers, G. J., Ripley, B., *et al.* (2002) The role of cerebrospinal fluid hypocretin measurement in the diagnosis of narcolepsy and other hypersomnias. *Arch Neurol* **59**: 1553–62.

Mileykovskiy, B. Y., Kiyashchenko, L. I. & Siegel, J. M. (2005) Behavioral correlates of activity in identified hypocretin/orexin neurons. *Neuron* **46**: 787–98.

Montplaisir, J., Billard, M., Takahashi, S. *et al.* (1978) Twenty-four-hour recording in REM-narcoleptics with special reference to nocturnal sleep disruption. *Biol Psych* **13**: 78–89.

Moscovitch, A., Partinen, M. & Guilleminault, C. (1993) The positive diagnosis of narcolepsy and narcolepsy's borderland. *Neurology* **43**: 55–60.

Mosko, S. S., Shampain, D. S. & Sassin, J. F. (1984) Nocturnal REM latency and sleep disturbance in narcolepsy. *Sleep* **7**: 115–25.

Nevsimalova, S., Prihodova, I., Kemlink, D., Lin, L. & Mignot, E. (2007) REM behavior disorder (RBD) can be one of the first symptoms of childhood narcolepsy. *Sleep Med* **8**: 784–6.

Nishino, S. & Mignot, E. (1997) Pharmacological aspects of human and canine narcolepsy. *Prog Neurobiol* **52**: 27–78.

Nishino, S. and Kanbayashi, T. (2005) Symptomatic narcolepsy, cataplexy and hypersomnia, and their implications in the hypothalamic hypocretin/ovexin system. *Sleep Med Rev* **9**: 269–310.

Nishino, S., Arrigoni, J., Valtier, D. *et al.* (1991) Dopamine D2 mechanisms in canine narcolepsy. *J Neurosci* **11**: 2666–71.

Nishino, S., Riehl, J., Hong, J. *et al.* (2000a) Is narcolepsy REM sleep disorder? Analysis of sleep abnormalities in narcoleptic Dobermans. *Neurosci Res* **38**: 437–46.

Nishino, S., Ripley, B., Overeem, S., Lammers, G. J. & Mignot, E. (2000b) Hypocretin (orexin) deficiency in human narcolepsy. *Lancet* **355**: 39–40.

Nishino, S., Bliesath, J., Honda, K. & Mignot, E. (2004) The occurrence of cataplexy in relation to proceeding REM sleep. *Sleep* **27**: A248.

Okura, M., Fujiki, N., Ripley, B. *et al.* (2001) Narcoleptic canines display periodic leg movements during sleep. *Psychiatry Clin Neurosci* **55**: 243–4.

Okura, M., Riehl, J., Mignot, E. & Nishino, S. (2000) Sulpiride, a D2/D3 blocker, reduces cataplexy but not REM sleep in canine narcolepsy. *Neuropsychopharmacology* **23**: 528–38.

Peyron, C., Tighe, D. K., van den Pol, A. N. *et al.* (1998) Neurons containing hypocretin (orexin) project to multiple neuronal systems. *J Neurosci* **18** : 9996–10015.

Peyron, C., Faraco, J., Rogers, W. *et al.* (2000) A mutation in a case of early onset narcolepsy and a generalized absence of hypocretin peptides in human narcoleptic brains. *Nat Med* **6**: 991–7.

Ribstein, M. (1976) Hypnagogic hallucinations. In *Narcolepsy*, eds C. Guilleminault, W. C. Dement & P. Passouant. New York: Spectrum.

Rosenthal, C. (1939) Uber das aufreten von halluzinatorisch-kataplektischem angstsyndrom, wachanfallen und ahnlichen storungen bei schizophrenen. *Mschr Psychiat* **102**: 11.

Saper, C. B., Chou, T. C. & Scammell, T. E. (2001) The sleep switch: hypothalamic control of sleep and wakefulness. *Trends Neurosci* **24**: 726–31.

Tafti, M., Rondouin, G., Basset, A. & Billiard, M. (1992) Sleep deprivation in narcoleptic subjects: effect on sleep stages and EEG power density. *Electroencephalogr Clin Neurophysiol* **83**: 339–49.

Takahashi, Y. & Jimbo, M. (1963) Polygraphic study of narcoleptic syndrome, with special reference to hypnagogic hallucinations and cataplexy. *Folia Psychiatr Neurol Jpn* Suppl. **7**: 343–7.

Vogel, G. (1960) Studies in psychophysiology of dreams III. The dream of narcolepsy. *Arch Gen Psychiatry* **3**: 421–8.

Yoshida, K., McCormack, S., Espana, R. A., Crocker, A. & Scammell, T. E. (2006) Afferents to the orexin neurons of the rat brain. *J Comp Neurol* **494**: 845–61.

Yoshida, Y., Fujiki, N., Nakajima, T. *et al.* (2001) Fluctuation of extracellular hypocretin-1 (orexin A) levels in the rat in relation to the light–dark cycle and sleep–wake activities. *Eur J Neurosci* **14**: 1075–81.

Zeitzer, J. M., Buckmaster, C. L., Lyons, D. M. & Mignot, E. (2004) Locomotor-dependent and -independent components to hypocretin-1 (orexin A) regulation in sleep-wake consolidating monkeys. *J Physiol* **557**: 1045–53.

Zhang, S., Zeitzer, J. M., Yoshida, Y. *et al.* (2004) Lesions of the suprachiasmatic nucleus eliminate the daily rhythm of hypocretin-1 release. *Sleep* **27**: 619–27.

Chapter 41

REM sleep and dreams: relationship to anxiety, psychosomatic, and behavioral disorders

Luigi Ferini-Strambi

Summary

Sleep disturbances are frequently associated with, and can comprise core features of, anxiety disorders. Studies using objective sleep recordings have demonstrated impaired sleep initiation and maintenance in persons with generalized anxiety disorder or panic disorder, but a normal latency to REM sleep. Increased phasic motor activity and eye movement density during REM sleep have been reported in combat veterans with post-traumatic stress disorder: moreover, nightmares and other symptomatic awakenings disproportionately arise from REM sleep.

One of the most consistent behavioral manifestations of sleep loss is the worsening of mood state. With prolonged sleep deprivation it is possible to observe an increase in self-reported feelings of depressed mood, anger, frustration, and anxiety. Interestingly, there is little evidence that waking stress leads to increased REM, although there have been reports of small elevations in REM following severe emotional upset. REM sleep might have some sort of calming effect.

The relationship between somatic distress and dream disturbance has been recently investigated: individuals who reported more incidents of both bad dreams and nightmares did report higher levels of somatic distress. However, REM sleep behavior disorder (RBD), a parasomnia characterized by complex and often violent motor behaviors that emerge from REM sleep and that are associated with violent and unpleasant dreams, represents a particular condition. A discrepancy between the aggressiveness displayed in dreams and the placid and mild-mannered temperament has been observed in patients with RBD.

Sleep, REM sleep, and anxiety disorders

The anxiety disorders in the *Diagnostic and Statistical Manual, 4th edition – text revised* (DSM-IV-R: API, 2000) are generalized anxiety, panic, post-traumatic stress, obsessive–compulsive, and phobic disorders. Sleep disturbances are frequently associated with, and can comprise, core features of anxiety disorders.

Post-traumatic stress disorder (PTSD) develops in some individuals after exposure to severely threatening stress and manifests with symptoms of re-experiencing the trauma, emotional numbing and avoidance behaviors, and heightened arousal. Specific criteria for the disorder related to sleep include nightmares with trauma-related content and difficulty initiating and maintaining sleep, which is the common definition of insomnia. The principal feature of generalized anxiety disorder (GAD) is chronic worry and tension. Impaired sleep initiation and maintenance are also symptom criteria for GAD. Panic disorder features recurring severe and unpredictable episodes of anxiety with crescendo-like onsets called "panic attacks," that are often complicated by anticipatory anxiety and phobic avoidance. Although not among the specific diagnostic criteria, panic disorder has also been associated in many studies with complaints of difficulty initiating and maintaining sleep. In addition, panic attacks can arise during sleep in many patients diagnosed with the disorder. Sleep disturbances can occur with, but seem to be less salient features of, obsessive–compulsive disorder (OCD) and specific and social phobic disorders.

In addition to frequently being a part of the presenting symptoms of anxiety disorders, insomnia is also a risk factor for their subsequent onset (Breslau *et al.*,

REM Sleep: Regulation and Function, eds. Birendra N. Mallick, S. R. Pandi-Perumal, Robert W. McCarley, and Adrian R. Morrison. Published by Cambridge University Press. © Cambridge University Press 2011.

1996). There is an overlap between interventions that target insomnia and other sleep disturbances and those that are used in treating anxiety disorders. Overlapping approaches include medications, and cognitive behavioral strategies that target worry, tension, and maladaptive cognitions. Optimal sequencing or integration of treatments targeting insomnia and sleep disturbance, however, are not well investigated.

Concerning polysomnographic data, an early study found impaired sleep maintenance and a reduced latency to REM sleep in a group with persons with OCD, which is consistent with a linkage between OCD and affective illness (Insel *et al.*, 1982). However, two more recent polysomnographic studies of persons with OCD failed to replicate these results, reporting instead that the sleep patterns of persons with OCD were essentially normal (Hohagan *et al.*, 1994; Robinson *et al.*, 1998).

Studies using objective sleep recordings demonstrated impaired sleep initiation and maintenance in persons with GAD (Saletu-Zyhlarz *et al.*, 1997), but a normal latency to REM sleep, in contrast to findings from major depression where REM-sleep latency is reduced.

Most but not all published studies of panic disorder that used objective methods of sleep recording (polysomnography, PSG) have found evidence of impaired sleep initiation and maintenance (Mellman, 2008).

Studies that have captured sleep panic attacks during polysomnographic recordings found that the episodes were preceded by either stage 2 or 3 of non-REM sleep. In particular, Mellman and Uhde (1989) specifically noted that sleep panic attacks originated during the transition from stage 2 into early slow-wave sleep, which is a period of diminishing arousal.

Evidence for abnormalities related to REM sleep in PTSD is consistent. Increased phasic motor activity and eye movement density during REM sleep have been reported in combat veterans with PTSD (Mellman, 2008). Nightmares and other symptomatic awakenings disproportionately arise from REM sleep. Breslau *et al.* (2004) reported more frequent transitions from REM sleep to stage 1 or wake in a community sample with either lifetime only (i.e., remitted) or current PTSD compared with trauma-exposed and trauma-unexposed controls. There is converging evidence for disruptions of REM-sleep continuity (symptomatic awakenings, increased awakening and arousals, and motor activity) and increased REM activation (eye movement density) with chronic PTSD. The limited number of studies that used objective recordings of sleep following trauma also suggest the relevance of REM-sleep disruption, in terms of short continuous periods of REM sleep before stage shifts or arousal (Habukawa *et al.*, 2007).

Effects of sleep deprivation on psychopathology

Total sleep deprivation

One of the most prominent and consistent behavioral manifestations of sleep loss is the worsening of mood state (Dinges *et al.*, 1997; Scott *et al.*, 2006). With a prolonged sleep deprivation, it is possible to observe an increase in self-reported feelings of depressed mood, anger, frustration, and anxiety (Caldwell *et al.*, 2004). In the absence of adequate sleep, negative reactions to adverse experiences appear to be significantly magnified, while positive reactions to pleasant events are often subdued (Zohar *et al.*, 2005). Sleep deprivation is associated not only with changes in mood, but also with alterations in brain function. As little as 24 hours of continuous wakefulness is correlated with significant reductions in glucose metabolism within the prefrontal cortex (Thomas *et al.*, 2000), a region of the brain crucial for personality, emotion regulation, and behavioral inhibition. Clinical psychopathological conditions such as mood disorders, psychosis, and antisocial behavior have all been linked to abnormalities of structure and function within the prefrontal cortex. Patients with unipolar depression frequently have abnormalities of brain volume within the prefrontal cortex and anterior cingulate gyrus (Beyer and Krishnan, 2002), and an altered functional activity within these regions, particularly reduced blood flow or metabolism within the prefrontal cortex, has been reported (Videbech, 2000). However, in some patients with mood disorders, sleep deprivation can have a seemingly paradoxical antidepressant effect, which correlates with normalization of metabolic activity within the anterior cingulate/prefrontal regions (Gillin *et al.*, 2001).

Also schizophrenia is closely linked with prefrontal dysfunction. Patients with schizophrenia often demonstrate deficits in executive functions, abilities which rely heavily on the integrative and working memory capacities of the frontal lobes (Stirling *et al.*, 2006). Patients suffering from schizophrenia show significantly reduced brain activity (Meyer-Lindenberg *et al.*,

2005) and reduced gray matter volume within the prefrontal cortex and anterior cingulate gyrus (Choi *et al.*, 2005). It has been demonstrated that these reductions correlate with the severity of both cognitive dysfunction and psychotic symptoms (Choi *et al.*, 2005).

Recently, some authors administered the Personality Assessment Inventory (PAI), a clinical measure of symptoms of psychopathology, to 25 healthy adults at rested baseline and again following 56 hours of continuous wakefulness (Kahn-Greene *et al.*, 2007). Comparisons showed a significant global increase in PAI psychopathology scores from baseline to sleep-deprived sessions, particularly for somatic complaints, anxiety, depression, and paranoia.

REM-sleep deprivation

It has been reported that during REM sleep the amygdaloid complex and the associated anterior cingulate cortex have a particularly elevated regional blood flow, suggesting a high level of activation in these regions (Maquet *et al.*, 1996). The authors speculated that this might be associated with emotionally charged memories and, as REM is closely coupled with dreaming, the emotional aspect of dreams. It is known that the amygdala is integral to the organism's ability to appraise dangerous situations, respond to threat or reward, and to predict the circumstances when these are likely to occur. Damage to the amygdala leads to defects in the recognition of emotion in others, and impairments to emotional learning and fear responses (Morris *et al.*, 1998). Other PET imaging studies of human REM have shown similar findings to those previously reported, but with greater changes in the paralimbic regions associated with the amygdala (Nofzinger *et al.*, 1997). It has been speculated that REM sleep integrates neocortical function with basal forebrain–hypothalamic motivational and reward systems (Nofzinger *et al.*, 1997).

However, REM sleep can be suppressed substantially and for many nights by most of the drugs that have been and are commonly used to treat depression, without any apparent effect of the REM loss. Some authors reported that the monoamine oxidase inhibitors (MAOIs), such as phenelzine, eliminated REM (after a few weeks of treatment) for many months in depressed or narcoleptic patients, without any adverse psychological effects (Landolt *et al.*, 1999; Wyatt *et al.*, 1971a,b). Other studies using phenelzine (Kupfer and Bowers, 1972) reported total or almost total (less than five minutes of REM per night) REM suppression, again without psychological ill effect. Most of the more modern tricyclic antidepressants and selective serotonin reuptake inhibitors (SSRIs) immediately and significantly reduce REM throughout the duration of treatment, which can last many weeks (Staner *et al.*, 1995). Again, there are no adverse mental effects other than some minor impairment to memory and these patients usually recover from their depression. Of course, such findings might suggest that these drugs largely affect REM control mechanisms rather than any underlying REM function.

REM sleep, dreams, and somatic distress

Somatic distress is operationally defined as heightened attention to, amplification of, and misinterpretation of both benign and functional somatic symptoms (Rief *et al.*, 1998). Subjects with somatic distress worry and ruminate about the implication of these physiological experiences. As a result, somatic distress is associated with depression, anxiety, neuroticism, negative affect, anxiety sensitivity, and poor coping (Watt and Stewart, 2000). A psychological predisposition for negative affect has been consistently shown to connect somatic distress to anxiety and depression. Somatizers also tend to catastrophically interpret bodily perceptions (Rief *et al.*, 1998) and demonstrate attentional biases towards both illness-related stimuli and threatening stimuli. To some extent, individuals high in somatic distress also tend to make somatic-based interpretations of common bodily sensations (e.g., my mouth was dry … there is something wrong with my salivary glands) and are more likely to be hypochondriacal (Noyes *et al.*, 2005). Subjects high in somatic distress often demonstrate heightened anxiety sensitivity, defined as the belief that anxiety symptoms (autonomic hyperarousal) will have dangerous or harmful consequences such as illness, loss of control, or more anxiety (Noyes *et al.*, 2005). Subjects high in anxiety sensitivity may also develop a fear of hyperarousal, in which anxiety itself becomes the anxiety-provoking stimulus. Internal bodily cues serve as conditioned stimuli for anxiety through interoceptive conditioning. For example, an individual with high anxiety sensitivity might misinterpret a heart palpitation associated with an anxious state as a heart attack, causing more anxiety, whereas a subject with a low anxiety sensitivity would consider the same heart palpitation as an unpleasant but transient symptom (Watt and Stewart, 2000).

There is little evidence that waking stress leads to increased REM, although there have been reports of small rises in REM following severe emotional upset (Cartwright *et al.*, 1967). REM sleep might have some sort of calming effect. For example, Smith and Lapp (1991) reported that students having undergone important and "challenging" examinations showed an increased REM density (number of REM bursts per minute of REM), but the authors did not discriminate between single and multiple REMs. The effect lasted for several nights afterwards. Although the authors attributed this to the intense learning situation, another explanation, of course, is that this effect on REM was associated with the acute stress of the examinations.

However, what is the relationship between somatic distress and dreaming? What is known about the pathogenesis of disturbed dreams (DD) or nightmares? Nightmares, as currently defined in two major nosologies (DSM-IV-R: API, 2000; ICSD-II: American Sleep Disorders Association, 2005), are characterized by awakenings primarily from REM sleep with clear recall of disturbing mentation. The emotional component of DD is typically fear related, although less frequently other emotions such as anger or disgust have also been reported (Zadra and Donden, 1993). Idiopathic nightmares, for which the cause is unknown, are also now distinguished from post-traumatic nightmares, which are more severe and distressing and often, but not necessarily, associated with PTSD. Both types of nightmares are distinguished from sleep terrors, which also involve fear-based arousals but which typically arise from non-REM sleep, are not accompanied by vivid and extensive dreams, and do not result in awakenings with clear recall of mentation.

Some community-based epidemiological studies indicate that 2 to 6% of respondents report weekly nightmares, a frequency generally thought to reflect moderately severe pathology (Nielsen and Levin, 2007). Frequent nightmares have been reported more prevalent in childhood and adolescence (DSM-IV-R: API, 2000), but a recent epidemiological study found relatively low prevalences in pre-schoolers (Simard *et al.*, 2008). Females at all ages consistently report nightmares more often than do males (Ohayon *et al.*, 1997), probably because women report both a greater quantity and a greater intensity of symptoms related to negative emotional disturbances, such as depression and anxiety, than do men (Nolen-Hoeksema, 1990).

Several studies indicate that nightmares are reactive to intense stress (Nielsen and Levin, 2007). Indeed, they are more frequently reported during periods of increased life stress (Barrett, 1996). Moreover, nightmares are more frequent and more prevalent in the psychiatric population. Disturbed dreams are associated with anxiety, heightened risk for suicide, dissociative phenomena, and PTSD (Nielsen and Levin, 2007). Links with problems in the expression and regulation of dysphoric emotions are suggested by the relationship of DD with both psychopathological traits and heightened physical and emotional reactivity (Levin and Fireman, 2002).

The association of nightmares with this wide spectrum of pathological symptoms and conditions, all of which are marked by considerable emotional distress, supports the contention that nightmare production is related to a general personality style characterized by intense reactive emotional distress (Blagrove *et al.*, 2004). A recent literature suggests that the waking distress engendered by DD, defined as DD distress, rather than DD frequency per se mediates the relationship between DD and waking psychological impairment. Nielsen and Levin (2007) proposed a model that posits that DD reflect transitory breakdowns in the naturally occurring emotion regulation capacities of REM sleep and/or dreaming. In this model, both DD frequency and distress are related but they are distinct components of the dreaming process, with different mechanisms. They propose that DD frequency is affected by transitory shifts in day-to-day stress levels, while DD distress is determined by a longer standing disposition to experience heightened distress and negative effect in response to emotional stimuli, particularly in the form of dysphoric imagery. Thus, DD without an accompanying high level of waking distress should have minimal impact on waking functioning, whereas even low incidence rates of DD with waking distress may be an important pathway for psychopathology, probably by sensitizing the dreamer to the fear component of the imagery.

The first empirical investigation of the relationship between somatic distress and dream disturbance has been recently investigated (Levin *et al.*, 2009). A total of 313 college undergraduates completed three measures of somatic distress (SCL-90-R Somatization Scale, Somatic Interpretations Questionnaire, and the Anxiety Sensitivity Index) and then monitored their DD incidence and distress for 21 consecutive days. It was predicted that high levels of somatic distress would

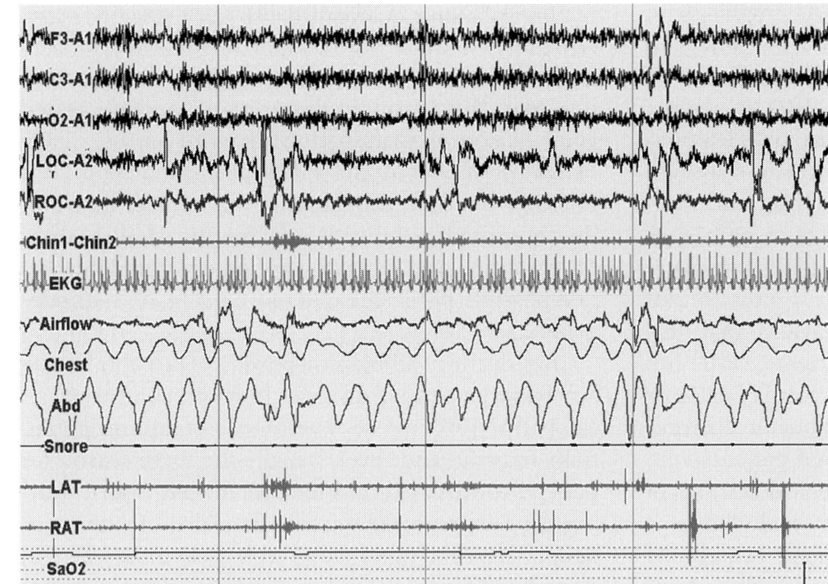

Figure 41.1 Polysomnography of a patient with REM sleep behavior disorder: REM sleep. (See plate section for color version.)

be associated with heightened levels of both DD incidence and distress. Although the results were somewhat mixed, individuals who reported more incidents of both bad dreams and nightmares did indeed report higher levels of somatic distress. However, these findings may have been compromised by method variance in which somatic distress was measured retrospectively, whereas nightmare and bad dream distress were measured prospectively. As retrospective reporting can be situationally biased based on present mood and is further subject to recall failures, the authors concluded that future studies should investigate this relationship utilizing prospective measures for both dream disturbances and somatic distress.

REM sleep behavior disorder and dreams with increased aggressiveness

REM sleep behavior disorder is characterized by complex and often violent motor behaviors that emerge from REM sleep and that are associated with dream mentation (ICSD-II: American Sleep Disorders Association, 2005). Patients typically seem to enact their dreams: they may talk, scream, gesture, move the arms often grasping, punching, or kicking a virtual object, and sometimes jump out of bed. Spontaneous awakening from episodes is not usual, but when this occurs, arousal is rapid and usually followed by a recall of a dream that generally matches the observed

behavior. For reasons not yet fully clarified, dreams of these patients tend to be unpleasant, stereotypical, action filled, and violent in nature. Video-PSG monitoring reveals a complete or intermittent loss of the physiological REM-sleep muscle atonia, as measured by surface electromyography (EMG) of the chin muscle, and an excessive EMG phasic activity during this stage (Figure 41.1).

Animal models of RBD showed that lesions of some regions of the brain stem are responsible for the emergence of the behaviors during REM sleep (Boeve *et al.*, 2007; Schenck and Mahowald, 2002).

REM sleep behavior disorder can occur in two forms, acute and chronic. The acute RBD has been observed in drug abusers (particularly with tricyclic antidepressants, monoamine inhibitors, or selective serotonin reuptake inhibitors) as well as during withdrawal from several substances (namely alcohol, meprobamate, nitrazepam, and pentazocine). The chronic form may be either idiopathic or secondary to various neurological disorders. Secondary RBD may be potentially triggered by any lesions involving the brain structures responsible for REM-sleep atonia, mostly located in the brain stem. REM sleep behavior disorder has been actually observed in cerebrovascular diseases, brain-stem tumors, Guillain-Barré syndrome, multiple sclerosis, and Machado–Joseph disease (Boeve *et al.*, 2007). REM sleep behavior disorder has been observed in association with two disorders not related to brain-stem impairment, as limbic encephalitis (Iranzo *et al.*, 2006) and with Morvan's syndrome (Liguori *et al.*, 2001). However, the most frequent association of RBD is with a group of neurodegenerative diseases called alpha-synucleinopathies, that include Parkinson's disease (PD), dementia with Lewy bodies (DLB), and multiple system atrophy (MSA) (Boeve *et al.*, 2007). In PD, muscle-tone abnormalities during REM sleep are frequent. Abnormalities in REM-sleep muscle atonia, regardless of the history of behavioral manifestations, was found in 58% of PD patients, while full RBD is present in approximately one-third of patients (Gagnon *et al.*, 2002). REM sleep behavior disorder may also be encountered in demented patients who show the clinical and neuropsychological features of DLB. Indeed, RBD has been recently included, as a suggestive feature, within the diagnostic criteria for DLB (McKeith, 2005). REM sleep behavior disorder is also extremely frequent in patients with MSA, being present in about 90% of them (Boeve *et al.*, 2007). When no neurological signs or central nervous system (CNS) lesions are found, RBD is currently defined as "idiopathic." This form accounts for up to 60% of the cases described in the literature. However, one prospective study performed on idiopathic RBD showed that 38% male RBD patients developed a Parkinsonian syndrome within four years from the RBD diagnosis. The study has been recently updated, showing that up to 65% idiopathic RBD patients eventually developed a Parkinsonian disorder and/or a dementia without Parkinsonism, about 13 years after the RBD onset (Schenck *et al.*, 2003).

A recent follow-up study of 93 RBD patients showed that 26 subjects developed a neurodegenerative disorder: a total of 14 patients developed PD, 7 developed DLB, 4 developed dementia that met clinical criteria for Alzheimer's disease, and 1 developed MSA (Postuma *et al.*, 2009): the estimated five-year risk of neurodegenerative disease was 17.7%, the ten-year risk was 40.6%, and the twelve-year risk was 52.4%.

However, in nearly 50% of patients, RBD remained idiopathic after 12 years. Therefore, the condition of idiopathic RBD is receiving increasing attention, as a possible prodrome in the development of a full-blown neurodegenerative disease (Fantini *et al.*, 2005a). Recent studies found several slight abnormalities associated to the motor dyscontrol during REM sleep. The latter include slowing of the electroencephalographic rhythms in both wakefulness and REM sleep,

neuropsychological abnormalities in specific functions, such as visuo-spatial constructional abilities and visuo-spatial learning, signs of autonomic impairment, olfactory deficit, subtle motor signs, and decreased color vision discrimination (Fantini *et al.*, 2006; Ferini-Strambi *et al.*, 2004; Postuma *et al.*, 2006). It is not known if these deficits will progress over time or if they are simple epiphenomena, but the whole body of observations strengthen the notion of idiopathic RBD as a possible prodrome of a more pervasive neurodegenerative disease.

Beside the psychological burden of possibly having a neurodegenerative disorder in its preclinical phase, idiopathic RBD per se represents a condition potentially harmful and this is usually the main reason for patients to seek medical attention. Indeed, injuries during sleep are reported by more than 75% of patients or bedpartners and they may include ecchymoses, lacerations, bone fractures, and even sub-dural haematomas (Ferini-Strambi *et al.*, 2005). Frequent and, obviously, unintentional injuries to bedpartners raise important medico-legal issues. It is not uncommon that the patient's spouse seek medical attention for traumatic lesions sustained during sleep, and inconvenience may occur when the health workers are not fully aware of this condition. Furthermore, the disorder may have a significant impact on the couple's life, since spouses often choose to sleep in a separate room for obvious safety reasons. Sometimes a psychiatric condition may be erroneously suspected and inappropriate treatments may be initiated, with an obvious impact on the patient and his or her family life. Other times, psychological factors are suspected, while the disorder is thought to be exquisitely neurologic.

Regardless of the extent of the sleep motor behaviors, patients with RBD experience frequent vivid and unpleasant dreams. Indeed, the vast majority of dreams tend to be stereotypical, action filled, and often violent in nature. Patients with RBD very commonly report dreams in which they are attacked by unfamiliar people or animals, and they either fight back in self-defence or attempt to flee (Ferini-Strambi *et al.*, 2005). Typical dreams may include an unfamiliar person entering the dreamer's house, a stranger threatening the dreamer or his relatives, or being attacked by animals. Fear and anger are the most commonly reported emotions associated to these dreams.

Fantini *et al.* (2005b) have evaluated the dream content and its relationship with the daytime aggressiveness in RBD. This study included 49 patients with polysomnographic-confirmed RBD and 71 healthy control volunteers matched for age, gender, and education. Subjects were asked to recall one or more recent dreams according to the Hall and Van de Castle method, and dreams that occurred within one year from the interview were included. The study found that a higher proportion of subjects in the RBD group (83.7%) were able to recall at least one dream, compared to same-age healthy subjects (49.3%). Ninety-eight (RBD) and 69 (controls) dreams were finally collected and analyzed. Compared to controls, patients with RBD reported a striking frequency of aggression, expressed by various indicators, namely a higher percentage of "dreams with at least one aggression" (66% vs. 15%), an increased "aggression/friendliness interactions" ratio (86% vs. 44%), an increased "aggressions/characters" (A/C) ratio (0.81 vs. 0.12). Further analysis of data showed that in both RBD and controls, the dreamer was personally involved in the aggression in about 90% of cases, while he was a witness in about 10% of cases. The characters involved in the aggression were largely males (96% males vs. 4% females) in the RBD group, while an equal representation of males and females was seen in the control group (55% males vs. 45% females). Physical aggression was the type of aggression far more represented in RBD dreams compared to controls' dreams (29.3% vs. 3.8%). Furthermore, dreams of RBD patients showed an overall higher percentage of physical activities and a reduced frequency of visual activity than dreams of controls. Another typical feature of RBD dreams was the very high frequency of animal characters (19% vs. 4%), almost invariably involved in aggressive interactions. Interestingly, none of the patients with RBD had a "dream with at least one element of sexuality," in contrast to what observed in control subjects (0% in RBD vs. 9% in controls). The latter is concordant with the observation that appetitive behaviors such as feeding or sexual, have never been observed as a manifestation of RBD, either in humans or in the animal model (Fantini and Ferini-Strambi, 2007).

Despite the increased aggressiveness in their dreams, patients with RBD don't show an increased daytime aggressiveness. No differences in daytime aggressiveness, as assessed by the total Aggression Questionnaire (AQ) scores, were found between RBD patients and controls. When looking at the subtypes of daytime aggressiveness, patients with RBD showed even less "physical aggressiveness" than control subjects (16.5 vs. 20.4), and no difference on "verbal aggressiveness, anger and hostility." This result corroborates early observations of a discrepancy between the aggressiveness displayed in dreams and the frequent placid and mild-mannered temperament in patients with RBD (Fantini *et al.*, 2005b).

According to the principle of continuity between dream content and waking mentation, dream subjects and emotions are in general continuous with the general level of well-being and with past or present emotional preoccupations and interests of the dreamers (Pesant and Zadra, 2006). In childrens' dream studies, it was found that children with more violence in their waking fantasies had more aggressive interactions in their dreams (Foulkes, 1967). Interestingly, in RBD patients, the amount of aggressiveness in dreams was found to inversely correlate with the measures of aggressiveness during the day. This inverse correlation could somewhat corroborate early theories of a compensatory nature of dreams, in which aspects of the personality neglected in waking life would be highlighted in dreams. Yet, the relationships between recurrent aggressive dreams and psychological measures in RBD patients have not been assessed. However, RBD patients show a high stereotypic dream content, namely a high occurrence of a human or animal aggressor threatening the dreamer or his entourage, in front of a variety of psychological profiles. The repetitive nature of dream content may suggest several linkages between dream content and the neural network for dreaming (Domhoff, 2001), and this could be particularly true in the case of RBD patients. According to the activation–synthesis model of dream generation, phasic discharges from brainstem generators activate either motor or perceptual, affective and cognitive pathways and these impulses are subsequently synthesized into dreams by the forebrain. (Hobson and McCarley, 1977). Thus, it may be hypothesized that such phasic motor activation induced by brain-stem locomotor pattern generators would be preferentially translated by the cortical imagery generators in activities such as fighting or running, rather than more static ones.

References

American Psychiatric Association (2000) *Diagnostic and Statistical Manual of Mental Disorders, 4th Ed (text revision, DSM-IV-R)*. Washington, DC: American Psychiatric Association Press.

American Sleep Disorders Association (2005) *ICSD-II, International Classification of Sleep Disorders: Diagnostic and Coding Manual*. Chicago, IL: American Academy of Sleep Medicine.

Barrett, D. (1996) *Trauma and Dreams*. Cambridge, MA: Harvard University Press.

Beyer, J. L. & Krishnan, K. R. (2002) Volumetric brain imaging findings in mood disorders. *Bipolar Disord* **4**: 89–104.

Blagrove, M., Farmer, L. & Williams, E. (2004) The relationship of nightmare frequency and nightmare distress to well-being. *J Sleep Res* **13**: 129–36.

Boeve, B. F., Silber, M. H., Saper, C. B. *et al.* (2007) Pathophysiology of REM sleep behavior disorder and relevance to neurodegenerative disease. *Brain* **130**: 2770–88.

Breslau, N., Roth, T. & Rosenthal, L. *et al.* (1996) Sleep disturbance and psychiatric disorders: a longitudinal epidemiological study of young adults. *Biol Psychiatry* **39**: 411–18.

Breslau, N., Roth, T., Burduvali, E. *et al.* (2004) Sleep in lifetime posttraumatic stress disorder: a community-based polysomnographic study. *Arch Gen Psychiatry* **61**: 508–16.

Caldwell, J., Caldwell, J., Brown. D, L, *et al.* (2004) The effects of 37 h of continuous wakefulness on the physiological arousal, cognitive performance, self-reported mood, and simulator flight performance of F-117A pilots. *Military Psychology* **16**: 163–81.

Cartwright, R. D., Monroe, L. & Palmer, C. (1967) Individual differences in response to REM sleep deprivation. *Arch Gen Psychiatr* **16**: 297–303.

Choi, J, Kang, D., Kim, J. *et al.* (2005) Decreased caudal anterior cingulate gyrus volume and positive symptoms in schizophrenia. *Psychiat Res: Neuroim* **139**: 239–47.

Dinges, D. F., Pack, F., Williams, K. *et al.* (1997) Cumulative sleepiness, mood disturbance, and psychomotor vigilance performance decrements during a week of sleep restricted to 4–5 h per night. *Sleep* **20**: 267–77.

Domhoff, G. W. (2001) A new neurocognitive theory of dreams. *Dreaming* **11**: 13–33.

Fantini, M. L., Ferini-Strambi, L. & Montplaisir, J. (2005a) Idiopathic REM sleep behavior disorder: toward a better nosological definition. *Neurology* **64**: 780–6.

Fantini, M. L., Corona, A., Clerici, S. *et al.* (2005b) Aggressive dream content without daytime aggressiveness in REM sleep behaviour disorder. *Neurology* **65**: 1010–15

Fantini, M. L., Postuma, R. B., Montplaisir, J. *et al.* (2006) Olfactory deficit in idiopathic REM sleep behavior disorder. *Brain Res Bull* **70**: 386–90.

Fantini, M. L. & Ferini-Strambi, L. (2007) REM-related dreams. In *REM Sleep Behavior Disorder: the New Science of Dreaming*, eds. P. McNamara & D. Barrett. Westport, CT: Greenwood Publishers, pp. 185–200.

Ferini-Strambi, L., Di Gioia, M. S., Castronovo, V. *et al.* (2004) Neuropsychological assessment in idiopathic REM sleep behavior disorder (RBD). Does the idiopathic form of RBD really exist? *Neurology* **62**: 41–5.

Ferini-Strambi, L., Fantini, M. L., Zucconi, M. *et al.* (2005) REM sleep behavior disorder. *Neurol Sci* **26** (Suppl 3): 186–92.

Foulkes, D. (1967) Dreams of the male child: four case studies. *J Child Psychol Psychiatry* **8**: 81–98.

Gagnon, J. F., Bédard, M. A., Fantini, M. L. *et al.* (2002) REM sleep behavior disorder and REM sleep without atonia in Parkinson's disease. *Neurology* **59**: 585–9.

Gillin, J. C., Buchsbaum, M., Wu, J. *et al.* (2001) Sleep deprivation as a model experimental antidepressant treatment: findings from functional brain imaging. *Depress Anxiety* **2**: 37–49.

Habukawa, M., Uchimura, N., Maeda, M. *et al.* (2007) Sleep findings in young adult patients with posttraumatic stress disorder. *Biol Psychiatry* **62**: 1179–82.

Hobson, J. A. & McCarley, R. W. (1977) The brain as a dream state generator: an activation-synthesis hypothesis of the dream process. *Am J Psychiatry* **134**:1335–48.

Hohagan, F., Lis, S., Krieger, S. *et al.* (1994) Sleep EEG of patients with obsessive-compulsive disorder. *Eur Arch Psychiatry Clin Neurosci* **243**: 273–8.

Insel, T., Gillin, J., Moore, A. *et al.* (1982) The sleep of patients with obsessive-compulsive disorder. *Arch Gen Psychiatry* **39**: 1372–7.

Iranzo, A., Graus, F., Clover, L. *et al.* (2006) Rapid eye movement sleep behavior disorder and potassium channel antibody-associated limbic encephalitis. *Ann Neurol* **59**: 178–81.

Jung, C. (1974) *Dreams*. Princeton, NJ: Princeton University Press.

Kahn-Greene, E. T., Killgore, D. B. & Kamimori, G. (2007) The effects of sleep deprivation on symptoms of psychopathology in healthy adults. *Sleep Med* **8**: 215–21.

Kupfer, D. J. & Bowers, M. B. (1972) REM sleep and central monoamine oxidase inhibition. *Psychopharmacology* **27**: 183–90.

Landolt, H. P., de Boer, L. P., Raimo, E. B. *et al.* (1999) Almost complete absence of REM sleep in a depressed patient during six months on Phenelzine. *Sleep Res Online* **2** (Suppl) **1**: 540.

Levin, R. & Fireman, G. (2002) Nightmares prevalence, nightmares distress, and self-reported psychological disturbance. *Sleep* **25**: 205–12.

Levin, R., Lantz, E., Fireman, G. *et al.* (2009) The relationship between disturbed dreaming and somatic distress. *J Nerv Ment Dis* **197**: 606–12.

Liguori, R., Vincent, A., Clover, L. *et al.* (2001) Morvan's syndrome: peripheral and central nervous system and cardiac involvement with antibodies to voltage-gated potassium channels. *Brain* **124**: 2417–26.

Maquet, P., Peters, J. M., Aerts, J. *et al.* (1996) Functional neuroanatomy of human repid eye movement sleep and dreaming. *Nature* **383**: 163–6.

McKeith, I. G. for the DLB Consortium (2005) Diagnosis and management of dementia with Lewy bodies: third report of the DLB Consortium. *Neurology* **65**: 1863–72.

Mellman, T. (2008) Sleep and anxiety disorders. *Sleep Med Clin* **3**: 261–8.

Mellman, T. & Uhde, T. (1989) Electroencephalographic sleep in panic disorder: a focus on sleep-related panic attacks. *Arch Gen Psychiatry* **46**: 178–84.

Meyer-Lindenberg, A. S., Olsen, R. K., Kohn, P. D. *et al.* (2005) Regionally specific disturbance of dorsolateral prefrontal-hippocampal functional connectivity in schizophrenia. *Arch Gen Psychiatry* **62**: 379–86.

Morris, J. S., Ohman, A. & Dolan, R. (1998) Conscious and unconscious emotional learning in the human amygdala. *Nature* **393**: 467–70.

Nielsen, T. & Levin, R. (2007) Nightmares: a new neurocognitive model. *Sleep Med Rev* **11**: 295–310.

Nofzinger, E. A., Mintun, M., Wiseman, M. B. *et al.* (1997) Forebrain activation in REM sleep: an FDG PET study. *Brain Res* **770**: 192–201.

Nolen-Hoeksema, S. (1990) *Sex Differences in Depression.* Stanford, CA: Stanford University Press.

Noyes, R. Jr, Watson, D. B., Letuchy, E. M. *et al.* (2005) Relationship between hypochondriacal concerns and personality dimensions and traits in a military population. *J Nerv Ment Dis* **193**: 110–18.

Ohayon, M., Morselli, P. L. & Guilleminault, C. (1997) Prevalence of nightmares and their relationship to psychopathology and daytime functioning in insomnia subjects. *Sleep* **20**: 340–8.

Pesant, N. & Zadra, A. (2006) Dream content and psychological well-being: a longitudinal study of the continuity hypothesis. *J Clin Psychol* **62**:111–21.

Postuma, R. B., Lang, A., Massicotte-Marquez, J. *et al.* (2006) Potential early markers of Parkinson disease in idiopathic REM sleep behavior disorder. *Neurology* **66**: 845–51.

Postuma, R. B., Gagnon, J. F., Vendette, M. *et al.* (2009) Quantifying the risk of neurodegenerative disease in idiopathic REM sleep behavior disorder. *Neurology* **72**: 1296–300.

Rief, W., Hiller, W. & Margraf, J. (1998) Cognitive aspects of hypochondriasis and the somatization syndrome. *J Abnorm Psychol* **107**: 587–95.

Robinson, D., Walsleben, J., Pollack, S. *et al.* (1998) Nocturnal polysomnography in obsessive-compulsive disorder. *Psychiatry Res* **80**: 257–63.

Saletu-Zyhlarz, G., Saletu, B., Anderer, P. *et al.* (1997) Nonorganic insomnia in generalized anxiety disorder: controlled studies on sleep, awakening and daytime vigilance utilizing polysomnography and EEG mapping. *Neuropsychobiology* **36**: 117–29.

Scott, J. P., McNaughton, L. & Polman, R. C. (2006) Effects of sleep deprivation and exercise on cognitive, motor performance and mood. *Physiol Behav* **87**: 396–408.

Schenck, C. H. & Mahowald, M. W. (2002) REM sleep behavior disorder: clinical, developmental, and neuroscience perspectives 16 years after its formal identification in *Sleep*. *Sleep* **25**:120–38.

Schenck, C. H., Bundlie, S. R. & Mahowald, M. W. (2003) REM behavior disorder (RBD): delayed emergence of parkinsonism and/or dementia in 65% of older men initially diagnosed with idiopathic RBD, and analysis of the minimum and maximum tonic and/or phasic electromyographic abnormalities found during REM sleep. *Sleep* **26**: Abstract Supplement: A316.

Simard, V., Nielsen, T., Tremblay, R. E. *et al.* (2008) Longitudinal study of bad dreams in preschool children: prevalence, demographic correlates, risk and protective factors. *Sleep* **31**: 62–70.

Smith, C. & Lapp, L. (1991) Increases in number of REMS and REM density in humans following an intensive learning period. *Sleep* **14**: 325–30.

Staner, L., Kerkhofs, M., Detroux, D. *et al.* (1995) Acute, subchronic and withdrawal sleep EEG changes during treatment with paroxetine and amitryptyline: a double blind randomised trial in major depression. *Sleep* **18**: 470–7.

Stirling, J., Hellewell, J., Blakey, A. *et al.* (2006) Thought disorder in schizophrenia is associated with both executive dysfunction and circumscribed impairments in semantic function. *Psychol Med* **20**: 1–10.

Thomas, M., Sing, H., Belenky, G. *et al.* (2000) Neural basis of alertness and cognitive performance impairments during sleepiness. I. Effects of 24 h of sleep deprivation on waking human regional activity. *J Sleep Res* **9**: 335–52.

Videbech, P. (2000) PET measurements of brain glucose metabolism and blood flow in major depressive disorder: a critical review. *Acta Psychiatr Scand* **101**: 11–20.

Watt, M. C. & Stewart, S. H. (2000) Anxiety sensitivity mediates the relationships between childhood learning experiences and elevated hypochondriacal concerns in young adulthood. *J Psychosom Res* **49**: 107–18.

Wyatt, R. J., Fram, D. H., Kupferm, D. J. *et al.* (1971a)
Total, prolonged drug induced REM sleep suppresssion
in anxious depressed patients. *Arch Gen Psychiat*
24: 145–55.

Wyatt, R. J., Fram, D. H. & Buchbinder R. (1971b)
Treatment of intractable narcolepsy with a monoamine
oxidase inhibitor. *New Eng J Med* **285**: 987–91.

Zadra, A. & Donden, D. C. (1993) Variety and intensity of
emotions in bad dreams and nightmares. *Can Psychol*
34: 294.

Zohar, D., Tzischinsky, O., Epstein, R. *et al.* (2005) The
effects of sleep loss on medical residents' emotional
reactions to work events: a cognitive-energy model. *Sleep*
28: 47–54.

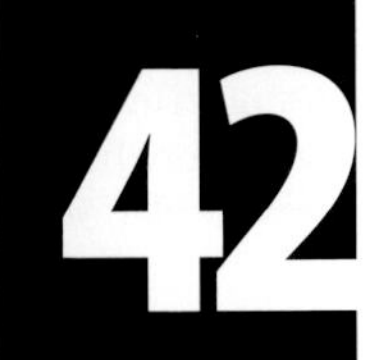

Chapter 42

REM sleep and emotion regulation

Martin Desseilles, Virginie Sterpenich, Thien Thanh Dang-Vu, and Sophie Schwartz

Summary

Despite substantial research focusing on the interaction between sleep and cognition, especially memory, the impact of sleep and sleep loss on affective and emotional regulation has comparatively attracted much less attention. This might be surprising considering that nearly all psychiatric and neurological disorders with impaired mood express co-occurring abnormalities of sleep, and that many sleep disorders are accompanied by mood disturbances, thus suggesting an intimate relationship between sleep and emotion. Yet, recent studies evaluating subjective as well as objective measures of mood and affect, combined with insights from clinical observations and neuroimaging research, offer new evidence for the emerging role of sleep in regulating emotional brain function. In this chapter, we review clinical and neuroimaging data that support the existence of such complex interactions between sleep and emotion regulation. We report that (1) sleep disorders are frequently associated with affective symptoms; (2) patients with mood disorders often present with sleep disturbances; (3) sleep deprivation may transitorily alleviate depressive symptoms; (4) dream experiences may be highly emotional; (5) brain regions involved in emotion processing and regulation, such as the limbic (e.g., amygdala, anterior cingulate cortex) and ventromedial prefrontal regions, are strongly activated during REM sleep; (6) subjective mood assessments exhibit a circadian modulation. New data also show that some hypothalamic neuropeptides (hypocretin/orexin) play a dual role in the stabilization of sleep–wake states and on mesolimbic dopamine activity, with significant effects on neural plasticity related to emotional learning, reward processing, and addiction. Together, these seemingly disparate observations converge to indicate a physiological interplay between sleep–wake and emotional brain functions serving the modulation, the preparation, and the optimization of waking behavior.

Emotional disturbances in sleep disorders

Insufficient sleep and sleep disorders are often accompanied by daytime complaints, several of them suggesting some form of emotional dysregulation. For example, patients with sleep-onset insomnia or with sleep-maintenance insomnia show increased vulnerability to stress and negative emotions (Waters *et al.*, 1993). Short sleep duration (less than five hours of sleep) is associated with suicidal ideation and attempts among adults in the general population (Goodwin and Marusic, 2008). Sleep deprivation raises anxiety levels, which is independently linked with suicidal ideation and suicide attempts in humans (Friedman *et al.*, 1999). There is also evidence that sleep disturbances may be linked to aggressive and impulsive behavior, as well as mood lability (Pakyurek *et al.*, 2002). In general, these results suggest that insomnia and chronic deprivation of sleep may influence mood, psychological distress, and emotional lability (Benca *et al.*, 1992).

Narcolepsy is another paradigmatic sleep disorder, which presents with an emotional component. Narcolepsy with cataplexy (NC) is a sleep–wake disorder characterized by excessive daytime sleepiness, nocturnal sleep disruption, and several manifestations of so-called "dissociated" or isolated rapid eye movement sleep (REM) features, such as muscle atonia (i.e., cataplexy), sleep paralysis, and hallucinations (Baumann and Bassetti, 2005). The pathognomic symptom of NC is cataplexy, which corresponds to short episodes of muscle tone loss with preserved consciousness triggered by emotions, most often by

REM Sleep: Regulation and Function, eds. Birendra N. Mallick, S. R. Pandi-Perumal, Robert W. McCarley, and Adrian R. Morrison. Published by Cambridge University Press. © Cambridge University Press 2011.

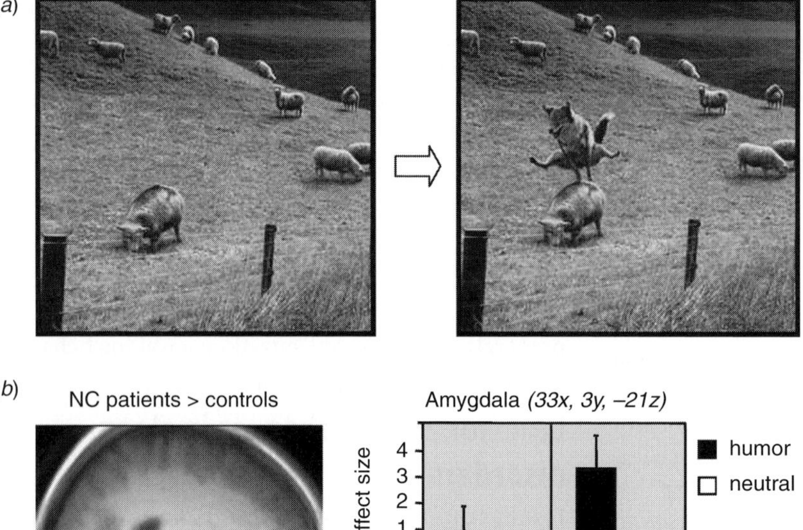

Figure 42.1 Amygdala response to humorous stimuli in narcolepsy–cataplexy (NC) patients. (*a*) Mini-sequence in which a neutral scene was followed by a second picture revealing a new element either neutral or humorous. Here a sequence judged as funny. (*b*) Increased amygdala response to humor in NC patients compared to controls. Parameter estimates show increased fMRI signal to humorous sequences in the patients but not in the controls. (Adapted from Schwartz *et al. Brain* 2008 with permission.) (See plate section for color version.)

laughing, joking, or playing games. Human narcolepsy is associated with a reduction or loss of a hypothalamic peptide called hypocretin or orexin (for a review see Desseilles *et al.*, 2008; Dang-Vu *et al.*, 2009). Interestingly, there is some overlap between brain activity patterns occurring during cataplexy and normal REM sleep (i.e., activation of the brain stem, thalamus, amygdala, and cingulate cortex; deactivation of the prefrontal cortex), suggesting similar brain generators for both conditions (Chabas *et al.*, 2007; Hong *et al.*, 2006; Maquet *et al.*, 1996; Schwartz and Maquet, 2002). A recent fMRI study revealed an increased amygdala (and reduced hypothalamic) response to emotionally positive stimuli (humorous pictures) in NC (Schwartz *et al.*, 2008) (Figure 42.1). Increased amygdala reactivity in NC was confirmed in another fMRI study in which patients could anticipate gains on a game-like task, together with altered responses in mesolimbic reward circuits and ventromedial prefrontal cortex (VMPFC) (Ponz *et al.*, 2010a). These findings are in line with recent animal data showing a link between the hypocretin/orexin system and the expression of motivated behaviors and addiction (Harris and Aston-Jones, 2006), and with the clinical observation that hypocretin-deficient NC patients rarely become addicted to highly addictive pharmacological treatments. Using an aversive conditioning paradigm, Ponz *et al.* (2010b) also demonstrated impaired emotional learning in NC patients, due to the absence of amygdala response to conditioned stimuli, together with an abnormal functional coupling between the amygdala and medial prefrontal cortex. These findings show that brain networks involved in the processing, evaluation, learning, and regulation of emotional signals might rely on neurotransmitters and neural pathways that contribute to the maintenance of sleep–wake states as well. These animal and human imaging data open a new avenue to the study of common brain systems that regulate both sleep, emotion, and reward brain functions.

Sleep alterations in mood disorders

The vast majority of psychiatric disorders, especially those involving mood perturbations, are associated with sleep abnormalities (Benca *et al.*, 1992). For example, sleep difficulties are common among persons with suicidal ideation, suicide attempts, and suicide completion. In depressed patients, in addition to sleep continuity disturbances and SWS deficits, several REM-sleep abnormalities have been reported

(Reynolds and Kupfer, 1987). In endogenous depression, reduced REM-sleep latency was found to co-occur with terminal insomnia, pervasive anhedonia, unreactive mood, and appetite loss. Interestingly, while increased REM-sleep density might be more severe in acute vs. remitted phases, reduced REM-sleep latency can persist even in remitted patients (Giles *et al.*, 1990). Sleep abnormalities might thus be biological markers of mood disorder susceptibility (Benca and Peterson, 2008). Vogel and colleagues hypothesized that an excessive amount of REM sleep and the ensuing decrease in REM-sleep pressure might cause major depression (Vogel *et al.*, 1990). As a consequence, partial REM-sleep deprivation and total sleep deprivation work by suppressing REM sleep and by increasing REM-sleep pressure. Interestingly, increased REM-sleep pressure through repetitive REM-sleep deprivation might be beneficial as an antidepressant treatment, especially for depressed subjects who are able to construct well organized dreams (Cartwright *et al.*, 2003). However, while several antidepressant treatments such as tricyclics increase REM-sleep pressure, REM-sleep suppression is not necessary for an antidepressant response since many antidepressant treatments do not reduce REM sleep (see also next section).

Post-traumatic stress disorder (PTSD) is an important psychiatric condition with major sleep disturbances, characterized by frequent nightmares and sleep initiation and/or maintenance insomnia due to recurrent, unwanted re-experiencing of a previous traumatic event. Interestingly, some studies suggested a link between REM-sleep activity (i.e., a more fragmented pattern of REM sleep and increased noradrenergic activity during REM sleep) in the acute aftermath of trauma and the subsequent development of PTSD (Mellman *et al.*, 2002). A recent behavioral study in healthy participants showed that REM sleep-rich late sleep contributes to the long-term consolidation of emotional memories, and suggests that sleep deprivation in the immediate aftermath of traumatic events could be a promising therapeutic measure to prevent PTSD (Wagner *et al.*, 2006). A recent hypothesis also suggests that REM sleep amplifies the abnormal activation of the amygdala and the deactivation of the medial frontal cortex that are observed at baseline in PTSD patients (Germain *et al.*, 2008).

Sleep problems are also reported in schizophrenia. While studies have not shown any differences between healthy subjects and schizophrenic patients for REM-sleep duration and REM-sleep density, decreased REM-sleep latency was found in several studies (Monti and Monti, 2005). In addition, schizophrenic patients do not show any REM sleep rebound after REM-sleep deprivation. It has also been suggested that some features of REM dreaming may overlap with clinical symptoms in schizophrenia, and that dreaming, in particular bizarre features in dreams, could be used as a model for psychosis (Scarone *et al.*, 2008).

Effects of sleep deprivation on emotional responses

We all know that after a night of poor-quality sleep, we may feel in a somewhat unusual mood. We may also react inappropriately, often impulsively, to unforeseen or emotional situations. Reduced emotional control is frequently observed after sleep deprivation in the form of irritability, impatience, childish humor, disregard of normal social conventions, and inappropriate interpersonal behaviors (Horne, 1993). Mood and emotion processing might actually be more affected by sleep deprivation than either cognitive or motor performance (Dinges *et al.*, 1997). Consistent with this observation, decision making that requires the processing of unexpected information, competing distraction, or emotions was found to be affected by sleep deprivation, unlike decision making involving rule-based, convergent, or logical tasks (for a review see Harrison and Horne, 2000). Using a gambling type of task, McKenna and colleagues (2007) recently showed that after one night of sleep deprivation, subjects take more risk than they ordinarily would when they are considering a gain, but less risk when considering a loss. The behavioral effects of sleep deprivation may thus include an (abnormal) augmentation of motivational or "drive-related" behaviors. In animals, REM-sleep deprivation has been reported to enhance appetite, sexual behavior, aggressiveness, and locomotor activity (Velazquez-Moctezuma *et al.*, 1989). In humans, sleep deprivation (in particular REM sleep) was shown to improve mood in patients with endogenous depression and increase appetite and sexual interest in normal subjects (McNamara, 1996). Because these behaviors are thought to involve activation of dopaminergic reward circuits, REM-sleep deprivation may enhance motivational behaviors through an action on dopaminergic functions.

To date, very few studies have investigated whether sleep deprivation inappropriately modulates emotional brain reactivity in humans. One study revealed enhanced amygdala response to emotional stimuli after one night of sleep deprivation, together with reduced functional connectivity between the amygdala and the medial prefrontal cortex (MPFC) (Yoo *et al.*, 2007). The MPFC is known to have an inhibitory influence on amygdala activity, and a disregulation of amygdala–MPFC connectivity is believed to significantly contribute to the neural underpinnings of anxiety and major depression (e.g., Davidson 2002; Johnstone *et al.*, 2007; Desseilles *et al.*, 2009). Using a gambling type of task, Venkatraman and colleagues (2007) provided the first evidence that 24 hours of sleep deprivation can modulate the neural systems associated with decision making. Following sleep deprivation, choices involving higher relative risk elicited greater activation in the right nucleus accumbens, consistent with an elevated expectation of the higher reward after the riskier choice was made. Concurrently, there was less activation for losses in the insular and orbitofrontal cortices suggesting blunted response to losses. By resetting limbic and mesolimbic reactivity to emotional challenges, a good night of sleep may regularize waking affective processing while fostering adapted behavioral responses.

Consolidation of emotional memory during sleep

Compared to the abundant data showing a role for sleep in non-emotional memory processes, the specific contribution of sleep physiology to the consolidation of emotional memories is less clear. Indeed, although several lines of evidence suggest a relationship between sleep and emotional processing, only a few studies investigated how sleep may determine the fate of emotional memories. Wagner *et al.* have contributed a series of behavioral studies demonstrating that REM sleep may enhance emotional memories (Wagner *et al.*, 2001, 2002), and that this emotional memory enhancement may persist for several years (Wagner *et al.*, 2006). Another study confirmed these findings by showing a decrement of memory selectively for highly arousing and negatively valenced pictures after 12 hours of wakefulness as compared to 12 hours of sleep (Hu *et al.*, 2006). On the other hand, Wagner *et al.* (2005) reported that cortisol blockade during sleep interferes with hippocampus-dependent declarative memory formation while it enhances amygdala-dependent emotional memory formation, thus suggesting that the natural cortisol rise during late sleep may dampen emotional memory formation. In consonance with the observation that sleep disturbances frequently follow traumatic experiences (Caldwell and Redeker, 2005), sleep deprivation immediately following a traumatic event has been suggested as a possible therapeutic tool to prevent the consolidation of emotional memories, and potentially thwart the progress of PTSD.

At the brain level, a few studies have started to provide some insights into the cerebral mechanisms underlying sleep-related emotional memory consolidation. Nishida *et al.* (2009) showed that the amount of REM sleep as well as concomitant right prefrontal theta power during a nap correlated with emotional memory facilitation. The authors suggested that increased prefrontal theta may represent the large-scale cooperation between subcortical limbic structures (including amygdala and hippocampal) and prefrontal regions, and that such synchronous activity within limbic and neocortical regions during REM sleep would modulate plastic changes essential for the modulation of affective experiences. A recent study by Sterpenich *et al.* (2007) used fMRI to directly test sleep-dependent emotional memory processing. Subjects who were sleep-deprived during the first night after exposure to arousing emotional pictures and who were retested 72 hours after encoding (including two nights of normal sleep), showed a lack of reduction in amygdala reactivity when re-exposed to these same emotional stimuli unlike subjects who were allowed to sleep during the first night after exposure to the emotional stimuli. The recruitment of the amygdala might allow the recollection of negative information despite the cognitive repercussion of sleep restriction, while retrieval performance deteriorated for neutral and positive stimuli after sleep deprivation. When retested six months after incidental encoding, recollection in the sleep group (compared to the sleep-deprived subjects) was associated with significantly larger responses and increased connectivity in a network encompassing the VMPFC, the extended amygdala, and the occipital cortex (Sterpenich *et al.*, 2009) (Figure 42.2). These results suggest that sleep during the first post-encoding night critically modulates the long-term systems-level consolidation of emotional memory.

Taken together, these results support a permissive role of sleep – and in particular REM sleep – in the functional brain changes that underlie the formation of enduring emotional memories in humans, and

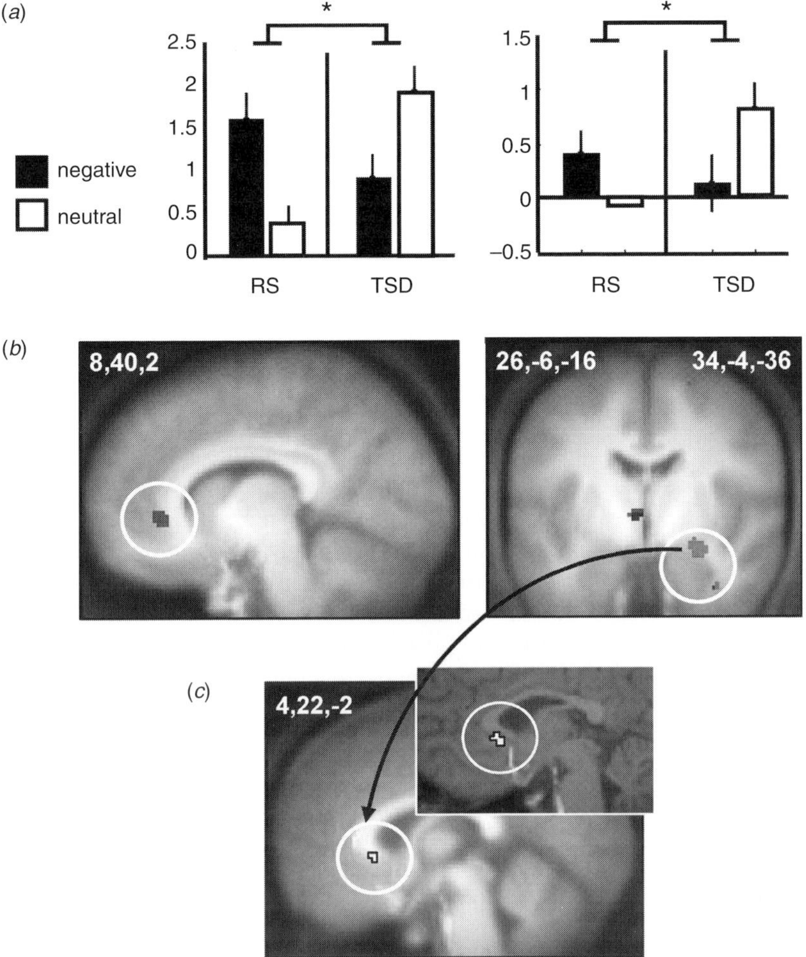

Figure 42.2 Effect of sleep on emotional memory after six months. Sterpenich's fMRI study was performed in three phases: encoding, first retrieval (after three days), and delayed retrieval (after six months). During the incidental encoding session, the subjects rated the valence of 40 negative, 40 positive, and 40 neutral pictures on a seven-point scale (–3, very unpleasant; 0, neutral; +3, very pleasant). During the post-encoding night, one half of the subjects were totally sleep deprived (TSD). The other participants went home and slept as usual (RS). After two additional nights, which allowed sleep-deprived participants to recover, subjects performed a first retrieval session during which 120 previously encoded pictures were presented, randomly mixed with 60 new ones. Six months after the encoding session, the subjects performed a second retest session during which the 120 initially encoded pictures were again mixed with 60 additional new ones. (a) Parameter estimates of activity in the MPFC and amygdala, showing increased activity for negative (black bars) than neutral (white bars) pictures for the RS compared to the TSD group after six months. (b) The amygdala (in red) was more activated by emotional stimuli during encoding, and the ventral medial PFC (in blue) showed a memory by delay interaction. (c) Ventral medial PFC was more connected to the amygdala for negative than neutral correctly recollected pictures and more so in the RS than TSD group (inset, enlarged prefrontal and temporal region in a representative subject). (Adapted from Sterpenich *et al. J Neurosci* 2009 with permission.) (See plate section for color version.)

that may involve a modulation of amygdala-mPFC functional connections.

REM dreaming and affective processing

Science seems to confirm the traditional belief that dreams are highly emotional. When compared to a real-life spectrum of emotions, the emotional content in dream reports tends to be predominantly negatively loaded with a high proportion of fear- or anxiety-related emotions (e.g., Valli and Revonsuo, 2009) (Figure 42.3). During wakefulness, the amygdala is known to respond to threatening stimuli, stressful situations, or novelty. Its high activity during REM sleep could reflect an elevated intensity of emotions

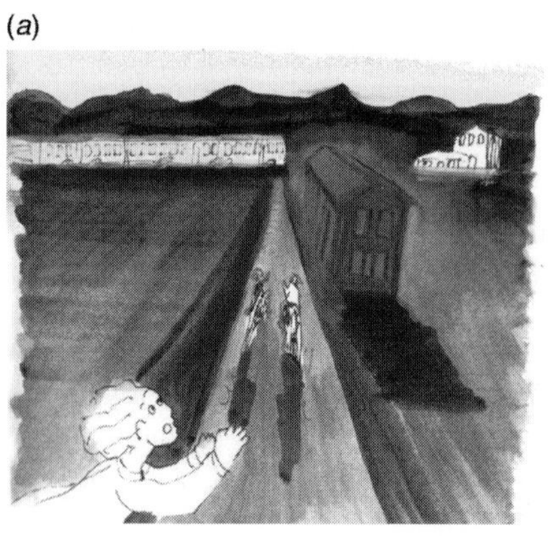

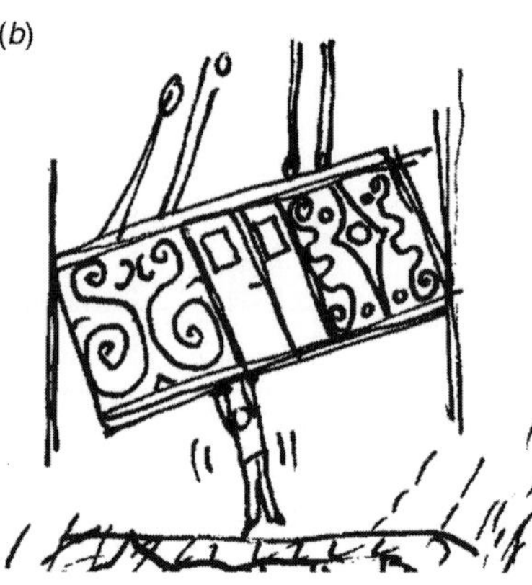

Figure 42.3 Examples of threatening situations associated with strong emotions in dreams. (*a*) Terrified, the dreamer tries to escape a danger by catching a train. (*b*) The dreamer is trapped in a space beneath an elevator, threatened to get crushed by the weight of the elevator. Drawings selected from a dream diary extensively analyzed elsewhere (S. Schwartz, Doctoral thesis). (See plate section for color version.)

in dreams (Maquet *et al.*, 1996; Maquet and Franck, 1997; Schwartz and Maquet, 2002).

Several theories suggest that dreaming may be beneficial for the regulation of emotional states (for a comprehensive review see Nielsen and Levin, 2007). Combining an evolutionary perspective of the function of dreaming with the empirical evidence concerning the frequency of emotionally negative dreams (e.g., nightmares and post-traumatic dreams), Revonsuo and Valli recently suggested that dreaming might serve to simulate responses to threatening events in a totally secure environment (Valli and Revonsuo, 2009). Such active rehearsal would enhance threat-avoidance skills and ultimately help the individual to respond in an adapted and efficient way to dangerous real-life events. A distinct but analogous theoretical explanation for the occurrence of negative emotions in dreams has been proposed by Nielsen and Levin (Levin and Nielsen, 2007; Nielsen and Levin, 2007). They proposed that bad dreams and nightmares would result from a "dysfunction in a network of affective processes that, during normal dreaming, serves the adaptive function of fear memory extinction" (Nielsen and Levin, 2007, p. 300). In short, the "affective network dysfunction" (AND) model stipulates that dreaming may promote the consolidation of fear extinction memories by (1) activating features of fear memories (largely independently from their episodic, real-world contexts); (2) reorganizing these features by creating novel simulated contexts in which the conditioned stimuli are presented without their pairing with the unpleasant unconditioned stimulus, but rather in non-fearful, contexts; and (3) allowing the experience of these modified emotional reactions to such recombined dream features that would foster the extinction of conditioned

responses. By identifying an affective network (i.e., hippocampus, amygdala, anterior cingulate, medial prefrontal cortex) whose dysfunction might account for different types of dysphoric dreaming (from occasional bad dreams to non-traumatic nightmares to replicative post-traumatic nightmares), the AND is a sophisticated model that integrates both cognitive and neural explanatory levels.

The suggested cathartic function of dreaming might also relate to the persistence of activity in medial prefrontal regions (MPFC) and orbitofrontal cortex during REM sleep (Maquet *et al.*, 1996; Nofzinger *et al.*, 1997), regions that are known to contribute inhibitory feedbacks on the amygdala. Moreover, the MPFC is also involved in the attribution of intentions, thoughts, and feelings to oneself and to others during wakefulness (Frith and Frith, 2003). We may speculate that MPFC activation during REM sleep may explain why dreamers often attribute thoughts, emotions, and intentions to the dreamed characters, an offline role-play that may ultimately facilitate the resolution of social or emotional conflicts. Conversely, deactivation in the dorsolateral prefrontal cortex (DLPFC) during REM sleep may explain why only very few dream reports represent an exact replay of full memory episodes (Fosse *et al.*, 2003; Schwartz, 2003). Taken together, these observations suggest that isolated episodic elements are reactivated during sleep (most likely via the activation of the hippocampus, limbic structures, and posterior cortical areas), although these elements do not form replicates of real-life episodes (because of the deactivation of the DLPFC among other possible causes). Future research may clarify whether and how exactly such role-play and re-experiencing of waking bits and pieces contribute to emotion regulation.

Chronobiology of emotions

While the previous sections highlighted some intricate links between sleep and emotion regulation, circadian modulations of affective processes suggest that chronobiological factors should also be considered. In healthy individuals, subjective mood exhibits a remarkable circadian rhythmicity (Birchler-Pedross *et al.*, 2009; Boivin *et al.*, 1997). One recent study suggested that mood changes after sleep deprivation may depend on morningness–eveningness chronotypes (Selvi *et al.*, 2007). Moreover, sleep abnormalities in depression have been found to relate to chronobiological disturbances (e.g., Germain and Kupfer, 2008; Lewy *et al.*, 2006; Wirz-Justice, 2008). Consistent with a circadian modulation of affective regulation, the most widely documented rapid-onset antidepressant therapy is sleep deprivation, which acts within 24 to 48 hours in 40 to 60% of depressed patients (Wu *et al.*, 2009). Indeed, one putative mechanism that may mediate such rapid antidepressant effects is the activation of the hypocretin/orexin system by sleep (or REM sleep) deprivation (Mignot, 2001). In line with this hypothesis, dampened diurnal variations in hypocretin-1 were observed in depression (Salomon *et al.*, 2003), and may thus underlie the contribution of sleep–wake physiology to the maintenance or treatment of depression (Benca *et al.*, 1992).

The vulnerability to the effect of sleep loss and its consequence on mood markedly differs between persons in a trait-like manner and may relate to some genetic predisposition (Van Dongen *et al.*, 2004). In particular, it was recently proposed that clock genes, which regulate circadian and seasonal rhythms, with allelic variants modulating individual rhythms at both the cellular and behavioral levels, may underlie these various phenotypes. In particular, in patients suffering from mood disorders, rare genetic variants of Period3 (Per3) were found to be associated with higher novelty seeking, marginally better response to antidepressant treatments (SSRIs), worse mood in the evening, worse family and spare-time social adjustment (Artioli *et al.*, 2007). In addition, Per3$^{5/5}$ variant is associated with morningness (Archer *et al.*, 2003), as well as with increased slow-wave activity during non-REM sleep, increased theta and alpha activity during wakefulness and REM sleep, and greater decrement of cognitive performance in response to sleep loss (Viola *et al.*, 2007). Moreover, Per3$^{5/5}$ might correlate with earlier age at onset of bipolar disorder (Benedetti *et al.*, 2008), which

is a predictor of worse evolution of the disease. A recent fMRI study revealed that, after staying awake all night, Per3$^{5/5}$ carriers showed widespread reduction of brain activity in prefrontal, temporal, parietal, and occipital areas, when compared to individuals with the short allele Per3$^{4/4}$ (Vandewalle *et al.*, 2009). While these data suggest that circadian genes impact strongly on sleep-loss vulnerability and cognition, it remains to be tested if the long variant directly impairs emotion regulation, independently of the effect of mood induced by sleep deprivation. "Chronobiotics" (i.e., the treatment of circadian rhythm disorders) such as melatonin administration might be used in order to prevent mood or emotional disruption in conditions where circadian regulation is compromised, such as sleep disorders, mental disorders, jet lag, or shift work.

It is well established that sleep- and circadian-related factors affect waking cognition. The studies reviewed in this chapter provide an emerging view that the neurobiology of sleep, REM sleep in particular, may promote the regulation of affective processes and optimize waking emotional functioning. Moreover, recent brain imaging findings as well as dream data suggest that an offline rehearsal and consolidation of emotional experiences may occur during sleep. Therefore, sleep may serve complementary and vital functions by fostering adapted defense mechanisms against past and future psychological (and physical) threats and by renewing our daily portion of motivation and good mood.

Acknowledgments

MD and TTD-V are supported by the Fonds National de la Recherche Scientifique (FNRS – Belgium). SS is supported by the Swiss National Science Foundation (#310000–114008 and #51NF40–104897) and the Pierre Mercier Foundation.

References

Archer, S. N., Robilliard, D. L., Skene, D. J. *et al.* (2003) A length polymorphism in the circadian clock gene Per3 is linked to delayed sleep phase syndrome and extreme diurnal preference. *Sleep* **26**(4): 413–15.

Artioli, P., Lorenzi, C., Pirovano, A. *et al.* (2007) How do genes exert their role? Period 3 gene variants and possible influences on mood disorder phenotypes. *Eur Neuropsychopharmacol* **17**(9): 587–94.

Baumann, C. R. & Bassetti, C. L. (2005) Hypocretins (orexins) and sleep-wake disorders. *Lancet Neurol* **4**(10): 673–82.

Benca, R. M., Obermeyer, W. H., Thisted, R. A. & Gillin J. C. (1992) Sleep and psychiatric disorders. A meta-analysis. *Arch Gen Psychiatry* **49**(8): 651–68; discussion 669–70.

Benca, R. M. & Peterson, M. J. (2008) Insomnia and depression. *Sleep Med* **9** Suppl 1: S3–9.

Benedetti, F., Dallaspezia, S., Colombo, C. *et al.* (2008) A length polymorphism in the circadian clock gene Per3 influences age at onset of bipolar disorder. *Neurosci Lett* **445**(2): 184–7.

Birchler-Pedross, A., Schroder, C. M., Munch, M. *et al.* (2009) Subjective well-being is modulated by circadian phase, sleep pressure, age, and gender. *J Biol Rhythms* **24**(3): 232–42.

Boivin, D. B., Czeisler, C. A., Dijk, D. J. *et al.* (1997) Complex interaction of the sleep-wake cycle and circadian phase modulates mood in healthy subjects. *Arch Gen Psychiatry* **54**(2): 145–52.

Caldwell, B. A. & Redeker, N. (2005) Sleep and trauma: an overview. *Issues Ment Health Nurs* **26**(7): 721–38.

Cartwright, R., Baehr, E., Kirkby, J., Pandi-Perumal, S. R. & Kabat, J. (2003) REM sleep reduction, mood regulation and remission in untreated depression. *Psychiatry Res* **121**(2): 159–67.

Chabas, D., Habert, M. O., Maksud, P. *et al.* (2007) Functional imaging of cataplexy during status cataplecticus. *Sleep* **30**(2): 153–6.

Dang-Vu, T. T., Desseilles, M., Schwartz, S. & Maquet P. (2009) Neuroimaging of narcolepsy. *CNS Neurol Disord Drug Targets* **8**(4): 254–63.

Davidson, R. J. (2002) Anxiety and affective style: role of prefrontal cortex and amygdala. *Biol Psychiatry* **51**(1): 68–80.

Desseilles, M., Balteau, E., Sterpenich, V. *et al.* (2009) Abnormal neural filtering of irrelevant visual information in depression. *J Neurosci* **29**(5): 1395–403.

Desseilles, M., Dang-Vu, T., Schabus, M. *et al.* (2008) Neuroimaging insights into the pathophysiology of sleep disorders. *Sleep* **31**(6): 777–94.

Dinges, D. F., Pack, F., Williams, K. *et al.* (1997) Cumulative sleepiness, mood disturbance, and psychomotor vigilance performance decrements during a week of sleep restricted to 4–5 hours per night. *Sleep* **20**(4): 267–77.

Fosse, M. J., Fosse, R., Hobson, J. A. & Stickgold, R. J. (2003) Dreaming and episodic memory: a functional dissociation? *J Cogn Neurosci* **15**(1): 1–9.

Friedman, S., Smith, L. & Fogel, A. (1999) Suicidality in panic disorder: a comparison with schizophrenic, depressed, and other anxiety disorder outpatients. *J Anxiety Disord* **13**(5): 447–61.

Frith, U. & Frith, C. D. (2003) Development and neurophysiology of mentalizing. *Philos Trans R Soc Lond B Biol Sci* **358**(1431): 459–73.

Germain, A., Buysse, D. J. & Nofzinger E. (2008) Sleep-specific mechanisms underlying posttraumatic stress disorder: integrative review and neurobiological hypotheses. *Sleep Med Rev* **12**(3): 185–95.

Germain, A. & Kupfer, D. J. (2008) Circadian rhythm disturbances in depression. *Hum Psychopharmacol* **23**(7): 571–85.

Giles, D. E., Roffwarg, H. P. & Rush, A. J. (1990) A cross-sectional study of the effects of depression on REM latency. *Biol Psychiatry* **28**(8): 697–704.

Goodwin, R. D. & Marusic, A. (2008) Association between short sleep and suicidal ideation and suicide attempt among adults in the general population. *Sleep* **31**(8): 1097–101.

Harris, G. C. & Aston-Jones, G. (2006) Arousal and reward: a dichotomy in orexin function. *Trends Neurosci* **29**(10): 571–7.

Harrison, Y. & Horne, J. A. (2000) The impact of sleep deprivation on decision making: a review. *J Exp Psychol Appl* **6**(3): 236–49.

Hong, S. B., Tae, W. S. & Joo, E. Y. (2006) Cerebral perfusion changes during cataplexy in narcolepsy patients. *Neurology* **66**(11): 1747–9.

Horne, J. A. (1993) Human sleep, sleep loss and behaviour. Implications for the prefrontal cortex and psychiatric disorder. *Br J Psychiatry* **162**: 413–19.

Hu, P., Stylos-Allan, M. & Walker, M. P. (2006) Sleep facilitates consolidation of emotional declarative memory. *Psychol Sci* **17**(10): 891–8.

Johnstone, T., van Reekum, C. M., Urry, H. L., Kalin N. H. & Davidson R. J. (2007) Failure to regulate: counterproductive recruitment of top-down prefrontal-subcortical circuitry in major depression. *J Neurosci* **27**(33): 8877–84.

Levin, R. & Nielsen, T. A. (2007) Disturbed dreaming, posttraumatic stress disorder, and affect distress: a review and neurocognitive model. *Psychol Bull* **133**(3): 482–528.

Lewy, A. J., Lefler, B. J., Emens, J. S. & Bauer, V. K. (2006) The circadian basis of winter depression. *Proc Natl Acad Sci USA* **103**(19): 7414–19.

Maquet, P. & Franck, G. (1997) REM sleep and amygdala. *Mol Psychiatry* **2**(3): 195–6.

Maquet, P., Peters, J., Aerts, J. *et al.* (1996) Functional neuroanatomy of human rapid-eye-movement sleep and dreaming. *Nature* **383**(6596): 163–6.

McKenna, B. S., Dicjinson, D. L., Orff, H. J. & Drummond, S. P. (2007) The effects of one night of sleep deprivation on known-risk and ambiguous-risk decisions. *J Sleep Res* **16**(3): 245–52.

McNamara, P. (1996) REM sleep: a social bonding mechanism. *New Ideas Psychol* **4**(1): 35–46.

Mellman, T. A., Bustamante, V., Fins, A. I., Pigeon W. R. & Nolan B. (2002) REM sleep and the early development of posttraumatic stress disorder. *Am J Psychiatry* **159**(10): 1696–701.

Mignot, E. (2001) A commentary on the neurobiology of the hypocretin/orexin system. *Neuropsychopharmacology* **25**(5 Suppl): S5–13.

Monti, J. M. & Monti, D. (2005) Sleep disturbance in schizophrenia. *Int Rev Psychiatry* **17**(4): 247–53.

Nielsen, T. & Levin, R. (2007) Nightmares: a new neurocognitive model. *Sleep Med Rev* **11**(4): 295–310.

Nishida, M., Pearsall, J., Buckner, R. L. & Walker, M. P. (2009) REM sleep, prefrontal theta, and the consolidation of human emotional memory. *Cereb Cortex* **19**(5): 1158–66.

Nofzinger, E. A., Mintun, M. A., Wiseman, M., Kupfer, D. J. & Moore, R. Y. (1997) Forebrain activation in REM sleep: an FDG PET study. *Brain Res* **770**(1/2): 192–201.

Pakyurek, M., Gutkovich, Z. & Weintraub, S. (2002) Reduced aggression in two inpatient children with the treatment of their sleep disorder. *J Am Acad Child Adolesc Psychiatry* **41**(9): 1025.

Ponz, A., Khatami, R., Poryazova, R. *et al.* (2010a) Abnormal activity in reward brain circuits in human narcolepsy with cataplexy. *Ann Neurol,* **67**(2), 190–200.

Ponz, A., Khatami, R., Poryazova, R. *et al.* (2010b) Reduced amygdala activity during aversive conditioning in human narcolepsy. *Ann Neurol* **67**(3), 394–8.

Reynolds, C. F., 3rd & Kupfer, D. J. (1987) Sleep research in affective illness: state of the art circa 1987. *Sleep* **10**(3): 199–215.

Salomon, R. M., Ripley, B., Kennedy, J. S. *et al.* (2003) Diurnal variation of cerebrospinal fluid hypocretin-1 (Orexin-A) levels in control and depressed subjects. *Biol Psychiatry* **54**(2): 96–104.

Scarone, S., Manzone, M. L., Gambini, O. *et al.* (2008) The dream as a model for psychosis: an experimental approach using bizarreness as a cognitive marker. *Schizophr Bull* **34**(3): 515–22.

Schwartz, S. (2003) Are life episodes replayed during dreaming? *Trends Cogn Sci* **7**(8): 325–7.

Schwartz, S. & Maquet, P. (2002) Sleep imaging and the neuro-psychological assessment of dreams. *Trends Cogn Sci* **6**(1): 23–30.

Schwartz, S., Ponz, A., Poryazova, R. *et al.* (2008) Abnormal activity in hypothalamus and amygdala during humour processing in human narcolepsy with cataplexy. *Brain* **131**(Pt 2): 514–22.

Selvi, Y., Gulec, M. Agargun, M. Y. & Besiroglu, L. (2007) Mood changes after sleep deprivation in morningness-eveningness chronotypes in healthy individuals. *J Sleep Res* **16**(3): 241–4.

Sterpenich, V., Albouy, G., Boly, M. *et al.* (2007) Sleep-related hippocampo-cortical interplay during emotional memory recollection. *PLoS Biol* **5**(11): e282.

Sterpenich, V., Albouy, G., Darsaud, A. *et al.* (2009) Sleep promotes the neural reorganization of remote emotional memory. *J Neurosci* **29**(16): 5143–52.

Valli, K. & Revonsuo, A. (2009) The threat simulation theory in light of recent empirical evidence: a review. *Am J Psychol* **122**(1): 17–38.

Van Dongen, H. P., Baynard, M. D., Maislin, G. & Dinges, D. F. (2004) Systematic interindividual differences in neurobehavioral impairment from sleep loss: evidence of trait-like differential vulnerability. *Sleep* **27**(3): 423–33.

Vandewalle, G., Archer, S. N., Wuillaume, C. *et al.* (2009) Functional magnetic resonance imaging-assessed brain responses during an executive task depend on interaction of sleep homeostasis, circadian phase, and PER3 genotype. *J Neurosci* **29**(25): 7948–56.

Velazquez-Moctezuma, J., Monroy, E. & Cruz, M. L. (1989) Facilitation of the effect testosterone on male sexual behavior in rats deprived of REM sleep. *Behav Neural Biol* **51**(1): 46–53.

Venkatraman, V., Chuah, Y. M., Huettel, S. A. & Chee, M. W. (2007) Sleep deprivation elevates expectation of gains and attenuates response to losses following risky decisions. *Sleep* **30**(5): 603–9.

Viola, A. U., Archer, S. N., James, L. M. *et al.* (2007) PER3 polymorphism predicts sleep structure and waking performance. *Curr Biol* **17**(7): 613–18.

Vogel, G. W., Buffenstein, A., Minter, K. & Hennessey, A. (1990) Drug effects on REM sleep and on endogenous depression. *Neurosci Biobehav Rev* **14**(1): 49–63.

Wagner, U., Gais, S. & Born, J. (2001) Emotional memory formation is enhanced across sleep intervals with high amounts of rapid eye movement sleep. *Learn Mem* **8**(2): 112–19.

Wagner, U., Fischer, S. & Born, J. (2002) Changes in emotional responses to aversive pictures across periods rich in slow-wave sleep versus rapid eye movement sleep. *Psychosom Med* **64**(4): 627–34.

Wagner, U., Degirmenci, M., Drosopoulos, S., Perras, B. & Born, J. (2005) Effects of cortisol suppression on sleep-associated consolidation of neutral and emotional memory. *Biol Psychiatry* **58**(11): 885–93.

Wagner, U., Hallschmid, M., Rasch, B. & Born, J. (2006) Brief sleep after learning keeps emotional memories alive for years. *Biol Psychiatry* **60**(7): 788–90.

Waters, W. F., Adams, S. G. Jr., Binks, P. & Varnado, P. (1993) Attention, stress and negative emotion in persistent sleep-onset and sleep-maintenance insomnia. *Sleep* **16**(2): 128–36.

Wirz-Justice, A. (2008). Diurnal variation of depressive symptoms. *Dialogues Clin Neurosci* **10**(3): 337–43.

Wu, J. C., Kelsoe, J. R., Schachat, C. *et al.* (2009) Rapid and sustained antidepressant response with sleep deprivation and chronotherapy in bipolar disorder. *Biol Psychiatry* **66**(3): 298–301.

Yoo, S. S., Gujar, N., Hu, P., Jolesz, F. A. & Walker, M. P. (2007) The human emotional brain without sleep – a prefrontal amygdala disconnect. *Curr Biol* **17**(20): R877–8.

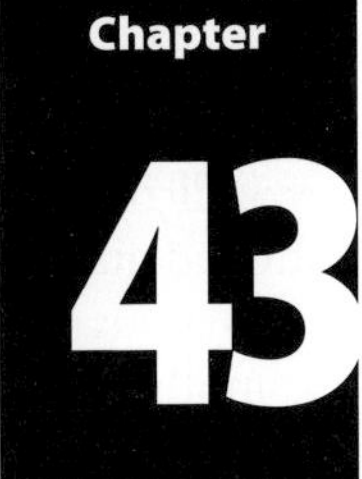

Neural modeling for cooperative/competitive regulation of REM sleep with NREM sleep and wakefulness

Akihiro Karashima, Yuichi Tamakawa, Yoshimasa Koyama, Norihiro Katayama, and Mitsuyuki Nakao

Summary

Recently, we proposed the model consists of a quartet of neuron groups: (1) sleep-active preoptic/anterior hypothalamic neurons (N-R group); (2) wake-active hypothalamic and brain-stem neurons exhibiting the highest rate of discharge during wakefulness and the lowest rate of discharge during paradoxical or REM sleep (WA group); (3) brain-stem neurons exhibiting the highest rate of discharge during REM sleep (REM group); and (4) basal forebrain, hypothalamic, and brain-stem neurons exhibiting a higher rate of discharge during both wakefulness and REM sleep than during NREM sleep (W-R group). In this chapter, we explain our revised model of sleep–wakefulness regulation in the rat, which includes a neural regulator quartet of NREM sleep, REM sleep, wakefulness, and a coregulator of REM sleep and wakefulness, whose parameters are tuned up so that the model reproduces some of the recent findings concerning the WA neurons. The physiological reality of the model structure is demonstrated by comparing the model neuron activities with the actual neuronal activities across state transition. Among the conceptual and mathematical models, one of the novel features of our model is involvement of the cholinergic W-R neuron group, which is assumed to contribute toward induction of wakefulness as well as REM sleep by selectively mediating autocatalytic activation with the WA or REM neurons. Through activity of this neuron group, the wakefulness–sleep flip-flop and the REM–NREM flip-flop interact with each other in our model. In fact pharmacological or physiological manipulations of REM sleep were shown to affect not only NREM sleep but wakefulness. Our successful modeling suggests that REM sleep is regulated cooperatively/competitively with NREM sleep and wakefulness by well orchestrated interactions among the aforementioned quartet of neural groups distributed in the hypothalamus and the brain stem with the aid of sleep-promoting substances. Finally, further possible updates in the model structure are described considering recent physiological findings.

Introduction

Our knowledge of the mechanism regulating sleep and waking states is continuously being updated. Examples of such updates include findings of the involvement of neurons in the ventrolateral preoptic hypothalamic area (VLPO) and the median preoptic nucleus (MnPN) in the regulation of non-rapid eye movement (NREM) sleep as well as rapid eye movement (REM) sleep (Sherin *et al.*, 1996; Suntsova *et al.*, 2002). The interactions of these neuron groups with those regulating wakefulness and REM sleep in the perifornical/posterior hypothalamic nuclei and the brain stem have been suggested to underlie the physiological mechanisms for maintenance and alternation of sleep and wakefulness (McGinty and Szymusiak, 2003; Saper *et al.*, 2001). In addition, possible involvement of the glutamatergic and GABAergic neuron groups in the brain stem adds new aspects to the regulatory mechanisms of REM sleep (Fuller *et al.*, 2007; Gvilia *et al.*, 2006a; Luppi *et al.*, 2007). So to speak, more light has been shed on glutamatergic neurons in the sublaterodorsal nucleus (SLD) in rats (peri-LCα in cats) as an essential physiological substrate of regulatory mechanism of REM sleep (Fuller *et al.*, 2007; Luppi *et al.*, 2007; Sakai *et al.*, 2001). Because the recent glutamatergic-GABAergic stories are mainly based on *c-fos* studies, Sakai's studies provide a part of their evidence in terms of neuronal activities (Fuller *et al.*,

2007; Luppi *et al.*, 2007). Nevertheless, they have not yet reached a unified story. There are some discrepancies in the involvement of the forebrain structure in REM-sleep regulation and the possible contribution of GABAergic inputs toward formation of REM-off activities (Fuller *et al.*, 2007; Luppi *et al.*, 2007; Sakai *et al.*, 2001). On the other hand, the aminergic–cholinergic story of REM–NREM regulation has been updated involving GABAergic systems (McCarley and Hobson, 1975; McCarley *et al.*, 1995; Mallick *et al.*, 2001; Pal and Mallick, 2006). Taken together, we are still on the way to complete understanding of the regulatory mechanism of REM sleep.

Mathematical models have improved our understanding of the neural mechanisms of sleep–wake control. Among these models, reciprocal-interaction models have portrayed the fundamental mechanism of the REM–NREM cycle, where the cholinergic and aminergic neuron groups are hypothesized to behave like a prey–predator system (McCarley and Hobson, 1975). This model was subsequently extended conceptually (McCarley *et al.*, 1995). Recently, we proposed the model consists of a quartet of neuron groups: (1) sleep-active preoptic/anterior hypothalamic neurons (N-R group); (2) wake-active hypothalamic and brain-stem neurons exhibiting the highest rate of discharge during wakefulness and the lowest rate of discharge during paradoxical or REM sleep (WA group); (3) brain-stem neurons exhibiting the highest rate of discharge during REM sleep (REM group); and (4) basal forebrain, hypothalamic, and brain-stem neurons exhibiting a higher rate of discharge during both wakefulness and REM sleep than during NREM sleep (W-R group) (Tamakawa *et al.*, 2006). Although the actual detail profiles of state-dependencies vary from neuron to neuron even within the same group, the model well reproduces the typical activities across state transitions of some sleep-related neurons in addition to the actual sleep and wakefulness patterns of rats as well as humans.

In this chapter, we explain our model of sleep-wakefulness regulation in the rat, which includes a neural regulator quartet of NREM sleep, REM sleep, wakefulness, and a coregulator of REM sleep and wakefulness, whose parameters are tuned up so that the model reproduces some of the recent findings concerning the WA neurons. The physiological reality of the model structure is demonstrated by comparing the model neuron activities with the actual neuronal activities across state transition, and by showing a possibility

that the model can reproduce the human sleep–wake rhythm only with alternation of model parameters. Our successful modeling suggests that the regulation of sleep and wakefulness is realized by well orchestrated interactions among the aforementioned quartet of neural groups distributed in the hypothalamus and the brain stem with the aid of sleep-promoting substances. In other words, the model suggests that REM sleep is regulated cooperatively/competitively with NREM sleep and wakefulness. Finally, further possible updates in the model structure are described considering recent physiological findings.

Neuron groups participating in regulation of sleep–wake states

Here we summarize the physiological understanding of the neural groups involved in changing and maintaining sleep–wake states. Although the following description includes hypotheses that have not yet been proven, their correctness is tentatively assumed here for the purposes of modeling. These neuron groups are categorized mainly by their discharge patterns, which alternate depending on sleep–waking states, i.e., REM-on, WA, N-R, and W-R. The REM-on and WA neurons, respectively, exhibit increased and reduced activities exclusively in REM sleep. The N-R neurons are activated in NREM sleep and REM sleep, but not during wakefulness. The W-R neurons exhibit higher activity during wakefulness and REM sleep than during NREM sleep. Thus, N-R and WA correspond to so-called "sleep-active" and "REM-off", respectively. Figure 43.1 schematically shows the localizations of each neuron group (Jones, 2000; McCarley *et al.*, 1995; McGinty and Szymusiak, 2003; Sakai and Crochet, 2003; Steriade and Hobson, 1976; Datta, 1995). Anatomical connections and putative functions of the REM-on, WA, N-R, and W-R neurons are not explained here. For details please refer to Appendix 43.1 and to our previous paper (Tamakawa *et al.*, 2006) and the other chapters in this book. Throughout the paper, abbreviated names of neurotransmitters are in parentheses next to the name of the neuron group, i.e., ACh: acetylcholine; nonACh: non-acetylcholine; NA: noradrenaline; 5HT: serotonin; Orx: orexin; and HA: histamine. Here, "nonACh" is used to represent "putatively glutamatergic or GABAergic," although the transmitter has not been precisely identified. Accordingly, each neuron is denoted by "nucleus or region": "discharge type" ("neurotransmitter").

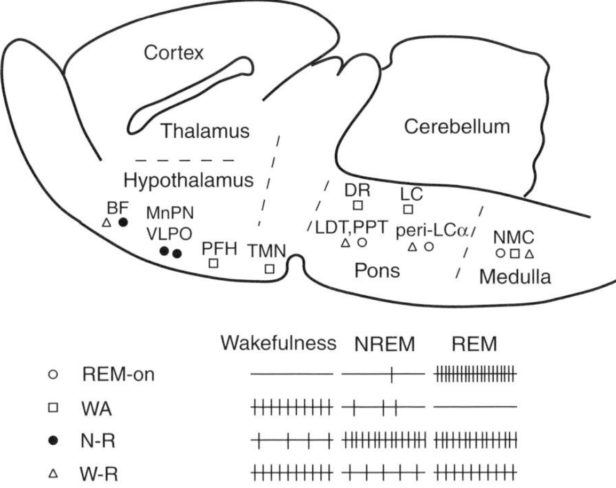

Figure 43.1 Locations of neuronal groups involved in the regulation of sleep and wakefulness and state dependency of their discharge patterns (Steriade and Hobson, 1976; McCarley *et al.*, 1995; Datta, 1995; Sakai and Crochet, 2003; McGinty and Szymusiak, 2003) (Adapted from Tamakawa *et al.*, 2006). Abbreviations of the nuclei are VLPO: ventrolateral preoptic hypothalamic area; MnPN: median preoptic nucleus; TMN: tuberomammillary nucleus; LC: locus coeruleus; DR: dorsal raphe nucleus; LDT: laterodorsal tegmental nucleus; PPT: pedunculopontine tegmental nucleus; peri-LCα: peri-locus coeruleus α; NMC: nucleus reticularis magnocellularis; PFH: perifornical lateral hypothalamus; and BF: basal forebrain. For the other abbreviations, see the introduction.

Neurons in the suprachiasmatic nucleus (SCN) send indirect projections to the sleep- and arousal-promoting systems in the brain stem (Aston-Jones *et al.*, 2001; Chou *et al.*, 2003; Deurveilher and Semba, 2005). In the model, the circadian modulators in N-R neurons are inhibitory for the active (dark) period and null for the rest (light) period; the modulator in WA neurons in the perifornical lateral hypothalamus is excitatory for the active period and null for the rest period. This circadian alternation of inhibitory/excitatory level in each neuron is assumed based on the circadian dependency of the extracellular orexin level (Yoshida *et al.*, 2001).

Various types of sleep-promoting substances (SPSs) have been considered to be involved in the homeostatic regulation of sleep and wakefulness. Two kinds of SPSs, SS1 and SS2, are also included to implement the homeostatic regulation of sleep and wakefulness. SS1 is accumulated during wakefulness, activates N-R neurons in VLPO, and is dissipated during sleep. In contrast, SS2 is accumulated during wakefulness and REM sleep, activates N-R neurons in the MnPN, and is dissipated during NREM sleep.

Modeling of regulatory mechanisms of sleep and wakefulness

Here, the constructed model of the mechanisms regulating sleep–wakefulness is explained. The model is composed of formal neurons, each of which represents the collective activities of neurons in the same group. The neuron groups included are *VLPO:N-R(GABA)*; *MnPN:N-R(GABA)*; *PFH:WA(Orx)*; *TMN:WA(HA)*; *BF:W-R(ACh)*; *LC:WA(NA)*; *DR:WA(5HT)*; *BS:REM-on(ACh)*; *BS:REM-on(nonACh)*; and *BS:W-R(ACh)*, where the model neuron is distinguished from the actual neurons by use of italic letters. Based on the physiological findings summarized above, these neurons are coupled to construct the model. In addition, auto-excitation mechanisms are introduced in *PFH:WA(Orx)*; *LC:WA(NA)*; *TMN:WA(HA)*; and *DR:WA(5HT)* neurons, because they exhibit spontaneous firing even in slice preparations of rat brain (Kamondi and Reiner, 1991; Liu *et al.*, 2002; Williams and Marshall, 1987; Yamanaka *et al.*, 2003). Two kinds of SPSs, *SS1* and *SS2*, are also included to implement the homeostatic regulation of sleep and wakefulness. *SS1* is accumulated during wakefulness, activates *VLPO: N-R(GABA)*, and is dissipated during sleep. In contrast, *SS2* is accumulated during wakefulness and REM sleep, activates *MnPN:N-R(GABA)*, and is dissipated during NREM sleep. Figure 43.2*a* depicts the model configuration in detail. The mathematical representation of the model is given in Appendix 43.1.

In modeling, some simplifications and tentative assumptions have been made, as follows. The REM-on and W-R neurons in the PFH are not distinguished from those in the brain stem, because no discharge patterns unique to them could be observed (Koyama *et al.*, 2003). The BF:N-R(GABA) neurons are not distinguished from those in the POA. The sleep-active neurons activated exclusively during NREM sleep in the preoptic/anterior hypothalamus are not explicitly included in the model since their function can be covered by the *VLPO:N-R(GABA)* and *MnPN:N-R(GABA)* neurons (for more detail see discussion). The REM-on(nonACh) and REM-on(GABA) neurons distributed in the brain stem are merged into *BS:REM-on(nonACh)*, as a result of which *BS:REM-on(nonACh)* can exert excitatory as well as inhibitory effects on target neurons. Therefore, REM-on inhibition is executed by *BS:REM-on(nonACh)* in the model. This, of course, does not conform to physiological findings. However, this would not be a crude simplification if the

439

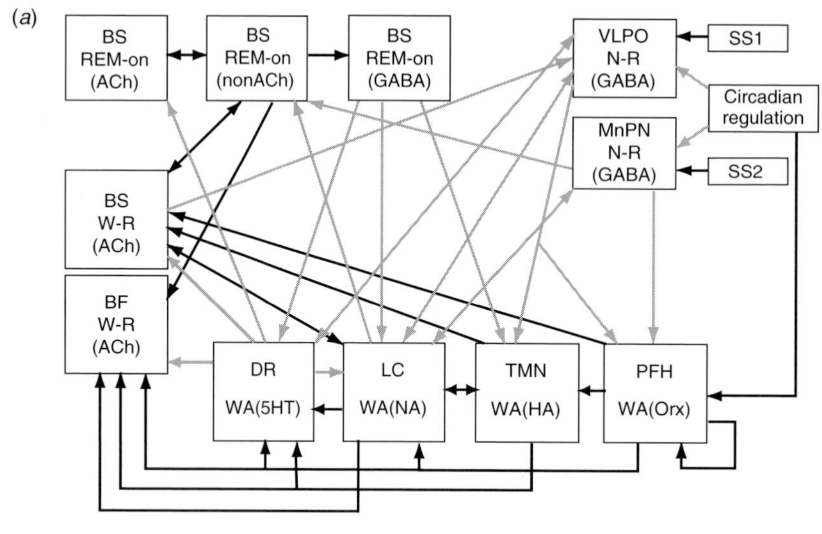

Figure 43.2 (a) Network model of mechanisms regulating sleep and wakefulness (adapted from Tamakawa *et al.*, 2006). Black and gray lines indicate excitatory and inhibitory connections, respectively. (b) Schematic representation of the model composed of the quartet of neuron groups: *WA, N-R, REM*, and *W-R*, where *W-R*={*BS:W-R(ACh), BF:W-R(ACh)*}, *N-R*={*VLPO:N-R(GABA), MnPN:N-R(GABA)*}, *REM*={*BS:REM-on(ACh), BS:REM-on(nonACh)*}, and *WA*={*PFH:WA(Orx), TMN:WA(HA), LC:WA(NA), DR:WA(5HT)*}. Couplings between the quartet of neuron groups schematize those in the detailed model to explicitly show their functions, with the inhibitory connection from *BS:W-R(ACh)* to *VLPO:N-R(GABA)* not shown for convenience of explanation. For abbreviations, see the text.

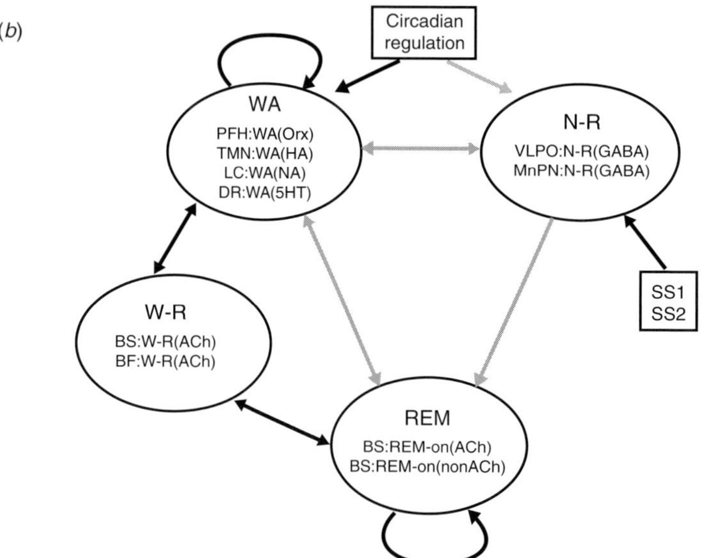

REM-on(GABA) neuron only reverses the sign of excitatory effect of the REM-on(nonACh) neuron. As noted above, the existence of REM-on(GABA) neurons is still controversial. Addressing this physiological issue is beyond the scope of this chapter; however, from the modeling point of view, whatever the mechanism underlying "REM-off activity" is, appropriate "REM-on" suppression is functionally needed although it does not have to be GABAergic. Therefore, such an "REM-on" inhibition is tentatively introduced as described above. Another controversy concerns the monoaminergic inhibition of BS:REM-on neurons. Because at least in the rat LDT the experimental results suggest the existence of

this inhibition (Sakai and Crochet, 2003; Thakker *et al.*, 1998), the *BS:REM-on* neurons are designed to undergo inhibitions by *LC:WA(NA)* and *DR:WA(5HT)* in the model. However, this inhibition alone does not play a decisive role in permitting REM sleep. This implementation also coincides with the idea that the cessation of monoaminergic activity is not sufficient for the induction of REM sleep (Sakai, 1988). Verification of this is left to future physiological studies.

As shown in Figure 43.2*b*, the model configuration can be represented by a quartet of neuron groups for purposes of understanding the operation of the model. The quartet comprises *WA, N-R, REM*, and

W-R, where *W-R*={*BS:W-R(ACh)*, *BF:W-R(ACh)*}, *N-R*={*VLPO:N-R(GABA)*, *MnPN:N-R(GABA)*}, *REM*= {*BS:REM-on(ACh)*, *BS:REM-on(nonACh)*}, and *WA*={*PFH:WA(Orx)*, *TMN:WA(HA)*, *LC:WA(NA)*, *DR:WA(5HT)*}. The couplings between the quartet of neuron groups schematize those in the detailed model to explicitly show their functions. That is, the *WA* neurons have mutual inhibitory couplings with the *REM* and *N-R* neurons. The *REM* neurons have mutual excitatory couplings with each other. The *WA* neuron group has auto-excitatory coupling. The *W-R* neurons have mutual excitatory couplings with the *REM* and *WA* neurons. The *N-R* neurons are activated by *SS1* and *SS2*, and inhibit the *REM* and *WA* neurons. Note that while the *WA*, *REM*, and *N-R* neurons have auto-excitatory mechanisms, each can be exclusively activated by mutual inhibitions between them.

Simulations of neuronal activities during REM sleep and state transitions in rats

Figure 43.3 shows a fundamental sleep–wakefulness pattern generated by the model whose parameter values are given in Appendix 43.1. A bidirectional state change between wakefulness and NREM sleep, and a state change from NREM sleep to wakefulness via REM sleep, are clearly observed. Here the sleep–wakefulness stages of the model are tentatively determined based on the activity levels of *TMN:WA(HA)*

and *BS:REM-on(ACh)* as members of the *WA* and *REM* groups, respectively: activity of *TMN:WA(HA)* > 0.6 defines wakefulness; activity of *BS:REM-on(ACh)* > 0.6 defines REM sleep; and otherwise NREM sleep occurs. When a state change from REM sleep to wakefulness takes place, sometimes a brief period of NREM sleep intervenes. This is because the transient state in which *WA* and *REM* neurons are both inactivated is forcibly categorized into one of the three states. Notably, this staging is nearly unaffected even if the other member in the respective group is selected. Most of the time courses of neuronal activity are faithfully reproduced in the model. In particular, the model closely mimics the complex pattern of MnPN neuron activity over sleep–waking states (Suntsova *et al.*, 2002) and the state dependency of DR:WA(5HT) neuron activity distinct from those of other WA neurons, i.e., the activity of DR:WA(5HT) survives during NREM sleep, but the other WA neurons do not (Lee *et al.*, 2005; Takahashi *et al.*, 2006, 2008).

For direct examination, the activities of the model neurons across state transitions are compared with those of actual neurons in rat PFH (Koyama *et al.*, 2003) and brain stem (Koyama *et al.*, 2001). In Figure 43.4 typical neuronal discharge patterns across state transitions are selected for comparison with those of simulation. The actual activities are those of the W-R and REM-on neurons in the brain stem and a WA neuron in the PFH. The W-R neuron is thought to be cholinergic, and one type of REM-on neuron is cholinergic and the other

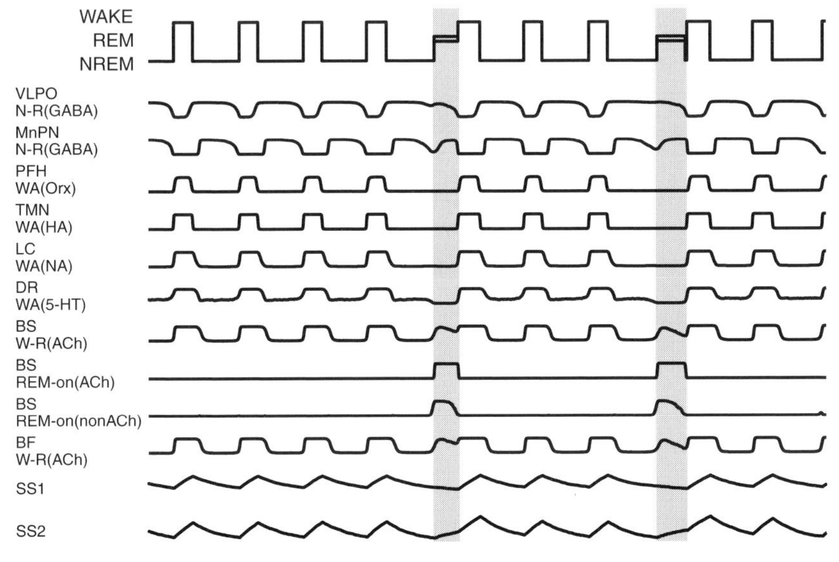

Figure 43.3 Simulated neuronal activities and levels of *SS1* and *SS2* associated with the state sequence of sleep and wakefulness in the inactive (light) period of the rat. Shaded periods indicate those of REM sleep. The model mimics the actual sleep–waking cycle of rats, which is characterized by the bidirectional state change between NREM sleep and wakefulness and unidirectional state changes from NREM sleep to REM sleep and from REM sleep to wakefulness.

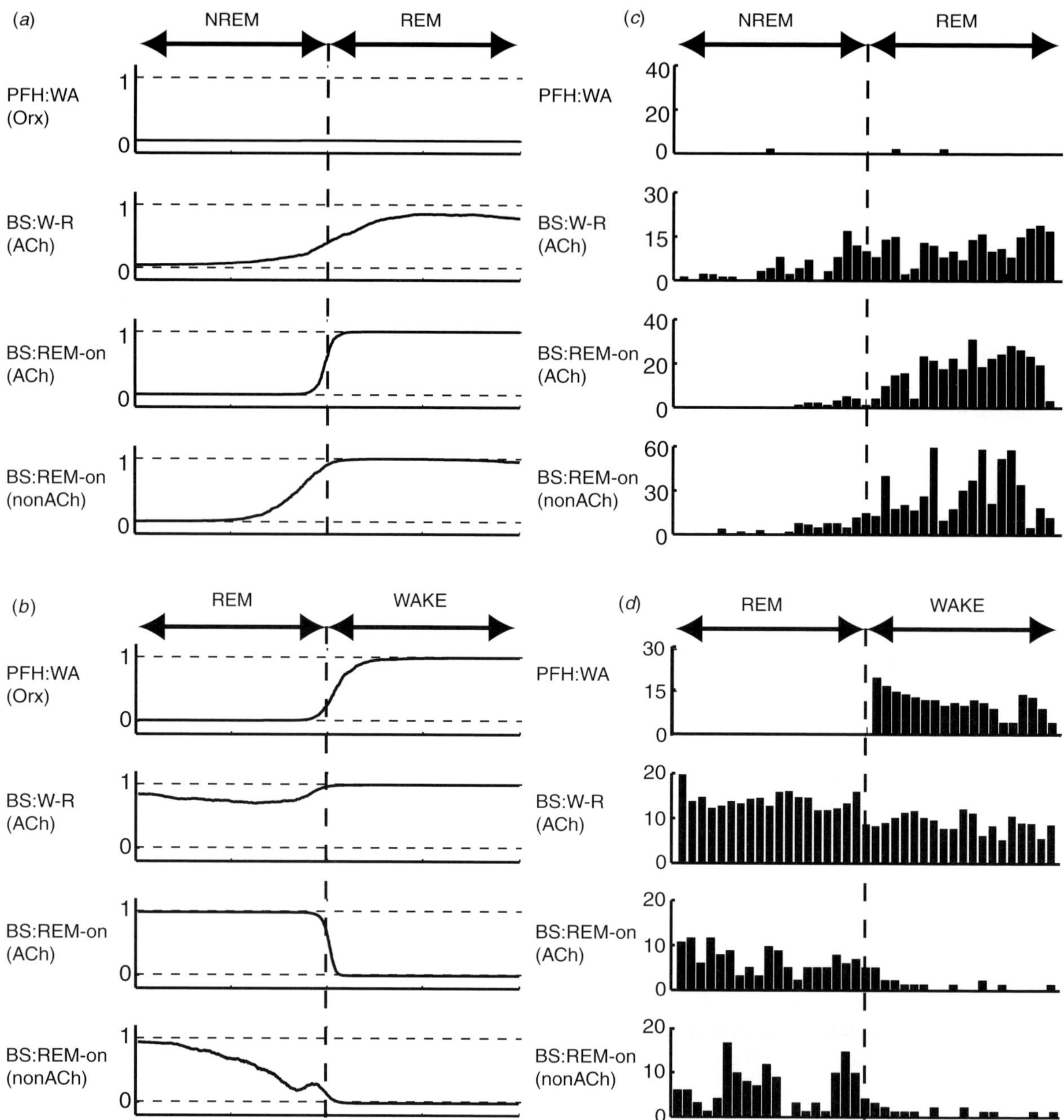

Figure 43.4 Comparisons between the model (left column) and actual (right column) neuronal activities across state transitions, where the vertical dotted line in each trace indicates the timing of state change (the actual neuronal activities are adapted from Tamakawa *et al.*, 2006). (*a*) From NREM sleep to REM sleep; (*b*) from NREM sleep to wakefulness; (*c*) from REM sleep to wakefulness; (*d*) from wakefulness to NREM sleep. The vertical axis indicates the count of neuronal spikes per two-second bin, 40 seconds before and after state transition is shown.

non-cholinergic; their neurotransmitters are conjectured based on spike waveform criteria (Koyama *et al.*, 1998). The WA neuron in the PFH is putatively an orexin neuron (Alam *et al.*, 2002; Koyama *et al.*, 2003; Lee *et al.*, 2005). Classification of neuronal discharge patterns was done according to the criteria described in the appendix of our previous paper (Tamakawa *et al.*, 2006).

Across the transition from NREM sleep to REM sleep, the W-R and cholinergic and non-cholinergic REM-on neurons in the brain stem begin to increase their discharge rates before the state change, although there are variations in when activation starts and how fast it grows. In contrast, the WA neuron is only minimally activated around the state change. In Figure 43.4*a*, some of the actual discharge patterns are compared with those of the model neurons, i.e., *PFH:WA(Orx); BS:W-R(ACh); BS:REM-on(ACh);* and *BS:REM-on(nonACh).* Naturally, the actual discharge patterns have short-term and long-term fluctuations. However, the activities of the model neurons mimic rough profiles of the actual neuronal discharge rates across the state transition from NREM sleep to REM sleep. Actually, there are some PFH:WA(Orx) neurons that exhibit brief activation across this transition (Tamakawa *et al.,* 2006, Fig. 6) in contrast to *PFH:WA(Orx)* in the model. This brief activation may reveal a background mechanism underlying the state change. The inhibitions exerted by *MnPN:N-R(GABA)* are weakened due to its reduced activity as NREM sleep nearly ends (see Figure 43.3). After the state change into REM sleep, inhibition by *MnPN:N-R(GABA)* is strengthened again. Because the *REM* neurons are subject to inhibition by *MnPN:N-R(GABA)* and the *REM* neurons exert inhibitory effects on the *WA* neurons, disinhibition followed by restored inhibition potentially induces brief activation of the *WA* neurons across the state transition. In the model, *PFH:WA(Orx)* does not exhibit such activation, since the balance between activation and inhibition differs from that for other *WA* neurons. Similarly, the observed variation in pattern of activity of PFH:WA(Orx) neurons could be explained by that in the balance between activation and inhibition.

In the transition from REM sleep to wakefulness, in contrast to the REM-on neurons, which decrease their discharge, the W-R neuron maintains activity, although with some variation. The WA neuron abruptly increases activity just after the state change. As shown in Figure 43.4*b*, the large fluctuations in actual activity patterns may prevent a direct comparison with model behavior. However, at least the overall profiles of actual neuronal activity patterns are shared by those of the model neuronal activities.

Model-based interpretation of regulatory mechanisms of REM sleep

The close accord in neuronal activities between the model and the actual data demonstrates the physiological accuracy of the model. In the following, cooperative/competitive mechanisms regulating REM sleep are explained in the light of operation of the model. Figure 43.5 illustrates the organization of the neural interactions associated with changes and maintenance of state in the model.

Suppressing REM-sleep induction after wakefulness

During wakefulness, the *N-R* neuron group is being activated by accumulation of *SS1* and *SS2*, and concurrently the *WA* and *REM* neurons are receiving inhibitions from the *N-R* neuron. When an *N-R* neuron activity completely suppresses the *WA* and *REM* neurons, i.e., turns them off, the state changes from wakefulness to NREM sleep, not to REM sleep.

Starting REM sleep after NREM sleep

During NREM sleep, *SS1* and *SS2* are dissipated. This gradually reduces *N-R* neuron suppression of the *WA* and *REM* neurons, which competitively determines which neuron group turns on next. That is, if reduction of suppression of the *REM* neuron reaches a threshold earlier than that of the *WA* neuron, the *REM* neuron turns on, due to mutual excitation between *REM-on(ACh)* and *REM-on(nonACh)* and between *REM-on(nonACh)* and *W-R(ACh)*. Otherwise, the *WA* neurons turn on as a result of their auto-excitability, as supported by the excitatory interconnections among *WA(NA), WA(HA),* and *WA(Orx)* and the mutual excitation between *WA(NA)* and *W-R(ACh)*.

Maintenance and termination of REM sleep

During NREM sleep, dissipation of *SS1* and *SS2* inactivates the *N-R* neurons. After the change to REM sleep, *SS1* continues to be dissipated, while *SS2* is accumulated progressively to reactivate *MnPN:N-R(GABA)*. Due to this, *MnPN:N-R(GABA)* increases suppression of the *REM* and *WA* neurons. REM sleep is being maintained by mutual excitation between *REM-on(ACh)* and *REM-on(nonACh)* and between *REM-on(nonACh)* and *W-R(ACh)*. However, augmented suppression by *MnPN:N-R(GABA)* weakens the *REM* neuron activities. Finally, the *REM* neurons are forced to turn off, which reactivates the *WA* neurons. This process is facilitated by disinhibition of *WA* neurons from *VLPO:N-R(GABA)* due to decrease in *SS1*. In this fashion, REM sleep is followed by wakefulness. Namely, at

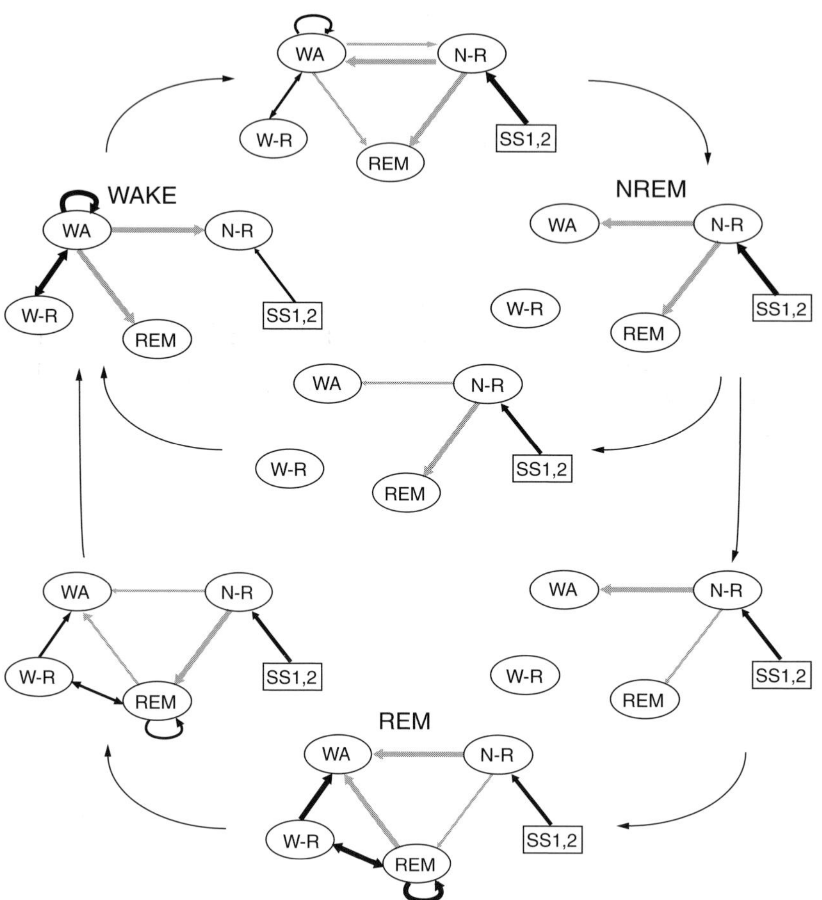

Figure 43.5 Organizations of interactions among the quartet of neuron groups in each state and across state transitions (revised from Tamakawa *et al.*, 2006). The inhibitory connection from *BS:W-R(ACh)* to *VLPO:N-R(GABA)* is not shown for convenience of illustration. Black and gray arrows indicate excitatory and inhibitory effects, respectively. Thickness indicates strength of the effect originating from the level of activation of the constituent neuron in each group.

the termination of REM sleep, turn-off of *REM* leads to turn-on of *WA*, which is different from the previously modeled mechanism that turn-on of *WA* leads to turn-off of *REM* (Tamakawa *et al.*, 2006). This alternation is responsible for the latest findings that silencing REM-on neurons is followed by reactivation of WA neurons (Takahashi *et al.*, 2006, 2008).

As illustrated above, the resulting neuronal activities and the organization of interactions are not always correlated. For example, coactivation of *MnPN:N-R(GABA)* and *BS:REM-on* during REM sleep appears inconsistent with the expected result of unidirectional inhibition by *MnPN:N-R(GABA)* of *BS:REM-on*. Actually, the mutual excitation between the *BS:REM-on* neurons and between *BS:REM-on* and *W-R* overcomes the inhibition by *MnPN:N-R(GABA)*. This is a model-based interpretation of the mechanism underlying the finding that, despite activation of the N-R neurons, REM sleep persists, as shown in Figure 43.1. In this fashion, the model structure

discloses a hidden mechanism realizing the complex state dependency of neuronal activity patterns briefly illustrated in Figure 43.1.

Modeling of human sleep and wakefulness rhythms

Human sleep and wakefulness are characterized by their concentration in phase and rhythmic, not random, REM–NREM alternation. In addition, the human sleep–wakefulness rhythm tends to exhibit bidirectional state change between REM sleep and NREM sleep, and almost unidirectional change from wakefulness to NREM sleep and REM sleep to wakefulness. In the present study, we can preserve the model structure used for rats and simulate the human sleep–wakefulness rhythm by tuning the model parameters. Concentrated sleep and wakefulness are realized by augmenting circadian modulations in the activities of *VLPO:N-R(GABA)*, *MnPN:N-R(GABA)*, and

PFH:WA(Orx). In order for REM–NREM alternation to continue without the intervention of wakefulness, the *WA* neurons should be sufficiently suppressed during sleep, and *MnPN:N-R(GABA)* alone is necessary to force the *REM* neurons to turn off. To satisfy the former condition, the rates of production and dissipation of *SS1* are reduced for human simulation. To meet the latter condition, inhibition by *MnPN:N-R(GABA)* of *REM-on(nonACh)* is enhanced. Additionally, the rate of production of *SS2* during REM sleep, k_r, and its rate of dissipation during NREM sleep, k_n, are increased so that *SS2* can change sufficiently faster than *SS1*, which allows several REM–NREM cycles to take place during a sleep period. The applied noise is reduced to obtain less random alternation between sleep and wakefulness. The modification of model parameters is described in the appendix. Figure 43.6 shows the simulated sleep–wakefulness rhythm. The major properties of the human sleep–wakefulness rhythm are clearly reproduced: (1) sleep starts with NREM sleep; (2) sleep ends with REM sleep; (3) sleep contains several REM–NREM cycles; and (4) the duration of REM sleep is progressively prolonged. Similar to the case of the rat, the state change from REM sleep to wakefulness is intervened by a brief period of NREM sleep. This is also due to the obligatory categorization of transient state.

The mechanisms underlying state changes are summarized, with special reference to how they differ from the rat model. Maintenance of each state is realized by the same mechanism as in the rat model. On the other hand, state changes are differently controlled, owing to the alteration of model parameters described above. Enhanced circadian regulation concentrates wakefulness and sleep along the time axis: wakefulness dominates when *N-R(GABA)/WA(Orx)* is inactivated/activated, and sleep dominates in the opposite case. The decreased rates of production/dissipation of *SS1* facilitate this concentration.

After the change to NREM sleep due to exclusive activation of the *N-R* neurons, *VLPO:N-R(GABA)* suppresses *LC:WA(NA)* until *SS1* is completely dissipated. In contrast, *SS2* is dissipated quickly during NREM sleep, which changes the state to REM sleep by reducing the inhibition of *BS:REM-on(nonACh)* exerted by *MnPN:N-R(GABA)*. This one-way state change from NREM sleep to REM sleep results from the organization of the human model, in which *MnPN:N-R(GABA)* can by itself completely suppress *BS:REM-on(nonACh)*. During REM sleep, *SS2* is accumulated quickly. The accumulated *SS2* changes the state to NREM sleep again by activating *MnPN:N-R(GABA)*. In this way, alternations between NREM sleep and REM sleep persist until the end of sleep. This cycle can end by state change from either NREM sleep or REM sleep to wakefulness. Nevertheless, because the suppression of *WA* neurons during REM sleep is stronger than during NREM sleep due to cooperative inhibition by *VLPO:N-R(GABA)* and *BS:REM-on(nonACh)*, the activity of *WA* neurons could be suppressed by the *REM* neurons longer than the *N-R* neurons if the activity of *VLPO:N-R(GABA)*

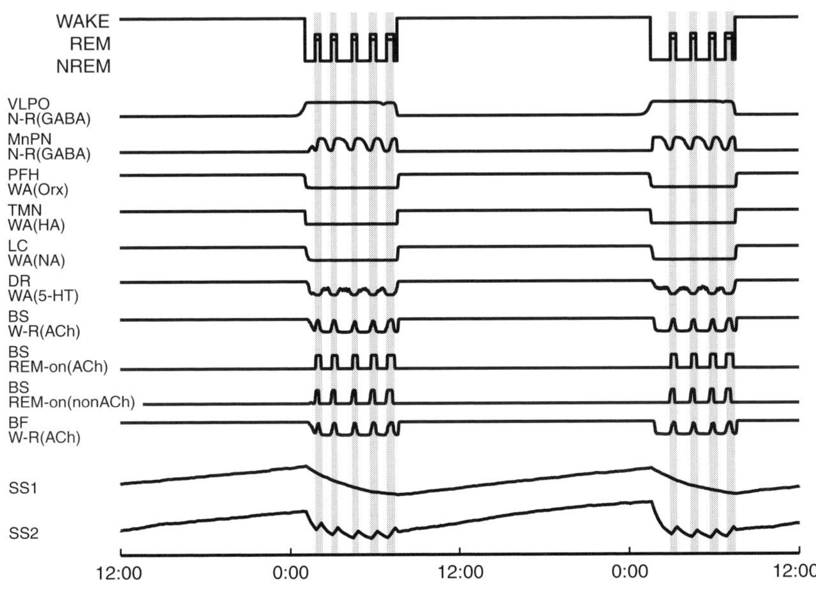

Figure 43.6 Simulation of the human sleep–wake cycle by tuning of the parameters of the rat model and introduction of a sinusoidal circadian input. Although neuronal activities and levels of *SS1* and *SS2* across sleep–wake cycles are not known, at least the sleep–waking pattern itself mimics the human one well.

decreases at a constant rate. Accordingly, REM sleep tends to end the cycle.

Possible further updates of model structure

The REM–NREM cycle was first modeled as a prey–predator system of cholinergic–aminergic neurons, i.e., the REM-on and WA neurons (McCarley and Hobson, 1975). In response to recent findings for sleep-active neurons and wake-related neurons, the GABAergic–glutamatergic system has been attracting researchers. In this context, Saper and his colleagues proposed the conceptual flip-flop (FF) model, which consists of double FFs: one for the sleep–wakefulness cycle and the other for the REM–NREM cycle (Saper *et al.*, 2001). Luppi *et al.* proposed a cascade model consisting of GABAergic–glutamatergic neurons including PAG and SLD (Luppi *et al.*, 2007). However, from the mathematical point of view, which mechanisms flips the FFs or induces state alternations in the cascade system is not known. In order to clarify these mechanisms, the contributions of modeling are essential.

Over the structural differences, most of the recently developed mathematical models share this double FF concept (Diniz Behn *et al.*, 2007; Phillips and Robinson, 2007). A simple FF realizes a bidirectional state transition, which does not necessarily agree with the properties of actual state transition, e.g., the state transitions from wakefulness to REM sleep and from REM sleep to NREM sleep seldom happen in the rat. Our model provides one possible quantitative implementation of such a peculiar multistable system, which is composed of interconnected multiple FFs and the SPSs that play various roles in homeostatic regulation. Among the conceptual and mathematical models, one of the novel features of our model is the involvement of the cholinergic W-R neuron group, which is assumed to contribute toward induction of wakefulness as well as REM sleep by selectively mediating autocatalytic activation with the WA or REM neurons (Tamakawa *et al.*, 2006). Through the activity of this neuron group, the wakefulness–sleep FF and the REM–NREM FF interact with each other in our model. In fact pharmacological or physiological manipulations of REM sleep were shown to affect not only NREM sleep but wakefulness (e.g., Bourgin *et al.*, 2000; Hagan *et al.*, 1999). The conceptual double FF model is characterized by the unidirectional coupling from the sleep–wakefulness FF to the REM–NREM FF, which is mediated by the aminergic systems (Saper *et al.*, 2001). This mechanism does not allow REM–NREM cycles to affect sleep–wakefulness cycles.

Our model needs further updates, considering the latest findings of the physiological properties of neuron groups involved in sleep–wakefulness regulation. In what follows, these findings are briefly summarized.

The preoptic hypothalamic area is one of most intensively investigated areas concerning induction and maintenance of sleep, which includes the VLPO and MnPN (McGinty and Szymusiak, 2003; Saper *et al.*, 2001). Recently, the VLPO is divided into the cluster and extension regions, which are tentatively called VLPOcl and VLPOex, respectively. *c-fos* expressions of VLPO neurons in relation to sleep–wake cycles suggest that the activity of the VLPOcl is related to the amount of NREM sleep and the VLPOex is related to the amount of REM sleep (Lu *et al.*, 2002). In addition, the anatomical study using anterograde tracer showed that the VLPOex has abundant projections to the GABAergic PAG neurons that are supposed to be involved in REM-sleep regulation (Lu *et al.*, 2006).

Concerning the possible functions of the MnPN neurons, recent studies suggest that they are involved in regulation of NREM sleep as well as REM sleep (Gvilia *et al.*, 2006a,b; Suntsova *et al.*, 2002). According to this discharge pattern across the transition from wakefulness to NREM sleep and the results of sleep deprivation, the MnPN neuron is thought to promote transitions to NREM sleep rather than consolidation of NREM sleep (Gvilia *et al.* 2006b). In addition to NREM sleep, the investigation of *c-fos* expression against REM-sleep restriction suggests that the MnPN neuron contributes to the homeostatic regulation of REM sleep (Gvilia *et al.*, 2006a). Besides the preoptic hypothalamic area, the NREM sleep-modulating area in the brain stem is suggested to mediate between regulation of NREM and REM sleep (Mallick *et al.*, 2004).

The recent unit-recording studies in the tuberomammillary nucleus (TMN) and the perifornical lateral hypothalamus (PFH) have renewed the knowledge concerning the functional relationship between the monoaminergic and peptidergic WA neurons (Lee *et al.*, 2005; Takahashi *et al.* 2006, 2008). Based on this knowledge, the orexin WA neuron is suggested to be mainly involved in induction of the waking state; the histamine WA neuron is suggested to contribute towards maintenance of a high level of vigilance. Instead, the noradrenergic and/or serotonergic neurons in the WA group might play a regulatory role of

REM sleep incorporating with the GABAergic REM-on neurons in the brain stem mentioned previously.

Updates of the model structure considering these latest findings are now going on, which will be presented elsewhere. We expect that our proposed framework of a quartet of neuron groups should still be valid in spite of these further updates.

Acknowledgments

This work was partly supported by "Academic Frontiers" Project for Private Universities (the Kansei Fukushi Research Center of Tohoku Fukushi University): matching fund subsidy from the Ministry of Education, Culture, Sports, Science, and Technology of Japan (2004–8). This work was also supported in part by Grant-in-Aid for Young Scientists (B), 20700346 and Scientific Research on Priority Areas, 21012001.

References

Alam, M. N., Gong, H., Alam, T. *et al.* (2002) Sleep–waking discharge patterns of neurons recorded in the rat perifornical lateral hypothalamic area. *J Physiol* **538**: 619–31.

Aston-Jones, G., Chen, S., Zhu, Y. & Oshinsky, M. L. (2001) A neural circuit for circadian regulation of arousal. *Nature Neurosci* **4**: 732–8.

Bourgin, P., Huitrón-Reséndiz, S., Spier, A. D. *et al.* (2000) Hypocretin-1 modulates rapid eye movement sleep through activation of locus coeruleus neurons. *J Neurosci* **20**: 7760–5.

Chou, T. C., Scammell, T. E., Gooley, J. J. *et al.* (2003) Critical role of dorsomedial hypothalamic nucleus in a wide range of behavioral circadian rhythms. *J Neurosci* **23**: 10,691–702.

Datta, S. (1995) Neuronal activity in the peribrachial area: relationship to behavioral state control. *Neurosci Biobehav Rev* **19**: 67–84.

Deurveilher, S. & Semba, K. (2005) Indirect projections from the suprachiasmatic nucleus to major arousal-promoting cell groups in rat: implications for the circadian control of behavioral state. *Neurosci* **130**:165–83.

Diniz Behn, C. G., Brown, E. N., Scammell, T. E. & Kopell, N. J. (2007) Mathematical model of network dynamics governing mouse sleep–wake behavior. *J Neurophysiol* **97**: 3828–40.

Fuller, P. M., Saper, C. B. & Lu, J. (2007) The pontine REM switch: past and present. *J Physiol* **584**: 735–41.

Gvilia, I., Turner, A., McGinty, D. & Szymusiak, R. (2006a) Preoptic area neurons and the homeostatic regulation of rapid eye movement sleep. *J Neurosci* **26**:3037–44.

Gvilia, I., Feng, X., McGinty, D. & Szymusiak, R. (2006b) Homeostatic regulation of sleep: a role of preoptic area neurons. *J Neurosci* **26**: 9425–33.

Hagan, J. J., Leslie, R. A., Pastel, S. *et al.* (1999) Orexin A activates locus coeruleus cell firing and increases arousal in the rat. *Proc Natl Acad Sci USA* **96**: 10,911–16.

Jones, B. (2000) Basic mechanisms of sleep–wake states. In *Principles and Practice of Sleep Medicine* (3rd edn.), eds. M. H. Kryger, T, Roth & W.C. Dement. Philadelphia: Saunders, pp.134–54.

Kamondi, A. & Reiner, P. B. (1991) Hyperpolarization-activated inward current in histaminergic tuberomammillary neurons of the rat hypothalamus. *J Neurophysiol* **66**: 1902–11.

Koyama, Y., Honda, T., Kusakabe, M., Kayama, Y. & Sugiura, Y. (1998) In vivo electrophysiological distinction of histochemically-identified cholinergic neurons using extracellular recording and labeling in rat laterodorsal tegmental nucleus. *Neurosci* **83**: 1105–12.

Koyama, Y., Takahashi, K. & Kayama, Y. (2001) Histamine is a transmitter to maintain tonic firing of mesopontine tegmental cholinergic neurons during wakefulness. In *Histamine Research in the New Millennium*, eds. T. Watanabe, H. Timmerman & K. Yanai. Amsterdam: Elsevier, pp.199–202.

Koyama, Y., Takahashi, K., Kodama, T. & Kayama, Y. (2003) State dependent activity of neurons in the perifornical hypothalamic area during sleep and waking. *Neurosci* **119**:1209–19.

Lee, M. G., Hassani, O. K. & Jones, B. E. (2005) Discharge of identified orexin/hypocretin neurons across the sleep–waking cycle. *J Neurosci* **25**: 6716–20.

Liu, R., Ding, Y. & Aghajanian, G. K. (2002) Neurokinins activate local glutamatergic inputs to serotonergic neurons of the dorsal raphe nucleus. *Neuropsychopharmacol* **27**: 329–40.

Lu, J., Bjorkum, A. A., Xu, M. *et al.* (2002) Selective activation of the extended ventrolateral preoptic nucleus during rapid eye movement sleep. *J Neurosci* **22**: 4568–76.

Lu, J., Sherman, D., Devor, M. & Saper, C. B. (2006) A putative flip-flop switch for control of REM sleep. *Nature* **441**: 589–94.

Luppi, P.-H., Gervasoni, D., Verret, L. *et al.* (2007) Paradoxical (REM) sleep genesis: the switch from an aminergic–cholinergic to a GABAergic–glutamatergic hypothesis. *J Physiol – Paris* **100**: 271–83.

Mallick, B. N., Kaur, S. & Saxena, R. N. (2001) Interactions between cholinergic and GABA-ergic neurotransmitters in and around the locus coeruleus for the induction and maintenance of rapid eye movement sleep in rats. *Neurosci* **104**: 467–85.

Mallick, B. N., Thankachan, S. & Islam, F. (2004) Influence of hypnogenic brain areas on wakefulness and REM sleep related neurons in the brain stem of freely moving cats. *J Neurosci Res* **75**:133–42.

McCarley, R. W. & Hobson, J. A. (1975) Neuronal excitability modulation over the sleep cycle: a structural and mathematical model. *Science* **189**: 58–60.

McCarley, R. W., Greene, R. W., Rainnie, D. G. & Portas, C. M. (1995) Brainstem neuromodulation and REM sleep. *Neurosci* **7**: 341–54.

McGinty, D. J. & Harper, R. M. (1976) Dorsal raphe neurons: depression of firing during sleep in cats. *Brain Res* **101**:569–75.

McGinty, D. & Szymusiak, R. (2003) Hypothalamic regulation of sleep and arousal. *Frontiers Biosci* **8**: 1074–83.

Pal, D. & Mallick, B. N. (2006) Role of noradrenergic and GABA-ergic inputs in pedunculopontine tegmentum for regulation of rapid eye movement sleep in rats. *Neuropharmacol* **51**:1–11.

Phillips, A. J. K. & Robinson, P. A. (2007)A quantitative model of sleep–wake dynamics based on the physiology of the brainstem ascending arousal system. *J Biol Rhythms* **22**: 167–79.

Sakai, K. (1988) Executive mechanism of paradoxical sleep. *Arch Ital Biol* **126**: 239–57.

Sakai, K. & Crochet, S. (2003)A neural mechanism of sleep and wakefulness. *Sleep Biol Rhythms* **1**: 29–42.

Sakai, K., Crochet, S. & Onoe, H. (2001) Pontine structures and mechanisms involved in the generation of paradoxical sleep. *Arch Ital Biol* **139**: 93–107.

Saper, C. B., Chou, T.C. & Scammell, T. E. (2001) The sleep switch: hypothalamic control of sleep and wakefulness. *Trends Neurosci* **24**: 726–31.

Sherin, J. E., Shiromani, P. J., McCarley, R. W. & Saper, C. B. (1996) Activation of ventrolateral preoptic neurons during sleep. *Science* **271**:216–19.

Steriade, M. & Hobson, J. (1976) Neuronal activity during the sleep-waking cycle. *Prog Neurobiol* **6**: 155–376.

Suntsova, N., Szymusiak, R., Alam, M. N., Guzman-Marin, R. & McGinty, D. (2002) Sleep–waking discharge patterns of median preoptic nucleus neurons in rats. *J Physiol* **543**: 665–77.

Takahashi, K., Lin, J. S. & Sakai, K. (2006) Neuronal activity of histaminergic tuberomammillary neurons during wake–sleep states in the mouse. *J Neurosci* **26**:10,292–8.

Takahashi, K., Lin, J. S. & Sakai, K. (2008) Neuronal activity of orexin and non-orexin waking-active neurons during wake–sleep states in the mouse. *Neurosci* **153**:860–70.

Tamakawa, Y., Karashima, A., Koyama, Y., Katayama, N. & Nakao, M. (2006) A quartet neural system model orchestrating sleep and wakefulness mechanisms. *J Neurophysiol* **95**: 2055–69.

Thakker, M. M., Strecker, R. E. & McCarley, R. W. (1998) Behavioral state control through differential serotonergic inhibition in the mesopontine cholinergic nuclei: a simultaneous unit recording and microdialysis study. *J Neurosci* **18**: 5490–7.

Williams, J. T. & Marshall, K. C. (1987) Membrane properties and adrenergic responses in locus coeruleus neurons of young rats. *J Neurosci* **7**: 3687–94.

Yamanaka, A., Muraki, Y., Tsujino, N., Goto, K. & Sakurai, T. (2003) Regulation of orexin neurons by the monoaminergic and cholinergic systems. *Biochem Biophys Res Commun* **303**: 120–9.

Yoshida, Y., Fujiki, N., Nakajima, T. *et al.* (2001) Fluctuation of extracellular hypocretin-1 (orexin A) levels in the rat in relation to the light–dark cycle and sleep–wake activities. *Eur J Neurosci* **14**: 1075–81.

Appendix 43.1

The model of rat sleep–wakefulness regulation

The model consists of ten formal neurons (X_1, …, X_{10}) and two sleep-promoting substances ($SS1$ and $SS2$). The mathematical expression and the parameter values are given as follows.

$$X_i = f_i(u_i), \quad (i = 1, \cdots, 10) \tag{A-1}$$

$$\frac{du_i}{dt} = -\frac{u_i}{\tau_i} + \sum_{j=1}^{10} W_{ij}X_j - \theta_i + 10\delta_{i1}(SS1 + C_1) + 10\delta_{i2}(SS2 + C_2) + 10\delta_{i3} \cdot C_3 + \xi_i, \tag{A-2}$$

$$f_i(u) = \frac{1}{1 + \exp\left(-\dfrac{u}{u_i}\right)}, \tag{A-3}$$

where the notations X_1, …, X_{10} represent the activities of VLPO:N-R(GABA), MnPN:N-R(GABA), PFH:WA(Orx), TMN:WA(HA), LC:WA(NA), DR:WA(5HT), BS:W-R(ACh), BS:REM-on(ACh), BS:REM-on(nonACh), and BF:W-R(ACh), respectively. In addition, SS1 and SS2 denote the SPSs modulating the activities of VLPO:N-R(GABA) and MnPN:N-R(GABA), respectively. W_{ij}, τ_i, θ_j, and μ_i are synaptic weights from the j-th neuron to the i-th, time constants, thresholds, and slope factors of the activation function f(u), respectively. δ_{ij} is Kronecker's delta, i.e., it takes the value 1 only if i = j, and otherwise is equal to 0. ξ_i is a 0-mean Gaussian noise whose standard deviation is 0.316. C_i (i = 1,2,3) is a circadian modulator; for the active period, C_1, C_2, and C_3 are −1.3, −1.05, and 0.1, respectively, while for the rest period they are null. The other parameter values are given as follows.

$$W_{ij} = \begin{bmatrix} 0 & 0 & 0 & 0 & -5 & -10 & -2 & 0 & 0 & 0 \\ 0 & 0 & 0 & 0 & -40 & 0 & 0 & 0 & 0 & 0 \\ -1.5 & -0.9 & 0.5 & 0 & 0 & 0 & 0 & 0 & 0 & 0 \\ -4 & 0 & 1.2 & 0 & 0.6 & 0 & 0 & 0 & -2 & 0 \\ -2 & -0.5 & 0.5 & 1.2 & 0 & -0.1 & 0.9 & 0 & -1.5 & 0 \\ -1 & 0 & 0.7 & 0.7 & 0.7 & 0 & 0 & 0 & -3 & 0 \\ 0 & 0 & 1.5 & 1.5 & 1.5 & -0.1 & 0 & 0 & 1.5 & 0 \\ 0 & 0 & 0 & 0 & 0 & -3 & 0 & 0 & 2 & 0 \\ 0 & -2.0 & 0 & 0 & -4.5 & 0 & 1 & 1.5 & 0 & 0 \\ 0 & 0 & 1.5 & 1.5 & 1.5 & -0.1 & 0 & 0 & 1.5 & 0 \end{bmatrix}$$

$\{\tau_i\} = \{1.5, 1.5, 1.5, 1.5, 1.5, 1.5, 2.25, 2.25, 1.5, 2.25\}$,
$\{\theta_i\} = \{0, 4, -0.4, -1.6, -0.5, -0.8, 1, 0.3, -0.3, 1\}$,
$\{\mu_i\} = \{1.5, 1.75, 0.25, 0.25, 0.5, 0.5, 0.5, 0.15, 0.25, 0.5\}$.

The dynamics of $SS1$ and $SS2$ are described as follows. $SS1$ is accumulated during wakefulness and otherwise dissipated. $SS2$ is accumulated during wakefulness and the REM state, and otherwise dissipated.

$$\frac{dSS1}{dt} = \delta_{wake}k_{wl} - \delta_{sleep}k_s \cdot SS1 - k_{c1} \cdot SS1 + \eta_1, \tag{A-4}$$

$$\frac{dSS2}{dt} = \delta_{wake}k_{w2} - \delta_{REM}k_r - \delta_{NREM}k_n \cdot SS2 \\ - k_{c2} \cdot SS2 + \eta_2, \tag{A-5}$$

where δ_{state} takes the value 1 if the network is in the specified state, and otherwise is 0. k_{w1}, k_{w2}, k_s, k_r, k_n, kc_1, and k_{c2} are the constants 0.15, 0.15, 0.015, 0.06, 0.01, 0.03, and 0.03, respectively. η_1 and η_2 are 0-mean Gaussian noise whose standard deviation is 0.3.

The equations are solved numerically by the 4-th order Runge–Kutta method with time resolutions of 0.01s for rats and 3.46s humans.

The model of human sleep–wakefulness regulation

To model human sleep–wakefulness regulation, some of the model parameters are modified as follows: W_{89}: 2→2.5, W_{95}: −5→−4.5. The circadian modulators are replaced by $2.2\left\{\sin\left(\frac{2\pi}{24}t\right)+1\right\}$ for C_1, $2.8\left\{\sin\left(2\pi\left(\frac{t}{24}+\frac{1}{50}\right)\right)+1\right\}$ for C_2, and $0.05\left\{\sin\left(\frac{2\pi}{24}t\right)+1\right\}$ for C_3. In addition, k_{w1}, k_{w2}, k_s, k_r, k_n, k_{c1}, and k_{c2} are the constants 0.015, 0.011, 0.012, 0.1, 0.06, 0.001, and 0.001, respectively. The standard deviations of η_1 and η_2 are 0.1.

Chapter

44

The selective mood-regulatory theory of dreaming: an adaptive, assimilative, and experimentally based theory of dreaming

Milton Kramer

Summary

REM sleep has the dream experience as a frequent if not inevitable concomitant. Questions arise about the construction, function, and meaning of this peculiar and puzzling experience. How are the dreams of the night organized? How do they relate to REM sleep and to each other across the night? How do they relate to waking consciousness? And, do they serve an adaptive function? I will describe the selective mood-regulatory theory of dreaming as an experimentally based attempt to answer these questions.

The beginning of our exploration of a function for dreaming is at the observation that dreaming and sleep disturbances may be related.

The core observation

The contribution of REM physiology

Freud (1955) proposed that the function of dreaming was to maintain the continuity of sleep, which is central to the restorative value of sleep (Stepanski, 2002). REM sleep provides three facts that support this idea that the function of REM/dreaming is to maintain the continuity of sleep. Firstly, the distribution of REM sleep across the night, more as the night goes on, is appropriate as the tendency to awaken increases the longer we sleep (Webb, 1969). Secondly, the typical REM period ends in a brief arousal, which we found in 90% of cases, and suggests a strong relationship between arousals and REM sleep. Lastly, Solms (1997) noted that brain-injured patients who reported the loss of dreaming also had a decreased continuity of sleep as a result of increased awakenings.

Many dream reports have no feeling in them, and in those that do a negative feeling is more common than a positive one (Kramer and Glucksman, 2006). Comparing a recalled dream, a nightmare, and a confabulated nightmare to each other showed that the recalled dream, one that hadn't disturbed sleep, had the most muted feeling while the actual and confabulated nightmare had more intense feelings (Taub *et al.*, 1978).

The intensity of dreaming

The intensity of dreaming has a developmental course across the REM period (Kramer *et al.*, 1975). The intensity increase in emotionality across the REM period is essentially linear between 2.5 and 30 minutes with a plateau between 20 and 30 minutes, which fits the eye movement periodicity of the REM period (Aserinsky, 1971; Johnson *et al.*, 1980). Aserinsky had speculated that dreaming might follow the ebb and flow of the REM period eye movements.

Dreaming and the emotional surge

The rise and fall in the intensity of content and affect across the dream period is in keeping with the possibility that during REM sleep there is a surge of emotion. I believe the dream serves to contain or attempt to contain that surge.

The variability and magnitude of alterations in heart rate, blood pressure, and respiration associated with REM sleep (Freemon, 1972) point to an accompanying emotional surge. However, efforts to connect dream content with the variability in autonomic function have been minimally successful at best (Pivik, 2000). Nevertheless, the autonomic functions during REM sleep are experiencing fluctuations consistent with an emotional surge occurring. If the integrative capacity of the dreamer is adequate, the affective intensity of the

---

REM Sleep: Regulation and Function, eds. Birendra N. Mallick, S. R. Pandi-Perumal, Robert W. McCarley, and Adrian R. Morrison. Published by Cambridge University Press. © Cambridge University Press 2011.

dream experience is contained, muted, and the dream then does not enter awareness. The result is that sleep is not disturbed and the function of dreaming is part of an assimilative process.

Dream function: containment of the emotional surge

To what is the attempt to control the emotional surge related? We compared individuals who reported having two nightmares a week to a group of vivid dreamers (Kramer *et al.*, 1984a). The two groups had the same content categories at about the same frequency. The integrative capacity of dreaming cannot be explained by the content of the dream. The ability to recall dreams does not reflect the capacity to integrate the emotional surge of dreaming as the vivid dreamers had a higher recall rate (89%) than the nightmare subjects (54%). We would expect a higher recall in the nightmare subjects if dream recall primarily occurs because the emotional surge is not contained.

Is a preoccupation with dreaming related to the ability to contain the emotional surge of REM sleep? Students with an interest in dreams believed they had more dreams than those without such an interest. In keeping a dream diary, they reported one-third fewer dreams than subjects who said they had no interest in dreams (Roth *et al.*, 1972). When poor sleepers are compared to good sleepers, the poor sleepers report a greater interest in dreams and in a diary study report about one-third more dreams (Arand *et al.*, 1972). The poor sleepers had more awakenings during the night than the good sleepers and awakening after a dream increases the likelihood of remembering it. Multiple awakenings during the night with increased dream recall may reflect a failure to contain the emotional surge during dreaming. Poor sleep may reflect an emotionally troubled state that has decreased the integrative capacity of the dreamer.

There does appear to be a predispositional factor, which may be determining of the capacity of the dreamer to contain the emotional surge of REM sleep. The nightmare subjects in the study noted earlier (Kramer *et al.*, 1984a) had higher scores on all the MMPI scales and on emotionally based scales of the Cornell Medical Index and had had more psychiatric hospitalizations. They reported that their nightmares were related to current troubling feelings, e.g., anger, sensitivity, and general emotion. The immediate emotional state of the person appears to be a determinant of the integrative capacity of their dreams on a given night.

The emotional responsivity of the dreamer to the dream experience is another factor reflecting the activity of the integrative function of dreaming. Others describe those with nightmares as more responsive and appearing more frightened during sleep, apparently in reaction to the dream experience (Kramer *et al.*, 1984a).

The integrative failure that is reflected in an increased responsivity in nightmare sufferers was confirmed in a study of Vietnam war veterans with chronic delayed post-traumatic stress disorder (CDPTSD) who have frequent nightmares (Kramer and Kinney, 1985). When they were given an above-threshold tone during sleep, they responded in 93% of trials while the control group responded only 52% of the times. They are more responsive and more emotionally troubled (Kramer *et al.*, 1984b). Predispositional factors, such as existing psychopathology, alter responsiveness. This integration failure may be due to an inability to contain "internal emotional forces." The CDPTSD patients had a higher awakening threshold than controls (Kramer and Kinney, 2003). If they were being hypervigilant, as they said they were, it was internally rather than externally directed. If it were externally directed, we would have expected lower rather than higher thresholds.

The CDPTSD subjects in the threshold study (Kramer and Kinney, 1985) failed to identify the external source of the awakening stimulus at a much higher rate than the control group, 92% of the time compared to 60% for the control group. This difference supports an internal focus of attention for the CDPTSD patients.

It appears that the emotional surge within an REM period is inextricably linked to the intensity of the dream experience (Kramer *et al.*, 1975) and probably to the intensity of physiological variables such as eye movements, heart rate, blood pressure, and respiration that occur during the dream period (Aserinsky, 1971; Freemon, 1972; Johnson *et al.*, 1980).

Mood before and after sleep

Introduction

The core observation in approaching the function of dreaming led to a view that the dream serves to protect the continuity of sleep by containing the repeated disruptions and emotional surges that occur across the night, regularly in REM sleep and perhaps irregularly from other sources. These observations draw our attention to the relationship of dreaming in particular and sleep in general to the emotional–affective state of the individual. There is an intimate relationship between sleep and how one feels. Prior wakefulness impacts sleep and sleep impacts subsequent wakefulness.

How depressed or anxious a person is before going to sleep has been shown to alter how well one sleeps (Rimon *et al.*, 1986; Rosa *et al.*, 1983). From a psychological perspective, the more intense emotional experiences of the day (Piccione *et al.*, 1977) and the thoughts a person has before going to sleep (Kramer *et al.*, 1982; Piccione *et al.*, 1976) are likely to appear in the dreams of the subsequent night. Sleep is clearly responsive to the experiences that precede it during the day.

The physiological and psychological aspects of sleep are also related to the waking activity of the next day. How well one performs on various psychomotor tasks following a night's sleep is influenced by even small alterations in the number of hours of prior sleep; decrements in performance can be shown with even a one-hour reduction in prior sleep (Wilkinson, 1968). Feeling states are predictive of performance (Lutz *et al.*, 1975) and feeling states are better predictors of performance during the day than hours of prior sleep (Johnson *et al.*, 1990). Mental activity in the morning is linked to the dreams of the prior night (Kramer *et al.*, 1982). There is a thematic continuity between the dreams of a night and the spontaneous verbal behavior of the following morning. Wakefulness is responsive to the experiences in sleep that preceded it. Sleep is linked to both prior and subsequent wakefulness in both its physiological and psychological aspects.

The possibility that sleep functions to alter the subjective state of the person seems plausible. An exploration of the sleep–mood and subjective state interaction should look at the relationship of both the psychology and physiology of sleep to waking mood and subjective state. Mood appears to vary from day to day, across the day and might well have a relationship to both dreams and sleep physiology.

The measurement of mood

The mood measurement device used in our studies was the Clyde Mood Scale (Clyde, 1963), a 48-item adjective checklist that yields scores on six subscales: friendly, aggressive, clear thinking, sleepy, unhappy, and dizzy (anxious). The subscales are independent, reliable, sensitive to change from night to morning, and repeated use does not lead to stereotypy (Kramer and Roth, 1973).

Mood difference across the night

We found that the intensity and variability of mood subscale scores decreased from night (pre-sleep) to morning (post-sleep) (Kramer, 2007). This was true in the laboratory, at home, across a wide age range (20–70), identically for both men and women, and whether the subject was in a hypnotic medication study or had been awakened for dream collection. We had expected that the mood subscale score for men and women would be different as their affective state (Cattell, 1973), sleep physiology (Williams *et al.*, 1974) and dream patterns (Winget and Kramer, 1979) are different. Nevertheless, if the night and morning mood differences can be related to the psychology and physiology of sleep, then sleep may play a role in mood regulation across the night.

Mood predictability across the night

Do the various aspects of mood vary systematically from night to morning and from day to day for each individual as does dreaming? We studied night and morning mood scores from 52 people, 40 women and 12 men, for 17 to 21 days (Kramer, 2007). We did two correlations. In the first, to capture the trait aspect of mood, we did a between-subject correlation of the averaged night scores to the averaged morning scores of each subscale. In the second, to capture the state aspect of mood, we did a within-subject correlation of night to morning mood for each mood subscale and then averaged the subscale correlations across subjects. The trait aspects of subscale mood mean correlations are quite high, with four of the six being above 0.88. Two correlations were low, sleepy r = 0.26, the only non-significant one, and dizzy (anxious) r = 0.62. The state aspects of mood subscale mean correlations were all quite low between r = 0.03 and r = 0.29, none of which were significant.

We clearly have evidence for a systematic night-to-morning mood subscale relationship at the trait level for five of the six mood subscales. However at the state level the variability is so high that none of the aspects of mood shows a systematic night-to-morning relationship. When we looked at the individual subscale correlations, we found 77, 25%, were significant. We found that 42 of the 52 subjects, 81%, had at least one significant correlation. The largest number of significant correlations is with the unhappy mood subscale in 22 of 52 subjects, 42%. The lowest number of significant correlations is with the sleepy subscale in 8 of 52 subjects, 15%.

The individual mood subscale scores showed a decline on 50% or more nights (64%, 59%, 62%, and 56%) for friendly, aggressive, unhappy, and clear thinking respectively; sleepy and anxious showed a decrease on fewer than 50% of the nights (49% and 47% respectively). The number of subjects showing a 50% decline or more on the aggressive mood subscale was 76%, for unhappy 74%, for friendly 69%, for clear thinking 63%, for sleepy 46%, and for anxious 41%.

We found a series of systematic relationships between pre- and post-sleep mood both between and within subjects.

Mood change and sleep deprivation

We did two sleep-deprivation studies to test whether the change in mood across the night was related to the intervening period of sleep. The first study was one night of sleep deprivation done in a group (Roth *et al.*, 1976a). We found that after the deprivation, the sleepy, aggressive, and friendly mood subscale scores were increased compared to baseline but recovered after one night of recovery sleep. The second sleep-deprivation study was done in the sleep laboratory with two consecutive nights of deprivation (Vaccarino *et al.*, 1981). With increased deprivation, the subjects showed increased scores on the sleepy and anxious mood subscales and a decreased score on the clear-thinking mood subscale.

Pre- and post-sleep mood is sensitive to even one night of sleep loss reflected in increased sleepy and anxious scores, and decreased clear-thinking scores. Changes in the friendly and aggressive scores may be more related to the social aspects of the experimental situation than to sleep loss. The decrease in the unhappy mood subscale score in normative studies remains to be explained (Kramer, 2007).

Mood change across the day

Mood change occurs across the day as well (Lysaght *et al.*, 1978) with the cheerful, energetic, and general activation subscales of the Pearson and Byars fatigue scale being maximal at noon and minimal at bedtime, and the reverse being true for the inert-fatigue and deactivation subscales. The changes across the day of the activation/deactivation subscales are phase advanced four hours on the diurnal temperature curve.

These changes in mood support the findings that the night–morning mood changes are different from those across the day although they are related. Most importantly, these mood patterns are not simple epiphenomenon of the diurnal temperature curve.

Mood and daytime performance

Does mood bear any relationship to significant daytime activity? In two studies we found that mood relates to daytime performance on psychomotor and cognitive tasks. In the first study (Lutz *et al.*, 1975; Roth *et al.*, 1976b) at three time points, 3.5, 10, and 22.5 hours, after ingesting an hypnotic, five of six mood subscales: sleepy (0.53) clear thinking (0.38), friendly (0.36), unhappy (0.33) and aggressive (0.18) showed a significant correlation with performance scores, both psychomotor and cognitive, averaged across the three time points. In a second study, subjects who were sleep deprived showed decrements in performance (Rosa *et al.*, 1981). Johnson and colleagues (1990) also have shown that post-sleep performance correlated better with morning mood than hours of prior sleep.

Mental content before, after, and during sleep

Introduction

Do dreams vary similarly to mood?

Dream differences between groups

Does dream content reflect differences in demographic variables? We found in a representative sample of adults in Cincinnati that in five demographic variables there were different and significant dream-content associations (Winget *et al.*, 1972). The sex of the dreamer had ten associated content differences, social class had six, age had four, and race and marital status three each. To illustrate, women had more characters and emotions in their dreams, while men had more aggression and achievement striving with success. Subjects in the lower social class had more characters in their dreams than those in the upper social class.

We have observed in both a laboratory and non-laboratory study (Kramer and Roth, 1979) that the dreams of schizophrenic and depressed patients were different. The schizophrenic patient has strangers as his unique character type and the depressed have family members as theirs.

The dream reflects psychological differences at the group level in both normal and psychopathological groups (Kramer and Roth, 1979). The mood state of the individual may be found to relate to these dream-content differences.

Dream differences between and within individuals

Is the dream organized at the individual level such that differences between individuals can be identified as well as between nights of an individual as we found in our studies of the relationship between pre- and post-sleep mood (see above)? We examined the question among dreams of normals and of schizophrenics (Kramer *et al.*, 1976) and found that the dreams of individuals are distinguishable one from the other, whether the person is mentally healthy or psychiatrically ill, and the dreams of an individual are different night to night. However, dreams from night to night are also linked (Kramer, 2007); as across 20 nights, the correlative level increases so that nights one to two have a content correlation of 0.05 and nights 19 to 20 a correlation of 0.80.

Dream differences across the night

If some processing change was occurring across the night, should the content of dreams be different from each other across the night? Given a set of dreams from a night, judges were unable to place them in their order of occurrence (Kramer *et al.*, 1976). However, we found (Kramer *et al.*, 1981) in a collection of dreams from different subjects that the number of words differed between REM period reports. Eight of 22 dream-content categories showed a change across the night with word length held constant. The mean content score of three of the significant content categories (total characters, single characters, and female characters) showed the inverted U-shaped change across REM periods with a numerical but non-significant decrease in REM period four. There is clear support for some sort of systematic dream-content change across the night (see below).

Dreams and waking thought

Are dreaming and waking thought related? If so, then the possibility is that the processing of content in dreams across the night might be relatable to prior and subsequent waking thought. We compared (Kramer, 2007) the content of Thematic Apperception Test (TAT) stories to the content of REM dreams and found that the intensity of the two fantasy productions was significantly correlated (r = 0.72). We felt this provided evidence for a trait relationship between waking and dreaming. We next examined (Kramer *et al.*, 1981) the relationship of the verbalized mental content immediately before and after sleep to the content of the intervening REM dreams and found that 9 of the 18 contents scored showed a significant correlation. This demonstrated a state relationship between waking and dreaming thought.

We explored the coherence within and connectedness between REM dreaming and waking (Kramer *et al.*, 1982). We found the pre- and post-sleep verbalizations of subjects thematically connected in 95% of individuals but the themes of REM dreams were only relatable to each other in 75% of subjects, a significant difference. Pre-sleep mentation was thematically connected to the subsequent night's dreams in 85% of individuals; post-sleep mentation was connected to the prior night's dreams in only 70% of people. Waking thought is more coherently organized than dreaming thought and dreams appear to be more reactive than proactive.

There is a thematic connection (Kramer, 2007) across the wake–sleep–wake continuum. The possibility of a functional interrelationship remains to be demonstrated.

The dreams' responsiveness to the emotional state of the dreamer

Introduction

I have repeatedly called attention to the organized nature of the dream report. (Kramer, 2007). The dream is also a highly responsive experience especially to the emotional state of the dreamer. We have done a series of studies to explore this relationship.

Emotionally significant waking (interpersonal) experiences influence dream content

We have described a series of seven studies that demonstrate that the principal emotional concern of the dreamer influences, i.e., is reflected in, the theme of the night's dreams (Kramer, 2007). (1) We have shown that the emotionally intense experiences of the day are what appear in dreams. (2) Specific emotionally capturing experiences such as beginning and ending an involving activity can be distinguished from each other in dream reports. (3) The pre-empting nature of the sleep-laboratory experience continues to be represented in dreams across time. (4) The interpersonal situation between dreamer and dream collector influences what is selected for reporting. (5) The emotional concern about who will observe and evaluate you can and does focus your dreams. (6) The sexual make up of a dream collection pair, same or different, influences the content of the dream experience and report. (7) Emotionally meaningful names presented during REM sleep are more likely to be incorporated into the dream experience than meaningless names. The emotionally responsive nature of the dream experience has, I believe, been convincingly demonstrated.

Medication treatment and affective change

We looked at an impersonal treatment that altered affect to see if dream content changed when affect changed (Kramer, 2007). We observed in depressed patients that after successful treatment with an anti-depressant medication their REM-dream content changed such that depression, hostility, anxiety, and intimacy in the dreams decreased, and heterosexuality and motility increased. Medication that affects the emotional affective dimension of the patient alters their dream content.

The relationship between mood and dreams

Introduction

We have shown that mood and sleep are related and that dreams are related to the individual's waking affective state as well as being reactive to the emotional state of the dreamer. If dreams contain or alter affective state, dream content and mood change ought to be related.

The mood change–dream content relationship

We studied two men in the sleep laboratory for 20 consecutive nights collecting from them pre- and post-sleep mood scores and their REM dreams (Kramer, 2007).

We found a series of significant relationships with the largest number of correlations being between the change (decrease) in the unhappy subscale score and an increase in characters in the dream. It was of considerable interest that the change that related most strongly to dream content change was the unhappy subscale. The unhappy subscale was one of three mood subscales, friendly and sleepy being the other two, that showed the most consistent change in sleep through studies. As discussed above, it was changes in the unhappy subscale that previously remained unexplained (Kramer, 2007). We repeated the study with 12 male subjects and found that mood change was significantly related to dream content (Kramer and Roth, 1980). The distribution of significant correlations across the mood subscales was not random and the unhappy subscale had significantly more correlations than the others. A significant relationship was found between three groups of content scales, i.e., characters, descriptive elements and activities, and mood change. The greatest number of correlations was between the character scales and the change in the unhappy mood subscale. How happy you feel on awakening in the morning depends mostly on whom you spent the night with in your dreams.

Affect is not directly and simply processed across the night (Kramer and Brik, 2002). We looked at the relationship between pre- and post-sleep mood and dream content. We found ten significant correlations between mood and dream content, two were with pre-sleep mood and eight were with post-sleep mood. We found no direct pass through relationship in which a pre-sleep aspect of mood correlated with an aspect of dream content and that content with the same aspect of mood post-sleep. Five of the ten significant correlations were between aspects of pre- and post-sleep mood and affect in the dream. The two pre-sleep correlations were between the dizzy (anxious) aspect of mood and dream confusion and sexual social interactions. There were three correlations with the post-sleep unhappy mood subscale score, namely dream sadness, confusion, and aggressive social interactions. The post-sleep friendly mood subscale score correlated with dream apprehension, anger, and aggressive social interactions. Post-sleep aggressive and clear-thinking aspects of mood had one dream content correlation each. Pre- and post-sleep mood is as connected to dream affect as to other dream contents. The connections were more proactive, eight of the correlations, than reactive, two correlations. How you feel in the morning is related to how you feel in your dreams and what happens in them.

A serious question has been raised by Strauch and Meier (1996) about the central role of affect in dreaming as only 50.2% of their dream reports contain a specific affect and an additional 23.4% a general feeling. In a study that looked at the change in dream affect in psychoanalytic treatment (Kramer and Glucksman, 2006), we found that only 58.3% had affect in the manifest content but 96% had affect if associations to the dream were included. We found that within a dream across time there was a systematic development of emotional intensity (Kramer *et al.*, 1975). It appears from our studies that affect is universally connected to the dream experience and could play a central role.

The relationship between mood and the physiology of sleep

Introduction

The possibility that mood changes could occur in relationship to the physiology of sleep, i.e., in sleep stages and total sleep time, invites an examination of their relationship.

Sleep deprivation and mood change

Total sleep deprivation studies were clearly linked to alterations in mood (Roth *et al.*, 1976a; Vaccarino *et al.*, 1981). The aspect of mood change (unhappy) most related to dreaming was not affected.

Mood change and sleep physiology

We did two studies to examine the relationship between mood change and sleep physiology. In the first study (Kramer, 2007), the changes across the night in the six mood subscales were correlated with five sleep variables, i.e., total sleep time, REM time, stage three/four time, stage two time, and number of awakenings. The largest number of significant correlations was between the change in the sleepy mood subscale score and total sleep time. Sleepy in previous studies (Kramer and Roth, 1980) was not related to the content of dreaming. In a replication study (Kramer *et al.*, 1976) pre- and post-sleep moods were assessed and seven sleep variables were scored. Awakenings were not scored but stage one time, sleep latency, and REM latency were added to the variables in the first study. We did a regression analysis using the seven sleep variables to predict the six mood subscale score changes. The two highest significant correlations (sleepy and friendly,

r = 0.42) were significantly different than the two lowest non-significant ones (unhappy and dizzy, r = 0.22). The non-REM aspects of sleep (stage two time, stage three/four time, and sleep latency) were predictive of the changes in the sleepy and friendly scores. The unhappy aspect of mood, the mood subscale most particularly related to dream content, was not related to the physiology of sleep.

We looked further at the relationship of the unhappy aspect of mood to REM sleep. We studied the relationship of the D scale score of the MMPI and the pre-sleep unhappy subscale score to the amount of REM sleep (Kramer *et al.*, 1972) and found no significant relationship. Unhappy mood is related to the content of dreaming and not the amount of REM sleep.

Dream content and sleep physiology are related to different aspects of mood change across the night. In two studies (Kramer, 2007), we found the distribution of significant correlations for dream-content categories and sleep variables to aspects of mood change across the night to be different. The 54 significant mood–dream correlations are primarily to the unhappy and secondarily to the friendly and aggressive aspects of mood change. The 26 significant sleep variables to mood subscale change correlations are primarily to the sleepy, dizzy, and clear-thinking aspects of mood.

The mood regulatory function of sleep

Sleep has a systematic relationship to mood change across the night. It appears that the physiology of sleep and the psychology of sleep are differentially related to various aspects of mood change across the night. The change in the sleepy aspect of mood relates to how much non-REM sleep one has had, while the change in the unhappy aspect of mood is a function of what one dreams about. The mood-regulatory function of sleep is suggested by the fact that pre-sleep mood is different than post-sleep mood. Specifically the mean level and variability of mood decreases across the night. It is as if a "funneling action" occurs, which decreases the intensity and variability of the various aspects of mood. The physiological and psychological activities during sleep appear to be "corrective" like a thermostat operating to move the mood level toward a central and lower point. The dream seems particularly involved with one aspect of mood, i.e., unhappy, and may be seen as a selective affective (mood) regulator, an "emotional thermostat" so to speak. Similarly, the physiological aspects of sleep, particularly non-REM sleep are related to changes in the sleepy aspects of mood also acting as a selective mood regulator.

The dream mechanism for mood change: emotional problem solving

Introduction

Dreaming should be related to the emotional state of the dreamer if dreaming is to protect sleep by absorbing the emotional surge that appears to accompany REM sleep. And indeed it is as previously described in the discussion of the mood change–dream content relationship. The question remains as to how the dream might change the affective state of the dreamer from pre-sleep to post-sleep?

It has been argued convincingly by Blagrove (1996) that adaptive problem solving of waking problems in sleep does not occur. He acknowledges that dreams may beneficially affect our waking moods. It is this change in mood that is the function for dreams that is being described in the mood-regulatory theory of dreaming.

Patterns of emotional problem solving

Two patterns of thematic dream development across the night are discernible (Kramer *et al.*, 1964), one of a progressive–sequential type in which an emotional problem is stated figuratively, worked on, and resolved; and the other of a repetitive–traumatic type in which the emotional problem is simply restated in different images or metaphors and no progress toward resolution occurs. The effectiveness of a night's dreaming in reducing the intensity and variability of mood occurs in about 60% of nights (Kramer, 2007). The variation for an individual in the effectiveness of a night's dreaming may be the result of the differential pattern of dreaming across the night. If one has experienced a progressive–sequential dream pattern, there may be a positive alteration in the emotional state of the dreamer. If the emotional problem one goes to sleep with is simply restated and not solved, a repetitive–traumatic dream pattern is experienced and a less successful night's dreaming has occurred. I am suggesting that it is through the mechanism of "emotional problem solving" (French, 1952) or failure to "problem solve" that the affective alteration in dreaming takes place or fails to occur. This thematic dream change

may be concomitant with the change in the intensity of unhappiness across the night and the appearance of the appropriate number and types of characters, descriptive elements, and activities in the dream. Dreamers show both patterns in approximately the same frequency (Kramer *et al.*, 1964), 60% / 40%, as I noted (Kramer, 2007) for the effectiveness of a night's dreams in changing waking affect across the night. People show both patterns, which underscores that there is not universal success in altering the residual emotional problems of the day. This could account for some of the variability in how a person feels on awakening in the morning.

Emotional problem solving: a comment

These patterns are elaborations or specifications of the general thesis that dreams may serve a problem solving function (French, 1952). It may be that through this effort at "emotional problem solving" that the success or failure to contain the emotional surge occurs. If successful, the arousal at the end of the REM period is for seconds and the dreamer returns to sleep with no memory of the arousal. If the emotional problem is not resolved, an awakening is more likely to occur and perhaps a nightmare. Difficulty in emotional problem solving during waking life is more often associated with the psychopathologically troubled who have been found to be more responsive to the arousal awakening at the end of an REM period and who report more bad dreams and nightmares (Kramer *et al.*, 1984a).

Given that sleep is generally a successful process, one would expect to find that the progressive-sequential pattern would be more common than the repetitive traumatic one. In the two subjects we studied in the sleep laboratory, 50% of their nights had the sequential pattern and 31% the repetitive pattern with the remainder a mixed pattern (Kramer *et al.*, 1964) It was on 63% of nights that the average mood intensity across the night decreased (Kramer, 2007). The current emotional and cognitive concerns of an individual are processed by a problem-solving mechanism across the wake–sleep–wake continuum and the resultant state is a determinant of performance the next morning.

In conclusion, the selective mood regulatory theory of dreaming is an example of an assimilative theory of dream function. In this theory, the dream functions to contain the emotional affective surge that may occur during sleep and that occurs regularly during REM sleep. If successful, one has no memory of dreaming and sleep proceeds essentially undisturbed. If unsuccessful or partially so, a dream recall occurs that, if conditions are right, becomes a disturbing dream or nightmare with a troubled awakening.

The experience of the recalled dream, which depends to a degree on a troubled state in the dreamer, opens the possibility for an extension of the assimilative, reductive view to encompass some degree of transformation and of accommodation as well. States of disturbance increase the likelihood of change. Dreaming that enters awareness can become the object of attention for the dreamer and lead to change in the dreamer, to an enhancement of self-knowledge.

References

Arand, D., Kramer, M., Czaya, J. & Roth, T. (1972) Attitudes toward sleep and dreams in good versus poor sleepers. *Sleep Res* **1**: 130.

Aserinsky, E. (1971) Rapid eye movement density and pattern in the sleep of normal young adults. *Psychophysiology* **8**: 361–75.

Blagrove, M. (1996) Problems with the cognitive psychological modeling of dreaming. *J Mind and Behav* **17**: 99–134.

Cattell, R. (1973) *Personality and Mood by Questionnaire*, 1st edn. San Francisco: Jossey-Bass Publishers.

Clyde, D. (1963) *Manual for the Clyde Mood Scale*. Miami, FL: Biometric Laboratory, University of Florida.

Freemon, F. (1972) *Sleep Research: a Critical Review*. Springfield, IL: Charles C. Thomas.

French, T. (1952) *The Integration of Behavior*. Chicago: University of Chicago Press.

Freud, S. (1955) *The Interpretation of Dreams*, 1st edn. New York: Basic Books.

Johnson, B., Kramer, M., Bonnet, M., Roth, T. & Jansen, T. (1980). The effect of Ketazolam on ocular motility during sleep. *Curr Ther Res* **28**: 792–9.

Johnson, L., Spinweber, C., Gomez, S. & Matteson, L. (1990) Daytime sleepiness, performance, mood, nocturnal sleep: the effect of benzodiazepine and caffeine on their relationship. *Sleep* **13**: 121–35.

Kramer, M. (2007) *The Dream Experience: A Systematic Exploration*. New York: Routledge, Taylor and Francis Group.

Kramer, M. & Brik, I. (2002) Affective processing by dreams across the night by dreams. *Sleep* (Suppl) **25**: A180–1.

Kramer, M. & Glucksman, M. (2006) Changes in manifest dream affect during psychoanalytic treatment. *J Am Acad Psychoanal Dynamic Psychiatry* **34**: 249–60.

Kramer, M. & Kinney, L. (1985) Vulnerability to developing delayed post-traumatic stress disorder: combat experience and psychological status. *Sleep Res* **14**: 131.

Kramer, M. & Kinney, L. (2003) Vigilance and avoidance during sleep in US Vietnam War veterans with posttraumatic stress disorder. *J Nerv Ment Dis* **191**: 685–7.

Kramer, M. & Roth, T. (1973) The mood-regulating function of sleep. In *Sleep 1972*, ed. W. Koella & P. Levin. Basel: S. Karger, pp. 563–71.

Kramer, M. & Roth, T. (1979) Dreams in psychopathology. In *Handbook of Dreams: Research, Theories and Applications*. ed. B. Wolman. New York: Von Norstrand Reinhold, pp. 361–87.

Kramer, M. & Roth, T. (1980) The relationship of dream content to night-morning mood change In *Sleep 1978*, eds. L. Popoviciu, B. Asigian & G. Bain. Basel: S. Karger, pp. 621–4.

Kramer, M., Whitman, R. M., Baldridge, B. J. & Lansky, L. M. (1964) Patterns of dreaming: the interrelationship of the dreams of a night. *J Nerv Ment Dis* **139**: 426–39.

Kramer, M., Roehrs, T. & Roth, T. (1972) The relationship between sleep and mood. *Sleep Res* **1**: 193.

Kramer, M., Roth, T. & Czaya, J. (1975) Dream development within a REM period. In *Sleep 1974*, eds. P. Levin & W. Koella. Basel: S. Karger pp. 406–8.

Kramer, M., Hlasny, R., Jacobs, G. & Roth, T. (1976) Do dreams have meaning? An empirical inquiry *Am J Psychiatry* **133**: 778–81.

Kramer, M., Roehrs, T. & Roth, T. (1976) Mood change and the physiology of sleep. *Compr Psychiatry* **17**: 161–5.

Kramer, M., McQuarrie, E. & Bonnet, M. (1981) Problem solving in dreaming: an empirical test. In *Sleep 1980*, ed. W. Koella. Basel: S. Karger, pp. 357–60.

Kramer, M., Roth, T., Arand, D. & Bonnet, M. (1981) Waking and dreaming mentation: a test of their interrelationship. *Neurosci Lett* **22**: 83–6.

Kramer, M., Moshiri, A. & Scharf, M. (1982) The organization of mental content in and between the waking and dreaming state. *Sleep Res* **11**: 106.

Kramer, M., Schoen, L. & Kinney, L. (1984a) Psychological and behavioral features of disturbed dreamers. *Psychiatr J Univ Ott* **9**: 102–6.

Kramer, M., Schoen, L. & Kinney, L. (1984b) The dream experience in dream disturbed Vietnam veterans. In *Post Traumatic Stress Disorders: Psychological and Biological Sequellae*, ed. B. Van der Kolk. Washington DC: American Psychiatric Press, pp. 81–95.

Lutz, T., Kramer, M. & Roth, T. (1975) The relationship between mood and performance. *Sleep Res* **4**: 152.

Lysaght, R., Roth, T., Kramer, M. & Salis, P. (1978) Variations in subjective state and body temperature across the day. *Sleep Res* 7: 308.

Piccione, P., Jacobs, G., Kramer, M. & Roth, T. (1977) The relationship between daily activities, emotions and dream content. *Sleep Res* **6**: 133.

Piccione, P., Thomas, S., Roth, T. & Kramer, M. (1976) Incorporation of the laboratory situation in dreams. *Sleep Res* **5**:120.

Pivik, T. (2000) Psychophysiology of dreams. In *Principles and Practice of Sleep Medicine*, 3rd edn, eds. M. Kryger, T. Roth & W. Dement. Philadelphia: W.B. Saunders, pp. 491–501.

Rimon, R., Fujita, M. & Takahata, N. (1986) Mood alterations and sleep. *Jpn J Psychiatry Neurol* **40**:153–9.

Rosa, R., Bonnet, M., Warm, J. & Kramer, M. (1981)The recovery of performance during sleep following sleep deprivation. *Sleep Res* **10**: 264.

Rosa, R., Bonnet, M. & Kramer, M. (1983) The relationship of sleep and anxiety in anxious subjects. *Biol Psychol* **16**: 119–26.

Roth, T., Kramer, M. & Trinder, J. (1972) Volunteers versus non-volunteers in dream research. *Psychophysiology* **9**: 116.

Roth, T., Kramer, M. & Lutz, T. (1976a) The effects of sleep deprivation on mood. *Psychiatric J Univ Ottawa* **1**: 136–9.

Roth, T., Kramer, M. & Lutz, T. (1976b) Intermediate use of triazolam: a sleep laboratory study. *J Int Med Res* **4**: 59–63.

Solms, M. (1997). *The Neuropsychology of Dreams: a Clinico-anatomical Study*. Mahwah, NJ: L. Erlbaum Associates.

Stepanski, E. (2002) The effect of sleep fragmentation on daytime function. *Sleep* **25**: 268–76.

Strauch, I. & Meier, B. (1996) *In Search of Dreams: Results of Experimental Dream Research*. Albany, NY: State University of New York Press.

Taub, J., Kramer, M., Arand, D. & Jacobs, G. (1978) Nightmare dreams and nightmare confabulations. *Compr Psychiatry* **19**: 285–91.

Vaccarino, P., Rosa, R., Bonnet, M. & Kramer, M. (1981) The effect of 40 and 64 hours of sleep deprivation on mood. *Sleep Res* **10**: 269.

Webb, W. (1969) Partial and differential sleep deprivation. In *Sleep: Physiology and Pathology: a Symposium*, ed. A. Kales A. Philadelphia: Lippincott, pp. 221–31.

Wilkinson W. (1968) Sleep deprivation: performance tests for partial and selective sleep deprivation. In *Progress in Clinical Psychology*, eds. I. Abt & B. Reis. New York: Grune and Stratton, pp. 28–43.

Williams, R., Karacan, I. & Hursch, C. (1974) *Electroencephalography (EEG) of Human Sleep: Clinical Applications*. New York: Wiley.

Winget, C. & Kramer, M. (1979) *Dimensions of Dreams*. Gainesville, FL: University Presses of Florida.

Winget, C., Kramer, M. & Whitman, R. (1972) Dreams and demography. *Can Psychiatr Assoc J* **17**:Suppl 2: SS203–8.

Index